Nutrition and Health

Series Editors

Adrianne Bendich
Wellington, FL, USA

Connie W. Bales
Durham VA Medical Center
Duke University School of Medicine
Durham, NC, USA

The Nutrition and Health series has an overriding mission in providing health professionals with texts that are considered essential since each is edited by the leading researchers in their respective fields. Each volume includes: 1) a synthesis of the state of the science, 2) timely, in-depth reviews, 3) extensive, up-to-date fully annotated reference lists, 4) a detailed index, 5) relevant tables and figures, 6) identification of paradigm shifts and consequences, 7) virtually no overlap of information between chapters, but targeted, inter-chapter referrals, 8) suggestions of areas for future research and 9) balanced, data driven answers to patient/health professionals questions which are based upon the totality of evidence rather than the findings of a single study.

Nutrition and Health is a major resource of relevant, clinically based nutrition volumes for the professional that serve as a reliable source of data-driven reviews and practice guidelines.

More information about this series at http://www.springer.com/series/7659

Jerrilynn D. Burrowes
Csaba P. Kovesdy • Laura D. Byham-Gray
Editors

Nutrition in Kidney Disease

Third Edition

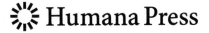 Humana Press

Editors
Jerrilynn D. Burrowes
School of Health Professions and
Nursing
Long Island University
Greenvale, NY
USA

Csaba P. Kovesdy
Division of Nephrology
University of Tennessee Health Science
Memphis, TN
USA

Laura D. Byham-Gray
School of Health Professions
Rutgers University–Newark
Newark, NJ
USA

Nutrition and Health
ISBN 978-3-030-44860-8   ISBN 978-3-030-44858-5   (eBook)
https://doi.org/10.1007/978-3-030-44858-5

This Humana imprint is published by the registered company Springer Nature Switzerland AG
The registered company address is: Gewerbestrasse 11, 6330 Cham, Switzerland

Jerrilynn dedicates this book to the millions of people worldwide with kidney disease who will benefit from the information embedded in these pages. The goal of this book is to improve the health and well-being of these individuals through optimal nutritional practices. Laura dedicates this book to her husband, Steven, and to her daughters, Erin and Jillian.

Foreword

To have been invited to write the foreword to the third edition of *Nutrition in Kidney Disease* is an honor and a privilege. The editors, Drs. Burrowes, Kovesdy, and Byham-Gray, are outstanding experts in the field of nutrition and kidney disease, which undoubtedly ensures the high standard of quality of the book.

Since its first edition in 2008, *Nutrition in Kidney Disease* has been recognized as a benchmark for practitioners and researchers interested in kidney disease and nutrition-related issues. The third edition has been updated and new chapters added that reflect the expanding knowledge in the field.

The book is organized into seven parts covering relevant topics concerning diet and nutrition across the full spectrum of kidney disease. The chapters have been written by highly respected researchers and professionals with vast experience in this area. One of the features that sets the book apart is the structure of the chapters. At the beginning of each chapter, the reader can find a list of the key words and points that will be addressed, thus providing a general overview of the most important information that will be covered in the pages that follow. Of special note is that the conclusion of each chapter, depending upon the theme addressed, offers information on how to apply the theoretical concepts in clinical practice.

In addition to the important issues discussed in the previous editions, this edition pays special attention to issues relating to the historical aspects of diet in the treatment of patients with chronic kidney disease, such as the low-protein diet that was first proposed more than 200 years ago, and also new topics that have been the recent focus of studies and discussions amongst researchers in this field. Of special importance here are the chapters on gut microbiota, advanced glycation end products, and dietary patterns. These chapters offer the reader both a general and current overview of the subject, while also highlighting those areas that are still in need of research.

A new chapter has been included on drug–nutrient interactions, a matter that is of critical importance in the treatment of chronic kidney disease considering the presence of numerous disorders in the metabolism of nutrients that can be aggravated by the improper use of various medicines employed in the treatment of the disease.

Recognizing that the complexity of a patient's diet in chronic kidney disease has an enormous psychological impact on their nutritional status and behavior, the editors have dedicated a number of chapters to this problem. These chapters propose strategies for improving the approach to communication employed by health care providers, particularly dietitians, to nutritional counseling with the intent of improving motivation and adherence by patients to dietary recommendations.

One of the last chapters ends the book on a high note, since it addresses the challenges faced by researchers in the area of nutrition and kidney diseases, while also covering the principles and processes that guide comparative effectiveness research.

I am certain that this book will continue to provide an effective learning experience and consolidate its reputation as the go-to source of reference for every health professional who is dedicated to the care of patients with kidney diseases and to research in this field.

Lilian Cuppari
Universidade Federal de São Paulo
São Paulo, Brazil

Preface

Approximately 10% of adults worldwide are believed to have chronic kidney disease (CKD), which is often associated with obesity, diabetes mellitus, hypertension, nephrotic syndrome, or advanced kidney failure. These conditions require intense nutritional support for the health, well-being, and longevity of the individual. Notwithstanding this need, people with CKD in many countries have no or very little access to dietitians. Moreover, it is alarming to note that most of these dietitians, particularly those outside of the USA, have limited access to cutting-edge, evidence-based information about the nutritional management of CKD. In countries where dietitians are available, many of them cannot obtain specific training regarding the nutritional needs of CKD patients. Therefore, this textbook is designed specifically to address the educational needs of dietitians around the world who seek current information about this topic. Thus, this edition will also be highly informative for nephrologists, nutrition scientists, nutritionists, researchers, and students whose research, practice, and education includes nutrition and kidney disease.

Organization and Content

This third edition of *Nutrition in Kidney Disease* is organized into seven parts with a variable number of chapters based on the breadth and depth of information. Part I addresses the differences in the epidemiology of CKD and renal replacement therapy worldwide, such as environmental, ethnic, cultural, political, and macroeconomic factors. Kidney function in health and disease and a comprehensive review of the history of dietary protein treatment for non-dialyzed CKD patients are also addressed. Part II includes a thorough review of the components of the nutrition assessment, which includes information about psychosocial issues affecting nutritional status in kidney disease and drug–nutrient interactions. In Parts III and IV, preventative strategies for common disorders associated with CKD such as hypertension, type 2 diabetes, obesity, and cardiovascular disease are provided, and current evidence-based treatment recommendations for the nutrition management of non-dialyzed, dialyzed, and transplanted adults are addressed. Part V presents the nutritional concerns of CKD populations with special needs (i.e., pregnancy, infancy, childhood, adolescence, and the elderly). The nutrition management of other disorders associated with kidney disease is covered in

Part VI; these include protein-energy wasting and the inflammatory response, bone and mineral disorders, nephrotic syndrome, nephrolithiasis, and acute kidney injury. Lastly, Part VII is devoted to cutting-edge research on topics of concern in nutrition in kidney disease such as the gut microbiome including pre- and probiotics, appetite regulation, advanced glycation end products, physical activity and structured exercise, and dietary patterns including plant-based diets. When appropriate, the new clinical practice guidelines in nutrition for individuals with CKD are integrated into the chapters. The textbook ends with a chapter for the practitioner that comprises an extensive and carefully selected list of resources that represent key information for the provision of high quality, evidence-based care to patients diagnosed with kidney disease.

Features

This textbook has a logical flow and format. Each part begins with an introduction that was written by the editors. Every chapter includes key points that are the learning objectives for the chapter and concludes with a summary. Up-to-date references are included for more in-depth review. Several chapters end with a case study that may be used to assess knowledge of the content area and to evoke critical thinking in the user within the context of didactic curricula. They provide thought-provoking, illustrative questions that will add to the student's learning and clinical application of the material. Answers to the case studies are provided at the end of select chapters.

Lastly, this textbook represents a collaborative effort between nationally and internationally recognized dietitians, professors, researchers, nephrologists, pharmacists, and exercise specialists in the field of kidney disease and clinical nutrition, thereby encouraging an interdisciplinary approach to providing care to this unique patient population across the globe. This collaborative effort should make this textbook marketable to many diversified audiences.

Greenvale, NY, USA   Jerrilynn D. Burrowes
Memphis, TN, USA   Csaba P. Kovesdy
Newark, NJ, USA   Laura D. Byham-Gray

Series Editor Page

The great success of the Nutrition and Health Series is the result of the consistent overriding mission of providing health professionals with texts that are essential because each includes: (1) a synthesis of the state of the science; (2) timely, in-depth reviews by the leading researchers and clinicians in their respective fields; (3) extensive, up-to-date fully annotated reference lists; (4) a detailed index; (5) relevant tables and figures; (6) identification of paradigm shifts and the consequences; (7) virtually no overlap of information between chapters, but targeted, inter-chapter referrals; (8) suggestions of areas for future research; and (9) balanced, data-driven answers to patients' as well as health professionals' questions which are based upon the totality of evidence rather than the findings of any single study.

The series volumes are not the outcome of a symposium. Rather, each editor has the potential to examine a chosen area with a broad perspective, both in subject matter as well as in the choice of chapter authors. The international perspective, especially with regard to public health initiatives, is emphasized where appropriate. The editors, whose trainings are both research and practice oriented, have the opportunity to develop a primary objective for their book, define the scope and focus, and then invite the leading authorities from around the world to be part of their initiative. The authors are encouraged to provide an overview of the field, discuss their own research, and relate the research findings to potential human health consequences. Because each book is developed de novo, the chapters are coordinated so that the resulting volume imparts greater knowledge than the sum of the information contained in the individual chapters.

Nutrition in Kidney Disease, Third Edition, edited by Jerrilynn D. Burrowes, PhD, RDN, CDN, FNKF; Csaba P. Kovesdy, MD; and Laura Byham-Gray, PhD, RDN, FNKF, is a very welcome and timely addition to the Nutrition and Health Series and fully exemplifies the series' goals. The highly acclaimed second edition of this volume was published in 2014; thus, an update of core chapters as well as the addition of new topics and case studies is warranted. The over-arching goal of the third edition is to provide clinically relevant and timely, objective guidance to the health professionals and advanced students who provide nutrition care for patients with renal insufficiency at all stages of the disease. The editors have been diligent in covering the newest research areas of medical nutrition therapy (MNT) and have added 12 new chapters, and many of the authors of key chapters found in the first as well as the second edition have returned to update their chapters. The unique inclusion of 17 case studies, each found in their relevant chapter as well as collected in a separate chapter, add further value to this excellent volume.

The editors of this informative text are international experts in their fields and have been recognized by their peers as outstanding contributors as evidenced by their degrees, affiliations, and honors. Dr. Burrowes earned her bachelor's degree from Fisk University in Nashville, TN; her MS degree in foods, nutrition, and dietetics from New York University; and her PhD in nutrition from New York University. Currently, Dr. Burrowes is Professor of Nutrition in the Department of Biomedical, Health and Nutritional Sciences at Long Island University, NY. She is a co-editor of the first and second editions of this volume, *Nutrition in Kidney Disease*, which were published in 2008 and in 2014, respectively, and she is currently the senior editor for the third edition. She is currently a Council Member of the International Society of Renal Nutrition and Metabolism (ISRNM) for the 2018–2020 term. For the past 8 years, Dr. Burrowes served as the Editor-in-Chief for the *Journal of Renal Nutrition*. She was also a member of the workgroup that developed the initial NKF-DOQI Clinical Practice Guidelines for Nutrition in Chronic Renal Failure (2000) and the workgroup that developed the joint NKF and Academy KDOQI/EAL Clinical Practice Guidelines in Nutrition in Chronic Kidney Disease (2020). Dr. Burrowes received the Recognized Renal Dietitian Award and the Joel D. Kopple Award from the NKF Council on Renal Nutrition and the Outstanding Service Award from the Renal Practice Group of the Academy of Nutrition and Dietetics.

Dr. Csaba P. Kovesdy, MD, FASN, earned his medical degree Summa cum Laude from the University of Pecs Medical School in Pecs, Hungary. He completed his residency in Internal Medicine at the Henry Ford Hospital in Detroit, Michigan, and a clinical fellowship in Nephrology at the Johns Hopkins Bayview Medical Center in Baltimore, Maryland. Dr. Kovesdy is an internationally recognized clinical researcher and renal outcomes investigator. He is the Fred Hatch Professor of Medicine in Nephrology and Director of the Clinical Outcomes and Clinical Trials Program at the University of Tennessee Health Science Center in Memphis, Tennessee, and Chief of Nephrology at the Memphis VA Medical Center in Memphis, Tennessee. Dr. Kovesdy's main research interests are centered on the epidemiology and outcomes of patients with pre-dialysis chronic kidney disease and end-stage renal disease (ESRD), with special emphasis on studying the role played by malnutrition and inflammation in driving poor outcomes in these populations. He has published his research in over 490 peer-reviewed articles as well as numerous abstracts and book chapters. He has been a member of the International Society of Renal Nutrition and Metabolism Council since 2012 and its Treasurer during 2014–2018, a Fellow of the American Society of Nephrology, and a member of the European Renal Association – European Dialysis and Transplant Association and the International Society of Nephrology.

Dr. Laura Byham-Gray received her bachelor of science in nutrition and dietetics from Mercyhurst University in Erie, Pennsylvania; her MS in food science and human nutrition from the University of Delaware; and her PhD in nutrition from the New York University, Steinhardt School of Education in the Department of Nutrition, Food Studies, and Public Health. She is

Professor and Vice Chair for Research in the Department of Clinical and Preventive Nutrition Sciences, School of Health Professions, Rutgers University. Prior to teaching, Dr. Byham-Gray practiced in the field of clinical nutrition with specialty practice in nutrition support and kidney disease for over 15 years. She received a NIDDK research grant that funded the development and validation of the predictive energy equation in hemodialysis, and she has recently completed another research-funded project from the Agency of Healthcare Research and Quality that explored protein-energy wasting in hemodialysis while integrating the patient perspective. Dr. Byham-Gray has held numerous elected and appointed positions at the national, state, and local levels of National Kidney Foundation (NKF), the American Society of Parenteral and Enteral Nutrition, and the Academy of Nutrition & Dietetics. Dr. Byham-Gray also chaired the Macronutrients Section of the joint NKF and Academy KDOQI/EAL Clinical Practice Guidelines in Nutrition in Chronic Kidney Disease. Dr. Byham-Gray has served as the associate editor for the National Kidney Foundation publication *The Journal of Renal Nutrition*. She has over 100 peer-reviewed articles and professional presentations related to kidney disease, dietetics practice, and clinical decision-making as well as management. Dr. Byham-Gray has served as the chief editor for three books: *Nutrition in Kidney Disease* (Springer Publications, 2008, 2014), and *A Clinical Guide to Nutrition Care in Kidney Disease* (Academy of Nutrition and Dietetics, 2013). She has received numerous awards, including the Presidential Citation for Outstanding Achievement from the University of Delaware, the Susan C. Knapp Excellence in Education Award, and the prestigious Joel D. Kopple Award.

Objectives and Organization of the Volume

The objectives of this comprehensive volume are to provide clinicians, dietitians, nutritionists, and related students, both graduate and advanced undergraduates, a broad review of the major aspects of kidney disease including the nutritional consequences and the nutritional needs of kidney disease patients during the various stages of this chronic, progressive disease. Additionally, there are chapters that address acute kidney diseases caused by injury and/or the formation of kidney stones. As the population globally ages and gets more overweight, the incidence of kidney disease will increase; diabetes and cardiovascular disease are also critical risk factors for kidney disease and kidney disease significantly increases the risk of each of these conditions; the multiple disease effects on nutritional requirements are examined in separate chapters. The editors of the third edition of *Nutrition in Kidney Disease* specifically designed this text to address the nutritional needs and management of kidney disease patients with regard to the issues facing both practicing and academic dietitians and the other members of the patient's clinical team. The volume contains seven parts and logically reviews the basics of each chapter's topic and then provides a detailed description of the effects of kidney disease (KD) in each of the areas that are reviewed.

Part I: Foundations for Clinical Practice and Overview

Part I contains three chapters that include discussions of the global demographics, clinical presentation and diagnostic criteria used to define chronic kidney disease (CKD), prevalence of use of renal replacement therapy globally, the major organizations that have been involved in setting the standards, the role of dietary protein in the progression of kidney disease, and the current recommendations for protein intake in patients with Stages 1–5 of CKD. Chapter 1 provides and in-depth examination of the prevalence of CKD in economically developed and underdeveloped nations around the world including an examination of the prevalence of patients with Stages 1–5 in these countries. On average, over 10% of most adult populations have CKD. The reasons for the differences between countries are reviewed including the prevalence of diabetes mellitus and hypertension as well as dietary habits, smoking, physical inactivity, socioeconomic status, birth weight, and genetic factors. The chapter also looks at renal replacement therapy (RRT) statistics and informs us that of all incident patients globally in 2016, 87.3% initiated RRT with hemodialysis, 9.7% started with peritoneal dialysis, and 2.8% received a preemptive kidney transplant. The chapter also discusses the recent guidelines for the care of senior adults with multiple chronic diseases including CKD. Chapter 2 reviews the history of dietary protein recommendations in non-dialyzed patients with CKD from the late 1800s through present day. The development of evidence-based guidelines and consensus statements during the last 20 years for dietary protein intake in CKD patients are presented using tables and figures, and the rationales for the uses of high protein diets in kidney disease patients are also addressed. The importance of well-controlled clinical nutrition studies and consequent recommendations for consumption of high-quality protein at reduced levels, along with essential amino acids, keto-acids, reduced salt intake, and other diet-specific data, are reviewed based upon the recommendations in the 115 references cited. There is a detailed discussion of the Modification of Diet in Renal Disease (MDRD) Study, which is the largest, most carefully conducted and most prominent, NIH funded, randomized, prospective controlled clinical trial of the effects of diet on progression of CKD.

Chapter 3 reviews the three major functions of healthy kidneys. Firstly, the kidneys precisely control the composition and volume of the body fluids, and, by doing so, these organs maintain the acid–base balance as well as the body's blood pressure by varying the excretion of water and solutes. Secondly, the kidneys remove various nitrogenous metabolic end products in the process of producing urine. In general, the kidneys filter plasma in the glomerulus to form a protein-free ultrafiltrate. This ultrafiltrate passes through the various tubular segments where reabsorption of essential constituents and secretion of unwanted products occur. Thirdly, as endocrine organs, the kidneys produce important hormones, such as renin, erythropoietin, and active vitamin D_3 (calcitriol). The kidneys also participate in the degradation of various endogenous and exogenous compounds prior to their release into the urine. In addition to carefully reviewing the physiology of the kidneys, the chapter includes a comprehensive discussion of the anatomy of the kidney, its structural unit, the nephron, and the function(s) of each of the components. Of great importance, the chapter describes the effects of kidney disease as well as related diseases such as diabetes on the structure and functions of the kidney so that we see how each disease impacts this organ. It is no wonder that we have evolved with two kidneys as these organs are critical to human life.

Part II: Components of Nutrition Assessment

Part II contains six practice-oriented chapters that review the steps involved in anthropomorphic and biochemical nutritional assessment of patients with kidney disease. Two new chapters look at the psychosocial aspects of nutritional status and the potential for drug–nutrient interactions. Chapter 4 defines anthropometry as the science that studies the comparative size, form, and proportion of the human body and its regional components. Body part measurements and their analyses are described in detail including weight, height, skinfold thickness, circumferences, and elbow and wrist breadths; depending upon the clinical condition such as CKD, subscapular and triceps skinfolds, arm and calf circumference, and other measurements may be included in the analyses. Studies using these measures in kidney disease patients are reviewed and the five tables provide guidelines and resources. Chapter 5 presents an overview of the role of the registered dietitian nutritionist (RDN) in managing patients diagnosed with CKD and those needing RRT as it relates to biochemical assessments. The current clinical practice guidelines for nutrition in CKD developed by the National Kidney Foundation (NKF) Kidney Disease Outcomes Quality Initiative (KDOQI) and the Academy of Nutrition and Dietetics (Academy) are reviewed. In addition, the International Society of Renal Nutrition and Metabolism (ISRNM) updates on biochemical assessment in patients diagnosed with CKD are discussed with regard to their purpose, strengths, and limitations. The objective biochemical criteria used to determine if a CKD patient has protein-energy malnutrition (PEM) or protein-energy wasting (PEW) are reviewed. The major biochemical assays used to assess nutritional status as well as KD stages are tabulated for the reader. Chapter 6 comprehensively discusses the Nutrition-Focused Physical Examination (NFPE) which was included as part of the overall Medicare assessment for ESRD and became widely used by RDNs in 2003. The revised 2014 SOP/SOPP for RDNs in Nephrology Nutrition direct the RDN to utilize the standardized NFPE on patients to assess for fat and muscle wasting; oral health conditions; hair, skin and nails; and signs of edema as well as conditions that impact nutritional status or impact the patient's ability to eat. The core competency standard of the NFPE is part of the accrediting standards in dietetic programs by the Accreditation Council for Education in Nutrition and Dietetics. CKD populations are often found to have signs of malnutrition including edema, ascites, weight loss, muscle weakness, muscle and fat wasting, reduced functional status, peripheral neuropathy, dry skin, ecchymosis, and pruritus. The practice-oriented chapter describes the preparation of the RDN prior to the NFPE, talking points, empathetic approaches, and systematic, thorough examination that does not disturb the patient unnecessarily. Specific nutrients that are adversely affected by RRT are outlined in detail.

Chapter 7 reviews the national standards used to determine the adequacy of the patient's diet and describes the methodologies used to collect patient information about their daily diet or frequency of consumption of foods. The national standards, however, were developed for healthy individuals and are not specific for patients with kidney disease or any other disease state often seen in CKD patients. Fortunately, in addition to describing standard dietary intake methodologies and values, the chapter explains the value of clearly determining protein and sodium status as these are critical issues for CKD patients. The five tables and figure and 125 targeted references provide clear guidance concerning the other nutrients that are important to determining the nutritional status of CKD, RRT, and kidney transplant patients.

Chapter 8 is a new chapter in this volume and looks at the major psychosocial issues that can affect the nutritional status of the patient with KD. The chapter examines the effects of depression, anxiety, loneliness, self-efficacy, food insecurity, limited health literacy, and social support. The chapter is sensitively written and reminds us that a newly diagnosed KD patient is frequently given new dietary restrictions and loss of freedom to enjoy preferred foods. Nutritionally relevant side effects from treatment and especially in patients with ESRD on hemodialysis is severe pain which affects 50% to 60%, and chronic fatigue that impacts 82% of patients. With respect to its effects on nutritional status, depression can undermine a patient's ability to adhere to dietary phosphorus (for example) and fluid restrictions. We also learn that there is a positive relationship between depression, malnutrition, and PEW in CKD patients. Food insecurity is reviewed and the role of poverty, lack of access to more healthful food, and the potential for racial bias are discussed. The other psychosocial aspects are reviewed and over 200 references are provided in this thoughtful chapter. Chapter 9, also a new chapter, provides a basic background in the metabolism and physiological effects of pharmaceuticals and describes the role of the liver and related organs, including the kidney, in the metabolism of drugs. Also, the chapter reviews common food–drug interactions and reviews the most common drugs prescribed for KD patients as well as transplant patients, and the potential for drug–nutrient as well as drug–herbal supplement interactions.

Part III: Preventative Strategies for Chronic Kidney Disease Among Adults

Chapter 10 examines the consequences of persistent high blood pressure (hypertension) and the potential to reduce this risk by making well-researched changes in dietary intakes. We learn that prolonged hypertension, along with diabetes mellitus, is the leading cause of CKD and prolonged uncontrolled hypertension is a major risk factor for ESRD and RRT. There are two diet programs that have been repeatedly shown to reduce blood pressure in hypertensive patients. The Dietary Approaches to Stop Hypertension (DASH) diet and the Mediterranean diet have each been shown to be effective in reducing blood pressure, and these programs have many similarities and some differences that are carefully reviewed in this chapter (see Chap. 31). The Kidney Disease Outcomes Quality Initiative (KDOQI) recommends all of the following be undertaken at the same time: weight loss in those who are overweight or obese and maintenance of weight in those with a body mass index (BMI) < 25 kg/m^2, adopting a DASH-type diet with the reduction of dietary sodium, increased physical activity, and reduction or moderate consumption of alcohol. Other nutrients are also reviewed with regard to reducing blood pressure, but also with specific recommendations for patients with CKD. Chapter 11 looks at the effects of diabetes on the development of nephropathy and clearly identifies the nutrition recommendations for patients with these concurrent comorbidities. Diabetic kidney disease (DKD) is the leading cause of ESRD in North America and affects Black, Hispanic, and Native American patients much more frequently than Caucasians. DKD is also a major risk factor for serious CVD and CVD death. The chapter, containing 115 relevant references, provides a detailed discussion of the MNT that is recommended for patients with both Type 1 and Type 2 diabetes who develop CKD. In addition to specific nutritional guidelines, the chapter also includes an informative table that reviews the most commonly used prescription drugs and their management during the stages of CKD.

Chapter 12 provides the reader with a broad overview of the epidemiology, basic science, and clinical aspects of obesity as it involves patients throughout the spectrum of CKD. Of importance, BMI can be used as a reasonably good indicator of total body fat content in CKD and dialysis patients. The prevalence of obesity continues to increase in patients at all stages of KD including transplantation and is obviously an additional burden on the patient's own kidneys as well as the transplanted kidney. In fact, population attributable risk analyses estimate that approximately one-fifth to one-fourth of kidney disease cases could be prevented by eliminating overweight and obesity; obesity also increases the risk for ESRD six fold compared to normal weight, age, and sex matched individuals. The chapter includes over 200 targeted references and 7 important tables and figures, as well as an extensive review of the pathology of the kidney as well as other organ responses associated with obesity, and reviews the effects of bariatric surgery on kidney functions in the obese patient. Chapter 13 reviews the multifaceted area of nutritional management of patients with CVD as well as KD. Both CKD and CVD share common risk factors, including obesity, reviewed in the preceding chapter, dyslipidemia, sedentary lifestyle, and both inadequate blood pressure control and diabetes control (see Chap. 11, and multiple dietary factors. CKD doubles the risk of developing CVD and increases the risk of stroke, atrial fibrillation, and cardiac failure. The chapter includes a full list of the diagnostic tests and criteria for CVD assessment especially in the KD patient. The nutritional needs of the patient with both diseases are reviewed throughout the progress of each of the diseases and modulation of recommendations are considered based upon the prescription drug(s) used; a relevant case study and related tables are included at the end of the chapter).

Part IV: Chronic Kidney Disease in Adults Treated By Renal Replacement Therapies

The five chapters in this part are focused on practice-based recommendations for care of the most seriously affected KD patients. Chapter 14 provides a detailed discussion of the five stages of CKD and the nutritional management of the patient with the primary goal of reducing the risk of progression of kidney disease. The chapter provides an historic perspective on the development of nutritional recommendations and reviews current guidelines as well as pointing to ongoing controversies regarding protein intake, guidelines in obese patients, major nutrient adjustments that are required in CKD Stage 5, and nutrient needs in transplant patients; nutritional requirements during the aging process that are altered by KD are also discussed. The diagnosis and treatment of anemia in CKD is described in detail. IgA nephropathy is reviewed with regard to a low-antigen diet and other relevant aspects of MNT. MNT programs to prevent malnutrition, electrolyte imbalances, dyslipidemia, and bone and mineral metabolism disorders are also discussed and a case study is included along with over 100 references and 7 helpful tables. Chapter 15 builds on the information in earlier chapters concerning the nutritional status of the hemodialysis (HD) patient and the effects of the types and frequency of dialysis, types of equipment used, the inflammatory status, and the PEW condition of the patient. Topics including anorexia, acidosis, fluid volume, and the specific nutrient effects of dialysis are reviewed. Recommendations are provided for nutrient intakes using conventional hemodialysis as well as nocturnal hemodialysis/short daily hemodialysis. Chapter 16 concentrates on the nutritional needs of the CKD patient who is receiving peritoneal dialysis (PD). We learn that the use of PD is increasing rapidly, thus the chapter's emphasis on this RRT is of importance especially as this is a new chapter topic for this volume. Patients who receive PD have many of the same nutritional issues seen in patients receiving HD. PD patients with low baseline serum albumin concentrations had a three-fold or higher adjusted risk of all-cause and cardiovascular mortality and 3.4-fold higher risk of infection-related mortality compared to HD patients. One difference between PD and HD is that PD is considered to be less catabolic than HD; however, certain patients may not get this benefit due to individual differences. The chapter includes recommendations for energy, protein, sodium, fluid, potassium, calcium, phosphorus, vitamin D, lipids, fiber, other vitamins and minerals, and trace elements intakes as well as a related case study and over 100 references.

Chapter 17, also a new chapter, goes beyond the standard dietary recommendations for RRT patients and reviews the nutritional interventions provided to the ESRD patient with PEW who cannot maintain their weight or balanced nutritional status with foods alone and must be given oral nutritional supplements, enteral or intradialytic parenteral nutrition. The chapter includes a concise discussion of the role of nutrition counseling in this very at-risk patient population, with emphasis on the continuum of care as the patient requires additional nutritional provision. The five tables and case study provide further specific guidance to the nutrition health professional. The final chapter in this part, Chap. 18, examines the importance of MNT through all stages of kidney transplantation (pre, peri, and post). The chapter includes a short history and current status of kidney transplantation in the USA. The purpose of the chapter is to provide an up-to-date and practical resource for registered dietitians, nutritionists, and other health professionals providing nutritional care to kidney transplant candidates and recipients. The chapter includes information on nutrition assessment, the nutritional impact of induction, and maintenance immunosuppressive medications, transplant-specific nutrition education, macro- and micronutrient recommendations, and common nutritional findings in the three phases of transplantation. We learn that in 2007, Federal legislation mandated that an RDN be a member of the transplant medical team. In 2017, a Framework for Standardized Transplant Specific Competencies was published for dietitians practicing in all solid organ transplants. The competencies highlight several key areas including transplant-specific MNT, the role of the transplant dietitian in each phase of transplant, quality and performance improvement, training including orientation and continuing education requirements for transplant dietitians, and general knowledge of transplant principles and regulations which are reviewed in this new chapter. There is a review of the current acceptable nutritional status of potential kidney transplant recipients and their use of MNT prior to surgery. Transplantation requires immunosuppression of the patient and this process increases the risk of infection and induction of mineral imbalances post surgery. The potential for worsening of diabetes following transplantation is also discussed. The nutritionally related adverse effects of the commonly used drugs during the three phases of transplantation are reviewed and the case study examines these phases in a patient evaluation.

Part V: Nutrition in CKD Among Special Needs Populations

Chapter 19 sensitively examines the unique nutritional requirements during a high-risk pregnancy complicated by CKD, while on dialysis, during breastfeeding, and post kidney transplantation. Currently, there is a paucity of data from well-controlled studies involving pregnant women with CKD; however, there are observational data that suggest a greater risk of pre-term and other birth complications and there may be a further loss of maternal kidney function. Both medications and nutrient intakes may need to be altered and therefore MNT by a clinical team trained to provide this intensive care is recommended. Dialysis adds an additional need for specialized care for both the pregnant woman and her fetus. The frequency of dialysis, type of dialysis, and content of the dialysate will require reformulation as the pregnancy progresses. These factors are covered in detail in the chapter. With regard to breastfeeding, it appears that few women breastfeed while on dialysis and post-transplant mothers are advised not to breastfeed due to the potential passage of immunosuppressive and other drugs to the infant. Chapter 20 describes the complexities of treating children, from infancy to early adulthood, that have CKD. The pediatric renal dietitian has expertise in childhood nutrition and growth combined with the experience in providing nutritional guidance to children with kidney dysfunctions. Congenital anomalies of the kidney and urinary tract account for about half of all causes of early childhood CKD and ESRD whereas glomerular diseases are more common in older children with CKD/ESRD. Normal growth is a critical issue in children with CKD. Poor nutritional status may contribute to reduced growth rate as well as PEW. Age at onset of KD, etiology and severity of the primary renal disorder, renal bone disease, fluid and electrolyte imbalance, metabolic acidosis, inflammation, anemia, abnormalities of the growth hormone-insulin growth factor axis, and suboptimal levels of sex hormones also influence growth and many of these factors are also influenced by nutritional status. According to the 2017 United States Renal Data System (USRDS) report, children receiving dialysis have a high prevalence of severe linear stunting, defined as less than the third percentile for length or height, compared to US norms. The chapter describes the numerous enzymes, growth factors, and hormones that are affected by the inflammation seen in pediatric CKD patients; most of these molecules are metabolic modulators that adversely affect normal hunger cues and further increase the risk of PEW and reduced growth rate. This comprehensive chapter, covering children from age 0–18, contains 179 relevant references, 10 helpful tables, and an important assessment form. Chapter 21 provides a broad overview of the effects of KD in the population over 65 years of age and the role of the nutrition specialist in the care of this at-risk patient population. Individuals 60 years of age and older have the highest prevalence of CKD and thus, not unexpectedly, the USRDS reports that adults older than 65 years of age are the most rapidly growing subset of the ESRD patient population. Furthermore, aging plus CKD are associated with increased frailty and debility, loss of physical function, cognitive changes, psychosocial factors, changes in sensory functions, and loss of appetite that can impact nutritional status and quality of life. The chapter begins with a description of the physical and physiological changes that result in decreased function of the kidneys that begin at about age 50 even in individuals with normal kidney function. New equations for determining kidney status in the elderly with KD are reviewed and tabulated; other chronic diseases common in CKD are also included such as diabetes and CVD. MNT is described in the context of aging as well as CKD and RRT. The case study highlights many of these complexities.

Part VI: Nutritional Management of Other Disorders that Impact Kidney Function

Chapter 22 concentrates on the effects of inflammation in CKD, PEW, and sarcopenia and provides nutritional guidance based upon the anti-inflammatory properties of certain dietary components. The chapter stresses data-driven clinical studies that have used well-recognized biomarkers of inflammation to define the state of malnutrition (seen in wasting and obesity) and sarcopenia in the CKD and RRT patient. There is a discussion of the role of the colon's microbiome, potentials for immunocompromise in HD, and other relevant conditions that increase inflammation and adversely affect nutritional status as kidney function diminishes. Diets and dietary components that can reduce inflammatory biomarkers are examined. The chapter includes 4 helpful tables and 2 important figures as well as over 90 references. Chapter 23 tackles the interrelationships between the loss of the kidney's function of synthesizing the active form of vitamin D; consequent effects of altering bone formation and resorption that result in, among other adverse effects, calcium deposition in blood vessels; dysregulation of mineral homeostasis, PTH, and phosphate; and, finally, significantly increased risk of major ESRD and/or CVD events. The chapter includes a detailed review of the multifaceted bone and mineral effects of CKD and the critical importance of controlling mineral intakes as well as awareness of potential drug–nutrient interactions. The 7 tables, case study, and over 100 references are of great use in understanding the complexities of bone abnormalities seen in advancing KD. Chapter 24 discusses nephrotic syndrome (NS) and the wide range of glomerular diseases that can cause this syndrome, the nutritional consequences, and recommended dietary changes to manage the syndrome. The NS includes primary (idiopathic), genetically inherited, or secondary causes including systemic disease or medication. Primary or idiopathic glomerular diseases that result in nephrotic syndrome include minimal change disease (MCD), membranous nephropathy, and focal segmental glomerulosclerosis (FSGS). The primary diagnosis of NS is loss of protein in the urine. There is a detailed description of the multifactorial effects of this protein loss over time. Protein and amino acid losses adversely affect muscle, platelets, lymphocytes, and bioactive molecules produced throughout the body's organs and tissues. Nutritional therapy in NS paradoxically includes decreased protein intake especially from meat and increased consumption of protein from plants. Dietary and pharmacological treatments are tabulated and the chapter includes over 100 references.

Chapter 25 is written by Dr. Han. The author recently (2019) edited an entire volume entitled *Nutritional and Medical Management of Kidney Stones* as part of the Nutrition and Health Series. The author provides a concise review of nephrolithiasis and current dietary recommendations. Nephrolithiasis (kidney stones, urolithiasis) is defined as the formation of stone-like structures in the urinary system caused by the precipitation of calcium, phosphate, urate, and other molecules. The current prevalence is estimated at about 9% and kidney stones are more prevalent in men than women, with a lifetime risk of 12% in men and 6% in women. Obesity and the metabolic syndrome are important risk factors for nephrolithiasis. The types of stones formed and their pathophysiology, symptoms and diagnosis, and genetic and dietary risk factors are reviewed. Dietary components including calcium, oxalate, protein, potassium, magnesium, phosphate, phytates, vitamins, and herbals as well as types of beverages are discussed. This comprehensive chapter includes 2 case studies, 9 informative, detailed tables, and 2 figures as well as over 180 targeted references. Chapter 26 describes the characteristics of acute kidney injury (AKI) including an abrupt reduction of kidney function over hours to days which results in failure to maintain electrolyte, acid–base, and fluid homeostasis. AKI can occur in up to 20% of all hospitalized patients. Several complications can occur in AKI including hyperkalemia, hyperphosphatemia, glucose intolerance, fluid overload, and azotemia (high blood nitrogen levels). Causes of AKI in individuals with prior normal kidney function can include physical kidney injury, burns, certain drugs, cancer treatment, infection, as examples. Urinary tract obstruction as seen in prostate disease is another cause. The importance of timely nutrition support has recently been recommended and is reviewed in detail including the use of enteral and parenteral nutrition support.

Part VII: Additional Nutritional Considerations in Kidney Disease

Chapter 27, a new chapter, examines the role of the gut microbiome in KD patients. The chapter begins with a basic description of the microbiome and its functions and we learn that nutrients can impact diversity, density, and functionality of the gut microbiota, while microbiota-derived metabolites connect the gut microbiota with distant organs, impacting health and disease. The chapter describes novel applications of nutritional strategies to modulate the dysfunctions of the gut microbiota often seen in CKD patients. The increased formation of urea in CKD adversely affects the microbiota and results in further formation of proinflammatory molecules. The potential usefulness of prebiotics and/or probiotics and synbiotics that contain both pre- and probiotics is reviewed with the caution that currently there are few well-controlled studies in this area. Chapter 28 is also a new chapter and looks at appetite regulation in KD. There is a detailed description of the role of the central nervous system and its interactions with the gastrointestinal system in appetite control. The hormones, enzymes, and other bioactive molecules are discussed and particular organs and tissues, such as the pancreas and adipose tissue, are examined to better understand their role in eating behaviors. In CKD, many of the key molecular factors are adversely affected resulting in loss of appetite, GI tract discomfort, adverse effects of medications on taste, as examples. The chapter includes over 100 targeted references. Chapter 29 is also a new chapter and discusses the relatively new area of research into the effects of advanced glycation end products (AGEs) in CKD. AGEs are formed internally and are sometimes used as biomarkers such as hemoglobin A1c for Type 2 diabetes status. AGEs have also been found in foods that have been exposed to high heat. The chapter reviews the increasing evidence that exogenous AGEs from diet have an important contribution to oxidative processes. Reduction of dietary AGE intake has been demonstrated to prevent or diminish pro-oxidant and pro-inflammatory responses in several recent clinical trials. The trials have demonstrated that dietary AGEs restriction may be of benefit to CKD patients. The chapter reviews the evidence that the kidneys are involved in maintaining AGE homeostasis. AGE-peptides undergo filtration followed by partial tubular reabsorption, and possibly also secretion after tubular uptake from the peritubular blood flow. Normal kidneys catabolize AGEs within the renal tubules. An elevation of AGEs in the urine is characteristic of reduction in kidney function and is markedly increased in CKD as well as before and after initiation of dialysis, especially HD. With regard to food sources of AGEs, the lower the cooking temperature, the lower the amount of AGEs generated. Cooking methods that use dry heat, such as broiling, searing, and frying, have been shown to cause the formation of the highest content of AGEs. An acidic pH has been shown to limit the formation of AGEs. Marinades made with vinegar for high-protein foods such as meats reduce the risk of AGE formation. The chapter includes reviews of clinical studies in diabetic and KD patients and contains over 50 related references including those with tables listing food AGE contents.

Chapter 30 begins with an assessment of the physical capabilities of the CKD patient. The CKD population is usually older, with increasingly common comorbidities such as diabetes, hypertension, and CVD. Frailty and low levels of physical function and activity are related to morbidity and mortality and are well-documented in people with CKD. Obesity is common; however, sarcopenic obesity is increasingly recognized. Even with these characteristics, the authors indicate, based upon clinical research, that physical activity can benefit the CKD patient. The chapter reviews several types of physical activity and exercise including aerobic, muscle strengthening, bone strengthening, balance, and flexibility. Several types of physical activity are discussed including combinations of endurance, resistance, flexibility, and balance exercises at least several days a week. Given the complexity of the disease conditions seen with CKD, a professional trainer who has experience with KD patients is recommended. Even though the chapter includes over 160 references, the authors indicate that it is widely acknowledged that there is a dearth of high-quality, adequately powered randomized clinical trials (RCT) in the exercise literature in CKD.

Chapters 31, 32, and 33 examine the roles of dietary patterns and dietary supplements (herbal and natural substances in Chapter 32 and vitamins and trace elements in Chap. 33) in patients with KD. Chapter 31 introduces the relatively new concept of dietary patterns. Dietary patterns reflect the daily intake of all foods over a prolonged period of time. The US National Kidney Foundation recommends plant-based diets for their cardioprotective benefits. These include the DASH diet and the Mediterranean diet, which are high in fiber; low in saturated fat and processed meats; contain sources of potassium, phosphorus, magnesium, and calcium; and have low levels of sodium (see Chap. 10). Meta-analyses have found that CKD patients who adhere to these diets have a decreased mortality risk; however, direct RCT have not been undertaken as yet. The observational data associating plant-based diets and reduced risk of CKD as well as slower disease progression are reviewed. Chapter 32 concentrates on the potential for herbal and other natural products sold as supplements that can either help or harm the CKD patient, especially those who cannot access dialysis. Specific herbs, fatty acids, and microbes are mentioned. The potential interactions with pharmaceutical medicines are discussed. Chapter 33 provides a detailed discussion of the changing essential nutrient needs of the KD and RRT patients. In addition to altered intake, metabolic changes in CKD patients may affect absorption, utilization, and excretion of micronutrients. Uremic toxicity, comorbidities, and finally the treatment of ESRD may all contribute to a heightened inflammatory status which affects the status of many micronutrients, especially those with antioxidant properties, such as vitamins C and E and minerals such as selenium. The chapter includes three examples of nutrient alterations in advanced CKD patients. Deficiency in vitamin K, an increased need for vitamin B6, and a reduced tolerance for vitamin A are reviewed. The chapter summarizes the studies that have looked at several single nutrient deficiencies such as thia-min, folate, and B12 as well as the bioactive molecule, homocysteine. Both essential and non-essential (sometimes toxic) minerals and trace elements are reviewed in CKD. The data is derived mainly from findings of deficiencies and/or toxicities and currently there are no RCT in this area that point to effects with long-term interventions.

Chapter 34, written by Dr. Burrowes, examines the need of the CKD patient to adhere to the dietary strategies that have been developed to main-tain kidney function during all stages of the disease. MNT is an integral com-ponent for successful treatment outcomes in patients with CKD. The chapter reviews both positive and negative factors that can influence a patient's ability to follow the recommended diet prescription. Factors that can improve adher-ence include social support from family and/or caregivers and dietitian/nutri-tionist and team's familiarity with the patient's culture, food habits, beliefs, and practices. Inhibitors of dietary adherence include the patient's lifestyle, attitude towards the disease, socioeconomic status, cultural barriers, and other factors. The chapter provides evidence-based recommendations from the American Heart Association that the renal RD and team can provide to the CKD patient, and the new areas of patient-centered web-based programs for behavioral modification as well as monitoring progress are reviewed. The chapter focuses on the complexity of the dietary program and the difficulties that the CKD patient faces especially as the disease worsens and concomitant conditions also become a significant issue in meeting the dietary program. Chapter 35 provides further guidance on improving patient adherence to their dietary requirements through effective communications and counseling. The chapter describes several methods that have been shown to increase KD patient adherence with their dietary prescriptions. The Transtheoretical Model used in identifying the stages of change is reviewed. Also, Cognitive Behavioral Therapy, Social Learning Theory, and Motivational Interviewing are examined as these have emerged as efficacious models for changing patient's food and lifestyle behaviors. Specific examples of questions and communication skills are provided in the text, case study, and relevant tables. Chapter 36, written by Dr. Byham-Gray, concentrates on the critical impor-tance of early dietary intervention in KD patients and the methodologies to conduct clinical research studies in this patient population. The chapter pro-vides a brief overview of the importance of documenting the initial nutri-tional status of the patient in order to verify the key clinical outcomes of any dietary intervention in CKD patients. As examples, bone disease, diabetes, dyslipidemias, hypertension, dialysis adequacy, and anemia are all either directly or indirectly related to nutritional status and/or intervention. Protein-energy malnutrition or PEW are independent contributors to mortality risk; however, it is unclear whether the malnutrition or wasting has worsened over a period of time or is the result of a suboptimal status at the time of CKD or dialysis initiation. The chapter includes a clear description of comparative effectiveness research and its related methodology, as well as a discussion of the research used to develop evidence-based National clinical guidelines and clinical research used to help assure a reduction in practice variation. Chapter 37 provides the kidney healthcare provider with an up-to-date compilation of relevant resource websites and citations, tables, and references. This chapter provides a compilation of professional resources that may be of benefit for the RDN and related practitioners. Its primary goal is to be an accessible reference for the practitioner who treats patients with CKD. The chapter is organized in four basic sections: (1) evidence-based practice guidelines in chronic kidney disease, (2) diet-related resources and food lists, (3) critical tools for conducting nutrition assessments and delivering quality care, and (4) internet websites and applications.

Conclusions

The above description of the volume's 37 chapters attests to the depth of information provided by the 58 highly respected chapter authors and volume editors. Each chapter includes complete definitions of terms with the abbreviations fully defined and consistent use of terms between chapters. Key features of the comprehensive volume include 134 detailed tables and informative figures; an extensive, detailed index; and more than 3350 up-to-date references that provide the reader with excellent sources of worthwhile practice-oriented information that will be of great value to nephrologists and related health providers, specialized nutrition practitioners, and clinical researchers, as well as graduate and medical students. In addition to specific data on foods and diets, the volume contains important sensitive chapters related to improving the success of CKD patients in adhering to their complex dietary programs.

In conclusion *Nutrition in Kidney Disease, Third Edition,* edited by Jerrilynn D. Burrowes, PhD, RDN, CDN, FNKF; Csaba P. Kovesdy, MD; and Laura Byham-Gray, PhD, RDN, FNKF, provides health professionals in many areas of kidney disease research and practice with the most current and well-referenced volume on importance of evidence-based nutritional interventions to assure the overall health of the individual with kidney disease throughout all stages of the disease. The volume serves the reader as the benchmark for integrating the complex interrelationships between nutritionally related risk factors such as hypertension, obesity, diabetes, and cardiovascular disease as well as genetic inherited kidney dysfunctions such as stone formation and nephron malformations. The new chapters of this valuable volume provide unique and concise data on drug–nutrient interactions; the psychosocial aspects of CKD and RRT; nutritional management of the newly diagnosed KD patient; the CKD patient with concurrent CVD; the hemodialysis patient and the peritoneal dialysis patient; the role of the microbiome, AGEs, and appetite regulation in KD; and the importance of examining dietary patterns in addition to single nutrients. Finally, the most relevant citations on all aspects of kidney function and diseases as well as recommended resources from National research centers and kidney disease organizations that provide reliable, up-to-date information based upon the totality of the research are included in this comprehensive volume. The broad scope as well as in-depth reviews found in each chapter makes this excellent volume a very welcome addition to the Nutrition and Health Series.

Adrianne Bendich, PhD, FACN, FASN

Series Editor Biography

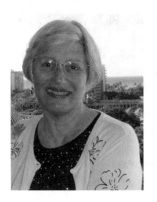

Adrianne Bendich, PhD, FASN, FACN has served as the Nutrition and Health Series Editor for more than 20 years and has provided leadership and guidance to more than 200 editors that have developed the 90 well-respected and highly recommended volumes in the series.

In addition to *Nutrition in Kidney Disease, Third Edition*, edited by Jerrilynn D. Burrowes, PhD, RDN, CDN, FNKF; Csaba P. Kovesdy, MD; and Laura Byham-Gray, PhD, RDN, FNKF, major new editions published from 2012–2020 include:

1. *Nutrition, Fitness, and Mindfulness*, edited by Dr. Jaime Uribarri and Dr. Joseph A. Vassalotti, 2020
2. *Vitamin E in Human Health*, edited by Peter Weber, Marc Birringer, Jeffrey B. Blumberg, Manfred Eggersdorfer, Jan Frank, 2019
3. *Handbook of Nutrition and Pregnancy, Second Edition*, edited by Carol J. Lammi-Keefe, Sarah C. Couch and John P. Kirwan, 2019
4. *Dietary Patterns and Whole Plant Foods in Aging and Disease*, edited as well as written by Mark L. Dreher, Ph.D, 2018
5. *Dietary Fiber in Health and Disease*, edited as well as written by Mark L. Dreher, Ph.D., 2017
6. *Clinical Aspects of Natural and Added Phosphorus in Foods*, edited by Orlando M. Gutierrez, Kamyar Kalantar-Zadeh and Rajnish Mehrotra, 2017
7. *Nutrition and Fetal Programming*, edited by Rajendram Rajkumar, Victor R. Preedy and Vinood B. Patel, 2017
8. *Nutrition and Diet in Maternal Diabetes*, edited by Rajendram Rajkumar, Victor R. Preedy and Vinood B. Patel, 2017
9. *Nitrite and Nitrate in Human Health and Disease, Second Edition*, edited by Nathan S. Bryan and Joseph Loscalzo, 2017
10. *Nutrition in Lifestyle Medicine*, edited by James M. Rippe, 2017
11. *Nutrition Guide for Physicians and Related Healthcare Professionals, Second Edition*, edited by Norman J. Temple, Ted Wilson and George A. Bray, 2016

12. *Clinical Aspects of Natural and Added Phosphorus in Foods*, edited by Orlando M. Gutiérrez, Kamyar Kalantar-Zadeh and Rajnish Mehrotra, 2016
13. *L-Arginine in Clinical Nutrition*, edited by Vinood B. Patel, Victor R. Preedy, and Rajkumar Rajendram, 2016
14. *Mediterranean Diet: Impact on Health and Disease,* edited by Donato F. Romagnolo, Ph.D. and Ornella Selmin, Ph.D., 2016
15. *Nutrition Support for the Critically Ill*, edited by David S. Seres, MD and Charles W. Van Way, III, MD, 2016
16. *Nutrition in Cystic Fibrosis: A Guide for Clinicians*, edited by Elizabeth H. Yen, M.D. and Amanda R. Leonard, MPH, RD, CDE, 2016
17. *Preventive Nutrition: The Comprehensive Guide for Health Professionals, Fifth Edition*, edited by Adrianne Bendich, Ph.D. and Richard J. Deckelbaum, M.D., 2016
18. *Glutamine in Clinical Nutrition*, edited by Rajkumar Rajendram, Victor R. Preedy and Vinood B. Patel, 2015
19. *Nutrition and Bone Health, Second Edition*, edited by Michael F. Holick and Jeri W. Nieves, 2015
20. *Branched Chain Amino Acids in Clinical Nutrition, Volume 2*, edited by Rajkumar Rajendram, Victor R. Preedy and Vinood B. Patel, 2015
21. *Branched Chain Amino Acids in Clinical Nutrition, Volume 1*, edited by Rajkumar Rajendram, Victor R. Preedy and Vinood B. Patel, 2015
22. *Fructose, High Fructose Corn Syrup, Sucrose and Health,* edited by James M. Rippe, 2014
23. *Handbook of Clinical Nutrition and Aging, Third Edition*, edited by Connie Watkins Bales, Julie L. Locher and Edward Saltzman, 2014
24. *Nutrition and Pediatric Pulmonary Disease*, edited by Dr. Youngran Chung and Dr. Robert Dumont, 2014
25. *Integrative Weight Management*, edited by Dr. Gerald E. Mullin, Dr. Lawrence J. Cheskin and Dr. Laura E. Matarese, 2014
26. *Nutrition in Kidney Disease, Second Edition,* edited by Dr. Laura D. Byham-Gray, Dr. Jerrilynn D. Burrowes and Dr. Glenn M. Chertow, 2014
27. *Handbook of Food Fortification and Health, Volume I,* edited by Dr. Victor R. Preedy, Dr. Rajaventhan Srirajaskanthan, Dr. Vinood B. Patel, 2013
28. *Handbook of Food Fortification and Health, Volume II,* edited by Dr. Victor R. Preedy, Dr. Rajaventhan Srirajaskanthan, Dr. Vinood B. Patel, 2013
29. *Diet Quality: An Evidence-Based Approach, Volume I,* edited by Dr. Victor R. Preedy, Dr. Lan-Ahn Hunter and Dr. Vinood B. Patel, 2013
30. *Diet Quality: An Evidence-Based Approach, Volume II,* edited by Dr. Victor R. Preedy, Dr. Lan-Ahn Hunter and Dr. Vinood B. Patel, 2013
31. *The Handbook of Clinical Nutrition and Stroke*, edited by Mandy L. Corrigan, MPH, RD Arlene A. Escuro, MS, RD, and Donald F. Kirby, MD, FACP, FACN, FACG, 2013
32. *Nutrition in Infancy, Volume I*, edited by Dr. Ronald Ross Watson, Dr. George Grimble, Dr. Victor Preedy and Dr. Sherma Zibadi, 2013
33. *Nutrition in Infancy, Volume II,* edited by Dr. Ronald Ross Watson, Dr. George Grimble, Dr. Victor Preedy and Dr. Sherma Zibadi, 2013

34. *Carotenoids and Human Health,* edited by Dr. Sherry A. Tanumihardjo, 2013
35. *Bioactive Dietary Factors and Plant Extracts in Dermatology,* edited by Dr. Ronald Ross Watson and Dr. Sherma Zibadi, 2013
36. *Omega 6/3 Fatty Acids,* edited by Dr. Fabien De Meester, Dr. Ronald Ross Watson and Dr. Sherma Zibadi, 2013
37. *Nutrition in Pediatric Pulmonary Disease*, edited by Dr. Robert Dumont and Dr. Youngran Chung, 2013
38. *Nutrition and Diet in Menopause*, edited by Dr. Caroline J. Hollins Martin, Dr. Ronald Ross Watson and Dr. Victor R. Preedy, 2013
39. *Magnesium and Health,* edited by Dr. Ronald Ross Watson and Dr. Victor R. Preedy, 2012
40. *Alcohol, Nutrition and Health Consequences*, edited by Dr. Ronald Ross Watson, Dr. Victor R. Preedy, and Dr. Sherma Zibadi, 2012
41. *Nutritional Health, Strategies for Disease Prevention, Third Edition*, edited by Norman J. Temple, Ted Wilson, and David R. Jacobs, Jr., 2012
42. *Chocolate in Health and Nutrition*, edited by Dr. Ronald Ross Watson, Dr. Victor R. Preedy, and Dr. Sherma Zibadi, 2012
43. *Iron Physiology and Pathophysiology in Humans*, edited by Dr. Gregory J. Anderson and Dr. Gordon D. McLaren, 2012

Earlier books included *Vitamin D, Second Edition*, edited by Dr. Michael Holick; *Dietary Components and Immune Function*, edited by Dr. Ronald Ross Watson, Dr. Sherma Zibadi, and Dr. Victor R. Preedy; *Bioactive Compounds and Cancer*, edited by Dr. John A. Milner and Dr. Donato F. Romagnolo; *Modern Dietary Fat Intakes in Disease Promotion*, edited by Dr. Fabien De Meester, Dr. Sherma Zibadi, and Dr. Ronald Ross Watson; *Iron Deficiency and Overload*, edited by Dr. Shlomo Yehuda and Dr. David Mostofsky; *Nutrition Guide for Physicians,* edited by Dr. Edward Wilson, Dr. George A. Bray, Dr. Norman Temple, and Dr. Mary Struble; *Nutrition and Metabolism,* edited by Dr. Christos Mantzoros; and *Fluid and Electrolytes in Pediatrics*, edited by Leonard Feld and Dr. Frederick Kaskel. Recent volumes include *Handbook of Drug-Nutrient Interactions,* edited by Dr. Joseph Boullata and Dr. Vincent Armenti; *Probiotics in Pediatric Medicine*, edited by Dr. Sonia Michail and Dr. Philip Sherman; *Handbook of Nutrition and Pregnancy*, edited by Dr. Carol Lammi-Keefe, Dr. Sarah Couch, and Dr. Elliot Philipson; *Nutrition and Rheumatic Disease*, edited by Dr. Laura Coleman; *Nutrition and Kidney Disease,* edited by Dr. Laura Byham-Grey, Dr. Jerrilynn Burrowes, and Dr. Glenn Chertow; *Nutrition and Health in Developing Countries,* edited by Dr. Richard Semba and Dr. Martin Bloem; *Calcium in Human Health,* edited by Dr. Robert Heaney and Dr. Connie Weaver; and *Nutrition and Bone Health*, edited by Dr. Michael Holick and Dr. Bess Dawson-Hughes.

Dr. Bendich is past President of Consultants in Consumer Healthcare LLC and is the editor of ten books, including *Preventive Nutrition: The Comprehensive Guide for Health Professionals, Fifth Edition,* co-edited with Dr. Richard Deckelbaum (www.springer.com/series/7659). Dr. Bendich serves on the Editorial Boards of the *Journal of Nutrition in Gerontology and Geriatrics* and *Antioxidants*, and has served as Associate Editor for *Nutrition, the International Journal*; served on the Editorial Board of the *Journal of*

Women's Health and Gender-based Medicine; and served on the Board of Directors of the American College of Nutrition.

Dr. Bendich was Director of Medical Affairs at GlaxoSmithKline (GSK) Consumer Healthcare and provided medical leadership for many well-known brands including TUMS and Os-Cal. She had primary responsibility for GSK's support for the Women's Health Initiative (WHI) intervention study. Prior to joining GSK, Dr. Bendich was at Roche Vitamins Inc. and was involved with the groundbreaking clinical studies showing that folic acid-containing multivitamins significantly reduced major classes of birth defects. She has co-authored over 100 major clinical research studies in the area of preventive nutrition. She is recognized as a leading authority on antioxidants, nutrition and immunity and pregnancy outcomes, vitamin safety, and the cost-effectiveness of vitamin/mineral supplementation.

Dr. Bendich received the Roche Research Award, is a Tribute to Women and Industry Awardee, and was a recipient of the Burroughs Wellcome Visiting Professorship in Basic Medical Sciences. She was given the Council for Responsible Nutrition (CRN) Apple Award in recognition of her many contributions to the scientific understanding of dietary supplements. In 2012, she was recognized for her contributions to the field of clinical nutrition by the American Society for Nutrition and was elected a *Fellow of ASN* (FASN). Dr. Bendich served as an Adjunct Professor at Rutgers University. She is listed in Who's Who in American Women.

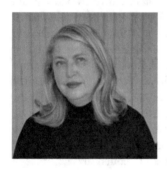

Connie W. Bales, PhD, RD is a Professor of Medicine in the Division of Geriatrics, Department of Medicine, at the Duke School of Medicine and Senior Fellow in the Center for the Study of Aging and Human Development at Duke University Medical Center. She is also Associate Director for Education/Evaluation of the Geriatrics Research, Education, and Clinical Center at the Durham VA Medical Center. Dr. Bales is a well-recognized expert in the field of nutrition, chronic disease, function, and aging. Over the past two decades, her laboratory at Duke has explored many different aspects of diet and activity as determinants of health during the latter half of the adult life course. Her current research focuses primarily on enhanced protein as a means of benefiting muscle quality, function, and other health indicators during geriatric obesity reduction and for improving perioperative outcomes in older patients. Dr. Bales has served on NIH and USDA grant review panels and is Past-Chair of the Medical Nutrition Council of the American Society for Nutrition. She has edited three editions of the *Handbook of Clinical Nutrition and Aging*, is Editor-in-Chief of the *Journal of Nutrition in Gerontology and Geriatrics* and is a Deputy Editor of *Current Developments in Nutrition*.

About the Volume Editors

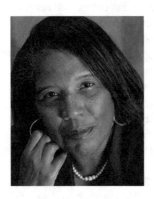

Jerrilynn D. Burrowes, PhD, RD, CDN, FNKF is Professor of Nutrition in the Department of Biomedical, Health and Nutritional Sciences at Long Island University (LIU) Post in Brookville, NY. Dr. Burrowes has numerous publications in refereed journals and she has been an invited speaker at several international, national, regional, and local professional meetings and conferences over the years on nutrition in kidney disease. She is a co-editor for the first and second editions of the textbook *Nutrition in Kidney Disease*, which were published by Humana Press in 2008 and Springer in 2014, and she is currently the senior editor for this third edition.

Dr. Burrowes has held many leadership and advisory roles in professional organizations and societies, and she has served on numerous association committees. She is currently a Council Member of the International Society of Renal Nutrition and Metabolism (ISRNM) for the 2018–2020 term. For the past 8 years, Dr. Burrowes served as the Editor-in-Chief for the *Journal of Renal Nutrition*. She was also a member of the workgroup that developed the initial NKF-DOQI Clinical Practice Guidelines for Nutrition in Chronic Renal Failure (2000) and the workgroup that developed the joint NKF and Academy KDOQI/EAL Clinical Practice Guidelines in Nutrition in Chronic Kidney Disease (2020). Dr. Burrowes received the Recognized Renal Dietitian Award and the Joel D. Kopple Award from the NKF Council on Renal Nutrition, and the Outstanding Service Award from the Renal Practice Group of the Academy of Nutrition and Dietetics.

Dr. Burrowes earned her bachelor's degree in biology/pre-medicine from Fisk University in Nashville, TN; her MS degree in foods, nutrition, and dietetics from New York University; and her PhD in nutrition from New York University.

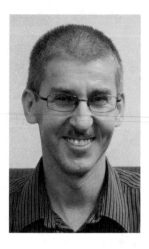

Csaba P. Kovesdy, MD is an internationally recognized clinical researcher and renal outcomes investigator. Dr. Kovesdy is the Fred Hatch Professor of Medicine in Nephrology and Director of the Clinical Outcomes and Clinical Trials Program at the University of Tennessee Health Science Center in Memphis, Tennessee, and Chief of Nephrology at the Memphis VA Medical Center in Memphis, Tennessee. Dr. Kovesdy earned his medical degree Summa cum Laude from the University of Pecs Medical School in Pecs, Hungary. He completed his residency in Internal Medicine at the Henry Ford Hospital in Detroit, Michigan, and a clinical fellowship in Nephrology at the Johns Hopkins Bayview Medical Center in Baltimore, Maryland.

Dr. Kovesdy's main research interests are centered on the epidemiology and outcomes of patients with pre-dialysis chronic kidney disease and ESRD, with special emphasis on studying the role played by malnutrition and inflammation in driving poor outcomes in these populations. He has published his research in over 490 peer-reviewed articles as well as numerous abstracts and book chapters. Dr. Kovesdy has been a member of the International Society of Renal Nutrition and Metabolism Council since 2012 and its Treasurer during 2014–2018, a Fellow of the American Society of Nephrology, and a member of the European Renal Association – European Dialysis and Transplant Association, and the International Society of Nephrology.

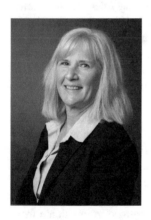

Laura D. Byham-Gray, PhD, RDN, FNKF is a Professor and Vice Chair for Research in the Department of Clinical and Preventive Nutrition Sciences, School of Health Professions at Rutgers University. Prior to teaching, Dr. Byham-Gray practiced in the field of clinical nutrition with specialty practice in nutrition support and kidney disease for over 15 years. She received a NIDDK research grant that funded the development and validation of the predictive energy equation in hemodialysis, and she has recently embarked on another research-funded project from the Agency of Healthcare Research and Quality with the plans to explore protein-energy wasting in hemodialysis while integrating the patient perspective.

Dr. Byham-Gray has held numerous elected and appointed positions at the national, state, and local levels of National Kidney Foundation, the American Society of Parenteral and Enteral Nutrition, and the Academy of Nutrition & Dietetics. Currently, she is chairing the Macronutrients Section of the joint NKF and Academy KDOQI/EAL Clinical Practice Guidelines in Nutrition in Chronic Kidney Disease. Dr. Byham-Gray has also served as the associate editor for the National Kidney Foundation publication *The Journal of Renal Nutrition*. She has over 100 peer-reviewed articles and professional presentations related to kidney disease, dietetics practice, and clinical decision-making as well as management. Dr. Byham-Gray has served as the chief editor for two books: *Nutrition in Kidney Disease* (Springer Publications, 2014) and *A Clinical Guide to Nutrition Care in Kidney Disease* (Academy of Nutrition and Dietetics, 2013). She has received numerous awards, including the Presidential Citation for Outstanding Achievement from the University of Delaware, the Susan C. Knapp Excellence in Education Award, and the prestigious Joel D. Kopple Award.

Dr. Byham-Gray received her bachelor of science in nutrition and dietetics from Mercyhurst University in Erie, Pennsylvania, her master of science in food science and human nutrition from the University of Delaware, and her PhD in nutrition from the New York University, Steinhardt School of Education in the Department of Nutrition, Food Studies, and Public Health.

Acknowledgment

We would like to thank Springer Publications and Dr. Adrianne Bendich for the opportunity to make this third edition of *Nutrition in Kidney Disease* a reality. We also gratefully acknowledge Ms. Diane Lamsback, Developmental Editor at Springer Nature, for her unwavering support and guidance throughout this project. She is the best of the best, and we thank her! Moreover, we express gratitude and appreciation to our contributors for their commitment and patience throughout this process.

Contents

Contributors

Shubha Ananthakrishnan, MD Division of Nephrology, Department of Medicine, UC Davis Medical Center, Sacramento, CA, USA

Carla Maria Avesani, PhD Nutrition Institute, Rio de Janeiro State University, Rio de Janeiro, Brazil

Department of Renal Medicine, Karolinska Institutet, and Baxter Novum, Stockholm, Sweden

Vinod K. Bansal, MD Division of Nephrology and Hypertension, Department of Medicine, Loyola University Healthcare, Maywood, IL, USA

Judith A. Beto, PhD, RDN Division of Nephrology and Hypertension, Department of Medicine, Loyola University Healthcare, Maywood, IL, USA

Annabel Biruete, PhD, RD Division of Nephrology, Department of Medicine, Indiana University School of Medicine, Indianapolis, IN, USA

Debra Blair, DCN, MPH, RD, LDN Rutgers, The State University of New Jersey, Clinical and Preventive Nutrition Sciences, School of Health Professions, Newark, NJ, USA

Natália Alvarenga Borges Institute of Nutrition, Rio de Janeiro State University (UERJ), Rio de Janeiro, RJ, Brazil

Jerrilynn D. Burrowes, PhD, RD Department of Biomedical, Health and Nutritional Sciences, School of Health Professions and Nursing, Long Island University-Post, Brookville, NY, USA

Laura D. Byham-Gray, PhD, RDN, FNKF Clinical and Preventive Nutrition Sciences, School of Health Professions, Rutgers University, Newark, NJ, USA

Winnie Chan, PhD, RD University of Birmingham, School of Sport, Exercise and Rehabilitation Sciences, Birmingham, UK

Charles Chazot NephroCare Tassin-Charcot, Sainte-Foy-lès-Lyon, France

Francis Dumler, MD Section of Nephrology, William Beaumont Hospital, Royal Oak, MI, USA

Meaghan Elger, MSc, RD, CD St. Michael's Hospital, Centre for Diabetes & Endocrinology, Toronto, ON, Canada

Antonette Flecha, PharmD SUNY Downstate Medical Center, Montefiore Medical Center, Transplant Surgery, Bronx, NY, USA

Allon N. Friedman, MD Department of Medicine, Indiana University School of Medicine, Indianapolis, IN, USA

Sana Ghaddar, PhD, RD, RN DaVita Health Care, Fremont, CA, USA

D. Jordi Goldstein-Fuchs, DSc, APN, NP-C, RD Department of Pediatric Nephrology, Lucile Packard Hospital Stanford, Palo Alto, CA, USA

Laryssa Grguric Formerly Nassau University Medical Center, Currently Working in Home Infusion for Coram/CVS Specialty Infusion Services, Miramar, FL, USA

Fitsum Guebre-Egziabher, MD, PhD Department of Nephrology, Dialysis and Hypertension, Hospices Civils de Lyon, Hôpital Edouard Herriot, Laboratoire CarMeN, INSERM u1060, Université Lyon-1, Lyon, France

Faculté de Médecine Lyon-Est, Université Lyon-1, Lyon, France

Haewook Han, PhD, RD, CSR, LDN, FNKF Atrius Health, Department of Nephrology, Boston, MA, USA

MS/DI Program Director, Tufts University Friedman School, Boston, MA, USA

Tufts Medical Center, Division of Nephrology, Boston, MA, USA

Diana Hao, Pharm D Solid Organ Transplant Pharmacy Service, UC Davis Medical Center, Sacramento, CA, USA

Katherine Schiro Harvey, MS, RDN, CD, CSR Renal Nutrition Services, Puget Sound Kidney Centers, Mountlake Terrace, WA, USA

Kathy K. Isoldi, PhD, RD Nutrition Department, Long Island University, Brookville, NY, USA

Kitty J. Jager, MD, PhD Department of Medical Informatics, Amsterdam Public Health Research Institute, Amsterdam UMC, University of Amsterdam, Amsterdam, The Netherlands

George A. Kaysen, MD, PhD Department of Medicine, Division of Nephrology, Genome University of California, Davis, and Biomedical Sciences Facility, Davis, CA, USA

Jaimon T. Kelly, PhD Griffith University, Menzies Health Institute Queensland, Gold Coast, QLD, Australia

Brandon Kistler, PhD, RD Department of Nutrition and Health Science, Ball State University, Muncie, IN, USA

Joel D. Kopple, MD Professor Emeritus of Medicine and Public Health, University of California, Los Angeles, CA, USA

The Lundquist Institute for Biomedical Innovation at Harbor-UCLA Medical Center, Torrance, CA, USA

Bengt Lindholm, MD, PhD Department of Renal Medicine, Karolinska Institutet, and Baxter Novum, Stockholm, Sweden

Denise Mafra Department of Clinical Nutrition, Federal University Fluminense, Niterói, Rio de Janeiro, Brazil

Linda McCann, RD, CSR Nephrology Nutrition Consultant/Speaker, Eagle, ID, USA

Anthony Meade, BSc, MND Royal Adelaide Hospital, Central Northern Adelaide Renal and Transplantation Service, Adelaide, Australia

Linda W. Moore, PhD, RDN, CCRP Department of Surgery, Houston Methodist Hospital, Houston, TX, USA

Christina L. Nelms, MS, RDN, LMNT PedsFeeds, LLC – Pediatric Renal Nutrition Consulting and Education, Kearney, NE, USA

University of Nebraska, Kearney, NE, USA

Marlies Noordzij, PhD Department of Medical Informatics, Amsterdam Public Health Research Institute, Amsterdam UMC, University of Amsterdam, Amsterdam, The Netherlands

Chhaya Patel, MA, RDN DaVita Dialysis, Program Manager Nutrition Services, Divisional Lead Dietitian for ORCA Division, Dietitian Council and EPIC Mentor, Walnut Creek, CA, USA

Daniel Pieloch, MS, RD, CPHQ, CCTC Robert Wood Johnson University Hospital, Transplant Center, RWJ Barnabas Health, New Brunswick, NJ, USA

Melissa Prest, DCN, RDN, CSR, LDN National Kidney Foundation of Illinois, Chicago, IL, USA

Wendy E. Ramirez, PharmD Evergreen Health Medical Center, Pharmacy, Kirkland, WA, USA

Alluru S. Reddi, MD, PhD Department of Medicine, Rutgers New Jersey Medical School, Newark, NJ, USA

Diane Rigassio Radler, PhD, RD Department of Clinical and Preventive Nutrition Sciences, Rutgers University, School of Health Professions, Newark, NJ, USA

Arti Sharma Parpia, MSc, RD St. Michael's Hospital, Toronto, ON, Canada

Alison L. Steiber, PhD, RDN Academy of Nutrition and Dietetics, Chicago, IL, USA

Vianda S. Stel, PhD Department of Medical Informatics, Amsterdam Public Health Research Institute, Amsterdam UMC, University of Amsterdam, Amsterdam, The Netherlands

Peter Stenvinkel, MD, PhD Department of Renal Medicine, Karolinska Institutet, Stockholm, Sweden

Jean Stover, RD, LDN DaVita Kidney Care, Philadelphia, PA, USA

Mandy Trolinger, MS, RD, PA-C Colorado Kidney Care, Lone Tree, CO, USA

Jaime Uribarri, MD Department of Medicine, Icahn School of Medicine at Mount Sinai, New York, NY, USA

Johnathan Voss, Pharm D, BCCCP, BCNSP John Peter Smith Hospital, Inpatient Pharmacy, Fort Worth, TX, USA

Bradley A. Warady, MD University of Missouri-Kansas City School of Medicine, Kansas City, MO, USA

Division of Nephrology, Dialysis and Transplantation, Children's Mercy Kansas City, Kansas City, MO, USA

Dana Whitham, MSc, RD St. Michael's Hospital, Centre for Diabetes & Endocrinology, Toronto, ON, Canada

Kenneth R. Wilund, PhD Department of Kinesiology and Community Health, University of Illinois, Urbana, IL, USA

William A. Wolfe, BS, MSW Women's Institute for Family Health of Philadelphia, Philadelphia, PA, USA

Jane Y. Yeun, MD Nephrology Section, Sacramento Veterans Administration Medical Center, Mather, CA, USA

Division of Nephrology, UC Davis Health, Sacramento, CA, USA

Jane Ziegler, DCN, RDN, LDN Department of Clinical and Preventive Nutrition Sciences, Rutgers University, School of Health Professions, Newark, NJ, USA

Part I
Foundations for Clinical Practice and Overview

Chronic kidney disease (CKD) is a global epidemic, with recent estimates suggesting that over 860 million people worldwide suffer from some form of kidney disease. With progressive loss of kidney function come hosts of complications, with nutritional derangements featuring prominently among conditions contributing to increased morbidity and mortality in patients with CKD and end-stage renal disease (ESRD). Nutritional management is quintessential in patients with all stages of CKD, but becomes especially important in those with more advanced stages, in whom it is used both to affect disease progression and to control metabolic complications such as hyperkalemia or hyperphosphatemia. The chapters in this section provide a general introduction to the disease states discussed in later parts of the book. Stel et al. describe the epidemiology of kidney disease, while Kopple and Burrowes summarize the history of nutritional interventions in CKD and provide a broad overview of its current applications and guideline recommendations. Finally, Reddi provides a general description of renal physiology and pathophysiology, which, together with the other two introductory chapters, helps to better contextualize subsequent chapters.

Chapter 1
Epidemiology and Changing Demographics of Chronic Kidney Disease in the United States and Abroad

Vianda S. Stel, Marlies Noordzij, and Kitty J. Jager

Keywords Epidemiology · Outcome · Chronic kidney disease · Renal replacement therapy Conservative care · Risk factors · Prevention

Key Points
- Large international differences exist in the incidence of renal replacement therapy (RRT) and in the prevalence of chronic kidney disease (CKD) and RRT across the world.
- There are many potential reasons for the international difference in the epidemiology of CKD and RRT, such as the variation of environmental, ethnic, cultural, political, and macro-economic factors.
- Since the start of RRT in the 1960s, the incidence of patients starting RRT has increased tremendously with a changing profile over time from predominantly young males with relatively few comorbidities to older, multi-comorbid individuals.
- People with CKD have a high mortality risk, and this risk is even higher in patients with end-stage kidney disease.
- The impact of reducing risk factors targeting both lifestyle factors (including physical inactivity, obesity, smoking, and salt intake) and specific noncommunicable diseases (such as diabetes and hypertension) on the development of CKD is still unclear.

Introduction

Chronic kidney disease (CKD) is increasingly recognized as a global public health problem; as many as 10–15% of the population worldwide is affected by CKD due to multiple causes [1, 2]. Globally, the prevalence of CKD increased by 87% between 1990 and 2016 to a total number of patients exceeding 275 million [3, 4].

Also, the prevalence of renal replacement therapy (RRT) for end-stage kidney disease (ESKD) has increased tremendously since its introduction in the 1960s. This rise can be explained by the fact that nowadays, older and sicker patients are being accepted for RRT when compared to the early days of

V. S. Stel · M. Noordzij · K. J. Jager (✉)
Department of Medical Informatics, Amsterdam Public Health Research Institute, Amsterdam UMC, University of Amsterdam, Amsterdam, The Netherlands
e-mail: k.j.jager@amsterdamumc.nl

© Springer Nature Switzerland AG 2020
J. D. Burrowes et al. (eds.), *Nutrition in Kidney Disease*, Nutrition and Health, https://doi.org/10.1007/978-3-030-44858-5_1

the treatment. In addition, patients survive longer on RRT, mostly because the quality of all RRT modalities has improved considerably over the past 50 years.

Worldwide, there is a large variation in the epidemiology of both CKD and RRT. The burden of CKD is also prominent and shows the fastest growth in low-income and middle-income countries [3]. It is evident that disparities in access to RRT exist. In low-income regions, especially in Africa and Asia, the access to RRT is limited, and prohibitive out-of-pocket expenditure is not uncommon [5–7].

In this chapter, we describe the changing demographics and outcomes among patients with CKD and those receiving RRT, and we discuss potential reasons for international differences in the epidemiology of CKD and RRT. In addition, we will discuss the prevention of five important risk factors for CKD as targeted by the World Health Organization (WHO) action plan, including physical inactivity, high salt intake, smoking, diabetes mellitus, and hypertension.

Chronic Kidney Disease

The Assessment and Definition of CKD Prevalence

According to the National Kidney Foundation Kidney Disease Outcomes Quality Initiative (NKF KDOQI) and Kidney Disease: Improving Global Outcomes (KDIGO) guidelines, CKD is defined by the presence of kidney damage or decreased kidney function for three or more months [8, 9]. Kidney damage refers to pathologic abnormalities which can, among others, be assessed by increased rates of urinary albumin excretion. Decreased kidney function refers to a decreased glomerular filtration rate (GFR) which is usually estimated (eGFR). The KDOQI guidelines recommend to do this by using serum creatinine and the Chronic Kidney Disease Epidemiology Collaboration formula (CKD-EPI). There are five CKD stages related to the level of kidney damage and kidney function (Table 1.1). As stated by the guidelines [8, 9], the persistence of the kidney damage or decreased kidney function should last for at least three months to distinguish CKD from acute kidney disease (named "chronicity criterion").

International comparison of CKD prevalence is challenging due to the different methods for the assessment of kidney dysfunction and the use of different definitions of CKD [10, 11]. Numerous studies reporting on CKD prevalence define CKD as eGFR <60 ml/min/1.73 m^2. Other studies define CKD as eGFR <60 ml/min/1.73 m^2 and/or the presence of albuminuria >30 mg/g or as the presence of albuminuria >30 mg/g alone or use absolute creatinine measurement. In addition, studies use various serum creatinine-based equations to estimate GFR such as the CKD-EPI formula, the Modification of Diet in renal Disease formula (MDRD), and the Cockcroft-Gault formula. So far, the chronicity criterion is rarely used in studies on CKD prevalence. Finally, sample selection methods vary across the studies and influence the representativeness of the sample. Hence, due to the heterogeneity of studies, the results of international comparisons of CKD prevalence should be interpreted with caution.

Table 1.1 GFR categories in CKD according to the KDIGO guidelines 2012

GFR category	GFR (ml/min/1.73 m^2)	Terms
G1	>90[a]	Normal or high
G2	60–89[a]	Mildly decreased
G3a	45–59	Mildly to moderately decreased
G3b	30–44	Moderately to severely decreased
G4	15–29	Severely decreased
G5	<15	Kidney failure

[a]In the absence of evidence of kidney damage neither GFR category G1 nor G2 fulfill the criteria for CKD

International Comparison of CKD Prevalence

Over the last decade, data on the burden of CKD have become increasingly available. These data contribute to our understanding of the scale of this public health problem. According to a meta-analysis, the global prevalence was 13.4% for CKD stages 1–5 and 10.6% for CKD stages 3–5 (Table 1.2) [12]. The majority of individuals having CKD are in stage 3 CKD (7.6%), and only few of them have ESKD (0.1%).

The burden of CKD varies substantially across the world. Within the United States in 2015–2016, 14–15% of the adult participants of the National Health and Nutrition Examination Survey (NHANES) study had CKD stages 1–4, representing 31–34 million people [13]. About half of them were categorized into CKD stages 3–4. The prevalence of CKD in Japan was similar to that in the United States [14]. In China, the estimate of the prevalence of CKD stages 3–5 was much lower, that is, 1.7% [15]. A study by the European CKD Burden Consortium also reported lower CKD prevalence estimates for Europe with large differences in CKD prevalence across countries, despite the use of one CKD definition and age and sex standardization to the European standard population [16]. The adjusted prevalence of CKD stages 3–5 varied from 1.0% to 5.9%. In Australia, CKD studies used to focus on screening of the population in individuals at high risk [17], and only recently, long-term surveillance was started to describe CKD prevalence of the general population not on RRT.

Although some developing countries (like South Africa, Senegal, and Congo) seem to have lower CKD prevalence estimates than developed countries (see Table 1.2) [12], several systematic reviews show that other developing countries have similar or even higher burden of CKD [12, 18]. For example, in Africa, the overall CKD prevalence from 21 medium-quality and high-quality studies was similar to that of the United States, that is, 13.9% [18]. In South Asian countries, the highest CKD prevalence was reported in Pakistan (21.2%) and the lowest in India (10.2%). Data on CKD prevalence in Latin America are scarce [19]. A small study in Mexico reported that 9.2% of the individuals had proteinuria, whereas in Chile 14.2% had proteinuria and 21% had a creatinine clearance <80 ml/min. A matter of great concern is the limited availability of high-quality data on CKD, in particular for developing countries [18].

CKD Prevalence in Subgroups

CKD prevalence rises substantially with age. Within the United States, the prevalence of CKD stages 1–4 in people over 70 years of age (44%) was eight times higher than in those aged 20–39 years (5.6%) [13]. In most countries, the prevalence of CKD was higher in females than in males [20].

Table 1.2 Mean prevalence of CKD split by geographical region with 95% confidence intervals

	Stages 1–5		Stages 3–5	
	N^a	Prevalence (%)	N^a	Prevalence (%)
S Africa, Senegal, Congo	5497	8.66 (1.31, 16.01)	1202	7.60 (6.10, 9.10)
India, Bangladesh	1000	13.10 (11.01, 15.19)	12,752	6.76 (3.68, 9.85)
Iran	17,911	17.95 (7.37, 28.53)	20,867	11.68 (4.51, 18.84)
Chile	0	NONE	27,894	12.10 (11.72, 12.48)
China, Taiwan, Mongolia	570,187	13.18 (12.07, 14.30)	62,062	10.06 (6.63, 13.49)
Japan, S Korea, Oceania	654,832	13.74 (10.75, 16.72)	298,000	11.73 (5.36, 18.10)
Australia	12,107	14.71 (11.71, 17.71)	896,941	8.14 (4.48, 11.79)
USA, Canada	20,352	15.45 (11.71, 19.20)	1,319,003	14.44 (8.52, 20.36)
Europe	821,902	18.38 (11.57, 25.20)	2,169,183	11.86 (9.93, 13.79)

Reproduced from Hill et al. [12], page 8, Table 1
[a]N is number of participants in the sample estimate

Within the United States, this was 16.0% (females) versus 12.4% (males) for CKD stages 1–4 [13]. A possible explanation for the higher CKD prevalence in women is their longer life expectancy combined with the natural decline of GFR with age. On the other hand, it may also be due to the potential overdiagnosis of CKD in women that may occur when using eGFR equations estimating kidney function [20]. Furthermore, the burden of CKD prevalence was the highest in Blacks and in persons with diabetes and hypertension [13].

Trends in CKD Prevalence

Papers reporting on time trends in CKD prevalence are scarce. In the United States, the unadjusted CKD prevalence for stages 3–4 as estimated by the CKD-EPI equation increased from the early 1990s (4.8%) to the early 2000s (6.4%). Interestingly, thereafter, it stabilized (around 6.9%) [13, 21]. The stabilization of the CKD prevalence was present in most subgroups defined by age, sex, and diabetic status. Also in Norway, the prevalence of CKD stages 1–5 estimated by the CKD-EPI equation remained stable for more than a decade from 1995 (11.1%) to 2008 (11.3%) [22]. In contrast, in the United Kingdom, the prevalence of CKD stages 3–5 estimated by the CKD-EPI equation declined over a 7-year period from 5.7% in 2003 to 5.2% in 2009/2010, despite the rising prevalence of obesity and diabetes in the general population [23].

Reasons for International Differences in CKD Prevalence

There are many factors which may contribute to the differences observed across countries and regions. For instance, regional differences in the prevalence of diabetes mellitus and hypertension as well as dietary habits, smoking, physical inactivity, socioeconomic status, birth weight, and genetic factors could lead to a difference in CKD prevalence [24–29]. The results of a European study indicated that, in general, countries with a higher prevalence of CKD also had a higher score on risk factors for CKD and vice versa (the average score on risk factors was based on the prevalence of diabetes mellitus, raised blood pressure, obesity, physical inactivity, current smoking, and salt intake) [24]. National and regional public health initiatives may contribute to differences in the prevalence of underlying causes of CKD, such as diabetes, hypertension, and obesity as well as the prevalence of CKD itself [24].

Part of the observed differences in CKD prevalence may also be a result of the heterogeneity of studies [10]. As mentioned earlier, studies may use different assessment and definitions of CKD, and the quality of the studies may differ. In addition, the age and sex distributions of general populations also have an influence on the CKD prevalence. Finally, the difference in CKD prevalence may partly be caused by differences in the selection of study samples. Some of these differences in methodology can be avoided by, for instance, using the same CKD definition and central measurement of serum creatinine and albuminuria in a reference laboratory. However, the sample may not be representative and may suffer from response bias. This problem cannot be solved.

Progression of CKD

So far, the knowledge on progression of CKD is rather limited. Studies on the progression of CKD in referred CKD patients have reported declines in the rates of eGFR from 0.35 to 5.16 ml/min per 1.73 m^2 per year [30–32]. Unfortunately, studies on eGFR progression are difficult to compare due to differences in the way CKD progression is expressed as well as the differences in factors influencing the progression of CKD progression, such as baseline eGFR, albuminuria, primary renal disease, and comorbidities. In general, studies found that younger age, male sex, and the presence of diabetes mellitus are associated with more rapid progression of CKD, even after adjustment for mortality risk [32–34].

Many studies have shown that individuals with CKD have a subsequent increased risk of all-cause and cardiovascular death [35, 36]. The results of meta-analyses have revealed that the cardiovascular mortality risk was about twice as high in patients with stage 3 CKD compared to individuals with normal kidney function [37, 38]. In stage 4 CKD, this risk was even three times higher. Of note, due to the high mortality risk, the majority of patients with CKD do not progress to advanced stages of CKD [39, 40]. In other words, in patients with CKD, the mortality risk is higher than the risk to develop ESKD, even in patients with stage 4 CKD. This seems to be even more pronounced in older persons with CKD. A study by Dalrymple [41] has shown that community-dwelling adults aged 65 years or older with CKD stages 3–5 are 13-fold more likely to die from any cause than to develop ESKD.

Renal Replacement Therapy (RRT)

RRT Epidemiology

The incidence of RRT for ESKD represents the number of new patients on RRT in a year. Around the world, there is a wide variation in the incidence of RRT, with the lowest rates in 2016 in South Africa (22 per million population (pmp)), Ukraine (36 pmp), Belarus (51 pmp), and Bangladesh (51 pmp) and the highest rates in Taiwan (493 pmp), the United States (378 pmp), and the Jalisco region of Mexico (355 pmp) [42]. Of all incident patients in 2016, 87.3% initiated RRT with hemodialysis, 9.7% started with peritoneal dialysis, and 2.8% received a preemptive kidney transplant.

Since the introduction of RRT in the 1960s, its incidence increased sharply and continuously. However, this pattern has changed in the period between 2003 and 2016. There has still been a marked increase in the incidence rate in some countries, for example, in Thailand (+19.4%), Malaysia (+13.2%), the Republic of Korea (+10.3%), Singapore (+8.8%), the Philippines (+8.7%), and the Jalisco region of Mexico (+7.5%). In the same time period, the incidence rate showed only a small increase or stabilized in many developed countries, including the United States (+2.2%), Japan (+2%), the United Kingdom (+1%), and Australia (+0.9%). Finally, there were some countries where the incidence rate has started to decrease, for example, Colombia (−2.8%), Austria (−1.5%), and Scotland (−1.4%) [42]. Figure 1.1 shows the trend for the incidence rate of RRT over the period from 2000 to 2016 for a selection of large renal registries on different continents.

The stabilizing or even decreasing incidence in some countries during recent years is mostly due to a stabilization of (or drop in) the number of dialysis patients, which could be explained by several potential factors. Firstly, it could be that more patients choose comprehensive conservative care over dialysis treatment. Secondly, better CKD management could lead to postponement of the initiation of RRT. Meanwhile, the incidence rate of kidney transplantation, including preemptive transplantations and those performed in the first 3 months of RRT, is still rising. This rise is mainly caused by a strong increase in the number of transplantations from both related and unrelated living donors, because transplantation with kidneys from deceased donors is still limited by the shortage of donor organs [48, 49].

Just like the incidence rate, the prevalence of RRT – representing the number of patients treated on the 31st of December of a year – shows a substantial variation between countries around the world.

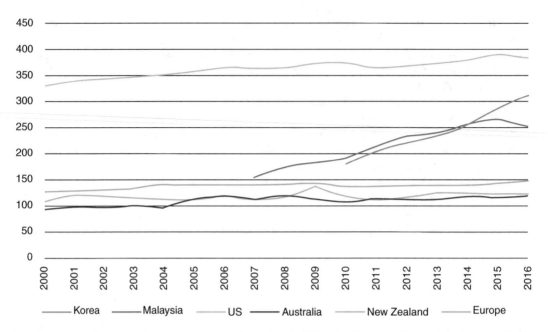

Fig. 1.1 The unadjusted incidence per million population (pmp) of RRT for ESKD in different parts of the world in the time period between 2000 and 2016. (Created with data from [42–47])

According to the international comparisons performed by the United States Renal Data System (USRDS), the ESKD prevalence in 2016 varied nearly 30-fold across the 36 countries that provided data [42]. The highest RRT prevalence was reported by Taiwan (3392 pmp), Japan (2599 pmp), and the United States (2196 pmp), whereas the lowest prevalence was reported by Bangladesh (117 pmp), South Africa (181 pmp), and Ukraine (188 pmp).

Among all patients prevalent on RRT on December 31, 2016, the largest group (63.1%) was treated with hemodialysis, of whom an overwhelming majority of 98% used in-center hemodialysis and 2% used home hemodialysis. Of the remaining patients, 7.0% received peritoneal dialysis, and almost one-third (29.6%) had a functioning kidney transplant. Again, there were large international differences with regard to the distribution of the RRT modalities, as is illustrated in Fig. 1.2.

Although the rapid increase of RRT incidence rates has come to an end in some parts of the world, the prevalence of RRT – representing the number of patients treated on the 31st of December of that year – is still rising in all countries (Fig. 1.3).

This continuing rise of the prevalence of RRT can be explained by the fact that both patient survival on RRT and graft survival after kidney transplantation have improved considerably over time as a result of better RRT strategies and techniques.

At the same time, the patient profile has changed from predominantly young males with relatively few comorbidities to older, multi-comorbid individuals. The causes of this change can be sought in the global epidemics of diabetes, obesity, and hypertension, together with an aging population and a greater acceptance of these patient groups onto RRT programs [49]. As a result of this more liberal acceptance policy, the mean age at the start of RRT has risen from 58.3 years in 1990 to 62.5 years in 2013 in the United States. Also, the share of diabetic patients in the RRT population has increased progressively. In 2016, a large variation was seen across countries in the percentages of incident patients with diabetes mellitus as the primary cause of ESKD, ranging from less than 16% in Norway, Latvia, and Romania to approximately 66% of patients in Malaysia, Singapore, and the Jalisco region of Mexico [42].

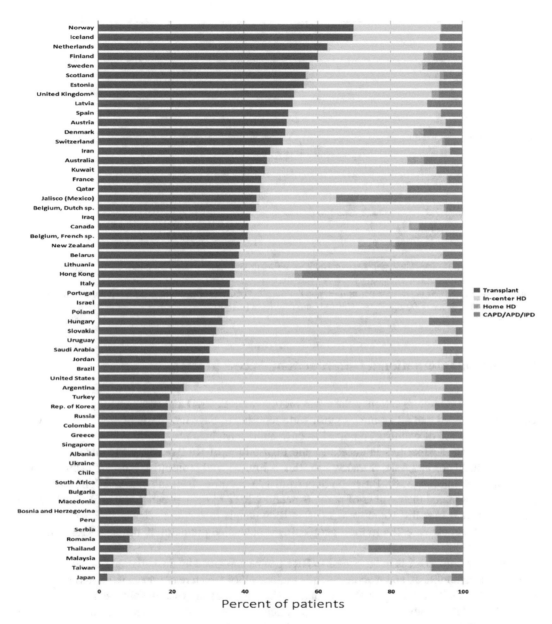

Fig. 1.2 Percentage distribution of type of renal replacement therapy modality used by ESKD patients, by country, in 2016. (Adapted from United States Renal Data System. 2018 USRDS annual data report: Epidemiology of kidney disease in the United States. National Institutes of Health, National Institute of Diabetes and Digestive and Kidney Diseases, Bethesda, MD, 2018. The data reported here have been supplied by the United States Renal Data System (USRDS). The interpretation and reporting of these data are the responsibility of the author(s) and in no way should be seen as an official policy or interpretation of the U.S. government)

The proportion of men treated with RRT is higher than the proportion of women. In contrast to the general population, the overall male-to-female ratio for RRT patients ranges between 1.2 and 1.4, whereas higher values of 2.0 or higher were observed for older subgroups. Recent data from Europe showed that this distribution has been stable for already 50 years in both incident and prevalent RRT patients and across all age categories and treatment modalities [50].

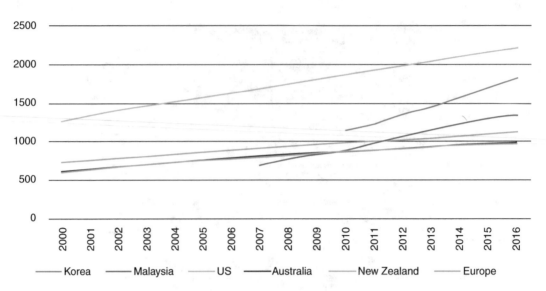

Fig. 1.3 The unadjusted prevalence per million population (pmp) of RRT for ESKD in different parts of the world in the time period between 2000 and 2016. (Created with data from [42–47])

Reasons for International Differences in Access to RRT

Globally, there is huge variation in the epidemiology of both CKD and RRT. A study by Crews and colleagues showed that all countries worldwide reported to have long-term hemodialysis services and that over 90% of countries reported to have short-term hemodialysis services [5]. It is, however, evident that disparities in access to and distribution of RRT exist. In low-income regions, especially in Africa and Asia, the access to RRT is limited, and prohibitive out-of-pocket expenditure is not uncommon [5, 6]. Based on data from 123 countries over the year 2010, Liyanage and colleagues estimated the number of patients needing RRT to be between 4.902 million and 9.701 million, whereas in reality there were 2.618 million people receiving RRT worldwide in that year, suggesting that at least 2.284 million people might have died prematurely because RRT could not be accessed [7].

International differences in the access to RRT can be explained by the variation of environmental, ethnic, cultural, political, and macroeconomic factors, all of which may impact the criteria of patient selection for RRT, the timing of RRT initiation, the choice of dialysis modality, dialysis treatment quality, cumulative dialysis times, and the prevalence of non-dialysis-related risk factors [51]. Of these factors, national wealth and health expenditure are believed to have the strongest influence on the incidence rate of RRT because they have a direct influence on healthcare organization and delivery at a national level. This is especially relevant because RRT is an extremely expensive treatment. In high-income countries, 1.3% of public health expenditure was spent on reimbursement for dialysis care, while this was 2.7% in upper-middle-income countries and 3.0% in lower-middle-income and low-income countries combined [52].

Information from renal registries offers the potential of a better understanding of the factors affecting the epidemiology of RRT. However, while most developed countries have established national RRT registries, population-based national renal registries are still unavailable for countries that altogether comprise at least half of the world's population [53]. This leaves a large part of the global ESKD population unidentified and healthcare providers uninformed about the size of the treatment challenges ahead.

RRT Prognosis and Outcomes

Mortality rises with increasing stage of CKD and is highest in patients on RRT. Remaining life expectancies of RRT patients are therefore substantially lower than in the age- and sex-matched general population: in dialysis patients, life expectancy is reduced to almost 30% and in transplant recipients to 60–70% of those in the general population [42, 43].

For those starting RRT between 2007 and 2011, unadjusted 5-year survival was 43% in the United States and 51% in Europe [42, 43]. Determinants of patient survival on RRT include age and sex, the cause of ESKD, timing of referral to a nephrologist, genetic factors, general population mortality, access to transplantation, and other aspects of quality of RRT care [54].

In the same period, 5-year survival of patients on dialysis was 41% in the United States and 42% in Europe [42, 43], but the Japanese Registry reported a much better survival of 60% for those starting dialysis in 2007 [55]. Also, other Asian registries provided good 5-year survival results on dialysis in this period with 52% in Malaysia [44], 54% in Taiwan [56], and 70% in Korea [45]. The Dialysis Outcomes and Practice Patterns Study (DOPPS) has shown that especially the first 3 months on hemodialysis convey a very high risk of death [57, 58]. Excess mortality concerns not only cardiovascular [59, 60] but also non-cardiovascular mortality [60, 61]. There is important international variation in the survival of dialysis patients [54]. The reasons for these differences are not fully understood. Only to a small extent can the differences be explained by patient age, sex, primary renal disease, and the presence of comorbid conditions [62, 63]. Another part seems to be attributable to variability in cardiovascular and all-cause background mortality in the general populations, but even if these and differences in treatment characteristics are taken into account, a major part of the variation in dialysis mortality across countries remains unexplained [64, 65]. Therefore, the question is to what extent these differences are due to patient selection. In countries with high transplantation rates, the older and less healthy patients will remain on dialysis, and this will result in lower dialysis population survival. This might explain part of the survival advantage of Japanese dialysis patients, as this country has very few transplant patients and thus keeps the healthiest patients on dialysis [54, 66]. Another interesting finding was that in general, the mortality of dialysis patients is higher in countries with high expenditure on healthcare [54]. This may suggest that a more liberal acceptance policy among richer nations together with different patterns of healthcare spending may contribute to a higher mortality of dialysis patients in these countries [54].

Patients receiving a kidney transplant have a better prognosis. Risk factors for death are manifold and include both patient and graft characteristics. The 5-year survival in those receiving a deceased donor kidney in the United States was 85%, and in Europe, it was 88%. Those receiving a kidney from a living donor had slightly better prospects: their survival probability was 92% in the United States and 94% in Europe [42, 43]. Compared with dialysis, there is less outcomes research on the international variation of outcomes in kidney transplantation. Nonetheless, a recent study in four countries (Australia, New Zealand, the United Kingdom, and the United States) found the best 1-year adjusted graft survival in Australia and the worst graft survival in the United Kingdom. In contrast, with respect to long-term kidney graft outcomes, the United States performed approximately 25% worse compared to the other countries. Case-mix differences and residual confounding were unlikely explanations, and the findings suggested that the differences might be due to potentially modifiable country-specific differences in care delivery and/or practice patterns [67].

Comprehensive Conservative Care

Whereas in developed countries the use of RRT has increased over the previous decades, the recent past conservative management as a treatment alternative for ESKD in elderly patients with multi-morbidity and poor prognosis has gained acceptance [68]. It has even been speculated that this increased acceptance may have contributed to the decline in the incidence of RRT as seen in some countries [68]. KDIGO has made a distinction between conservative care that is the result of limited resources (choice-restricted conservative care) and conservative care due to unrecognized kidney failure and medically advised conservative care (comprehensive conservative care). The latter is planned patient-centered holistic care for stage 5 CKD not including dialysis. It should include interventions to delay the progression of kidney disease and decrease the risk of adverse events, shared decision-making, active symptom management, advance care planning, psychological support, social and family support, and cultural and spiritual domains of care [69].

Data related to conservative care are scarce. A community-based cohort study of more than 1.8 million adults in Canada showed that over a median follow-up period of 4.4 years, the incidence of treated ESKD was 0.18% and that of untreated ESKD 0.17% [70]. In patients with eGFR 15–29 ml/min/1.73m^2, adjusted rates of untreated kidney failure were more than fivefold higher among people older than 85 years of age compared with young adults [70]. This does not imply that these elderly were all receiving comprehensive conservative care. In a large number of them, ESKD may have gone unrecognized. Australian investigators observed similar findings. For each individual starting RRT for ESKD, there was another person dying from ESKD without having received RRT [71].

In contrast to RRT, the incidence and prevalence of comprehensive conservative care are not known. A survey among nephrologists in 11 European countries found that in 2009, up to 15% of patients with ESKD received comprehensive conservative care and that the presence of severe clinical conditions, vascular dementia, and a low physical functional status as well as patient preference were important factors in the decision-making not to start RRT [72]. According to a survey that was sent to all 71 adult renal units in the United Kingdom in 2013, comprehensive conservative care was practiced in almost all UK units, but its scale and organizations varied widely [73]. In a Spanish single-center study in the same period, comprehensive conservative care was selected in 39% of the ESKD cases [74].

Randomized controlled trials (RCTs) comparing the outcomes of comprehensive conservative care and dialysis have not been published. Current evidence therefore comes from observational studies. A number of systematic reviews were performed with respect to survival outcomes. The most comprehensive one to date reported that the one-year survival of elderly patients on hemodialysis, peritoneal dialysis, and comprehensive conservative management was 78.4%, 77.9%, and 70.6%, respectively [75]. The difference between survival on dialysis and that on comprehensive conservative management increased with follow-up time [75]. A meta-analysis including three studies [76–78] showed that patients choosing dialysis had half the risk of death compared to those opting for conservative management (pooled adjusted hazard ratio 0.53 (95%CI 0.30–0.91)) [79]. In line with this, another recent paper reported a 3-year mortality risk in an elderly cohort that was twice as high in comprehensive conservative care compared to dialysis (adjusted hazard ratio 2.18 (95% CI 1.39–3.40)). Nevertheless, the paper also showed that survival after 3 years of comprehensive conservative management was common [80]. Several studies reported loss of survival benefit with dialysis in the presence of high comorbidity [76, 77, 81] and in the very elderly [82].

However, it is likely that in all these studies the choice for comprehensive conservative management or dialysis suffers from confounding by indication, which hampers the interpretation of study findings. Furthermore, many of these comparisons may suffer from lead-time bias. Finally, publication bias may hamper valid conclusions. It can therefore be concluded that the literature does not allow a confident estimate of the relative survival benefits of these treatments [75]. Only RCTs will be able to provide us with valid answers to this question, and hopefully, an ongoing RCT in the UK will help to shed some light on this (https://doi.org/10.1186/ISRCTN17133653).

Prevention of Important Risk Factors for CKD

The prevention of important risk factors for CKD may prevent or delay the development of CKD and its complications. The WHO developed a Global Action Plan for the Prevention and Control of Noncommunicable Diseases (NCDs) 2013–2020 (Fig. 1.4) [83]. This action plan aims at reducing the global burden of NCDs by targeting both lifestyle factors and specific NCDs. The plan yields nine public health targets, five of which are important risk factors for CKD including diabetes, hypertension, physical inactivity, high salt intake, and smoking. Although these nine public health targets do not include CKD, the plan does acknowledge the link between NCDs such as diabetes and hypertension and CKD. Of note, lowering one risk factor for CKD may also influence the other risk factors for CKD.

In order to prevent or delay the progression of CKD, screening for kidney disease in people with diabetes and hypertension is now generally recommended. Additionally, the treatment of both diabetes and hypertension appears to have improved with increased prescription rate for glycemic control medication, angiotensin-converting enzyme inhibitors (ACEi), and antihypertensive medication [84–87]. However, the impact of the improved treatment of diabetes and hypertension on the development of CKD and its complications is, with the current knowledge, difficult to establish. To give an example, the decrease in the incidence of RRT for ESKD due to diabetes mellitus in several countries [42] could be partly explained by a slower progression of CKD (better prevention) but also by a change in RRT initiation practices.

 A 25% relative reduction in risk of premature mortality from cardiovascular diseases, cancer, diabetes, or chronic respiratory diseases.

 At least 10% relative reduction in the harmful use of alcohol, as appropriate, within the national context.

 A 10% relative reduction in prevalence of insufficient physical activity.

 A 30% relative reduction in mean population intake of salt/sodium.

 A 30% relative reduction in prevalence of current tobacco use in persons aged 15+ years.

 A 25% relative reduction in the prevalence of raised blood pressure or contain the prevalence of raised blood pressure, according to national circumstances.

 Halt the rise in diabetes and obesity.

 At least 50% of eligible people receive drug therapy and counselling (including glycaemic control) to prevent heart attacks and strokes.

 An 80% availability of the affordable basic technologies and essential medicines, including generics, required to treat major noncommunicable diseases in both public and private facilities.

Fig. 1.4 The nine global voluntary targets from the WHO Global Action Plan for the Prevention and Control of NCDs 2013–2020. Reprinted from the nine global voluntary targets from the WHO Global Action Plan for the Prevention and Control of NCDs 2013–2020. (Reprinted from Global action plan for the prevention and control of noncommunicable diseases 2013–2020, World Health Organization, Voluntary Global Targets, page 5, Copyright (2013))

Several studies have shown that the implementation of nationwide lifestyle measures such as physical inactivity, smoking, and salt intake can reduce the prevalence of risk factors for CKD [88–90]. Implemented lifestyle measures in the general population are, for example, campaigns to increase physical activity (e.g., exercise 30 minutes per day and 10,000 steps per day), a law that forbid smoking in public spaces and workspace, and salt restriction in bread and processed food. Unfortunately, only few studies have investigated the impact of these and other lifestyle measures on kidney outcomes. A systematic review has described the effect of salt reduction on both hypertension and proteinuria in people with CKD [91], whereas another review has reported on the association between smoking cessation and kidney function [92]. There is a need for these kinds of studies using hard renal outcomes such as the start of renal replacement therapy.

As a final comment, it is worthwhile to mention that the effect of the public health policies targeting NCDs may likely differ largely among countries which is caused by substantial international differences in the prevalence of CKD, the prevalence of the risk factors of CKD, and the public health policies targeting NCDs.

Conclusion

Substantial differences exist in the incidence of RRT and in the prevalence of CKD and RRT across the world. Both the prevalence of CKD and RRT are among the highest in the United States. Since the start of RRT in 1960s, the incidence of patients starting RRT has increased tremendously with a changing profile over time from predominantly young males with relatively few comorbidities to older, multi-comorbid individuals. In some countries, the incidence of RRT is now stabilizing or even declining. Unfortunately, many patients with ESKD, in particular in developing countries, do not have access to RRT. As a result of limited resources, these patients may receive choice-restricted conservative care. In some high-income countries, comprehensive conservative care in elderly patients with multi-morbidity and poor prognosis seems to gain more acceptance.

There are many potential reasons for the international difference in the epidemiology of CKD and RRT, such as the variation of environmental, ethnic, cultural, political, and macroeconomic factors. Among those factors, national wealth and health expenditure are believed to have the strongest influence on the incidence rate of RRT. In general, countries with a higher prevalence of CKD may also have a higher prevalence of risk factors for CKD, such as diabetes mellitus, hypertension, and obesity.

People with CKD have a high mortality risk, and this risk is even higher for patients with ESKD. Because of these serious adverse outcomes, it is important to prevent or delay CKD. The World Health Organization developed a Global Action Plan for the Prevention and Control of Noncommunicable Diseases (NCDs) aimed at reducing the global burden of NCDs by targeting both lifestyle factors including physical inactivity, obesity, smoking, and salt intake and specific NCDs such as diabetes and hypertension. The impact of this global action plan on the development of CKD and its complications is still unclear.

References

1. Eckardt K-U, Coresh J, Devuyst O, Johnson RJ, Köttgen A, Levey AS, et al. Evolving importance of kidney disease: from subspecialty to global health burden. Lancet. 2013;382:158–69.
2. Levin A, Tonelli M, Bonventre J, Coresh J, Donner JA, Fogo AB, et al. Global kidney health 2017 and beyond: a roadmap for closing gaps in care, research, and policy. Lancet. 2017;390:1888–917.

3. Xie Y, Bowe B, Mokdad AH, Xian H, Yan Y, Li T, et al. Analysis of the Global Burden of Disease study highlights the global, regional, and national trends of chronic kidney disease epidemiology from 1990 to 2016. Kidney Int. 2018;94:567–81.
4. GBD 2017 Disease and Injury Incidence and Prevalence Collaborators. Global, regional, and national incidence, prevalence, and years lived with disability for 354 diseases and injuries for 195 countries and territories, 1990–2017: a systematic analysis for the Global Burden of Disease Study 2017. Lancet. 2018;392:1789–858.
5. Crews DC, Bello AK, Saadi G, World Kidney Day Steering Committee. Burden, access, and disparities in kidney disease. Kidney Int. 2019;95:242–8.
6. Bello AK, Levin A, Tonelli M, Okpechi IG, Feehally J, Harris D, et al. Assessment of Global Kidney Health Care Status. JAMA. 2017;317(18):1864–81.
7. Liyanage T, Ninomiya T, Jha V, Neal B, Patrice HM, Okpechi I, et al. Worldwide access to treatment for end-stage kidney disease: a systematic review. Lancet. 2015;385:1975–82.
8. National Kidney Foundation. KDOQI clinical practice guideline for diabetes and CKD: 2012 update. Am J Kidney Dis. 2012;60(5):850–86.
9. KDIGO. 2012 Clinical Practice Guideline for the evaluation and management of chronic kidney disease. Kidn Int Suppl. 2012;3(1):1–P150.
10. Brück K, Jager KJ, Dounousi E, et al. on behalf of the European CKD Burden Consortium. Methodology used in studies reporting chronic kidney disease prevalence: a systematic literature review. Nephrol Dial Transplant. 2015;30:iv6–iv16.
11. Stanifer JW, Muiru A, Jafar TH, Patel UD. Chronic kidney disease in low- and middle-income countries. Nephrol Dial Transplant. 2016;31(6):868–74.
12. Hill NR, Fatoba ST, Oke JL, Hirst JA, O'Callaghan CA, Lasserson DS, et al. Global prevalence of chronic kidney disease – a systematic review and meta-analysis. PLoS One. 2016;11(7):e0158765.
13. Centers for Disease Control and Prevention. Chronic kidney disease surveillance system—United States. website. http://www.cdc.gov/ckd.
14. Imai E, Horlo M, Watanabe T, Iseki K, Yamagata K, Hara S, et al. Prevalence of chronic kidney disease in the Japanese general population. Clin Exp Nephrol. 2009;13(6):621–30.
15. Zhang L, Wang F, Wang L. Prevalence of chronic kidney disease in China: a cross-sectional survey. Lancet. 2012;379:815–22.
16. Brück K, Stel VS, Gambaro G, Hallan S, Völzke H, Ärnlöv J, et al. on behalf of European CKD Burden Consortium. CKD prevalence varies across the European general population. J Am Soc Nephrol. 2016;27:2135–47.
17. Venuthurupalli SK, Hoy WE, Healy HG, Cameron A, Fassett RG. CKD screening and surveillance in Australia: past, present, and future. Kidney Int Rep. 2018;3(1):36–46.
18. Stanifer JW, Jing B, Tolan S. The epidemiology of chronic kidney disease in sub-Saharan Africa: a systematic review and meta-analysis. Lancet Glob Health. 2014;2(3):E174–81.
19. Cusumano AM González Bedat MC. Chronic kidney disease in Latin America: time to improve screening and detection. Clin J Am Soc Nephrol. 2008;3(2):594–600.
20. Carrero JJ, Hecking M, Chesnaye NC, Jager KJ. Sex and gender disparities in the epidemiology and outcomes of chronic kidney disease. Nat Rev Nephrol. 2018;14:151–64.
21. Murphy D, McCulloch CE, Lin F, Banerjee T, Bragg-Gresham JL, Eberhardt MS, et al. Trends in prevalence of chronic kidney disease in the United States. Ann Intern Med. 2016;165(7):473–81.
22. Hallan SI, Øvrehus MA, Romundstad S. Long-term trends in the prevalence of chronic kidney disease and the influence of cardiovascular risk factors in Norway. Kidney Int. 2016;90(3):665–73.
23. Aitken GR, Roderick PJ, Fraser S, Mindell JS, O'Donoghue D, Day J, et al. Change in prevalence of chronic kidney disease in England over time: comparison of nationally representative cross-sectional surveys from 2003 to 2010. BMJ Open. 2014;4:e005480.
24. Stel VS, Brück K, Fraser S, Zoccali C, Massy ZA, Jager KJ. International differences in chronic kidney disease prevalence: a key public health and epidemiologic research issue. Nephrol Dial Transplant. 2017;32(Suppl_2):ii129–35.
25. Chrysohoou C, Panagiotakos DB, Pitsavos C, Skoumas J, Zeimbekis A, Kastorini CM, et al. Adherence to the Mediterranean diet is associated with renal function among healthy adults: the ATTICA study. J Ren Nutr. 2010;20:176–84.
26. Stengel B, Tarver-Carr ME, Powe NR, Eberhardt MS, Brancati FL. Lifestyle factors, obesity and the risk of chronic kidney disease. Epidemiology. 2003;14:479–87.
27. Vart P, Gansevoort RT, Coresh J, Reijneveld SA, Bültmann U. Socioeconomic measures and CKD in the United States and The Netherlands. Clin J Am Soc Nephrol. 2013;8:1685–93.
28. Silverwood RJ, Pierce M, Hardy R, Sattar N, Whincup P, Ferro C, et al. Low birth weight, later renal function, and the roles of adulthood blood pressure, diabetes, and obesity in a British birth cohort. Kidney Int. 2013;84:1262–70.
29. Böger CA, Gorski M, Li M, Hoffmann MM, Huang C, Yang Q, et al. CKDGen Consortium: association of eGFR related loci identified by GWAS with incident CKD and ESRD. PLoS Genet. 2011;7:e1002292.

30. Jones C, Roderick P, Harris S, Rogerson M. Decline in kidney function before and after nephrology referral and the effect on survival in moderate to advanced chronic kidney disease. Nephrol Dial Transplant. 2006;21:2133–43.
31. de Goeij MC, Liem M, de Jager DJ, Voormolen N, Sijpkens YW, Rotmans JI, et al. Proteinuria as a risk marker for the progression of chronic kidney disease in patients on predialysis care and the role of angiotensin-converting enzyme inhibitor/angiotensin II receptor blocker treatment. Nephron Clin Pract. 2012;121:c73–82.
32. Bruck K, Jager KJ, Zoccali C, Bello AK, Minutolo R, Ioannou K, et al. Different rates of progression and mortality in patients with chronic kidney disease at outpatient nephrology clinics across Europe. Kidney Int. 2018;93:1432–41.
33. Eriksen BO, Tomtum J, Ingebretsen OC. Predictors of declining glomerular filtration rate in a population-based chronic kidney disease cohort. Nephron Clin Pract. 2010;115:c41–50.
34. Levin A, Djurdjev O, Beaulieu M, Er L. Variability and risk factors for kidney disease progression and death following attainment of stage 4 CKD in a referred cohort. Am J Kidney Dis. 2008;52:661–71.
35. Coresh J, Turin TC, Matsushita K, Sang Y, Ballew SH, Appel LJ, et al. Decline in estimated glomerular filtration rate and subsequent risk of end-stage renal disease and mortality. JAMA. 2014;311(24):2518–31.
36. Tonelli M, Wiebe N, Culleton B, House A, Rabbat C, Fok M, et al. Chronic kidney disease and mortality risk: a systematic review. J Am Soc Nephrol. 2006;17:2034–47.
37. Matsushita K, van der Velde M, Astor BC, Woodward M, Levey AS, de Jong PE, et al. on behalf of the Chronic Kidney Disease Prognosis Consortium. Association of estimated glomerular filtration rate and albuminuria with all-cause and cardiovascular mortality in general population cohorts: a collaborative meta-analysis. Lancet. 2010;375(9731):2073–81.
38. van der Velde M, Matsushita K, Coresh J, Astor BC, Woodward M, Levey A, et al. on behalf of the Chronic Kidney Disease Prognosis Consortium. Lower estimated glomerular filtration rate and higher albuminuria are associated with all-cause and cardiovascular mortality. A collaborative meta-analysis of high-risk population cohorts. Kidney Int. 2011;79(12):1341–52.
39. Keith DS, Nichols GA, Gullion CM, Brown JB, Smith DH. Longitudinal follow-up and outcomes among a population with chronic kidney disease in a large managed care organization. Arch Intern Med. 2004;164(6):659–63.
40. Foley RN, Murray AM, Li S, Herzog CA, McBean AM, Eggers PW, et al. Chronic kidney disease and the risk for cardiovascular disease, renal replacement, and death in the United States Medicare population, 1998 to 1999. J Am Soc Nephrol. 2005;16(2):489–95.
41. Dalrymple LS, Katz R, Kestenbaum B, Shlipak MG, Sarnak MJ, Stehman-Breen C, et al. Chronic kidney disease and the risk of end-stage renal disease versus death. J Gen Intern Med. 2011;26(4):379–85.
42. United States Renal Data System. 2018 USRDS annual data report: epidemiology of kidney disease in the United States. Bethesda: National Institutes of Health, National Institute of Diabetes and Digestive and Kidney Diseases; 2018.
43. ERA-EDTA Registry. ERA-EDTA Registry Annual Report 2016. Amsterdam UMC, location AMC, Department of Medical Informatics, Amsterdam, 2018.
44. Seng WH, Meng OL, Chau KT, Ganeshadeva YALM. Chapter 3: Death and survival on dialysis. In: Wong HS, Goh BL, eds. 24th report of the Malaysian Dialysis and Transplant Registry 2016. Kuala Lumpur; 2018.
45. Korean ESRD Registry. ESRD Registry Report 2018. Availbale at http://www.ksn.or.kr/rang_board/list.html?code=sinchart_eng.
46. ANZDATA Registry. 41st Report, Chapter 1: incidence of end stage kidney disease. Adelaide: Australia and New Zealand Dialysis and Transplant Registry; 2018. Available at: http://www.anzdata.org.au.
47. ANZDATA Registry. 41st Report, Chapter 2: prevalence of end stage kidney disease. Adelaide: Australia and New Zealand Dialysis and Transplant Registry; 2018. Available at: http://www.anzdata.org.au.
48. Van de Luijtgaarden MW, Jager KJ, Segelmark M, Pascual J, Collart F, Hemke AC, et al. Trends in dialysis modality choice and related patient survival in the ERA-EDTA Registry over a 20-year period. Nephrol Dial Transplant. 2016;31:120–8.
49. Pippias M, Jager KJ, Kramer A, Leivestad T, Sánchez MB, Caskey FJ, et al. The changing trends and outcomes in renal replacement therapy: data from the ERA-EDTA Registry. Nephrol Dial Transplant. 2016;31:831–41.
50. Antlanger M, Noordzij M, van de Luijtgaarden M, Carrero JJ, Palsson R, Finne P et al. Sex Differences in Kidney Replacement Therapy Initiation and Maintenance. Clin J Am Soc Nephrol. 2019;14(11):1616–25. https://doi.org/10.2215/CJN.04400419.
51. Ploos van Amstel S, Noordzij M, Warady BA, Cano F, Craig JC, Groothoff JW, et al. Renal replacement therapy for children throughout the world: the need for a global registry. Pediatr Nephrol. 2018;33:863–71.
52. Van der Tol A, Lameire N, Morton RL, Van Biesen W, Vanholder R. An international analysis of dialysis services reimbursement. Clin J Am Soc Nephrol. 2019;14:84–93.
53. Liu FX, Rutherford P, Smoyer-Tomic K, Prichard S, Laplante S. A global overview of renal registries: a systematic review. BMC Nephrol. 2015;16:31.
54. Kramer A, Stel VS, Caskey FJ, Stengel B, Elliott RF, Covic A, et al. Exploring the association between macroeconomic indicators and dialysis mortality. Clin J Am Soc Nephrol. 2012;7:1655–63.
55. Masakane I, Nakai S, Ogata S, Kimata N, Hanafusa N, Hamano T, et al. An overview of regular dialysis treatment in Japan (As of 31 December 2013). Ther Apher Dial. 2015;19:540–74.

56. Wu M-S, Wu I-W, Hsu K-H. Survival analysis of Taiwan renal registry data system (TWRDS) 2000–2009. Acta Nephrol. 2012;26:104–8.
57. Robinson BM, Zhang J, Morgenstern H, et al. Worldwide, mortality risk is high soon after initiation of hemodialysis. Kidney Int. 2014;85:158–65.
58. Noordzij M, Jager KJ. Increased mortality early after dialysis initiation: a universal phenomenon. Kidney Int. 2013;85:12–4.
59. Foley RN, Parfrey PS, Sarnak MJ. Clinical epidemiology of cardiovascular disease in chronic renal disease. Am J Kidney Dis. 1998;32(suppl 3):S112–9.
60. De Jager DJ, Grootendorst DC, Jager KJ, van Dijk PC, Tomas LM, Ansell D, et al. Cardiovascular and noncardiovascular mortality among patients starting dialysis. JAMA. 2009;302:1782–9.
61. Sarnak MJ, Jaber BL. Mortality caused by sepsis in patients with end-stage renal disease compared with the general population. Kidney Int. 2000;58:1758–64.
62. Goodkin DA, Bragg-Gresham JL, Koenig KG, Wolfe RA, Akiba T, Andreucci VE, et al. Association of comorbid conditions and mortality in hemodialysis patients in Europe, Japan, and the United States: the Dialysis Outcomes and Practice Patterns Study (DOPPS). J Am Soc Nephrol. 2003;14:3270–7.
63. Van Manen JG, Van Dijk PC, Stel VS, Dekker FW, Clèries M, Conte F, et al. Confounding effect of comorbidity in survival studies in patients on renal replacement therapy. Nephrol Dial Transplant. 2007;22:187–95.
64. Yoshino M, Kuhlmann MK, Kotanko P, Greenwood RN, Pisoni RL, Port FK, et al. International differences in dialysis mortality reflect background general population atherosclerotic cardiovascular mortality. J Am Soc Nephrol. 2006;17:3510–9.
65. Van Dijk PC, Zwinderman AH, Dekker FW, Schön S, Stel VS, Finne P, et al. Effect of general population mortality on the north-south mortality gradient in patients on replacement therapy in Europe. Kidney Int. 2007;71:53–9.
66. Robinson BM, Akizawa T, Jager KJ, Kerr PG, Saran R, Pisoni RL. Factors affecting outcomes in patients reaching end-stage kidney disease worldwide: differences in access to renal replacement therapy, modality use, and haemodialysis practices. Lancet. 2016;388:294–306.
67. Merion RM, Goodrich NP, Johnson RJ, McDonald SP, Russ GR, Gillespie BW, et al. Kidney transplant graft outcomes in 379 257 recipients on 3 continents. Am J Transplant. 2018;18:1914–23.
68. Kurella Tamura M. Recognition for conservative care in kidney failure. Am J Kidney Dis. 2016;68:671–3.
69. Davison SN, Levin A, Moss AH, et al. Executive summary of the KDIGO Controversies Conference on Supportive Care in Chronic Kidney Disease: developing a roadmap to improving quality care. Kidney Int. 2015;88:447–59.
70. Hemmelgarn BR, James MT, Manns BJ, O'Hare AM, Muntner P, Ravani P, et al. Rates of treated and untreated kidney failure in older vs younger adults. JAMA. 2012;307:2507–15.
71. Australian Institute of Health and Welfare 2016. Incidence of end-stage kidney disease in Australia 1997–2013. Cat. no. PHE 211. Canberra: AIHW.
72. van de Luijtgaarden MW, Noordzij M, van Biesen W, Couchoud C, Cancarini G, Bos WJ, et al. Conservative care in Europe--nephrologists' experience with the decision not to start renal replacement therapy. Nephrol Dial Transplant. 2013;28:2604–12.
73. Okamoto I, Tonkin-Crine S, Rayner H, Murtagh FE, Farrington K, Caskey F, et al. Conservative care for ESRD in the United Kingdom: a national survey. Clin J Am Soc Nephrol. 2015;10:120–6.
74. Teruel JL, Burguera Vion V, Gomis Couto A, Rivera Gorrín M, Fernández-Lucas M, Rodríguez Mendiola N, et al. Choosing conservative therapy in chronic kidney disease. Nefrologia. 2015;35:273–9.
75. Foote C, Kotwal S, Gallagher M, Cass A, Brown M, Jardine M. Survival outcomes of supportive care versus dialysis therapies for elderly patients with end-stage kidney disease: a systematic review and meta-analysis. Nephrology (Carlton). 2016;21:241–53.
76. Shum CK, Tam KF, Chak WL, Chan TC, Mak YF, Chau KF. Outcomes in older adults with stage 5 chronic kidney disease: comparison of peritoneal dialysis and conservative management. J Gerontol A Biol Sci Med Sci. 2014;69:308–14.
77. Chandna SM, Da Silva-Gane M, Marshall C, Warwicker P, Greenwood RN, Farrington K. Survival of elderly patients with stage 5 CKD: comparison of conservative management and renal replacement therapy. Nephrol Dial Transplant. 2011;26:1608–14.
78. Brown MA, Collett GK, Josland EA, Foote C, Li Q, Brennan FP. CKD in elderly patients managed without dialysis: survival, symptoms, and quality of life. Clin J Am Soc Nephrol. 2015;10:260–8.
79. Wongrakpanich S, Susantitaphong P, Isaranuwatchai S, Chenbhanich J, Eiam-Ong S, Jaber BL. Dialysis therapy and conservative management of advanced chronic kidney disease in the elderly: a systematic review. Nephron. 2017;137:178–89.
80. Morton RL, Webster AC, McGeechan K, Howard K, Murtagh FE, Gray NA, et al. Conservative management and end-of-life care in an Australian Cohort with ESRD. Clin J Am Soc Nephrol. 2016;11:2195–203.
81. Murtagh FEM, Marsh JE, Donohoe P, Ekbal NJ, Sheerin NS, Harris FE. Dialysis or not? A comparative survival study of patients over 75 years with chronic kidney disease stage 5. Nephrol Dial Transplant. 2007;22:1955–62.

82. Verberne WR, Geers AB, Jellema WT, Vincent HH, van Delden JJ, Bos WJ. Comparative survival among older adults with advanced kidney disease managed conservatively versus with dialysis. Clin J Am Soc Nephrol. 2016;11:633–40.
83. WHO. Global action plan for the prevention and control of noncommunicable diseases 2013–2020. Geneva: WHO; 2013.
84. Remuzzi G, Macia M, Ruggenenti P. Prevention and treatment of diabetic renal disease in type 2 diabetes: The BENEDICT study. J Am Soc Nephrol. 2006;17(Suppl 2):S90–S7.
85. Golan L, Birkmeyer JD, Welch HG. The cost-effectiveness of treating all patients with type 2 diabetes with angiotensin-converting enzyme inhibitors. Ann Intern Med. 1999;131:660–7.
86. Levey AS, Schoolwerth AC, Burrows NR, Williams DE, Stith KR, McClellan W, Centers for Disease Control and Prevention Expert Panel. Comprehensive public health strategies for preventing the development, progression, and complications of CKD: report of an expert panel convened by the Centers for Disease Control and Prevention. Am J Kidney Dis. 2009;53:522–35.
87. Turner G, Wiggins K, Johnson D, et al. Cari guidelines: primary prevention of chronic kidney disease: blood pressure targets. Kidney Health Australia: Westmead; 2012.
88. Laine J, Kuvaja-Kollner V, Pietila E, Koivuneva M, Valtonen H, Kankaanpää E. Cost-effectiveness of population-level physical activity interventions: a systematic review. Am J Health Promot. 2014;29:71–80.
89. Bibbins-Domingo K, Chertow GM, Coxson PG, Moran A, Lightwood JM, Pletcher MJ, et al. Projected effect of dietary salt reductions on future cardiovascular disease. N Engl J Med. 2010;362:590–9.
90. Bala MM, Strzeszynski L, Topor-Madry R, Cahill K. Mass media interventions for smoking cessation in adults. Cochrane Database Syst Rev. 2013;(6):CD004704.
91. McMahon EJ, Campbell KL, Bauer JD, Mudge DW. Altered dietary salt intake for people with chronic kidney disease. Cochrane Database Syst Rev. 2015;(2):CD010070.
92. Orth SR, Hallan SI. Smoking: a risk factor for progression of chronic kidney disease and for cardiovascular morbidity and mortality in renal patients—absence of evidence or evidence of absence? Clin J Am Soc Nephrol. 2008;3:226–36.

Chapter 2
History of Dietary Protein Treatment for Non-dialyzed Chronic Kidney Disease Patients

Joel D. Kopple and Jerrilynn D. Burrowes

Keywords Chronic kidney disease · Low-protein diets · Supplemented very-low-protein diets Essential amino acids · Ketoacid analogs of essential amino acids · End-stage kidney disease · Uremia Uremic toxins · Progression of kidney disease · Glomerular filtration rate

Key Points
- Protein-modified diets have been recommended for the management of patients with chronic kidney disease (CKD) since the last half of the 1800s. Currently, almost all diets recommended for non-dialyzed CKD patients (stages 3–5) include some degree of protein restriction.
- In patients with CKD, low-protein diets reduce the accumulation of uremic toxins in the body, particularly when CKD is advanced (i.e., stages 4 and 5).
- Low-protein diets (LPDs) generally are also lower in potassium, phosphorus, and often sodium content. These diets may delay the need for chronic hemodialysis, peritoneal dialysis, or kidney transplantation, at least by reducing the severity of uremic toxicity and possibly also by slowing the rate of loss of glomerular filtration rate (GFR).
- It has been recommended that non-dialyzed stage 3–5 CKD patients should be prescribed either (1) a LPD providing 0.55–0.60 g protein/kg body weight (BW)/day with about 50% high biological value (HBV) protein or (2) a very-low-protein diet (VLPD) providing 0.28–0.43 g of protein/kg BW/day supplemented with additional ketoacid/amino acid analogs (a mixture of four essential amino acids (histidine, lysine, threonine, and tryptophan), the calcium salts of ketoacid analogs of four other essential amino acids (isoleucine, leucine, phenylalanine, and valine), and the hydroxyacid analog of methionine to meet the protein requirements of 0.55–0.60 g/kg BW/day.
- The most recent clinical practice guidelines on nutrition in CKD patients from the National Kidney Foundation (NKF) Kidney Disease Outcomes Quality Initiative (KDOQI) and the Academy of Nutrition and Dietetics recommend for nondiabetic stage 3–5 CKD patients either the abovementioned LPD or a VLPD that provides 0.28–0.43 g protein/kg body weight/day that is supplemented with a sufficient amount of essential amino acids and ketoacid analogs to meet the protein requirements of 0.55–0.60 g/kg body weight/day.
- For CKD patients with large urinary protein losses, it seems reasonable to add 1 g of additional HBV protein to the diet for each gram of urine protein excretion above 5 g/day.

J. D. Kopple (✉)
Professor Emeritus of Medicine and Public Health, University of California, Los Angeles, CA, USA

The Lundquist Institute for Biomedical Innovation at Harbor-UCLA Medical Center, Torrance, CA, USA
e-mail: jkopple@lundquist.org

J. D. Burrowes
Department of Biomedical, Health and Nutritional Sciences, School of Health Professions and Nursing, Long Island University-Post, Brookville, NY, USA

© Springer Nature Switzerland AG 2020
J. D. Burrowes et al. (eds.), *Nutrition in Kidney Disease*, Nutrition and Health,
https://doi.org/10.1007/978-3-030-44858-5_2

Introduction

Dietary protein restriction has been recommended for the treatment of patients with chronic kidney disease (CKD) since at least the latter half of the nineteenth century [1]. Interestingly, and continuing to the present day, there have been two different views advanced regarding the benefits of protein restriction for CKD patients: (1) protection of the health and function of the diseased kidney and (2) preservation or improvement of the overall health of the patient. For over 100 years, the views of workers in this field have often fluctuated widely between these two potential benefits of low-protein diets (LPDs). This chapter will review the history of dietary protein recommendations in non-dialyzed patients with CKD from the late 1800s through present day. In addition, evidence-based guidelines and consensus statements published within the last 20 years that address recommendations for dietary protein intake (DPI) in CKD patients will be presented. Moreover, a brief discussion about high-protein diets and kidney disease is addressed.

Dietary Protein Intake in CKD from the Late 1800s to 1950s

In 1869, Beale found that blood and urine urea levels were directly related to the quantity of meat ingested [2]. By decreasing meat intake, blood urea would decrease, and the amount of urea and constituents in urine would also fall. This was an important goal because renal urea excretion was thought to increase the workload and therefore stress on the diseased kidney. However, it is now known that renal excretion of urea consumes almost no energy [3, pp. 622–633]. Beale also recognized that reducing protein intake could improve the clinical status of patients with kidney disease [2]. There was a contrary view held by some researchers that higher protein intakes would have a stimulatory or strengthening effect on the kidney [4]. It is possible that support for this latter theory was provided by the observations that kidney weight of rats correlated directly with their protein intake and blood urea levels [5, 6]. These latter observations might also have been considered to support the abovementioned view that a higher protein intake, by engendering greater urea excretion, increased the workload of the kidney.

In 1914, a prominent German physician, Franz Volhard, postulated that there were two causes of the clinical manifestations of kidney failure: the retention of compounds, including urea, which are normally excreted in the urine and that cause the "pure" uremic syndrome, and symptoms caused by the kidney disease itself [7, 8]. Today, we might ascribe these latter symptoms as the systemic manifestations of the renal disease itself or of the illness that caused the renal disease. Examples of these latter conditions would include hypertension, nephrotic syndrome, cardiovascular disease, and the nonrenal sequelae of such illnesses as diabetes mellitus or lupus erythematosus. In 1918, Volhard recommended a LPD, particularly vegetarian, and 2000 kcal/day [8, 9]. He contended that this diet could decrease serum urea levels, reduce uremic symptoms, and possibly prolong survival.

In the second, third, and fourth decades of the twentieth century, a number of investigators conducted studies in small animals (e.g., rats and rabbits) who had either no underlying kidney disease or specific induced kidney injury, such as Masugi glomerulonephritis or bipolar clamped kidneys [10–12]. They found that high-protein diets per se could induce progressive kidney disease in these animals or could accelerate the progression of kidney disease in animals with underlying kidney disease. The kidneys of rats with no previous kidney disease that were fed high-protein diets developed proteinuria and abnormal urine sediment and displayed interstitial fibrosis and glomerular scarring. Hypertension was not uncommon. Some studies indicated that LPDs prevented or ameliorated these effects [11, 12]. Not all investigators confirmed that high-protein diets caused injury to the normal kidney of rodents [13]. One group of investigators reported that three factors influenced the development and progression of kidney disease: (1) a high-protein diet, (2) the source of the protein fed (beef liver was reported to be particularly injurious to the kidney), and (3) the duration of feeding the diet [11]. Usually, little effort was made in these studies to control the intake of other nutrients including sodium, phosphorus, and potassium. Interestingly, Newburgh and Curtis [11] found that feeding urea to rats did not cause renal injury, suggesting that the mechanisms of the renal injury from high-protein diets were not an increased workload from the urea excretion.

In the 1930s and particularly the 1940s, several sets of studies reported benefits of LPDs for people with CKD [14–16]. These benefits included reduction in serum urea, improvement in uremic symptoms, and slowing of the progression of kidney failure. Kempner employed a low-salt, rice-fruit-sugar diet for treatment "in all serious instances of acute and chronic nephritis, in heart failure that does not respond to the customary treatment with salt restriction and drugs, and in arteriosclerotic and hypertensive vascular disease with cardiac, cerebral, retinal or renal involvement" [14]. Kempner reported that this diet provided about 2000 kcal with not more than 5 g fat, 150 mg Na, 200 mg Cl, and about 20 g protein. Some patients with severe uremia and/or fluid overload underwent dramatic improvement with the loss of edema fluid, reduced blood pressure, and reduced uremic symptoms [14].

Other investigators described clinical benefits in advanced CKD patients with diets providing 10–25 g protein/day. These diets sometimes were preceded by a period of treatment with no protein intake [15, 16]. These physicians emphasized the importance of providing adequate calories to maintain protein mass and the difficulty of attaining adequate energy intake in patients with severely advanced CKD [14–16]. In these studies, which were carried out in the era before dialysis or transplantation, there appeared to be greater interest in treating patients with acute rather than chronic kidney failure, presumably because of the better long-term prognosis of the former patients [15, 16].

Thomas Addis added substantially to this body of literature [17]. His studies in subtotally nephrectomized rats confirmed that LPDs reduced the increase in their renal mass and were associated with less proteinuria, hematuria, and cylindruria and lower blood urea nitrogen (BUN). Addis concluded that the osmotic workload from the urea, the major osmolyte in urine, and also chloride and sodium, the next two most abundant urinary osmolytes, increased the workload of the diseased kidney with reduced functional mass. By decreasing urea production, a LPD would reduce the renal workload, thereby protecting the kidney from hypertrophy and ultimately further renal damage [17].

Addis's theories were not supported by the following observations. As indicated above, urea feeding did not appear to damage the kidney [11]. Renal oxygen consumption does not increase during osmotic diuresis [18, 19]. Most of the energy expenditure by the kidney is due to renal tubular reabsorption of solutes, particularly sodium and chloride, and is not associated with excretion of osmolytes or concentration of urine [20]. Third, Addis did not perform convincing pathological correlations with his dietary studies; his outcome measures included kidney size, urinalyses, and blood urea. In addition, he did not conduct controlled clinical trials of different protein diets in humans with kidney disease [17]. Investigators were unsure whether other nutrients that are associated with the protein content of the diet might be the nephrotoxic factors [1].

Many of the major investigators and thought leaders in renal physiology and renal disease in the late 1930s, 1940s, and early 1950s did not accept the thinking of Addis and other researchers who contended that LPDs would slow the loss of kidney function. These thought leaders argued that severely protein-restricted diets might engender malnutrition [1, 3, 21, 22]. Studies of small numbers of patients with acute nephritis did not indicate that high-protein or low-protein diets altered the urinary sediment or change their clinical course [23]. Probably influenced by these previous thinkers, in the 1950s, Merrill focused on the role of diet to reduce uremic toxicity and improve metabolism while maintaining acceptable nutritional status [24]. He did recommend diets restricted in protein (to about 0.50–0.60 g protein/kg/day), phosphorus, and other minerals when the glomerular filtration rate (GFR) had declined to where retention of substantial amounts of nitrogenous products and other chemicals led to accumulation in the blood. Merrill recognized the importance of high biological value (HBV) protein and the protein-sparing effects of a high energy intake. He clearly was familiar with many of the relevant principles of clinical nutrition and incorporated this thinking into his dietary recommendations for CKD patients [24].

Interestingly, although the mechanistic theories of Addis concerning how LPDs might protect the diseased kidney were not confirmed, some of his theories are prototypes of theories that are in favor with many investigators today. This is particularly true with regard to why LPDs may be protective of rats and probably humans with CKD [25, 26]. For example, in rats with CKD, a normal or high-protein diet increases GFR which, in turn, leads to increased glomerular filtration of solutes and hence increased solute absorption, e.g., sodium and chloride, by the remaining functional renal tubules; as indicated above, this will increase their workload. Higher-protein diets in rats also cause glomerular afferent arterial vasodilation, alters the glomerular basement membrane physiology, and increases single nephron blood flow and glomerular blood pressure. These diets also increase oxidative stress, inflammation, and protein deposition in the kidney. Higher protein intakes, by increasing acid production, may stimulate biochemical processes that promote fibrosis. In addition, higher protein intakes can also increase proteinuria in the diseased kidney, which itself is pathogenic. In CKD rats with reduced functioning nephrons, even a usual protein diet will engender these responses. Moreover, the protein and phosphorus contents of the diet are usually directly related, and higher phosphorus intakes are also associated with progressive kidney damage [27].

Dietary Protein Intake in CKD in the 1960s and 1970s

Starting in the early 1960s, there was an outpouring of studies of low-protein, low-phosphorus diets for the treatment of people with CKD (see below). What led to this outpouring of research is not entirely clear. We suspect that it may have been related to the exciting reports showing that chronic dialysis could keep people with end-stage kidney disease (ESKD) alive for extended periods of time. Also, successful kidney transplantation began to be reported at almost the same time. Hence, people with ESKD, which heretofore was considered to be a quickly and invariably fatal condition, suddenly could be kept alive for many years. This led to a reevaluation among healthcare workers of the syndrome of advanced CKD and its possible treatments, since it no longer was a terminal condition. One result was the exploration of potential treatments to keep advanced CKD patients alive and in a better metabolic, nutritional, and clinical state until they developed the need for renal replacement therapy (RRT; i.e., chronic dialysis treatment or kidney transplantation). At this time, there was virtually no discussion of using LPDs to slow progression of kidney disease. However, diets low in protein and minerals, especially sodium, potassium, and phosphorus, were considered to delay the need for RRT by maintaining advanced CKD patients in a healthier metabolic and physiological state and, thereby, reducing uremic symptoms.

In 1963, Giordano published a study in which advanced CKD patients were prescribed a diet providing almost no protein that was supplemented with primarily essential amino acids (EAAs), minerals, and food sources of energy [28]. He contended that uremic patients were able to reutilize endogenous or exogenous urea for protein synthesis, maintain positive nitrogen (N) balance, and manifest a reduction in uremic symptoms with a LPD that provided 23 g of HBV protein per day and adequate calories. However, this diet was hard to follow because it was unpalatable [28].

One year later, Giovannetti and Maggiore [29] reported the benefits of a very-low-protein diet (VLPD) providing about 1.0–1.5 g nitrogen per day that, after a period of days, was supplemented with about 12.7 g/day of the eight EAAs (omitting histidine) or about 1.5–2.2 g/day of nitrogen from egg protein and amino acids or albumen. This diet was given to eight patients with severe stage 5

CKD, six of whom, with urea clearances of 1.8–4.0 mL/min, were able to live without dialysis for up to 10 months. Patients sometimes required initial hemodialysis to improve their uremic symptoms to the point where they could ingest their entire VLPD. This diet contained 2000–3000 kcal from butter, lard, vegetable oil, sugar, honey, maize starch and special wheat starch, and select fruits and vegetables with the least amount of nitrogen (i.e., low biological value (LBV) proteins). Plasma urea improved dramatically. After undergoing rather markedly negative N-balance with the unsupplemented VLPD, the patients' N-balance became positive when the EAAs or egg protein was added [29]. This diet was sometimes referred to as the G-G diet [30]. Despite these findings, the use of the G-G diet was not widespread among patients with uremia in many countries, including the United States, because it was not well accepted by patients and it was likely to cause protein-energy malnutrition [31]. Low-protein, wheat starch products were developed during this time to satisfy dietary energy needs without providing additional protein, but many patients did not accept these products or other high-calorie, low-protein foods [32].

Although chronic hemodialysis therapy was just beginning to become available in the early 1960s for the overwhelming proportion of people with advanced CKD or ESKD, a protein-restricted diet that provided adequate amounts of amino acids, energy, and other essential nutrients was the only therapeutic option that was widely available to alleviate symptoms and to prolong life [29]. During this period of time, there was essentially no consideration of whether these diets could delay the progression of CKD.

In 1965, Berlyne and Shaw [33] modified the G-G diet to incorporate the preferences of British patients with advanced uremia. The Manchester modification of the G-G diet, as it was called, contained 18 g of protein plus 250 mg L-methionine and provided 2300 kcal (1300 kcal as liquid glucose, protein from spaghetti and biscuits, and 1000 kcal from cream and oil) [33]. Kluthe et al. [34, 35] developed a German modification of the G-G diet that included potatoes and eggs, which together provided a combination of proteins that were of HBV. This diet provided 20–25 g of protein/day with 40% LBV and 60% HBV. Energy was supplied by butter/margarine for a total of 2000 kcal/day [34, 35].

In 1968, Kopple et al. [32] conducted a prospective, randomized comparison study in far advanced CKD patients in which they received either a high-calorie 20-g protein diet with 13 g of HBV protein or an isocaloric 40-g mixed protein diet. (Calorie intake was maintained at about 35 kcal/kg/day in both groups.) The 40-g mixed protein diet contained at least 1.5 times the minimal daily requirement of each EAA. The 20-g protein diet contained about 14 g of HBV protein supplied from two whole eggs. Kopple et al. [32] found that both diets relieved uremic symptoms to a similar degree. There was a major decrease in serum urea nitrogen (SUN) with both diets, although the SUN decreased further with the 20-g protein diet. However, patients were able to maintain body weight better with the 40-g mixed protein diet. Moreover, this latter diet was more acceptable to patients because of the greater variety of food choices. On the other hand, patients ingesting the 20-g protein diet lost weight; they were dissatisfied with the diet and displayed poor dietary adherence. The researchers concluded that chronically uremic patients may have better outcomes with a 40-g protein diet with at least 1.5 times the minimal daily requirement of EAA [32].

In a subsequent study, Kopple and Coburn [31] compared a 20-g protein diet (about 0.30 g protein/kg/day) with 67% HBV protein to a 40-g protein diet (about 0.60 g/kg/day) with 79% HBV protein in uremic patients. Calorie intake was maintained between 33 and 40 kcal/kg/day in both diets with the use of such high-calorie, low-protein foods as wheat starch bread, low-protein puddings, candies, and liquid glucose. Results showed that N-balance was consistently positive in uremic patients who received the 40-g protein diet and was usually negative with the 20-g protein diet. Nitrogen balance was significantly more positive with the 40-g protein diet than with the 20-g protein diet. Moreover, mean body weight increased only with the 40-g protein diet [31]. Other studies support the nutritional adequacy of the 0.60 g protein/kg/day in stage 4 and 5 CKD patients who are not hypercatabolic and do not have large amounts of proteinuria [36].

Essential Amino Acid and Ketoacid-Supplemented Very-Low-Protein Diets

In order to maximally reduce uremic toxicity while maintaining good nutritional status, Bergstrom and coworkers [37] developed a diet that provided about 16–20 g protein/day from foods that were supplemented with EAA. For the amount of protein and amino acids included, this diet should provide a much lower amount of potassium, phosphorus, and probably sodium and various other compounds (e.g., creatinine, purines, pyrimidines, food additives) that is found in foodstuffs that contain similar amounts of protein. Norée and Bergstrom [38] treated uremic patients in Sweden for an average of 8.4 months with an unselected protein-poor diet (16–20 g/day) plus oral EAAs including histidine. Patients demonstrated a reduction in uremic symptoms that persisted for the several months that patients followed this diet; patients maintained N-balance with this diet. Moreover, patients with low serum albumin, total protein, and total iron binding capacity (TIBC) at baseline showed an increase in these values after 1 month of EAA supplementation that persisted during treatment. The authors concluded that uremic symptoms can be resolved, protein depletion counteracted, and nutritional status improved with this EAA-supplemented very-low-protein diet (SVLPD) [38]. By modifying the composition of the EAA supplement, these investigators were able to obtain more normal plasma and intracellular muscle free amino acid concentrations in advanced CKD patients [39, 40]. To our knowledge, they did not conduct studies on the effect of this EAA SVLPD on progression of CKD or survival in advanced CKD patients.

In another effort to provide adequate protein nutrition to advanced CKD patients while minimizing uremic toxicity, researchers began to examine the use of alpha ketoacid (KA) or alpha hydroxyacid analogs of EAA (Fig. 2.1). With the exception of lysine and threonine, humans can reversibly transaminate the EAA at the alpha amino carbon to form the respective EAA analog. Thus, these KAs and hydroxyacids offer the benefit that they provide amino acid precursors without the nitrogen load (i.e., the alpha amino (NH_2) moiety) (see Fig. 2.1). To the extent to which they are aminated, these compounds provide a sink for amino nitrogen which therefore reduces the generation of urea and other nitrogen-containing potential toxins. Initially, it was thought that the substantial amounts of urea are hydrolyzed in vivo, and the amino groups released from urea can be used for amination of KAs and hydroxyacids for synthesis of new amino acids [28, 42]. Subsequent research indicated that only small amounts of urea are hydrolyzed. Hence, reduction in urea synthesis, decreased amino acid degradation, and recycling of the amino groups in the amino acids, rather than urea reutilization, appear to be the main causes for net reduction in urea appearance with these diets [43, 44].

In addition to reducing the nitrogen load and generation of potential uremic toxins, KAs and hydroxyacid supplements of EAAs offer other potential advantages. The KA analog of leucine, alpha-ketoisocaproic acid, appears to reduce protein degradation in skeletal muscle [45]; leucine itself is reported to increase muscle protein synthesis [46]. These actions may both promote anabolism and reduce synthesis of urea and other toxic nitrogenous compounds. Since the KAs and hydroxyacids are strong acids, they are usually provided as calcium salts. As such, they have an alkalinizing effect, which might contribute to the ability of SVLPDs to slow the progression of kidney failure (see below). A recent review discusses the potential role of KAs and hydroxyacids in greater detail [41].

Walser was the first person to extensively use combinations of KAs and hydroxyacid analogs to reduce uremic toxicity in advanced CKD patients [47–49]. After several years of experimentation with different combinations and quantities of KAs and hydroxyacid analogs, he used a mixture of the KA analogs of four EAAs, valine, leucine, isoleucine, and phenylalanine, the hydroxyacid of methionine, all given as the calcium salts, plus the other four EAAs, tryptophan, lysine, threonine, and histidine, and the semi-EAA, tyrosine, to treat advanced CKD patients [47–49]. Roughly 16–20 g of this KA/EAA mixture was fed to advanced CKD patients who were also prescribed a diet providing about

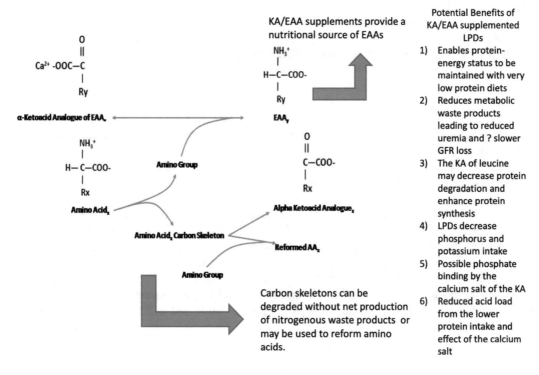

Fig. 2.1 Reversible transamination of a ketoacid (KA) analog of an amino acid (AA) and an AA. The R denotes the side chain of the AA, and the subscripts (x) and (y) refer to different AAs or KAs. Transamination is catalyzed by aminotransferase enzymes (i.e., transaminases). During this process, there is a substitution of the amino group with either a keto group (forming a KA) or a hydroxy group (yielding a hydroxyacid). The α amino group of the essential AA (EAA) is commonly transferred to a ketoglutarate or oxalo-acetate to generate the AAs glutamate or aspartate, respectively. Glutamate, a major recipient of these amino groups, can be oxidatively deaminated to generate NH_3 and regenerate a ketoglutarate. The KA formed by transamination can be degraded by oxidation. KA or hydroxyacid analogs of the EAAs, except lysine or threonine, can be transaminated to form their respective EAA. GFR glomerular filtration rate, LPD low-protein diet. (Reprinted with permission from Shah et al. [41])

20 g/day of protein of miscellaneous quality. Walser and his colleagues demonstrated that the KAs and the hydroxyacid were readily transaminated to their respective amino acids. This SVLPD maintained N-balance, reduced uremic symptoms, and appeared to be safe [47–50]. However, not all patients accepted this rigorous, unusual diet.

As clinical experience increased, Walser also reported that many CKD patients ingesting this diet seemed to experience a slowing in their rate of loss of GFR [47–49]. These anecdotal findings were initially received with surprise and much skepticism. But as Walser continued to report these anecdotal observations, other investigators began to study this question.

By the 1970s, use of EAA and KA supplements had become more widespread for the treatment of chronic renal failure [48]. Numerous studies were conducted by other investigators in the following two decades to examine the effectiveness of these EAA/KA SVLPDs on nutritional status, progression of renal disease and postponement of dialysis [38, 50–54]. It was argued that supplementing a protein-restricted diet with a mixture of EAAs and KAs prevented the need for a large amount of HBV protein and allowed patients the flexibility to choose from a wider variety of foods [55]. It also ensured that adequate EAAs were ingested [56]. However, the 0.60 g protein/kg/day diet was also shown to maintain N-balance in CKD patients and provided the recommended dietary allowances for EAAs

[31, 36, 57]. This diet should provide about 50% HBV protein and will still contain about as much miscellaneous quality protein as did the SVLPD.

Alvestrand et al. [52] treated a group of patients with severe renal insufficiency with 18 g of protein of mixed biological value supplemented with EAAs or KAs to postpone the need to start dialysis. The patients were treated for an average of 215 days until they received dialysis therapy or a kidney transplant. After commencing the diet, uremic symptoms disappeared, serum urea decreased, and after more than 3 months of dietary therapy, they reported N-balance was more positive than in patients fed a poorly controlled 40-g protein diet. They also concluded that this EAA or KA SVLPD could be an alternative to early dialysis therapy without endangering life expectancy. The authors emphasized that the success of conservative dietary therapy (i.e., very-low-protein diet supplemented with EAAs or KAs) is dependent on the patient's adherence to the prescribed diet, which involves proper nutrition education, counseling, and close supervision from a registered dietitian (RD) or international equivalent [52].

Mitch et al. [50] treated 24 advanced CKD patients with 20–30 g of mixed quality protein, less than 600 mg of phosphorus, and 18 g of an EAA-KA mixture per day for a mean of 20 months. Each patient received intensive nutrition education. Fifty-nine percent of patients displayed a reduced rate of increase in serum creatinine levels; no patients showed a more rapid rise in serum creatinine. These findings supported the contention that an EAA/KA SVLPD can retard the rate of progression of CKD. Dialysis was postponed by an accumulated total of 13 patient years. Moreover, nutritional status, as assessed by body weight, N-balance, serum albumin, and serum transferrin, was maintained [50].

The Modification of Diet in Renal Disease (MDRD) Study

As a result of a number of clinical trials in CKD patients that suggested LPDs or SVLPDs might slow the rate of progression of renal failure, the United States National Institutes of Health (NIH) funded the Modification of Diet in Renal Disease (MDRD) Study, which is the largest, most carefully conducted, and most prominent randomized, prospective controlled clinical trial of the effects of diet on progression of CKD [58]. The MDRD Study examined the effects of (Study 1) a usual protein and phosphorus diet (1.3 g protein/kg/day) vs. a low-protein, low-phosphorus diet (0.58 g protein/kg/day) and (Study 2) the low-protein, low-phosphorus diet (0.58 g protein/kg/day) vs. an EAA/KA SVLPD and very-low-phosphorus diet (0.3 g miscellaneous protein/kg/day that was supplemented with 0.28 g/kg/day of EAA and KA). True measured GFR of the patients was 25–55 ml/min/1.73m^2 in Study 1 and 13–24 ml/min/1.73m^2 in Study 2. Patients in Study 1 and Study 2 were also randomized independently to treatment with moderate vs. more strict blood pressure control (mean arterial blood pressure, 107 vs. 92 mm Hg). The key questions addressed were whether dietary protein restriction or strict blood pressure control would slow the progressive loss of GFR and whether such treatments were safe for the patient.

Five hundred and eighty-five patients were evaluated in Study 1 and 255 patients in Study 2 for a mean follow-up of 2.2 years. The results were inconclusive. In Study 1, the projected mean decline in GFR at 3 years between the diet groups or between the blood pressure groups was not significantly different. As compared to the usual protein diet and the moderate blood pressure treatment, the low-protein group and the low-blood-pressure group underwent a significantly more rapid decline in GFR during the first 4 months after randomization and a significantly slower decline thereafter. In Study 2, patients prescribed the EAA/KA SVLPD had a marginally slower decrease in GFR than did patients prescribed the LPD ($p = 0.07$) [58].

Although many nephrologists concluded from the MDRD Study that an LPD providing 0.58 g protein/kg/day or an SVLPD had no effect on slowing of GFR in CKD patients, several factors may have inadvertently prejudiced the MDRD Study from finding a difference in GFR loss between the two diets. First, the mean follow-up of 2.2 years may have been too short to adequately assess the effects of the low protein intakes. Both in Study 1 and especially in Study 2, the rate of GFR decline with the lower vs. the higher protein intakes tended to be slower at the time the study ended. In Study 2, the slower decline of GFR with the SVLPD vs. the LPD was almost statistically significant ($p = 0.07$). As indicated above, in Study 1, the GFR with the LPD decreased significantly more rapidly during the first 4 months and significantly more slowly for the rest of the follow-up period [58]. Most likely, the initial greater fall in GFR with the LPD probably reflected a decrease in nephron hyperfiltration; the decrease in nephron hyperfiltration is a known physiological effect of LPDs. In fact, the possibility that this might occur was extensively discussed during the planning of the MDRD Study, but at the time the MDRD Study was designed, data that LPDs reduce renal hyperfiltration in CKD patients had not yet been published. If the decision had been made that the key method of analysis of the rate of decline in GFR would start after the first 4 months of treatment, the conclusion from the MDRD Study would be that LPDs do significantly retard the rate of progression of renal failure. Another limitation of the MDRD Study was that there was no comparison of an EAA/KA SVLPD to a normal protein intake.

Other problems with the MDRD Study were that about 23% (59 of 255) patients in Study 2 had polycystic kidney disease, a nonglomerular genetic disease that may be particularly resistant to the effects of protein restriction [59]. Also, some CKD patients exhibit slow or no decline in GFR with no specific intervention other than perhaps treatment of blood pressure [60]. No attempt was made to exclude these patients from the MDRD Study. Moreover, the tryptophan content of the EAA/KA supplement was increased in order to reduce the possibility that this diet was insufficient in tryptophan content and might induce malnutrition. At that time, it was not realized that tryptophan is a metabolic precursor of indoxyl sulfate, which appears to be a nephrotoxin that might increase the rate of CKD progression [61]. Indeed, in the MDRD feasibility study, where additional tryptophan was not given, the EAA/KA SVLPD was associated with a slower decline in GFR than the EAA SVLPD ($p < 0.01$), but not more slowly than with the 0.58 g protein/kg/day diet ($p = 0.15$).

Secondary analyses of data from the MDRD Study support the conclusion that a LPD has a beneficial effect on the rate of GFR decline, proteinuria, and onset of ESKD [62, 63]. Each 0.2 g/kg/day decrease in protein intake was associated with a decline in the rate of GFR loss and a decrease in risk of end stage or death [64]. Although long-term (10-year) follow-up of the EAA/KA SVLPD group revealed a higher risk of death [63], interpretation of this finding is unclear since these patients only had access to the EAA/KA supplement for about the first 2.2 years of this 10-year follow-up.

Following publication of the results of the MDRD Study, a number of research studies continued to support and some nephrologists and dietitians continued to promote the treatment of advanced CKD patients with a LPD and EAA/KA SVLPDs. Many clinical trials with EAA/KA SVLPDs were conducted in CKD patients [54, 65–70]. Some of these trials were randomized, progressive, and controlled although in smaller numbers of patients. However, some, but not all of these trials, reported a reduction in the rate of loss of GFR [66, 70]. Few patients appeared to develop protein-energy wasting (PEW) [71]. In those studies where PEW was described in some patients, it was not clear that patients were carefully managed with regard to their dietary energy and protein intake.

Several meta-analyses were conducted on the effects of diet on progression of CKD in nondiabetic and diabetic adults. In meta-analyses where the time until the start of RRT was used as the criteria for reduction in progression of CKD, EAA/KA SVLPDs and LPDs were shown to significantly slow progression [71–73]. A meta-analysis by Fouque and Aparicio [56] using eight randomized controlled trials (RCTs) with 763 patients prescribed LPDs and SVLPDs (stages 3 and 4) and 751 controls showed a 31% reduction in renal death (95% CI: 0.55–0.85). A recent meta-analysis in nondiabetic adults with CKD indicated that in comparison to normal protein intakes, EAA/KA SVLPDs increased the time to starting RRT but LPDs had little or no effect [71]. In the one meta-analysis where a reduction in the rate of decline of GFR was used as the criterion, a statistically significant reduction in the rate of progression of CKD was also observed with LPDs and SVLPDs [74]. However, the rate of slowing was only 0.53 ml/min/1.73 m² per year, which was not considered to be clinically important.

One must bear in mind that these analyses did not exclude CKD patients who did not adhere to the LPDs and SVLPDs. It is possible that the reduction in progressive renal failure would have been more pronounced if the analyses had been restricted to patients who adhered to their prescribed diets. Such an analysis would be very difficult if not impossible to conduct because patients who adhere more closely to LPDs or SVLPDs might be more likely to take their medicines as prescribed, to live a healthier lifestyle, and to have other characteristics that might influence progression of CKD, independent of their diet.

The findings from these two sets of meta-analyses may not be in conflict. Whether LPDs and SVLPDs do or do not slow the loss of GFR, the decreased intake of protein, potassium, phosphorus, and possibly sodium with these latter diets may sufficiently reduce uremic toxicity in far advanced CKD patients, so that nephrologists may delay the inauguration of RRT [75, 76]. The study by Brunori et al. [77] provides evidence to this effect. These investigators studied elderly, nondiabetic CKD patients who, at the start of the study, were >70 years of age and had a GFR, defined as the mean of their serum creatinine and urea clearances, of 5–7 ml/min. Patients were randomly assigned to either start chronic dialysis therapy (n = 56 patients) or receive treatment with a 0.30 g protein/kg/day vegan diet supplemented with EAA/KA (n = 56 patients). The latter patients continued on the SVLPD until they exhibited signs indicating a need for dialysis therapy. Median follow-up was 26.5 months, and the median time that patients followed the SVLPD was 10.7 months. Forty of the SVLPD patients began dialysis treatment due to fluid overload or hyperkalemia. There was no difference in survival between the two groups, although hospitalization was significantly lower in the SVLPD patients as compared to the dialysis patients (p <0.01), with 41% of hospitalizations due to their dialysis access site [77].

LPDs and SVLPDs may also be used to delay the need for thrice-weekly hemodialysis or daily chronic peritoneal dialysis (CPD) in patients approaching ESKD [78, 79]. By reducing accumulation of toxins with these diets, patients may begin RRT with once or twice weekly dialysis therapy. EAA/KA SVLPD therapy has also been used in some far advanced CKD patients to successfully avoid the need for emergency placement of a vascular access for urgent dialysis. In these patients, uremia was controlled with a SVLPD for sufficient time to allow a surgically created vascular fistula or graft to mature and be used [80]. Clearly, there is a need for more studies to examine whether dietary therapy can safely delay the need for dialysis therapy in advanced CKD patients.

In a recent systematic review of controlled trials, Rhee et al. [81] compared the clinical management of CKD patients with different levels of dietary protein intake. The risk of progression to ESKD was significantly reduced, and the trend toward all-cause mortality was also lower in patients who received the LPD (<0.80 g/kg/day) compared to a higher-protein diet (>0.80 g/kg/day). Moreover, the SVLPD (<0.40 g/kg/day) as compared to a dietary protein intake <0.80 g/kg/day was associated with greater preservation of kidney function after 1 year and a significant reduction in the rate of progression to ESKD [81]. The optimal protein intake that may slow the progression of renal damage is unknown, but the authors are of the opinion that a EAA/KA SVLPD and possibly a 0.60 g protein/kg/day diet are probably effective in slowing CKD progression [82, 83]. These diets will not engender PEW as long as there is adequate intake of calories, protein, and other essential nutrients. Sufficient EAAs must be given either by ensuring adequate HBV protein, provided with the 0.60 g protein/kg/day diet, or as pure EAAs or their KA or hydroxyacid precursors ingested with the SVLPD.

It is the authors' opinion that intensive nutrition education, monitoring and evaluation, and an assessment of dietary adherence by the RD (or international equivalent), which occurred in the MDRD Study and in a number of other clinical trials of dietary therapy for CKD patients, are warranted for patients who are prescribed LPDs. Moreover, this surveillance by the RD is necessary to reduce the risk of PEW in this population.

Variations in Low-Protein Diets

Some investigators involved with the MDRD Study concluded that a diet providing 0.75 g protein/kg/day, which they rounded out to 0.80 g protein/kg/day, was as effective as lower-protein diets at retarding progression of kidney failure and maintaining adequate nutrition [84]. These conclusions were largely based on a post hoc analysis of the MDRD Study data and particularly a linear regression analysis of total protein (or total protein plus the EAA/KA supplement). It has been argued that examination of this regression analysis is likely to indicate that a 0.60 g protein/kg/day diet might lower progression of CKD more effectively. This latter diet appears to maintain nutritional status well and to generate less uremic toxicity compared to higher protein intakes [31, 36]. For CKD patients who may not be able to ingest adequate calories with the 0.60 g protein/kg/day diet or who find this diet too difficult to follow, it may be necessary to prescribe a higher-protein diet. However, even under these latter circumstances, we do not recommend a diet providing more than 0.80 g protein/kg/day for patients who have stage 4 or 5 CKD.

The original N-balance studies and clinical assessments of nutritional status with the EAA/KA SVLPDs that were carried out by Walser and associates evaluated a 0.30 or 0.40 g protein/kg/day diet supplemented with about 0.28–0.30 g EAA/KA/kg/day [48, 49, 65]. This diet was demonstrated to maintain N-balance and nutritional status [49]. Similar quantities of the EAA/KAs were employed in the MDRD Study. However, in recent years, the amount of the EAA/KA supplement that is often used and recommended is closer to about 0.12 g/kg/day [55, 66, 67, 69, 85, 86]. To our knowledge, the nutritional adequacy of this lower quantity of EAA/KAs has not been evaluated. We suspect that a major incentive for reducing the dosages of EAA/KAs is the relatively high cost of this supplement. Although a high incidence of PEW has not been reported with these lower doses, this may reflect the fact that most CKD patients prescribed the SVLPDs ingest higher amounts of dietary protein.

Recently, there has been much discussion regarding the potential benefits of vegan or vegetarian diets for CKD patients [70, 87]. These diets have been recommended for people without CKD, those with mild CKD, those with more advanced CKD prescribed the EAA/KA SVLPDs, those receiving chronic hemodialysis or peritoneal dialysis, and renal transplant recipients. The potential advantages of these diets are nicely summarized by Kalantar-Zadeh and Moore [87]. Potential benefits of these diets include the following: (1) Epidemiological studies indicate that people who appear to have normal kidney function and whose diets consist of a high plant content (e.g., the Mediterranean diet) live longer. (2) Diets higher in nuts, low-fat dairy products, and legumes and lower in red meat and processed meat are associated with a lower incidence of CKD [88]. (3) These diets can be associated with lower sodium intake and higher potassium intake, which may lead to reduced hypertension and oxidative stress. (4) The higher nitrate content of plant-based diets also may reduce blood pressure. (5) Dietary phosphorus content and intestinal phosphorus absorption may decrease somewhat, probably due to the higher phytate content of these diets [89].

A high plant-based diet may present an alkaline load that, by alkalinizing the kidney and urine, is reported to reduce the rate of progression of CKD. Some evidence suggests that animal fat may promote albuminuria, and choline and carnitine found in meat may increase production of potentially toxic trimethylamine, trimethylamine N-oxide, and other compounds in the gastrointestinal tract [90, 91]. A potential disadvantage of the vegetarian diet is that plant foods are often higher in potassium. For patients ingesting 0.60 g protein/kg/day, some vegetarian diets and particularly a vegan diet might provide inadequate amounts of some EAAs. Thus, it would seem that those at greatest risk of adverse events with a vegetarian/vegan diet may be advanced CKD patients who are not receiving dialysis treatment and who are ingesting diets providing about 0.60 g protein/kg/day. It is emphasized that no randomized prospective, controlled clinical trials have examined the health benefits and safety of vegetarian diets in CKD patients, except for studies that have assessed the ability of such diets to alkalinize urine [92].

Low-Protein Food Products

In the 1960s, food manufacturers began to produce high-calorie, low-protein food products in order to satisfy the energy needs of CKD patients prescribed LPDs. Low-protein wheat starch flour was one of the first products produced to make bread, muffins, cookies, cakes, and pancakes. For example, a 40-g slice of low-protein bread supplied 0.20 g protein and 115 calories compared to a regular slice of bread that provides 2 g of protein and 65 calories. The calorie content of the low-protein bread could be increased with the addition of butter/margarine and jelly/jam. However, because of the lack of gluten in the wheat starch flour, few patients (and dietitians) were able to make an acceptable bread product that was palatable and easy to handle. Low-protein pasta was also developed since it could be prepared with cream, butter, herbs, and other seasonings to increase the calorie content and the flavor. These products made it possible for patients to reduce their intake of LBV protein which, in turn, allowed them to consume more HBV proteins. Another available product was a powdered carbohydrate, protein-free supplement which could be added to any liquid such as water, soup, juice, or soft drinks.

Today, low-protein food products have become more widely available and palatable, which should increase patient adherence. Flavis® (Dr. Schar) (Lyndhurst, NJ) (https://www.flavis.com/en) is one food manufacturer that has entered the low-protein food market. They have a wide selection of low-protein pastas, breads, cookies, and snacks. Cambrooke Therapeutics (Ayer, MA) (https://www.cambrooke.com/), another manufacturer of low-protein food products, has developed more than 35 low-protein foods in 12 different food categories, specifically for the renal diet.

Dietary Protein Therapy in the Present Day

Evidence-Based Guidelines and Consensus Statements on Dietary Protein Intake in CKD

Since the early 2000s, several professional organizations have developed guidelines and consensus statements that include recommendations for protein intake in patients with stage 3–5 CKD (Table 2.1). In 2000, the evidence-based National Kidney Foundation (NKF) KDOQI Clinical Practice Guidelines for Nutrition in Chronic Renal Failure (hereafter referred to as the KDOQI Nutrition Guidelines) were published [93]. These guidelines were the basis for nutrition management of adult predialysis patients (CKD stages 4–5) for almost two decades. The KDOQI Nutrition Guidelines recommended that in patients with chronic renal failure (i.e., GFR <25 mL/min/1.73 m^2), 0.60 g of protein/kg/day should be considered. However, for patients who will not accept this protein recommendation or who are unable to maintain adequate dietary energy intake with this LPD, a protein intake of up to 0.75 g/kg/day may be prescribed. Moreover, ≥50% of the dietary protein should come from HBV sources [93].

In 2006, the Australia and New Zealand Renal Guidelines Taskforce published evidence-based practice guidelines for the nutritional management of CKD [94]. The taskforce determined the amount of dietary protein per day that is appropriate to optimize nutritional status and to prevent malnutrition in CKD patients. For patients with stage 3 CKD and patients with stage 4 CKD, they recommend 0.75–1.0 g/kg body weight (BW)/day. However, they state that the latter group should consume adequate calories and more than 50% HBV protein. As mentioned above, many researchers in this field think there is no therapeutic advantage to these higher protein intakes and recommend lower-protein diets, particularly for people with stage 4 CKD [31, 32, 36, 37, 47–49, 52, 70]. To our knowledge, there were no recommendations made for dietary protein intake of non-dialyzed stage 5 CKD patients (see Table 2.1) [94].

Table 2.1 Daily dietary protein recommendations in non-dialyzed patients with CKD

Guideline	Patients	Protein intake recommendation
NKF/KDOQI Clinical Practice Guidelines for Nutrition in Chronic Renal Failure [93]	GFR <25 mL/min	0.60 g/kg/day 0.75 g/kg/day (for non-adherent patients) ≥50% HBV protein
Australian-New Zealand Clinical Practice Guidelines [94]	Stage 3 (GFR 30–59 ml/min)	0.75–1.0 g/kg IBW/day
	Stage 4 (GFR 15–29 ml/min)	0.75–1.0 g/kg IBW with adequate kilojoule intake >50% HBV
ESPEN Guideline on Enteral Nutrition: Adult Renal Failure [95]	GFR 25–70 mL/min	0.55–0.60 g PRO (2/3 HBV)/kg/day
	GFR < 25 mL/min	0.55–0.60 g PRO/kg/day (2/3 HBV) OR ~ 0.30 g/kg/day supplemented with EAA or EAA/KA
	eGFR <20 mL/min	0.30–0.50 g/kg BW/day with KA (when available) to meet PRO requirements
Fresenius Kabi [85]	Stage 3a: eGFR 45–59[a]	0.80 g/kg/day (KAA not required)
	Stage 3b: eGFR 30–44[a]	0.60–0.70 g/kg/day + optional: 1 tablet/5 kg BW/day (depending on the biological value of dietary protein)
	Stage 4: eGFR 15–29[a]	0.60 g/kg/day + optional: 1 tablet/5 kg BW/day (depending on the biological value of dietary protein) OR 0.30–0.40 g/kg/day +1 tablet/5 kg BW/day
	Stage 5: eGFR <10–15 (not on dialysis)	0.60 g/kg/day + optional: 1 tablet/5 kg BW/day (depending on the biological value of dietary protein) OR 0.30–0.40 g/kg/day +1 tablet/5 kg BW/day
KDIGO [96]	GFR < 30 mL/min/1.73m^2	0.80 g/kg/day
	Adults at risk of progression	Avoid >1.3 g/kg/day
Australian KHA-CARI Guidelines [97]	Early CKD (stages 1–3)	0.75–1.0 g/kg/day with adequate calorie intake <0.60 g/kg/day is not recommended because of the risk of malnutrition
ISRNM [98]	All CKD	0.60–0.80 g/kg/day (without signs of malnutrition) ≥50% HBV +1.0 g/kg/day (presence of illness)
National Institute for Health and Care Excellence [99]	Stages 3–5	Do not prescribe low-protein diets (i.e., <0.60–0.80 g/kg/day) to patients with CKD
Italian Society of Nephrology [86]	All CKD	LPD: 0.60 g/kg/day (animal sources + protein-free products) Vegan diet: 0.70 g/kg/day (plant sources) VLPD: 0.30–0.40 g/kg/day (plant sources + protein-free products + EAA + KA)
KDOQI Guidelines: 2020 Update [100]	Stages 3–5	0.55–0.60 g/kg BW/day OR 0.28–0.43 g dietary protein/kg BW/day with additional KA/AA analogs to meet protein requirements (total: 0.55–0.60 g /kg BW/day)
	Stage 3–5 (with diabetes)	0.60–0.80 g/kg BW/day

(continued)

Table 2.1 (continued)

Guideline	Patients	Protein intake recommendation
Special populations		
NKF/KDOQI Guidelines for Hypertension and Antihypertensive Agents in CKD [101]	Stages 1–2	1.4 g/kg/day (~ 18% of kcal)
	Stages 3–4	0.60–0.80 g/kg/day (~ of 10% kcal)
KDOQI Clinical Practice Guidelines and Clinical Practice Recommendations for Diabetes and Chronic Kidney Disease [102]	All diabetics with CKD	0.80 g/kg/day and ≤20% of total kcal
Canadian Diabetes Association Guidelines [103]	All diabetes with CKD	0.80 g/kg/day; avoid intakes <1.3 g/kg/day

Abbreviations: *IBW* ideal body weight, *NKF-KDOQI* National Kidney Foundation Kidney Disease Outcomes Quality Initiative, *MHD* maintenance hemodialysis, *PD* peritoneal dialysis, *eGFR* estimated glomerular filtration rate, *HBV* high biological value, *ESPEN* Enteral Society for Parenteral and Enteral Nutrition, *EAA* essential amino acids, *KA* ketoanalogs, *KAA* keto/amino acids, *ISRNM* International Society of Renal Nutrition and Metabolism, *CKD* chronic kidney disease, *LPD* low-protein diet, *KDOQI* Kidney Disease Outcomes Quality Initiative, *BW* body weight
[a]With increasing serum creatinine

The Australia and New Zealand Renal Guidelines Taskforce specified under what circumstances IBW, actual body weight, or adjusted body weight should be used to determine protein requirements. Clinicians should aim for weight to be within a body mass index (BMI) of 20–25 kg/m^2 if GFR is between 15 and 59 mL/min. The taskforce recommended that if the patient is obese (BMI >30 kg/m^2), IBW can be adjusted using the following formula:

$$\text{Adjusted body weight} = \left[\left(\text{actual weight} - \text{ideal weight} \right) \times 0.25 \right] + \text{IBW}$$

Actual body weight should be used when (1) weight is within reasonable range of ideal or standard body weight (recommended BMI range), (2) recent weight change has not occurred, (3) the patient is not malnourished, and (4) the patient has been slightly overweight or underweight almost all of his/her life. *Adjusted body weight* should be used when patients are overweight or obese, using clinical judgment [94].

More recently, two American organizations, the NKF and the Academy of Nutrition and Dietetics, convened a workgroup to update and expand the nutrition guidelines for CKD patients. This document is the current KDOQI clinical practice guidelines [100]. For metabolically stable non-dialyzed patients (stage 3–5 CKD) without diabetes mellitus, the workgroup recommends a LPD that provides 0.55–0.60 g dietary protein/kg BW/day or an SVLPD that provides 0.28–0.43 g dietary protein/kg BW/day plus additional EAAs/KAs to provide a total protein intake of 0.55–0.60 g/kg BW/day [100]. These recommended dietary protein intakes seem reasonable to us. However, for metabolically stable patients with diabetes mellitus and stage 3–5 CKD, the KDOQI workgroup considers it reasonable to prescribe 0.60–0.80 g protein/kg BW/day [100]. For CKD patients with large urinary protein losses, it seems reasonable to add 1 g of additional HBV protein to the diet for each gram of urine protein excretion above 5 g/day. (Refer to Chaps. 15 and 16 for dietary protein recommendations for adult maintenance hemodialysis patients and peritoneal dialysis patients, respectively.)

It has been argued that patients who are prescribed and who adhere to LPDs have increased risk of developing PEW [90–94, 100, 104–108] (Fig. 2.2). A number of studies indicate that in almost all clinically stable non-dialyzed CKD patients, the 0.60 g protein/kg/day diet is nutritionally adequate if patients ingest sufficient calories, about 30–35 kcal/kg/day. This energy intake is not always easy for advanced CKD patients to attain. It is common for CKD patients with GFR levels of 25–35 ml/min/1.73 m^2 to lose weight [109, 110], probably (at least partly) because they ingest inadequate amounts of calories [36, 109]. CKD patients must be carefully monitored and managed to ensure that

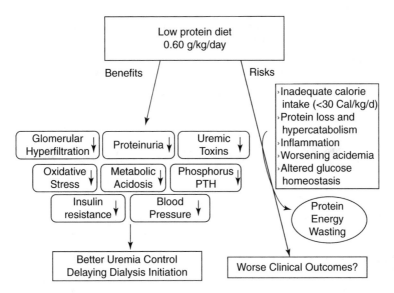

Fig. 2.2 Diagram of the role of low-protein diet in management of chronic kidney disease. Reduction in phosphorus intake and blood pressure levels are probably due to the lower phosphorus and sodium content of low-protein diets. Reduced insulin resistance has been occasionally described in reports of the responses to supplemented very-low-protein diets. (Modified with permission from Ko et al. [108])

energy intake is adequate and that they do not lose weight or develop PEW. As stated previously, CKD patients require frequent nutrition education, monitoring and evaluation, and an assessment of dietary adherence by an RD (or international equivalent). This continuous surveillance is aimed at identifying risk factors for and preventing PEW in patients prescribed LPDs and SVLPDs.

High-Protein Diets and Kidney Disease

Low-carbohydrate, high-protein diets are the fad today for people seeking weight loss; examples of this diet are the Atkins diet and the ketogenic diet [111]. The effects of these types of diets on the kidneys in people with normal kidney function are inconclusive. In the short term, a high-protein diet in people with normal kidney function may not cause deterioration of the kidneys; however, the long-term effects have not been examined fully. On the other hand, in people with preexisting kidney disease or a family history of kidney disease, caution should be taken before consuming a high-protein diet (i.e., more than 1.2 g/kg/day). Studies suggest that a high-protein diet in people with preexisting kidney damage may result in progressive damage, possibly by increasing renal blood flow and intra-glomerular pressure, which then leads to higher GFR [112, 113]. Such diets also promote greater accumulation of toxic protein-derived nitrogenous metabolites [107, 108] (Fig. 2.3). Therefore, it is the recommendation of the authors that before a low-carbohydrate, high-protein diet is considered for weight loss, individuals should be evaluated for preexisting kidney disorders to prevent further damage.

The mechanisms underlying the effects of a high-protein diet on the progression of CKD has been examined. Protein metabolism leads to the production of nitrogenous end products such as urea, ammonia, uric acid, and strong acids that are excreted by the kidneys and concentrated in the urine at levels higher than in plasma. After consumption of protein or an infusion of amino acids, there is a rapid reversible increase in GFR that is dependent on inhibition of tubuloglo-merular feedback that involves the renin-angiotensin system and nitric oxide that is possibly

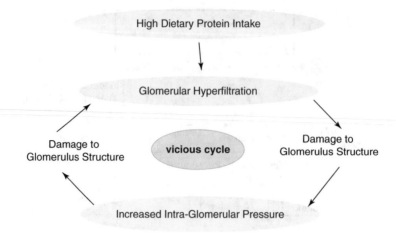

Fig. 2.3 Diagram of the effect of a high-protein diet on kidney function. (Reprinted with permission from Ko et al. [108])

influenced by vasopressin and glucagon. Hyperfiltration creates a vicious cycle because of the workload on the remaining nephrons in terms of filtration and reabsorption of sodium and other electrolytes, glucose, amino acids, and small proteins. This continued process resulting from a high-protein diet is considered one of the mechanisms leading to kidney failure [114]. As indicated above, a recent epidemiological study indicates that diets higher in red meat and processed meat and lower in nuts, low-fat dairy products, and legumes are associated with a higher incidence of CKD [88].

Conclusion

Protein-modified diets and particularly LPDs have been recommended for the management of patients with CKD since the last half of the 1800s. The characteristics of these diets have varied greatly. The potential benefits attributed to these diets include the following: (1) Protein-restricted diets reduce the accumulation of uremic toxins in the body and the severity of uremic toxicity, particularly when CKD is advanced. (2) LPDs facilitate the reduction in potassium, phosphorus, and possibly sodium intake. (3) LPDs may slow the progression of CKD and the loss of GFR; however, not all nephrologists believe LPDs have this effect. (4) Certain food sources of protein or certain amino acids or amino acid precursors may be less harmful or more beneficial to the kidney.

There are basically two types of protein-restricted diets currently recommended for CKD patients. One is a LPD that provides 0.55–0.60 g protein/kg BW/day with about 50% HBV protein. Meeting energy needs or improving patient acceptance may require the protein content of this diet to be increased up to 0.75 g/kg/day. The other diet is a SVLPD that provides about 0.28–0.43 g protein/kg BW/day that is supplemented with a mixture of four essential amino acids (histidine, lysine, threonine, and tryptophan) and the calcium salts of the ketoacid analogs of four other essential amino acids (isoleucine, leucine, phenylalanine, and valine) and the hydroxyacid analog of methionine to meet the total protein requirements of 0.55–0.60 g/kg BW/day. These diets may delay the need for RRT (i.e., chronic hemodialysis, peritoneal dialysis, or kidney transplantation) by reducing the severity of uremic toxicity and possibly also by slowing the rate of loss of GFR.

References

1. Kopple JD. History of dietary protein therapy for the treatment of chronic renal disease from the mid 1800s until the 1950s. Am J Nephrol. 2002;22(2/3):278–83.
2. Beale JS. Kidney diseases, urinary deposits, and calculous disorders: their nature and treatment. Philadelphia: Lindsay and Blakiston; 1869. p. 85.
3. Smith HW. The kidney. Structure and function in health and disease. New York: Oxford University Press; 1951.
4. Warner JH. The therapeutic perspective: medical practice, knowledge and identify in America, 1820–1885. Cambridge, MA: Harvard University Press; 1986. p. 91–2.
5. Watson CW, Lyon G. A preliminary note on the influence of a meat diet on the kidneys. J Physiol. 1906;34:19–21.
6. MacKay EM, MacKay LL, Addis T. Factors which determine renal weight. V. The protein intake. Am J Phys. 1928;86:459–65.
7. Volhard F, Fahr T. Die Brightsche Nierenkrankheit: Klinik, Pathologie und Atlas. Berlin: Springer; 1914.
8. Heidland A, Gerabek W, Sebekova K. Franz Volhard and Theodor Fahr: achievements and controversies in their research in renal disease and hypertension. J Hum Hypertens. 2001;15:5–16.
9. Volhard F. Die Doppelseitigen Hamatogenen Nierenerkrankungen (Brightsche Krankheit) im Handbuch der inneren Hamwege, Berlin: Springer-Verlag Berlin Heidelberg GMBH; 1918. pp. 1149–1722.
10. Newburgh LH, Clarkson S. Renal injury produced in rabbits by diets containing meat. Arch Intern Med. 1923;323:850–69.
11. Newburgh LH, Curtis AC. Production of renal injury in the white rat by the protein of the diet: dependence of the injury on the duration of feeding and on the amount and kind of protein. Arch Intern Med. 1928;42:801–21.
12. Farr LE, Smadel JE. The effect of dietary protein on the course of nephrotoxic nephritis in rats. J Exp Med. 1939;70:615–27.
13. Jackson H Jr, Riggs MD. The effect of high protein diets on the kidneys in rats. J Biol Chem. 1926;67:101–7.
14. Kempner W. Treatment of hypertensive vascular disease with rice diet. Am J Med. 1948;4:545–77.
15. Borst JGG. Protein katabolism in uraemia: effects of protein-free diet, infections, and blood transfusions. Lancet. 1948;1:824–8.
16. Bull GM, Joekes AM, Lowe KG. Conservative treatment of anuric uraemia. Lancet. 1949;2:229–34.
17. Addis T. Glomerular nephritis, diagnosis and treatment. New York: Macmillan; 1948.
18. Bucht H, Werke L, Josephson B. The oxygen consumption of the human kidney during heavy tubular excretory work. Scand J Clin Lab Invest. 1949;1:277–84.
19. Clark JK, Barker HG. Studies of renal oxygen consumption in man. 1: the effect of tubular loading (PAH), water diuresis, and osmotic (mannitol) diuresis. J Clin Invest. 1951;30:745–50.
20. Arendshorst WJ, Navar LG. Renal circulation and glomerular hemodynamics. In: Schrier RW, editor. Diseases of the kidney and urinary tract. 7th ed. Philadelphia: Lippincott Williams & Wilkins; 2001. p. 59–60.
21. Fishberg AM. Hypertension and nephritis. 4th ed. Philadelphia: Lea & Febiger; 1939.
22. Peters JP, Van Slyke DD. Quantitative clinical chemistry. Interpretations. Vol. 1. Baltimore: Williams & Wilkins; 1946.
23. Naeraa A. Studies on urinary sediment. III: effect of high protein diet upon the course of nephritis, with special reference to the urinary sediment. Acta Med Scand. 1938;95:359.
24. Merrill JP. The treatment of renal failure. Therapeutic principles in the management of acute and chronic uremia. New York: Grune & Stratton; 1955. p. 134–53.
25. Cortinovis M, Ruggenenti P, Remuzzi G. Progression, remission and regression of chronic renal disease. Nephron. 2016;134:20–4.
26. Zhong J, Yang H-C, Fogo AB. A perspective on chronic kidney disease progression. Am J Physiol Renal Physiol. 2017;312:F375–84.
27. Da J, Xie X, Wolf M, Disthabanchong S, Wang J, Zha Y, et al. Serum phosphorus and progression of CKD and mortality: a meta-analysis of cohort studies. Am J Kidney Dis. 2015;66(2):258–65.
28. Giordano C. Use of exogenous and endogenous urea for protein synthesis in normal and uremic subjects. J Lab Clin Med. 1963;62:231–46.
29. Giovannetti S, Maggiore Q. A low-nitrogen diet with proteins of high biological value for severe chronic uremia. Lancet. 1964;1:1000–3.
30. Di Iorio B, De Sato NG, Anastasio P, Perma A, Pollastro R, Di Micco L, et al. The Giordano-Giovannetti diet. J Nephrol. 2013;26(Suppl 22):S143–52.
31. Kopple JD, Coburn J. Metabolic studies of low protein diets in uremia. I. Nitrogen and potassium. Medicine. 1973;52:583–9.
32. Kopple JD, Shinaberger JH, Coburn JW, Rubin ME. Protein nutrition in uremia: a review. Am J Clin Nutr. 1968;21(5):508–15.

33. Berlyne G, Shaw AB, Nilwarangkur S. Dietary treatment of chronic renal failure: experiences with modified Giovannetti diet. Nephron. 1965;2:129–47.
34. Kluthe R, Quirin H, Oechslen D, Wenig A. "Kartoffel-Ei-Diät" bei fortgeschrittener Niereninsuffizienz. Med Klin. 1967;62(26):1020–2.
35. Kluthe R, Oechslen D, Quirin H, Jesdinsky HJ. Six years experience with a special low protein diet. In: Kluthe R, Berlyne G, Burton B, editors. Uremia: an international conference on pathogenesis diagnosis and therapy. Stuttgart: George Thieme; 1972. p. 250–6.
36. Kopple JD, Monteon FJ, Shaib JK. Effect of energy intake on nitrogen metabolism in nondialyzed patients with chronic renal failure. Kidney Int. 1986;29:734–42.
37. Bergstrom J, Furst P, Norée LO. Treatment of chronic uremic patients with protein-poor diet and oral supply of essential amino acids. I. Nitrogen balance studies. Clin Nephrol. 1975;3:187–940.
38. Norée LO, Bergstrom J. Treatment of chronic uremic patients with protein-poor diet and oral supply of essential amino acids. II. Clinical results of long-term treatment. Clin Nephrol. 1975;3(5):195–203.
39. Alvestrand A, Ahlberg M, Furst P, Bergstrom J. Clinical results of long-term treatment with a low protein diet and a new amino acid preparation in patients with chronic uremia. Clin Nephrol. 1983;19:67–73.
40. Bergstrom J, Ahlberg M, Alvestrand A, Furst P. Amino acid therapy for patients with chronic renal failure. Infusionsther Klin Ernahr. 1987;14(Suppl 5):8–11.
41. Shah AP, Kalantar-Zadeh K, Kopple JD. Is there a role for ketoacid supplements in the management of CKD? Am J Kidney Dis. 2015;65(5):659–73.
42. Richards P, Metcalfe-Gibson A, Ward EE, Wrong O, Houghton BJ. Utilisation of ammonia nitrogen for protein synthesis in man, and the effect of protein restriction and uraemia. Lancet. 1967;2(7521):845–9.
43. Tom K, Young VR, Chapman T, Masud T, Akpele L, Maroni BJ. Long-term adaptive responses to dietary protein restriction in chronic renal failure. Am J Phys. 1995;268(4 pt 1):E668–77.
44. Varcoe R, Halliday D, Carson ER, Richards P, Tavill AS. Efficiency of utilization of urea nitrogen for albumin synthesis by chronically uraemic and normal man. Clin Sci Mol Med. 1975;48(5):379–90.
45. Mitch WE, Walser M, Sapir DG. Nitrogen sparing induced by leucine compared with that induced by its keto analogue, alpha-ketoisocaproate, in fasting obese man. J Clin Invest. 1981;67(2):553–62.
46. Buse MG, Reid SS. Leucine. A possible regulator of protein turnover in muscle. J Clin Invest. 1975;56(5):1250–61.
47. Walser M, Coulter AW, Dighe S, Crantz FR. The effect of keto-analogues of essential amino acids in severe chronic uremia. J Clin Invest. 1973;52(3):678–90.
48. Walser M. Ketoacids in the treatment of uremia. Clin Nephrol. 1975;3:180–6.
49. Mitch W, Walser M. Nitrogen balance of uremic patients receiving branched-chain ketoacids and the hydroxy-analogue of methionine as substitutes for the respective amino acids. Clin Nephrol. 1977;8(2):341–4.
50. Mitch WE, Walser M, Steinman TI, Hill S, Zeger S, Tungsanga K. The effect of a keto acid-amino acid supplement to a restricted diet on the progression of chronic renal failure. N Engl J Med. 1984;311:623–9.
51. Heidland A, Kult J, Rockel A, Heidbreder E. Evaluation of essential amino acids and keto acids in uremic patients on low-protein diet. Am J Clin Nutr. 1978;31:1784–92.
52. Alvestrand A, Ahlberg M, Fürst P, Bergstrom J. Clinical experiences with amino acid and keto acid diets. Am J Clin Nutr. 1980;33:1654–9.
53. Gretz N, Korb E, Strauch M. Low-protein diet supplemented by ketoacids in chronic renal failure: a prospective controlled study. Kidney Int. 1983;24:S263–7.
54. Barsotti G, Morelli E, Giannoni A, Guiducci A, Lupetti S, Giovannetti S. Restricted phosphorus and nitrogen intake to slow the progression of chronic renal failure: a controlled trial. Kidney Int. 1983;24(Suppl 16):S278–84.
55. Aparicio M, Bellizzi V, Chauveau P, Cupisti A, Ecder T, Fouque D, et al. Do ketoanalogues still have a role in delaying dialysis initiation in CKD predialysis patients? Semin Dial. 2013;26(6):714–9.
56. Fouque D, Aparicio M. Eleven reasons to control the protein intake of patients with chronic kidney disease. Nat Clin Pract Nephrol. 2007;3(7):383–92.
57. Kopple JD, Sorensen MK, Coburn JW, Gordon S, Rubini ME. Controlled comparison of 20-gm and 40-gm protein diets in the treatment of chronic uremia. Am J Clin Nutr. 1968;21:553–64.
58. Klahr S, Levy AS, Beck GJ, Caggiula AW, Hunsicker L, Kusek JW, et al. and MDRD Study Group. The effects of dietary protein restriction and blood pressure control on the progression of chronic renal disease. N Engl J Med. 1994;330:877–84.
59. Klahr S, Breyer JA, Beck GJ, Dennis VW, Hartman JA, Roth D, et al. Dietary protein restriction, blood pressure control, and the progression of polycystic kidney disease. Modification of Diet in Renal Disease Study Group. J Am Soc Nephrol. 1995;5(12):2037–47.
60. Walser M. Progression of chronic renal failure in man. Kidney Int. 1990;37(5):1195–210.
61. Niwa T, Nomura T, Sugiyama S, Miyazaki T, Tsukushi S, Tsutsui S. The protein metabolite hypothesis, a model for the progression of renal failure: an oral sorbent lowers indoxyl sulfate levels in undialyzed uremic patients. Kidney Int. 1997;52:S23–8.

62. Levey AS, Greene T, Sarnak MJ, Wang X, Beck GI, Kusek JW, et al. Effect of dietary protein restriction on the progression of kidney disease: long-term follow-up of the Modification of Diet in Renal Disease (MDRD) study. Am J Kidney Dis. 2006;48:879–88.

63. Menon V, Kopple JD, Wang X, Beck GJ, Collins AJ, Kusek JW, et al. Effect of a very low protein diet on outcomes: long-term follow-up of the Modification of Diet in Renal Disease (MDRD) study. Am J Kidney Dis. 2009;53:208–17.

64. Levey AS, Greene T, Beck GJ, Caggiula AW, Kusek JW, Hunsicker LG, et al. Dietary protein restriction and the progression of chronic renal disease: what have all of the results of the MDRD study shown? J Am Soc Nephrol. 1999;10:2426–39.

65. Walser M, Hill SB, Ward L, Magder L. A crossover comparison of progression of chronic renal failure: ketoacids versus amino acids. Kidney Int. 1993;43(4):933–9.

66. Malvy D, Maingourd C, Pengloan J, Bargros P, Nivet H. Effects of severe protein restriction with ketoanalogues in advanced renal failure. J Am Coll Nutr. 1999;18(5):481.

67. Prakash S, Pande DP, Sharma S, Sharma D, Bal CS, Kulkarni H. Randomized, double-blind, placebo-controlled trial to evaluate efficacy of ketodiet in predialytic chronic renal failure. J Ren Nutr. 2004;14(2):89–96.

68. Teplan V, Schuck O, Knotek A, Hajny J, Horackova M, Kvapil M. Enhanced metabolic effect of erythropoietin and keto acids in CRF patients on low-protein diet: Czech multicenter study. Am J Kidney Dis. 2003;41(3 Suppl 1):S26–30.

69. Aparicio M, Chauveau P, De Precigout V, Bouchet JL, Lasseur C, Combe C. Nutrition and outcome on renal replacement therapy of patients with chronic renal failure treated by a supplemented very low protein diet. J Am Soc Nephrol. 2000;11(4):708–16.

70. Garneata L, Stancu A, Dragomir D, Stefan G, Mircescu G. Ketoanalogue-supplemented vegetarian very low-protein diet and CKD progression. J Am Soc Nephrol. 2016;27(7):2164–76.

71. Hahn D, Hodson EM, Fouque D. Low protein diets for non-diabetic adults with chronic kidney disease. Cochrane Database Syst Rev. 2018;(10):CD001892. https://doi.org/10.1002/14651858.CD001892.pub4.

72. Fouque D, Laville M, Boissel JP. Low protein diets for chronic kidney disease in non-diabetic adults. Cochrane Database Syst Rev. 2006;(2):CD001892.

73. Pedrini MT, Levey AS, Lau J, Chalmers TC, Wang PH. The effect of dietary protein restriction on the progression of diabetic and nondiabetic renal diseases: a meta-analysis. Ann Intern Med. 1996;124(7):627–32.

74. Kasiske BL, Lakatua JD, Ma JZ, Louis TA. A meta-analysis of the effects of dietary protein restriction on the rate of decline in renal function. Am J Kidney Dis. 1998;31(6):954–61.

75. Kopple JD, Gordon S, Wang M, Swendseid ME. Factors affecting serum and urinary guanidinosuccinic acid levels in normal and uremic subjects. J Lab Clin Med. 1977;90:303–11.

76. Heerspink HJL, Navis G, Ritz E. Salt intake in kidney disease—a missed therapeutic opportunity? Nephrol Dial Transplant. 2012;27(9):3435–42.

77. Brunori G, Viola BF, Parrinello G, De Biase V, Como G, Franco V, et al. Efficacy and safety of a very low protein diet when postponing dialysis in the elderly: a prospective randomized multicenter controlled study. Am J Kidney Dis. 2007;49(5):569–80.

78. Caria S, Cupisti A, Sau G, Bolasco P. The incremental treatment of ESRD: a low-protein diet combined with weekly hemodialysis may be beneficial for selected patients. BMC Nephrol. 2014;15:172.

79. Bolasco P, Cupisti A, Locatelli F, Cari S, Kalantar-Zadeh K. Dietary management of incremental transition to dialysis therapy: once-weekly hemodialysis combined with low-protein diet. J Ren Nutr. 2016;26(6):352–9.

80. Duenhas M, Goncalves E, Dias M, Leme G, Laranja S. Reduction of mortality related to emergency access to dialysis with very low protein diet supplements with ketoacids (VLPD+KA). Clin Nephrol. 2013;79(5):387–93.

81. Rhee CM, Ahmadi S-F, Kovesdy CP, Kalantar-Zadeh K. Low protein diet for conservative management of chronic kidney disease: a systematic review and meta-analysis of controlled trials. J Cachexia Sarcopenia Muscle. 2018;9:235–45.

82. Bellizzi V, Calella P, Carrero JJ, Fouque D. Very low-protein diet to postpone renal failure: pathophysiology and clinical applications in chronic kidney disease. Chron Dis Transl Med. 2018;4:45e5.

83. Hanafusa N, Lodebo BT, Kopple JD. Current uses of dietary therapy for patients with far-advanced CKD. Clin J Am Soc Nephrol. 2017;12(7):1190–5.

84. Levey AS, Adler S, Caggiula AW, England BK, Greene T, Hunsicker LG, et al. Effects of dietary protein restriction on the progression of advanced renal disease in the modification of diet in renal Disease study. Am J Kidney Dis. 1996;27(5):652–63.

85. Aparicio M, Bellizzi V, Chauveau P, Cupisti A, Ecder T, Fouque D, et al. Keto acid therapy in predialysis chronic kidney disease patients: final consensus. J Ren Nutr. 2012;22:S22–4.

86. Bellizzi V, Cupisti A, Locatelli F, Bolasco P, Brunori G, Cancarini G, et al. Low-protein diets for chronic kidney disease patients: the Italian experience. BMC Nephrol. 2016;17(1):77.

87. Kalantar-Zadeh K, Moore LW. Does kidney longevity mean healthy vegan food and less meat or is any low-protein diet good enough? J Ren Nutr. 2019;29(2):79–81.

88. Haring B, Selvin E, Liang M, Coresh J, Grams ME, Petruski-Ivleva N, et al. Dietary protein sources and risk for incident chronic kidney disease: results from the Atherosclerosis Risk in Communities (ARIC) Study. J Ren Nutr. 2017;27(4):233–42.

89. Watanabe MT, Barretti P, Caramori JCT. Attention to food phosphate and nutrition labeling. J Ren Nutr. 2018;28(4):e29–31.

90. Black AP, Anjos JS, Cardozo I, Carmo FL, Dolenga CJ, Nakao LS, et al. Does low-protein diet influence the uremic toxin serum levels from the gut microbiota in nondialysis chronic kidney disease patients? J Ren Nutr. 2018;28(3):208–14.

91. Pignanelli M, Bogiatzi C, Gloor G, Allen-Vercoe E, Reid G, Urquhart BL, et al. Moderate renal impairment and toxic metabolites produced by the intestinal microbiome: dietary implications. J Ren Nutr. 2019;29(1):55–64.

92. Goraya N, Simoni J, Jo C-H, Wesson DE. Comparison of treating metabolic acidosis in CKD stage 4 hypertensive kidney disease with fruits and vegetables or sodium bicarbonate. CJASN. 2013;8(3):371–81.

93. National Kidney Foundation. KDOQI clinical practice guidelines for nutrition in chronic renal failure. Am J Kidney Dis. 2000;35(suppl 2):S1–S104.

94. Dietitians Association of Australia. Evidence based practice guidelines for the nutritional management of chronic kidney disease. Nutrition Dietetics. 2006;63(Suppl. 2):S35–45.

95. Cano N, Fiaccadori E, Tesinsky P, Toigo G, Druml W, Kuhlmann M, et al. ESPEN guidelines on enteral nutrition: adult renal failure. Clin Nutr. 2006;25:295–310.

96. Kidney Disease: Improving Global Outcomes (KDIGO) CKD Work Group. KDIGO 2012 clinical practice guideline for the evaluation and management of chronic kidney disease. Kidney Int Suppl. 2013;3:1–150.

97. Johnson DW, Atai E, Chan M, Phoon RKS, Scott C, Toussant ND, et al. KHA-CARI guideline: early chronic kidney disease: detection, prevention and management. Nephrology. 2013;18:340–50.

98. Ikizler TA, Cano NJ, Franch H, Fouque D, Himmelfarb J, Kalantar-Zadeh K, et al. Prevention and treatment of protein energy wasting in chronic kidney disease patients: a consensus statement by the International Society of Renal Nutrition and Metabolism. Kidney Int. 2013;84:1096–107.

99. National Clinical Guideline Centre. Chronic kidney disease. Early identification and management of chronic kidney disease in adults in primary and secondary care. London: National Institute for Health and Care Excellence (NICE); 2014; p. 59 (Clinical guideline no. 182).

100. Ikizler TA, Burrowes J, Byham-Gray L, Campbell K, Carrero JJ, Chan W, et al. KDOQI Nutrition in CKD Guideline Work Group. KDOQI clinical practice guideline for nutrition in CKD: 2020 update. Am J Kidney Dis. 2020; in press.

101. National Kidney Foundation. K/DOQI clinical practice guidelines on hypertension and antihypertensive agents in chronic kidney disease. Am J Kidney Dis. 2004;43(Suppl 2):S1–S290.

102. National Kidney Foundation. KDOQI Clinical Practice Guidelines and clinical practice recommendations for diabetes and chronic kidney disease. Am J Kidney Dis. 2007;49:S1–S180.

103. Whitman D. Nutrition for the prevention and treatment of chronic kidney disease in diabetes. Can J Diabetes. 2014;38:344–8.

104. Kopple JD, Zhu X, Lew N, Lowrie EG. Body weight-for-height relationships predict mortality in maintenance hemodialysis patients. Kidney Int. 1999;56:1136–48.

105. Kalantar-Zadeh K, Kopple JD, Kilpatrick RD, McAllister CJ, Shinaberger CS, Gjertson DW, et al. Association of morbid obesity and weight change over time with cardiovascular survival in hemodialysis population. Am J Kidney Dis. 2005;46:489–500.

106. Johnson DW. Dietary protein restriction as a treatment for slowing chronic kidney disease progression: the case against. Nephrology. 2006;11:58–62.

107. Kalantar-Zadeh K, Moore LW, Tortorici AR, Chou JA, St-Jules DE, Aoun A, et al. North American experience with low protein diet for nondialysis-dependent chronic kidney disease. BMC Nephrol. 2016;17:90.

108. Ko GJ, Obi Y, Tortoricci AR, Kalantar-Zadeh K. Dietary protein intake and chronic kidney disease. Curr Opin Clin Nutr Metab Care. 2017;20(1):77–85.

109. Kopple JD, Greene T, Chumlea WC, Hollinger D, Maroni BJ, Merrill D, et al. Relationship between nutritional status and GFR: results from the MDRD study. Kidney Int. 2000;57:1688–703.

110. Ku E, Kopple JD, Johansen KL, McCulloch CE, Go AS, Xie D, et al. CRIC Study Investigators. Longitudinal weight change during CKD progression and its association with subsequent mortality. Am J Kidney Dis. 2018;71(5):657–65.

111. Jasni SK, Osman NA, Tajola'aurus NS. Effectiveness of the Atkins diet as a treatment of weight reduction. J Nat Sci Res. ISSN 2225–0921 (Online). 2013;3(13):30. Accessed from: https://iiste.org/Journals/index.php/JNSR/article/view/9057.

112. Tirosh A, Golan R, Haman-Boehm I, Henkin Y, Schwarzfuchs D, Rudich A, et al. Renal function following three distinct weight loss dietary strategies during 2 years of a randomized controlled trial. Diabetes Care. 2013;36:2225–32.

113. Marckmann P, Osther P, Pedersen AN, Jespersen B. High-protein diets and renal health. J Ren Nutr. 2015;25(1):1–5.

114. Fouque D, Mitch WE. Dietary approaches to kidney disease. In: Skorecki K, Chertow GM, Marsden PH, Taal MW, Yu ASL, editors. Brenner and Rector's the kidney. 10th ed. Philadelphia: Elsevier; 2016. p. 1956.

Chapter 3
Kidney Function in Health and Disease

Alluru S. Reddi

Keywords Nephron · Glomerulus · Renal function · Chronic kidney disease · Nephrotic syndrome Nephritic syndrome · Diabetic nephropathy · Podocytopathies · IgG4-related diseases

Key Points
1. Describe the gross and microscopic structure of the kidney.
2. Discuss the various functions of the normal kidney.
3. Define and discuss the various renal syndromes, such as acute kidney injury, chronic kidney disease, nephrotic and nephritic syndromes, tubulointerstitial diseases, vascular diseases of the kidney, podocytopathies, and IgG4-related diseases.

Introduction

The kidneys perform three major functions. As regulatory organs, the kidneys precisely control the composition and volume of the body fluids and maintain acid-base balance as well as blood pressure by varying the excretion of water and solutes. As excretory organs, the kidneys remove various nitrogenous metabolic end products in the urine. In general, the kidneys filter plasma in the glomerulus to form a protein-free ultrafiltrate. This ultrafiltrate passes through the various tubular segments where reabsorption of essential constituents and secretion of unwanted products occur. As endocrine organs, the kidneys produce important hormones, such as renin, erythropoietin, and active vitamin D_3 (calcitriol). In addition, the kidneys participate in the degradation of various endogenous and exogenous compounds. In order to understand these functions, it is essential to examine the gross and microscopic structure of the kidneys.

The editors acknowledge Kishore Kuppasani's contribution to this chapter in *Nutrition in Kidney Disease*, *Second Edition*, Nutrition and Health, DOI https://doi.org/10.1007/978-1-62,703-685-6_1, © Springer Science+Business Media New York 2014

A. S. Reddi (✉)
Department of Medicine, Rutgers New Jersey Medical School, Newark, NJ, USA
e-mail: reddias@njms.rutgers.edu

© Springer Nature Switzerland AG 2020
J. D. Burrowes et al. (eds.), *Nutrition in Kidney Disease*, Nutrition and Health,
https://doi.org/10.1007/978-3-030-44858-5_3

Anatomy of the Kidney

The kidneys are paired, bean-shaped structures located retroperitoneally in the lumbar region, one on either side of the vertebral column [1–3]. The lateral edge of the kidney is convex, while the medial aspect is concave with a notch called the hilum. The hilum receives the blood and lymphatic vessels, the nerves, and the ureter. The hilum contains a cavity, the renal sinus, where the ureter expands to form the renal pelvis. The normal adult kidney is about 10–12 cm long, 5–7 cm wide, and 2–3 cm thick, and it weighs 125–170 g.

Each kidney is composed of the parenchyma and the collecting system. The parenchyma consists of an outer cortex and an inner medulla. The medulla is divided into an outer (toward the cortex) and an inner medulla (toward the pelvis). The collecting system includes the calyces, the renal pelvis, and the ureters. The major calyces unite to form the renal pelvis. The renal pelvis drains into the ureter, which connects the kidney to the bladder.

The basic structural and functional unit of the kidney is the nephron. There are about 600,000 (range 300,000–1,400,000) nephrons in each kidney. Each nephron contains specialized cells that filter the plasma and then selectively remove, reabsorb, and secrete a variety of substances into the urine. The nephron consists of a renal corpuscle, the proximal tubule, the loop of Henle, and the distal tubule. The collecting duct is not part of the nephron because it is embryologically derived from the ureteric bud, whereas the nephron is derived from the metanephric blastema. However, the collecting duct is commonly included in the nephron because of its related function.

Renal Corpuscle

The renal corpuscle consists of the glomerulus and Bowman's capsule. Generally, the term "glomerulus" is widely used for the entire corpuscle. The glomerulus is composed of a capillary network lined by an inner thin layer of endothelial cells, a central region of mesangial cells surrounded by collagen-like mesangial matrix, and an outer layer of visceral epithelial cells. The endothelial and epithelial cells are separated by the glomerular basement membrane (GBM).

The GBM is a dense fibrillar structure, which is the only anatomic barrier between blood and urine. Biochemical studies of the GBM showed that it contains predominantly type IV collagen, proteoglycans, and laminin. Collagen provides the structural framework, whereas proteoglycans, such as heparan sulfate, confer a negative charge to the GBM. Because of this negative charge, filtration of albumin is curtailed. Bowman's capsule, which is a double-walled cup surrounding the glomerulus, consists of an outer layer of parietal epithelial cells. Between the visceral epithelial and parietal epithelial cells is a space called Bowman's space. The glomeruli are located exclusively in the cortex, which undergo pathologic changes in several disease conditions.

The endothelial cells line the glomerular capillaries, and they are separated by large (70 nm) fenestrations. These fenestrations limit filtration of only cellular elements such as erythrocytes but not water or proteins. The epithelial cells, also called podocytes, represent the visceral layer of Bowman's capsule. The podocytes have foot processes that cover the GBM. These foot processes are separated by a thin diaphragmatic structure called the slit diaphragm or slit pore.

The renal corpuscle is responsible for the ultrafiltration of the blood, which is the first step in urine formation. In this process, medium- and small-sized molecules are allowed to pass through into Bowman's space, while large-size molecules, such as proteins, are left behind. To enter Bowman's space, the ultrafiltrate must pass through the fenestrae of the endothelial cells, the layers of the basement membrane, and the slit diaphragms of the foot processes. Podocytes synthesize several cytoskeleton (e.g., actin, synaptopodin) and slit diaphragm (e.g., nephrin, podocin) proteins as well as angiogenic factors such as vascular endothelial growth factor. Discussion of these factors in the maintenance of glomerular capillary integrity is beyond the scope of this chapter.

In the last 10–15 years, there has been considerable interest in podocyte biology in various hereditary and acquired glomerular diseases. Only pathophysiological abnormalities in podocytes can cause both functional and structural abnormalities, and these abnormalities have been classified as podocytopathies, and a brief discussion of these podocytopathies is presented at the end of this chapter.

Proximal Tubule

Bowman's capsule continues as the proximal tubule, which is lined by cuboidal or columnar cells with a brush border on their luminal surface. The brush border consists of millions of microvilli, which markedly increase the surface area available for the absorption of solutes and water through cells (transcellular transport) or between cells (paracellular transport) or both. The proximal tubule reabsorbs about 60% of the ultrafiltrate. Several electrolytes (Na^+, K^+, Cl^-, HCO_3^-, Ca^{2+}, HPO_4^{3-}), amino acids, glucose, and water are reabsorbed in the proximal tubule. Also, secretion of organic acids and bases occurs in the proximal tubule. The proximal tubule is susceptible to insults such as renal ischemia and nephrotoxins, resulting in altered kidney function.

Thin Limb of Henle's Loop

The proximal tubule continues into the medulla as the thin descending limb of Henle's loop. The loop then bends back and becomes the thin ascending limb of Henle's loop. The thin descending limb is more permeable to water and less permeable to NaCl. As a result, water moves into the interstitium and makes the ultrafiltrate more concentrated than in the proximal tubule. In contrast, the thin ascending limb is impermeable to water but permeable to NaCl. Therefore, the ultrafiltrate becomes dilute and the medullary interstitium hypertonic. Thus, the thin descending and ascending limbs participate in the countercurrent multiplication of the urinary concentration process.

Distal Tubule

The distal tubule includes the thick ascending limb of Henle's loop and the distal convoluted tubule. The thick limb runs from the medulla into the cortex up to its parent glomerulus, where it forms the macula densa, a component of the juxtaglomerular apparatus that secretes renin. The thick ascending limb of Henle's loop is responsible for the reabsorption of Na^+, K^+, and Cl^- in the ratio of 1:1:2. The reabsorption of these electrolytes is dependent on the Na/K-ATPase located in the basolateral membrane. NaCl reabsorption also occurs in the distal convoluted tubule. Both segments of the distal tubule are normally impermeable to water, and thus, the fluid formed in the distal tubule is hypotonic. The impermeability of the distal tubule to water, combined with active transport of Na^+ and Cl^- out of the thick ascending limb, makes the medullary interstitium hypertonic. The distal tubule is connected to the collecting duct by the connecting tubule.

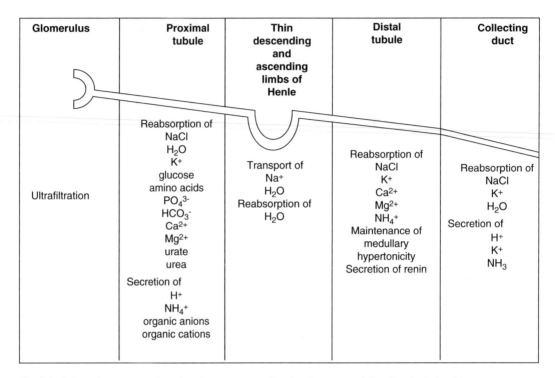

Fig. 3.1 Schematic representation of nephron segments showing the structural-functional relationships

Collecting Duct

Depending on its location in the kidney, the collecting duct can be divided into the cortical, outer medullary, and inner medullary portions. The epithelium of the collecting ducts contains two types of cells: principal (65%) and intercalated (35%) cells. The principal cell is the predominant type of cell lining the collecting duct system. In the cortical collecting duct, principal cells are responsible for K^+ secretion and Na^+ reabsorption. This function is regulated by aldosterone. Intercalated cells are involved in H^+ and HCO_3^- secretion. Transport of water occurs in all segments of the collecting duct in the presence of the antidiuretic hormone or vasopressin. Figure 3.1 summarizes the functions of various segments of the nephron.

Interstitium

The renal interstitium, a space between tubules, is comparatively sparse. It increases from the cortex to the medulla. In humans, the fractional volume of the cortical interstitium ranges from 12% in younger individuals to 16% in older subjects. In the medulla, the interstitial volume increases from the outer to the inner medulla in the range of 4% to approximately 30%.

Two types of interstitial cells have been described in the cortex: type 1 cortical interstitial cell, which resembles a fibroblast, and type 2 interstitial cell with mononuclear or lymphocyte-like structure. Between the cells is a space that contains collagen and fibronectin. It is believed that the peritubular fibroblast-like interstitial cells secrete erythropoietin. Type 2 interstitial cells are believed to represent bone marrow-derived cells. Three types of interstitial cells have been described in the medulla. None of these cells are the site of erythropoietin; however, some cells (type 1 medullary interstitial cell) contain lipid droplets, which are believed to have hypotensive effects. All medullary interstitial cells synthesize proteoglycans that are present in the interstitium.

Blood Supply

Each kidney is usually supplied by one renal artery arising from the abdominal aorta. After or before entering the hilum, the renal artery divides into an anterior and a posterior branch; both of them give rise to a total of five segmental arteries. The segmental arteries are end arteries, and occlusion of a single artery results in infarction of the area supplied. These segmental branches form the interlobar arteries in the renal sinus, which follow the curvature of the kidneys to form arcuate arteries. From these arteries arise interlobular arteries that course radially through the cortex toward its surface. The interlobular arteries give rise to the afferent arterioles, which divide into five to eight lobules and form the glomerular capillaries. The loops of these capillaries reunite to form the efferent arteriole of the glomerulus. The efferent arteriole leaves the glomerulus as a short unbranched segment before it branches into capillaries. These capillaries, which supply blood to the proximal and distal tubules of the cortex, are known collectively as the peritubular capillary network. The efferent arterioles of glomeruli located in the juxtamedullary cortex and near the medullary region not only supply blood to their own tubules but also run deep into the medulla. These long, thin vessels are called arteriolae rectae, or straight arterioles. They form a loop with straight venules or venulae rectae of the medulla to form the vasa recta of the kidney. Thus, the blood supply to the medulla is entirely derived from the efferent arterioles of the juxta-medullary glomeruli. The capillaries of the outer cortex converge to form the stellate veins which drain into the interlobular veins, then into the arcuate and interlobar veins, and finally into the renal vein.

Clinical Evaluation of Kidney Function

Currently, determination of serum creatinine and blood urea nitrogen (BUN) concentrations and estimation of glomerular filtration rate (GFR) remain the most important tests to assess kidney function in clinical practice. GFR can be measured directly by radioisotope methods or indirectly from serum creatinine concentration as estimated GFR (eGFR), using a predictive equation. Although serum creatinine concentration of 0.8–1.2 mg/dL and a BUN concentration of 10 mg/dL are considered normal, their values vary with muscle mass and protein intake as well as the functional status of the liver. Therefore, an eGFR is recommended for evaluation of kidney function. Most clinical laboratories provide both serum creatinine and eGFR to the physician for assessment of kidney function. An eGFR of 60 ml/min/1.73 m^2 or less is considered chronic kidney disease (CKD). In addition to eGFR, urinalysis provides an assessment of glomerular, tubular, and interstitial functions of the kidney. The presence of albuminuria, hematuria, and red blood cell (RBC) casts in a well-performed urinalysis indicates significant glomerular disease. Determination of urine pH and urine osmolality is helpful in assessing the kidney's ability to acidify as well as concentrate or dilute the urine. A renal biopsy is needed to assess the pathology of the kidney in disease states.

Kidney Function in Disease States

When GFR is decreased due to functional or structural damage to the kidney, a variety of functions and also the structure of the kidney are altered. These functional and structural disturbances are briefly discussed below.

Fluid, Electrolyte, and Acid-Base Disturbances

When GFR is below normal but not low enough, the kidneys try to maintain relatively normal fluid, electrolyte, and acid-base balance. However, when GFR is severely decreased, the kidneys retain Na^+, water, K^+, Mg^{2+}, PO_4^{3-}, and H^+, resulting in edema, either hyponatremia or hypernatremia, hyperkalemia, hypermagnesemia, hyperphosphatemia, and severe metabolic acidosis. Hypocalcemia results from decreased calcitriol production by the kidney. Patients also develop hypertension (HTN) due to retention of Na^+ and water. Anemia and bone disease are commonly seen in patients with low GFR.

Acute Kidney Injury

Acute kidney injury (AKI) is defined as an abrupt decrease in renal function, resulting in accumulation of nitrogenous (creatinine and BUN) and nonnitrogenous waste products. Before 2004, at least 35 definitions of AKI were reported, which were not standardized or validated. In 2004, the Acute Dialysis Quality Initiative group proposed the RIFLE system based on the increase in serum creatinine and urine output. This system classified AKI into three severity categories (R = risk, I = injury, F = failure) and two clinical categories (L = loss, E = end-stage renal disease). According to this classification, AKI is described as an abrupt (within 48 h) reduction in kidney function defined as an absolute increase in serum creatinine level of 0.3 mg/dL or a 50% increase in serum creatinine level from baseline or a reduction in urine output of <0.5 ml/kg/h for >6 h [4, 5]. The RIFLE system was subsequently modified by the acute kidney injury group, and classified AKI into three stages. Subsequently, the Kidney Disease Improving Global Outcomes (KDIGO) workgroup took these modifications and developed a unified definition of AKI, as shown in Table 3.1.

Table 3.1 Staging of AKI by KDIGO workgroup [4]

Stage	Serum creatinine	Urine output
1	≥1.5–1.9 times baseline or >0.3 mg/dl increase	<0.5 ml/kg/h for 6–12 h
2	≥2.0–2.9 times baseline	<0.5 ml/kg/h for ≥12 h
3	≥3.0 times baseline or increase of serum creatinine to ≥4.0 mg/dl or RRT or, in patients <18 years, decrease of eGFR to <35 ml per min per 1.73 m²	<0.3 ml/kg/h for ≥24 h or anuria for >12 h

Abbreviation: *RRT* renal replacement therapy, *eGFR* estimated glomerular filtration rate

Studies have shown that even a small increase in serum creatinine levels is associated with increased morbidity and mortality in patients with AKI. For example, it was reported that an increase in serum creatinine by ≥ 0.5 mg/dL was associated with a 6.5-fold increase in hospital mortality, while an increase in serum creatinine of 0.3–0.4 mg/dL was associated with only 70% increase in mortality risk. Even the length of the hospital stay was prolonged by AKI [6].

The causes of AKI are divided into three major categories: prerenal, renal, and postrenal. Prerenal AKI is due to decreased renal perfusion, caused by hypovolemia, decreased effective arterial blood volume, renal artery disease, and/or altered intrarenal hemodynamics. These patients are usually volume depleted. A variety of intrinsic renal disorders due to an acute insult to the renal vasculature, glomerulus, tubules, or interstitium can cause AKI. Acute tubular necrosis remains the major form of AKI due to renal ischemia and exposure to nephrotoxins, such as drugs or contrast material. Postrenal AKI is due to obstruction to the urinary system by either intrinsic or extrinsic masses.

Treatment of AKI includes volume repletion in hypovolemic conditions and elimination of the causative agent or disease process. Some patients may require hemodialysis or other renal replacement therapies, such as continuous venovenous hemodialysis. AKI is usually a reversible process; however, it is a risk factor for progression to CKD in a small percentage of patients (See Chap. 26).

Chronic Kidney Disease

CKD was first defined by KDOQI guidelines in 2002 based on eGFR and classified into five stages [7]. Subsequently, these guidelines were reviewed by KDIGO workgroup in 2012 and reintroduced a modified definition and classification [8, 9]. According to this workgroup, CKD is defined as abnormalities of kidney structure or function (GFR <60 ml/min/1.73 m^2) for >3 months with implications for health. The abnormalities in kidney structure include albuminuria, urine sediment abnormalities, electrolyte and other abnormalities due to tubular disorders, abnormalities detected by histology, structural abnormalities detected by imaging, and history of kidney transplantation. From these kidney structural abnormalities, the cause of CKD can be identified. Therefore, the KDIGO classification of CKD is based on *cause, eGFR,* and *albuminuria,* as shown Table 3.2. The cause is based on presence or absence of systemic disease and location within the kidney of pathologic-anatomic location. The disease categories fall into four groups: (1) glomerular diseases, (2) tubulointerstitial diseases, (3) vascular diseases, and (4) cystic and congenital diseases. In the new classification, the term stage is replaced by G (GFR), and albuminuria is classified into A1 (albuminuria stage 1) to A3.

According to the US renal data system [10], the overall prevalence of CKD, using the KDOQI classification [7], in the US adult general population is 14.8% in 2013–2016 and remained stable in the last two decades. The prevalence is highest in CKD stage 3. The prevalence of albuminuria did not change much since 2001 [10]. The prevalence of CKD among diabetics has decreased from 43.6% (2001–2004) to 36% in 2013 to 2016. In contrast, a similar decrease was not seen in subjects with HTN, and the prevalence remains at 31%. The prevalence of CKD is much higher in women than men, which attributed to longer life expectancy of women and overdiagnosis of CKD with eGFR equation [11]. However, kidney function deteriorates much faster in men than women, and they develop end-stage renal disease (ESRD) much earlier than women.

There are several risk factors for the progression of CKD, including hypertension, diabetes, hyperlipidemia, excessive protein intake, smoking, anemia, and genetic predisposition to kidney disease. CKD is one of the major risk factors for cardiovascular disease. Conservative management of CKD includes (1) control of blood pressure (<130/80 mm/Hg for patients with no proteinuria and <120/80 mm/Hg for those with proteinuria >1 g/day), using dietary sodium restriction <100 mEq/L and antihypertensive agents such as angiotensin-converting enzyme inhibitors (ACE-Is) or angiotensin receptor blockers (ARBs) as well as a low-dose diuretic; (2) maintenance of HbA$_{1c}$ ~7% in type 2

Table 3.2 Classification of CKD [8]

GFR categories		
GFR category	GFR (ml/min/1.73 m^2)	Terms
G1	≥90	Normal or high
G2	60–90	Mildly decreased
G3a	45–59	Mildly or moderately decreased
G3b	30–44	Moderately to severely decreased
G4	15–29	Severely decreased
G5	<15	Kidney failure

Albuminuria categories				
Category	AER (mg/24 h)	ACR (approximate equivalent) mg/mmol	mg/g	Terms
A1	<30	<3	<30	Normal to mildly increased
A2	30–300	3–30	30–300	Moderately increased
A3	>300	>30	>300	Severely increased

Abbreviations: *GFR* glomerular filtration rate, *CKD* chronic kidney disease, *AER* albumin excretion rate, *ACR* albumin/creatinine ratio

diabetic patients; (3) restriction of protein intake <0.8 g/kg/day; (4) maintenance of low-density lipoprotein (LDL) cholesterol <100 mg/dL; (5) maintenance of hemoglobin ~10–12 g/dL and control of bone disease; and (6) smoking cessation. Dialysis or kidney transplantation is required if the patient progresses to ESRD. Dietary management with fruits and vegetables is becoming an area of great interest in patients with CKD.

Nephrotic Syndrome

This syndrome is characterized by proteinuria >3.5 g/day, hypoalbuminemia, edema, hyperlipidemia, and lipiduria. The nephrotic syndrome is caused by (1) either primary (idiopathic) or secondary (known) glomerular diseases; (2) drugs, such as nonsteroidal anti-inflammatory drugs, heroin, and gold; and (3) bacterial, viral, and parasitic infections. Among secondary glomerular diseases, diabetes is the leading cause of nephrotic syndrome in adults (see below). The primary glomerular diseases that cause nephrotic syndrome are minimal change disease, focal segmental glomerulosclerosis, membranous nephropathy, and membranoproliferative glomerulonephritis.

Proteinuria is caused by losses of charge and size in the GBM. Also, a decrease in protein (nephrin, podocin, α-actinin) or mutation in genes that encode these proteins in slit diaphragm and cytoskeleton of podocytes can cause proteinuria. Hypoalbuminemia is due to renal loss of albumin and increased catabolism. Both hypoalbuminemia and increased salt and water retention lead to edema formation. Recently, it has been proposed that an increase in Na$^+$ reabsorption by the epithelial sodium channel (ENaC) located in the late distal convoluted tubule and cortical collecting duct is responsible for accumulation of Na$^+$ and edema formation in nephrotic syndrome. Hyperlipidemia is secondary to increased hepatic synthesis and decreased degradation of lipoproteins.

The patients with nephrotic syndrome are at risk for thrombotic complications, infections, cardiovascular disease, and skeletal abnormalities. Management of nephrotic syndrome includes salt and water restriction in edematous patients; ACE-Is or ARBs for proteinuria and control of hypertension; low-protein diet to improve serum albumin level, proteinuria, and renal function; vaccination to prevent infection from encapsulated organisms; prevention of thrombosis by avoiding prolonged immobilization and volume depletion; and control of hyperlipidemia. Anticoagulation is recommended in patients whose serum albumin levels are <2.0 g/dL and with high risk for thromboembolic complications (e.g., patients with membranous nephropathy). Immunosuppressive therapy is reserved for patients with primary renal diseases. Elimination of the secondary cause usually improves nephrotic syndrome (See Chap. 24).

Nephritic Syndrome

The nephritic syndrome, also called glomerulonephritis, is characterized by hematuria, RBC casts, hypertension, renal insufficiency, and varying degrees of proteinuria. Based upon the etiology and pathogenic mechanisms, this syndrome can present as (1) asymptomatic hematuria or proteinuria, (2) acute nephritis to rapidly progressive glomerulonephritis (RPGN), and finally (3) chronic sclerosing glomerulonephritis. There are several primary (e.g., RPGN) and secondary (e.g., systemic lupus erythematosus) causes of nephritic syndrome. Treating the underlying cause by conservative (acute nephritis) or aggressive (RPGN) management and control of blood pressure remain the mainstay of therapy in patients with nephritic syndrome. A substantial number of patients present with renal insufficiency, requiring renal replacement therapy.

Tubulointerstitial Diseases

Tubulointerstitial diseases (TIDs) are a group of clinical disorders that affect principally the tubules and interstitium. Pathologically, TIDs are characterized by tubular epithelial injury, atrophy, hyperplasia or hypertrophy, and fibrosis. Initially, the glomeruli and blood vessels are usually spared [12]. The tubulointerstitium is affected in all forms of renal disease. Based upon the morphologic changes and the rate of deterioration of renal function, TIDs can be classified into acute TID or acute interstitial nephritis or chronic TID or chronic interstitial nephritis. Acute TID manifests as sudden onset of renal failure within days to weeks (1 day to 2 months), hematuria, mild proteinuria, white blood cell (WBC) casts, and at times eosinophiluria or eosinophilia. It is usually caused by drugs and infections. The accurate diagnosis is made by renal biopsy. Acute TID is caused by drugs, infections, or immune disorders. Treatment includes removing the causative agent or in some cases steroids. Renal replacement therapy may be necessary in some patients.

Chronic TIDs are caused by a variety of drugs; infections; vascular, metabolic, immune, and hematologic diseases; urinary tract obstruction; and heavy metals. In some cases, the cause is unknown. Clinical manifestations include hypertension, renal insufficiency, hyperkalemia, anemia (both hyperkalemia and anemia are disproportional to the degree of renal insufficiency), inability to concentrate urine, and Fanconi syndrome. Urinalysis shows mild proteinuria and absence of RBC casts. Glomeruli are affected secondarily. Pathologic findings of the kidney include progressive scarring of the interstitium, tubular atrophy, and infiltration with lymphocytes and macrophages. Removal of the offending agent or treatment of the underlying cause and control of blood pressure with dietary sodium restriction and antihypertensive agents and correction of anemia as well as bone disease remain the mainstay of therapy in patients with chronic TIDs.

Vascular Diseases

Renal artery stenosis, hypertensive nephrosclerosis, vasculitis affecting the medium and small renal arteries, renal vein thrombosis as a complication of nephrotic syndrome, and several thrombotic microangiopathic diseases such as hemolytic uremic syndrome and thrombotic thrombocytopenic purpura are some of the vascular diseases that cause altered kidney function. Appropriate management is required to prevent the progression of kidney disease.

Diabetic Nephropathy

As stated previously, diabetes is the leading secondary cause of nephrotic syndrome in adults and deserves special attention. Also, 35–44% of both types of diabetic patients eventually develop ESRD. In order to prevent the progression of kidney disease and also delay the onset of ESRD, it is essential to follow the natural history and clinical course of diabetic nephropathy. It appears that there are two pathways for progression of diabetic nephropathy: One is proteinuric, and the other is non-proteinuric pathways. In the majority of type 1 and possibly type 2 diabetic patients, the kidney disease progresses (proteinuric pathway) through five distinct stages. Stage 1 (early hypertrophy-hyperfunction) corresponds to the onset of diabetes, which is characterized by enlarged kidneys and increased GFR. These changes can be reversed by good glycemic control. Stage 2 (normoalbuminuria) develops 2–5 years after onset of the disease and involves an increase in GFR and the development of some structural changes in the kidney. GFR improves with good glycemic control. Stage 3 (incipient nephropathy) takes 6–15 years to develop and is characterized by the presence of microalbuminuria (30–300 mg/day), which is the first clinical sign of diabetic nephropathy. There are progressive changes in the kidney, and patients develop hypertension. In addition to glycemic control, lowering blood pressure to <130/80 mm Hg with an ACE-I or ARBs has been proven to be extremely beneficial in preventing the progression of kidney disease to other stages of diabetic nephropathy. Stage 4 (overt nephropathy) occurs 15 to 20 years later and is characterized by clinically detectable proteinuria. Patients develop nephrotic syndrome, and hypertension becomes worse, resulting in gradual decrease in GFR (GFR decreases by 1 ml/min/month). Some type 1 and type 2 diabetic patients develop CKD without any microalbuminuria or proteinuria. These patients are usually referred to as non-proteinuric subjects with CKD. The progression of CKD in these patients follows a non-proteinuric pathway. How CKD progresses in non-proteinuric subjects is unclear at this time. Strict blood pressure control with two to four antihypertensives, if needed, stabilizes GFR in both proteinuric and non-proteinuric patients. Despite good glycemic and blood pressure control, some patients invariably progress to stage 5 (ESRD), requiring either maintenance dialysis or kidney transplantation for survival. Restriction of protein, Na^+, and phosphate in the diet has been shown to be beneficial in patients with CKD stages 3–5. Thus, glucose control, blood pressure control, and low-protein diet play a significant role in the management of diabetic nephropathy.

Despite classic studies on several pathways of diabetic nephropathy, recent work on podocyte biology has attracted much attention because podocytopenia occurs in diabetes [13, 14]. In Pima Indians with type 2 diabetes, reduced number of podocytes correlated strongly with albuminuria, decreased GFR, and glomerulosclerosis [14]. Podocytes are terminally differentiated cells, and their loss implies that they are not replaced. As a result, the glomerular capillary function is lost. In addition to podocytopenia, there is loss of slit diaphragm proteins such as nephrin, causing albuminuria in diabetes. Thus, podocyte dysfunction may contribute to diabetic kidney disease but also its progression.

Podocytopathies

In addition to acting as a filtration barrier, podocytes have the following functions: (1) maintain the shape of underlying glomerular capillaries, (2) produce extracellular matrix proteins, and (3) produce angiogenic cytokines such as vascular endothelial growth factors [13, 14]. Any disease that causes abnormalities in one or more of these functions results in podocyte injury, leading to functional and structural changes in the kidney. Several kidney diseases are associated with podocyte injury. These include minimal change disease, focal segmental glomerulosclerosis, membranous nephropathy, membranoproliferative glomerulonephritis, diabetic nephropathy, and lupus podocytopathy that is unrelated to immunologic lupus nephritis. Mutations in genes that encode slit diaphragm proteins such as nephrin and podocin cause nephrotic syndrome of the Finnish type and steroid-resistant nephrotic syndrome, respectively.

There are no specific therapeutic options for management of podocytopathies. Drugs that are available for use include steroids, cyclosporine, tacrolimus, rituximab, abatacept, and fibroblast growth factor. The efficacy of cyclin-dependent kinase inhibitors and glycogen synthase kinase-3 inhibitors is being investigated.

IgG4-Related Diseases

IgG4-related renal disease is a recently described disease that is receiving much attention among nephrologists. Originally described as autoimmune pancreatitis, the IgG4 disease has been described in every organ of the body, including the kidney [15, 16]. The most common manifestation in the kidney is TID [12]. Histologic features of TID include plasma cell-rich infiltrate, eosinophils in some cases, and immune complex deposits along the tubular basement membrane. Interstitial fibrosis is common. Immunostaining shows the presence of IgG4 in granular pattern.

Although IgG4-related renal disease is mostly TID, glomeruli are also affected in some cases [15, 16]. The common glomerular lesions are idiopathic membranous nephropathy, membranoproliferative glomerulonephritis, IgA nephropathy, and mesangioproliferative immune complex GN. IgG4-related plasma cell arteritis has also been described in the kidney. It can also present as acute kidney injury or CKD. Imaging studies of the kidney may show enlargement as well as masses mimicking renal carcinoma.

In patients with IgG4-related renal or systemic disease, serum levels of IgG and IgG4 are elevated. Antinuclear autoantibodies are usually positive, but antibodies to double-stranded DNA are absent, thus excluding the diagnosis of lupus nephritis.

The treatment choice of IgG4-related kidney disease is corticosteroids. Two treatment regimens have been tried. The Japanese experience suggests prednisone 0.6 mg/kg for 2–4 weeks followed by tapering to 5 mg/day for 3–6 months. The maintenance dose is 2.5–5 mg/day for 3 years. Another treatment regimen is that of Mayo Clinic experience. Prednisone is started at 40 mg/day for 4 weeks and then tapering to nothing over a period of 12 weeks.

Corticosteroid-sparing therapy during the remission period has been suggested using drugs such as methotrexate, azathioprine, mycophenolate mofetil, cyclophosphamide, and rituximab. Bortezomib, a proteasome inhibitor, has also been tried.

Conclusion

This chapter has provided a brief review of gross and microscopic anatomy of the kidney and its functions in health and disease. A variety of commonly seen renal abnormalities have been discussed that require nutritional and pharmacologic intervention alone or in combination for management.

References

1. Reddi AS. Structure and function of the kidney. In: Reddi AS, editor. Essentials of renal physiology. New Jersey: College Book Publishers; 1999. p. 21–43.
2. Kriz W, Elgar M. Renal anatomy. In: Feehally J, Floege J, Tonelli M, Johnson RJ, editors. Comprehensive clinical nephrology. 6th ed. Edinburgh: Elsevier; 2019. p. 3–14.
3. Fenton RA, Praetorious J. Anatomy of the kidney. In: Skorecki K, Taal MW, Chertow GM, Marsden PA, Taal MW, Yu ASL, editors. Brenner and Rector's The Kidney, vol. 1. 10th ed. Philadelphia: Elsevier; 2016. p. 42–82.e8.
4. Kidney Disease: Improving Global Outcomes (KDIGO) Acute Kidney Injury Work Group. KDIGO clinical practice guideline for acute kidney injury. Kidney Int Suppl. 2012;2:1–138.
5. Hoste EAJ, Kellum JA. Definitions, classifications, epidemiology, and risk factors of acute kidney injury. In: Turner N, Lameire N, Goldsmith DJ, et al., editors. Oxford textbook of clinical nephrology. 4th ed. Oxford, UK: Oxford University Press; 2016. p. 1831–43.
6. Chertow GM, Burdick E, Honour M, Bonventre JV, Bates DW. Acute kidney injury, mortality, length of stay, and costs in hospitalized patients. J Am Soc Nephrol. 2005;16:3365–70.
7. Levey AS, Coresh J, Balk E, Kausz T, Levin A, Steffes MW, et al. National Kidney Foundation guidelines for chronic kidney disease: evaluation, classification, and stratification. Ann Intern Med. 2003;139:137–47.
8. Kidney Disease: Improving Global Outcomes (KDIGO) CKD Work Group. KDIGO 2012 clinical practice guideline for the evaluation and management of chronic kidney disease. Kidney Int Suppl. 2013;3:1–150.
9. Upadhyay A, Inker LA, Levey AS. Chronic kidney disease: definition, classification, and approach to management. In: Turner N, Lameire N, Goldsmith DJ, et al., editors. Oxford textbook of clinical nephrology. 4th ed. Oxford: Oxford University Press; 2016. p. 743–154.
10. Saran R, Robinson B, Abbott KC, Agodoa LYC, Bragg-Gresham J, Balkrishnan R, et al. US Renal Data System 2018 Annual Data Report: epidemiology of kidney disease in the United States. Am J Kidney Dis. 2019;73(3 Suppl 1):Svii–Sxxii, S1–S772.
11. Carrero JJ, Hecking M, Chesnaye NC, Jager KJ. Sex and gender disparities in the epidemiology and outcomes of chronic kidney disease. Nature Rev Nephrol. 2018;14:151–64.
12. Kelly CJ, Neilson EG. Tubulointerstitial diseases. In: Skorecki K, Taal MW, Chertow GM, Marsden PA, Taal MW, Yu ASL, editors. Brenner and Rector's The Kidney, vol. 1. 10th ed. Philadelphia: Elsevier; 2016. p. 1209–1230.e7.
13. Singh L, Singh G, Dinda AK. Understanding podocytopathy and its relevance to clinical nephrology. Indian J Nephrol. 2015;25:1–7.
14. Lin JS, Susztak K. Podocytes: the weakest link in diabetic kidney disease? Curr Diab Rep. 2016;16(5):25.
15. Cornell LD. IgG4-related kidney disease. Curr Opin Nephrol Hypertens. 2011;21:279–88.
16. Salvadori M, Tsalouchos A. Immunoglobulin G4-related kidney diseases: an updated review. World J Nephrol. 2018;7:29–40.

Part II
Components of the Nutritional Assessment

Nutrition screening is the first step in the nutrition care process (NCP) that is designed to detect actual and potential risks for protein-calorie malnutrition (PCM) and/or protein-energy wasting (PEW). The next step in the NCP for patients who are at moderate or high risk for PCM or PEW is the nutrition assessment, which is an integral part of care for patients with chronic kidney disease. An accurate assessment of nutritional status is critical for managing and treating chronic kidney disease. This section includes an in-depth review of the components of the nutrition assessment and addresses psychosocial issues affecting nutritional status in patients with kidney disease and drug-nutrient interactions.

The ABCDs of the nutrition assessment are presented in this section of the book. The "A," which stands for *A*nthropometry, is described by Dumler as the component of the nutrition assessment that is a simple, reliable, and easily available practical method for evaluating body composition. Anthropometry requires precise techniques of measurement and the use of proper equipment to provide accurate, reproducible data. Strengths and limitations of the various body composition methods and standardized sites for these measurements are presented.

In the next chapter, Ghaddar presents the "B" component of the nutrition assessment—an evaluation of *B*iochemical data that provides objective information about the patient's nutritional and metabolic status. There are, however, limitations to the use of biochemical data in the CKD population, which Ghaddar addresses in this chapter. Positive and negative acute phase reactants in relation to CKD as well as the method used to assess dietary protein intake in stable patients are discussed. Ghaddar includes a table of select biochemical parameters that are routinely used in the dialysis setting as part of the patient's plan of care and a brief explanation for abnormal values.

The "C" component of the nutrition assessment stands for the *C*linical assessment. In this chapter, Ziegler discusses the nutrition-focused physical examination (NFPE) and clinical assessment in patients with CKD. A brief history of the NFPE and its inclusion in the standards of professional performance for renal dietitians are addressed. The NFPE is an essential component of the nutrition assessment that is used to determine the patient's nutritional status and the factors that may impact the consumption of an adequate diet. Specific techniques for performing the exam are provided. Ziegler includes a table of physical findings related to micronutrient deficiencies in CKD with references for additional readings.

The last component of the nutrition assessment is "D," which stands for *D*ietary assessment. In this chapter, Moore provides a comprehensive review of dietary assessment methodologies—from the commonly used 24-hour recall, 3-day food record, and food frequency questionnaire to more sophisticated methods such as the Automated Self-Administered 24-hour Recall and the Automated Multiple-Pass Method. In addition, use of biomarkers in assessing dietary intake is also addressed. Several tables are included in the chapter, one of which presents practice guidelines in CKD and the dietary intake methodologies recommended in each one.

The chapter by Wolfe addresses various psychosocial issues that affect nutritional status in patients with CKD such as depression, anxiety, loneliness, self-efficacy, food insecurity, limited health literacy, and the availability of social support and its impact on nutritional status. The strategies that may mitigate these factors are also discussed. Lastly, Flecha et al. provide a detailed discussion about drug-nutrient interactions including herbal supplements and their effects on immunosuppressants in renal transplant recipients.

Chapter 4
Anthropometric Assessment in Kidney Disease

Francis Dumler

Keywords Height · Weight · Body mass index · Skinfold thickness · Circumference measurements and ratios · Conicity index · Bone breaths · Frame size · Sarcopenia · National Health and Nutrition Examination Survey III

Key Points
- Understand the importance of anthropometry as a practical and simple tool for quantification of body composition.
- Become familiar with body measurements at the core of the evaluation of clinical nutritional status using anthropometry.
- Develop a better understanding of body mass index, its limitations, and available alternatives for better discrimination between muscle and fat components of body mass.
- Use of anthropometric parameters for evaluating the risk of cardiovascular disease in chronic kidney disease patients as well as the general population.
- Provide selective tables from the *Anthropometric Reference Data for Children and Adults* published by the National Health Statistics Reports as an appendix.
- Inclusion of URL addresses for those needing in-depth anthropometric technical information.

Introduction

An adequate nutritional status is essential to maintaining an optimal level of health. Prolonged and ongoing illnesses, such as chronic kidney disease (CKD), are characterized by a persistent inflammatory state that negatively impacts nutritional status. Conversely, a diminished nutritional status may facilitate worsening of the disease process and its comorbidities, thereby creating a vicious cycle. Thus, monitoring nutritional status and body composition is imperative to the appropriate management of CKD [1].

Anthropometry is the science that studies the comparative size, form, and proportion of the human body and its regional components. There is a relationship between body dimensions and its composition, particularly fat, and to a lesser extent, muscle mass. A fundamental concept in its application is the intimate relationship between morphology and functional capacity. Anthropometry is an integral element of medical anthropology and epidemiology, forensics, biomechanics, and

---

F. Dumler (✉)
Section of Nephrology, William Beaumont Hospital, Royal Oak, MI, USA

© Springer Nature Switzerland AG 2020
J. D. Burrowes et al. (eds.), *Nutrition in Kidney Disease*, Nutrition and Health,
https://doi.org/10.1007/978-3-030-44858-5_4

ergonomics. In clinical practice, anthropometry is used in the assessment of body composition and nutritional status and to evaluate the relationship between anthropometric parameters and risk and outcomes. It is also employed to assess the impact of genetics, the environment, and stress on the human physique.

Composition analyses technologies are continuously evolving particularly for specific assessments of bone, fat, muscle, and water content and their distribution. These techniques include, in addition to anthropometry, bioimpedance analysis, dual-energy X-ray absorbtiometry, quantitative magnetic resonance, magnetic resonance imaging and spectroscopy, and positive emission tomography [2, 3]. Strengths and limitations of these techniques may be found in Table 4.1.

Anthropometry is a simple, reliable, and easily available practical method for measuring regional fatness. Anthropometric parameters are important in evaluating body composition and assessing nutritional status. Anthropometric parameters are also important in the estimation of cardiovascular risk in chronic kidney disease patients and the general population at large.

Table 4.1 Body composition methods

Method	Components evaluated	Strengths	Limitations
Skinfold thickness	Subcutaneous fat thickness in specific sites of the body	Reliable method for assessing regional fatness	Most skinfold calipers have an upper limit of 45–60 mm, limiting use in moderately overweight subjects. Measurement reliability depends on technicians' skill and experience level
Bioelectrical impedance analysis (BIA) and bioelectrical impedance spectroscopy (BIS)	Total body water, which is converted to fat-free mass(FFM) assuming 73% of body water is FFM	Cheap, safe, quick, requires minimal patient participation and technician expertise Define body composition in subject groups, and monitor individual changes over time Allows estimation of body cell mass	Validity is population-specific and influenced by sex, age, height, disease state, and race Compared to DXA, it underestimates FFM in normal-weight individuals and overestimates FFM in obese individuals
Dual-energy X-ray absorptiometry (DXA)	Total and regional body fat, lean mass (LM), bone mineral density	High accuracy and reproducibility for all age groups Noninvasive, quick, and no subject performance needed; it is not confounded by disease states or growth disorders	Small amount of radiation exposure Fat mass estimates are confounded by trunk thickness Expensive apparatus
Ultrasound	Tissue layer thickness (skin, adipose, muscle)	Highly repeatable, readily available, portable and quick Noninvasive and no radiation Accurate and precise Estimates fat thickness in multiple sites of the body Capable of measuring the thickness of muscle and bone	Requires a skilled, experienced technician Measurement procedures and techniques are not yet standardized Inherent confounders such as fascia can complicate the interpretation of results Higher cost than field methods
Magnetic resonance imaging (MRI) and computed tomography (CT)	Total and regional fat (including subcutaneous and visceral), skeletal muscle, organs and other internal tissues, lipid content in the muscle and liver	High accuracy and reproducibility MRI does not involve exposure to radiation	Expensive, lengthy procedure limited to normal and moderately overweight individuals Very large body sizes do not fit in the field of view High radiation exposure with CT

Adapted from Aragon et al. [3]. Open Access, BioMed Central

Anthropometric Techniques

A comprehensive description of anthropometric techniques is beyond the scope of this chapter. There are two excellent sources describing these techniques in great detail: the National Health and Nutrition Examination Survey (NHANES) Anthropometry Manual and the second edition of *Applied Body Composition Assessment* [4, 5]. The dimensional components of classic anthropometry include weight, height, skinfold thickness, circumferences, and elbow and wrist breadths. Standardized sites for these measurements are shown in Tables 4.2, 4.3, 4.4, and 4.5. A variety of computed measurements may be derived from the primary data using population-specific (linear) or generic (quadratic) equations [6–9]. By convention, all measurements are made on the right side of the body. Limb amputation, disease, malformation, or a functioning arteriovenous access will require taking measurements on the opposite side. All measures should be done posttreatment in dialysis patients.

Anthropometric methods have been used in large-scale studies, including the NHANES and the Korean NHANES [10, 11]. Anthropometric techniques are currently applied to the study and management of metabolic and nutrition disease processes in various populations around the world [12, 13]. The availability of these data provides the clinician with a reference frame when evaluating individual patients.

More relevant to CKD, anthropometry was a significant component of both the Modification of Diet in Renal Disease (MDRD) and the Hemodialysis (HEMO) clinical trials [14, 15]. Based on these studies, it is suggested that weight, height, subcapsular and triceps skinfolds, and arm and calf circumference be part of the nutrition evaluation in CKD patients.

Recently, there has been a developing interest in the evaluation of sarcopenia [16, 17]. Particular populations at risk include the elderly [18], those with sarcopenic obesity [19], and individuals afflicted with chronic inflammatory conditions including chronic kidney [20, 21] and cardiovascular diseases [22].

Table 4.2 Standardized sites for skinfold measurements

Site	Fold direction	Anatomical reference	Measurement
Chest	Diagonal	Axilla and nipple	Fold taken between the axilla and nipple as high as possible
Subcapsular	Diagonal	Inferior angle of scapula	Fold taken along natural cleavage line of skin below inferior angle of the scapula
Midaxillary	Horizontal	Xiphisternal junction	Fold taken on midaxillary line at level of xiphisternal junction
Suprailiac	Oblique	Iliac crest	Fold taken posteriorly to midaxillary line and superiorly to the iliac crest along natural cleavage of skin
Abdominal	Horizontal	Umbilicus	Fold taken 3 cm lateral and 1 cm inferior to center of the umbilicus
Triceps	Vertical (midline)	Acromial process of scapula and olecranon process of ulna	Distance between lateral projection of acromial process and inferior margin of olecranon process measured on lateral aspect of the arm with the elbow flexed 90°. Midpoint is marked on lateral side of the arm. Fold is lifted 1 cm above marked line.
Biceps	Vertical (midline)	Biceps brachii	Fold is lifted over the belly of the biceps brachii at the level marked for the triceps and on line with anterior border of the acromial process and the antecubital fossa
Thigh	Vertical (midline)	Inguinal crease and patella	Fold is lifted on anterior aspect of the thigh midway between the inguinal crease and proximal border of the patella. Body weight is shifted to left foot.
Calf	Vertical (midline)	Maximal calf circumference	Fold is lifted at level of maximal calf circumference on medical aspect of the calf with the knee and hip flexed 90°

Adapted with permission from Heyward and Wagner [5]. Chapter 4: Skinfold Method, p. 58

Table 4.3 Standardized sites for circumference measurements (trunk)

Site	Anatomical reference	Position	Measurement
Neck	Laryngeal prominence	Perpendicular	Measure just inferior to laryngeal prominence (Adam's apple).
Shoulder	Deltoid muscles and acromion processes of the scapula	Horizontal	Apply tape snugly over maximum bulges of the deltoid muscles, inferior to acromion processes. Record measurement at end of normal expiration.
Chest	Fourth costosternal joints	Horizontal	Apply tape snugly around the torso at level of fourth costosternal joints. Record at end of normal expiration.
Waist	Narrowest part of the torso, level of the "natural" waist between the ribs and iliac crest	Horizontal	Apply tape snugly around the waist at level of narrowest part of the torso. An assistant is needed to position the tape behind the client. Take measurement at end of normal expiration.
Abdominal	Maximum anterior protuberance of the abdomen, usually at the umbilicus	Horizontal	Apply tape snugly around the abdomen at level of greatest anterior protuberance. An assistant is needed to position the tape behind the client. Take measurement at end of normal expiration.
Hip (buttocks)	Maximum posterior extension of the buttocks	Horizontal	Apply tape snugly around the buttocks. An assistant is needed to position the tape on opposite side of the body.

Adapted with permission from Heyward and Wagner [5]. Chapter 5: Additional Anthropometric Methods, p. 69

Table 4.4 Standardized sites for circumference measurements (limbs)

Site	Anatomical reference	Position	Measurement
Arm (biceps)	Acromion process of scapula and olecranon process of ulna	Perpendicular to long axis of the arm	With arms hanging freely at sides and palms facing thighs, apply tape snugly around the arm at level marked for triceps and biceps skinfolds
Forearm	Maximum girth of the forearm	Perpendicular to long axis of the forearm	With arms hanging down away from the trunk and forearm supinated, measure the maximum girth of the proximal part of the forearm
Wrist	Styloid processes of the radius and ulna	Perpendicular to long axis of the forearm	With elbow flexed and forearm supinated, measure just distal to the styloid processes of the radius and ulna
Thigh (proximal)	Gluteal fold	Horizontal	Measure around the thigh just distal to the gluteal fold
Thigh (mid)	The inguinal crease and proximal border of the patella	Horizontal	With knee flexed 90° (right foot on bench), measure at level between the inguinal crease and proximal border of the patella
Thigh (distal)	Femoral epicondyles	Horizontal	Measure proximal to the femoral epicondyles
Knee	Patella	Horizontal	Measure around the knee at mid-patellar level with knee relaxed in slight flexion
Calf	Maximum girth of the calf muscle	Perpendicular to long axis of the leg	Measure maximum girth of the calf while sitting on end of table with legs hanging freely
Ankle	Malleoli of the tibia and fibula	Perpendicular to long axis of the leg	Measure minimum circumference of the leg, just proximal to the malleoli

Adapted with permission from Heyward and Wagner [5]. Chapter 5: Additional Anthropometric Methods, p. 70

Sarcopenia has been defined in various ways depending on methodologies used. The European Working Group on Sarcopenia in Older People has recently published an updated revised consensus on definition and diagnosis. Low muscle strength and content are distinctive of sarcopenia, and poor physical performance is indicative of severe compromise [23].

Table 4.5 Standardized sites for bony breadth measurements

Site	Anatomical reference	Position	Measurement
Biacromial (shoulder)	Lateral borders of the acromion (scapula)	Horizontal	Position: standing, arms hanging vertically, shoulders relaxed, downward, and slightly forward. Apply blade tips to lateral borders of acromion processes. Measure from the rear
Chest	Sixth ribs on midaxillary line	Horizontal	Position: standing with the arms slightly abducted. Apply blade tips on the sixth ribs at the midaxillary line. Measure at end of normal expiration
Bi-iliac	Iliac crests	Forty-five degree downward angle	Position: standing, arms folded across the chest, apply blade tips at a 45° downward angle, at maximum breadth of the iliac crest. Measure from the rear
Bitrochanteric	Greater trochanter of the femur	Horizontal	Position: standing, arms folded across the chest. Apply blade tips with considerable pressure to compress soft tissues. Measure maximum distance between trochanters from the rear
Knee	Femoral epicondyles	Diagonal or horizontal	Position: sitting and the knee flexed to 90°. Apply blade tips firmly on lateral and medial femoral epicondyles
Ankle (bi-malleolar)	Malleoli of the tibia and fibula	Oblique	Position: standing and weight evenly distributed. Apply blade tips to the most lateral part of lateral malleolus and most medial part of the medial malleolus. Measure from the rear at an oblique plane
Elbow	Epicondyles of the humerus	Oblique	Position: elbow flexed 90°, the arm raised horizontal, the forearm supinated. Apply blade tips firmly to the medial and lateral humeral epicondyles at an angle that bisects the right angle at the elbow
Wrist	Styloid process of the radius and ulna (snuff box)	Oblique	Position: elbow flexed 90°, upper arm vertical and close to the torso, forearm pronated. Apply blade tips firmly at an oblique angle to the styloid processes of the radius (at proximal part of anatomical snuff box) and ulna

Adapted with permission from Heyward and Wagner [5]. Chapter 5: Additional Anthropometric Methods, p 71

Muscle mass content using dual-energy X-ray absorptiometry (DXA) is recommended in clinical practice. Computed tomography (CT) and magnetic resonance (MR) are also used, albeit in more elaborate clinical studies [23, 24]. In field work, or when DXA is not available, muscle mass is measured using bioimpedance analysis (BIA) and/or by anthropometry (sum of skinfold thickness, mid-calf and mid-arm circumference) [25].

Weight and Height Measurements

Body weight is usually stable varying less than 0.5% to 1% within a 6- to 10-week timeframe. A change of 5% or more suggests a gain/loss of water or tissue mass. A 10% or greater loss of body weight over a 6-month period is considered clinically significant and warrants full evaluation. Body weight is measured using a *precision body scale* calibrated to 0.1 kg. Body height is best measured standing up with a straight back and neck using a height meter or stadiometer. A bar attached to the weight scale may be used if none is available. For patients with spine curvatures, or who are unable to stand, body height is derived from knee height or arm span lengths. Knee height is measured sitting or lying down with the knee at 90° using a caliper under the sole and the blade pressing down against the thigh about 5 cm behind the patella. Arm span is measured from the tip of the longest finger on each hand while standing erect against a wall with arms fully stretched horizontally. Of note, knee height and arm span change very little with age and should be used in the elderly when appropriate.

Body mass index (BMI), expressed as kg/m^2, defines the relationship between weight and height which correlates to overall body fat content (thinness or thickness). However, it is not a measure of percent body fat. BMI does not take into account body shape. For the same weight and height, an individual may have relatively more muscle and less fat mass than another with more fat and less muscle mass. Yet, in both circumstances, BMI will be the same. Body fat in different parts of the body have a different biology. This has led to consider further measures that may better relate to body shape (hence distribution of fat and muscle mass). These include waist circumference, waist-to-hip ratio, and conicity index [26, 27].

Waist circumference is a surrogate for abdominal obesity and visceral adipose tissue. Waist circumference is strongly associated with visceral fat in patients with CKD [28]. However, others have found waist circumference to be poorly correlated with visceral adipose tissue as measured by computed tomography in non-dialysis CKD patients [29]. There is a direct correlation between waist circumference and C-reactive protein [30–32]. Studies suggest that increased visceral, but not subcutaneous, fat is independently associated with risk of progression of CKD, cardiovascular events, and all-cause mortality [33–37]. The predictive value of triglycerides and cholesterol for survival and atherosclerotic complications in hemodialysis patients is dependent on waist circumference [38].

In a study of overweight patients with hypertension, abdominal obesity persisted as a risk factor even after adjustment for dyslipidemia, elevated blood glucose levels, and other variables associated with renal insufficiency. Even after adjustment for multiple covariates including BMI, higher mortality rates were noted for all waist circumference categories compared with the reference population [39–42]. These findings suggest that waist circumference may be a simple and inexpensive tool to be used in epidemiological studies. Because waist circumference is a function of both height and abdominal fat, some recommend factoring by height or height square for a tighter correlation to cardiovascular risk factors.

The predictive value of waist-to-hip or waist-to-height ratio has also been evaluated in several studies. Waist-to-hip ratio, but not BMI, is related to cardiac events in patients with CKD. In the general population, there is an association between waist-to-hip ratio, but not BMI, and incident CKD and mortality [43, 44]. Abdominal adiposity measured as waist circumference or waist-to-hip ratio, irrespective of general adiposity, is a more important determinant of CKD and cardiovascular risk in adults than BMI [45–48]. Relying exclusively on BMI may underestimate the importance of obesity as a risk factor for developing kidney disease and as a cardiovascular disease risk factor in patients with established CKD.

The conicity index (waist circumference/[0.109 × square root of weight/height]) is a measure of visceral fat that evaluates the deviation from a cylindrical shape to a double-cone shape with a common base at the waist. The conicity index is an independent predictor of systemic inflammation, cardiovascular risk, and glomerular filtration rate in pre-dialysis patients [49]. In a recent study of the Framingham population, the conicity index had the most discriminatory accuracy for the 10-year cardiovascular event when compared with other obesity indices. The waist-to-hip ratio was also found to have a relatively good discriminatory power [50, 51].

Skinfold and Circumference Measurements

Skinfold thickness has been extensively used for estimation of fat mass. The thickness at a given location is assumed to be the sum of the two layers of skin and the subcutaneous mass contained in between (Table 4.2). Single or multiple sites may be selected depending on need and circumstances [4]. The summation of skinfold thickness values provides an assessment of subcutaneous fat content. The internal adipose component is derived from the abdominal circumference. Results are comparable to those obtained by CT and MRI at selected sites. Discrepancies in other areas are attributed to irregular fat tissue deposition or distortion from the supine position during CT or MRI data acquisition [5].

The distribution of subcutaneous and visceral fat is similar within each gender. About 30% to 50% of body fat is located in the subcutaneous compartment. Visceral body fat distribution varies considerably between body compartments. Aging is associated with changes in lean and fat mass content [52, 53]. Older individuals with similar body density have proportionally less subcutaneous fat than younger ones. As individuals get heavier, subcutaneous fat increases while visceral fat decreases. This highlights the importance of using appropriate reference standards [53].

Mid-arm, mid-thigh, and mid-calf circumferences (Tables 4.3 and 4.4), when combined with skinfold thickness, allow estimation of skeletal muscle mass. This measurement can be further refined by making adjustments for bone thickness. Muscle mass measured by anthropometry may be expressed as muscle area or circumference. Fat-free mass decreases with aging due to loss of skeletal muscle and visceral organ tissues. Geriatric-based equations are therefore recommended when evaluating an older population [4, 5].

Frame Size

There is a direct relationship between skeletal breadths and the bone and muscle components of free mass. Estimation of frame size using skeletal breadths (Table 4.5) can help differentiate a higher weight due to a larger musculoskeletal mass from that of a larger fat mass. Previous studies have shown that wrist, ankle, and elbow breadths are a good predictor of frame size [54]. Frame size may be helpful in determining if a higher body weight is related to greater bone and muscle mass rather than increased fat content.

Reference Data

As described earlier, availability of adequate reference standards is critical to the correct application and interpretation of anthropometry in evaluating nutritional status and body composition. The NHANES III provides the most comprehensive dataset [10, 53]. Anthropometric measurements were obtained from 19,593 survey participants and included weight, height, recumbent length, circumferences, limb lengths, and skinfold thickness measurements. The *Anthropometric Reference Data for Children and Adults* published by the National Health Statistics Reports includes weighted population means, standard error of the means, and selected percentiles of body measurement values. As measurements vary by sex, age, and ethnicity or race, results are reported by subgroups [53].

Many anthropometry techniques and methodologies have been described in this chapter. However, from a clinical perspective, the most significant components are weight, height, skinfold thickness, and limb circumferences. These measurements are easy to obtain and have been used in the MDRD and HEMO studies, and the reference population is well defined by the NHANES III dataset. Individual patient percentiles can be easily assigned from the reference tables [53].

Conclusion

Anthropometry is one of the oldest approaches for quantifying body composition. It is the most practical tool for use in the field and clinical settings that provides an index of nutritional status and risk for malnutrition. In addition, it is a useful instrument for evaluating the risk potential for developing kidney and cardiovascular disease, progression of kidney failure, morbidity, and mortality. Finally, anthropometry is a simple, inexpensive, and noninvasive way of prospectively monitoring nutritional status, risk assessment, and response to treatment strategies.

References

1. Dumler F. Body composition modifications in patients under low protein diets. J Ren Nutr. 2011;21:76–81.
2. Lemos T, Gallagher D. Current body composition measurement techniques. Curr Opin Endocrinol Diabetes Obes. 2017;24:310–4.
3. Aragon AA, Schoenfeld BJ, Wildman R, Kleiner S, VanDussseldorp T, Taylor L, et al. International society of sports nutrition position stand: diets and body composition. J Int Soc Sports Nutr. 2017;14:16–35.
4. National Health and Nutrition Examination Survey (NHANES) Anthropometry Procedures Manual. 2017. Available from https://wwwn.cdc.gov/nchs/data/nhanes/2017-2018/manuals/2017_Anthropometry_Procedures_Manual.pdf.
5. Heyward VH, Wagner DR. Applied body composition assessment. 2nd ed. Champaign: Human Kinetics; 2004.
6. Jackson AS, Pollock ML, Ward A. Generalized equations for predicting body density of women. Med Sci Sports Exerc. 1980;12:175–82.
7. Jackson AS, Pollock ML. Generalized equations for predicting body density of men. Br J Nutr. 1978;40:497–504.
8. Peterson MJ, Xzerwinski SA, Siervogel RM. Development and validation of skinfold-thickness prediction equations with a 4-compartment model. Am J Clin Nutr. 2003;77:1186–91.
9. Al-Gindan YY, Hankey CR, Govan L, Gallagher D, Heymsfield SB, Lean MEJ. Derivation and validation of simple anthropometric equations to predict adipose tissue mass and total fat mass with MRI as the reference method. Br J Nutr. 2015;114:1852–67.
10. National Health and Nutrition Examination Survey Homepage. http://www.cdc.gov/nchs/nhanes.htm.
11. Kweon S, Kim Y, Jamg M-J, Kim Y, Kim K, Choi S, et al. Data resource profile: the Korea National Health and Nutrition Examination Survey (KNHANES). Int J Epidemiol. 2014;43:69–77.
12. Liang X, Chen X, Li J, Yan M, Yang Y. Study on body composition and its correlation with obesity. A Cohort Study in 5121 Chinese Han participants. Medicine. 2018;97(21):e10722.
13. Feeney EL, O'Sullivan A, Nugent AP, McNully B, Walton J, Flynn A, et al. Patterns of dairy food intake, body composition and markers of metabolic health in Ireland: results from the National Adult Nutrition Survey. Nutr Diabetes. 2017;7:e243. https://doi.org/10.1038/nutd.2016.54. PMID https://www.ncbi.nlm.nih.gov/pubmed/28218736#.
14. Kopple JD, Greene T, Chumlea WC, Hollinger D, Maroni BJ, Merrill D, et al. Relationship between nutritional status and the glomerular filtration rate: results from the MDRD study. Kidney Int. 2000;57:1688–703.
15. Chumlea WC, Dwyer J, Bergen C, Burkart J, Paranandi L, Frydrych A, et al. Nutritional status assessed from anthropometric measures in the HEMO study. J Ren Nutr. 2003;13:31–8.
16. Beaudart C, Zaaria M, Reginster J-Y, Bruyère O. Health outcomes of sarcopenia: a systematic review and meta-analysis. PLoS One. 2017;12(1):e0169548. https://doi.org/10.1371/journal.pone.0169548. PMID: https://www.ncbi.nlm.nih.gov/pubmed/28095426.
17. Bruyère O, Beaudart C, Ethgen O, Reginster J-Y, Locquet M. The health economics burden of sarcopenia: a systematic review. Maturitas. 2019;119:61–9.
18. Sanchez-Garcia S, Garcia-Peña C, Duque-Lopez MX, Juarez-Cedillo T, Cortes-Nuñez AR, Reyes-Beaman S. Anthropometric measures and nutritional status in a healthy elderly population. BMC Public Health. 2007;7:2–11.
19. Sanada K, Chen R, Willcox B, Ohara T, Wen A, Takenaka C, et al. Association of sarcopenic obesity predicted by anthropometric measurements and 24-y all-cause mortality in elderly men: the Kuakini Honolulu Heart Program. Nutrition. 2018;46:97–102.
20. Pereira R, Cordeiro AC, Avesani CM, Carrero JJ, Lindholm B, Amparo FC, et al. Sarcopenia in chronic kidney disease on conservative therapy: prevalence and association with mortality. Nephrol Dial Transplant. 2015;30:1718–25.
21. Moorthi RN, Avin KG. Clinical relevance of sarcopenia in chronic kidneydisease. Curr Opin Nephrol Hypertens. 2017;26:219–28.
22. Atkins JL, Whincup PH, Morris RW, Lennon LY, Papacosta O, Wannamethee SG. Sarcopenic obesity and risk of cardiovascular disease and mortality: a population-based cohort study of older men. JAGS. 2014;62:253–60.
23. Cruz-Jentoft A, Bahat G, Bauer J, Boirie Y, Bruyère O, Cederholm T, et al. Sarcopenia: revised European consensus on definition and diagnosis. Age Ageing. 2019;48:16–31.
24. Giglio J, Kamimura MA, Souza NC, Bichels AV, Cordeiro AC, Pinho N, et al. Muscle mass assessment by computed tomography in chronic kidney disease patients: agreement with surrogate methods. Euro J Clin Nutr. 2017;73:46–53.

25. Giglio J, Kamimura MA, Lamarca F, Rodriguez J, Santin F, Avesani CM. Association of sarcopenia with nutritional parameters, quality of fife, hospitalization, and mortality rates of elderly patients on hemodialysis. J Ren Nutr. 2018;28:197–207.
26. Taylor RW, Jones IE, Williams SM, Goulding A. Evaluation of waist circumference, waist-to-hip ratio, and the conicity index as screening tools for high trunk fat mass, as measured by dual-energy X-ray absorptiometry, in children aged 3–19 years. Am J Clin Nutr. 2000;72:490–5.
27. Valdez R, Seidell JC, Ahn YI, Weiss KM. A new index of abdominal adiposity as an indicator of risk for cardiovascular disease. A cross population study. Int J Obes Relat Metab Disord. 1993;17:77–82.
28. Sanches FMR, Avesani CM, Kamimura MA, Lemos MM, Axelsson J, Vasselai P, et al. Waist circumference and visceral fat in CKD: a cross-sectional study. Am J Kidney Dis. 2008;52:66–73.
29. Velludo CM, Kamimura MA, Sanches FM, Lemos MM, Canziani ME, Pupim LB, et al. Prospective evaluation of waist circumference and visceral adipose tissue in patients with chronic kidney disease. Am J Nephrol. 2010;31(12):104–9.
30. Forouhi NG, Sattar N, McKeigue PM. Relation of C-reactive protein to body fat distribution and features of the metabolic syndrome in Europeans and South Asians. Int J Obes Relat Metab Disord. 2001;25:1327–31.
31. Saijo Y, Kiyota N, Kawasaki Y, Miyazaki Y, Kashimura J, Fukuda M, et al. Relationship between C-reactive protein and visceral adipose tissue in healthy Japanese subjects. Diabetes Obes Metab. 2004;6:249–58.
32. Brinkley TE, Hsu FC, Beavers KM, Church TS, Goodpaster BH, Stafford RS, et al. Total and abdominal adiposity are associated with inflammation in older adults using a factor analysis approach. J Gerontol A Biol Sci Med Sci. 2012;67(10):1099–106. https://doi.org/10.1093/gerona/gls077.
33. Elsayed EF, Sarnak MJ, Tighiouart H, Griffith JL, Kurth T, Salem DN, et al. Waist-to-hip ratio, body mass index, and subsequent kidney disease and death. Am J Kidney Dis. 2008;52:29–38.
34. Kovesdy CP, Czira ME, Rudas A, Ujszaszi A, Rosivall L, Novak M, et al. Body mass index, waist circumference and mortality in kidney transplant recipients. Am J Transplant. 2010;10:2644–51.
35. Kramer H, Shoham D, McClure LA, Durazo-Arvizu R, Howard G, Judd S, et al. Association of waist circumference and body mass index with all-cause mortality in CKD: the REGARDS (Reasons for Geographic and Racial Differences in Stroke) study. Am J Kidney Dis. 2011;58:177–85.
36. Jacobs EJ, Newton CC, Wang Y, Patel AV, McCullough ML, Campbell PT, et al. Waist circumference and all-cause mortality in a large US cohort. Arch Intern Med. 2010;170:1293–301.
37. Zoccali C, Postorino M, Marino C, Pizzini P, Cutrupi S, Tripepi G, et al. Waist circumference modifies the relationship between the adipose tissue cytokines leptin and adiponectin and all-cause and cardiovascular mortality in hemodialysis patients. J Intern Med. 2011;269:172–81.
38. Postorino M, Marino C, Tripepi G, Zoccali C, CREDIT Working Group. Abdominal obesity modifies the risk of hypertriglyceridemia for all-cause and cardiovascular mortality in hemodialysis patients. Kidney Int. 2011;79:765–72.
39. Postorino M, Marino C, Trippi G, Zoccali C, CREDIT Working Group. Abdominal obesity and all-cause and cardiovascular mortality in end-stage renal disease. J Am Coll Cardiol. 2009;53:1265–72.
40. Emerging Risk Factors Collaboration. Separate and combined associations of body-mass index and abdominal adiposity with cardiovascular disease: collaborative analysis of 58 prospective studies. Lancet. 2011;377:1085–95.
41. Tanamas S, Ng WL, Backholer K, Hodge A, Zimmer P, Peeters A. Quantifying the proportion of deaths due to body mass index- and waist circumference-defined obesity. Obesity. 2016;24:735–42.
42. Cho GJ. Differential relationship between waist circumference and mortality according to age, sex, and body mass index in Koreans with age of 30–90 years; a nationwide health insurance database study. BMC Med. 2018;16:131. https://www.ncbi.nlm.nih.gov/pubmed/30092838.
43. Burton JO, Gray LJ, Webb DR, Davies MJ, Khunti K, Crasto W, et al. Association of anthropometric obesity measures with chronic kidney disease risk in a non-diabetic patient population. Nephrol Dial Transplant. 2012;27(5):1860–6. https://doi.org/10.1093/ndt/gfr574.
44. Sezer S, Karakan S, Acar NO. Association of conicity index and renal progression in pre-dialysis chronic kidney disease. Ren Fail. 2012;34:165–70.
45. Ashwell M, Gibson S. Waist-to-height ratio as an indicator of 'early health risk': simpler and more predictive than using a 'matrix' based on BMI and waist circumference. BMJ Open. 2016;6:e010159.
46. Emdin C, Khera AV, Natarajan P, Klarin D, Zekavat SM, Hsiao AJ, et al. Genetic association of waist-to-hip ratio with cardiometabolic traits, type 2 diabetes, and coronary heart disease. JAMA. 2017;317:626–63.
47. Egeland GM, Igland J, Vollser SE, Sulo G, Eide GE, Tell GS. High population attributable fractions of myocardial infarction associated with waist–hip ratio. Obesity. 2016;24:1162–9.
48. Sezer S, Karakan S, Odgen CL. Association of conicity index and renal progression in pre-dialysis chronic kidney disease. Ren Fail. 2012;34:165–70.
49. Hsieh SD, Muto T. The superiority of waist-to-height ratio as an anthropometric index to evaluate clustering of coronary risk factor among non-obese men and women. Prev Med. 2005;40:216–20.

50. Motamed M, Perumal D, Fhea M, Zamani F, Ashrafi H, Haghjoo M, et al. Conicity index and waist-to-hip ratio are superior obesity indices in predicting 10-year cardiovascular risk among men and women. Clin Cardiol. 2015;38:527–34.
51. Gallagher D, Visser M, De Meersman RE, Sepulveda D, Baumgartner RN, Pierson RN, et al. Appendicular skeletal muscle mass: effects of age, gender, and ethnicity. J Appl Physiol. 1997;83:229–39.
52. Atlantis E, Martin SA, Haren MT, Taylor AW, Wittert GA, for the Florey Adelaide Male Aging Study. Lifestyle factors associated with age-related differences in body composition: the Florey Adelaide Male Aging Study. Am J Clin Nutr. 2008;88:95–104.
53. Fryar CD, Kruzon-Moran D, Gu Q, Ogden CL. Anthropometric reference data for children and adults: United States, 2015–2016. National Health Statistics Reports # 122, December 20, 2018. https://www.cdc.gov/nchs/data/nhsr/nhsr122-508.pdf.
54. Frisancho R. New standard of weight and body composition by frame size and height for assessment of nutritional status of adults and the elderly. Am J Clin Nutr. 1984;40:808–19.

Chapter 5
Biochemical Nutritional Assessment in Chronic Kidney Disease

Sana Ghaddar

Keywords Nutritional assessment · Biochemical parameters · Chronic kidney disease · C-reactive protein · Albumin · Prealbumin · Metabolic acidosis · Oxidative stress · Malnutrition · Uremia · Protein-energy wasting · Protein-energy malnutrition · Protein catabolic rate · Normalized protein catabolic rate · Protein nitrogen appearance · Renal nutrition therapy

Key Points
- Discuss the role of the registered dietitian nutritionist (RDN) in managing patients diagnosed with chronic kidney disease (CKD) as it relates to biochemical assessments.
- Discuss the latest NKF-KDOQI/AND guidelines and the ISRNM updates on biochemical assessments in patients diagnosed with CKD.
- Identify objective biochemical assessment parameters and their functions, and discuss their strengths and limitations.

Introduction

Chronic kidney disease (CKD) is defined as a gradual loss of the structural and functional characteristics of the kidneys for more than 3 months. This gradual loss in kidney function irreversibly and negatively affects various metabolic pathways that maintain body homeostasis. These vital pathways regulate fluid, electrolyte and acid-base balance, energy and protein metabolism, and excretion of metabolic wastes [1].

Chronic kidney disease is characterized by five stages. When kidney function progressively decline across those stages, the dysfunction of the various metabolic pathways and associated signs and symptoms intensify. Signs such as hypoalbuminemia, malnutrition, hyperlipidemia, volume overload, hypertension, hyperkalemia, metabolic abnormalities, bone and mineral disorders, and anemia are commonly noted with advanced stages. Uremia is another symptom this patient population experiences with worsening kidney function. Uremia occurs as a result of the buildup of nitrogenous waste of both endogenous and exogenous protein metabolism. It causes anorexigenic symptoms, such as decreased

The editors acknowledge David B. Cockram's contribution to this chapter in *Nutrition in Kidney Disease*, *Second Edition*, Nutrition and Health, DOI 10.1007/978-1-62703-685-6_1, © Springer Science+Business Media New York 2014.

S. Ghaddar (✉)
DaVita Health Care, Fremont, CA, USA

© Springer Nature Switzerland AG 2020
J. D. Burrowes et al. (eds.), *Nutrition in Kidney Disease*, Nutrition and Health,
https://doi.org/10.1007/978-3-030-44858-5_5

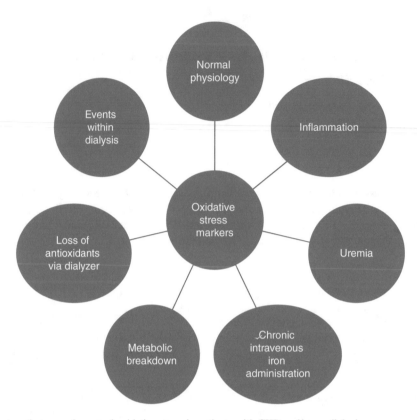

Fig. 5.1 Factors that cause increased oxidative stress in patients with CKD and/or on dialysis

sense of smell, altered taste, xerostomia, impaired appetite, nausea, and vomiting. In addition to the above, patients with CKD often present with comorbid conditions that put them at a high risk of increased levels of oxidative stress (Fig. 5.1). They face daily challenges related to their disease management, given the restrictive nature of the recommended renal diet, polypharmacy, food availability, and socioeconomic and/or physical constraints [2].

Suboptimal nutritional status, especially protein energy wasting (PEW), is commonly observed in patients with CKD, with worsening results reported in those presenting with more advanced stages (especially when estimated glomerular filtration rate (eGFR) is < 45 ml/min/1.73 m^2 BSA) and those undergoing renal replacement therapies (RRT) [3, 4]. Suboptimal nutritional status is significantly associated with increased rate of hospitalization, morbidity, and mortality in this patient population. Based on the United States National Health and Nutrition Examination Survey III (U.S. NHANES III) data, malnutrition was a significant and an independent outcome among patients ≥ 60 years old presenting with eGFR < 30 ml/min/1.73 m^2 and those requiring RRT [5].

Globally, 2.62 million patients received dialysis treatments in 2010, with the projected need for dialysis most likely doubling by 2030 [6]. The total cost of treatment for patients diagnosed with earlier stages of CKD (i.e., stages 1–3) was reported to be significantly higher than that associated with the more advanced stages (i.e., stages 4–5). In 2013, Medicare spending for CKD patients ≥ 65 years old and who have CKD exceeded $50 billion, representing 20% of all Medicare spending in this age group [7]. Additionally, CKD is recognized by the federal government as one of the significant and preventable health problems that the United States faces and is included in the Healthy People 2020 agenda. One of the goals of Healthy People 2020 is to reduce the incidence of CKD and "associated complications, disability, death, and economic costs." Healthy People 2020 focuses on building a healthier nation. Its objective is to "identify the most significant preventable threats to health and to establish national goals to reduce these threats," and its vision is to "have a society in which all people live long, healthy lives" [8]. Given the above, it is saddening to note that less than half of the high-risk population (i.e., those diagnosed with hypertension and/or diabetes mellitus) were screened for kidney disease [9], yet more than half of the patients diagnosed with advanced stages of CKD and those on dialysis present with at least three comorbid conditions (i.e., type 2 diabetes mellitus, hypertension, and hyperlipidemia) [1], with reported hospital days of 12.8 per patient-year [10]. This CKD patient population self-reported lower quality of life scores as compared to the general population [10]. Therefore, early screening and detection for CKD, controlling and treating the underlying comorbid condition(s), and optimizing those patients' nutritional status may significantly control progression of CKD, reduce the rates of hospitalization and mortality, reduce cost, and improve quality of life.

The registered dietitian nutritionists (RDNs) play an important role in the interdisciplinary care team as experts in proactively identifying abnormal biochemical and nutritional parameters shown to negatively impact overall metabolic and nutritional needs. They are also skilled in providing appropriate individualized nutritional therapies that aim at improving patients' health and wellbeing and at decreasing progression of CKD [1, 9, 11, 12].

This chapter presents an overview of the role of the RDN in managing patients diagnosed with CKD as it relates to biochemical assessments. It covers the latest clinical practice guidelines for nutrition in chronic kidney disease developed by the National Kidney Foundation (NKF) Kidney Disease Outcomes Quality Initiative (KDOQI) and the Academy of Nutrition and Dietetics [1]. In addition, the International Society of Renal Nutrition and Metabolism (ISRNM) updates on biochemical assessment in patients diagnosed with CKD, their function, and their strengths and limitations will also be addressed.

Biochemical Assessment of Nutritional Status

Assessment of biochemical parameters provides an objective evaluation on patients' overall nutritional status. Most nutrition-related biochemical parameters are routinely done as part of patients' monthly assessments and plan of care. When it comes to evaluating patients' nutritional status, the RDNs focus on indicators that help identify whether the patients are adequately nourished, malnourished, protein and/or energy malnourished, or protein and/or energy wasted. Malnutrition includes over- and undernutrition; it reflects imbalances in nutrients, such as protein, calories, fat, vitamin(s), and mineral(s), as well as electrolyte(s) and fluid. Malnutrition can also reflect suboptimal nutritional status, which can be either excessive intake or deficient intake of any identified nutrient. Protein-energy malnutrition (PEM) is defined as malnutrition of both protein and energy. Protein-energy wasting (PEW), on the other hand, is defined by the ISRNM workgroup as "a state of nutritional and metabolic derangements in patients with CKD characterized by simultaneous loss of systematic body protein and energy stores, leading ultimately to loss of muscle and fat mass and cachexia." PEW was first introduced and defined by the ISRNM workgroup in 2007 [4, 13], and objective criteria to identify patients presenting with the PEW syndrome were then developed in 2015 [4]. When assessing the patient, it is important to differentiate between protein wasting, which refers to insufficient protein levels, and energy wasting, which refers to insufficient caloric intake.

It has been heavily emphasized by the ISRNM workgroup that the health care team distinguishes between PEW and malnutrition when assessing the health and nutritional status of patients diagnosed with CKD. Though malnutrition is often associated with a patient's nutritional intake, PEW is significantly correlated with factors associated with the pathophysiological mechanisms seen in CKD, which may or may not be dependent on patients' nutrient intake related to anorexia and/or dietary availability and restriction [4]. Management and prevention of PEW include individualized and continuous nutritional counseling, providing adequate dialysis therapy, preventing or correcting muscle wasting, and managing patients' comorbid conditions (e.g., metabolic acidosis, diabetes, infection, congestive heart failure, and/or depression). Oral or parenteral nutritional supplements, along with appetite stimulants and muscle-enhancing agents, should be considered when evaluating patients who are unable to sustain protein and energy stores with the traditional therapeutic approaches [4].

The commonly reported causes for the suboptimal nutritional status in patients with CKD, especially those with advanced stages and/or those undergoing dialysis, are non-nutrition related and may or may not be a true reflection of patients' overall nutritional intake [3]. The KDOQI workgroup panel recommends that a comprehensive assessment is conducted by the RDN to rule out any underlying cause(s) that result in the observed altered nutritional status. This should be followed by providing individualized medical and nutritional interventions developed by the interdisciplinary health care team as part of patient's plan of care. The comprehensive assessment encompasses an assessment of anthropometric, dietary, and biochemical parameters [1]. Assessment of anthropometric parameters and dietary recommendations are reviewed in other chapters of this text book.

The KDOQI workgroup recommends that the biochemical assessment includes parameters routinely done as part of the patient's workup; additional parameters may be recommended for confirmatory purposes, as needed [1]. The ISRNM workgroup proposed assessing the following biochemical parameters as part of the clinical diagnosis of PEW: serum albumin level < 3.8 g/dL, serum prealbumin (transthyretin) < 30 mg/dL, and serum total cholesterol < 100 mg/dL. Additional assessment criteria include identifying any significant decline and/or changes in body mass, muscle mass, and dietary intake [4] (Table 5.1).

The biochemical parameters routinely assessed in the dialysis setting as part of patients' plan of care include: (1) For protein and nutritional status and intake: serum albumin, blood urea nitrogen (BUN), normalized protein catabolic rate (nPCR), and total cholesterol; (2) for dialysis clearance and accumulation of urea in blood: Kt/V and BUN; (3) for fluid balance: sodium, interdialytic weight gains, target weight, and post weight trends; (4) for electrolyte balance: sodium and potassium; (5) for bone mineral disorder: calcium, phosphorus, intact parathyroid hormone, and alkaline phosphatase; (6) for diabetes control: blood glucose and hemoglobin A1C; (7) for metabolic acidosis/alkalosis: serum bicarbonate; (8) for anemia or a possible bleed: hemoglobin, hematocrit, ferritin, iron panel, and total iron binding protein; and (9) for a possible presence of inflammation and/or infection: ferritin and

Table 5.1 ISRNM diagnostic criteria for protein-energy wasting

Category	Criteria	Suggested Threshold
Serum chemistry	Serum albumin	<3.8 g/dL by bromocresol green (BCG) method
	Serum prealbumin	<30 mg/dL (maintenance dialysis only)
	Serum cholesterol	<100 mg/dL
Body mass	Body mass index	<23 kg/m^2 (edema-free dry weight)
	Unintentional weight loss	5% over 3 months or 10% over 6 months
	Body fat percentage	<10%
Muscle mass	Muscle wasting	5% over 3 months or 10% over 6 months
	Mid-arm muscle area	Decrease by >10% in reference to 50th percentile of reference population
	Creatinine appearance	No specific threshold recommended Influenced by both muscle mass and meat intake
Dietary intake		Unintentional intake for >2 months:
	Protein intake	Stage 2–5 CKD: unintentional low DPI <0.6 g/kg/day Dialysis patients: unintentional low DPI <0.8 g/kg/day for at least 2 months
	Energy intake	<25 kcal/kg/day for at least 2 months

Adapted from Obi et al. [4]
Abbreviation: *DPI* dietary protein intake

white blood cell count (WBC). Additional confirmatory tests include C-reactive protein (CRP), erythrocyte sedimentation rate (ESR), and prealbumin (transthyretin) (Table 5.2).

Table 5.2 Assessment of selected biochemical parameters

Biochemical parameters	Assessment	
Albumin	Negative acute phase reactant protein Produced by the liver Half-life = 14–21 days	
	Normal	Optimal nutritional status Chronic starvation Anorexia nervosa (with body mass index (BMI) <12)
	Low	Fluid overload, malnutrition, chronic inflammation, infection, dental disorder, hepatic failure, nephrotic syndrome, advanced chronic kidney disease, patients on renal replacement therapy (RRT), especially patients on peritoneal dialysis due to excessive peritoneal losses, alcoholism, depression (related to decreased intake), falsely low in older adults who have sedentary lifestyle
Prealbumin (transthyretin)	Negative acute phase reactant protein Produced by the liver Half-life = ~ 2 days	
	Increases	Recent improvement in nutritional status
	Low	Recent/acute malnutrition, inflammation and/or infection, liver disease
Transferrin	Negative acute phase reactant protein Produced by the liver Half-life = ~ 2 days	
	High	High demand of iron by the body Iron deficiency Chronic blood loss
	Low	Iron overload Chronically low (seen in patients with chronic inflammation independent of iron status)
Potassium	Electrolyte responsible for cardiac conduction and muscle contraction	
	High	Decline in renal function Hypoaldosteronism Increased cellular destruction and tissue catabolism Increased potassium intake Certain medications Metabolic acidosis
	Low	Low K intake Intake of K-wasting diuretic medication
Bicarbonate	Acid-base balance	
	Acidosis $HCO3^-$ < 24 (<22: patients on MHD)	May cause bone resorption and osteopenia, increased risk of hyperkalemia, increased protein catabolism
	Alkalosis $HCO3^-$ > 26	May cause nausea, numbness, prolonged muscle cramps, muscle twitching, hand tremors, and dizziness (and if severe → confusion)
	High	Prolonged vomiting
	Low	Kidney failure Excessive lactic acid production Hypoxemia Very low blood pressure Ketoacidosis Prolonged diarrhea

(continued)

Table 5.2 (continued)

Biochemical parameters	Assessment	
Blood urea nitrogen (BUN)	Direct indicator of protein breakdown Indirect indicator of protein status Should be interpreted with other nutritional biochemical parameters	
	High	Decline in kidney function Increase in protein intake or increased endogenous or exogenous protein metabolism Inadequate dialysis in patients on RRT Falsely elevated in the presence of dehydration
	Low	Older patients Decline in dietary protein intake Optimal renal residual function (BUN: low to normal level)
Normalized protein catabolic rate (nPCR)	Indirect estimate of protein intake	
	High	Falsely elevated in the presence of increased endogenous protein metabolism (that is in the presence of an active inflammation or infection), chronically low protein intake
	Low	Decreased protein intake
Serum total cholesterol	Assessment of overall nutritional status, when evaluated with other nutritional biochemical markers	
	High	Increased saturated fat intake
	Low	Protein energy wasting Hypoalbuminemia Low BMI Reduced dietary protein intake

Abbreviation: *MHD* maintenance hemodialysis; *RRT* renal replacement therapy

Negative Acute Phase Reactant (APR) Proteins: Serum Albumin, Prealbumin (Transthyretin), and Transferrin

Serum Albumin

Serum albumin (Salb) is a protein that has a half-life of about 14–21 days. It maintains oncotic pressure within the capillary as well as fluid balance. In addition, it serves as a carrier molecule for various minerals, hormones, and fatty acids. Salb is impacted by various bodily responses; therefore, it is essential that the clinicians conduct a thorough assessment when using Salb to evaluate a patient's nutritional status and nutritional requirements.

Salb is one of the acute phase reactant (APR) proteins; its level is negatively impacted by stress. When the body senses stress, an inflammatory process gets initiated, which then activates the production of cytokines; circulating cytokines suppress the synthesis of Salb [14–16]. A concept of "stress-induced hypoalbuminemia" has been introduced in the acute clinical setting to identify those patients whose Salb levels are below optimum due to the stress induced by their health status (infectious and/or inflammatory states), independent of their protein and nutritional intake [17].

Decreased Salb level is commonly seen in patients presenting with advanced stages of CKD and those undergoing renal replacement therapy (RRT); the level is negatively correlated with the number of years on dialysis. Patients diagnosed with advanced stages of CKD present with higher inflammatory markers as compared to the general healthy population; therefore, maintaining an optimal Salb level continues to be a challenge for the clinicians and patients [4, 14].

Salb alone is a weak reflection of patients' protein and nutritional intake. A meta-analysis that included 63 studies and 2125 patients [18] and a 1-year case-control study that included 15 healthy individuals who presented with anorexia nervosa [19] showed that Salb can remain normal in individuals who present with a starvation state (body mass index (BMI) < 12 kg/m^2) or in those who present with anorexia nervosa, respectively. When the body senses a state of chronic starvation in an attempt to maintain homeostasis and meet cellular energy and protein demands, it becomes capable of efficiently using the endogenous protein stores when exogenous protein intake is inadequate.

Salb level can also be falsely low due to the variations in hydrostatic and oncotic pressures related to changes in body positions, which is especially seen in the elderly who have a sedentary lifestyle [20]. Other factors reported to negatively impact Salb concentration are dental disorders [21], urinary or peritoneal losses, alcoholism, and/or depression. Depression is reported to negatively affect interest in food and overall caloric intake [22].

Though assessment of Salb alone may not be a reliable indicator of patients' nutritional intake, the KDOQI evidence summary stated that a low Salb level is a sensitive measure of nutritional status [1]. Salb is a reliable measure used to identify patients who are at risk of PEW, as defined by the 7-point subjective global assessment (SGA) score in patients undergoing maintenance hemodialysis (MHD). A Salb level of less than 3.8 g/dL is reported as one of the diagnostic criteria for the PEW syndrome [4]. Salb concentration is also the strongest predictor of mortality in patients diagnosed with CKD [1, 3, 4] and in those undergoing MHD [23–25] and peritoneal dialysis (PD) [1, 26]. A Salb level less than or equal to 3.5 g/dL was significantly associated with higher odds of mortality over 10 years among patients undergoing MHD [27].When combined with appropriate management of patient's underlying conditions, a high-protein diet combined with nutritional supplements, as appropriate, has been shown to positively impact patients' nutritional status and serum albumin level [1].

Serum Prealbumin (Transthyretin)

Serum prealbumin (prealb, also known as transthyretin) is another marker used to assess patients' nutritional status. Prealb is also produced by the liver and, similar to Salb, its level is negatively impacted by inflammation and liver disease. Unlike Salb that has a half-life of up to 21 days, serum prealb has a relatively shorter half-life of about 2 days. Therefore, serum prealb is considered a sensitive indicator of acute changes in patients' protein-energy status. It can change rapidly as a response to altered nutritional status and can be used to assess the effectiveness of, and response to, the nutritional intervention provided [18].

Serum prealb is a negative acute phase reactant protein. It can be used to assess a recent decline in nutritional status related to the presence of a recent active infection, inflammation, or illness. Serum prealb concentration is significantly negatively correlated with nPCR; its decline negatively impacts lean muscle and fat tissue index and is associated with an increase in CRP, interleukin-6 (IL-6), and other inflammatory markers. Low serum prealb is predictive of 3-year mortality in patients undergoing MHD [17] and is independently correlated with increased mortality and hospitalization related to infection [1, 15, 28].

Since prealb is metabolized and excreted by the kidneys; a careful assessment of the trend in prealb levels should be considered for patients who present with decreased residual kidney function and those undergoing MHD. Therefore, it is recommended that a series of prealb measurements be done and the results compared to the patient's baseline level [22]. Serum prealb level can be low in patients diagnosed with hyperthyroidism, independent of their nutritional status or acute conditions. Moreover, since prealb functions as a transport protein for thyroxin, prealb molecules become saturated with the elevated thyroxine levels providing a false low reading. Similarly, the level can be low in patients presenting with a low serum thyroxine level [29]. Therefore, a careful assessment of serum prealb in combination with other biochemical and anthropometric parameters is recommended when assessing patients' nutritional status.

Serum Transferrin

Serum transferrin is also a negative acute phase reactant protein that is synthesized by the liver. Its serum level is affected by the patient's liver function, blood count, rate of erythropoiesis, red blood cell (RBC) half-life, iron stores, and rate of iron utilization. Traditionally, serum transferrin level has been considered one of the parameters used to assess nutritional status; however, recently, it has been shown to be a non-reliable marker for nutritional status [17]. Since the main function of transferrin is to transport iron within the circulation, its level tends to be more of an indication of circulating iron status than of nutritional status [17, 18].

Serum transferrin concentration increases when there is a higher demand for iron to produce RBC. Therefore, we see an increase in serum transferrin level in individuals presenting with iron deficiency, with chronic blood loss (as in the case of bleeding), and/or with shortened RBC half-life (as in the case of infection and inflammation) [17]. On the other hand, low serum transferrin is seen in individuals who present with iron overload. Serum transferrin level tends to be normal and/or to trend toward the lower end of the normal range in patients presenting with a decrease in iron demand. Examples are healthy and stable individuals who have stable iron demand and adequate iron stores [17, 30, 31].

In patients who present with uremia, as in the case of those diagnosed with advanced stages of CKD and those on RRT, the body's demand for iron is often higher than that of the general population. However, due to the elevated inflammatory state commonly seen in this patient population, some patients present with a serum transferrin level that is chronically low or trending toward the lower end of the normal range, independent of their actual body iron stores. Therefore, a careful assessment of the patient's status should be considered when interpreting the results.

Positive Acute Phase Reactants (APR): Inflammatory Markers

Approximately 8.4 million adults in the United States are diagnosed with both diabetes and CKD. In addition to the cardiovascular risks associated with diabetes, CKD also increases risks of cardiovascular events, increased circulating inflammatory markers, and premature mortality [32, 33]. These conditions trigger acute or chronic inflammation, as well as an acute phase response of the body's host defense and adaptive mechanisms. Increased inflammatory markers are positively correlated with increased APR proteins [15, 16, 30, 34–36]. The presence of inflammation is defined as a substantial change (at least 25%) in the usual level of any of the various APR proteins produced by the hepatocytes [35]. Additionally, chronic inflammation associated with CKD is defined when CRP level increases to above 5 mg/L for at least 3 months; a normal CRP level is < 1 mg/L [36]. An increase in CRP level is reported to negatively correlate with nutritional status and with a decrease in Salb and prealb concentrations [1, 15, 16, 34–36]. Examples of positive APRs are interleukin (IL)-6 (a major inducer of most APR), CRP, IL-1beta, tumor necrosis factor (TNF)-alpha, interferon gamma, fibrinogen (which has a substantial effect on the erythrocyte sedimentation rate (ESR), alpha-1 antitrypsin, haptoglobin, IL-1 receptor antagonist, hepcidin, ferritin, and procalcitonin [35].

The acute phase response induces a number of behavioral, physiological, biochemical, and nutritional changes in response to the increased production of cytokines. These biological changes are fever, anemia of chronic disease, anorexia, drowsiness, lethargy, muscle wasting, increased production of corticotropin-releasing hormone, amyloidosis, altered serum concentrations of various minerals such as iron, copper, and zinc and, when produced in large amounts, can lead to septic shock [36]. All of the above negatively impact patients' overall nutritional status, regardless of their protein intake. Therefore, a thorough comprehensive assessment is warranted to provide both appropriate medical and nutrition assessment and therapy in this patient population.

Electrolytes

Serum Potassium

Serum potassium (K) is the most abundant intracellular cation (98% of total body K stores), with only 2% found in the intracellular space. The body stores about 50–75 mEq of K per kilogram (kg) of body weight, which accounts for at least 3000 mEq. Maintaining Na/K balance between the intracellular and extracellular space is essential, and it is controlled by the Na/K-ATPase pump found in the cell membrane. The Na/K-ATPase pump transports Na + out of the cell and K+ into the cell at a ratio of 3:2. This balance in concentration maintains an optimal action potential essential for normal muscle and neural function. Any imbalance in serum K level results in a dysfunction of that action potential and thus may cause muscle paralysis and potentially life-threatening cardiac arrhythmias. Serum K level is often impacted by the correlation among the following three factors: K intake, distribution of K across the cell membrane, and urinary K excretion [37–39].

Ingested K is absorbed from the intestine and excreted in the urine through the kidneys. If K is ingested in large amounts in healthy individuals, the excess K is absorbed by the muscle and liver cells via the Na/K-ATPase pumps and is facilitated by both insulin and beta-2-adrenergic receptors. However, some of the ingested K remains in the extracellular space [39]. Elevated extracellular (serum) K level stimulates the release of aldosterone, which activates Na + channels in the luminal membrane in an attempt to increase K excretion via the kidneys and normalize serum level. When the kidneys are functioning properly, K excretion is increased with higher K intake, the phenomenon known as K adaptation. With the decline in kidney function, the K adaptive mechanism is lost, leading to hyperkalemia (elevated serum K level) [39].

Hyperkalemia can result in patients presenting with decreased kidney function, hypoaldosteronism, increased cellular destruction (hemolysis), and tissue catabolism (K leaks out of the cells) [40, 41] and with the ingestion of high K foods and beverages, K-containing salt substitutes, and certain medications (e.g., K-sparing diuretics, angiotensin-converting enzyme (ACE) inhibitors, angiotensin receptor blockers (ARBs), triamterene, nonsteroidal anti-inflammatory drugs (NSAIDs), among others) [42]. Hyperkalemia is also common in patients presenting with metabolic acidosis in attempt to buffer the excess serum H+ ion. A transcellular shift happens to maintain an acid-base balance, in which H+ moves into the intracellular space in exchange with K+ [43, 44] (see Table 5.2).

Hyperkalemia can cause muscle weakness, paralysis, cardiac conduction abnormalities, cardiac arrhythmias, and metabolic acidosis [45]. Therefore, given the life-threatening physiological changes associated with hyperkalemia, a tight control of serum K level becomes essential. The RDN works closely with the patients on managing serum K levels, especially those diagnosed with advanced CKD (stages 4 and 5), and those who are dialysis dependent. The RDN provides individualized nutritional counseling on food and beverage items that would manage serum K level. The RDN also provides recommendations on adjusting the dialysate K bath for patients who are dialysis dependent.

Metabolic Acidosis

Metabolic acidosis is defined as an excess production of acids in the body, coupled with impairment in the kidneys' ability to excrete acids and to reabsorb and regenerate bicarbonate (base). Metabolic acidosis results when serum bicarbonate level drops to 24 mmol/L or below in patients diagnosed with stages 3–5 CKD. A serum bicarbonate level maintained between 22 and 26 mmol/L is considered acceptable for patients undergoing maintenance dialysis [1].

In healthy individuals, metabolic acidosis is caused by the inability of serum bicarbonate to buffer the excessive production of acids, as in the case of excessive lactic acid production with the lack of oxygen from prolonged anaerobic physical activity. Metabolic acidosis can also result from intestinal loss of bicarbonate due to prolonged diarrhea, very low blood pressure coupled with low O_2 supply to the cells and tissues (hypoxemia and hypoxia), and/or with ketoacidosis in patients with type 1 diabetes mellitus. The lungs and the kidneys play a major role in compensating for the presence of acidosis in the body. The lungs compensate by promoting a rapid and deep respiration (Kussmaul respiration to expel CO2), and the kidneys compensate through a much slower process by increasing the production of bicarbonate ion (HCO_3^-: a base) and increasing the excretion of hydrogen ions [46, 47].

Metabolic acidosis increases the catabolism of muscle protein; impairs contractibility of the myocardium, which increases the risk of heart failure; reduces respiratory reserves; aggravates secondary hyperparathyroidism, bone resorption, and osteopenia; increases the risk of hyperkalemia; reduces the expression of insulin-like growth factor and growth hormone receptor [46, 47]; and may increase the risk of systematic inflammation, hypotension, and malaise [46]. Metabolic acidosis also reduces the synthesis of amino acids and increases its oxidation rate [47]. Moreover, it is significantly correlated with a faster decline in residual kidney function [46–52] and increased mortality rate among patients diagnosed with CKD [46].

Correcting for metabolic acidosis is significantly correlated with improvement in nutritional biochemical parameters [1], such as improving SGA scores [1, 53], Salb level [1, 48, 54, 55], serum prealb [1, 55], and nPCR [1, 45], as well as slowing down CKD progression as measured by albuminuria [47] and GFR [50–52]. Correcting metabolic acidosis can be achieved either by the intake of oral bicarbonate supplementation in patients who are not on dialysis or by adjusting the bicarbonate level in the dialysate bath in patients undergoing RRT. Some patients in this latter group may still need to take additional oral bicarbonate supplementation to achieve an optimal acid-base balance. Though it is sodium-based, sodium bicarbonate supplementation did not cause significant fluid retention [1]. An intake of 1800 mg of oral bicarbonate supplementation daily did not have any effect on patients' fluid status [48, 49].

Dietary modification, such as increasing consumption of fruits and vegetables, decreases serum acids by about 50% [1, 47, 49, 56]. Decreased renal acid load slows down the progression of the decline in kidney function in patients diagnosed with earlier stages of renal disease. Since most fruits and vegetables are high in K, and given the nature of the renal diet that is limited in K (for patients with advanced stages of CKD and those undergoing MHD), low-K food choices should be considered. It is worth noting that in case a higher dietary protein intake is recommended as part of the patient's individualized medical nutrition therapy, close monitoring of the patient's acid-base status should be considered, and an adjustment in the bicarbonate level may be indicated. A high protein intake is inversely correlated with serum bicarbonate level [57].

Assessment of Nutritional Status

The use of selected biochemical parameters to assess nutritional intake can provide objective data, can be used to estimate the patient's overall protein intake, is feasible, and is routinely done as part of the patient's monthly laboratory assessment. These include blood urea nitrogen (BUN), normalized protein catabolic rate (nPCR), serum creatinine, and serum total cholesterol.

Blood Urea Nitrogen and Protein Catabolic Rate

Blood Urea Nitrogen

Blood urea nitrogen (BUN) is a biochemical parameter that can be used as an indicator of the amount of protein breakdown by the liver and thus an indirect measurement of the patient's protein intake. Urea, a breakdown of protein, is filtered out of the blood via the kidneys and into the urine. In the normal healthy population, BUN level should be stable and within normal range. A decline in kidney function leads to an accumulation of urea in the blood, therefore any acute change in BUN may be indicative of an acute increase of protein intake (exogenous) or protein metabolism (endogenous) [22].

In patients with advanced stages of CKD and in those receiving RRT, BUN can provide an estimate of dietary protein intake [22]. Monthly screening of pre-dialysis BUN is a routine practice in the outpatient hemodialysis setting. BUN should be assessed in combination with other biochemical parameters, as results can be falsely interpreted if assessed as a sole indicator of dietary protein intake. BUN can be within the lower range, independent of dietary protein intake, in patients who still have some residual kidney function. On the other hand, it can be falsely elevated in the presence of dehydration, inadequate dialysis, and/or increased endogenous protein catabolism. A patient's baseline pre-dialysis BUN should be assessed and compared with subsequent values; any abrupt changes in the level should be investigated. A gradual reduction in BUN level is often seen in older patients, which can be correlated with the decline in dietary protein intake.

Protein Nitrogen Appearance/Protein Catabolic Rate

Protein nitrogen appearance (PNA), also referred to as protein catabolic rate (PCR), can provide an objective indication of net protein metabolism, though its use to assess protein intake in patients diagnosed with CKD has not been fully supported in the literature [1]. PCR has been routinely used in the clinical setting to indirectly estimate protein intake; it is estimated by measuring the rate of increase in serum urea nitrogen between two hemodialysis treatments in clinically stable patients using urea kinetic modeling. PCR is thought to reflect the amount of protein catabolized in excess of the amount of protein synthesized per day. Unfortunately, the level can be limited (over- or underestimated) in patients who present with catabolic or anabolic states and/or in those with residual renal function. PCR overestimates protein intake with an intake < 1 g/kg of body weight and underestimates protein intake when the intake is > 1 g/kg of protein per day [58].

Clinically in the dialysis setting, PCR is typically normalized so that protein intake can be compared to estimated protein requirements (i.e., intake is usually normalized to either the actual or the adjusted body weight (ABW) reported to the laboratory), independent of body mass. This normalized protein intake value is expressed as normalized protein catabolic rate (nPCR). Therefore, inaccuracy in reporting a patient's target or desired weight provides an inaccurate nPCR value [59]. Normalization of PCR to body weight may be misleading in obese, malnourished, and edematous individuals if target or ABW is not carefully established and accurately reported to the laboratory. In patients presenting with edema, an assessment of serum sodium (Na) level combined with a thorough clinical assessment can assist clinicians in establishing an accurate estimation of target weight. For patients who are over- or underweight, the RDN can use any of the available standardized formulas to calculate ABW.

nPCR is normalized by dividing PCR by $V/0.58$. V is the patient's urea volume calculated by either urea kinetics using bioelectrical impedance analysis (BIA) or anthropometric equations and is an estimate of fat-free body mass, whereas the 0.58 factor is the proportion of V as a fraction of total body weight [1].

nPCR may fluctuate based on a patient's overall health and nutritional status. The 2020 KDOQI workgroup reported that nPCR is a significant predictor of Salb concentration and mortality in patients undergoing MHD; this correlation was not studied in other stages of CKD [1]. A decrease in nPCR is often seen in patients who present with a low Salb level or in those who present with uremic syndromes related to inadequate dialysis. Patients who receive adequate dialysis present with better urea clearance and control of uremic symptoms, an improved overall appetite and protein intake, and thus a higher nPCR level [1].

nPCR should be assessed with other biochemical indicators when evaluating patients' overall nutritional and health status. In a stable individual, nPCR provides an estimation of daily protein intake; for example, nPCR of 1.4 may indicate a protein intake of 1.4 grams of protein per kg of body weight. In well-dialyzed patients, nPCR <1.2 g/kg/day may indicate poor protein intake or may be a sign of onset of an acute illness. The KDOQI expert panel recommends maintaining nPCR >1.2 g/kg/day [1].

nPCR should be carefully evaluated as its level can be falsely elevated, thus providing an overestimation of a patient's actual protein intake. Examples are patients who present with increased catabolism, such as those presenting with active inflammation or infection, and those who present with a protein intake that is chronically below the daily recommendation. In such cases, the increase is possibly due to endogenous protein catabolism in an attempt to meet the protein needed for normal daily repair. A rapid increase in nPCR over a short period of time may indicate either an active inflammatory status, an increased endogenous protein catabolism, and/or a reflection of the patient's most recent protein intake that may not reflect usual dietary habits. In the latter example, examining the trend in the patient's serum prealb (if readily available), CO2, BUN, and Salb may help the RDN to interpret any recent changes in dietary protein intake. For example, a rapid elevation in nPCR coupled with a sudden decrease in serum CO2 and an increase in prealb level, if available, may indicate a recent increase in protein intake. Serum CO2 is inversely correlated with dietary protein intake in the CKD population [57]. On the other hand, nPCR can be falsely low (underestimating dietary protein intake) in patients presenting with anabolic states. Examples are patients recovering from infections or growing children. Therefore, a careful assessment of dietary protein habits combined with other nutrition-related biochemical parameters should be considered in order to accurately assess patient's nutritional status and provide individualized dietary therapy.

Serum Creatinine, Creatinine Clearance, and Creatinine Index

Serum creatinine (SCr) is an indicator of muscle mass and is routinely measured as part of the patient's monthly plan of care. SCr is a by-product produced by endogenous (muscle mass) and exogenous (protein intake) protein metabolism and is excreted by the kidneys. In the normal healthy population, SCr level is usually higher in those presenting with higher muscle mass. The level is affected by changes in kidney function and, to a lesser extent, by the intake of high biological value (HBV) protein (i.e., animal products). SCr is used as a screening indicator of residual renal function; a decline in residual function results in an increase in SCr concentration. A urine Cr test is also used to provide a measurement of urinary excretion of Cr, which is used to calculate creatinine clearance (CrCl) obtained by a 24-hour urine collection. CrCl provides a more accurate assessment of renal function as compared to SCr if done by itself. The concentration can be falsely elevated with dehydration, increased muscle mass, an abrupt increase in protein intake, and/or an intake of certain medications or dietary supplements such as creatine [60].

SCr and CrCl values provide a guidance for the RDN to individualize daily protein recommendations for patients diagnosed with earlier stages of CKD who are not receiving RRT. A low-protein diet (0.6–0.8 gram of protein per kg of ABW) is recommended to preserve remaining kidney function in this patient population, especially among patients who present with GFR < 60 ml/min/1.73m^2 [1].

Creatinine index, which is calculated utilizing kinetic modeling, is another marker that can provide information on protein malnutrition; it is used to estimate somatic protein mass. However, the clinical usefulness of this index has not been established [60].

Serum Total Cholesterol

Low serum total cholesterol level is identified as one of the markers of PEW, in addition to hypoalbuminemia, low BMI, and reduced dietary protein intake. All of the above are reported to be positively correlated with increased mortality rates in patients presenting with CKD, especially those presenting with advanced stages and in those undergoing maintenance dialysis therapy. Though cardiovascular disease (CVD) mortality rate in the CKD population continues to be high, the cause for such mortality was reported not to be related to hyperlipidemia, as shown to be the case in the general population [3, 61]. On the contrary, hyperlipidemia, along with increased body weight, has been reported to be correlated with longevity in patients undergoing MHD: the phenomena known as "obesity and cholesterol paradoxes" or "reverse epidemiology" [3]. Conversely, both low BMI and low serum total cholesterol levels were consistently correlated with increased mortality risk in this patient population, as explained by the "endotoxin-lipoprotein hypothesis" [36]. Patients with CKD often present with a gradual loss of body fat and with decreased serum cholesterol level throughout the progression of their disease. Hypocholesterolemia reflects a general decline in serum lipoprotein levels and is often associated with malnutrition, a condition commonly seen in this patient population. Circulating lipoproteins neutralize the endotoxins coming from the gastrointestinal tract, resulting in even lower anti-inflammatory production of cytokines and adiponectin, which are both reported to have a protective effect against CV-related mortality. Additionally, a fall in lipoprotein concentration below optimal level, as seen in the presence of hypocholesterolemia, results in decreased ability to bind with lipopolysaccharides, which are reported to have a role in removing circulating endotoxins. The end result is increased risk of cardiovascular events [36].

Conclusion

Patients with CKD often present with multiple comorbid conditions, which place them at increased risk of inflammation and associated malnutrition. Additionally, these patients are at increased risk of uremia, metabolic acidosis, decreased protein and energy intake, increased rate of protein catabolism and malnutrition, and progression of CKD—all of which are reported to significantly and negatively impact their nutritional status and quality of life, and to increase the rate of hospitalization and mortality.

Early screening for, and diagnosis of, CKD and providing individualized medical and nutritional therapies are essential to slow down the progression of the disease and its associated side effects. This can be accomplished by utilizing an interdisciplinary team approach. RDNs play an important role in the interdisciplinary care team; they are expert at providing medical nutrition therapy that is tailored to the individual's needs and nutritional status. This includes, but is not limited to, managing malnutrition, inflammation, uremia, metabolic acidosis, weight, and disorders of lipid and bone metabolism. The RDN monitors patients' nutritional status at least every 1–3 months or more frequently based on the patients' status. They are also expert at identifying whether the patient presents with inadequate nutrient intake, PEM or PEW, and mineral and electrolyte imbalances or whether the patient presents with an illness that may worsen their nutritional status.

Several assessment tools are available for the RDN to consider when assessing the patients and planning their tailored medical nutrition therapy (MNT). Objective parameters provide information about patients' overall nutritional and metabolic status; however, each also has its own limitation. Therefore, a comprehensive assessment of biochemical parameters should be considered when planning an individualized MNT for this patient population. A strong negative correlation exists between Salb, prealb, body weight, total cholesterol level, nPCR and metabolic acidosis, and rates of morbidity, hospitalization, and mortality. Additionally, there is a strong and positive correlation between decreased nutritional status and acute inflammatory markers in this patient population, which places them at increased risk for malnutrition/wasting and associated side effects. All of which leads to further malnutrition, decreased quality of life, and increased rate of depression.

References

1. Ikizler TA, Burrowes J, Byham-Gray L, Campbell K, Carrero JJ, Chan W, et al. KDOQI Nutrition in CKD Guideline Work Group. KDOQI clinical practice guideline for nutrition in CKD: 2020 update. Am J Kidney Dis. 2020; in press.
2. Kidney Disease: Improving Global Outcomes (KDIGO). Chapter 1. Definition and classification of CKD. Kidney Int. 2013;3:S19–62.
3. Kovesdy CP, Kalantar-Zadeh K. Why is protein–energy wasting associated with mortality in chronic kidney disease? Semin Nephrol. 2009;29(1):3–14.
4. Obi Y, Qader H, Kovesdy CP, Kalantar-Zadeh K. Latest consensus and update on protein-energy wasting in chronic kidney disease. Curr Opin Clin Nutr. 2015;18(3):254–62.
5. Garg AX, Blake PG, Clark WF, Clase CM, Haynes RB, Moist LM. Association between renal insufficiency and malnutrition in older adults: results from the NHANES III. Kidney Int. 2001;60(5):1867–74.
6. The global burden of kidney disease and the sustainable development goals [Internet]. World Health Organization. World Health Organization; 2018 [cited 2019Aug23]. Available from: https://www.who.int/bulletin/volumes/96/6/17-206441/en/.
7. National Institute of Diabetes and Digestive and Kidney Diseases. U.S. Department of Health and Human Services; 2016 [cited 2019Aug23]. Available from: https://www.niddk.nih.gov/health-information/health-statistics/kidney-disease.
8. Chronic Kidney Disease [Internet]. Chronic Kidney Disease | Healthy People 2020. [cited 2019Sep08]. Available from: https://www.healthypeople.gov/2020/topics-objectives/topic/chronic-kidney-disease/objectives.
9. Saran R, Robinson B, Abbott K, Agodoa L, Albertus P, Ayanian J, et al. US renal data system 2015 annual data report: epidemiology of kidney disease in the United States. Am J Kidney Dis. 2016;67(3):A7–8.
10. Obrador G, Curhan G, Motwani S. Epidemiology of Chronic Kidney Disease. Retrieved from https://www.uptodate.com/contents/epidemiology-of-chronic-kidney-disease. 2018.
11. Collins AJ, Foley RN, Herzog C, Chavers BM, Gilbertson D, Ishani A, et al. Excerpts from the US renal data system 2009 annual data report. Am J Kidney Dis. 2010;55:S1. https://doi.org/10.1053/j.ajkd.2009.10.009.
12. Sum SS-M, Marcus AF, Blair D, Olejnik LA, Cao J, Parrott JS, et al. Comparison of subjective global assessment and protein energy wasting score to nutrition evaluations conducted by registered dietitian nutritionists in identifying protein energy wasting risk in maintenance hemodialysis patients. J Ren Nutr. 2017;27:325–32.
13. Fouque D, Kalantar-Zadeh K, Kopple J, Cano N, Chauveau P, Cuppari L, et al. A proposed nomenclature and diagnostic criteria for protein–energy wasting in acute and chronic kidney disease. Kidney Int. 2008;73(4):391–8.
14. Kumar N, Henderson H, Cameron BD, McCullough PA. Malnutrition, obesity, and undernutrition in chronic kidney disease. Oxford Med Online. 2018; https://doi.org/10.1093/med/9780199592548.003.0106_update_001.
15. Molfino A, Heymsfield S, Zhu F, Kotanko P, Levin N, Dwyer T, Kaysen G. Prealbumin is associated with visceral fat mass in patients receiving hemodialysis. J Ren Nutr. 2013;23:406–10.
16. Jones C, Akbani H, Croft D, Worth D. The relationship between serum albumin and hydration status in hemodialysis patients. J Ren Nutr. 2002;12:209–12.
17. Bharadwaj S, Ginoya S, Tandon P, Gohel TD, Guirguis J, Vallabh H, et al. Malnutrition: Laboratory markers vs nutritional assessment. Gastroenterol Rep. 2016;4(4):272–80.

18. Lee JL, Oh ES, Lee RW, Finucane TE. Serum albumin and prealbumin in calorically restricted, nondiseased individuals: a systematic review. Am J Med. 2015;128(9):1023.e1–22.
19. Haluzík M, Kábrt J, Nedvídková J, Svobodová J, Kotrlíková E, Papežová H. Relationship of serum leptin levels and selected nutritional parameters in patients with protein-caloric malnutrition. Nutrition. 1999;15(11–12):829–33.
20. Petersen PH, Felding P, Hørder M, Tryding N. Effects of posture on concentrations of serum proteins in healthy adults. Dependence on the molecular size of proteins. Scand J Clin Lab Inv. 1980;40(7):623–8.
21. Akar H, Akar GC, Carrero JJ, Stenvinkel P, Lindholm B. Systemic consequences of poor oral health in chronic kidney disease patients. Clin J Am Soc Nephrol. 2010;6(1):218–26.
22. Bansal S, Cho M, Beddhu S, Schwab S, Lam A. Assessment of nutritional status in hemodialysis patients. Retrieved from https://www.uptodate.com/contents/assessment-of-nutritional-status-in-hemodialysis-patients#! 08 Oct 2018.
23. de Mutsert R, Grootendorst D, Indemans F, Boeschoten E, Krediet R, Dekker F. Association between serum albumin and mortality in dialysis patients is partly explained by inflammation, and not by malnutrition. J Ren Nutr. 2009;19:127–35.
24. Gurreebun F, Hartley G, Brown A, Ward M, Goodship T. Nutritional screening in patients on hemodialysis: is subjective global assessment an appropriate tool? J Ren Nutr. 2017;17:114–7.
25. de Roij van Zuijdewijn CL, ter Wee PM, Chapdelaine I, Bots ML, Blankestijn PJ, van den Dorpel MA, et al. A comparison of 8 nutrition-related tests to predict mortality in hemodialysis patients. J Ren Nutr. 2015;25:412–9.
26. Leinig C, Moraes T, Ribeiro S, Riella M, Olandoski M, Martins C, Pecoits-Filho R. Predictive value of malnutrition markers for mortality in peritoneal dialysis patients. J Ren Nutr. 2011;21:176–83.
27. Araújo I, Kamimura M, Draibe S, Canziani M, Manfredi S, Avesani C, et al. Nutritional parameters and mortality in incident hemodialysis patients. J Ren Nutr. 2006;16:27–35.
28. Fiedler R, Jehle P, Osten B, Dorligschaw O, Girndt M. Clinical nutrition scores are superior for the prognosis of haemodialysis patients compared to lab markers and bioelectrical impedance. Nephrol Dial Transplant. 2009;24:3812–7.
29. Raguso CA, Dupertuis YM, Pichard C. The role of visceral proteins in the nutritional assessment of intensive care unit patients. Curr Opin Clin Nutr. 2013;6(2):211–6.
30. Adamson JW. Normal Iron physiology. Semin Dial. 1999;12:219–23.
31. Cavill I. Iron status as measured by serum ferritin: the marker and its limitations. Am J Kidney Dis. 1999;34:S12–7.
32. Provenzano M, Coppolino G, Faga T, Garofalo C, Serra R, Andreucci M. Epidemiology of cardiovascular risk in chronic kidney disease patients: the realsilent killer. Reviews in Cardiovascular Medicine. 2019;20(4):209.
33. Zelnick LR, Weiss NS, Kestenbaum BR, Robinson-Cohen C, Heagerty PJ, Tuttle K, et al. Diabetes and CKD in the United States population, 2009–2014. Clin J Am Soc Nephrol. 2017;12(12):1984–90.
34. Lakshmi BS, Devi NH, Suchitra MM, Srinivasa Rao PVLN, Kumar VS. Changes in the inflammatory and oxidative stress markers during a single hemodialysis session in patients with chronic kidney disease. Ren Fail. 2018;40:534–40.
35. Kovesdy CP, Kopple JD, Kalantar-Zadeh K. Inflammation in renal insufficiency. Retrieved from https://www.uptodate.com/contents/inflammation-in-renal-insufficiency (25 Sept 2017).
36. Kushner I, Furst D, Romain P. Acute phase reactant. Retrieved from https://www.uptodate.com/contents/acute-phase-reactants. 12 July 2017.
37. Giebisch GH, Wang WH. Potassium transport – an update. J Nephrol. 2010;23 Suppl 16:S97.
38. Youn JH, McDonough AA. Recent advances in understanding integrative control of potassium homeostasis. Annu Rev Physiol. 2009;71:381.
39. Mount DB, Zandi-Nejad K. Disorders of potassium balance. In: Brenner and Rector's the Clausen T, Everts ME. Regulation of the Na,K-pump in skeletal muscle. Kidney Int 1989;35:1.
40. Sever MS, Erek E, Vanholder R, Kantarci G, Yavuz M, Turkmen A, et al. Serum potassium in the crush syndrome victims of the Marmara disaster. Clin Nephrol. 2003;59:326.
41. Perkins RM, Aboudara MC, Abbott KC, Holcomb JB. Resuscitative hyperkalemia in noncrush trauma: a prospective, observational study. Clin J Am Soc Nephrol. 2007;2:313.
42. Chang AR, Sang Y, Leddy J, Yahya T, Kirchner HL, Inker LA, et al. Antihypertensive medications and the prevalence of hyperkalemia in a large health system. Hypertension. 2016;67:1181.
43. Rose BD, Post TW, Adrogué HJ, Madias NE. PCO2 and [K+]p in metabolic acidosis: certainty for the first and uncertainty for the other. J Am Soc Nephrol. 2004;15:1667.
44. Aronson PS, Giebisch G. Effects of pH on potassium: new explanations for old observations. J Am Soc Nephrol. 2011;22:1981.
45. Mount DB. Clinical manifestations of hyperkalemia in adults [Internet]. UpToDate. 2017 [cited 2019Aug24]. Available from: https://www.uptodate.com/contents/clinical-manifestations-of-hyperkalemia-in-adults.
46. Kovesdy CP. Pathogenesis, consequences, and treatment of metabolic acidosis in chronic kidney disease. Retrieved from https://www.uptodate.com/contents/pathogenesis-consequences-and-treatment-of-metabolic-acidosis-in-chronic-kidney-disease. 13 No 2018.

47. Goraya N, Simoni J, Jo C, Wesson D. Dietary acid reduction with fruits and vegetables or bicarbonate attenuates kidney injury in patients with a moderately reduced glomerular filtration rate due to hypertensive nephropathy. Kidney Int. 2012;81:86–93.
48. de Brito-Ashurst I, Varagunam M, Raftery M, Yaqoob M. Bicarbonate supplementation slows progression of CKD and improves nutritional status. J Am Soc Nephrol. 2009;20:2075–84.
49. Goraya N, Simoni J, Jo C, Wesson D. Treatment of metabolic acidosis in patients with stage 3 chronic kidney disease with fruits and vegetables or oral bicarbonate reduces urine angiotensinogen and preserves glomerular filtration rate. Kidney Int. 2014;86:1031–8.
50. Scialla J, Appel L, Astor B, Miller E, Beddhu S, Woodward M, Parekh R, Anderson C. Net endogenous acid production is associated with a faster decline in GFR in African Americans. Kidney Int. 2012;82:106–12.
51. Kanda E, Ai M, Kuriyama R, Yoshida M, Shiigai T. Dietary acid intake and kidney disease progression in the elderly. Am J Nephrol. 2014;39:145–52.
52. Banerjee T, Crews D, Wesson D, Tilea A, Saran R, Ríos-Burrows N, et al. High dietary acid load predicts ESRD among adults with CKD. J Am Soc Nephrol. 2015;26:1693–700.
53. Szeto CC, Wong TY, Chow KM, Leung CB. Oral sodium bicarbonate for the treatment of metabolic acidosis in peritoneal dialysis patients: a randomized placebo-control trial. J Am Soc Nephrol. 2003;14:2119–26.
54. Movilli E. Correction of metabolic acidosis increases serum albumin concentrations and decreases kinetically evaluated protein intake in haemodialysis patients: a prospective study. Nephrol Dial Transplant. 1998;13:1719–22.
55. Verove C, Maisonneuve N, Azouzi AE, Boldron A, Azar R. Effect of the correction of metabolic acidosis on nutritional status in elderly patients with chronic renal failure. J Renal Nutr. 2002;12:224–8.
56. Goraya N, Simoni J, Jo C, Wesson D. A comparison of treating metabolic acidosis in CKD stage 4 hypertensive kidney disease with fruits and vegetables or sodium bicarbonate. J Am Soc Nephrol. 2013;8:371–81.
57. Gennari FJ, Greene VL, Wang X, Levey AS. Effect of dietary protein intake on serum total CO2 concentration in chronic kidney disease: modification of diet in renal disease study findings. J Am Soc Nephrol. 2005;1:52–7.
58. Lorenzo V, de Bonis E, Rufino M, Hernández D, Rebollo S, Rodríguez A, et al. Caloric rather than protein deficiency predominates in stable chronic haemodialysis patients. Nephrol Dial Transplant. 1995;10:1885–9.
59. Virga G, Viglino G, Gandolfo C, Aloi E, Cavalli P. Normalization of protein equivalent of nitrogen appearance and dialytic adequacy in CAPD. Perit Dial Int. 1996;16:S185–9.
60. Desmeules S, Levesque R, Jaussent I, Leray-Moragues H, Chalabi L, Canaud B. Creatinine index and lean body mass are excellent predictors of long-term survival in haemodiafiltration patients. Nephrol Dial Transplant. 2004;19(5):1182–9.
61. Longenecker JC. Traditional cardiovascular disease risk factors in dialysis patients compared with the general population: the CHOICE study. J Am Soc Nephrol. 2002;13(7):1918–27.

Chapter 6
Nutrition-Focused Physical Examination and Assessment in Chronic Kidney Disease

Jane Ziegler

Keywords Chronic kidney disease · Nutrition-focused physical examination · Micronutrient deficiencies · Physical findings

> **Key Points**
> - Review current standards of practice/standards of professional performance and other regulatory requirements for the nutrition-focused physical assessment.
> - Describe the nutrition-focused physical examination techniques.
> - Integrate the nutrition-focused physical examination findings into assessment and plan of care for patients with chronic kidney disease.

History of the Nutrition-Focused Physical Examination

The initial Medicare Conditions for Coverage for end-stage renal disease (ESRD) were available in 1976 [1] directing registered dietitian/nutritionists (RDN) to perform a nutrition-focused physical examination (NFPE) as part of their assessment. However, most NFPE practices by the RDN began with the introduction of the subjective global assessment (SGA) in the 1980s [2–4]. It was not until the 1990s that the NFPE became more widely used in assessment practices and was introduced into the nutrition care process in 2003 [4, 5]. Components of the NFPE were first included in the Academy of Nutrition and Dietetics' (Academy) 2012 Revised Standards of Practice in Nutrition Care and Standards of Practice/Standards of Professional Performance (SOP/SOPP) for RDNs that are now part of the SOP/SOPP for RDNs in both adult and pediatric populations [6, 7]. The revised 2014 SOP/SOPP for RDNs in Nephrology Nutrition also contain the required NFPE core standards of practice indicators for NFPE [8].

These SOP/SOPP standards [6–8] direct the RDN to utilize NFPE on patients to assess for fat and muscle wasting; oral health conditions; hair, skin and nails; and signs of edema as well as conditions that impact nutritional status or impact the patient's ability to eat. The nutrition profes-

The editors acknowledge Mary Pat Kelly's contribution to this chapter in *Nutrition in Kidney Disease*, *Second Edition*, Nutrition and Health, DOI https://doi.org/10.1007/978-1-62703-685-6_1, © Springer Science+Business Media New York 2014.

J. Ziegler (✉)
Department of Clinical and Preventive Nutrition Sciences, Rutgers University, School of Health Professions, Newark, NJ, USA
e-mail: ziegleja@shp.rutgers.edu

© Springer Nature Switzerland AG 2020
J. D. Burrowes et al. (eds.), *Nutrition in Kidney Disease*, Nutrition and Health, https://doi.org/10.1007/978-3-030-44858-5_6

sion has also added the required core competency standard of the NFPE as part of the accrediting standards in dietetic programs by the Accreditation Council for Education in Nutrition and Dietetics (ACEND) [9].

If RDNs do not perform a thorough NFPE, the nutrition assessment is not complete and, as a result, malnutrition and other conditions which impact eating ability may go undiagnosed. RDNs should be utilizing the NFPE on patients to identify malnutrition as well as to identify any condition that may impact nutritional status, impair dietary intake, or reflect nutritional conditions [4]. The NFPE is the comprehensive physical examination conducted by the RDN involving inspection and palpation and, in some instances, percussion and auscultation of physical features [4]. The NFPE should be targeted to the patient's condition but refers to the inspection for clinically manifested nutrient deficiencies; measurement of anthropometrics and body composition and vital signs; assessment of skin, nails, and hair; edema, lymph nodes, and cranial nerves (taste, smell, dysphagia screening); muscle and fat wasting; and head, neck, and orofacial examination [4]. Abdominal, heart, and lung assessment may be performed in select populations as findings may impact nutrition diagnoses and plan of care. Results from the NFPE can then be combined with the medical and dietary history findings in developing the nutrition diagnosis.

The NFPE is essential for the identification of signs and symptoms that may reflect macro- and micronutrient deficiencies and influence ingestion and digestion [10–12]. Of particular concern in the chronic kidney disease (CKD) population is that malnutrition is a major concern with signs of malnutrition including edema, ascites, weight loss, muscle weakness, muscle and fat wasting, reduced functional status, peripheral neuropathy, dry skin, ecchymosis, and pruritus [13, 14]. The 2012 consensus statement on the characteristics of adult malnutrition by the Academy and the American Society of Parenteral and Enteral Nutrition (ASPEN) [15, 16] integrates select NFPE components into a nutrition assessment to detect malnutrition. It highlights the importance of adequate training on physical examination techniques to perform accurately and evaluate patient examination findings for a nutrition diagnosis [15]. However, the NFPE has not been widely used among nutrition clinicians due to the lack of education and training, inexperience or lack of confidence and/or lack of a full appreciation of its role in assessing nutritional status. The NFPE is an essential component of a comprehensive nutrition assessment to determine the patient's nutritional status and factors that may impact the patient's ability to consume an adequate diet.

The purpose of this chapter is to review the importance of the NFPE as part of the comprehensive nutrition assessment in determining the nutritional status of a patient. The NFPE will assist in confirming the presence of malnutrition and other conditions which may affect the patient's ability to consume an adequate diet. This chapter will also review the specific techniques used in the examination of nutrition-focused physical findings in the patient with CKD to include examination of the skin, hair, nails and the orofacial area.

The Nutrition-Focused Physical Examination (NFPE)

The medical history including the nutrition history and the NFPE provide the foundation for the nutritional care and intervention in the patient with CKD. These clinical skills of history taking and NFPE are fundamental to the practice of clinical nutrition and patient care. Clinical skills include a combination of talk and touch that are used to interpret and apply the information through the use of diagnostic reasoning and critical thinking. A NFPE requires a systematic approach to assure that all needed data are collected and reviewed. As such, the history and physical examination do not have to be completed in a special sequence as the needs of the patient take first priority. However, a systematic approach helps to prevent missing the observation and collection of important information in making a nutrition diagnosis. A primary aim is to perform the NFPE so the process flows smoothly, minimizing the number of times the patient has to change position and to conserve the energy of the patient. Depending on the setting and the patient's condition or abilities, adaptations of the examination may be necessary.

Getting Started with the Nutrition-Focused Physical Examination

Prior to beginning the NFPE, it is important to review the health/medical record to collect past medical and surgical history, medications and dietary supplements, diagnostic testing, biochemical values, current conditions, and concerns which may impact nutritional status or dietary intake. Specific diet and nutrition questions completed as part of the nutrition assessment will be helpful as you begin the examination process. Specifically, ask for changes in appetite as well as the number of meals and/or snacks consumed daily. Ask about ability to chew and swallow, the presence of dry mouth, and any changes in taste and smell. Note the chief complaint and any other acute medical conditions as well as chronic conditions. Take note of any dental concerns, use of dentures, history of oral surgery, or any conditions that may increase the risk of difficulty chewing or dysphagia. Medications that affect the oral health (xerostomia, bleeding) should be noted as well [17, 18].

Some common supplies needed to perform an examination by the RDN are the following:

- Examining gloves
- Cotton-tipped applicators
- Gauze squares
- Pen light
- Tongue blades

Prior to starting the NFPE, be sure to gather the equipment and arrange nearby for convenience. Open wrapped items in advance of the NFPE and delay gloving until you begin your examination.

General Inspection

The first step in the NFPE is to greet the patient allowing for observation of any problematic issues. You can observe the patient for manner or affect, dress, level of apprehension, skin tone and facial expressions, grooming, mobility and gait, head positioning, and stature. Shaking the patient's hand allows the assessment of hand strength, which is a measure of functional status. All these observations contribute to your overall examination and impression of the patient and provide clues to potential issues that may affect nutritional status or dietary intake [4]. The renal system can affect many aspects of the physical examination which may be more notable with significant disease progression [19].

Anthropometric Data and Body Composition

Actual measured weight and height should be collected along with a history of weight changes including both long-term and recent weight changes [17, 20]. Ongoing weight measurements, monitored over time, are helpful to determine overall health status. Adjustments to the weight status should be made for suspected influence of edema, ascites, and/or polycystic organs [20]. The use of validated body composition methods in individuals with CKD includes waist circumference and body mass index (BMI) and body compartment estimates. No reference standard for assessing body composition in CKD patients is available, and studies have not found differences in body composition analysis between methods. Dual-energy X-ray absorptiometry (DXA), bioelectrical impedance (BIA), creatinine kinetics (CK), and computed tomography (CT) can be used to assess body composition among CKD patients [20].

Assessment of Fluid Status

Observe the patient for the appearance of hypovolemia or fluid overload. In a dehydrated state, the eyes may appear to be sunken or hollow, and the mucous membranes appear dry. Pinching the skin located over the anterior chest wall can determine if reduced skin turgor or elasticity exists. Although a somewhat insensitive measure of fluid status, these indicators may be most pronounced in circumstances of vomiting or diarrhea. A patient with fluid overload may be breathless due to pulmonary edema or pleural effusions as well as present with more obvious signs of peripheral edema. Observe for pitting edema in the legs at the base of the spine especially in patients confined to the bed. Begin palpating the legs at the ankle area and observe the highest level at which edema can be recognized. In severe cases, edema can be observed in the scrotum or labia [19].

Skin, Hair, and Nails

Observe the patient's skin for color, texture, temperature, and other characteristics. Skin should be an appropriate color for ethnicity, smooth and slightly warm to the touch. The patient with advanced CKD may look unwell with skin pallor. In marked uremia, the skin may appear yellow; however, this is a feature that occurs late in the disease process. Scratch marks on the skin may indicate the presence of pruritus [17–19].

Inspect and palpate the scalp and hair to determine texture, hair distribution, and quantity as well as pattern of hair loss, if any. The hair should be evenly distributed, and the scalp should be free of any lesions or scales. Inquire about changes in hair texture, structure and strength including broken or brittle hairs, and pigment changes. Hair loss/changes can be associated with deficiencies in protein, vitamin C, iron, or zinc [19, 21].

Pallor of the palmar creases of the hand can be suggestive of anemia. Nails should be convex in shape and smooth upon palpation, and the nail bed should be pink. Inspect the nails for Muehrcke's lines, a possible sign of hypoalbuminemia seen in nephrotic syndrome [19, 22]. Lindsey's nails of CKD are recognized by the proximal half of the nail being white and the distal half red or brown [19, 23]. Spooning of nails or koilonychia (concave nail) may be indicative of iron deficiency [19, 24].

Eyes

To assess the palpebral conjunctival color of the eyes, ask the patient to look up and gently depress the lower lids to expose the sclera and conjunctiva. Inspect for color and any abnormal findings. Palpebral conjunctival pallor may indicate anemia which is common in CKD. Normal conjunctiva is pink beneath a pale anterior rim [25]. Skin colored or beige nodules or lesions on or near the eye lids (xanthelasma) may be associated with lipid disorders [26].

Muscle and Fat Wasting

Both obesity and muscle wasting are commonly seen in patients with CKD and may occur simultaneously [27]; therefore, muscle and fat stores should be assessed by observation and palpation. Muscle wasting or muscle atrophy refers to a loss of substance and quality of the muscle [3, 18, 28]. The upper body may be more accessible and less affected by edema [29, 30]. Assess both sides of the body to differentiate between nutrition-related wasting and those conditions such as a stroke that may present with variations in muscle tone on each side of the body [30]. Muscle stores can be assessed in several areas. The temple region should appear flat or slightly bulging in a well-nourished state. Lightly palpate the temple region to assess tone and bulk of the temporalis muscle [3, 15, 18, 30]. A scooped or depressed temple region is indicative of muscle wasting. The muscle surrounding the clavicle bone area should feel firm and appear well-defined. Muscle wasting is palpable as stringy muscles and reduced muscle mass. The acromion area in a well-nourished individual appears as a rounded shoulder with firm muscle surrounding the shoulder and neck; however, in an obese individual, it may be difficult to differentiate muscle wasting due to excessive fat tissue. In muscle wasting, the acromion process may slightly protrude and, in more extensive wasting, the shoulder joint appears square and bones appear more prominent. The scapular bone area is another site to assess for muscle loss. In a well-nourished individual, the scapula should not appear apparent, but if wasting is present, depressions around the scapula may appear. Depressions between the scapula and spine also appear noticeable. The interosseous muscles on the dorsal aspect of the hand can be assessed for muscle wasting. In a well-nourished individual, this muscle should appear as a flat or mild bulge between the index finger and thumb. This area becomes depressed, and bones appear prominent in muscle wasting. The lower extremities can be assessed in three areas: the quadriceps, the patellar region, and the posterior calf area. Muscles should be well rounded and developed and the kneecap should not be prominent. As wasting occurs, the quadriceps develop a depression on the inner thigh, the kneecap becomes prominent with little muscle surrounding it, and the calf muscle becomes thin with minimal definition [3, 15, 18, 28, 30].

Fat stores are assessed in the orbital region, the midaxillary line, and the arm. The orbital fat stores are palpated below the eye and, in a well-nourished individual, they should appear as slightly bulged. Fat wasting appears as a slight to deep depression around the eye. Skin may appear loose and dark circles can appear. Upon palpation of the midaxillary line, ribs should not be evident, and the iliac crest should not be protruding. Fat wasting is identified by ribs being apparent and the iliac crest being more prominent. Lastly, the upper arm region is assessed under the triceps muscles. Ample fat tissue should be palpated when the skinfold is rolled between the fingers. As fat wasting occurs, this pinch of skin becomes less obvious and fingers may actually be almost touching [15, 28, 30].

Orofacial Examination

In addition to assessing fat and muscle stores in the orofacial region, an examination of the cranial nerves, the muscles of mastication, the temporomandibular joint (TMJ), and the oral cavity as well as screening for dysphasia risk is important in the prevention and treatment of malnutrition [17, 18].

Head and Face

Inspect external characteristics of the facial structures and assess for symmetry. Observe nasolabial folds for symmetry and flattening of the fold on one side of the face may indicate weakness and suggestive of potential swallowing concerns. Palpate the TMJ while the mouth is open and closed to observe for pain or tenderness and any clicking sounds that may interfere with biting and chewing [17, 18].

Cranial Nerve (CN) Assessment

Trigeminal Nerve (CN V)

The trigeminal nerve has both sensory and motor functions. The trigeminal nerve has three branches or divisions including the ophthalmic branch, which supplies sensation and function to the forehead, cornea, and conjunctiva. The maxillary branch supplies the skin in the middle of the face as well as the upper part of the palate and nasopharynx. The mandibular branch supplies the skin of the mandible and muscles of mastication (temporalis, masseter, and pterygoid muscles). Sensation is tested using the cotton-tipped applicator sequentially across the forehead, cheek, and lower mandible using both ends of the applicator, testing for correct sensation and while comparing sides. The motor functions of the trigeminal nerve are tested by examining the muscles of mastication. While the patient clenches, the temporalis and masseter muscles are palpated to assess for the tone, muscle bulk, pain, or tenderness [17, 18, 31].

Facial Nerve (CN VII)

The facial nerve primarily provides motor function to the face. The initial observation of the facial features can provide early evidence of asymmetrical expression (flattening of the nasolabial fold). Testing of the facial nerve can be achieved by asking the patients to wrinkle their forehead; to smile while showing their teeth, puffing out their cheeks; and to purse their lips. Assess opening of the mouth and jaw strength by having the patients open their mouth against resistance from your hand on their mandible. Weakness, limited jaw opening, pain, or tenderness may indicate difficulty biting, chewing and swallowing, and maintaining food and fluid within the oral cavity [17, 18, 31].

Glossopharyngeal Nerve (CN IX) and Vagus Nerve (CN X)

The glossopharyngeal nerve and the vagus nerve are tested together. The glossopharyngeal nerve primarily innervates the muscles of the tongue and pharynx. The vagus nerve, in addition to other motor functions, innervates the muscles of the pharynx and larynx. To evaluate these nerves together, press a tongue blade lightly on the tongue and observe the uvula and the rise of the soft palate and positioning of the tonsillar pillars. The uvula should not deviate to one side or the other and the rise of the palate should be symmetrical. A quick dysphagia screening can be performed by asking the patients to clear their throat and then perform a dry swallow [17, 18, 31]. Hoarseness or a wet cough can be indicative of the need for additional evaluation by a speech language pathologist.

Spinal Accessory Nerve (CN XI)

The spinal accessory nerve innervates the sternocleidomastoid and upper part of the trapezius muscles. Clinical examination of this nerve involves asking the patients to shrug their shoulders while applying resistance. Clinical significance for testing this CN is to assess head positioning and ability of the patients to maintain their head over their shoulders to minimize risk of choking when eating [17, 18, 31].

Hypoglossal Nerve (CN XII)

The hypoglossal nerve provides motor innervation to the tongue. When examining the tongue, carefully inspect for atrophy or asymmetry. Ask the patient to protrude the tongue. If the tongue deviates to one side or the other, the ability to chew, form a bolus, and swallow may be impaired. Strength of the tongue can be assessed by having the patient press the tongue against each cheek while the examiner applies pressure to the outside of the cheek [17, 18, 31].

Examination of the Oral Cavity

The oral cavity consists of three types of mucosa. These include masticatory mucosa and lining mucosa, which include the buccal and labial mucosa, and the specialized mucosa of the dorsal tongue. The masticatory mucosa is located on the hard palate and gingiva, and is a keratinized stratified squamous epithelium. A nonkeratinized stratified squamous epithelium composes the mucosal lining of most of the oral cavity including the buccal and labial mucosa and the soft palate [32, 33]. The cells of the oral cavity mucosa have a rapid turnover of 3–7 days; therefore, micronutrient deficiencies may manifest rapidly in the area of the lips and the oral mucosa [32, 34–37]. Although physical signs are nonspecific, other parameters such as diet history and biomarkers are useful for confirming physical findings. However, barriers exist in the reliability and specificity of these biomarkers for many nutrients. The oral examination should be prefaced with questions regarding any changes in taste and smell, any burning sensations in the mouth or on the tongue, and pain and location of the pain as well as any bleeding of the gingiva. If the patient is wearing dentures, ask that they remove the dentures. Gloves, tongue depressor, cotton gauze square, and a light source are needed for the intraoral examination [17, 18].

The oral examination begins with observation of the lips for signs of cracking, fissuring, lesions, and color changes. Invert the lips to observe color and wetness and any abnormal findings. Mucosal alterations, periodontal inflammation, gingival bleeding, and dentition should be assessed. Use the tongue depressor to move the cheeks laterally to allow for examination of the gingiva, teeth, and sulci. The dorsal and ventral surfaces of the tongue are examined by asking the patient to protrude the tongue, move it from side to side, and touch the tip of the tongue to the hard palate – observing for abnormalities and function concerns. Use a handheld light source and gloved hands, grasp the tip of the tongue with a cotton gauze pad, and move the tongue to observe all sides for any abnormalities. The examiner should also observe the floor of the mouth for wetness or pooling of saliva [17, 18].

Oral Manifestations of CKD

The oral cavity is often referred to as a mirror of systemic health, and it is one of the first locations to manifest signs of systemic disease and nutritional deficiencies [32–37]. A variety of common manifestations in the oral cavity that occur in the CKD population include altered taste, gingival hyperplasia, xerostomia, parotitis, enamel hypoplasia, mucosal lesions including hairy leukoplakia, lichenoid reactions, ulcerations, angular cheilitis, and candidiasis [38, 39].

Uremic stomatitis can occur due to markedly elevated levels of urea and other nitrogenous wastes in the blood of patients with CKD. Uremic stomatitis can come on suddenly and presents as white plaques primarily seen on the buccal mucosa and floor of the mouth and tongue. Symptoms include pain, unpleasant taste, burning sensations, and a uremic odor in the patient's breath [39, 40].

Dry mouth or xerostomia occurs frequently and is a significant complaint in the CKD population. Several conditions contribute to dry mouth including medications, inflammation, dehydration, mouth breathing, and also restricted fluid intake. Uremic patients can experience dry mouth from retrograde parotitis, metabolic abnormalities, and use of diuretics [39, 41].

Taste Changes

A metallic taste is often described in the CKD population due to the presence of urea in the saliva and its subsequent breakdown to ammonia and carbon dioxide by bacterial urease, which then contributes to this altered taste. The change in taste may also be a result of metabolic disturbances, use of medications, and changes in the salivary flow and its composition. High levels of urea and dimethyl and trimethyl amines and low levels of zinc have been associated with decreased taste perception in uremic patients [39, 41].

Due to bleeding tendencies as a result of abnormal thrombocyte function and a decrease in platelet factor III, mucosal petechiae and ecchymosis may be observed. The use of anticoagulants during hemodialysis may also cause these symptoms [39, 42].

Renal osteodystrophy is a frequent long-term complication of renal disease; it is a spectrum of bone metabolism disorders associated with different pathogenic pathways. Bone demineralization with trabeculation and cortical loss, giant cell radiotransparencies, or metastatic calcifications of the soft tissues may result. As a result, the oral cavity can show marked jaw enlargement with malocclusion, enamel hypoplasia, severe destruction of the periodontal tissues, tooth mobility, and drifting of teeth [39, 43].

Candidiasis can also contribute to poor oral health presenting as angular cheilitis, pseudomembranous, or erythematous ulceration or as a chronic atrophic infection [39, 44]. A variety of oral mucosal lesions, in particular white patches and ulceration, lichenoid reactions, and oral hairy leukoplakia can occur due to immunosuppressive drugs. White patches of skin, uremic frost, is due to the collection of urea crystals on the epithelial surfaces following perspiration. These patches are occasionally seen intraorally due to saliva evaporation [39, 45].

Periodontal Disease

Gingival hyperplasia, increased levels of plaque, calculus, gingival inflammation, and increased prevalence and severity of destructive periodontal diseases are common in CKD. Common medications used in CKD such as calcium channel blockers and calcineurin inhibitors can lead to gingival hyperplasia. Gingival overgrowth related to these medications can be severe and may require surgical resection. Improved oral hygiene may decrease the incidence or delay the onset of gingival hyperplasia. Gingival bleeding, petechiae, and ecchymosis result from platelet dysfunction, and they are due to the effects of anticoagulants in CKD patients. Periodontal problems with attachment loss, recession, and deep pockets can occur [39–46].

Orofacial Physical Findings Associated with Specific Nutrient Deficiencies

Malnutrition is a serious problem in CKD, but disordered micronutrient status is less well recognized [47, 48]. CKD predisposes individuals to inadequate intake of vitamins and minerals due to diet recommendations, medication interactions, impaired absorption, altered metabolism, comorbidities, treatments, and excessive loss in urine or dialysate. Risk of micronutrient deficiencies increases with age. Suboptimal intake of micronutrients may also contribute to chronic complications such as cardiovascular disease and inflammation. Many risk factors in CKD contribute both to malnutrition and inadequate micronutrient status. Vitamin and mineral deficiencies are the main concern; however, toxicity of micronutrients or their metabolites are potential issues [49–55].

Diet

Dietary restrictions in CKD aiming to reduce protein, phosphate, or potassium intake may predispose individuals to micronutrient deficiencies. It has been found that micronutrient deficiency in the diet is prevalent in the CKD population [49, 56]. Nutrients with specific relevance to the orofacial region include most B vitamins, as well as vitamins A, D, C, and E. Minerals including calcium, fluoride, iron, and zinc also may demonstrate oral manifestations if deficiency occurs [32, 37].

Absorption

Micronutrient homeostasis is related to normal absorption in the gastrointestinal tract. The majority of water-soluble vitamins are absorbed in the intestine via a specific carrier-mediated process. In animal models of CKD, the expression of carriers for thiamin and folic acid has been shown to be significantly reduced [39, 57]. Intestinal absorption of other water-soluble vitamins, riboflavin, pyridoxine, and biotin is also impacted by CKD. Intestinal losses of these vitamins may be another avenue of compromised micronutrient status [39, 58–60].

Losses

All stages of CKD involve micronutrient losses. In early stages of CKD, micronutrient loss in the urine is due to the use of diuretics as well as limited reabsorption [61, 62]. In ESRD, micronutrients are removed by dialysis. Data are limited on micronutrient losses due to the different types of dialysis, differing supplementation routines, and individual differences [63, 64].

Medications

Medications interact with micronutrient absorption and metabolism. Drugs may directly affect nutrient metabolism, micronutrient homeostasis, or appetite [65, 66].

Micronutrients Most Affected in CKD with Observable Physical Findings

Vitamin C

Loss of vitamin C in a single dialysis treatment is observed to be approximately 28–60% [39, 63, 67–70]. In addition to the loss in dialysis, vitamin C is readily oxidized to dehydroascorbic acid during the dialysis treatment. One concern with vitamin C supplementation is the potential for hyperoxaluria since oxalate is a major metabolite of vitamin C [71]. Oxalate levels in dialysis patients are twice as high as normal and, with supplementation of vitamin C, the level of oxalate in the blood can be as much as seven times higher. Newer advances in renal replacement therapy appear to prevent complications from high blood oxalate levels. In addition to the loss of vitamin C in dialysis, the intake of vitamin C in CKD patients is likely to be low due to potassium restrictions [67]. Vitamin C deficiency is associated with gingival edema and bleeding and loose teeth [32, 72–74].

Thiamin

Thiamin deficiency has been associated with cardiomyopathy or Wernicke's encephalopathy, both traditionally linked to alcoholism. Thiamin deficiency may be the cause of unexplained encephalopathy in the CKD population with the primary symptom being that of disturbed consciousness [75–78]. There does not appear to be data to suggest a thiamin deficiency in the CKD population; however, there is some evidence that this population could be at risk of insufficient or deficient thiamin concentrations [67]. Thiamin deficiency does not typically produce classic oral manifestations [32, 37, 79], although there have been limited reports of appearance of vesicles and ulcerations of the oral mucosa [32, 80].

Pyridoxine

Losses of pyridoxine during dialysis remain controversial; however, mean intake of pyridoxine has been found to be significantly lower than the Dietary Reference Intakes for age and sex. Moreover, serum pyridoxine levels are at suboptimal levels for many [81, 82]. In addition to lower dietary intakes of pyridoxine reported in the CKD population, prescribed medications may interfere with the action or metabolism of pyridoxine and increase the possibility of a deficiency [67]. Symptoms of a pyridoxine deficiency include angular stomatitis, mucosal ulceration, atrophic glossitis, and gingival erythema [32, 72, 79, 80] in addition to a burning tongue [83].

Folic Acid

Folic acid is weakly bound to plasma proteins; therefore, significant loses are observed during dialysis. Plasma concentrations of folic acid have been found to be reduced by 37% after dialysis [64]. Dietary restriction of potassium contributes to a low intake of folate. Medications can also interfere with folic acid [67]. In advanced CKD, altered folic acid metabolism and/or excretion may contribute to low plasma levels and deficiency status [84]. Oral epithelial cells depend on folic acid as it is a cofactor in DNA synthesis [32]. Deficiency of folic acid results in symptoms of angular cheilitis, stomatitis, atrophic glossitis, and burning sensations [32, 33, 37, 79, 85].

Physical Findings Related to Micronutrient Deficiencies

Micronutrient deficiencies are usually described as a single deficiency or as multiple nutrient deficiencies. Table 6.1 reviews some of the nutrition-related clinical and physical changes as a result of micronutrient deficiencies. However, some of these findings may not be diet-related, and other

Table 6.1 Physical findings related to micronutrient deficiencies

	Abnormal physical findings	Possible nutrient deficiency
Skin [10, 11, 17–19, 21–24, 26, 35, 36, 63, 69, 70, 72, 75, 86–91]	Petechiae, bruising	Vitamin C or K
	Skin that appears swollen or red. Blisters or lesions may be evident (dermatitis)	Essential fatty acid Zinc Vitamin B_6, riboflavin, niacin, vitamins A and C
	Scaly, flaky skin (xerosis)	Essential fatty acid, vitamin A
	Pallor	Iron, folate and/or vitamin B_{12}, biotin, copper
Hair [19, 21, 87, 89–91]	Thinning or loss of hair (alopecia), dull/lack luster	Protein, zinc, essential fatty acids, selenium, biotin, copper
	Corkscrew hair	Vitamin C, copper
	Depigmentation	Protein, copper, selenium
Nails [19, 22–24, 89–91]	Spoon-shaped nails (koilonychia)	Iron
	Pale or white nail bed	Vitamins A and C
	Flaky	Magnesium
	Splinter hemorrhage	Vitamin C
	Beau's transverse lines	Protein
Eyes [25, 26]	Pale conjunctiva	Iron, folate, and/or vitamin B_{12}
Orofacial area [32–55, 87, 89–91]	Angular stomatitis Cheilosis	Riboflavin, niacin, vitamin B_6, iron
	Glossitis Magenta tongue	Riboflavin, niacin, vitamins B_6 and B_{12}, folate, and/or iron
	Pallor	Iron
	Bleeding gums and mucosa	Vitamins C and B_{12}
	Taste disturbances	Zinc
	Mouth lesions	Zinc
	Xerostomia	Zinc
	Aphthous stomatitis	Vitamin B_{12}, folate
	Candidiasis	Vitamin C, iron
	Stomatopyrosis Dysesthesia	Iron, vitamin B_{12}, folate, magnesium
	Tooth loss Dental caries	Vitamins B_{12} and C Excessive fermentable carbohydrate intake

factors such as drug-nutrient interactions, nutrient-nutrient interactions, increased requirements, disease process, altered absorption, digestion, metabolism, and excretion of nutrients may contribute to deficiencies.

Conclusion

Confirm abnormal physical findings during the NFPE with the patient's medical history, diet history, medication/supplements interactions, diagnostic testing, and biochemical markers to determine any nutrition-related problems. From this, the RDN can then make the nutrition diagnosis(es) and develop interventions and monitoring plans to address the abnormal findings and/or refer to the appropriate health care practitioners. The NFPE is another tool used to support the nutrition assessment and the care of the patient. As integral members of the interprofessional team caring for patients with CKD,

RDNs incorporate physical findings as part of the comprehensive nutrition assessment to diagnose malnutrition and other nutritional factors that impact food intake.

References

1. Federal Register. Fed Register (41 FR 22501). 3 June 1976.
2. Baker JP, Detsky AS, Wesson DE, Wolman SL, Stewart S, Whitewell J, et al. Nutrition Assessment: a comparison of clinical judgment and objective measurements. N Engl J Med. 1982;306(16):969–72.
3. Detsky AS, McLaughlin JR, Baker JP, Johnston N, Whittaker S, Mendelson RA, et al. What is subjective global assessment of nutritional status? JPEN J Parenter Enteral Nutr. 1987;11(1):8–13.
4. Touger-Decker R. Physical assessment skills for dietetics practice. The past, the present, and recommendations for the future. Top Clin Nutr. 2006;21(3):190–8.
5. Academy of Nutrition and Dietetics. Nutrition care process. https://www.eatrightpro.org/practice/practice-resources/nutrition-care-process. Published 2003. Accessed 30 May 2019.
6. Academy of Nutrition and Dietetics: Revised 2017 Standards of Practice in Nutrition Care and Standards of Professional Performance for Registered Dietitian Nutritionists. https://jandonline.org/article/S2212-2672(17)31625-8/fulltext. Accessed 30 May 2019.
7. Academy of Nutrition and Dietetics: Revised 2015 Standards of Practice and Standards of Professional Performance for Registered Dietitian Nutritionists (Competent, Proficient, and Expert) in Pediatric Nutrition. https://jandonline.org/article/S2212-2672(14)01831-0/fulltext. Accessed 30 May 2019.
8. Academy of Nutrition and Dietetics and National Kidney Foundation: Revised 2014 Standards of Practice and Standards of Professional Performance for Registered Dietitian Nutritionists (Competent, Proficient, and Expert) in Nephrology Nutrition https://jandonline.org/article/S2212-2672(14)00547-4/fulltext. Accessed 30 May 2019.
9. Accreditation Council for Education in Nutrition and Dietetics. Accreditation Council for Education in Nutrition and Dietetics Accreditation Standards. https://www.eatrightpro.org/acend/accreditation-standards-fees-and-policies/2017-standards. Accessed 30 May 2019.
10. Litchford M. Putting the nutrition-focused physical assessment into practice in long-term care. Ann Longterm Care. 2013;21(11):1–12.
11. Kight MA, Kelly MP, Castillo S, Migliore V. Conducting physical examination rounds for manifestations of nutrient deficiency or excess: an essential component of JCAHO assessment performance. Nutr Clin Pract. 1999;14:93–8.
12. Touger-Decker R, Mobley C. Position of the academy of nutrition and dietetics: oral health and nutrition. J Acad Nutr Diet. 2013;113(5):693–01.
13. Aurora P. Chronic kidney disease. 2019. https://emedicine.medscape.com/article/238798-overview#a3. Accessed 30 May 2019.
14. Kuhlmann MKKA, Wittwer M, Horl WH. OPTA- malnutrition in chronic renal failure. Nephrol Dial Transplant. 2007;22(suppl 3):iii13–9.
15. White JV, Guenter P, Jenson G, Malone A, Schofield M. Consensus Statement: Academy of Nutrition and Dietetics and American Society for Parenteral and Enteral Nutrition: characteristics recommended for the identification and documentation of adult malnutrition (undernutrition). JPEN J Parenter Enteral Nutr. 2012;36:275–83.
16. Tappenden KA, Quatrara B, Parkhurst ML, Malone A, Fanjiang G, Ziegler T. Critical role of nutrition in improving quality of care: an interdisciplinary call to action to address adult hospital malnutrition. JPEN J Parenter Enteral Nutr. 2013;37(4):482–97.
17. Eden MH, Khale Y, Napenas JJ. Introduction to oral manifestations of systemic diseases: evaluation of the patient. Atlas Oral Maxillofac Surg Clin North Am. 2017;25:85–92.
18. Scrivani SJ, Spierings ELH. Classification and differential diagnosis of oral and maxillofacial pain. Oral Maxillofac Surg Clin North Am. 2016;28:233–46.
19. Dhaun N, Kluth D. The renal system. In: Innes JA, Dover AR, Fairhurst K, editors. Macleod's clinical examination. 14th ed. New York: Elsevier Ltd; 2018. p. 237–50.
20. National Kidney Foundation Kidney Disease Outcomes Quality Initiative and the Academy of Nutrition and Dietetics clinical practice guidelines for nutrition in chronic kidney disease: 2019 update. Am J Kidney Dis (In press).
21. Finner AM. Nutrition and hair: deficiencies and supplements. Dermatol Clin. 2013;31:167–72.
22. Meuhrcke R. The fingernails in chronic hypoalbuminaemia. Br Med J. 1956;1:1327–8.
23. Lindsay PG. The half-and-half nail. Arch Intern Med. 1967;119:583–7.

24. Tosti A, Baran R, Dawber P. The nails in systemic disease and drug-induced changes. In: DeBerker DAR, Baran R, Dawber RPR, editors. Handbook of diseases of the nails and their management. Osney Mead, Oxford: Blackwell Science; 1995. p. 91.
25. Sheth TN, Choudhry NK, Bowes M, Detsly A. The relation of conjunctival pallor to the presence of anemia. J Gen Intern Med. 1997;12:102–6.
26. LeBlond RF, DeGowin RL, Brown DD, editors. DeGowin's diagnostic examination. 9th ed. San Francisco: McGraw-Hill; 2009.
27. Johansen KL, Lee C. Body composition in chronic kidney disease. Curr Opin Nephrol Hypertens. 2015;24(3):268–75.
28. Secker DJ, Jeejeebboy RN. How to perform subjective global nutritional assessment in children. J Acad Nutr Diet. 2012;112:424–31.
29. Keys A. Caloric undernutrition and starvation, with notes on protein deficiency. J Am Med Assoc. 1948;138(7): 500–11.
30. Fischer M, Jevenn A, Hipskind P. Evaluation for muscle and fat loss as diagnostic criteria for malnutrition. Nutr Clin Pract. 2015;30(2):243–7.
31. Damodara O, Rizk E, Rodriguez J, Lee G. Cranial nerve assessment: a concise guide to clinical examination. Clin Anat. 2014;27:25–30.
32. Tolkachjov SN, Bruce AJ. Oral manifestations of nutritional disorders. Clin Dermatol. 2017;35:441–52.
33. Dreizen S. Oral indications of the deficiency states. Postgrad Med. 1971;49:97–102.
34. Touger-Decker R, Mobley C. Academy of nutrition and dietetics position of the academy of nutrition and dietetics: oral health and nutrition. J Acad Nutr Diet. 2013;113:693–701.
35. Rigassio-Radler D, Lister T. Nutrient deficiencies associated with nutrition-focused physical findings of the oral cavity. Nutr Clin Pract. 2013;28(6):710–21.
36. Jensen GL, Binkley J. Clinical manifestations of nutrient deficiency. JPEN J Parenter Enteral Nutr. 2002;26:S29–33.
37. Thomas DM, Mirowski GW. Nutrition and oral mucosal diseases. Clin Dermatol. 2010;28:426–31.
38. Proctor R, Kumar N, Stein A, Moles D, Porler S. Oral and dental aspects of chronic renal failure. J Dent Res. 2005;84:199–208.
39. Kuravatti S, David MP, Indira AP. Oral manifestations of chronic kidney disease-an overview. Int J Contemp Med Res. 2016;3(4):1149–52.
40. Neville BW, Damm DD, Allen CM. Oral manifestations of systemic diseases. In: Oral and macillofacial pathodogy. 2nd ed. USA: WB Saunders Company; 2012. p. 705–36.
41. Asha V, Latha S, Pai A, Srinivas K, Ganapathy KS. Oral manifestations in diabetic and nondiabetic chronic renal failure patients on hemodialysis. J Indian Acad Oral Med Radiol. 2012;24:274–9.
42. Chuang SF, Sung JM, Kuo SC, Huang JJ, Lee SY. Oral and dental manifestations in diabetic and nondiabetic uremic patients receiving hemodialysis. Oral Surg Oral Med Oral Pathol Oral Radiol Endod. 2005;99:689–95.
43. Kalyvas D, Tosios KI, Leventis MD, Tsiklakis K, Angelopoulos AP. Localized jaw enlargement in renal osteodystrophy: report, a case and review of the literature. Oral Surg Oral Med Oral Pathol Oral Radiol Endod. 2004;97: 68–74.
44. Shaun A, Summers A, Tilakaratne WM, Fortune F, Ashman N. Renal disease and the mouth. Am J Med. 2007;120:568–75.
45. De Rossi SS, Click M. Dental considerations for the patient with renal disease receiving hemodialysis. J Am Dent Assoc. 1996;127:211–9.
46. Craig RG. Interactions between chronic renal disease and periodontal disease. Oral Dis. 2008;14:1–7.
47. Fissell RB, Bragg-Gresham JL, Gillespie BW, Goodkin DA, Bommer J, Saito A, et al. International variations in vitamin prescription and association with mortality in the Dialysis Outcomes and Practice Patterns Study (DOPPS). Am J Kidney Dis. 2004;344:293–9.
48. Tonelli M, Wiebe N, Hemmelgarn B, Klarenbach S, Field C, Manns B, et al. Trace elements in hemodialysis patients: a systematic review and meta-analysis. BMC Med. 2009;7:25.
49. Jankowska M, Rutkowski B, Debska-Slizien A. Vitamins and microelement bioavailability in different stages of chronic kidney disease. Nutrients. 2017;9:282–9.
50. Rutkowski B, Slominska E, Szolkiewicz M, Smolenski RT, Striley C, Rutkowski P, et al. N-methyl-2-pyridoxine-5-carboxamide: a novel uremic toxin? Kidney Int Suppl. 2003;63:S19–21.
51. Coburn SP, Reynolds RD, Mahuren JD, Schaltenbrandd WE, Wang Y, Ericson KL, et al. Elevated plasma 4-pyridoxic acid in renal insufficiency. Am J Clin Nutr. 2002;75:57–64.
52. Bruck K, Stel VS, Gambaro G, Hallan S, Volzke H, Arnlov J, et al. CKD prevalence varies across the European general population. J Am Soc Nephrol. 2016;27:2135–47.
53. Mills KT, Xu Y, Zhang W, Bundy JD, Chen CS, Kelly TN, et al. A systematic analysis of worldwide population-based data on the global burden of chronic kidney disease in 2010. Kidney Int. 2015;88: 950–7.

54. Mendonca N, Hill TR, Granic A, Davies K, Collerton J, Mathers JC, et al. Micronutrient intake and food sources in the very old: analysis of the Newcastle 85+ study. Br J Nutr. 2016;116:751–61.
55. Inzitari M, Doets E, Bartali B, Benetou V, Di Bari M, Visser M, et al. Nutrition in the age-related disablement process. J Nutr Health Aging. 2011;15:599–604.
56. Bossola M, Di Stasio E, Viola A, Leo A, Carlomagno G, Monteburini T, et al. Dietary intake of trace elements, minerals, and vitamins of patients on chronic hemodialysis. Int Urol Nephrol. 2014;46:809–15.
57. Bukhari FJ, Moradi H, Gollapudi P, Ju Kim H, Vaziri ND, Said HM. Effect of chronic kidney disease on the expression of thiamin and folic acid transporters. Nephrol Dial Transplant. 2011;26:2137–44.
58. Vaziri ND, Said HM, Hollander D, Barbari A, Patel N, Dang D, et al. Impaired intestinal absorption of riboflavin in experimental uremia. Nephron. 1985;41:26–9.
59. Barbari A, Vaziri ND, Benavides I, Chen YT, Said H, Pahl MV. Intestinal transport of pyridoxine in experimental renal failure. Life Sci. 1989;45:663–9.
60. Said HM, Vaziri ND, Oveisi F, Hussienzadha S. Effect of chronic renal failure on intestinal transport of biotin in the rat. J Lab Clin Med. 1992;120:471–5.
61. Mydlík M, Derzsiová K, Zemberová E. Influence of water and sodium diuresis and furosemide on urinary excretion of vitamin B(6), oxalic acid and vitamin C in chronic renal failure. Miner Electrolyte Metab. 1999;25:352–6.
62. Larkin JR, Zhang F, Godfrey L, Molostvov G, Zehnder D, Rabbani N, et al. Glucose-induced down regulation of thiamine transporters in the kidney proximal tubular epithelium produces thiamine insufficiency in diabetes. PLoS One. 2012;7:e53175.
63. Sirover WD, Liu Y, Logan A, Hunter K, Benz RL, Prasad D, et al. Plasma ascorbic acid concentrations in prevalent patients with end-stage renal disease on hemodialysis. J Ren Nutr. 2015;25:292–300.
64. Heinz J, Domröse U, Westphal S, Luley C, Neumann KH, Dierkes J. Washout of water-soluble vitamins and of homocysteine during haemodialysis: effect of high-flux and low-flux dialyzer membranes. Nephrology (Carlton). 2008;13:384–9.
65. Jankowska M, Trzonkowski P, Debska-Slizien A, Marszałł M, Rutkowski B. Vitamin B6 status, immune response and inflammation markers in kidney transplant recipients treated with polyclonal anti-thymocyteglobulin. Transplant Proc. 2014;46:2631–5.
66. Jankowska M, Marszałł M, Debska-Slizien A, Carrero JJ, Lindholm B, Czarnowski W, et al. Vitamin B6 and the immunity in kidney transplant recipients. J Ren Nutr. 2013;23:57–64.
67. Steiber AL, Kopple JD. Vitamin status and needs for people with stages 3–5 chronic kidney disease. J Ren Nutr. 2011;21:355–68.
68. Jankowska M, Debska-Slizien A, Łysiak-Szydłowska W, Rutkowski B. Ascorbic acid losses during single hemodialysis session. Ann Acad Med. 2003;33:289–93.
69. Wang S, Eide TC, Sogn EM, Berg KJ, Sund RB. Plasma ascorbic acid in patients undergoing chronic haemodialysis. Eur J Clin Pharmacol. 1999;55:527–32.
70. Bakaev VV, Efremov AV, Tityaev II. Low levels of dehydroascorbic acid in uraemic serum and the partial correction of dehydroascorbic acid deficiency by haemodialysis. Nephrol Dial Transplant. 1999;14:1472–4.
71. Canavese C, Marangella M, Stratta P. Think of oxalate when using ascorbate supplementation to optimize iron therapy in dialysis patients. Nephrol Dial Transplant. 2008;23:1463–4.
72. Jen M, Yan AC. Syndromes associated with nutritional deficiency and excess. Clin Dermatol. 2010;28:669–85.
73. Li R, Byers K, Walvekar RR. Gingival hypertrophy: a solitary manifestation of scurvy. Am J Otolaryngol. 2008;29:426–8.
74. Nishida M, Grossi SG, Dunford RG, Ho AW, Trevisan M, Genco RJ. Dietary vitamin C and the risk for periodontal disease. J Periodontol. 2000;71(8):1215–23.
75. Moradi H, Said HM. Functional thiamine deficiency in end-stage renal disease: malnutrition despite ample nutrients. Kidney Int. 2016;90:252–4.
76. Ueda K, Takada D, Mii A, Tsuzuku Y, Saito SK, Kaneko T, et al. Severe thiamine deficiency resulted in Wernicke's encephalopathy in a chronic dialysis patient. Clin Exp Nephrol. 2006;10:290–3.
77. Barbara PG, Manuel B, Elisabetta M, Giorgio S, Fabio T, Valentina C, et al. The suddenly speechless florist on chronic dialysis: the unexpected threats of a flower shop? Diagnosis: Dialysis related Wernicke encephalopathy. Nephrol Dial Transplant. 2006;21:223–5.
78. Hung SC, Hung SH, Tarng DC, Yang WC, Chen TW, Huang TP. Thiamine deficiency and unexplained encephalopathy in hemodialysis and peritoneal dialysis patients. Am J Kidney Dis. 2001;38:941.
79. Schlosser BJ, Pirigyl M, Mirowski GW. Oral manifestations of hematologic and nutritional diseases. Otolaryngol Clin North Am. 2011;44:183–203vii.
80. Nolan A, McIntosh WB, Allam BF, Lamey PJ. Recurrent aphthous ulceration: vitamin B1, B2, and B6 status and response to replacement therapy. J Oral Pathol Med. 1991;20(8):389–91.
81. Kopple JD, Mercurio K, Blumenkrantz MJ, Jones MR, Tallos J, Roberts C, et al. Daily requirement for pyridoxine supplements in chronic renal failure. Kidney Int. 1981;19(5):694–704.

82. Podda GM, Lussana F, Moroni G, Faloni EM, Lombardi R, Fontana G, et al. Abnormalities of homocysteine and B vitamins in the nephrotic syndrome. Thromb Res. 2007;120(5):647–52.
83. Bapurao S, Raman L, Tullpulle PG. Biochemical assessment of vitamin B6 nutritional status in pregnant women with orolingual manifestations. Am J Clin Nutr. 1982;36:581–6.
84. Hannisdal R, Ueland PM, Svardal A. Liquid chromatography-tandem mass spectrometry analysis of folate and folate catabolites in human serum. Clin Chem. 2009;55:1147–54.
85. Drage LA, Rogers RS III. Clinical assessment and outcome in 70 patients with complaints of burning or sore mouth symptoms. Mayo Clin Proc. 1999;74:223–8.
86. Esper DH. Utilization of nutrition-focused physical assessment in identifying micronutrient deficiencies. Nutr Clin Pract. 2015;30(2):194–202.
87. Walters RW, Grichnik JM. Follicular hyperkeratosis, hemorrhage, and corkscrew hair. Arch Dermatol. 2006;142:658.
88. Ashouria N, Mousdicas N. Pellagra like-dermatitis. N Engl J Med. 2006;354(15):1614.
89. Jankowska M, Szupryczynska N, Debska-Slizien A, Borek P, Kaczkan M, Rutkowski B, Malgorzewicz S. Dietary intake of vitamins in different options of treatment in chronic kidney disease: is there a deficiency? Transplant Proc. 2016;48:1427–30.
90. Holden RM, Vincent K, Morton AR, Clase C. Fat-soluble vitamins in advanced CKD/ESKD: a review. Semin Dial. 2012;25(3):334–43.
91. Tucker BM, Safadi S, Friedman AN. Is routine multivitamin supplementation necessary in US chronic adult hemo-dialysis patients? A systematic review. J Ren Nutr. 2015;25(3):257–64.

Chapter 7
Dietary Assessment in Kidney Disease

Linda W. Moore

Keywords Dietary intake assessment · Dietary record · Food frequency questionnaire · Recommended dietary allowance · Chronic kidney disease · Acute kidney injury · Hemodialysis · Kidney transplantation · Biomarkers

---

Key Points
- An overview of the Dietary Reference Intakes and suggestions that these approaches to dietary intake assessment may have applicability to kidney diseases.
- Historical approaches to dietary intake assessment have provided only moderate correlation to biomarkers of dietary intake.
- Multiple methods and multiple days of dietary intake assessment should be considered when evaluating dietary intake in an individual as well as in groups.

Introduction

Understanding the dietary intake of people with kidney disease is fundamental to addressing their treatment or the prevention or slowing the progression of kidney disease. Several recent guidelines on chronic kidney disease (CKD) vary on recommendations for assessing the dietary intake of patients (Table 7.1) [1–8]. Whether the approach to assessing dietary intake is considered warranted is not discussed in these guidelines, so perhaps it is not an issue of the reliability of dietary intake assessment methods but rather one of the origin of the guidelines. For example, the guidelines from the joint National Kidney Foundation Kidney Disease Outcomes Quality Initiative and the Academy of Nutrition and Dietetics Clinical Practice Guidelines for Nutrition in CKD are written to be multidisciplinary and include guidelines for dietitians [1]. However, many of the other guidelines for CKD are physician-specific, and obtaining the dietary record is not included in their guidelines, perhaps because physicians do not normally collect this information. In contrast, assessment of dietary intake is a significant practice of dietetics, and dietitians routinely evaluate dietary intake in assessing the nutritional status of patients.

L. W. Moore (✉)
Department of Surgery, Houston Methodist Hospital, Houston, TX, USA
e-mail: LWMoore@houstonmethodist.org

© Springer Nature Switzerland AG 2020

J. D. Burrowes et al. (eds.), *Nutrition in Kidney Disease*, Nutrition and Health,
https://doi.org/10.1007/978-3-030-44858-5_7

Table 7.1 Assessment of dietary intake recommended in practice guidelines for chronic kidney disease

Guideline	Publication year	Target population	Targeted nutrients	Recommended assessment methodology
EBPG guideline on Nutrition [2]	2007	Adults requiring maintenance hemodialysis	Protein, energy	Dietary records (24-hr recall, 3- or 7-day food record) or food questionnaires
KDOQI Guideline for Diabetes and CKD [7]	2007	People with diabetes having stages 1–5 CKD	Protein for stages 1–4 CKD	Not specified
Medical Services Commission, British Columbia [6]	2008	Adults ≥19 years of age at increased risk for CKD (diabetes, hypertension, family history of kidney disease, or ethnicity as First Nations, Pacific Islanders, African descent, Asian) or already have CKD	Not specified	Not specified
Chronic Kidney Disease, National Collaborating Centre for Chronic Disease [8]	2008	People with CKD not requiring dialysis or transplant, ≥16 years of age	Potassium, phosphate, protein, calorie, salt intake (unspecified amounts)	Not specified
KDOQI Pediatric Nutrition [3]	2009	Children, stages 2–5 CKD	Protein, energy, vitamins (thiamin, riboflavin, niacin, pantothenic acid, pyridoxine, biotin, cobalamin, ascorbic acid, retinal, a-tocopherol, vitamin K, vitamin D, folic acid), minerals (copper, zinc, calcium, and phosphorus), and amino acids (carnitine)	Not specified
US Department of Veterans Affairs [5]	2014	Adult incident or prevalent patients (not requiring dialysis or transplant) with eGFR 30–60 mL/min having evidence of kidney damage	Protein, potassium, sodium, phosphorus	Food recall records for patients with malnutrition
Academy of Nutrition and Dietetics [4]	2018	Adults, stages 1–5D CKD	Protein, energy	Diet recall (food records or 24-hour recall), FFQ
KDOQI Nutrition in CKD Guideline Work Group [1]	2020	Adults, stages 1–5D CKD	Protein, energy	Interviews and diaries; 24-hr recall, 3-day food record (including one weekend day and/or one dialysis day, if applicable)

Abbreviations: *5D* stage 5 including dialysis, *FFQ* food frequency questionnaire, *KDOQI* Kidney Disease Outcomes Quality Initiative, *GFR* glomerular filtration rate, *EBPG* evidence-based practice guideline, *CKD* chronic kidney disease, *US* United States, *mL/min* milliliters per minute

Purpose and Utility of Dietary Intake Assessment

The intent of dietary intake assessment is to aid in understanding the eating patterns and practices of individuals or groups for education, for nutritional status assessment and disease risk, and for research. As an educational tool, the dietary intake assessment serves as a type of evaluation pre- and post-education or pre- and post-event evaluation (e.g., the diagnosis of disease, occurrence of an acute injury). Soliciting dietary intake information regarding the time prior to the diagnosis of a condition (the diet history) forms a baseline understanding for the educational session—a sort of pretest. Once the education sessions begin, additional dietary intake assessments provide a status of individual or group understanding and food opportunity (the ability to obtain or interest in obtaining or consuming the recommended foods). Fundamental to behavior change is understanding the difference between a food or a food pattern previously practiced and the one being recommended. Dietary intake records help to reinforce the education.

Eating practices and patterns are related to nutritional status and disease risk. The discovery of most vitamins and essential nutrients came about as certain foods were demonstrated to be antidotes to common diseases. For example, citrus fruits for treatment or prevention of scurvy resulted in the knowledge that foods missing from the diet resulted in disease and, ultimately, the discovery of ascorbic acid (vitamin C) as the essential missing nutrient [9, 10]. These discoveries resulted in the assessment of dietary intake as a surrogate for nutritional status. In contrast to missing nutrients, examining dietary intake also provided information on dietary excesses for understanding how foods consumed in excess were contributing to disease conditions (e.g., overweight/obesity, heart disease, diabetes, kidney disease).

Methodology of Dietary Intake Assessment

Dietary intake assessment is performed in different ways. A recollection of food intake may be obtained for either a previous 24-h period (e.g., the 24-h recall) or over a longer period of time (e.g., the Food Frequency Questionnaire (FFQ)). Both of these methods require the person to remember what foods they consumed. Alternatively, a food diary is a prospective food record and may be collected for a period of days or longer. Each method has advantages and disadvantages as well as applicability. Comparing dietary intake to recommended intake will be different with each instrument.

The Food and Nutrition Board of the Institute of Medicine (IOM) joined with Canadian scientists to establish reference values for nutrient intakes of healthy US and Canadian individuals and populations [11]. These reference values replace previous publications of Recommended Dietary Allowances (RDA) used in the USA and Recommended Nutrient Intakes used in Canada and are now referred to as the Dietary Reference Intakes (DRIs). The DRIs are intended for dietary planning [12] and assessment [13] of both individuals and groups and take into account the distribution of nutrient requirements and usual intake. According to the DRIs, the RDA is the dietary intake that would meet the needs of almost all healthy individuals (97–98%) of a particular age or sex. The RDA is based on the estimated average requirement (EAR) and is two standard deviations above the EAR. The EAR is the average daily nutrient intake required to meet the needs of half of the healthy population of a particular age or sex and provides insight into the proportion of a group that will experience inadequate nutrient intake [14]. Assessment of estimated energy requirement (EER) is different from EAR in that the EER is the estimated energy intake (EI) that would be required to maintain body weight (e.g., the body weight of someone who has a body mass index (BMI) between 18.5 and 25 kg/m^2) according to their life stage, sex, and activity level. The adequate intake (AI) is the mean intake of a nutrient or food component in a group of healthy people and is used as a reference when no RDA is available (e.g., dietary fiber or omega-3 fatty acids).

The tolerable upper intake level (UL) of a nutrient has been described as the highest average nutrient intake that is likely to cause no health risk. Another consideration in dietary assessment is the distribution of nutrients. An Acceptable Macronutrient Distribution Range (AMDR) for adults is available for individuals for carbohydrate (45–65% of energy), protein (10–35% of energy), and fat (20–35% of energy). Together, these terms represent the DRIs and provide more than one assessment of dietary intake. For example, assessing whether an individual or a group meet the AI level but exceed the UL is a new opportunity for dietary intake assessment. These terms and definitions represent current guidance on dietary assessment and will be referred to in subsequent sections of this chapter. A description of the tools currently used in dietary intake assessment, how they are analyzed, and where they are applied to DRIs are reviewed below.

24-H Recall

Typically used as a quick assessment of dietary intake, the 24-h recall requires that the individual be able to remember what was consumed on the day prior to the interview day. Memory can be aided by the presence of another family member or someone residing with the person being interviewed. The interviewer who is leading the recall may also utilize prompts to aid in the recall of foods (e.g., time of day, the setting during which the food was consumed) and portion sizes (e.g., visuals such as food models, measuring tools, or representative serving utensils). The 24-h recall is easy to implement and quick to analyze for macronutrients (as described in "Diet Record or Diary" below). It is often used in the clinic or research setting for individuals and for groups.

For a more thorough nutrient analysis, data from the 24-h recall are analyzed by using proprietary nutrient analysis software (see a list of examples in "Diet Record or Diary" section), by entering foods into the free online Nutrient Data Laboratory service from the US Department of Agriculture's Agricultural Research Library [15], or by using food lists such as the "Choose Your Foods: Food Lists for Diabetes" from the Academy of Nutrition and Dietetics (Academy) [16]. An example of the use of the Academy's lists of Food Choices is shown in Tables 7.2 and 7.3. The lists of food choices contain crude estimates of macronutrient distribution across foods by grouping the foods into categories (e.g., starch, fruit, dairy, non-starchy vegetables, meats and meat substitutes, and fats). Combination foods (e.g., lasagna, casseroles, desserts) are accounted for by including all the food groups represented by the combination food. Another method of collecting and analyzing the 24-h recall is the automated, self-administered 24-h recall (ASA24®) reviewed below [17].

Automated Multiple-Pass Method

A method for collecting a 24-h recall from in-person interviews or over the telephone is the computerized Automated Multiple-Pass Method (AMPM) [18, 19]. The process of the AMPM incorporates five discussions called "passes" of foods consumed the previous day (Fig.7.1) [19]. First, the participant is asked for a *quick list* of all foods eaten the previous day; a series of questions are then asked to probe for potential *forgotten foods* (such as snacks, nonalcoholic beverages, sweets). The third pass is a series of questions regarding the *time and occasion* that foods were eaten, and it is used to sort foods into groups by eating occasion. The fourth pass is a *detailed review* of the foods to obtain descriptions and amounts and also to include additions to the foods. The fifth and *final review* is another opportunity to list foods not recalled earlier.

Incorporating the system into a computer model has allowed the interview to be automated, and it standardizes the probing methods. According to Raper et al., the AMPM contains more than 2400 questions, 21,000 response options, and 500,000 potential pathways [19]. The system allows for pre-filled responses, which reduces the interviewer and respondent burden if an item was detailed in the first (*quick list*) pass. For example, identifying the type of juice as orange would not require that information to be asked in the fourth (*detailed* review) pass. Instead, the *detailed* review pass could focus on identifying whether the item was 100% juice and if it was calcium-fortified. The AMPM has been used in the National Health and Nutrition Examination Survey (NHANES) since 2001 and is administered by trained interviewers [20].

The Automated Self-Administered 24-H Recall (ASA24®)

Collaborations between the United States Department of Agriculture (USDA), the National Cancer Institute, and Baylor College of Medicine (Houston, TX) have transformed the AMPM methodology into an Internet-based automated self-administered 24-h recall (ASA24®) [17, 21]. The tool is available on the National Cancer Institute's website [17]. Respondents are guided by the ASA24 through the five

Table 7.2 Crude dietary analysis spreadsheet for total kilocalories, carbohydrate, protein, and fat using food groups to estimate intake

	A	B	C	D	E	F	G
1	a	Starch	Fruit	Milk[b]	Nonstarch-vegetable	Meat/substitute[c]	Fat
2	Breakfast						
3							
4	Lunch						
5							
6	Dinner						
7							
8	Snack						
9							
10	*Total*	=Sum(B2:B9)	=Sum(C2:C9)	=Sum(D2:D9)	=Sum(E2:E9)	=Sum(F2:F9)	=Sum(G2:G9)
11							
12		Carbohydrate	Protein	Fat			
13	Grams	=(15*B10) + (15*C10) + (12*D10) + (5*E10)	=(2*B10) + (8*D10) + (2*E10) + (7*F10)	=(0.5*B10) + (2*F10) + (5*G10)			
14	kcal	=4*B13	=4*C13	=9*D13			
15	Total kcal	=Sum(B14:D14)					
16	kcal%	=(B14/B15)*100	=(C14/B15)*100	=(D14/B15)*100			
17	Keep ratio at:[d]	50–55%	15–20%	30% or less			

Adapted with permission from the Academy of Nutrition and Dietetics, Choose Your Foods: Lists for Diabetes, Copyright 2014

[a]To activate this table in a spreadsheet, select cells A1:H16, copy and paste into spreadsheet software; remove the * in cell A1 after pasting. Add the number of servings of each food group at each meal time (e.g., see Table 7.1) and then read the results in rows 13–16

[b]Assumes nonfat milk product is used. If milk product with fat is used, an equivalent number of fat exchanges should be added to column H for that meal

[c]Assumes a lean meat exchange is used. If a higher fat content is used, an equivalent number of fat exchanges should be added to column H for that meal

[d]Recommended levels to use as reference. Adjust as desired; not linked to any formulae

Table 7.3 Example of crude dietary analysis spreadsheet for total kilocalories, carbohydrate, protein, and fat using food groups to estimate intake and showing number of food servings or choices for each food group listed by meal category

	A	B	C	D	E	F	G
1		Starch	Fruit	Milk	Nonstarch vegetable	Meat/substitute	Fat
2	Breakfast	2	1	1	0	1	2
3							
4	Lunch	3	2	1	2	2	2
5							
6	Dinner	3	2	0	2	3	3
7							
8	Snack	1	1	0.5	0	0	0
9							
10	*Total*	9	6	2.5	4	6	7
11							
12		Carbohydrate	Protein	Fat			
13	Grams	275	88	52			
14	kcal	1100	352	464			
15	Total kcal	1916					
16	kcal%	57	18	24			
17	Keep ratio at	50–55%	15–20%	30% or less			

Adapted with permission from the Academy of Nutrition and Dietetics, Choose Your Foods: Lists for Diabetes, Copyright 2014

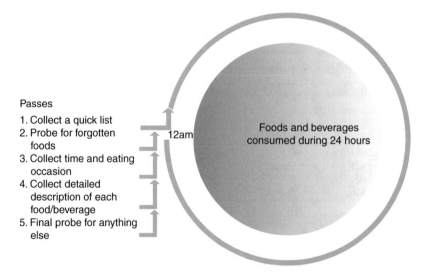

Passes
1. Collect a quick list
2. Probe for forgotten foods
3. Collect time and eating occasion
4. Collect detailed description of each food/beverage
5. Final probe for anything else

12am

Foods and beverages consumed during 24 hours

Fig.7.1 The steps in obtaining a 24-h dietary intake using the Automated Multiple-Pass Method, from midnight to midnight on the previous day

passes of the AMPM with over 10,000 food pictures of eight different portion size equivalents. An optional module for collecting dietary supplement information is also available on the portal. The ASA24 consists of two portals: one for respondents where both English and Spanish tools are located and a researcher portal where data analyses are available. The software is freely available to researchers, clinicians, and students [17]. The automation of the ASA24 eases the ability to obtain and analyze a 24-h dietary recall utilizing the proven accuracy of the AMPM. Researchers recently compared the ASA24 to the interviewer-led AMPM in over 1000 participants from three healthcare systems across the USA [22]. They found equivalency between the two dietary recall methods with participants favoring the ASA24.

The dietary intake data captured by the ASA24® are analyzed based on the Food and Nutrient Database for Dietary Surveys (FNDDS) from the Agricultural Research Service of the USDA [15]. The FNDDS is used to analyze the data from the *What We Eat in America* survey [23], which is the source of dietary intake information used for the NHANES [24]. The FNDDS is a database of nutrient values from foods based on the USDA National Nutrient Database for Standard Reference and is updated approximately every 2 years in association with the NHANES survey. The researcher portal of the ASA24 is designed for professional users (researchers, clinicians, educators) and allows them to set parameters for a study or series and obtain dietary analyses [17]. The professional then reports the results to respondents.

Food Frequency Questionnaire

A FFQ may be considered an adaptation of the diet history. It is typically a general list of structured questions aimed at eliciting food items commonly or uncommonly consumed and settings where foods are consumed in order to obtain a sense of usual food intake. A FFQ may also be aimed at elucidating special or specific foods or food groups, depending on the purpose of the questionnaire. FFQs are widely used by epidemiologists in large cohort studies due to their ease of use and their ability to reduce variance across individual participants and because they are relatively inexpensive to implement. Additionally, compared to diet records, the FFQ is noted to be more applicable when evaluating specific food intakes than the diet record, which may be more suitable to evaluating nutrient intakes [25, 26]. Two of the most commonly used FFQs were developed separately by Block [27, 28] and Willett [29, 30] and have been used in many epidemiologic trials. Many FFQs are adaptations of the Block or Willett designs.

Block FFQ

The Block FFQ was developed with data obtained from 24-h recalls collected in NHANES II [27, 31]. The food items selected for the FFQ were based on the contribution of foods represented in the 24-h recalls and the energy represented by those foods. Portion sizes from the 24-h recalls were used to represent the portion sizes offered in the FFQ as "small," "medium," or "large." The Block FFQ was used in the Women's Health Trial Feasibility Study. Three 4-day diet records that were collected during a 1-year period prior to administration of the FFQ were compared with the Block FFQ [28]. Correlations ranged from 0.5 to 0.7 between the 24-h recalls and the FFQ [27, 28]. The Block Health Habits and History Questionnaire is another version of the full-length Block FFQ that contains approximately 100 food items [31].

Diet History Questionnaire

The Diet History Questionnaire (DHQ), which was developed by the National Cancer Institute, is based on the Block FFQ where some of the questions were redesigned using a cognitive evaluation of the question format and grouping [32]. The DHQ has been compared to both the Block FFQ and Willett FFQ [33], and it appears to perform similarly with regard to assessing diet-disease risk.

However, the DHQ and Block FFQ may provide better information on absolute intakes than the Willett FFQ. Yet, in a biomarker study measuring doubly labeled water (a biomarker for energy expenditure) and urinary nitrogen excretion (a biomarker for protein intake), the DHQ was shown to underestimate dietary energy and protein intakes [34, 35]. Currently, the DHQ (DHQIII) is a questionnaire that consists of 135 food items and 26 dietary supplement questions that may be used to assess dietary intake over the previous year (with or without portion size information) or over the past month (with or without portion size estimates) [36].

Willett FFQ

The Willett FFQ (or the Harvard Food Frequency Questionnaire) was designed to provide a simple method for ranking the intake of food items representative of dietary intake over the previous year [29] and has been used in the Nurses' Health Study [30, 37] and the Health Professionals Follow-Up Study [38, 39]. The validation of the Willett FFQ has been performed by comparing results of two FFQ reports taken at 1-year intervals to two 7-day diet records completed within approximately 2–3 months of the FFQ [26, 39]. Correlation between the diet record and the Willett FFQ ranged from 0.5 to 0.7[26, 30, 39].

FFQ Data Analysis

The portion size of a food consumed is multiplied by the frequency of consumption to obtain the nutrient totals in the FFQs. Totals are generally reported as an amount per period (often standardized to estimate daily consumption equivalents or monthly consumption equivalents). Many FFQs have also been adapted to provide information on how the foods consumed apply to food guidance such as MyPyramid (reported as MyPyramid equivalents per day), the Healthy Eating Index, the Overall Nutrition Quality Index, a prudent vs. Western dietary pattern, servings of food in food groups, or other guidelines, as applicable [26, 36, 40–43].

Diet Record or Diary

The diet record or diary is a prospective record of food consumed. The participant records food and beverage intake throughout the day as the food is consumed, preferably at the end of each meal or snack. The record is maintained on paper or electronic device/system, and it is usually submitted to a reviewer after an agreed number of days' collection. Multiple-day diet records are used for both dietary intake assessments and as a self-monitoring tool for dietary intervention programs [44, 45]. Attainment of dietary goals has been improved by participant engagement in diet record keeping [45–50].

To confirm the accuracy of the content, a professional with expertise in diets, such as a registered dietitian, dietetic technician, or trained dietary interviewer, usually reviews the diet record. Similar to the methods used in the 24-h recall, the reviewer will typically query the participant on portion size, the content of combination foods (e.g., Was the lasagna vegetable, beef, or turkey?), more detail on foods that might be more than the standard food item (e.g., Was the orange juice fortified with calcium?), or how the food was prepared (e.g., Was the food prepared at home or purchased at a restaurant?). The amount of time spent on the review process will depend on the goal for the record keeping. If the goal is weight loss or gain, then a review that would provide information on macronutrient intake will suffice and could be as simple as that outlined in Tables 7.2 and 7.3 where the evaluation is only of food choices and number of servings to calculate macronutrient content. These tables are based on the Academy's and the American Diabetes Association publication series "Choose Your Foods" which are food lists for meal planning that can be used for teaching patients with diabetes, kidney disease, or weight management needs [16]. Table 7.2 depicts the formulaic layout in a type of spreadsheet software for tracking the number of food choices and resulting macronutrients of an individual's daily intake. Table 7.3 depicts the appearance of the spreadsheet once the data have been entered. These tables are provided for readers to develop a quick-analysis tool using the formulae and layout shown in Table 7.2.

Alternatively, if the goal is to assess dietary intake of a micronutrient (e.g., sodium, potassium, or phosphorus), the review process may be more detailed. Analyses of these data may require proprietary computer software, such as that available from Food Processor (ESHA Research, Salem, OR) [51], FoodWorks (The Nutrition Company, Long Valley, NJ) [52], NutriBase (CyberSoft, Phoenix, AZ) [53], andNutritionistPro™ (Axxya Systems, Stafford, TX) [54], or accessing the free Nutrient Data Laboratory service from the US Department of Agriculture's Agricultural Research Library [15]. Another variable in choosing the diet record analysis methodology is the setting or purpose of the diet record. Working with an individual or with groups or on a research project will contribute to the decision on which systems to use for analysis as well as the methodology.

Currently, most of the proprietary nutrient analysis software programs provide comparison to the DRIs or the ability to program for DRI assessment. As shown in the "Application of Dietary Intake Assessment to Dietary Guidelines" section, this evaluation requires a computational approach and is an excellent addition to professional nutrition software programs. As more is learned about the DRIs and how to apply them, demand for these features will likely increase. What is not available from the professional nutrition software programs is the ability for clients to enter their food intake into a mobile application that links back to the professional software used by the nutrition practitioner. Currently, only the ASA24® provides that capability.

Application of Dietary Intake Assessment to Dietary Guidelines

Dietary Intake Assessment of Individuals

As indicated in previous sections of this chapter, assessing usual dietary intake is challenging and varies by the method used and frequency of assessment. Multiple records appear to be more informative than one method or record alone. Assessments of usual intake should include variations on the day of the week to account for day-to-day variability. Likewise, assessments should exclude holidays or special occasions because individuals tend to eat differently on these special days.

In the individual setting, estimating that the probability an individual is consuming a diet that is within their target level can be accomplished by comparing the EAR to the individual's mean and standard deviation (SD) of usual intake of the nutrient [13]. This concept is illustrated for dietary protein, phosphorus, and magnesium intake in Table 7.4 [55]. It is not recommended to use the RDA as a measure of nutrient intake adequacy because intakes below the RDA cannot be assumed to be inadequate for an individual [13]. This is partly because the RDA exceeds the actual requirement for all individuals except 2–3% of the population.

If an individual's mean usual intake of a nutrient is largely different than the median requirement (the EAR) and the difference is positive, then it may be assumed that the individual's intake of that nutrient is adequate (or inadequate if the difference is largely negative). A rule of thumb recom-

Table 7.4 Examples of dietary protein, phosphorus, and magnesium intake for healthy adult (19–70+ years of age) men and women and the probability that the dietary intake is adequate

Protein intake (g/kg/day)[a]	Phosphorus intake (mg/day)	Magnesium—men (mg/day)[b]	Magnesium—women (mg/day)[b]	z-Score[c]	Probability of adequacy (%)[d]
0.50	461	278	210	−2.06	2
0.53	485	293	222	−1.64	5
0.56	506	305	231	−1.28	10
0.58	520	314	237	−1.04	15
0.62	549	331	251	−0.53	30
0.66	580	350	265	0	50[d]
0.74	640	386	293	1.04	70
0.76	654	395	299	1.28	85
0.79	675	407	308	1.64	95
0.82	699	422	320	2.06	98[e]

[a]Without additional amino acid supplements
[b]The age group for magnesium represented in the table is 31–70+ years
[c]z-Score represents the standard deviation (SD) units above or below the mean and is calculated for these data using the following equation: z = (estimated dietary intake − EAR)/SD, where EAR is the estimated average requirement of the nutrient. SD units for these nutrients are provided in the Dietary Reference Intakes: The Essential Guide to Nutrient Requirements [55]
[d]The 50% probability of adequacy is the EAR for the nutrient and represents the amount required by half of the healthy population in the age and sex group represented in the table. Dietary protein and phosphorus requirements are not different between males and females
[e]Represents two SDs above the EAR and is considered the recommended dietary allowance (RDA) that would meet the needs of almost all (97–98%) of the age and sex group represented in the table

mended by the IOM is that, for individuals, intakes below the EAR *need to be increased* and those between the EAR and the RDA *probably should be increased* [13, 56]. A more detailed description of this approach and guidance on the approach for nutrients for which no EAR has been established is available from the IOM's Dietary Guidelines website [11, 13] and a recent practice paper of the Academy [56].

Dietary Intake Assessment of Groups

The dietary intake of groups of people is important on many levels. From a public health level, the dietary intake of a population (e.g., a country, city, community, school, household; members of healthcare provider groups; people having a medical diagnosis; people having a particular lifestyle) can provide information relevant to planning for food supply needs, healthcare needs and risks, and programs to improve healthcare outcomes. Nonetheless, retrieving such dietary intake information on groups is difficult. In the USA, the NHANES provides extensive information on the dietary intake of the noninstitutionalized US population, and it has served as the reference resource for the DRIs [11]. The survey is also capable of providing information on the dietary intake of groups of people with certain medical conditions, but the analytical methodology is critical to obtaining the most accurate information.

To estimate the proportion of a group that is below the DRI, dietary intake information from more than 1 day is required because the distribution of intakes will vary between individuals and between days. In NHANES, for example, it is possible to evaluate the mean dietary intake or the dietary intake from a single 24-h recall. The dietary data are collected on multiple days of the week, and the large sample sizes available account for between-subject variability. This information may provide insight into the dietary intake of a group of people (e.g., an age group, a socio-economic group, a group with a certain medical condition), but it is not possible to evaluate how the group compares to the DRIs without evaluating the usual intake of the group. To estimate the usual intake of a group from the NHANES data, both days of the dietary intake record are required [57, 58]. The recommendation for a minimum of 2 nonconsecutive days to estimate the usual dietary intake is based on the need to account for the within-subject variability that is common for individuals.

In general, whether using the NHANES data or developing new dietary intake data, 2 or 3 consecutive days of dietary intake are recommended for estimating the usual intake of a group [13, 59]. The distribution of intake should be part of the dietary assessment technique. Since the spread or distribution of usual intake of most nutrients is wider than the distribution of the requirement, it is not appropriate to compare the mean of the usual intake to the mean of the requirement. Comparing means would result in an overestimation of the group proportion who are consuming adequate or inadequate (e.g., the tail probabilities) nutrients. Methods used for handling the issues of distribution have been described by the National Research Council [60], the Iowa State University [57], and also a webinar series hosted by the National Cancer Institute [58]. These methods vary slightly from each other, but each indicates that the inter- and intrasubject variability, as well as the range of distribution of the nutrient requirement, must be accounted for when making comparisons to other groups, to the DRIs or other clinical guidelines, or to a health condition. The EAR cut-point method, recommended by the IOM and the National Research Council, is one example that can be applied when the variability of the intake of the nutrient is ≤60% [55]. This method is illustrated in Table 7.4 for dietary protein, phosphorus, and magnesium intake.

Murphy et al. have outlined precautions important for dietary assessment of groups [61]. These precautions include:

- Avoid comparing group mean intake to the RDA because the prevalence of inadequacy would be missed; it is essential to know about the tail probabilities.
- Avoid comparing the mean intake of a group to the EAR because 50% would have an inadequate intake. It is better to compare the distribution of intakes to determine the proportion of a group below the EAR—the prevalence of inadequacy.
- Use multiple, nonconsecutive-day dietary intake information and adjust for variability [58, 61].
- Use validated dietary intake collection methods to avoid systematic errors [56, 58, 61].

Evidence

Whether dietary intake assessment tools can provide accurate results has been tested by several methods, some of which are listed here and discussed below:

- Direct observation—performed with participants housed in a research or similar setting, receiving prepared and tare-weighed meals compared to self-reported records of what was consumed
- Comparison of one dietary assessment tool to another
- Evaluation of subgroups to determine if characteristics identify those more or less likely to accurately record or recall their intake
- Comparison of the dietary intake assessment tool to a biomarker or series of biomarkers

Assessment of the 24-H Recall, the AMPM

The AMPM was validated in men and women, in different ethnicities, and for macronutrients as well as many micronutrients [62–68]. Conway et al. [62] measured macronutrient intake from a single 24-h dietary recall using the AMPM and compared reported intake to direct observation of intake in 45 men between the ages of 21 and 65 years with a mean BMI of 27.6 kg/m^2 (range, 20.8–39.2 kg/m^2). No relationship was demonstrated between BMI and precision of the dietary recall ($r^2 = 0.01$, $p = 0.44$). Observed EI from protein was 14.4 ± 0.4% compared to recall at 14.3 ± 0.4%. Mean total EI observed was 3294 ± 111 kcal/day compared to recall at 3541 ± 124 kcal/day.

A similar study design was used by Conway et al. [63] to evaluate the accuracy of a single 24-h dietary recall of women. A group of 49 women, ages 21–63 years, with mean BMI of 29.7 kg/m^2 (range, 20.0–44.6 kg/m^2) were included in the analysis. The observed EI from protein was 15.9 ± 0.6% compared to recall at 15.6 ± 0.6% ($p < 0.02$). Mean total observed EI was 2214 ± 91 kcal compared to recall 2376 ± 91 kcal ($p < 0.05$). These investigators found that the actual intake of women was within 10% of the recalled intake 95% of the time. They concluded that the AMPM was an accurate method for 24-h recall of dietary intake.

Rumpler et al. [67] utilized the AMPM in 12 healthy volunteers to evaluate the degree of reporting error (under- or overreporting) in two 24-h recalls. They assumed the difference between the reported (AMPM) and measured food intake as bias and were interested in determining both the average and variance in bias. The group mean difference in AMPM and measured food intake was found to be similar, but individual differences were observed. For example, the absolute within-person difference in reporting error averaged 18% for protein, 23% for carbohydrate, and 15% for fat. They concluded that group estimates of macronutrients contained small average bias using the AMPM, but estimates for individuals may contain significant bias and be less accurate. These investigators proposed that some of the bias may be related to how foods are grouped in the AMPM analysis and that foods producing the greatest reporting error might be adjusted in the analysis.

Assessment of the FFQ

Studies performed to test the comparability of FFQs have shown that the FFQs correlate modestly with each other but vary on their correlations with the 24-h recall or the diet record. Wirfalt et al. [68] determined that the energy-adjusted correlation coefficient between a reduced Block FFQ and the mean of three 24-h recalls was 0.47 for dietary fat and carbohydrate intake, but not for the Willett FFQ. Likewise, neither FFQ appeared to be associated with the 24-h dietary recall for protein intake. Subar et al. [33] compared the DHQ, Block FFQ, and Willet FFQ to each other and to four 24-h recalls. In this study, the DHQ and the Block FFQ correlated moderately with the 24-h recalls ($r = 0.5$), but the Willett FFQ correlation to the 24-h recall was about 0.3–0.4. After adjusting to EI, all three of the FFQs had correlations of 0.5–0.6 with the 24-h recall [33].

Comparison of the Willet FFQ to a 7-day diary indicated a correlation of approximately 0.3 for energy and protein between the two dietary intake assessment tools, which did not change significantly when the data were energy adjusted (Spearman's $\rho \approx 0.34$) [69]. However, when the low-energy reporters were excluded, the correlation between the two tools decreased significantly (Spearman's $\rho = 0.22$).

Use of Biomarkers in Assessing Dietary Intake

A biomarker has been defined as "a characteristic that is objectively measured and evaluated as an indicator of normal biological processes, pathogenic processes, or pharmacologic responses to a therapeutic intervention" [70]. Biomarkers are recognized as useful in clinical trials for measuring efficacy and, as such, play an important role in research as well as in clinical management. Dietary biomarkers serve as indicators of response to dietary intake and have been used to measure the accuracy of dietary intake assessment [71, 72]. Similar to the issues relating biomarkers to drug metabolism, the correlation of biological levels (e.g., from tissue, blood, urine) of a dietary biomarker is dependent on individual variations in dietary intake, in the nutrient's kinetic action, nutrient–nutrient interactions, biomarker selection, biomarker sample collection, analytic methods, accuracy of the dietary intake assessment tools and of dietary composition tables, and statistical handling of the data [35, 72–74].

A biomarker is often considered a "gold standard"—however, the application of particular biomarkers to dietary intake assessment must be well quantified and understood. For example, the use of urine urea nitrogen (UUN) excretion is considered the biomarker for dietary protein intake (DPI). However, the use of UUN should also account for kidney function because the clearance of urea in people with kidney disease (not just kidney failure) is altered. Adjusting for this variation, however, is possible [75, 76] and increases the applicability for comparing UUN excretion to DPI in the population.

Doubly Labeled Water and Urine Urea Nitrogen for Assessment of Dietary Energy and Protein Intake

The AMPM and DHQ were used to assess dietary measurement error in the Observing Protein and Energy Nutrition (OPEN) study [34, 35]. Subjects ($n = 484$), aged 40–69, had three in-person visits over a period of 3 months where they completed the DHQ twice, provided two 24-h recalls (one at visit 1 and again at visit 3), were dosed with doubly labeled water at visit 1, and completed two 24-h urine collections between visits 1 and 2 (9 days apart). Doubly labeled water is used to determine total energy expenditure (TEE), and UUN excretion is used to determine protein catabolism. In this study, approximately 21% of men and women were underreporters of EI using the 24-h recall (the AMPM), and 49% were underreporters using the DHQ. Similarly, about 12% were underreporters of DPI using the AMPM, and 35% were underreporters using the DHQ. Underreporting of EI increased as BMI increased in both men and women but was less in the AMPM vs. the DHQ and was not apparent for DPI in the AMPM. These data suggest a greater accuracy of the AMPM than the DHQ for assessing dietary intake, that underreporting is present in about 21% of subjects, and that underreporting increases at higher BMIs.

To further evaluate the ability of the AMPM to be used in large, diverse samples, Moshfegh et al. [77] studied 525 people between the ages of 30 and 69 years, with a BMI range of 18–44, over a 7-week period. They compared the reported EI to TEE by using the doubly labeled water technique. The protocol consisted of three 24-h dietary recalls (one in-person interview and two telephone follow-up interviews interspersed across a 2-week period), one in-person visit where doubly labeled water was consumed, two more in-person visits where urine samples were collected, and a final in-person visit where resting energy expenditure (REE) was measured. The EI/TEE was 100% in normal weight men and 94% in normal weight women. However, as weight increased (overweight to obese), this ratio decreased: 86% and 80%, respectively, in men and 85%

and 79%, respectively, in women. More overweight and obese participants were found to be low EI reporters (19.4% and 34.0% of men, 24.7% and 35.3% of women). The EI/REE was a mean of 1.43 for the sample with an average physical activity level of 1.61 (95% CI: 1.15, 2.25). The investigators concluded that the AMPM is valid for evaluation of EI in group samples and extrapolation to the population level. They postulated that the reported EI by overweight and obese individuals could be accurate but not reflective of TEE due to eating less on the days of 24-h recall since the subjects knew the schedule of the interview visits. Further studies need to be performed in overweight and obese subjects to improve the reporting or interpretation of reported dietary intake in these subgroups.

Association of Urinary Sodium Levels with Dietary Intake

The AMPM was compared to 24-h urine sodium in a group of 465 healthy adult men and women, aged 30–69 years, and found to have a mean reporting accuracy ≥0.85 in all sub-groupings. In this study, the dietary sodium intake collected using the AMPM was compared to a 24-h urine collected for the same time period. The accuracy of dietary sodium intake reports in men was a mean of 0.93 (95% CI, 0.89–0.97) and in women was a mean of 0.90 (95% CI, 0.87–0.90). Younger women (30–49 years old) had a slightly lower reporting accuracy (0.85; 95% CI, 0.81–0.90), while older women (50–69 years old) had a reporting accuracy of 0.95 (95% CI, 0.90–1.01). The high correlation between the AMPM and 24-h urinary sodium in this study implies that the AMPM is an accurate estimate of dietary sodium intake in healthy adult men and women. Adjustments for level of kidney function have not been studied to determine if the 24-hour urine would accurately reflect dietary sodium intake in people with CKD. Furthermore, recent discovery of sodium reservoirs in the skin suggest the urinary sodium output may be altered by this phenomenon [78]. To date, no clinical methods for detecting the skin-sodium reserve have been developed.

Plasma Ascorbic Acid, Carotenoids, and Vitamin A Levels for Assessing Dietary Intake

Evaluation of antioxidant status has used blood levels of vitamins C, E, and A to reflect dietary and/or supplement use [79]. However, the correlation of these nutrients to dietary intake is only modest. Correlation coefficients of 0.12–0.53 for blood levels of vitamin C and 0.1–0.5 for blood levels of carotenoids to dietary intake are typical [72, 79, 80], even when combined as integrated biomarkers [81].

Association of Serum Uric Acid Levels and Urinary Isoflavones with Dietary Intake

NHANES III (1988–1994) was used by Choi et al. [82] to evaluate the association of serum uric acid levels with dietary intake. They noted a positive association of serum uric acid level with increasing intake of meats and seafood and a negative association with increased intake of dairy foods. Similarly, the NHANES (1999–2002) was used to demonstrate that urinary isoflavone levels could be used as a biomarker of isoflavone intake [83]. Adults reporting an average consumption of 3.1 mg/day of dietary isoflavone had a geometric mean urinary isoflavone concentration of 5.0 ng/mL.

Applications to Kidney Disease Settings

Dietitians working in kidney disease in the late 1970s and 1980s had a unique opportunity to learn about the usefulness of dietary intake assessment. A first-of-its-kind national study was taking place in the relatively newly funded end-stage renal disease program. The National Cooperative Dialysis Study (NCDS) was funded to determine the effect of dialysis prescription on patient morbidity [84]. The NCDS is most renowned for the measurement and monitoring of the dialysis prescription (evolved to what is currently referred to as Kt/V) and its adequacy. But dietitians involved in the NCDS learned something in addition to monitoring the dialysis prescription—they learned how to monitor the dietary protein prescription. Dietitians working in the NCDS and hemodialysis units at this time were uniquely afforded an in-depth understanding of the intake and metabolism of dietary protein in people receiving chronic hemodialysis [75, 85]. These dietitians also learned that assessing DPI of dialysis patients is similar to pharmacokinetics. How so? Pharmacokinetics is basically a measurement of the time required for a drug to appear in the blood and its rate of disappearance. The NCDS was monitoring how urea nitrogen was removed (the rate of disappearance) from the blood by dialysis and re-accumulated (the rate of appearance) between dialysis sessions [84]. In stable patients, the accumulation of urea nitrogen between dialysis sessions was the result of dietary nitrogen intake. So, even in people with no kidney function (and, therefore, no measureable urinary nitrogen excretion), it was possible to determine the DPI. This process became known as urea kinetics and protein catabolic rate (PCR) [84–86]. Researchers had the gold standard for DPI assessment in people with kidney disease—a biomarker.

As will be described in the sections below, the DPI of patients with kidney disease has been assessed in multiple reports and related to the PCR. However, no statistical adjustments for the distribution of the DPI or PCR have been described to date in the CKD population, and both DPI and PCR are known to have inter- and intrasubject variability. Only group-mean comparisons were available in the reports shown. Additionally, the EI comparison to basal metabolic rate (BMR) or to REE has rarely been described in this population.

The recommended dietary intake of people with kidney disease differs for some nutrients from that of healthy individuals [1, 4, 55]. Guidelines for kidney disease are based on the level of kidney function and the type of treatment for kidney replacement therapy [1, 4, 87]. Dietary assessment approaches as well as some recommendations follow in the sections below.

Acute Kidney Injury

Patients with acute kidney injury (AKI) are at risk for being in a hypercatabolic state, usually due to the underlying disease [88–91]. According to the Kidney Disease: Improving Global Outcomes (KDIGO) AKI work group, AKI is defined as an increase in serum creatinine ≥0.3 mg/dL within 48 h or increase in serum creatinine ≥1.5 times the baseline that is known to have occurred within the previous 7 days or a decrease in urine volume < 0.5 mL/kg/h over 6 h [87]. AKI can be present well before acute kidney failure (AKF) occurs where renal replacement therapy (RRT) will be required. This is important because the dietary intake of people with early or milder AKI (e.g., not requiring RRT) may have a critical impact on their outcome. Additionally, a report on 309 cases of AKF indicated that approximately 58% of the cases demonstrated moderate to severe malnutrition at the time of the AKF diagnosis, that 57% of the cases were housed in the medical ward of the hospital (compared to 43% in intensive care units), and that compromised nutritional status was associated with increased mortality in these cases [92]. Once the patient requires nutrition support, while important to provide adequate protein, energy, vitamins, and minerals to attenuate the hypercatabolism, the dietary intake assessment per se becomes an evaluation of the nutrition support provided and not the oral dietary intake. At this juncture, adjustments for kidney function and/or kidney replacement therapy should be applied. This situation warrants evaluating the biomarkers of protein and energy metabolism to determine if adequate support is being provided [90, 91, 93]. Recent practice guidelines for AKI make four recommendations related to nutrition, but no recommendation was made regarding assessment of the adequacy of nutrition support [87].

Chronic Kidney Disease

CKD encompasses the reduced or mild kidney dysfunction described by the NKF [94] as stages 1 and 2 (or where solute filtration may be adequate but kidney damage is present from nephrocalcinosis or microalbuminuria, for example), moderate CKD (stages 3a and 3b [95], where kidney function is ~30–60% of normal), and severe CKD (stages 4 and 5, where kidney function is <30% of normal or where dialysis or a kidney transplant is required to sustain life). These descriptions of the levels or stages of kidney function provide insight into the changes that might be necessary for altering dietary intake. The stages also identify that the assessment techniques will vary and become more complex as CKD advances.

Nondialysis CKD

A review of dietary assessment methods in nondialysis CKD identified a mixture of methodologies for collecting, evaluating, and reporting dietary intake in nondialysis CKD (Table 7.5) [43, 96–106].

Small Studies

Automated, Multiple-Pass Method

The AMPM was utilized to assess the baseline intake and the intake during two intervention periods of a randomized, controlled, crossover study of 31 participants with eGFR $\geq$43 ml/min/1.73m^2. The investigation was performed to determine the effect of increasing the dietary phosphorus from inorganic sources on the urinary albumin excretion and FGF23 levels [97].The AMPM was performed twice during each of the three periods (baseline, increased inorganic dietary phosphorus, and increased organic phosphorus). Participants and investigators were blinded as to the period in which they consumed the high inorganic phosphorus. The AMPM was used to determine the background dietary phosphorus. The study demonstrated a 500-mg/d higher urinary phosphorus excretion

Table 7.5 Reported dietary protein and energy intake in nondialysis kidney disease assessed using diet records, prior to dietary intervention

Author	N	Dietary assessment method	Kidney function (mL/min)	Dietary protein intake (g/kg/day)	Dietary energy intake (kcal/kg/day)
Chang et al. [96]	31	3-day record	75[a]	0.88[b]	21.1[b]
Bernhard et al. [102]	26	3-day record	26[a]	1.13	31.7
Dussol et al. [98]	25	Willett FFQ	89[c]	1.09	22.8[b]
Dussol et al. [98]	22	Willett FFQ	82[c]	1.00	21.3[b]
Fassett et al. [101]	113	4-day record	41[d]	0.9	21.4
Hansen et al. [99]	14	3-day record	94[c]	1.2	29.6
Hansen et al. [99]	15	3-day record	92[c]	1.1	30.8
Meloni et al. [100]	37	3-day record	44[c]	1.52	37.8[b]
Meloni et al. [100]	32	3-day record	48[c]	1.6	38.0[b]
Mircescu et al. [103][e]	53	3-day record	16[a]	0.62[e]	32.3[e]
Rotily et al. [97]	31	Willett FFQ	NR	1.22	28
Rotily et al. [97]	34	Willett FFQ	NR	1.22	22.9
Rotily et al. [97]	31	Willett FFQ	NR	1.40	30.7

NR not reported
[a]Calculated as eGFR
[b]Estimated from total dietary energy intake normalized to reported baseline body weight
[c]GFR measured as clearance of diethylene triamine penta-acetic acid
[d]Calculated as clearance of creatinine
[e]Patient selection was from a group already restricting dietary protein intake

during the high-inorganic-phosphorus diet than during the low-inorganic-phosphorus diet. No effect on microalbuminuria was detected, but a trend appeared when two participants who had been non-adherent to the meals were excluded from analyses. FGF23 did not change, but intact parathyroid hormone concentration was increased during the high-inorganic-phosphorus diet period.

FFQ

When dietitians examined the intake of people enrolling in trials to use diet as a method for preventing kidney disease progression, baseline data on DPI and DEI indicated variability in intakes (see Table 7.5). Rotily et al. [98] performed dietary intake assessment in a group (*n* = 96) of idiopathic calcium stone formers using the Willett FFQ. The FFQ was used to assess baseline dietary intake. Urinary data were available from 24-h urine collections. Urinary GI alkali (the sum of gastrointestinal absorption of sodium, potassium, calcium, magnesium, and chloride with the product of phosphorus and a constant of 1.8) and urinary creatinine excretion had a significant, positive correlation to animal protein intake from the FFQ ($r = 0.54$ and 0.50, respectively). Urinary potassium, oxalate, and calcium oxalate saturation also correlated with animal protein intake ($r = 0.44, 0.45$, and 0.44, respectively). A significant, negative correlation was seen between urinary oxalate excretion and DEI ($r = -0.43$). Whereas this was a small study, it depicted a relationship between dietary intake and urinary biomarkers of nephrolithiasis in patients who would be considered having stage 1 or stage 2 CKD. Dussol et al. [99] used the Willett FFQ to evaluate the dietary energy intake (DEI) and DPI of 47 patients with type 1 or type 2 diabetes with nephropathy. Both DPI and PCR were measured, but no correlation was shown. The DPI vs. PCR at baseline in the usual protein intake group was 1.13 vs. 1.09 g/kg/day (a 3.7% error); at month 12, 1.18 vs. 1.1 (a 7.3% error); and at month 24, 1.03 vs. 1.02 (<1% error). The DPI vs. PCR at baseline in the low-protein group was 1.08 vs. 1.0 g/kg/day (8% error); at month 12, 1.02 vs. 0.84 (21% error); and at month 24, 1.10 vs. 0.87 (21% error).

Diet Record

Evaluation of the dietary intake of 29 nondialysis patients with insulin-dependent diabetic nephropathy used 3-day diet records at baseline and at two 4-week intervals was reported by Hansen et al. [100]. In this study, a relative difference in DPI correlated to relative change in albuminuria (Spearman's $\rho = 0.51, p < 0.01$).

Meloni et al. [101] randomly assigned 69 nondialysis patients with diabetes to a low-protein or free-protein diet to examine whether the low-protein diet would slow the progression of kidney disease and monitor for malnutrition over a 12-month period. The study utilized 3-day diet records of nonconsecutive days measured quarterly. At baseline, the groups had similar dietary protein (1.6 ± 0.7 and 1.5 ± 0.4 g/kg/day, low-protein vs. free-protein, respectively). The participants randomized to low protein reported $0.72 \pm 0.3, 0.66 \pm 0.2, 0.66 \pm 0.3$, and 0.68 ± 0.4 g protein/kg/day at the follow-up visits, whereas the free-protein group reported $1.4 \pm 0.7, 1.41 \pm 0.6, 1.36 \pm 0.3$, and 1.38 ± 0.3 g protein/kg/day at follow-up visits. No biomarker confirmation of the dietary protein was assessed; however, the urinary protein excretion was statistically significantly reduced in the low-protein group from baseline (2.4 ± 1.1 to 1.3 ± 0.5 g/24 h, $p < 0.01$) compared to no change in the free-protein group (2.6 ± 0.8 to 2.4 ± 1.0 g/24 h).

Fassett et al. [102] evaluated dietary intake using a 4-day diet record (including 1 weekend day) in 113 patients with CKD entering the Lipid lowering and Onset of Renal Disease (LORD) trial. The diary instructions included pictorial references to portion sizes of commonly consumed foods to aid in accuracy. The diary was to be recorded prospectively but "as close to their next pathology visit as possible"—3 months from the time that diary instructions were provided [102]. Valid reporting was assessed as a ratio of the EI to estimated REE of 1.27. This study determined that 70.8% of subjects underreported their EI. No mention of adjustment for intrasubject variability was indicated in this report, and no PCRs were available for assessing the accuracy of the DPI recording.

Bernhard et al. [103] evaluated a 3-day diet record and compared DPI to protein nitrogen appearance (PNA; 1.13 vs. 1.11 g/kg/day; a < 2% error) at baseline.

Mircescu et al. [104] utilized a 3-day diet record every 2 weeks during a 12-week baseline phase prior to randomizing subjects to a low-protein vs. very-low-protein diet with ketoacid analogs [104]. The baseline phase was used to assess compliance (±10% of recommended DPI and DEI) prior to randomization. The authors only report on those subjects who qualified (57/167 evaluated) to be randomized.

Large Cohort and Cross-Sectional Studies

Automated, Multiple-Pass Method

Data from NHANES 2001–2008 have been evaluated to determine the mean dietary intake of people with CKD [105–107]. NHANES used the AMPM for dietary intake assessment [18], and the authors applied the MDRD equation for estimating kidney function and staged the kidney function according to the NKF criteria [94, 108]. Mean DEI and DPI were lower in those with CKD compared to those without CKD, even after adjusting for age. Evaluations of the difference from recommended intakes require additional analyses of the intra- and intersubject distributions and have not been reported as yet.

FFQ

The Block FFQ was used to estimate usual dietary intake at baseline over the previous year in the Multiethnic Study of Atherosclerosis. Foods were grouped to estimate the effect of animal vs. plant foods on microalbuminuria in people with eGFR <60 mL/min compared to ≥60 mL/min. Participants were excluded if they had known cardiovascular disease or diabetes. People consuming a diet high in low-fat dairy foods or a pattern of high intake of whole grains and fruits had independently lower odds for microalbuminuria and a lower urinary albumin-to-creatinine ratio. These baseline data also indicated that people consuming a diet high in nondairy animal products had a higher mean albumin-to-creatinine ratio.

Dialysis

The FFQ in Dialysis

The Willett FFQ was used to evaluate the dietary intake in a group of hemodialysis patients who were awaiting kidney transplantation [26, 109]. No statistical comparisons of the FFQ results were made with biomarkers measured (body composition, serum lipids, PCR). The investigators indicated that since the FFQ was an estimate of long-term dietary intake and the PCR was a near-term assessment, it would be inappropriate to compare the two. Instead, they used the FFQ and biomarkers to demonstrate, separately, the differences in dietary intake and body composition between normal-weight, overweight, and obese individuals on chronic hemodialysis waiting for kidney transplantation.

A dialysis-specific FFQ was developed by Bross et al. using the Block FFQ methodology [96, 110, 111]. Researchers accessed information from a subset of hemodialysis patients participating in the Nutrition and Inflammation in Dialysis Patients (NIED) cohort study in Southern California to develop the Dialysis-FFQ. Participants maintained a 3-day diet record that included the last dialysis day of the week and two subsequent days. Paper records were reviewed with the participants by a trained dietitian and converted to electronic data where food items were ranked according to types of foods and nutrients provided. The Dialysis-FFQ is a 100-item questionnaire, estimated to take 30–40 min to complete and intended to represent the food intake during the previous 3-month period. It can be accessed through NutritionQuest.com (Berkley, CA) [112] and is available as either a scannable, paper, or electronic form. This hemodialysis-specific FFQ was developed in a target population consisting of mostly ethnic minorities (43% were African American and 38% were Hispanic) and should be tested in broader hemodialysis populations for wider validity. However, the process represents an important step in gathering representative usual intake of hemodialysis patients.

More recently, Delgado et al. [113] utilized the Block FFQ in hemodialysis patients and calibrated it to self-reported 24-hour intakes that were subsequently entered into the ASA24®. Dietitians instructed patients on completing a 3-day food record and then entered the diary into the ASA24. This was an interesting approach; however, it omits an important feature of the ASA24—the multiple-pass method of information collection has been proven to strengthen the validity of self-reporting. The investigators used information from the 3-day food record to then reenter data into the ASA24 that excluded foods not listed on the Block FFQ (referred to as the Block FFQ-restricted). The purpose of the approach was to develop a method for calibrating the Block FFQ to self-reported intakes. The investigators determined that the 3-day food records restricted to the Block FFQ compared well to the full 3-day records and provided linear regression equations that could be used to implement their approach in future assessments. Their premis was that the Block FFQ is easier to manage than full food records and could be made more accurate by the regression equations.

Diet Records in Dialysis

Diet records or diaries have been utilized in several dialysis studies. The NCDS used a dietary intake record to compare the DPI to the calculated PCR and to compare phosphorus and potassium intake to DPI [84, 114]. At that time (ca. 1978), a mixed diet from 683 diet records indicated a strong correlation of dietary phosphorus to DPI ($r = 0.847$) and of dietary potassium to DPI ($r = 0.754$). Whether these correlations would hold in today's mixed diet (given that an increased number of foods may have added phosphorus) [115, 116] would need to be determined. However, this was useful information at the time in that it supported the decision to use urea as the surrogate biomarker for dialysis adequacy; urea is a reliable marker of protein catabolism, and protein intake is correlated to phosphorus and potassium intake. Subjects in the NCDS maintained 5-day food records (including a weekend) at five different time points during the 1-year study [114]. The correlation of DPI to PCR in the NCDS study was 0.443, $p < 0.01$.

More recently, the HEMO study utilized annual 2-day diet diary-assisted recalls that included 1 dialysis day and 1 nondialysis day over the 7-year study period in 1397 maintenance hemodialysis patients [117, 118]. The diet was recorded by the patient, reviewed with the dietitian, and then analyzed for energy and protein. In this study, the DPI correlated with the PCR ($r = 0.17$, $p < 0.0001$) but not to serum albumin, creatinine, or cholesterol. However, no statistical relationship was evident between DPI and PCR for the group of people age 50–64 years.

Chauveau et al. [119] compared dietary recall of DPI to PCR in 99 maintenance hemodialysis patients using a 7-day record. Subjects maintained the food record and reviewed the records with a dietitian during dialysis sessions. The correlation of DPI to PCR increased during the week ($r^2 = 0.26$, 0.49, and 0.57 for the first, second, and third dialysis sessions, respectively).

Imani et al. [120] examined the dietary intake of 36 participants with ESRD receiving chronic peritoneal dialysis. Dietary intake was assessed using 3-day diet records at baseline, week 5, and week 10 of the study. The study was performed to test the effect of a ginger supplement (1000 mg) vs. placebo on serum glucose, inflammation, and oxidative stress. The diet records were kept during two days of the week and one day of the weekend. The records were entered into nutrition analysis software (Nutritionist IV, N-squared Computing, San Bruno, CA). The serum glucose was significantly reduced in the ginger group (-2 ± 0.9 mmol/L) vs. placebo (0.6 ± 0.7 mmol/L; $p < 0.05$) despite sustained carbohydrate intake of 223 ± 16, 222 ± 15, and 222 ± 16 g/d at baseline, week 5, and week 10, respectively.

Transplantation

The FFQ in Kidney Transplantation

Guida et al. [121] have reported use of the Willett FFQ in kidney transplant recipients during the first year posttransplant. The FFQ was completed at baseline (time of transplant surgery) and at 1-year posttransplant. Adherence was assessed as having 90% compatibility between the FFQ and the diet recommendations during the first 90 days posttransplant. For analytical purposes, those considered nonadherent were compared to the group having success with the dietary protocol. Biomarkers of urinary excretion of sodium and urea from 24-h urine collections were used to confirm findings (data not shown). DEI, DPI, and dietary sodium were decreased or maintained in the adherent group compared to increases in the nonadherent group. These results were confirmed by decreased body weight in the adherent group vs. increased body weight in the nonadherent group.

Diet Records in Kidney Transplantation

A 3-day food record was used to determine baseline dietary intake in a prospective study of the effect of dietary changes on serum lipid profile in a group of 23 male and female stable kidney transplant recipients [122]. Decreasing the dietary fat intake from 41% to 33% of total energy consumed was associated with a significant reduction (13%, $p < 0.01$) in serum total cholesterol levels in men over a 6-month period, but not in women.

A 3-day food record was also used in reporting dietary guideline adherence of 90 kidney transplant recipients in Taiwan [123]. This cross-sectional study observed that 81% of the participants were consuming excessive total dietary fat, that only 1.1% consumed adequate dietary fiber, and that the majority had poor adherence to the dietary guidelines.

Evaluation of 44 stable kidney transplant recipients, using 3-day food record (including 1 weekend day) maintained at four time points during the first year posttransplant, identified that women increased their DPI and DEI significantly compared to no change over the year in men [124]. This dietary change was accompanied by a mean increase in BMI by 1.9 kg/m^2 in women (a mean weight gain of 5.4 kg or 10.6%). Whole-body bone densitometry indicated a 12% mean increase in body fat mass, a 7% increase in lean body mass, and a 1.4% increase in bone mass in these women over the year, while men had a significant reduction in mean body fat mass (8%) and bone mass (2.3%) and a 1% increase in lean body mass (not significant).

A 7-day diet record was maintained by 106 stable kidney transplant recipients (with abnormal glucose tolerance) at the time of transplantation and at 1 and 2 years posttransplantation [125]. Three random days from each food record (including 1 weekend day) were used for the dietary intake assessments. Subjects were randomized to receive either aggressive risk factor modification for coronary vascular disease or standard posttransplant care. No correlations to biomarkers were reported.

Recommendations for Kidney Disease

The concepts relating dietary intake assessment methodologies and correlation to biomarkers or outcomes in the general population are useful for evaluating these tools in kidney disease. The presentation of information provided in this chapter from the kidney disease literature outlines areas where improvement or alternate methodologies may be considered, such as:

- Apply the statistical methodologies suggested for accounting for dietary intake distribution and determine the characteristics of patients with kidney disease who are at risk for inadequate intake using these methods.
- Evaluate the level of DPI, DEI, or other nutrients that is associated with malnutrition or other outcomes in this population using current dietary assessment tools and methodologies.
- Assess the efficacy of multiple days and multiple methods of intake assessment when evaluating dietary intake in individuals and/or groups of people with CKD (by stage of CKD).
- Determine the utility of available data sets for answering some of the questions regarding dietary intake assessment in CKD using new statistical approaches or queries that were not assessed in the original evaluation of the data sets to provide further insight for future trials.

As new research agendas are considered, it is important to express appreciation for all of the effort and expense provided by individual investigators, kidney disease programs and centers, and the patients who offer themselves to this work. Their efforts have helped to define and design the research that has and will answer many questions in kidney disease.

Acknowledgments   Gillian Gorski, a clinical nutrition student at the University of Houston, Houston, Texas, provided valuable assistance with the bibliography and review of papers.

References

1. Ikizler TA, Burrowes J, Byham-Gray L, Campbell K, Carrero JJ, Chan W, et al. KDOQI Nutrition in CKD Guideline Work Group. KDOQI clinical practice guideline for nutrition in CKD: 2020 update. Am J Kidney Dis. 2020; in press.
2. Fouque D, Vennegoor M, Ter Wee P, Wanner C, Basci A, Canaud B, et al. EBPG Guideline on Nutrition. Nephrol Dial Transplant. 2007;22:ii45–87.
3. KDOQI Work Group. KDOQI clinical practice guideline for nutrition in children with CKD: 2008 update. Am J Kidney Dis. 2009;53:S11–S104.
4. Chronic Kidney Disease. Chicago: Academy of Nutrition and Dietetics; 2018; Available at: https://www.andeal.org/topic.cfm?menu=5303. Last accessed 6 Jan 2020.
5. The Management of CKD Working Group. Management of chronic kidney disease (CKD) in primary care. US Department of Veterans Affairs; 2008; Available at: http://www.healthquality.va.gov/Chronic_Kidney_Disease_Clinical_Practice_Guideline.asp. Last accessed 5 July 2019.
6. Chronic kidney disease – Identification, evaluation and management of patients. Ministry of Health British Columbia 2014; Available at: http://www.bcguidelines.ca/guideline_ckd.html. Last accessed 5 July 2019.
7. KDOQI Work Group. KDOQI clinical practice guidelines and clinical practice recommendations for diabetes and chronic kidney disease. Am J Kidney Dis. 2007;49:S12–S154.
8. Chronic kidney disease in adults: assessment and management. Clinical guideline [CG182]. National Institute for Health and Clinical Excellence; 2015; Available at: https://www.nice.org.uk/guidance/cg182. Last accessed 5 July 2019.
9. Baron JH. Sailors' scurvy before and after James Lind – a reassessment. Nutr Rev. 2009;67:315–32.
10. Magiorkinis E, Beloukas A, Diamantis A. Scurvy: past, present and future. Eur J Intern Med. 2011;22:147–52.
11. Food and Nutrition Board, Institute of Medicine, National Academy of Sciences. Dietary reference intakes. National Academies Press; Available at: https://www.nal.usda.gov/fnic/dietary-reference-intakes. Last accessed 5 July 2019.
12. Food and Nutrition Board, Institute of Medicine, National Academy of Sciences. Dietary reference intakes: Applications in Dietary Planning. National Academies Press; 2003; Available at: https://www.nap.edu/catalog/10609/dietary-reference-intakes-applications-in-dietary-planning. Last accessed 5 July 2019.
13. Food and Nutrition Board, Institute of Medicine, National Academy of Sciences. Dietary reference intakes: Applications in Dietary Assessment. National Academies Press; 2000; Available at: https://www.nap.edu/catalog/9956/dietary-reference-intakes-applications-in-dietary-assessment. Last accessed 5 July 2019.
14. Food and Nutrition Board, Institute of Medicine, National Academy of Sciences. Dietary reference intakes for energy, carbohydrate, fiber, fat, fatty acids, cholesterol, protein, and amino acids. Washington, DC: National

Academies Press; 2005; Available at: https://www.nap.edu/catalog/10490/dietary-reference-intakes-for-energy-carbohydrate-fiber-fat-fatty-acids-cholesterol-protein-and-amino-acids. Last accessed 5 July 2019.

15. USDA Food and Nutrient Databases. Beltsville, MD: Agricultural Research Service, Food Surveys Research Group; 2018 [updated January 29, 2019]; Available at: http://ndb.nal.usda.gov/ndb/. Last accessed 5 July 2019.

16. Choose Your Foods: Food Lists for Diabetes. Chicago: Academy of Nutrition and Dietetics and American Diabetes Association; 2014.

17. ASA24 Automated self-administered 24-hour dietary assessment tool. National Cancer Institute, Division of Cancer Control & Population Sciences; 2019 [updated February 1, 2019]; Available at: https://epi.grants.cancer.gov/asa24/. Last accessed 5 July 2019.

18. Moshfegh AJ. USDA automated multiple-pass method. Beltsville: USDA Agricultural Research Service; 2016. [updated September 8, 2016]; Available at: https://www.ars.usda.gov/northeast-area/beltsville-md-bhnrc/beltsville-human-nutrition-research-center/food-surveys-research-group/docs/ampm-usda-automated-multiple-pass-method/. Last accessed 5 July 2019.

19. Raper N, Perloff B, Ingwersen L, Steinfeldt L, Anand J. An overview of USDA's dietary intake data system. J Food Comp Anal. 2004;17:545–55.

20. Dwyer J, Ellwood K, Moshfegh AJ, Johnson CL. Integration of the continuing survey of food intakes by individuals and the National Health and Nutrition Examination Survey. J Am Diet Assoc. 2001;101:1142–3.

21. Zimmerman TP, Hull SG, McNutt S, Mittl B, Islam N, Guenther PM, et al. Challenges in converting an interviewer-administered food probe database to self-administration in the National Cancer Institute automated self-administered 24-hour recall (ASA24). J Food Comp Anal. 2009;22S:548–51.

22. Thompson FE, Dixit-Joshi S, Potischman N, Dodd KW, Kirkpatrick SI, Kushi LH, et al. Comparison of interviewer-administered and automated self-administered 24-hour dietary recalls in 3 diverse integrated health systems. Am J Epidemiol. 2015;181:970–8.

23. What We Eat in America. Washington, DC: United States Department of Agriculture; 2018 [updated July 31, 2018]; Available at: https://www.ars.usda.gov/northeast-area/beltsville-md-bhnrc/beltsville-human-nutrition-research-center/food-surveys-research-group/docs/wweianhanes-overview/. Last accessed 5 July 2019.

24. About the National Health and Nutrition Examination Survey. Atlanta: Centers for Disease Control and Prevention; 2017 [updated September 15, 2017]; Available at: http://www.cdc.gov/nchs/nhanes/about_nhanes.htm. Last accessed 6 Mar 2019.

25. Hunter DJ, Sampson L, Stampfer MJ, Colditz GA, Rosner B, Willett WC. Variability in portion sizes of commonly consumed foods among a population of women in the United States. Am J Epidemiol. 1988;127:1240–9.

26. Hu FB, Rimm E, Smith-Warner SA, Feskanich D, Stampfer MJ, Ascherio A, et al. Reproducibility and validity of dietary patterns assessed with a food-frequency questionnaire. Am J Clin Nutr. 1999;69:243–9.

27. Block G, Hartman AM, Dresser CM, Carroll MD, Gannon J, Gardner L. A data-based approach to diet questionnaire design and testing. Am J Epidemiol. 1986;124:453–69.

28. Block G, Woods SM, Potosky A, Clifford C. Validation of a self-administered diet history questionnaire using multiple diet records. J Clin Epidemiol. 1990;43:1327–35.

29. Willett WC, Stampfer MJ, Underwood BA, Speizer FE, Rosner B, Hennekens CH. Validation of a dietary questionnaire with plasma carotenoid and alpha-tocopherol levels. Am J Clin Nutr. 1983;38:631–9.

30. Willett WC, Sampson L, Stampfer MJ, Rosner B, Bain C, Witschi J, et al. Reproducibility and validity of a semiquantitative food frequency questionnaire. Am J Epidemiol. 1985;122:51–65.

31. Block Questionnaires. NutritionQuest; 2019; Available at: http://www.nutritionquest.com. last accessed 5 July 2019.

32. Subar A, Thompson F, Smith A, Jobe J, Ziegler R, Potischman N, et al. Improving food frequency questionnaires: a qualitative approach using cognitive interviewing. J Am Diet Assoc. 1995;95:781–8.

33. Subar AF, Thompson FE, Kipnis V, Midthune D, Hurwitz P, McNutt S, et al. Comparative validation of the Block, Willett, and National Cancer Institute food frequency questionnaires. Am J Epidemiol. 2001;154:1089–99.

34. Subar A, Kipnis V, Troiano R, Midthune D, Schoeller D, Bingham S, et al. Using biomarkers to evaluate the extent of dietary misreporting in a large sample of adults: the OPEN study. Am J Epidemiol. 2003;158:1–13.

35. Kipnis V, Subar AF, Midthune D, Freedman LS, Ballard-Barbash R, Troiano RP, et al. Structure of dietary measurement error: results of the OPEN biomarker study. Am J Epidemiol. 2003;158:14–21.

36. Diet History Questionnaire III. Bethesda: National Cancer Institute, Cancer Control and Population Science Branch, Risk Factor Monitoring Branch; [updated June 28, 2019]; Available at: https://epi.grants.cancer.gov/dhq3/. Last accessed 6 Mar 2019.

37. The Nurses' Health Study. Nurses Health Study; Available at: https://www.nurseshealthstudy.org/. Last accessed 6 Mar 2019.

38. Harvard School of Public Health: Health Professionals Follow-up Study. 2018; Available at: https://sites.sph.harvard.edu/hpfs/. Last accessed 5 July 2019.

39. Rimm EB, Giovannucci EL, Stampfer MJ, Litin LB, Willett WC. Reproducibility and validity of an expanded self-administered semiquantitative food frequency questionnaire among male health professionals. Am J Epidemiol. 1992;135:1114–26.

40. Chiuve SE, Sampson L, Willett WC. Adherence to the overall nutrition quality index and risk of total chronic disease. Am J Prev Med. 2011;40:505–13.

41. Millen AE, Midthune D, Thompson FE, Kipnis V, Subar AF. The National Cancer Institute diet history questionnaire: validation of pyramid food servings. Am J Epidemiol. 2006;163:279–88.

42. Mayer-Davis EJ, Vitolins MZ, Carmichael SL, Hemphill S, Tsaroucha G, Rushing J, et al. Validity and reproducibility of a food frequency interview in a multi-cultural epidemiologic study. Ann Epidemiol. 1999;9:314–24.

43. Nettleton JA, Steffen LM, Palmas W, Burke GL, Jacobs DR Jr. Associations between microalbuminuria and animal foods, plant foods, and dietary patterns in the multiethnic study of atherosclerosis. Am J Clin Nutr. 2008;87:1825–36.

44. Burke LE, Warziski M, Starrett T, Choo J, Music E, Sereika S, et al. Self-monitoring dietary intake: current and future practices. J Renal Nutr. 2005;15:281–90.

45. Burke LE, Conroy MB, Sereika SM, Elçi OU, Styn MA, Acharya SD, et al. The effect of electronic self-monitoring on weight loss and dietary intake: a randomized behavioral weight loss trial. Obesity. 2011;19:338–44.

46. Hollis JF, Gullion CM, Stevens VJ, Brantley PJ, Appel LJ, Ard JD, et al. Weight loss during the intensive intervention phase of the weight-loss maintenance trial. Am J Prev Med. 2008;35:118–26.

47. Acharya SD, Elci OU, Sereika SM, Styn MA, Burke LE. Using a personal digital assistant for self-monitoring influences diet quality in comparison to a standard paper record among overweight/obese adults. J Am Diet Assoc. 2011;111:583–8.

48. Helsel DL, Jakicic JM, Otto AD. Comparison of techniques for self-monitoring eating and exercise behaviors on weight loss in a correspondence-based intervention. J Am Diet Assoc. 2007;107:1807–10.

49. Johnson F, Wardle J. The association between weight loss and engagement with a web-based food and exercise diary in a commercial weight loss programme: a retrospective analysis. Int J Behav Nutr Phys Act. 2011 ;8:83.

50. Beasley JM, Riley WT, Davis A, Singh J. Evaluation of a PDA-based dietary assessment and intervention program: a randomized controlled trial. J Am Coll Nutr. 2008;27:280–6.

51. Food Processor. ESHA Research; [updated February 2019]; Available at: http://www.esha.com/. Last accessed 5 July 2019.

52. FoodWorks. The Nutrition Company; Available at: http://www.nutritionco.com/index.htm. Last accessed 6 Mar 2019.

53. NutriBase. CyberSoft, Inc.; Available at: http://www.nutribase.com/. Last accessed 5 July 2019.

54. Nutritionist Pro. Axxya Systems; Available at: http://www.nutritionistpro.com/. Last accessed 5 July 2019.

55. Food and Nutrition Board, Institute of Medicine, National Academy of Sciences. Dietary reference intakes: the essential guide to nutrient requirements. Washington, DC: The National Academies Press; 2006. Available from: https://www.nap.edu/catalog/11537/dietary-reference-intakes-the-essential-guide-to-nutrient-requirements.

56. Murphy SP, Barr SI. Practice paper of the American Dietetic Association: using the dietary reference intakes. J Am Diet Assoc. 2011;111:762–70.

57. Nusser SM, Carriquiry AL, Dodd KW, Fuller WA. A semiparametric transformation approach to estimating usual daily intake distributions. J Am Stat Assoc. 1996;91:1440–9.

58. Kirkpatrick SI, Dodd KW, Tooze J, Bailey RL, Freedman L, Midthune D et al. Measurement error webinar series. Risk factor monitoring and methods, National Cancer Institute, National Institutes of Health; 2012; Available at: https://epi.grants.cancer.gov/events/measurement-error/. Last accessed 5 July 2019.

59. Moshfegh AJ, Goldman J, Cleveland L. What we eat in America, NHANES 2001–2002: usual nutrient intakes from food compared to dietary reference intakes. U.S. Department of Agriculture, Agricultural Research Service; 2005; Available at: https://www.ars.usda.gov/research/publications/publication/?seqNo115=184176. Last accessed 5 July 2019.

60. National Research Council. Nutrient adequacy. Assessment using food consumption surveys. Washington, DC: National Academy Press; 1986.

61. Murphy SP, Guenther PM, Kretsch MJ. Using the dietary reference intakes to assess intakes of groups: pitfalls to avoid. J Am Diet Assoc. 2006;106:1550–3.

62. Conway J, Ingwersen L, Moshfegh A. Accuracy of dietary recall using the USDA five-step multiple-pass method in men: an observational validation study. J Am Diet Assoc. 2004;104:595–603.

63. Conway J, Ingwersen L, Vinyard B, Moshfegh A. Effectiveness of the US Department of Agriculture 5-step multiple-pass method in assessing food intake in obese and nonobese women. Am J Clin Nutr. 2003;77:1171–8.

64. Blanton CA, Moshfegh AJ, Baer DJ, Kretsch MJ. The USDA automated multiple-pass method accurately estimates group total energy and nutrient intake. J Nutr. 2006;136:2594–9.

65. Ard JD, Desmond RA, Allison DB, Conway JM. Dietary restraint and disinhibition do not affect accuracy of 24-hour recall in a multiethnic population. J Am Diet Assoc. 2006;106:434–7. https://doi.org/10.1016/j.jada.2005.12.006.
66. Bailey RL, Dodd KW, Gahche JJ, Dwyer JT, McDowell MA, Yetley EA, et al. Total folate and folic acid intake from foods and dietary supplements in the United States: 2003–2006. Am J Clin Nutr. 2010;91:231–7.
67. Rumpler WV, Kramer M, Rhodes DG, Moshfegh AJ, Paul DR. Identifying sources of reporting error using measured food intake. Eur J Clin Nutr. 2007;62:544–52.
68. Wirfalt AKE, Jeffery RW, Elmer PJ. Comparison of food frequency questionnaires: the reduced Block and Willett questionnaires differ in ranking on nutrient intakes. Am J Epidemiol. 1998;148:1148–56.
69. Brunner E, Stallone D, Juneja M, Bingham S, Marmot M. Dietary assessment in Whitehall II: comparison of 7 d diet diary and food-frequency questionnaire and validity against biomarkers. Br J Nutr. 2001;86:405–14.
70. Biomarkers Definitions Working Group. Biomarkers and surrogate endpoints: preferred definitions and conceptual framework. Clin Pharmacol Ther. 2001;69:89–95.
71. Bingham SA. Biomarkers in nutritional epidemiology. Public Health Nutr. 2002;5:821–7.
72. Jenab M, Slimani N, Bictash M, Ferrari P, Bingham S. Biomarkers in nutritional epidemiology: applications, needs and new horizons. Hum Genet. 2009;125:507–25.
73. Day N, McKeown N, Wong M, Welch A, Bingham S. Epidemiological assessment of diet: a comparison of a 7-day diary with a food frequency questionnaire using urinary markers of nitrogen, potassium and sodium. Int J Epidemiol. 2001;30:309–17.
74. Kipnis V, Midthune D, Freedman L, Bingham S, Day NE, Riboli E, et al. Bias in dietary-report instruments and its implications for nutritional epidemiology. Public Health Nutr. 2002;5:915–23.
75. Sargent JA, Gotch FA. Mass balance: a quantitative guide to clinical nutritional therapy. I. The predialysis patient with renal disease. J Am Diet Assoc. 1979;75:547–51.
76. Maroni BJ, Steinman T, Mitch W. A method for estimating nitrogen intake of patients with chronic renal failure. Kidney Int. 1985;27:58–61.
77. Moshfegh AJ, Rhodes DG, Baer DJ, Murayi T, Clemens JC, Rumpler WV, et al. The US Department of Agriculture automated multiple-pass method reduces bias in the collection of energy intakes. Am J Clin Nutr. 2008;88:324–32.
78. Titze J, Luft FC. Speculations on salt and the genesis of arterial hypertension. Kidney Int. 2017;91:1324–35.
79. Dragsted L. Biomarkers of exposure to vitamins A, C, and E and their relation to lipid and protein oxidation markers. Eur J Nutr. 2008;47:3–18.
80. Holmes MD, Powell IJ, Campos H, Stampfer MJ, Giovannucci EL, Willett WC. Validation of a food frequency questionnaire measurement of selected nutrients using biological markers in African-American men. Eur J Clin Nutr. 2007;61:1328–36.
81. Jin Y, Gordon MH, Alimbetov D, Chong MF-F, George TW, Spencer JPE, et al. A novel combined biomarker including plasma carotenoids, vitamin C, and ferric reducing antioxidant power is more strongly associated with fruit and vegetable intake than the individual components. J Nutr. 2014;144:1866–72.
82. Choi H, Liu S, Curhan G. Intake of purine-rich foods, protein, and dairy products and relationship to serum levels of uric acid: the Third National Health and Nutrition Examination Survey. Arthritis Rheum. 2005;52: 283–9.
83. Chun O, Chung S, Song W. Urinary isoflavones and their metabolites validate the dietary isoflavone intakes in US adults. J Am Diet Assoc. 2009;109:245–54.
84. Sargent JA, Lowrie EG. Which mathematical model to study uremic toxicity? National Cooperative Dialysis Study. Clin Nephrol. 1982;17:303–14.
85. Sargent JA, Gotch FA, Henry RR, Bennett N. Mass balance: a quantitative guide to clinical nutritional therapy. II. The dialyzed patient. J Am Diet Assoc. 1979;75:551–5.
86. Wineman RJ, Sargent JA, Piercy L. Nutritional implications of renal disease. II. The dietitian's key role in studies of dialysis therapy. J Am Diet Assoc. 1977;70:483–7.
87. Kidney Disease: Improving Global Outcomes Workgroup. KDIGO clinical practice guideline for acute kidney injury. Kidney Int. 2012;2:1–138.
88. Saadeh E, Ikizler TA, Shyr Y, Hakim RM, Himmelfarb J. Recombinant human growth hormone in patients with acute renal failure. J Ren Nutr. 2001;11:212–9.
89. Chima CS, Meyer L, Hummell AC, Bosworth C, Heyka R, Paganini EP, et al. Protein catabolic rate in patients with acute renal failure on continuous arteriovenous hemofiltration and total parenteral nutrition. J Am Soc Nephrol. 1993;3:1516–21.
90. Moore LW, Acchiardo S, Smith SO, Gaber AO. Nutrition in the critical care settings of renal diseases. Adv Ren Replace Ther. 1996;3:250–60.
91. Brown RO, Compher C, American Society for Parenteral Enteral Nutrition Board of Directors. A.S.P.E.N. Clinical guidelines: nutrition support in adult acute and chronic renal failure. J Parenter Enteral Nutr. 2010;34:366–77.

92. Fiaccadori E, Lombardi M, Leonardi S, Rotelli CF, Tortorella G, Borghetti A. Prevalence and clinical outcome associated with preexisting malnutrition in acute renal failure: a prospective cohort study. J Am Soc Nephrol. 1999;10:581–93.

93. McClave SA, Taylor BE, Martindale RG, Warren MM, Johnson DR, Braunschweig C, et al. Guidelines for the provision and assessment of nutrition support therapy in the adult critically ill patient: Society of Critical Care Medicine (SCCM) and American Society for Parenteral and Enteral Nutrition (A.S.P.E.N.). JPEN J Parenter Enteral Nutr. 2016;40:159–211.

94. Kidney Disease: Improving Global Outcomes Workgroup. KDIGO 2012 clinical practice guideline for the evaluation and management of chronic kidney disease. Kidney Int Suppl. 2013;3:i-150.

95. Levin A, Stevens P, Work Group. KDIGO guideline for CKD classification and management – proposed. New York: KDIGO; 2011; Available at: http://www.kdigo.org/clinical_practice_guidelines/CKD.php. Last accessed 31 Oct 2012.

96. Bross R, Noori N, Kovesdy CP, Murali SB, Benner D, Block G, et al. Dietary assessment of individuals with chronic kidney disease. Semin Dial. 2010;23:359–64.

97. Chang AR, Miller ER III, Anderson CA, Juraschek SP, Moser M, Whie K, et al. Phosphorus additives and albuminuria in early stages of CKD: a randomized controlled trial. Am J Kidney Dis. 2017;69:200–9.

98. Rotily M, Leonetti F, Iovanna C, Berthezene P, Dupuy P, Vazi A, et al. Effects of low animal protein or high-fiber diets on urine compostion in calcium nephrolithiasis. Kidney Int. 2000;57:1115–23.

99. Dussol B, Iovanna C, Raccah D, Darmon P, Morange S, Vague P, et al. A randomized trial of low-protein diet in type 1 and in type 2 diabetes mellitus patients with incipient and overt nephropathy. J Ren Nutr. 2005;15:398–406.

100. Hansen HP, Christensen PK, Tauber-Lassen E, Klausen A, Jensen BR, Parving H-H. Low-protein diet and kidney function in insulin-dependent diabetic patients with diabetic nephropathy. Kidney Int. 1999;55:621–8.

101. Meloni C, Morosetti M, Suraci C, Pennafina MG, Tozzo C, Taccone-Gallucci M, et al. Severe dietary protein restriction in overt diabetic nephropathy: benefits or risks? J Ren Nutr. 2002;12:96–101.

102. Fassett RG, Robertson IK, Geraghty DP, Ball MJ, Coombes JS. Dietary intake of patients with chronic kidney disease entering the LORD trial: adjusting for underreporting. J Ren Nutr. 2008;17:235–42.

103. Bernhard J, Beaufrere B, Laville M, Fouque D. Adaptive response to a low-protein diet in predialysis chronic renal failure patients. J Am Soc Nephrol. 2001;12:1249–54.

104. Mircescu G, Garneata L, Stancu SH, Capusa C. Effects of a supplemented hypoproteic diet in chronic kidney disease. J Ren Nutr. 2007;17:179–88. https://doi.org/10.1053/j.jrn.2006.12.012.

105. Moore LW, Parrott JS, Rigassio-Radler D, Byham-Gray L, Gaber AO. The effect of menses on the measurement of proteinuria and estimation of dietary intake in US females. J Am Diet Assoc. 2011;111:A15.

106. Moore LW, Byham-Gray LD, Scott Parrott J, Rigassio-Radler D, Mandayam S, Jones SL, et al. The mean dietary protein intake at different stages of chronic kidney disease is higher than current guidelines. Kidney Int. 2013;83:724–32.

107. Moore LW, Byham-Gray L, Parrott JS, Radler D, Jones SL, Mandayam SA, et al. Dietary protein intake in chronic kidney disease from the National Health and Nutrition Examination Survey. J Am Soc Nephrol. 2011;22:175A.

108. Coresh J, Selvin E, Stevens L, Manzi J, Kusek J, Eggers P, et al. Prevalence of chronic kidney disease in the United States. J Am Med Assoc. 2007;298:2038–47.

109. Guida B, Trio R, Nastasi A, Laccetti R, Pesola D, Torraca S, et al. Body composition and cardiovascular risk factors in pretransplant hemodialysis patients. Clin Nutr. 2004;23:363–72.

110. Kalantar-Zadeh K, Kovesdy CP, Bross R, Benner D, Noori N, Murali SB, et al. Design and development of a dialysis food frequency questionnaire. J Ren Nutr. 2011;21:257–62.

111. Kalantar-Zadeh K, Kopple JD, Deepak S, Block D, Block G. Food intake characteristics of hemodialysis patients as obtained by food frequency questionnaire. J Ren Nutr. 2002;12:17–31.

112. Block questionnaire – 2008 FFQ for dialysis patients. NutritionQuest; 2019; Available at: http://www.nutrition-quest.com. Last accessed 5 July 2019.

113. Delgado C, Ward P, Chertow GM, Storer L, Dalrymple L, Block T, et al. Calibration of the brief food frequency questionnaire among patients on dialysis. J Ren Nutr. 2014;24:151–156.e151.

114. Schoenfeld PY, Henry RR, Laird NM, Roxe DM. Assessment of nutritional status of the National Cooperative Dialysis Study population. Kidney Int. 1983;23:S80–8.

115. Uribarri J. Phosphorus homeostasis in normal health and in chronic kidney disease patients with special emphasis on dietary phosphorus intake. Semin Dial. 2007;20:295–301.

116. Murphy-Gutekunst L. Hidden phosphorus: where do we go from here? J Ren Nutr. 2007;17:e31–6.

117. Greene T, Beck GJ, Gassman JJ, Gotch FA, Kusek JW, Levey AS, et al. Design and statistical issues of the hemodialysis (HEMO) study. Control Clin Trials. 2000;21:502–25.

118. Burrowes JD, Cockram DB, Dwyer JT, Larive B, Paranandi L, Bergen C, et al. Cross-sectional relationship between dietary protein and energy intake, nutritional status, functional status, and comorbidity in older versus younger hemodialysis patients. J Ren Nutr. 2002;12:87–95.

119. Chauveau P, Grigaut E, Kolko A, Wolff P, Combe C, Aparicio M. Evaluation of nutritional status in patients with kidney disease: usefulness of dietary recall. J Ren Nutr. 2007;17:88–92.
120. Imani H, Tabibi H, Najafi I, Atabak S, Hedayatti M, Rahmani L. Effects of ginger on serum glucose, advanced glycation end products, and inflammation in peritoneal dialysis patients. Nutrition. 2015;31:703–7.
121. Guida B, Trio R, Laccetti R, Nastasi A, Salvi E, Perrino NR, et al. Role of dietary intervention on metabolic abnormalities and nutritional status after renal transplantation. Nephrol Dial Transplant. 2007;22:3304–10.
122. Lopes IM, Martin M, Errasti P, Martinez JA. Benefits of a dietary intervention on weight loss, body composition, and lipid profile after renal transplantation. Nutrition. 1999;15:7–10.
123. Lin I-H, Wong T-C, Nien S-W, Chou Y-T, Chiang Y-J, Wang H-H, et al. Dietary compliance among renal transplant recipients: a single-center study in Taiwan. Transplant Proc. 2019;51:1325–30.
124. El Haggan W, Vendrely B, Chauveau P, Barthe N, Castaing F, Berger F, et al. Early evolution of nutritional status and body composition after kidney transplantation. Am J Kidney Dis. 2002;40:629–37.
125. Orazio LK, Isbel NM, Armstrong KA, Tamarskyj J, Johnson DW, Hale RE, et al. Evaluation of dietetic advice for modification of cardiovascular disease risk factors in renal transplant recipients. J Ren Nutr. 2011;21:462–71.

Chapter 8
Psychosocial Issues Affecting Nutritional Status in Kidney Disease

William A. Wolfe

Keywords End-stage renal disease · Chronic kidney disease · Nutrition · Malnutrition · Depression · Anxiety · Loneliness · Food insecurity · Limited health literacy · Self-efficacy · Social support

Key Points
- Research on psychosocial factors affecting nutritional status in CKD has historically been focused primarily on depression.
- Additional psychosocial factors affecting nutritional status include anxiety, loneliness, self-efficacy, food insecurity, limited health literacy, and social support.
- Collectively, these additional factors may constitute a more holistic foundation for interventions to improve nutrition in CKD patients.

Introduction

Under the rubric of the psychosocial dimension, multiple factors have been demonstrated to affect and also have a strong potential of affecting the nutritional status of patients with kidney disease. Among these are depression, anxiety, loneliness, self-efficacy, food insecurity, limited health literacy, and the relative availability of various forms of social support (Table 8.1). The aim of this chapter is to first provide an overview which broadens the perspective on psychosocial factors that can affect nutritional status in chronic kidney disease (CKD). A second aim is to suggest strategies for mitigating psychosocial factors that detrimentally impact nutrition and bolster those which can help to optimize it. As will be revealed through the overview, research on psychosocial factors has been uneven, and many knowledge gaps remain in fully understanding their impact on the nutritional status of patients with CKD.

Depression

Research on psychosocial issues affecting chronic kidney disease (CKD) patients in general, and their effects on nutritional status in particular, has been dominated by a focus on depression. Estimates on the prevalence of depression in patients with CKD have varied. For example, in a study of 103

W. A. Wolfe (✉)
Women's Institute for Family Health of Philadelphia, Philadelphia, PA, USA

© Springer Nature Switzerland AG 2020
J. D. Burrowes et al. (eds.), *Nutrition in Kidney Disease*, Nutrition and Health,
https://doi.org/10.1007/978-3-030-44858-5_8

Table 8.1 Psychosocial factors that affect nutritional status in patients with chronic kidney disease

Factor	Definition
Depression	Classically entails feelings of sadness, despair, and lack of optimism about the future, which can clearly undermine adherence to any medical regiment
Anxiety	Classical symptoms have included nervousness, restlessness, and feelings of uneasiness. Potential independent effects of anxiety on nutrition, apart from depression, has been a neglected area of research
Loneliness	Defined as unpleasant feelings of isolation due to unmet human needs, loneliness has likewise been neglected as a psychosocial factor in the nutritional status of CKD patients. It has unmeasured and potentially profound implications as an exacerbating factor in nutrition
Self-efficacy	Self-efficacy, simplistically defined as the confidence to complete a task, is a modifiable psychosocial factor which research has shown can affect nutritional issues with CKD patients. Several studies have laid out blueprints for interventions for dialysis patients, which could potentially enhance patients' self-efficacy and in turn their nutritional status
Food insecurity	Emerging research shows that food insecurity is another largely overlooked factor in the nutritional status of CKD patients, which also has potential implications for mental health issues (anxiety and depression) and medication compliance (e.g., buying food vs. filling prescriptions). It remains an unmet issue
Limited health literacy	Statistics reveal that 50% of ESRD patients struggle with some degree of limited health literacy (LHL). Evidence shows that LHL has multidimensional ramifications for CKD patients, including their nutritional status. Renal dietitians also face special challenges meeting the needs of patients with LHL due to time constraints
Social support	Social support, defined as the perception that one is cared for, is a well-established mediating factor in medical outcomes, including the nutritional status of CKD patients. Given the unique high frequency and long duration of dialysis clinic staffs' face-to-face contact with patients, it may represent a largely untapping source of creative social support to improve nutritional outcomes

in-center dialysis patients, 34% were found to be mild-to-moderately depressed, 12.6% moderate-to-severely depressed, and 7.8% severely depressed [1]. In a systematic review and meta-analysis of studies on depression, Palmer et al. [2] estimated a 39.3% prevalence in CKD, although its true incidence has been noted to be unknown [3]. This variation in estimates has been attributed to differences in the tools used for measuring depression [4] and stages of CKD examined [5]. The increased prevalence of depression among CKD patients stands in contrast to the general population, where reports show an incidence of between 5% to 9% in women and 2% to 3% in men [6].

The reasons for this increased prevalence of depression among CKD patients can be readily understood in light of the many life changes that come with a diagnosis of CKD, the side effects from treatment, and the inevitable decline in physical functioning that occurs over time. For many patients, depressive symptoms begin with a feeling that they have lost control of their life when the diagnosis is first made [7]. Among the usual ways, this is initially experienced through new dietary restrictions and loss of freedom to enjoy preferred foods. As to the side effects from treatment, and especially patients with end-stage renal disease (ESRD) on in-center hemodialysis, there is severe pain which affects 50–60% [8] and chronic fatigue that impacts 82% [9]. Research has also associated the progressive deterioration in physical functioning [10] as a contributing factor in depression in CKD patients [11]. In addition to its emotional ramifications for patients, depression has been found to be an independent predictor of nonadherence with blood pressure medications [12], a higher risk for hospitalization [13], faster decline in the estimated glomerular filtration rate (eGFR), earlier initiation of dialysis therapy [14], and premature death [15].

With respect to its effects on nutritional status, mounting evidence is showing that depression can undermine a patient's ability to adhere to dietary and fluid restrictions. For example, recommendations for the management of hyperphosphatemia from the National Kidney Foundation Kidney Disease Outcomes Quality Initiative (KDOQI) call for patients to limit their dietary intake of phosphorus [16]. Research has shown that depression can make accomplishing this more difficult. In a study of 49 dialysis patients who were considered nonadherent, Akman et al. [17] found that depressed patients had twice the likelihood of nonadherence with dietary phosphorus restrictions than those who were not depressed.

Phosphate binder medication has been characterized as the cornerstone in the management of hyperphosphatemia [18] with a targeted phosphorus level of 3.5–5.5 mg/dL [19]. Studies have shown that 74% of patients are unable to consistently adhere to their binder regiment [20], and depression has been found to be a contributing factor. Tracy and colleagues [21] discovered that higher levels of depression were associated with poorer phosphate binder adherence. An Iranian study of 159 dialysis patients linked higher depression scores with nonadherence to binders [22].

Thrice-weekly hemodialysis treatment is the third strategy in hyperphosphatemia management, with a weekly goal of removing 1800–3000 mg of phosphorus per treatment [23]. Its effectiveness depends on patients being able to consistently attend treatments; however, 35% of patients miss treatments and 32% shorten them [24]. Studies have found that depression is strongly associated with missed treatments. Aebel-Groesch and associates [25] looked at 54,441 dialysis patients screened for depression from 2000 clinics and found a significantly higher rate of missed treatments among those who were depressed, compared to patients not depressed. Weisbord [26] examined 286 dialysis patients with moderate-to-severe depression and found it was independently associated with missed treatments. Most recently, Salmi and colleagues [27] in a cross-sectional analysis of data from the Dialysis Outcomes and Practice Patterns Study (DOPPS) involving 8501 patients from 20 countries, discovered that the 4493 patients who missed treatments over a 4-month period were more likely to be struggling with depression.

While excessive intradialytic weight gain (IDWG) has often been viewed as reflecting a good appetite in dialysis patients [28], it is more critically a major risk factor for long-term adverse cardiovascular outcomes [29]. Recommendations have long called for patients to limit their fluid intake to 1000–2000 mL/day [16], which is known to be among the most difficult challenge they face. Consistent with its widespread adverse effects, depression has been documented to be closely associated with nonadherence in CKD patients. Taskapan et al. [30] examined the potential associations between psychiatric disorders such as depression and compliance with fluid restrictions. They found that IDWGs were significantly higher in depressed patients compared to those not depressed. In a cross-sectional study, Khalil and associates [31] examined the relationship between depressive symptoms and fluid and dietary adherence in 100 dialysis patients and found that moderate-to-severely depressed patients were more likely to be nonadherent with fluid restrictions. This evidence was supported by another cross-sectional study that included 100 dialysis patients in which depression was independently associated with an inability to consistently comply with fluid restrictions [32].

KDOQI guidelines [16] also suggest limiting daily potassium intake, and research has shown that depression can also adversely affect patients' adherence with this recommendation. Sensky et al. [33] looked at the associations between psychosocial variables, including depression and dietary compliance in 45 patients, and discovered that higher pre-dialysis serum potassium was associated with depression. Similarly, in a cross-sectional study of 80 patients in three dialysis clinics in Lima, Peru, Valderrama and colleagues [34] found that more severe depressive symptoms were associated with higher pre-dialysis serum potassium levels.

Lastly, there is a generalized relationship between depression, malnutrition, and protein-energy wasting (PEW) in CKD patients. Kimmel and associates [35] highlighted anorexia secondary to depression which can limit patients' protein and caloric intake and evolve into a vicious cycle of progressive undernutrition. More specific to serum albumin, the traditional marker of patients' protein status, Koo et al. [36] found that higher depressive scores were correlated with all nutritional markers, including serum albumin. Finally, in non-CKD populations, a bidirectional relationship has been found between depression and malnutrition, with micronutrient deficiencies resulting from the latter, worsening mental health symptoms over time [37].

Anxiety

The five subtypes of anxiety disorders that exist on a continuum from normal to pathologic are generalized anxiety, obsessive-compulsive disorder, panic disorders, post-traumatic stress disorder, and social anxiety disorder [38]. Cohen and associates [39] have described anxiety as a "disruptive feelings of uncertainty, dread and fearfulness" (p. 2250). Somatic symptoms can include dizziness, palpitations, nervousness, chest pain, avoidance, difficulties breathing, fear of losing control, and fear of dying [40].

The true prevalence of anxiety among CKD patients is unknown but has been estimated to be as high as 69.3% [41] and to vary by renal replacement therapy [42]. In a 16-month study of dialysis patients, anxiety was found to increase over time [43]. This high incidence of anxiety among CKD patients is contrasted with the general population, where the rate is 7.7% in women and 4.6% in men [44].

The reasons for this increased prevalence of anxiety among CKD patients can be understood by what they have to experience regularly, especially those on in-center dialysis. For example, Feroze and associates [45] interviewed 179 dialysis patients and discovered they often experience anxiety from such routine treatment-related events as having a new person connecting them to the hemodialysis machine and hearing alarm bells sounds. Additional treatment experiences that can contribute to anxiety are dialysis-induced hypotensive episodes, which may result in muscle cramping, dizziness, and a loss of consciousness. Studies have found that these unpredictable events may occur 15–30% of the time during treatment, with a 50% frequency among the elderly and diabetic patients [46]. Concerns about safety in dialysis facilities is a third factor that can add to patients' anxiety, and questions about it have been increasing [47, 48]. Research has found that 50% of patients have anxiety related to clinic safety [45], and an equal number worry that a dialysis staff might make a mistake during their treatment [49]. Finally, there is the anxiety stemming from CKD patients having to confront their own mortality and probable shortened life span [50]. Investigations have discovered a high rate of death anxiety among these patients [51, 52].

In contrast to the voluminous research on depression and its associations with outcomes in CKD patients, including nutritional issues, there has been virtually no research exclusively on anxiety. The studies that have included anxiety as a variable have almost always been combined with a focus on depression [53, 54]. This lack of specific attention to anxiety prompted Lowe et al. [55] to characterize it as the "stepchild" of affective disorders (p. 266). Several explanations have been made for this relative neglect of anxiety. First, since anxiety symptoms often coincide with depressive symptoms, there has been a tendency to perceive them as representing depression rather than as an independent condition [56]. Another possible reason for less attention to anxiety in CKD patients is that there are fewer validated measures compared to the numerous measures for depression [57]. Cukor and associates [56] have raised concerns about the ability of the commonly used Hospital Anxiety and Depression Scale to accurately measure anxiety disorders in dialysis patients. In a recent comparison of screening instruments for assessing anxiety, 40–60% of dialysis patients with anxiety were missed [58]. In addition, it has long been known that anxiety is more difficult to detect during clinical interviews [59]. This was illustrated in a meta-analysis of studies on primary care physicians' ability to detect anxiety disorders, in which only one-third of the cases were correctly diagnosed [60].

Notwithstanding the hurdles to recognize and accurately diagnose anxiety disorders, there has been an emphasis on the importance of understanding the effects of anxiety disorders on outcomes, compared to depression [61–64]. A study which assessed the association between generalized anxiety disorder (GAD) and depression of 2740 adult patients' functional status and disability days, GAD and depressive symptoms were found to have different and independent effects [57]. Consistent with efforts for more specificity, subtypes of panic disorders have been found to be differentially associated with the severity and clinical properties of such comorbidities as suicide attempts, sleep disorders, and a sense of mastery [65]. Finally, although the distinctive effects of anxiety on the nutritional status of CKD patients will have to await future research, it has been suggested that many seemingly irrational behaviors of patients (e.g., nonadherence to dietary recommendations) may actually be the expression of underlying anxiety [39].

Loneliness

Loneliness is a psychosocial issue defined as unpleasant feelings of isolation due to unmet human relationship needs [66]; it has become the focus of ever-increasing investigations because of its associations with many negative health outcomes. For example, loneliness has been tied to increased risky sexual behaviors [67], unintended pregnancy [68], reduced physical inactivity [69], higher cholesterol levels [70], increased blood pressure [71], and heightened risk of depression [72].

In elderly patients, loneliness has been linked with several negative developments and outcomes including a decline in cognitive function [73], feelings of hopelessness and poor self-care capacity [74], and increased suicide risk [75]. A decreased resistance to infection is another adverse development that has been linked to loneliness [76], with a suggested mediating pathway being the growing evidence on the close relationship between loneliness and immune dysregulation [77, 78]. More relevant to the immediate focus of concern, research strongly supports an association between loneliness, depression, anorexia, and malnutrition in the elderly [79–82]. The detrimental effects of a solitary life on nutritional status is further evidenced in studies showing that when the elderly live alone, there is often a reduced motivation to cook [83] and less food is eaten during mealtimes [84].

Research on the relationship between the nutritional status of CKD patients and loneliness has been sporadic. In an earlier study, Bergstrom [85] mentioned loneliness as contributing to low protein intake in CKD patients due to anorexia. Most recently, Stevenson and associates [86] conducted interviews with dialysis patients about adapting to the renal diet and found that many experienced feelings of "isolation from family and friends" (p. 411).

Evidence suggests that loneliness may be a pervasive, yet largely overlooked factor that can detrimentally affect the nutritional status of CKD patients. First is the well-established fact that strong feelings of social isolation tend to ensue from a diagnosis of ESRD and its treatments [87]. Second is the predominately geriatric ESRD population with 176,579 patients being over 65 years of age and 118,537 older than 75 [88]. Relevant to this age group, a cross-sectional study of individuals 60–80 years old in Eastern Europe found that 30–50% were severely lonely [89]. In the United States, 43% of persons over age 65 felt subjectively lonely on a regular basis [90]. In many instances, this is likely due to the death of a spouse. In terms of the ramifications of spousal death for nutritional issues, research has found that older men who lose a spouse can be particularly vulnerable to undernutrition because they tend to have fewer close relationships outside of their spouse, and they often lack cooking skills [91]. Consistent with this evidence, a study of older men who live alone found they were more likely not to have eaten for 1 or 2 days [92]. As to older women who are widowed, studies have discovered they can become nutritionally at risk because there is a tendency for them not to cook for themselves when they no longer have someone to cook for [93, 94].

The gradual deterioration in physical functioning that occurs with ESRD is another factor that can exacerbate social isolation and loneliness. Research has shown that loneliness becomes much more common among individuals with debilitating chronic conditions because it severely limits their mobility and social engagement [95].

Additional overlooked factors that can contribute to loneliness among older CKD patients are the broad changes that have occurred in families over time. Among the most important of these is the disappearance of the large extended family living in the same community as the elderly. Research shows that a large portion of adult children now live more than an hour away from their aging parents, and 80% of this is attributed to moving away due to the job market [96]. A greater geographic distance now characterizes many intergenerational family relationships [97]. Living in less proximity to their aging parents has resulted in a reduced frequency of contact from adult children to provide tangible and emotional support [98], which has been linked to increased loneliness and depression among older adults [99].

Finally, based on evidence from non-CKD populations, a widely prevalent loneliness-associated anorexia among older CKD patients could, theoretically, be interfacing with the anorexia associated with aging [100] and anorexia stemming from uremic toxins [101], which may further aggravate malnutrition and protein-energy wasting (PEW).

Food Insecurity

The United States Department of Agriculture (USDA) [102] defines food insecurity as a lack of consistent access to enough food for a healthy life. There are four different levels of food security: (1) High food security defined as no reported indicators of food access; (2) marginal security denotes the existence of one or two indicators such as anxiety over food or shortages; (3) low food insecurity reflects a reduced quality, variety, and desirability of food in the diet; and (4) very low food security refers to the presence of multiple indicators of disrupted eating patterns and reduced food intake. Additional data by Colman-Jensen and associates [103] has shown that in 2017, (1) 11.8% of United States' households were food insecure and 4.8% (5.8 million households) had very low food security, and (2) the rate of food insecurity among whites was 8.8%, 18.8% among Hispanics, and 21.8% among African Americans.

Ever-increasing attention has focused on food insecurity because of its links with a diverse array of adverse health developments including obesity [104], markers of cardiovascular disease [105], type 2 diabetes [106], and unwanted pregnancy [107]. A recent investigation by Seligman and associates [108] also found that food insecurity is associated with an increased risk of hospital admissions for hypoglycemia and that exhaustion of a food budget is the primary driver. Moreover, the relationship between food insecurity and poor health can be bidirectional, in that negative health outcomes stemming from food insecurity can themselves increase the severity of food insecurity [109].

As would intuitively be expected, food insecurity is a major risk factor for malnutrition in the elderly [110]. In a study by Wolfe and associates [111] on the experiences of older Americans with food insecurity, the following sampling of quotes were obtained: "With all my expenses…sometimes I have to go to bed without eating. Right now I don't have groceries here. I have to wait for my daughter to offer or give me something"; "I have to wait for the check that I get weekly so that I can go and buy some food" (p. 2763). Consistent with research, surveys have found that elderly African Americans are 4.2 times more likely to struggle with food insecurity than elderly white individuals [112].

Food insecurity is also a complex phenomenon whose negative effects often extend well beyond food and dietary concerns to include mental health issues. For example, a recent Australian study found that food insecurity is associated with an increased risk of depression in disadvantaged urban areas [113]. In an investigation by Whitaker and others [114], which looked at food insecurity and the risk for depression and anxiety among mothers of young children, the percentage of women with both mental health problems increased as food insecurity worsened. Most recently, an investigation examined the psychological distress of African Americans struggling with food insecurity ($n = 4003$) and found a six-fold odds of higher psychological distress [115].

Another consequence of food insecurity beyond dietary issues can be compliance with medications. Given the economic constraints that come with food insecurity, research has found that patients often have to choose between paying for food or medications [116, 117]. Individuals struggling with food insecurity are also more likely to delay getting prescriptions refilled, compared with those who are food secured [118, 119].

Turning to food insecurity and the nutritional status of CKD patients, only one study has focused explicitly on its relationship with malnutrition. The investigation by Wilson and colleagues [120] looked at the presence of food insecurity in 98 dialysis patients, of whom 44% were white and 56% African American. Being African American was found to be a significant predictor of food insecurity, and 64% of the patients were mildly to moderately malnourished and 13.3% severely malnourished.

A master's thesis on nutrition by Coleman [121] at the University of Cincinnati examined the use of oral nutritional supplements in 85 dialysis patients as a function of food insecurity; 90.6% of the study's participants were African American. Serum albumin levels were used to assess nutritional status. The investigation showed that 47% of the patients had some degree of food insecurity, and a significant association was found between food insecurity and the need for oral supplements. Again, food insecurity was found to be more highly prevalent among African American dialysis patients.

The only other explicit attention to food insecurity and nutritional issues with CKD has been on its possible role in racial disparities of ESRD. In a cross-sectional analysis of data from the National Health and Nutrition Examination Survey (NHANES) 2003–2008 ($N = 9126$), Crews and associates [122] suggested that food insecurity may contribute to disparities in kidney disease, especially among individuals with diabetes and hypertension. In a subsequent probability sample of NHANES III data ($N = 34,955$), Banerjee and colleagues [123] concluded that food insecurity was independently associated with a higher likelihood of developing ESRD. Lastly, Banerjee et al. [124] linked food insecurity to a faster progression to ESRD via its close association with poverty and the consequent inability of individuals to afford a healthier diet of fruits and vegetables.

Finally, given the paucity of attention to the dynamics between food security and nutrition, several questions can be suggested for future investigations. First, based on findings from studies of food insecurity with non-CKD populations, to what extent could the high incidence of food insecurity among CKD patients in general, and African American patients in particular, be a contributing factor to both malnutrition and PEW? Research might also focus on the persistent problem of medication nonadherence among these patients and to what extent food insecurity might be forcing them to make a choice between paying for food or medications. Lastly, given the evidence from non-CKD populations that food insecurity can engender depression, to what degree could food insecurity-linked depression with CKD patients be a contributing factor in this widely prevalent mental health problem?

Limited Health Literacy

The National Academy of Medicine defined health literacy as the degree to which individuals have the capacity to obtain, process, and understand basic health information and services needed to make appropriate health decisions [125]. An estimated 90 million Americans have limited health literacy (LHL) [126], which is associated with having less education, older age, and lower income [127]. There has been ongoing interest in LHL because of its links to a diverse array of adverse health outcomes including an increased risk for hospitalization [128], lower adherence to medication [129], increased emergency room visits [130], higher rates of diabetes complications [131], and an elevated risk of mortality [132].

LHL can also have psychosocial implications for an individual's mental health; it has been shown to be associated with an increased risk for depression [133], and people struggling with it often harbor feelings of shame [134]. Not surprisingly, LHL can adversely affect patients' interactions with health professionals. Patients can often be intimidated by their interaction with health professionals because of shame, and they are less likely to ask questions or admit they do not understand information provided by their health-care provider [135].

In patients with CKD, it has been estimated that as high as 50% of patients struggle with some degree of LHL [136]. Consistent with its broad ramifications for health issues, LHL has also been shown to affect outcomes in CKD patients. For instance, LHL has been found to restrict patients' knowledge of kidney disease [137]; it is associated with missed dialysis treatments [138], decreased likelihood of patients being referred for kidney transplantation [139], a lower GFR [140], and an increased risk of death [141].

One of the major thrusts of research associated with LHL and nutrition in CKD has been to provide a better understanding of the learning difficulties of patients. Doak and Doak [142] conducted an assessment of reading materials for the renal diet and discovered that it is well beyond the reading level of 55% of patients. Kalista-Richards [143] emphasized the importance of matching reading materials with CKD patients' learning abilities. Lambert et al. [144] found that most patients' experiences with the renal diet feel it is overwhelming, frustrating, and a very emotional journey.

Recent studies have looked at the use of various technologies, such as computers and mobile application devices, to aid with the learning difficulties of CKD patients. Connelly et al. [145] conducted a pilot study to explore the usefulness of a dietary intake monitoring application (DIMA) with 12 dialysis patients who had varying levels of health literacy. The investigators discovered that the subjects used the DIMA much more at the end of the study as they did in the beginning, and that it was useful in modifying dietary behaviors. Welch et al. [146] undertook a 6-week pilot intervention using a Daily Activity Monitoring Application (DAMA) to self-monitor diet and fluid intake with 24 dialysis patients. While the DAMA was found to have a potential to facilitate dietary and fluid self-monitoring, additional refinement and testing were deemed needed. Lastly, Sevick and associates [147] conducted a randomized trial of a technology-supported behavioral intervention to reduce dietary sodium in 179 adult dialysis patients over a 16-week period. While the investigators found that the technology intervention was feasible and acceptable to patients, the patients' fluid weight gains did not change, and the desired behavioral changes observed at 8 weeks were not sustained.

Final areas of research focused on are the challenges renal dietitians face trying to overcome the extra hurdle represented by patients' LHL. For example, Morton De Souza [148], in discussing practical strategies for enhancing learning with low literacy patients, pointedly mentioned the increased workload on dietitians and time constraints. Most recently, Lambert, Mansfield, and Mullan [149] uncovered a major theme of frustration with dietitians that is linked directly to the learning difficulties of patients and inadequate time to properly provide education.

Self-Efficacy

Self-efficacy is a psychosocial concept which has been defined as the confidence in one's ability to succeed with a given task or situation [150]. The strength of self-efficacy is particularly important because an individual is not only more likely to initiate a new behavior but continue until success is achieved [151]. Moreover, self-efficacy is not a generalized response but is very specific to a given behavior. It has been pointed out, for example, that a patient might feel very efficacious about taking prescribed medication but have no confidence in the ability to follow recommended dietary changes [152].

Self-efficacy has become a central focus in research because of its links to a diverse array of health outcomes including the ability to cope with cancer [153], duration of breastfeeding [154], predictor of eating disorders [155], and level of physical activity [156]. Consistent with these broad implications, self-efficacy has also been found to be associated with CKD outcomes. Kauric-Klein et al. [157] examined the impact of an education intervention on blood pressure self-efficacy in a group of dialysis patients and found it was associated with lower diastolic blood pressure. In a randomly selected study of 50 dialysis patients in the Philippines, Balaga et al. [158] found an inverse relationship between hemoglobin levels and self-efficacy.

Self-efficacy and nutritional parameters in CKD patients have also been explored. Rosenbaum [159] found that a higher perceived self-efficacy enabled dialysis patients to better resist the urge to drink excessively. Bradly et al. [160] also documented that patients with higher self-efficacy averaged lower weekend IDWGs. Several studies have examined the relationship between dietary sodium intake and self-efficacy in CKD patients and have found a pattern of evidence suggesting that younger-aged CKD patients are more likely to have a lower self-efficacy for restricting intake, compared to older patients [161–164]. The results of the studies suggest that age-specific dietary education strategies may need to be developed to improve adherence.

Fewer studies have been conducted on the relationship between self-efficacy and adherence to dietary phosphorus and potassium restrictions. Elliott et al. [165], for example, conducted a cross-sectional survey of 95 dialysis patients, in three clinics, which looked at modifiable factors associated with dietary adherence. Among the factors found to be associated with adherence were an individual's level of self-efficacy and health beliefs. These findings prompted the investigators to suggest that clinicians may obtain better results with phosphorus control if they focus not only on dietary education but also on individual patient's self-efficacy beliefs. Focusing specifically on serum potassium, Zrinya et al. [166] similarly linked greater self-efficacy with better dietary adherence.

Social Support

Social support has been defined as the perception that one is cared for, and there are two basic forms [167, 168]. First is informational/education support, which entails the provision of tangible assistance such as helping a person to learn and understand something important to his/her well-being. Secondly, there is emotional support which involves listening and extending empathy, warmth, and nurturance to another person.

Over the last several decades, social support has become a central focus in health-related research and clinical practice because of its mediating role in an almost endless array of outcomes and behaviors. These include anxiety [169], depression [170], falls in older adults [171], low birth weight [172], risky sexual behaviors [173], and type 2 diabetes in adults [174].

Consistent with its widespread impact, social support has also been found to be a mediating variable in several outcomes for CKD patients. For example, low social support was recently found to be a factor in late-life depression of ESRD patients [175]. In a study which explored the perceived effects of support on depression and anxiety in hemodialysis patients, Lilympak et al. [176] found increased support from friends was linked with a 57% reduction in anxiety. Symister and Friend [177] reported that higher social support decreased depression in CKD patients by improving their self-efficacy which, in turn, enhances optimism. A Turkey-based study of 73 dialysis patients by Karadag and associates [178] found that those with lower levels of perceived support from family were more likely to experience severe fatigue, compared to patients with higher perceived support. In another study, Plantinga et al. [179] found that the availability of social support was significantly associated with a reduced risk of hospitalization in CKD patients. Finally, and most importantly, Thong and associates [180] concluded that the level of social support predicts survival in dialysis patients.

Social support from family, friends, and the dialysis staff has been found to be associated indicators of nutritional status in dialysis patients. Boyer and associates [181] linked support from family with better adherence to phosphate binders. In an Italian observational study conducted by Cicolini et al. [182] of 72 dialysis patients, those with stronger family support were found to have lower phosphate and serum potassium levels. The effects of an education program focused on IDWG by the dialysis clinic staff were evaluated in 26 dialysis patients who were noncompliant with their fluid restrictions. The program consisted of teaching and weekly reinforcements from staff about diet and fluids. Following the 2-month intervention, investigators found a significant decrease in IDWG (from 2.64 kg to 2.21 kg), and adherence to fluid restrictions increased from 47% to 71% [183].

Potential Strategies for Mitigating Psychosocial Factors That Negatively Impact Nutrition and Bolstering Those Which Can Help Enhance It

Depression

The earliest reports on depression as a serious problem accompanying CKD were published in the mid-1960s [184], well before the federal legislation that created the ESRD program in 1972. Over the next five decades, hundreds of reports have been published on the prevalence of depression and its ramifications in dialysis patients. Mounting evidence has also surfaced in recent years showing that depression can undermine the patient's ability to adhere to the renal diet [17, 21, 22, 30–34, 36]. Research has shown that diligent efforts by patients to comply with the renal diet may cause mild depression, which can lead to relapses in adherence [185].

Despite overwhelming evidence on the profound implications of depression in dialysis patients, reports continue to show that it remains largely unrecognized and untreated in the vast majority of these patients [186]. An investigation by Watnick and colleagues [187] discovered that almost half of the patients starting dialysis were depressed, but only 16% were receiving treatment for depression. A previously unrecognized partial explanation for this was recently uncovered in a study by Pena-Polanco and associates [188], which found that, in some instances, dialysis companies are simply unwilling to provide treatment for depression. No explanation for this was offered by the companies, and the study's investigators concluded that it "represents a major obstacle to the systematic provision of therapy" [p. 302]. This dismal outlook prompted Chilcot and Hudson [189] to ask, "Is successful treatment of depression in dialysis patients an achievable goal?"(p. 1).

Notwithstanding its persistent neglect, evidence shows that depression can be successfully treated when it is made a priority. For example, a study of depressed dialysis patients compared the effectiveness of the antidepressant paroxetine with agomelatine [190]. By the twelfth week of treatment, depression scores of patients prescribed agomelatine were lower. Non-pharmacological interventions for depression in dialysis patients have also been examined. Cukor and associates [191] looked at the effectiveness of a psychosocial intervention for depression involving individualized cognitive behavioral therapy and found an 89% reduction in symptoms at the end of the treatment period. Koo and associates [192] found that therapeutic interventions for depression resulted in improved nutritional status in dialysis patients. Finally, research has shown that social workers are among the most under-utilized health professionals in dialysis facilities who can successfully provide psychotherapeutic interventions for depression in dialysis patients [193–196]. An investigation by Prescott [197] found that the majority of dialysis patients prefer to seek and receive treatment for such mental health issues as depression from their clinic social worker.

Anxiety

Because it has been largely neglected in investigations, the full extent to which anxiety adversely affects nutritional status of CKD patients is unknown. The Brief Anxiety Symptom Inventory [198] is a self-administered tool which has been used successfully to assess depression in hospitalized patients and can be used with dialysis patients. Research has shown that some patients will benefit from pharmacotherapy alone, but most will benefit from a combination of individualized psychotherapeutic support [199]. Once again, dialysis clinic social workers are an underutilized resource for helping patients with anxiety.

Loneliness

Available evidence reviewed in this chapter suggests that loneliness may be largely overlooked, but it is a significant factor that adversely affects the nutritional status of CKD patients. Because loneliness has been found to be an independent risk factor for malnutrition in older people [200], it may have profound implications for patients on dialysis, given that the majority are over 65 years of age [88]. However, because loneliness is not routinely identified as a nutritional risk factor by dietitians, there is the need to determine its prevalence in CKD patients. The UCLA Loneliness Scale [201] is the most commonly used self-reported tool for assessing loneliness in medical patients.

The professional literature has recommended various types of interventions to reduce social isolation and loneliness in older individuals including social support groups, reminiscence therapy, videoconferencing, and animal companionship [202]. The feasibility of any of these interventions for dialysis patients is unknown. Additional pragmatic strategies can be suggested to help lessen the potentially adverse nutritional ramifications from loneliness. For instance, a simple initiative that dietitians can take with older patients who live alone is to encourage available family members to occasionally call and have a meal with them. Advising patients to reach out and rebuild old social networks has also been suggested as a strategy to counter loneliness and social isolation [203]. Older patients could also be advised to take advantage of free socialization opportunities at local senior centers in the community. Finally, in some dialysis clinics, there is a greater awareness of and sensitivity to the potential detrimental effects of loneliness. As a result, efforts are being made to encourage mutual peer support among and between patients themselves [204–206]. Hughes et al. [207] found that a major benefit from such support includes empathy and an understanding with patients that they are not alone in their suffering.

Food Insecurity

Food insecurity is not routinely assessed in CKD patients by renal dietitians, but evidence reveals it may be more of a serious problem than typically assumed. A first step in any intervention is to determine the presence of food insecurity. A quick assessment tool [208] consisting of the following two questions has been developed and is widely utilized in health-care settings:

- QUESTION: How often during the past 12 months were you worried that food would run out before money was gotten to buy more? RESPONSES: Often true, sometimes true, or never true.
- QUESTION: How often during the past 12 months did the food that was purchased didn't last and you didn't have enough money to buy more? RESPONSES: Often true, sometimes true, or never true.

When food insecurity is detected, the dietitian can suggest the following actions to help mitigate the potential adverse effects of food insecurity on nutritional status. For example, dietitians can give patients information on lower cost foods they can purchase that are appropriate for the renal diet. A referral to Meals on Wheels services is another practical action that can be taken with older patients. There are also food banks in most communities which dietitians can inform patients about and where almost anyone struggling with food insecurity can go to supplement inadequate supplies during a given month.

Finally, a position paper by the Academy of Nutrition and Dietetics [209] has suggested that dietitians have an important role to play in combatting food insecurity. They can support legislative and regulatory processes that promote uniform, adequately funded food and nutrition assistance programs for vulnerable populations.

Limited Health Literacy

It has been established that patients with LHL mostly fail to adhere to medical recommendations as a result of not fully understanding the medical information provided [210]. In discussing interventions to help patients with LHL improve their nutritional status, a number of education strategies and methods have been found to be effective with patients in general, and particularly in those with LHL. First, it is universally recognized that written health information materials should match the patient's reading level [211]. Avoiding medical jargon and using plain language are also well-established practices [212]. For patients who struggle with remembering verbal instructions, visual aids that include pictures have been found to be effective in increasing comprehension, in addition to reducing the amount of reading required [213]. Asking open-ended questions and limiting the number of topics discussed in a session is another method that has been shown to work with learning-challenged patients [134]. In addition, a tailored educational approach involving collaboration with patients has been found to be more effective than a didactic approach [214]. The teach-back educational method has also been shown to have positive effects in a wide range of health outcomes with improving patients' understanding and adherence [215]. This basically involves patients repeating back information in their own words so health professionals can assess their level of understanding and add/correct information as necessary. Finally, evidence has shown that single and isolated teaching sessions are often insufficient to ensure that patients fully understand a health-related task, making frequent reinforcement necessary to achieve optimal adherence [216–218]. Reinforcement appears to be particularly important with CKD patients because many have LHL and struggle with cognitive impairment and depression, both of which affect the ability to recall information [219]. Thus, as Ramsdell and Annis [220] have succinctly stated, educating CKD patients is "a continuing repetitive process" (p. 217).

Studies have shown that when renal dietitians are able to implement these educational strategies and methods with learning-challenged CKD patients, they can be more effective at addressing nutritional issues. For instance, the benefits of matching educational materials and patients' reading levels were recently illustrated in a study by Duffrin et al. [221] with African American dialysis patients who had a fourth-grade reading level. Through matching language with these patients' reading level, investigators were able to validate an assessment tool to accurately measure food intake.

Several investigators have demonstrated that when renal dietitians spend more time and/or have more frequent contact with patients, it greatly enhances comprehension and adherence. For example, in a study by Ford and associates [222], which examined the effectiveness of an additional 20–30 minutes of diet education per month with patients, serum phosphorus and calcium/phosphorus levels were significantly lowered in the experimental group of patients, compared to the control group. In an investigation by Morey et al. [185], they asked the question whether more dietetic time could enhance nutritional outcomes. Patients in the experimental group received an increased frequency of dietetic education/counseling interventions, which resulted in significantly lower serum phosphate levels compared to those in the control group. Confirming that CKD patients need more frequent reinforcements to optimize outcomes, those in the experimental group returned to their baseline serum phosphate levels soon after the intervention ended [185]. Karavetian and Ghaddar [223] conducted a cluster-based randomized trial to examine the effects of self-management dietary counseling on hyperphosphatemia. Patients in the experimental group received two additional 20-minute counseling sessions each week throughout the 8-week study period. Posttest analysis revealed significant improvements in serum phosphorus levels in the experimental group, but no improvement in the two control groups. Finally, there is the earlier investigation by Milas and associates [224] on compliance with a low protein diet. They found that ongoing praise and encouragement from dietitians were instrumental in helping pre-dialysis patients maintain their level of motivation for dietary adherence. (Refer to Chap. 34 for section on "Dietary Adherence.")

Given that a lack of information on educational strategies does not appear to be the main obstacle to dietitians being more effective with learning-challenged patients, coalescing evidence would suggest that it is the pragmatic issue of time. For example, a seminal investigation by Burrowes, Russell, and Rocco [225] examined factors affecting dietitians' ability to implement the NKF-KDOQI Nutrition Guidelines for Adults and found that time was a major impediment. Hand and associates [226] next looked explicitly at the variable of time in relationship to dietitians being able to follow the NKF-KDOQI Guidelines for frequency and method of dietary assessment and again discovered that time is a significant limiting factor. Hand and Burrowes [227] subsequently conducted a survey of 3382 renal dietitians to assess perceptions of their roles and responsibilities and found that the expanded administrative responsibilities imposed on them have taken away valuable face-to-face clinical time with patients. More recently, Hand, Albert, and Sehgal [228] conducted a cross-sectional study to quantify how dietitians spend their time in dialysis facilities. They found that only 25% of the dietitian's time is available for direct patient care, which may be insufficient to improve nutritional status [228]. Some concluding evidence on how limited time is adversely affecting the effectiveness of dietitians comes from a study by Wood and Gills [229] who explored dietitians' day-to-day engagement with LHL patients. The following quote from a participant in the study serves to illustrate the frustrating experience dietitians have trying to achieve the best outcomes:

> You only have so much time to do the assessment, the plan you know, to provide some recommendations and then you're off on your way….If they don't understand it and they're not seeing you for another month then a whole month goes by without any change being made. (p. 54)

Finally, as has been argued elsewhere, inherent in the ever-decreasing time that dietitians have for individual patients is their inadequate staffing in dialysis facilities; this may be the most fundamental obstacle to ultimately achieve optimal nutritional outcomes [230, 231]. Additional support for this comes from a *Report to Congress on Medical Nutrition Therapy* [232],which declared that the "dietitian ratio [is] one of the most important measures in determining the adequacy of nutrition therapy in dialysis centers" (p. 17).

Self-Efficacy

The basic assumption of the self-efficacy theory is that an individual's belief in his/her own capabilities to produce desired effects by their own actions is the most important determinants of the behaviors they choose to engage in, as well as how much they persevere in the face of obstacles and challenges [233]. Self-efficacy has become a central focus in health promotion because of its profound impact on behaviors. Potential blueprints for interventions to enhance self-efficacy with CKD patients come from several reports. First, a Taiwan study by Tsay [234] examined the effects of a self-efficacy training program on fluid compliance in a group of dialysis patients. The training consisted of 12 educational sessions each lasting 1 hour on such topics as the pathophysiology of renal failure, medications, complications, nutrition, and fluid restrictions. The investigators found that patients in the experimental self-efficacy training group significantly decreased their IDWG more than patients in the control group. Aliasgharpour and Shemali [235] also investigated the effects of a self-efficacy promotion training program on body weight changes in patients undergoing hemodialysis. After 2 months, patients in the intervention group significantly reduced their IDWG, compared to those in the control group [235].

Studies have also looked at the impact of empowerment on enhancing patients' self-efficacy, and they likewise serve as potential roadmaps for intervention. For instance, Moattari and associates [236] conducted a randomized controlled trial on the effects of empowerment on clinical and laboratory indicators in dialysis patients. Components of empowerment included self-management, education, and enhanced goal-setting and problem-solving. Significant improvements following empowerment were observed in systolic/diastolic blood pressure, IDWGs, and hemoglobin levels in the intervention group compared to the control group [236]. Tsay and Hung [237] also examined the effectiveness of an empowerment program on self-care, self-efficacy, and depression in a randomized control trial that included 25 dialysis patients in the intervention group and 25 in the control group. Data collected 6 weeks following the intervention revealed a significantly greater improvement in self-care and self-efficacy with patients exposed to the empowerment program compared to those not exposed to the program [237].

Social Support

Robust evidence shows that the availability of social supports, including from patients' family and dialysis staff, can enhance adherence with various nutritional parameters such as serum phosphorus [180, 181] and IDWG [182]. Increasing social support from patients' families may not always be an achievable goal, but bolstering it from dialysis staff is achievable. In this case, and compared to health-care professionals who provide medical services to patients with other chronic conditions, the interdisciplinary team in dialysis facilities would appear to be in a uniquely strategic position to increase the availability of different forms of support. This is because of the frequency of face-to-face contact with patients (e.g., three times a week, for 3–5 hours each day) and its long duration (e.g., often for years). Capitalizing on this extended and frequent interaction would appear to offer many opportunities to develop innovative approaches to further optimize nutritional outcomes. Evidence of this potential comes from a cross-sectional study by Yokoyama and associates [238] which examined the effects of perceived encouragement from dialysis staff on adherence to fluid restrictions in 72 dialysis patients. Using the Staff Encouragement Scale to assess patients' perceptions, encouragement was found to be positively and significantly associated with better fluid adherence.

Conclusion

In forays on psychosocial factors that impact patients with CKD in general, and their nutritional status in particular, the predominate focus has been on depression. There is a growing consensus that the psychosocial dimension entails many more factors that are understudied yet play an important role in the overall health of these patients [239]. This chapter has endeavored to broaden the perspective on psychosocial factors that can affect the nutritional status of CKD patients. Consistent with the growing body of evidence, a recent investigation by Johansson et al. [240] found that energy and protein intake in older ESRD patients is independently associated with psychosocial issues. However, as the overview of research in this chapter reveals, many knowledge gaps remain in fully understanding the impact of these factors on this nutritionally vulnerable population in which, as Bergstrom and Lindholm [241] have noted, malnutrition can be a direct cause of death in elderly patients. Thus, as Norton and associates [242] have suggested, a better understanding of the psychosocial determinants and appreciation of their underlying associations with meaningful clinical outcomes could help practitioners striving to achieve more optimal outcomes.

References

1. Johnson S, Dwyer A. Patient perceived barriers to treatment of depression and anxiety in hemodialysis. Clin Nephrol. 2008;69:201–6. Available from: https://doi.org/10.5414/cnp69201.
2. Palmer S, Vecchio M, Craig JC, Tonelli M, Johnson DW, Nicolucci A, et al. Prevalence of depression in chronic kidney disease: systematic review of meta-analysis of observation studies. Kidney Int. 2013;84:179–91.
3. Ossareh S, Tabrizian S, Zehbarjardi M, Joodat RS. Prevalence of depression in maintenance hemodialysis patients and its correlation with adherence and medications. Iran J Kidney Dis. 2014;8(6):467–74.
4. Chilcot J, Wellsted D, Da Silva-Gane M, Farrington K. Depression on dialysis. Nephrol Clin Pract. 2008;108(4):c256–64.
5. Cameron JI, Whiteside C, Katz J, Devins GM. Differences in quality of life across renal replacement therapies: a meta-analysis comparison. Am J Kidney Dis. 2000;35(4):629–37. Available from: https://doi.org/10.1016/S0272-6386(00)70009-6.
6. Kessler RC, Berglund P, Demler O, Jin R, Koretz D, Merikangas KR, et al. The epidemiology of major depressive disorder: results from the National Comorbidity Survey Replication (NCS-R). JAMA. 2003;289(23):3095–105. Available from: https://doi.org/10.1001/jama.289.23.3095.
7. Chiaranal C. The lived experience of patients receiving hemodialysis treatment for End-Stage Renal Disease: a qualitative study. J Nurs Res. 2016;24(2):101–8. Available from: https://doi.org/10.1097/jnr.0000000000000100.
8. Santoro D, Satta E, Messina S, Costantino G, Savica V, Bellinghieri G. Pain in end-stage renal disease: a frequent and neglected clinical problem. Clin Nephrol. 2013;79(Suppl 1):S2–S11.
9. Jhamb M, Weisbord SD, Steel JL, Unruh M. Fatigue in patients receiving maintenance dialysis: a review of definitions, measures and contributing factors. Am J Kidney Dis. 2008;52(2):353–65. Available from: https://doi.org/10.1053/j.ajkd.2008.05.005.
10. Sutcliffe BK, Bennett PN, Fraser SF, Mohebbi M. The deterioration in physical function of hemodialysis patients. Hemodial Int. 2018;22(2):245–53. Available from: https://doi.org/10.1111/hdi.12570.
11. Kittiskulnam P, Sheshadri A, Johansen KL. Consequences of CKD on functioning. Semin Nephrol. 2016;36(4):305–18. Available from: https://doi.org/10.1016/j.semmephrol.2016.05.007.
12. Kauric-Klein Z. Depression and medication adherence in patients on hemodialysis. Curr Hypertens Rev. 2017;13(2):138–43. Available from: https://doi.org/10.2174/1573402113666171129182611.
13. Lopes AA, Bragg J, Young E, Goodkin D, Mapes D, Combe C, et al. Depression as a predictor of morbidity and hospitalization among hemodialysis patients in the United States and Europe. Kidney Int. 2002;62(1):199–207.
14. Tsai YC, Chiu YW, Hung CC, Hwang SJ, Tsai JC, Wang SL, et al. Association of symptoms of depression with progression of CKD. Am J Kidney Dis. 2012;60(1):54–61. Available from: https://doi.org/10.1053/j.ajkd.2012.02.325.
15. Kimmel PL, Peterson RA. Depression in end-stage renal disease patients treated with hemodialysis: tools, correlates, outcomes and needs. Semin Dial. 2005;18(2):91–7. Available from: https://doi.org/10.1111/j.1525-139x.2005.18209.x.
16. Ikizler TA, Burrowes J, Byham-Gray L, Campbell K, Carrero JJ, Chan W, et al. KDOQI Nutrition in CKD Guideline Work Group. KDOQI clinical practice guideline for nutrition in CKD: 2020 update. Am J Kidney Dis. 2020; in press.
17. Akman B, Uyar M, Afsar B, Sezer S, Ozdemir FN, Haberal M. Adherence, depression and quality of life on a renal transplantation waiting list. Transpl Int. 2007;20(8):682–7. Available from: https://doi.org/10.1111/j.1432-2277.2007.00495.x.
18. Umeukeje EM, Mixon AS, Cavanaugh KL. Phosphate-control adherence in hemodialysis patients: current perspectives. Patient Prefer Adherence. 2018;12:1175–91. Available from: https://doi.org/10.2147/PPA.S145648.
19. National Kidney Foundation. K/DOQI Clinical practice guidelines for bone metabolism and disease in chronic kidney disease. Am J Kidney Dis. 2003;42(Suppl 3):S1–S201.
20. Karamanidou C, Clatworthy J, Weinman J, Horne R. A systematic review of the prevalence and determinants of nonadherence to phosphate binding medication in patients with end-stage renal disease. BMC Nephrol. 2008;9:2. Available from: https://doi.org/10.1186/1471-2369-9-2.
21. Tracy HM, Green C, McCleary J. Noncompliance in hemodialysis as measured with MBHL. Psychol Health. 1987;1(4):411–23.

22. Ossareh S, Tabrizian S, Joodat RS. Prevalence of depression in maintenance hemodialysis patients and its correlation with adherence to medication. Iran J Kidney Dis. 2014;8:467–74.

23. Waheed AA, Pedraza F, Lenz O, Isakova T. Phosphate control in end-stage renal disease: barriers and opportunities. Nephrol Dial Transplant. 2013;28(12):2961–8. Available from: https://doi.org/10.1093/ndt/gft244.

24. Denhaerynek K, Manhaeve D, Dobbels F, Garzoni D, Nolte C, De Geest S. Prevalence and consequences of nonadherence to hemodialysis regiments. Am J Crit Care. 2007;16(3):225–35.

25. Aebel-Groesch K, Dunn D, Major A, Mayes S, Njord L, Benner O, Tentori F. Hospitalization and missed dialysis treatments are common in hemodialysis patients with depressive symptoms. Davita Clinical Research. Available from https://www.davitaclinicalresearch.com/publication/hospitalization-missed-dialysis-treatment. Accessed 12 Dec 2018.

26. Weisbord SD, Mor MK, Sevick A, Shields AM, Rollman BL, Palevsky PM, et al. Associations of depressive symptoms and pain with dialysis adherence, health resources utilization, and mortality in patients receiving chronic hemodialysis. Clin J Am Soc Nephrol. 2014;9(9):1594–602.

27. Salmi IA, Larkina M, Subramanian L, Subramanian L, Morgenstern H, Jacobson SH, et al. Missed hemodialysis treatments: international variation, predictors, and outcomes in the Dialysis Outcomes and Practice Patterns Study (DOPPS). Am J Kidney Dis. 2018;72(5):634–43.

28. Testa A, Beaud JM. The other side of the coin: interdialytic weight gain as an index of good nutrition. Am J Kidney Dis. 1998;31:830–4. Available from: https://doi.org/10.1016/S0272-6386(98)70052-6.

29. Fischbach M, Zaloszyc A, Schroff R. The interdialytic weight gain: a simple marker of left ventricular hypertrophy in children on chronic haemodialysis. Pediatr Nephrol. 2015;30(6):859–63.

30. Taskapan H, Ates F, Kaya B, Emul M, Kaya M, Taskapan C, Sabin I. Psychiatric disorders and large interdialytic weight gain in patients in chronic haemodialysis. Nephrology (Carlton). 2005;10(1):15–20.

31. Khalil AA, Frazier SK, Lennie TA, Sawaya BP. Depressive symptoms and dietary adherence in patients with end-stage renal disease. J Ren Care. 2011;37(1):30–9. Available from: https://doi.org/10.1111/j.1755-6686.2011.00202.x.

32. Alosaimi FD, Asiri M, Alswayt S, Almodameg S. Psychosocial predictors of nonadherence to medical management among patients on maintenance dialysis. Int J Nephrol Renovasc Dis. 2016;9:263–72. Available from: https://doi.org/10.2147/IJNRD.S121548.

33. Sensky T, Leger C, Gilmour S. Psychosocial and cognitive factors associated with adherence to dietary and fluid restriction regimens by people on chronic haemodialysis. Psychother Psychosom. 1996;65(1):36–42.

34. Garcia-Valderrama FW, Fajardo C, Guevara R, Gonzalez-Perez V, Hurtado A. Poor adherence to diet in hemodialysis: role of anxiety and depression. Nefrologia. 2002;22(3):245–52.

35. Kimmel PL, Weihs K, Peterson RA. Survival in hemodialysis patients: the role of depression. J Am Soc Nephrol. 1993;4(1):12–27.

36. Koo JR, Yoon JW, Kim SG, Lee YK, Oh KH, Kim GH, et al. Association of depression with malnutrition in chronic hemodialysis patients. Am J Kidney Dis. 2003;41(5):1037–42.

37. Kvamme JM, Gronli O, Florholmen J, Jacobsen BK. Risk of malnutrition is associated with mental health symptoms in community living elderly men and women: the Tromso Study. BMC Psychiatry. 2011;11:112. Available from: https://doi.org/10.1186/1471-244x-11-112.

38. Barlow DH. Anxiety and its disorders. New York: Guilford Press; 1988.

39. Cohen SD, Cukor D, Kimmel PL. Anxiety in patients treated with hemodialysis. Clin J Am Soc Nephrol. 2016;11(12):2250–5. Available from: https://doi.org/10.2215/CJN.02590316.

40. Gelenberg AJ. Psychiatric and somatic markers of anxiety: identification and pharmacologic treatment. Prim Care Companion J Clin Psychiatry. 2000;2(2):49–54.

41. Squalli-Houssaini T, Ramouz I, Fahi Z, Tahiri A, Sekkat FZ, Ouzeddoun N, et al. Effects of anxiety and depression in haemodialysis adequacy. Nephrol Ther. 2005;1(1):31–7.

42. Karaminia R, Tavallaii SA, Lorgard-Dezfuli-Nejad M, Moghani Lankarani M, et al. Anxiety and depression: a comparison between renal transplant recipients and hemodialysis patients. Transplant Proc. 2007;39(4):1082–4. Available from: https://doi.org/10.1016/j.transproceed.2007.03.088.

43. Cukor D, Coplan J, Brown C, Peterson RA, Kimmel PL. Course of depression and anxiety diagnosis in patients treated with hemodialysis: a 16-month follow-up. Clin J Am Soc Nephrol. 2008;3(6):1752–8.

44. Kessler RC, Petukhova M, Sampson NA, Zaslavsky AM, Wittchen HU. Twelve-month and lifetime prevalence and lifetime Morbid Risk of anxiety and Mood Disorders in the United States. Int J Methods Psychiatr Res. 2012;21(3):169–84. Available from: https://doi.org/10.1002/mpr.1359.

45. Feroze U, Martin D, Kalantar-Zadeh K, Kim JC, Reina-Patton A, Kopple JD. Anxiety and depression in maintenance dialysis patients: preliminary data of a cross-sectional study and brief literature review. J Ren Nutr. 2012;22(1):207–10. Available from: https://doi.org/10.1053/j.jrn.2011.10.009.

46. Sulowicz W, Radziszewski A. Pathogenesis and treatment of diabetic hypotension. Kidney Int. 2006;70(Suppl 104):S36–9. Available from: https://doi.org/10.1038/sj.ki.5001975.

47. Pippias M, Tomson CRV. Patient safety in chronic kidney disease: time for nephrologists to take action. Nephrol Dial Transplant. 2014;29(1):474–5. Available from: https://doi.org/10.1093/ndt/gft364.
48. Kliger AS. Maintaining safety in the dialysis facility. Clin J Am Soc Nephrol. 2015;10(4):688–95.
49. Garrick R, Kliger A, Stefanchik B. Patient and facility safety in hemodialysis opportunities and strategies to develop a culture of safety. Clin J Am Soc Nephrol. 2012;7(4):680–8. Available from: https://doi.org/10.2215/CJN.06530711.
50. Feroze U, Martin D, Reina-Patton A, Kalantar-Zadeh K, Kopple JD. Mental health, depression and anxiety in patients on maintenance dialysis. Iran J Kidney Dis. 2010;4(3):173–80.
51. Dewina A, Emaliyawati E, Praptiwi A. Death anxiety level among patients with chronic renal failure undergoing hemodialysis. J Nurs Care. 2018. Available from: https://doi.org/10.24198/jnc.v1i1.15757.
52. Shafaii M, Payami M, Amini K, Pahlevan S. The relationship between death anxiety and quality of life in hemo-dialysis patients. J Hayat. 2017;22(4):325–38.
53. Kutner NG, Fair PL, Kutner MH. Assessing depression and anxiety in chronic dialysis patients. J Psychosom Res. 1985;29(1):23–31. Available from: https://doi.org/10.1016/0022-3999(85)90005-4.
54. Lee YJ, Kim MS, Cho S, Kim SR. Association of depression and anxiety with reduced quality of life in patients with predialysis chronic kidney disease. Int J Clin Pract. 2013;67(4):570–9. Available from: https://doi.org/10.1111/ijcp.12020.
55. Lowe B, Decker O, Muller S, Brähler E, Schellberg D, Herzog W, et al. Validation and standardization of the Generalized Anxiety Disorder Screener (GAD-7) in the general population. Med Care. 2008;46(3):266–74.
56. Cukor D, Coplan J, Brown C, Friedman S, Newville H, Safier M, et al. Anxiety disorders in adults treated by hemo-dialysis: a single-center study. Am J Kidney Dis. 2008;52(1):128–36. Available from: https://doi.org/10.1053/j.ajkd.2008.02.300.
57. Spitzer RL, Kroenker K, Williams JBW, Lowe B. A brief measure for assessing generalized anxiety disorders. Arch Intern Med. 2006;166(10):1092–7. Available from: https://doi.org/10.1001/archinte.166.10.1092.
58. Preljevic VT, Osthus TBH, Sandvik L, Opjordsmoen S, Nordhus IH, Os I, et al. Screening for anxiety and depression in dialysis patients: comparison of the Hospital anxiety and Depression Scale and the Beck Depression Inventory. J Psychosom Res. 2012;73(2):139–44.
59. Kroenke K, Spitzer RL, Williams JB, Monahan PO, Lowe B. Anxiety disorders in primary care: prevalence, impairment, comorbidity and detection. Ann Intern Med. 2007;146:317–25.
60. Olariu E, Forero CG, Castro-Rodriguez J-I, Rodrigo-Calvo MT, Álvarez P, Martín-López LM, et al. Detection of anxiety disorder in primary care: a meta-analysis of assisted and unassisted diagnoses. Depress Anxiety. 2015;32(7):471–84. Available from: https://doi.org/10.1002/da.22360.
61. Eysenck MW, Fajkowska M. Anxiety and depression: toward overlapping and distinctive features. Cogn Emot. 2018;32(7):1391–400. Available from: https://doi.org/10.1080/026999931.2017.1330255.
62. Beuke CJ, Fischer R, McDowall J. Anxiety and depression: why and how to measure their separate effects. Clin Psychol Rev. 2003;23(6):831–48. Available from: https://doi.org/10.1016/S0272-7358(03)00074-6.
63. Baldwin DS, Evans DL, Hirschfeld RM, Kasper S. Can we distinguish anxiety from depression? Psychopharmacol Bull. 2002;36(Suppl 2):158–65.
64. Nitschke JB, Heller W, Imig JC, McDonald RP, Miller GA. Distinguishing dimensions of anxiety and depression. Cogn Ther Res. 2001;25(1):1–22.
65. Pattyn T, Van Den Eede F, Lamers F, Veltman D, Sabbe BG, Penninx BW. Identifying panic disorder subtypes using factor mixture modeling. Depress Anxiety. 2015;32(7):509–17. Available from: https://doi.org/10.1002/da.22379.
66. Ryan AK, Willits FK. Family ties, physical health and psychological well-being. J Aging Health. 2007;19:907–20.
67. Hubach RD, DiStefano AS, Wood MM. Understanding the influence of loneliness on HIV risk behavior in young men who have sex with men. J Gay Lesbian Soc Serv. 2012;24(4):371–95. Available from: https://doi.org/10.1080/10538720.2012.721676.
68. Sable MR, Washington CC, Schwartz LR, Jorgenson M. Social well-being in pregnant women: intended versus unintended pregnancies. J Psychosoc Nurs Ment Health Serv. 2007;45(12):24–31.
69. Hawkley LC, Thisted RA, Cacioppo JT. Loneliness predicts reduced physical activity: cross-sectional and longi-tudinal analyses. Health Psychol. 2009;28(3):354–63. Available from: https://doi.org/10.1037/a0014400.
70. Whisman MA. Loneliness and the metabolic syndrome in a population-based sample of middle-aged and older adults. Health Psychol. 2010;29(5):550–4. Available from: https://doi.org/10.1037/a0020760.
71. Hawkley LC, Masi CM, Berry JD, Cacioppo JT. Loneliness is a unique predictor of age-related differences in systolic blood pressure. Psychol Aging. 2006;21(1):152–64.
72. Kara M, Mirici A. Loneliness, depression and social support of Turkish patients with chronic obstructive pulmo-nary disease and their spouses in Turkey. J Nurs Scholarsh. 2004;36(4):331–6.
73. Tilvis RS, Kahonen-Vare MH, Jolkkonen J, Valvanne J, Pitkala KH, Strandberg TE. Predictors of cognitive decline and mortality of aged people over a 10-year period. J Gerontol A Biol Sci Med Sci. 2004;59(3):268–74.

74. Cohen-Manfield J, Parpura-Gill A. Loneliness in older persons: a theoretical model and empirical findings. Int Psychogeriatr. 2007;19(2):279–94. Available from: https://doi.org/10.1017/S1041610206004200.

75. Wiktorsson S, Runeson B, Skoog I, Ostling S, Waern M. Attempted suicide in the elderly: characteristics of suicide attempters 70 years and older and a general population comparison. Am J Geriatr Psychiatry. 2010;18(1):57–67.

76. Miller G. Social neuroscience. Why loneliness is hazardous to your health. Science. 2011;331(6014):138–40. Available from: https://doi.org/10.1126/science.331.6014.138.

77. Cacioppo JT, Cacioppo S, Capitanio JP, Cole SW. The neuroendocrinology of social isolation. Annu Rev Psychol. 2015;66:733–67. Available from: https://doi.org/10.1146/annurev-psych-010814-015240.

78. Jaremka LM, Fagundes CP, Glaser R, Bennett JM, Malarkey WB, Kiecolt-Glaser JK. Loneliness predicts pain, depression and fatigue: understanding the role of immune dysregulation. Psychoneuroendocrinology. 2013;38(8):1310–7. Available from: https://doi.org/10.1016/j.psyneuen.2012.11.016.

79. Ramic E, Pranjic N, Batic-Mujanovic O, Karic E, Alibasic E, Alic A. The effect of loneliness on malnutrition in elderly population. Med Arh. 2011;65(2):92–5.

80. Schilp J, Wijnhoven HA, Deeg DJ, Visser M. Early determinants for the development of undernutrition in an older general population: longitudinal aging study Amsterdam. Br J Nutr. 2011;106(5):708–17. Available from: https://doi.org/10.1017/S0007114511000717.

81. Hanna KL, Collins PF. Relationship between living alone and food and nutrient intake. Nutr Rev. 2015;73(9):594–611. Available from: https://doi.org/10.1093/nutrit/nuv024.

82. Cacioppo JT, Hughes ME, Waite LJ, Hawkley LC, Thisted RA. Loneliness as a specific risk factor for depressive symptoms: cross-sectional and longitudinal analyses. Psychol Aging. 2006;21(1):140–51.

83. Alpass FM, Neville S. Loneliness and depression in older males. Aging Ment Health. 2003;7(3):210–6.

84. Loeher JL, Robinson CO, Roth DL. The effect of the presence of others on caloric intake in homebound older adults. J Gerontol A Biol Sci Med Sci. 2005;60(11):1475–8.

85. Bergstrom J. Nutrition and mortality in hemodialysis. J Am Soc Nephrol. 1995;6(5):1329–41.

86. Stevenson J, Tong A, Gutman T, Campbell KL, Craig JC, Brown MA, et al. Experiences and perspectives of dietary management among patients on hemodialysis: an interview study. J Ren Nutr. 2018;28(6):411–26. Available from: https://doi.org/10.1053/j.jrn.2018.02.005.

87. Bayhakki, Hatthakit U. Lived experiences of patients on hemodialysis: a meta-synthesis. Nephrol Nurs J. 2012;39(4):293–304.

88. United States Renal Data System. 2018 USRDS annual data report: epidemiology of kidney disease in the United States. National Institutes of Health, National Institutes of Diabetes and Digestive and Kidney Diseases, Bethesda, 2018. https://www.usrds.org/2018/view/Default.aspx. Assessed 14 Jan 2019.

89. Hansen T, Slagsvold B. Late-life loneliness in 11 European countries: results from the generations and gender survey. Soc Indic Res. 2016;124:1–20. Available from: https://doi.org/10.1007/a10433-017-0421-8.

90. Perissinotto CM, Stijacic CM, Canzer I, Covinsky KE. Loneliness in older persons: a predictor of functional decline and death. Arch Intern Med. 2012;172(14):1078–83. Available from: https://doi.org/10.1001/archinternmed.2012.1993.

91. Hughes G, Bennett KM, Hetherington MM. Old and alone: barriers to healthy eating in older men living on their own. Appetite. 2004;43(3):269–76.

92. Frongillo EA, Rauscherback BS, Roe DA, Williamson DF. Characteristics related to elderly persons' not eating for 1 or more days: implications for meal programs. Am J Public Health. 1992;82(4):600–2.

93. Quandt SA, McDonald J, Arcury TA, Bell RA, Vitolins MZ. Nutritional self-management of elderly widows in rural communities. Gerontologist. 2000;40(4):86–96.

94. Heuberger R, Wong H. The association between depression and widowhood and nutritional status in older adults. Geriatr Nurs. 2014;35(6):428–33. Available from: https://doi.org/10.1016/j.gerinurse.2014.06.011.

95. Honigh-de Vlaming R, Haverman-Nies A, Groeniger I, de Groot L, van 't Veer P. Determinants of trends in loneliness among Dutch older people over the period 2005-2010. J Aging Health. 2014;26(3):422–40. Available from: https://doi.org/10.1177/0898264313518066.

96. Sage Minder. Elderly loneliness. Available: https://www.sageminder.com/seniorhealth/mentalhealth/elderlyloneliness.aspx. Assessed 10 Dec 2018.

97. Silverstein M, Bengtson VL. Intergenerational solidarity and the structure of adult child-parent relationships in American families. Am J Sociol. 1997;103(2):429–60.

98. Ha JH, Carr D. The effect of parent-child geographic proximity on widowed parents' psychological adjustment and social integration. Res Aging. 2005;27(5):578–610. Available from: https://doi.org/10.1177/0164027505277977.

99. Tosi M, Grundy E. Intergenerational contacts and depressive symptoms among older parents in Eastern Europe. Aging Ment Health. 2018;12:1–7. Available from: https://doi.org/10.1080/13607863.2018.1442412.

100. Morley JE, Thomas DR. Anorexia and aging: pathophysiology. Nutrition. 1999;15(6):499–503.

101. Bergstrom J. Anorexia and malnutrition in hemodialysis patients. Blood Purif. 1992;10:35–9.

102. United States Department of Agriculture. Definitions of food scarcity. https://www.ers.usda.gov/topics/food-nutrition-assistance/food-security-in-the-us/definitions-of-food-security.aspx. Assessed 6 May 2020.
103. Coleman-Jensen A, Rabbitt MP, Gregory CA, Singh A. Household food security in the United States in 2018. U.S. Department of Agriculture. https://www.ers.usda.gov/publications/pub-details/?pubid=94848. Assessed 6 May 2020.
104. Laraia BA. Food insecurity and chronic disease. Adv Nutr. 2013;4(2):203–12. Available from: https://doi.org/10.3945/an.112.003277.
105. Gowda C, Hadley C, Aiello AE. The association between food insecurity and inflammation in the U.S. adult population. Am J Public Health. 2012;102(8):1579–88. Available from: https://doi.org/10.2105/AJPH.2011.300551.
106. Seligman HK, Bindman AB, Vittinghoff E, Kanaya AM, Kushel MB. Food insecurity is associated with diabetes mellitus: results from the National Health Examination and Nutrition Examination Survey (NHANES) 1999-2002. J Gen Intern Med. 2007;22(7):1018–23.
107. Patel SA, Surkin PJ. Unwanted childbearing aid food insecurity in the United States. Matern Child Nutr. 2016;12(2):362–72. Available from: https://doi.org/10.1111/mcn.12143.
108. Seligman HK, Bolger AF, Guzman D, Lopez A, Bobbins-Domingo K. Exhaustion of food budgets at month's end and hospital admissions for hypoglycemia. Health Aff (Millwood). 2014;33(1):116–23.
109. McGee M. Screening for food insecurity in Canadians. Global Health Magazine. April 18, 2018. https://juxtamagazine.org/2018104/18/screening-for-food-insecurity-in-Canadians. Assessed 21 Jan 2019.
110. Donini LM, Scardella P, Piombo L, Neri B, Asprino R, Proietti AR, et al. Malnutrition in elderly: social and economic determinants. J Nutr Health Aging. 2013;17(1):9–15. Available from: https://doi.org/10.1007/s12603-012-0374-8.
111. Wolfe WS, Frongillo EA, Valois P. Understanding the experience of food insecurity by elders suggests ways to improve its measurement. J Nutr. 2003;133(9):2762–9.
112. Ziliak JP, Gundersen C. The health consequences of senior hunger in the United States: evidence from the 1999-2004 NHANES. August 2017. Available from: https://www.feedingamerica.org/sites/default/files/research/senior-hunger-research/senior-health-consequences-2014.pdf.
113. Ramsey R, Giskes K Turrell G, Gallegos D. Food insecurity among adults residing in disadvantaged urban areas: potential health and dietary consequences. Public Health Nutr. 2011;15(2):227–237. Queensland University of Technology School of Public Health. https://pdfs.semanticscholar.org/0cae/b6d304d56692576b2857f969ff-1084f3ece4.pdf.
114. Whitaker RC, Phillips SM, Orzol SM. Food insecurity and risk of depression and anxiety in mothers and behavior problems in their preschool-age children. Pediatrics. 2006;118(3):e859–68. Available from: https://doi.org/10.1542/peds.2006-0239.
115. Allen NL, Becerra BJ, Becerra MB. Associations between food insecurity and the severity of psychological distress among African-Americans. Ethn Health. 2018;23(5):511–20. Available from: https://doi.org/10.1080/13557858.2017.1280139.
116. Sattler EL, Lee JS. Persistent food insecurity is associated with levels of cost-related medication and adherence in low-income older adults. J Nutr Gerontol Geriatr. 2013;32(1):41–58. Available from: https://doi.org/10.1080/21551197.2012.722888.
117. Berkowitz SA, Seligman HK, Choudry NK. Treat or eat: food insecurity, cost-related medication underuse and unmet needs. Am J Med. 2014;127(4):303–310.e3. Available from: https://doi.org/10.1016/j.amjmed.2014.01.002.
118. Billimek J, Sorkin DH. Food insecurity processes of care and self-reported medication underuse in patients with type 2 diabetes: results from the California Heart Interview Survey. Health Serv Res. 2012;47(6):2159–68. Available from: https://doi.org/10.1111/j.1475-6773.2012.01463.x.
119. Kushel MB, Gupta R, Gee L, Haas JS. Housing instability and food insecurity as barriers to health care among low-income Americans. J Gen Intern Med. 2006;21(1):71–7. Available from: https://doi.org/10.1111/j.1525-1497.2005.00278.x.
120. Wilson G, Molaison EF, Pope J, Hunt AE, Connell CL. Nutritional status and food insecurity in hemodialysis patients. J Ren Nutr. 2006;16(1):65–8. Available from: https://doi.org/10.1053/j.jrn.2005.10.009.
121. Coleman ME. Oral supplements and serum albumin levels in dialysis patients as function of feed security. University of Cincinatti, 2011. https://etd.ohiolink.edu/!etd.send_file?accession=ucin1384851154&disposition=inline. Assessed 6 May 2020.
122. Crews DC, Kuczmarski MF, Grubbs V, Hedgeman E, Shahinian VB, Evans MK, et al. Effects of food insecurity on chronic kidney disease in lower-income Americans. Am J Nephrol. 2014;39:27–35.
123. Banerjee T, Crews DC, Wesson DE, Dharmarajan S, Saran R, Ríos Burrows N, et al. Food insecurity CKD and subsequent ESRD in U.S. adults. Am J Kidney Dis. 2017;70(1):38–47. Available from: https://doi.org/10.1053/j.ajkd.2016.10.035.

124. Banerjee T, Liu Y, Crews DC. Dietary patterns and CKD progression. Blood Purif. 2016;41:117–22. Available from: https://doi.org/10.1159/000441072.
125. Institute of Medicine. Health literacy: a prescription to end confusion. Washington, D.C.: The National Academic Press; 2004.
126. Paasche-Orlow MK, Parker RM, Gazmararian JA, Nielsen-Bohlman LT, Rudd RR. The prevalence of limited health literacy. J Gen Intern Med. 2005;20:175–84.
127. Fraser SD, Roderick PJ, Casey M, Taal MW, Yuen HM, Nutbean D. Prevalence and associations of limited health literacy in chronic kidney disease: a systemic review. Nephrol Dial Transplant. 2013;28(1):129–37.
128. Baker DW, Parker RM, Williams MV, Clark WS. Health literacy and the risk of hospital admission. J Gen Intern Med. 1998;13(12):791–8.
129. Kripalani S, Gatti ME, Jacobson TA. Association of age, health literacy and medication management strategies with cardiovascular medication adherence. Patient Educ Couns. 2010;81(2):177–81. Available from: https://doi.org/10.1016/j.pec.2010.04.030.
130. Schumacher JR, Hall AG, Davis TC, Arnold CL, Bennett RD, Wolf MS, Carden DL. Potentially preventable use of emergency services: the role of low health literacy. Med Care. 2013;51(8):654–8. Available from: https://doi.org/10.1097/MLR.0b013e3182992c5a.
131. Schillinger D, Grumbach K, Piette J. Association of health literacy with diabetes outcomes. JAMA. 2002;288(4):475–82. Available from: https://doi.org/10.1001/jama.288.4.475.
132. Baker DW, Wolf MS, Feinglass J, Thompson JA, Gazmararian JA. Health literacy and mortality among elderly persons. Arch Intern Med. 2007;167(14):1503–9.
133. Gazmararian J, Baker D, Parker R, Blazer DG. A multivariate analysis of factors associated with depression: evaluating the role of health literacy as a potential contributor. Arch Intern Med. 2002;160(21):3307–14.
134. Parikh NS, Parker RM, Nurss JR, Baker DW, Williams MV. Shame and health literacy: the unspoken connection. Patient Educ Couns. 1996;27(1):33–9.
135. Easton P, Entwistle VA, Williams B. How the stigma of low health literacy can impair patient-professional spoken interactions and affect health insights from a qualitative investigation. BMC Health Serv Res. 2013;13:319. Available from: http://www.biomedcentral.com/1472-6963/13/319.
136. Jain D, Green JA. Health literacy in kidney disease: review of the literacy and implications for clinical practice. World J Nephrol. 2016;5(2):147–51.
137. Wright JA, Wallston KA, Elasy TA, Ikizier TA, Cavanaugh KL. Development and results of a kidney disease knowledge survey given to patients with CKD. Am J Kidney Dis. 2011;57(3):387–95.
138. Green JA, Mor MK, Shields AM, Sevick MA, Arnold RM, Palevsky PM, et al. Association of health literacy with dialysis adherence and health resource utilization in patients receiving maintenance hemodialysis. Am J Kidney Dis. 2013;62(1):73–80. Available from: https://doi.org/10.1053/j.ajkd.2012.12.014.
139. Grubbs V, Gregory SE, Perez-Stable EJ, Hsu CY. Health literacy and access to kidney transplantation. Clin J Am Soc Nephrol. 2009;4(1):195–200. Available from: https://doi.org/10.2215/cjn.03290708.
140. Ricardo AC, Yang W, Lash JP. Limited health literacy is associated with low glomerular filtration in Chronic Renal Insufficiency Cohort (CRIC) study. Clin Nephrol. 2014;81(1):30–7. Available from: https://doi.org/10.5414/cn108062.
141. Cavanaugh KL, Wingard RL, Hakim EM, Eden S, Shintani A, Wallston KA, et al. Low health literacy associates with increased mortality in ESRD. J Am Soc Nephrol. 2010;21(11):1979–85. Available from: https://doi.org/10.1681/ASN.2009111163.
142. Doak LG, Doak CC. Literacy levels of renal education materials. J Ren Nutr. 1993;3(4):191–4. Available from: https://doi.org/10.1016/S1051-2276(12)80094-X.
143. Kalista-Richards M. The dynamics of education: making a match. J Ren Nutr. 1998;8(2):88–94. Available from: https://doi.org/10.1016/s1051-2276(98)90048-6.
144. Lambert K, Mansfield K, Mullan J. How do patients and carers make sense of renal dietary advice? A qualitative exploration. J Ren Care. 2018;44(4):238–50. Available from: https://doi.org/10.1111/jorc.12260.
145. Connelly K, Siek KA, Chauday B, Jones J, Astroth K, Welch JL. An offline mobile nutrition monitoring intervention for varying-literacy patients receiving hemodialysis: a pilot study examining usage and usability. J Am Med Inform Assoc. 2012;19(5):705–12. Available from: https://doi.org/10.1136/amiajnl-2011-000732.
146. Welch JL, Astroth KS, Perkins SM, Johnson CS, Connelly K, Siek KA, et al. Using a mobile application to self-monitor diet and fluid intake among adults receiving hemodialysis. Res Nurs Health. 2013;36(3):284–98. Available from: https://doi.org/10.1002/nur.21539.
147. Sevick MA, Piraino BM, St Jules DR, et al. No difference in average interdialytic weight gain observed in a randomized trial with a technology-supported behavioral intervention to reduce dietary sodium intake in adults undergoing hemodialysis in the United States: preliminary outcomes of the BalanceWise Study. J Ren Nutr. 2016;26(3):149–58. Available from: https://doi.org/10.1053/j.jrn.2015.11.006.

148. Mortin De Souza DL. Practical strategies for enhancing patient education in hemodialysis clinics. J Ren Nutr. 2004;14(4):253–62. Available from: https://doi.org/10.1053/j.jrn.2004.08.003.

149. Lambert K, Mansfield K, Mullan J. Qualitative exploration of the experiences of renal dietitians and how they help patients with end-stage kidney disease to understand the renal diet. Nutr Diet. 2018. Available from: https://doi.org/10.1111/1747-0080.12443.

150. Bandura A. Social foundation of thought and action: a social cognitive theory. Prentice Hall: Englewood Cliff, New Jersey; 1986.

151. Bandura A. Self efficacy: the exercise of control. New York: WH.Freeman; 1997.

152. Clark NM, Dodge JA. Exploring self-efficacy as a predictor of disease management. Health Educ Behav. 1999;26(1):72–89. Available from: https://doi.org/10.1177/109019819902600107.

153. Moshar CE, DuHamel KN, Smith MY. Self-efficacy for coping with cancer in a multiethnic sample of breast cancer patients: associations with barriers to pain management and disease. Clin J Pain. 2010;26(3):227–34.

154. Blyth R, Creedy DK, Dennis C-L, Moyle W, Pratt J, De Vries SM. Effect of maternal confidence on breastfeeding duration: an application of the Breastfeeding Self-Efficacy Theory. Birth. 2018;46(1):121–8.

155. Linde JA, Jeffery RW, Levey RL, Sherwood NE, Utter J, Pronk NP, et al. Binge eating disorder, weight control self-efficacy and depression in overweight men and women. Int J Obes Relat Metab Disord. 2004;28(3):418–25.

156. McAuley E, Blissmer B. Self-efficacy determinants and consequences of physical activity. Exerc Sport Sci Rev. 2000;28(2):85–8.

157. Kauric-Klein Z, Peters RM, Yarandi HN. Self efficacy and blood pressure self-care behaviors in patients on chronic hemodialysis. West J Nurs Res. 2017;39(7):886–905. Available from: https://doi.org/10.1177/0193945916661322.

158. Balaga PA. Self-efficacy and self-care management of chronic renal failure patients. Asian J Health. 2012;2:111–29. Available from: https://pdfs.semanticscholar.org/090e/d57759f55ad0352edca46a5bf53807f418e2.pdf. http://dx.doi.org/10.7828/ajoh.v2i1.121.

159. Rosenbaum M, Smira KB. Cognitive and personality factors in the delay of gratification of hemodialysis patients. J Pers Soc Psychol. 1986;51:357–64.

160. Brady BA, Tucker CM, Alfino PA, Tarrant DG, Finlayson GC. An investigation of factors associated with fluid adherence among hemodialysis patients: a self-efficacy theory based approach. Ann Behav Med. 1998;19:339–43.

161. Kugler C, Vilamick H, Haverich A, Maes B. Nonadherence with diet and fluid restrictions among adults having hemodialysis. J Nurs Scholarsh. 2005;37(1):25–9.

162. Chan YM, Zalilah MS, Hii SZ. Determinants of compliance behaviors among patients undergoing hemodialysis in Malaysia. PLoS One. 2012;7(8):e41362. Available from: https://doi.org/10.1371/journal.pone.0041362.

163. Clark-Cutaia MN, Ren D, Hoffman LA, Burke LE, Sevick MA. Adherence to hemodialysis dietary sodium recommendations: influence of patient characteristics, self-efficacy and perceived barriers. J Ren Nutr. 2014;24(2):92–9. Available from: https://doi.org/10.1053/j.jrn.2013.11.007.

164. Park KA, Choi-Kwon S, Sim YM, Kim SB. Comparison of dietary compliance and dietary knowledge between older and younger Korean hemodialysis patients. J Ren Nutr. 2008;18(5):415–23. Available from: https://doi.org/10.1053/j.jrn.2008.04.004.

165. Elloitt JO, Ortman C, Almaani S, Lee YH, Jordan K. Understanding the associations between modifying factors, individual health beliefs and hemodialysis patients' adherence to a low-phosphorus diet. J Ren Nutr. 2015;25(2):111–20. Available from: https://doi.org/10.1053/j.jrn.2014.08.006.

166. Zrinyi M, Juhasz M, Balla J, Katona E, Ben T, Kakuk G, Pall D. Dietary self-efficacy: determinants of compliance behaviours and biochemical outcomes in haemodialysis patients. Nephrol Dial Transplant. 2003;18(9):1869–73. Available from: https://doi.org/10.1093/ndt/gfg307.

167. Langford CPH, Bowsher J, Maloney JP. Social support: a conceptual analysis. J Adv Nurs. 1997;25(1):95–100. Available from: https://doi.org/10.1046/j.1365-2648.1997.1997025095.x.

168. Hefner J, Eisenberg D. Social support and mental health among college students. Am J Orthopsychiatry. 2009;79(4):491–9. Available from: https://doi.org/10.1037/a0016918.

169. Uchino BN. Social support and health: a review of physiological processes potentially underlying links to disease outcomes. J Behav Med. 2006;29(4):377–87. Available from: https://doi.org/10.1007/s10865-006-9056-5.

170. Evans M, Donelle L, Hume-Loveland L. Social support and online postpartum discussion groups. Patient Educ Couns. 2012;87(3):405–10. Available from: https://doi.org/10.1016/j.pec.2011.09.011.

171. Nicholson NR. A review of social isolation: an important but under-assessed condition in older adults. J Prim Prev. 2012;33(2–3):137–52. Available from: https://doi.org/10.1007/s10935-012-0271-2.

172. Feldman P, Dunkel-Schetter C, Sandman C, Wadhwa P. Maternal support predicts birth weight and fetal growth on human pregnancy. Psychosom Med. 2000;62(5):715–25.

173. Mazzaferro KE, Murray PJ, Ness RB, Bass DC. Depression, stress and social support as predictors of high-risk sexual behaviors and STIs in young women. J Adolesc Health. 2006;39(4):601–3. Available from: https://doi.org/10.1016/j.jadohealth.2006.02.004.

174. Griffith LS, Field BJ, Lustman PJ. Life stress and social support in diabetes: association with glycemic control. Int J Psychiatry Med. 1990;20(4):365–72.

175. Amado L, Poveda V, Ferreira R, et al. Depression in late-life patients with end-stage renal disease under online haemodiafiltration is associated with low social support, muscle mass and creatine serum levels. J Clin Nephrol Ren Care. 2016;2(1):1–5.

176. Lilympaki I, Makri A, Vlantousi K, Kputelekos I, Babatsikpu F, Polikandrioti M. The effect of perceived social support in the level of anxiety and depression in hemodialysis patients. Mater Sociomed. 2006;28(5):361–5.

177. Symister P, Friend R. The influence of social support and problematic support on optimism and depression in chronic illness: a prospective study evaluating self-esteem as a mediator. Health Psychol. 2003;22(2):123–9. Available from: https://doi.org/10.1037/0278-6133.22.2.123.

178. Karadag E, Kilic SP, Metin O. Relationship between fatigue and social support in hemodialysis patients. Nurs Health Sci. 2013;15(2):164–71. Available from: https://doi.org/10.1111/nhs.12008.

179. Plantinga LC, Fink NE, Harrington-Levey R, Finkelstein FO, Hebah N, Powe NR, et al. Association of social support with outcomes in incident dialysis patients. Clin J Am Soc Nephrol. 2010;5(8):1480–8. Available from: https://doi.org/10.2215/CJN.01240210.

180. Thong MSY, Kaptein AA, Krediet RT, Boeschoten EW, Dekker DW. Social support predicts survival in dialysis patients. Nephrol Dial Transplant. 2007;22:845–50.

181. Boyer CB, Friend R, Chlouverakis G, Kaloyanides G. Social support and demographic factors influencing compliance of hemodialysis patients. J Appl Soc Psychol. 1990;20(22):1902–18.

182. Cicolini G, Palma E, Simonetta C, Di Nicola M. Influence of family carers on haemodialyzed patients' adherence to dietary and fluid restrictions: an observation study. J Adv Nurs. 2012;68(11):2410–7.

183. Barnett T, Li Yoong T, Pinikahana J, Si-Yen T. Fluid compliance among patients having haemodialysis: can an educational programme make a difference? J Adv Nurs. 2008;61(3):300–6.

184. Shea EJ, Bogdan DF, Freeman RB, Schreiner GE. Hemodialysis for chronic renal failure. IV Psychological considerations. Ann Intern Med. 1965;62:558–63.

185. Morey B, Walker R, Davenport A. More dietetic time, better outcome? Nephron Clin Pract. 2008;109:c173–80. Available from: https://doi.org/10.1159/000145462.

186. Hackett ML, Jardine MJ. We need to talk about depression and dialysis: but what questions should we ask and does anyone know the answers? Clin J Am Soc Nephrol. 2017;12(2):222–4. Available from: https://doi.org/10.2215/CJN.13031216.

187. Watnick S, Kirwin P, Mahnensmith R, Concato J. The prevalence and treatment of depression among patients starting dialysis. Am J Kidney Dis. 2003;41:105–10.

188. Pena-Polanco JE, Mor MK, Tohme FA, Fine MJ, Palevsky PM, Weisbord SD. Acceptance of antidepressant treatment by patients on hemodialysis and their renal providers. Clin J Am Soc Nephrol. 2017;12(2):298–303. Available from: https://doi.org/10.2215/cjn.07720716.

189. Chilcot J, Hudson JL. Is successful treatment of depression in dialysis patients an achievable goal? Semin Dial. 2018:1–5. Available from: https://doi.org/10.1111/sdi.12755.

190. Chen J, Xie S. Agomelatine versus paroxetinein treating depression and anxiety symptoms in patients with chronic kidney disease. Neuropsychiatr Dis Treat. 2018;14:547–52.

191. Cukor D, Halen NV, Asher DR, Coplan JD, Weedon J, Wyka KE, et al. Psychosocial intervention improves depression, quality of life and fluid adherence in hemodialysis. J Am Soc Nephrol. 2014;25:196–2006. Available from: https://doi.org/10.1681/ASN.2012111134.

192. Koo JR, Yoon JY, Joo MH, Lee HS, Oh JE, Kim SG, et al. Treatment of depression and effect of antidepression treatment on nutritional status in chronic hemodialysis patients. Am J Med Sci. 2005;329(1):1–5. Available from: https://doi.org/10.1097/00000441-200501000-00001.

193. Jackson K. Nephrology social work: caring for the emotional needs of dialysis patients. Soc Work Today. 2014;14(5). https://www.socialworktoday.com/archive/091514p20.shtml.

194. Center for Dialysis Care. Dialysis social work services. http://www.cdcare.org/patient-resources/dialysis-social-work-services/. Accessed 6 May, 2020.

195. Waedian J, Sun F. Treating depression among end-stage renal disease patients: lessons from cognitive behavioral classes. J Nephrol Soc Work. 2011;35(Summer):17–24.

196. Johnstone S. Wellnee programming: nephrology social work expands its role in renal disease management. Nephrol News Issues. 2005;19:59–71.

197. Prescott M. Managing mental illness in the dialysis treatment environment: a team approach. Nephrol News Issues. 2006;20(13):32–41.

198. Derogatis LR, Melisaratos N. The brief symptom inventory: an introduction. Psychol Med. 1983;13(3):595–605.

199. Andrews G, Craemer M, Crino R, Hunt C, Lampe L, Page A. The treatment of anxiety disorders: clinician's guide and patient manuals. 2nd ed. Cambridge: Cambridge University Press; 2003.

200. Boulos C, Salameh P, Barberger-Gateau P. Social isolation and risk for malnutrition among older people. Geriatr Gerontol Int. 2017;17(2):286–94. Available from: https://doi.org/10.1111/ggi.12711.
201. Russell D. UCLA Loneliness Scale (Version 3): reliability, validity and factor structure. J Pers Assess. 1996;66:20–40.
202. Landeiro F, Barrows P, Leal J. Reducing social isolation and loneliness in older people: a systematic review protocol. BMJ Open. 2007;7(5):e013778. Available from: https://doi.org/10.1136/bmjopen-2016-013778.
203. Price B. Approaches to counter loneliness and social isolation. Nurs Older People. 2015;27(7):31–5. Available from: https://doi.org/10.7748/NOP.27.7.e722.
204. Satoe JNT, Jedeloo S, Van Staa A. Effective peer-to-peer support for young people with end-stage renal disease: a mixed methods evaluation of Camp Cool. BMC Nephrol. 2013;14:279. http://www.biomedcentral.com/1471-2369/14/279
205. St Clair Russell J, Southerland S, Huff E, Thomson M, Meyer K, Lynch J. A peer-to-peer mentoring program for in-center hemodialysis: a patient-centered quality improvement program. Nephrol Nurs J. 2018;45:481–96.
206. Taylor F, Gutteridge R, Willis C. Peer support for CKD patients and carers: overcoming barriers and facilitating access. Health Expect. 2016;19:617–30. Available from: https://doi.org/10.1111/hex.12348.
207. Hughes J, Wood E, Smith G. Exploring kidney patients' experiences of receiving individual peer support. Health Expect. 2009;12(4):396–406. Available from: https://doi.org/10.1111/j.1369-7625.2009.00568.x.
208. Gundersen C, Engelhard E, Crumbaugh AS, Seligman HK. Brief assessment of food security accurately identifies high-risk US adults. Public Health Nutr. 2017;20(8):1367–71. Available from: https://doi.org/10.1017/S1368980017000180.
209. Holben D. Position of the American Dietetic Association: food insecurity in the United States. J Am Diet Assoc. 2010;110:1368–77. Available from: https://doi.org/10.1016/j.jada.2010.07.015.
210. Lindquist LA, Go L, Fleisher J, Jain N, Friesema E, Baker DW. Relationship of health literacy to intentional and unintentional non-adherence of hospital discharge medications. J Gen Intern Med. 2012;27(2):173–8.
211. Zarcadoolas C, Pleasant A, Greer DS. Understanding health literacy: an expanded model. Health Promot Int. 2005;20(2):195–203. Available from: https://doi.org/10.1093/heapro/dah609.
212. Castro CM, Wilson C, Wang F, Schillinger D. Babel babble: physicians' use of unclarified medical jargon with patients. Am J Health Behav. 2007;31(Suppl 1):S85–95.
213. Houts PS, Doak CC, Doak LG, Loscalzo MJ. The role of pictures in improving health communication: a review of research on attention, comprehension, recall and adherence. Patient Educ Couns. 2006;61(2):173–90. Available from: https://doi.org/10.1016/j.pec.2005.05.004.
214. Norris SL, Engelgau MM, Narayan KMV. Effectiveness of self-management training in type 2 diabetes: a systematic review of randomized controlled trials. Diabetes Care. 2001;24(3):561–87.
215. Ha Dinh TT, Bonner A, Clark R, Ramsbotham J, Hines S. The effectiveness of the teach-back method on adherence and self-management in health education for people with chronic disease: a systematic review. JBI Database System Rev Implement Rep. 2016;14(1):210–47. Available from: https://doi.org/10.11124/jbisrir-2016-2296.
216. Baker DW, DeWalt DA, Schillinger D, Hawk V. The effect of progressive, reinforcing telephone education and counseling versus brief education intervention on knowledge, self-care behaviors and heart failure. J Card Fail. 2011;17(10):789–96.
217. Sudore RL, Schillinger D. Interventions to improve care for patients with limited health literacy. J Clin Outcomes Manag. 2009;16(1):20–9.
218. Roberts NJ, Ghiassi R, Partridge MR. Health literacy in COPD. Int J Chron Obstruct Pulmon Dis. 2008;3(4):499–507. Available from: https://doi.org/10.2147/COPD.S1088.
219. Rock PL, Rosier JP, Riedel WJ, Blackwell AD. Cognitive impairment in depression: a systematic review and meta-analysis. Psychol Med. 2014;44(10):2029–40. Available from: https://doi.org/10.1017/S0033291713002535.
220. Ramsdell R, Annis C. Patient education: a continuing repetitive process. ANNA J. 1996;23(2):217–21.
221. Duffrin C, Carraway-Stage VG, Briley A, Christiano C. Validation of a dietary intake tool for African American dialysis patients with low literacy. J Ren Care. 2015;41(2):126–33. Available from: https://doi.org/10.1111/jorc.12104.
222. Ford JC, Pope JF, Hunt AE, Gerald B. The effect of diet education on the laboratory values and knowledge of hemodialysis patients with hyperphosphatemia. J Ren Nutr. 2004;14(1):36–44. Available from: https://doi.org/10.1053/j.jrn.2003.09.008.
223. Karavetian M, Ghaddar S. Nutritional education for the management of osteodystrophy in patients on haemodialysis: a randomized controlled trial. J Ren Care. 2013;39(1):19–30. Available from: https://doi.org/10.1111/j.1755-6686.2012.00327.x.
224. Milas NC, Nowalk MP, Akpele L, Castaldo L, Coyne T, Doroshenko L, et al. Factors associated with adherence to the dietary protein intervention in the Modification of Diet in Renal Disease Study. J Am Diet Assoc. 1995;95(11):1295–300.

225. Burrowes JD, Russell GB, Rocco MV. Multiple factors affect renal dietitians' use of the NKF-K/DOQI Adult Nutrition Guidelines. J Ren Nutr. 2005;15(4):407–26.
226. Hand RK, Steiber A, Burrowes J. Renal dietitians lack time and resources to follow the NKF KDOQI Guidelines for frequency and method of diet assessment: results of a survey. J Ren Nutr. 2013;23(6):445–9. Available from: https://doi.org/10.1053/j.jrn.2012.08.010.
227. Hand RK, Burrowes JD. Renal dietitians' perceptions of roles and responsibilities in outpatient dialysis facilities. J Ren Nutr. 2015;25(5):404–11. Available from: https://doi.org/10.1053/j.jrn.2015.04.008.
228. Hand RK, Albert JM, Sehgal AR. Quantifying the time used for renal dietitian's responsibilities: a pilot study. J Ren Nutr. 2019. Available from: https://doi.org/10.1053/j.jrn.2018.11.007. [epub ahead of print].
229. Wood J, Gillis DE. Exploring dietitians' engagement with health literacy: concept and practice. Can J Diet Pract Res. 2015;76(2):51–5.
230. Wolfe WA. Moving the issue of renal dietitian staffing forward. J Ren Nutr. 2012;22(5):515–20.
231. Wolfe WA. Adequacy of dialysis clinic staffing and quality of care: a review of evidence and areas of needed research. Am J Kidney Dis. 2011;58(2):166–76.
232. Thompson TG. Report to congress on medical nutrition therapy 2004. Available from: https://www.cms.gov/Medicare/Coverage/InfoExchange/Downloads/Report-to-Congress-Medical-Nutrition-Therapy.pdf. Assessed 6 May 2020.
233. Bandura A. Towards a unifying theory of behavioral change. Psychol Rev. 1977;84(2):195–215.
234. Tsay SL. Self-efficacy training for patients with end-stage renal disease. J Adv Nurs. 2003;43(4):370–5.
235. Aliasgharpour M, Shomali M, Moghaddam MZ, Faghihzadeh S. Effect of a self-efficacy promotion training programme on the body weight changes in patients undergoing haemodialysis. J Ren Care. 2012;38(3):155–61. Available from: https://doi.org/10.1111/j.1755-6686.2012.00305.x.
236. Moattari M, Ebrahimi M, Sharifi N, Rouzbeh J. The effect of empowerment on the self-efficacy, quality of life and clinical and laboratory indicators of patient treated with hemodialysis: a randomized controlled trial. Health Qual Life Outcomes. 2012;10:115. Available from: https://doi.org/10.1186/1477-7525-10-115.
237. Tsay SL, Hung LO. Empowerment of patients with end-stage renal disease- a randomized controlled trial. Int J Nurs Stud. 2004;41(1):59–65. Available from: https://doi.org/10.1016/S0020-7489(03)00095-6.
238. Yokoyama Y, Suzukamo Y, Hotta O, Yamazaki S, Kawaguchi T, Hasegawa T, et al. Dialysis staff encouragement and fluid control and adherence in patients on hemodialysis. Nephrol Nurs J. 2009;36(3):289–97.
239. Cukor D, Cohen SD, Paterson RA, Kimmel PL. Psychosocial aspects of chronic diseases: ESRD as a paradigmatic illness. J Am Soc Nephrol. 2007;18(12):3042–55. Available from: https://doi.org/10.1681/ASN.2007030345.
240. Johansson L, Hickson M, Brown EA. Influence of psychosocial factors in energy and protein intake of older people on dialysis. J Ren Nutr. 2013;23(5):348–55.
241. Bergstrom J, Lindholm B. Malnutrition, cardiac disease and mortality: an integrated point of view. Am J Kidney Dis. 1998;32(5):834–41.
242. Norton JM, Moxey-Mims MM, Eggers PW, et al. Social determinants of racial disparities in CKD. J Am Soc Nephrol. 2016;27(9):2576–95. Available from: https://doi.org/10.1681/ASN.2016010027.

Chapter 9
Drug-Nutrient Interactions

Antonette Flecha, Johnathan Voss, and Diana Hao

Keywords Pharmacokinetics · Absorption · Bioavailability · Distribution · Volume of distribution
Metabolism · Elimination · Clearance · Half-life · Area under the time-concentration curve (AUC)
Pharmacodynamics · Precipitant agent · Object agent · Ex vivo bio-inactivations (type I interaction)
Absorption phase-associated interaction (type II interaction) · Physiologic action-associated interaction (type III interaction) · Elimination phase-associated interaction (type IV interaction)

Key Points
- Most drug-nutrient interactions can be described using the principles of pharmacokinetics and pharmacodynamics.
- A precipitant agent – a compound that alters the pharmacokinetic or pharmacodynamics properties of the object agent – may be either the drug or nutrient in a drug-nutrient interaction.
- One definition that has been proposed to describe a clinically significant drug-nutrient interaction requires an interaction to lead to a 20% change in a pharmacokinetic or pharmacodynamic property.
- Type I interactions (ex vivo bio-inactivation) occur outside of the body and is most commonly seen between compounds in parenteral nutrition.
- Type II interactions (absorption phase-associated interaction) can be broken down into three subtypes: type IIA (enzyme function modification), type IIB (transport protein modification), and type IIC (complexation, binding, and/or other deactivating process that occurs in the gastrointestinal tract); treatment of hyperphosphatemia due to chronic kidney disease or end-stage renal disease is an example of an intentional type IIC drug-nutrient interaction.
- Type III interactions (physiologic action-associated interaction) occur when the precipitant agent alters the distribution, systemic metabolism or transport, or penetration to specific organs or tissues of the object compound.
- Type IV interactions (elimination phase-associated interactions) describe modulation, antagonism, or impairment of renal or enterohepatic elimination of the object agent.

A. Flecha
SUNY Downstate Medical Center, Montefiore Medical Center, Transplant Surgery, Bronx, NY, USA

J. Voss
John Peter Smith Hospital, Inpatient Pharmacy, Fort Worth, TX, USA

D. Hao (✉)
Solid Organ Transplant Pharmacy Service, UC Davis Medical Center, Sacramento, CA, USA
e-mail: dhao@ucdavis.edu

© Springer Nature Switzerland AG 2020
J. D. Burrowes et al. (eds.), *Nutrition in Kidney Disease*, Nutrition and Health,
https://doi.org/10.1007/978-3-030-44858-5_9

- Enteral nutrition supplied as tube feeding has important interactions with many medications, including phenytoin, warfarin, and levothyroxine. In patients receiving continuous tube feeding, these interactions may be mitigated by holding tube feeds for 1 hour before and 1 hour after medication administration.
- Gastric emptying is reduced by high-fat foods, which may increase the absorption of acid stable medications or decrease the absorption of medications that are broken down in acidic environments.

Introduction

The causes of drug-nutrient interactions are often multifactorial but can be narrowed down into four general types of interactions: physical, chemical, physiologic, or pathophysiologic [1]. As interactions between drugs and nutrients lead to alterations in the pharmacokinetic or pharmacodynamic parameters of either the drug or nutrient involved, it is important to understand the basic principles of pharmacokinetics and pharmacodynamics. The term pharmacokinetics (often referred to simply as kinetics) refers to the methods of describing the disposition of a drug or nutrient in the body. The pharmacokinetics of a compound can be broken down into four basic principles: absorption, distribution, metabolism, and excretion.

Absorption refers to the process of a compound being absorbed from the site of introduction – often the gastrointestinal (GI) tract – to be incorporated into the human body. Absorption can be described using the term bioavailability, which refers to the proportion of the compound administered that becomes available in the systemic circulation. Intravenous administration of medications or nutrients, by definition, provides 100% bioavailability. Using the enteral route of administration often leads to a lower bioavailability due to incomplete absorption or loss of the compound during absorption. The rate of absorption is also an important pharmacokinetic parameter and is usually estimated using t_{max}, the time from administration to achieve peak serum concentration. For orally administered medications, this can provide an estimate of the intestinal transit time.

Distribution refers to the extent of dispersal throughout the body of the compound after administration. This parameter is described using the term volume of distribution (V_d). The V_d describes the theoretical volume that would be necessary to contain the administered medication to provide the serum concentration measured. A compound with a V_d of around 5 liters will be mostly concentrated in the blood (since this is the typical blood volume of an average adult). It is possible for the V_d to be larger than the total body volume (approximately 42 L), and this usually relates to a compound that is highly distributed in the tissue. In general, compounds with a high V_d are more lipophilic, less ionized, and less highly protein bound than compounds with a low V_d. Overall, the distribution of drugs is not known to be affected by nutrients and vice versa, so this pharmacokinetic parameter is relatively unimportant in terms of determining the significance of a specific drug-nutrient interaction.

Metabolism and *elimination* are best thought of as variations of the same goal – to remove the effects of the substance in question. Metabolism often refers to the conversion of a substance into a different form than how it is introduced into the body so that it may be further eliminated. This process most often takes place in the hepatocytes of the liver through two primary processes: activity of the cytochrome P450 system of enzymes and conjugation with compounds such as glutathione. Many interactions with medications occur due to interactions with cytochrome P450 enzymes and will be described later. Metabolism via conjugation is not often the source of an interaction. *Elimination* refers to the ultimate removal of the substance in question from the body. This can be through metabolism followed by elimination via either the GI tract or urinary tract. Elimination can also occur directly from the urinary tract with excretion of the active compound directly into the urine. Both metabolism and excretion contribute to the pharmacokinetic property known as the clearance or elimination rate. The most common parameter used to describe the elimination rate of a compound is the half-life

$(t_{1/2})$ – the time it takes for the serum concentration of a substance to decrease to half its original concentration. In general, a compound is largely eliminated from the body after five half-lives as only 3.125% of the initial amount of the compound would still be present in the body.

To bring together these concepts, the parameter area under the time-concentration curve (AUC) is often used to refer to the overall exposure to the compound in question. This parameter is affected by most of the pharmacokinetic parameters, most notably the bioavailability, the clearance, and sometimes the rate of absorption for orally administered compounds.

Pharmacodynamics refers to the physiologic effects of a medication or nutrient on the body. This may refer specifically to the actions of a medication on a specific receptor throughout the body or to activity in a specific tissue. Many interactions involve the antagonism of one compound on another at the site of action. In this case, the compound that causes the interaction is referred to as the precipitant agent [1]. The agent that is affected after the addition of the precipitant agent is referred to as the object agent. As in this definition, an interaction can occur with the addition of the precipitant agent. It is also possible for an interaction to be discovered upon the discontinuation of a medication or nutrient or upon a dose change of a medication or nutrient.

While there is potential for interactions between medications and nutrients, not all interactions will be clinically significant. A clear consensus has not been established, but one definition of a clinically significant drug-nutrient interaction states that a 20% change in a pharmacokinetic or pharmacodynamic parameter from baseline is clinically significant [1]. For example, if a patient has been on a stable regimen of phenytoin that provides a therapeutic baseline serum concentration of 15 mcg/mL and is then started on continuous enteral nutrition due to becoming critically ill and requiring mechanical ventilation, then the introduction of the precipitant agent (enteral nutrition in this example) would have to cause a decrease in the serum phenytoin concentration of at least 3 mcg/mL to be considered significant.

Types of Interactions

Four major types of drug-nutrient interactions have been identified [2]. They include ex vivo bio-inactivations (type I), absorption phase-associated interactions (type II), physiologic action-associated interactions (type III), and elimination phase-associated interactions (type IV).

Ex vivo *bio-inactivations* are interactions that occur outside of the body. In terms of drug-nutrient interactions, ex vivo bio-inactivations often occur between components in parenteral nutrition (e.g., the destabilizing nature of Fe^{3+} when added to a parenteral nutrition admixture containing lipid emulsion) and when medications are given in conjunction with enteral nutrition (e.g., fluoroquinolones) [3–5]. It is also possible for an ex vivo bio-inactivation to occur if a drug is given at the same time as certain foods, but this is less common. The best way to avoid this type of drug-nutrient interaction is to avoid the combination of the offending agents by using alternatives when possible or simply by separating the administration of the interacting compounds by a few hours.

Absorption phase-associated interactions only affect medications or nutrients delivered orally or enterally. These types of drug-nutrient interactions can be broken down into three types based on the effect of the precipitant on different processes related to absorption: enzyme function modification (type A), transport protein modification (type B), and complexation, binding, and/or other deactivating processes that may occur in the GI tract (type C) [2]. Of note, separating the administration times of the interacting agents will minimize the consequences of a type II interaction.

A common and important type IIA interaction involves the precipitant agent of grapefruit juice and its effects on the absorption of many different medications [6]. The mechanism of this interaction involves the inhibition of the function of a cytochrome P450 enzyme known as CYP3A4 in the intestinal lumen. As this enzyme is usually responsible for breaking down numerous medications, inhibition of its effects within enterocytes will lead to more of the object agent being available for absorption, causing an increase in drug exposure. This may be most notable for cyclosporine, tacrolimus, and felodipine given the possible negative consequences from increased exposure to these compounds [7–9]. Of note, CYP3A4 is also present in the liver, but inhibition of the enzyme in the liver leads to increased exposure due to a decreased rate of metabolism. This interaction is not demonstrated with grapefruit juice so its CYP3A4 inhibition occurs exclusively in enterocytes [8, 9].

A noteworthy type IIB interaction involves inhibition of the intestinal type 2 intestinal apical carnitine/organic cation transporter (OCTN2). This enzyme is responsible for the uptake of carnitine as well as important medications such as levofloxacin, spironolactone, and valproic acid [10, 11]. In particular, chronic use of valproic acid may lead to impaired absorption of carnitine leading to carnitine deficiency in susceptible individuals [12–15]. Another noteworthy type IIB interaction involves the inhibition of the PEPT1 intestinal uptake transporter by zinc, which is contained in many over-the-counter cold remedies. This transporter is responsible for the uptake of many cephalosporin antibiotics, so co-administration of these medications with zinc may lead to decreased absorption and, therefore, inadequate treatment of infection, although this has not been demonstrated as significant in clinical practice [16, 17].

Important type IIC interactions involve the oral administration of antibiotics with polyvalent metal cations. The polyvalent cations chelate some medications leading to a decrease in the overall absorption of the object agent. This has most notably been seen with fluoroquinolones and tetracyclines when co-administered with iron-, calcium-, magnesium-, or aluminum-containing products or tube-feed formulations [6, 18–23]. This interaction would lead to decreased absorption of the affected agents, which could lead to underexposure to the antibiotic and consequently a failure to completely treat an infection and/or the development of drug resistance. This interaction can be avoided by separating the administration of polyvalentcation-containing products (e.g., antacids) by at least 2 hours. Of note, this interaction also includes foods high in polyvalent cations such as dairy products.

Physiologic action-associated interactions occur after the absorption of at least one of the interacting agents has completed the absorption phase. The mechanism of this type of interaction involves a change in the distribution, systemic metabolism or transport (as opposed to transport within the GI tract), or penetration to specific organs or tissues of the object compound. One important difference between this type of interaction and absorption phase-associated interactions involves how they are managed: to avoid an absorption phase-associated interaction, the precipitant and object agents may be administered separate from each other by several hours. This approach is not expected to influence the incidence of a physiologic action-associated interaction, and a dose adjustment of the object agent is indicated to mediate the interaction. A classic example of this type of interaction is the "cheese reaction." In this reaction, if a patient currently on a monoamine oxidase inhibitor (MAOI) were to consume a food with a high amount of tyramine, a pressor effect is noted, leading to extremely elevated blood pressures. This occurs as tyramine induces the release of natural vasopressors (e.g., norepinephrine, epinephrine) which are traditionally metabolized by monoamine oxidase in the periphery; however, with the inhibition of monoamine oxidase from nonselective MAOIs, significant hypertension may result [24–26]. Of note, this reaction is not as clinically important as it once was as nonselective MAOIs are rarely used in clinical practice and foods are now processed more efficiently than when the "cheese effect" was first described, leading to a decrease in the overall tyramine content in foods of concern (e.g., aged cheeses, beer) [27]. While nonselective MAOIs are rarely used in clinical practice, linezolid and isoniazid have some MAOI properties, so caution may be warranted in regard to tyramine exposure in patients on these medications [28, 29].

Lastly, *elimination phase-associated interactions* involve the modulation, antagonism, or impairment of renal or enterohepatic elimination. This form of interaction may be mediated by competition between drugs and nutrients for tissue-specific transport proteins for elimination. This is most clearly seen with the increased reabsorption of lithium in the renal tubules in patients on a sodium-restricted diet [30].

Important Drug-Nutrient Interactions

Continuous Enteral Nutrition

Critically ill patients often require administration of enteral nutrition in a continuous fashion to prevent the development of caloric and protein deficits while also decreasing the potential for feeding intolerance [31]. There are some medications that are noted to interact with continuous enteral nutrition that may pertain to any patient regardless of baseline renal function: phenytoin, warfarin, and levothyroxine [32]. It is unknown if these interactions involve physical incompatibilities with tube-feeding formulations and impaired dissolution into solution leading to inadequate absorption, or if there is adsorption of these medications to the enteral access devices themselves, although a combination of these mechanisms is most likely.

Phenytoin, a sodium-channel-blocking antiepileptic, demonstrates a significant decrease in absorption – up to 80% when the oral solution is used in combination with continuous enteral nutrition [33]. In one study of neurosurgical patients on seizure prophylaxis, normal daily maintenance doses of 300–400 mg/day had to be increased to doses of 800–1200 mg/day, and therapeutic levels were still not obtained [34]. This was confirmed to be related to continuous tube-feeding administration as many of the patients included developed phenytoin toxicity after the continuous enteral nutrition regimen was discontinued.

Warfarin, a vitamin K antagonist anticoagulant, is widely used for the treatment of venous thromboembolism and for the prevention of stroke in patients with atrial dysrhythmias and mechanical valves. When co-administered with continuous enteral tube feeding, it has been noted that doses significantly above that of a patient's home regimen may be necessary to maintain a therapeutic prothrombin time (PT) and international normalized ratio (INR) [35, 36]. The mechanism of this interaction is vitamin K independent given the low quantity of vitamin K contained in most tube-feeding formulations. This interaction is more likely related to sequestration of warfarin in the tube feeding via interactions with the macromolecular fraction of enteral feeds, possibly by directly binding to protein components [37, 38].

Levothyroxine is a thyroid hormone used as a replacement in patients with hypothyroidism. With initiation of continuous enteral nutrition and administration of previously therapeutic doses of levothyroxine, it has been noticed that thyroid-stimulating hormone levels have increased, indicating the development of hypothyroidism. This is believed to be related to adsorption of levothyroxine to enteral access devices, and an empiric increase in the previous levothyroxine dose by 25 mcg may be an effective mitigation strategy for this drug-nutrient interaction [39]. Regardless, thyroid hormone levels should be monitored closely in this patient population.

One approach to mitigate these interactions to a degree is withholding of enteral nutrition before and after medication administration. This was first shown to be effective with phenytoin in the same report in which phenytoin doses were increased drastically to achieve a therapeutic serum phenytoin concentration [34]. In this study, tube feeds were held 2 hours before and 2 hours after phenytoin administration. Withholding of tube feeds 1 hour before and after medication administration has been shown to be adequate in the case of phenytoin, warfarin, and levothyroxine [33, 39, 40]. This strategy would likely prove effective in enhancing absorption of many enterally administered medications if an interaction with enteral feeding is suspected, although medications that require food for adequate absorption would not demonstrate this benefit [1]. Of note, the overall best time frame for withholding of tube feeding is not well known, and there are certainly risks associated with this practice. For example, with medications administered multiple times a day (e.g., phenytoin), withholding tube feeds around each dose would clearly lead to an inability to attain the patient's goal for calorie and protein delivery, leading to a deficit that is likely to be detrimental. To avoid this issue, the tube-feeding rate may be adjusted so that the same total volume of tube feeding is provided throughout the day, but this may lead to an increased risk in the complications associated with provision of tube feeding including aspiration, hyperglycemia, diarrhea, and other GI-related adverse effects [1]. If GI intolerance occurs, mitigation strategies include the addition of a prokinetic medication (keeping in mind that metoclopramide is cleared by the kidneys so dose adjustment may be necessary), adjustment of the current enteral nutrition formulation to a more dense formula so that lower total volumes would need to be administered to reach nutrition goals, electively underfeeding the patient for a short period of time, or adjusting the associated medication to an intravenous formulation if available. For phenytoin, warfarin, levothyroxine, fluoroquinolones, and tetracyclines, we recommend holding tube feeds for 1 hour before and 1 hour after medication administration if enteral delivery of these medications is necessary; however, to decrease complications related to nutrition goal attainment and GI tolerance, these medications should not be given more than twice daily. In the case of ciprofloxacin and tetracyclines, intravenous administration may be preferred, since interactions with these medications and polyvalent cations are likely to be significant even with the withholding of enteral nutrition for 1 hour before and hour after medication administration.

See Fig. 9.1 for a schematic of the steps and factors associated with oral drug absorption.

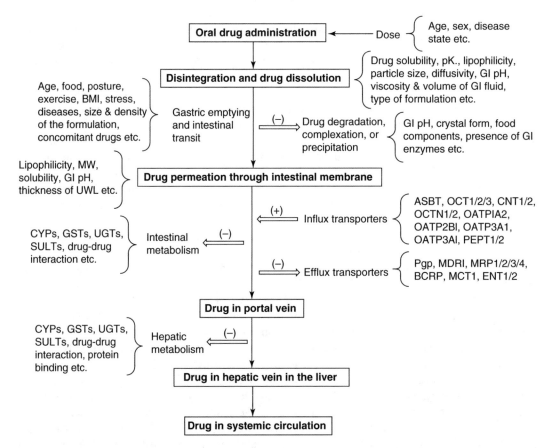

Fig. 9.1 Drug pharmacokinetics. Schematic diagram of the steps and factors associated with oral drug absorption. Molecular weight (MW), unstirred water layer (UWL), cytochrome P450 (CYP), UDP-glucuronosyltransferase (UGT), glutathione S-transferase (GST), sulfotransferase (SULT), apical sodium-dependent bile acid transporter (ASBT), organic cation transporter (OCT), concentrative nucleotide transporter (CNT), electroneutral organic cation transporter (OCTN), organic anion transporting polypeptide (OATP), peptide transport protein (PEPT), P-glycoprotein (P-gp), multidrug resistance protein (MDR), multidrug resistance-associated protein (MRP), breast cancer resistance protein (BCRP), monocarboxylate transporter protein (MCT), equilibrative nucleoside transporter (ENT). (+) and (−) indicate an increase or a decrease in the rate and/or extent of drug absorption. (Reprinted from Abuhelwaet al. [44]. Copyright 2017, with permission from Elsevier)

Medication and Food Timing Considerations

Some medications may have alterations in their absorption in relation to food consumption. Specifically, absorption may be impaired or enhanced often related to alterations in gastric and intestinal transition times, although type IIC (chelation) reactions are also of concern. In general, high-fat foods slow gastric emptying leading to an increased exposure to the acid environment found in the stomach. This will decrease overall absorption of medications that are broken down in acid environments (e.g., digoxin) but may increase absorption of medications that are acid stable (e.g., carbamazepine) since a longer transit time provides more time for absorption to occur [41]. Usually with this occurrence, overall exposure to the medication (the AUC) may be increased, but the peak concentration (C_{max}) will be lower due to slowed progression through the gastrointestinal tract and prolonged absorption. Because of this association, some medications are recommended to be given with food to decrease side effects associated with high peak concentrations (e.g., orthostasis associated with carvedilol administration) [42]. Other causes of slowed gastric emptying include provision of large volumes of fluid in a short period of time, high protein concentrations, acidic foods, and medication effects (e.g., anticholinergic agents, opiates, and octreotide). For some medications (e.g., posaconazole, rivaroxaban, ziprasidone, and some antiretrovirals), adequate absorption relies upon being administered with food or after consuming a meal [41]. In regard to timing of food and administration of medications, our recommendation is to follow the recommendations of the package insert of medications and/or to consult with a pharmacist to assist with timing of medications in relation to meals.

Renal Disease Considerations

Certain organs dictate which nutrients can be metabolized by the body. When those organs are compromised, or failing, such as in renal failure, those nutrients may not be metabolized appropriately and tend to build up, and simple electrolytes such as potassium can become toxic and life-threatening. Hyperkalemia can cause fatal arrhythmias and needs to be monitored and managed appropriately. If a patient is on certain medications for hypertension such as enalapril, which is an angiotensin converting enzyme (ACE) inhibitor, or losartan, which is an angiotensin receptor blocker (ARB) – both of which increase potassium – and they consume excess dietary potassium and/or have renal insufficiency, there can be dire consequences.

When a patient suffers from renal insufficiency, clearance of phosphate starts to decline. If the amount of dietary phosphate isn't changed, it will begin to accumulate in the patient's body; initially they have no symptoms, but in more severe cases they develop pruritus. Hyperphosphatemia can be treated with calcium carbonate or prescription treatment such as calcium acetate, or sevelamer, with meals to bind to consumed phosphate in a purposefully induced type IIC chelation interaction.

Renal Transplant Considerations

Tacrolimus and cyclosporine are calcineurin inhibitors used to prevent allograft rejection after transplantation. Almost all renal transplant recipients are on either medication after receiving a renal transplant, along with other immunosuppressive agents. Tacrolimus and cyclosporine are hepatically metabolized by the cytochrome P450 system, specifically by the CYP3A4 isoenzyme. If a transplant patient on either of those medications were to drink grapefruit juice or pomegranate juice, this can cause an increase in the levels of tacrolimus or cyclosporine. At supratherapeutic levels, tacrolimus can cause tremors and seizures, and both medications are nephrotoxic in excessive doses. Foods can also pose a problem; patients on immunosuppressants need to avoid raw and undercooked meats and unpasteurized milk or cheese as they may contain *Listeria* or other bacteria that an immunocompromised patient cannot fight off. Transplant patients should also be educated to avoid all herbal products as they may interact with their immunosuppressive regimen.

Herbal Product Considerations

It is also important to know that certain herbal/nutrient products that patients believe have health benefits can be toxic. Products sold without a prescription can be unsafe, even lethal, and oftentimes interact with prescription medications. Table 9.1 presents important herbal/nutrient interactions that are known in the medical community. Unfortunately, there is often a misconception that if a product can be purchased without a prescription, it must be harmless. It is important to ask every patient not only what medications he/she takes, including over-the-counter medications, but also if he/she is taking any herbal products as they are often thought of as innocuous homeopathic remedies void of interactions with other therapies.

Conclusion

Drug-nutrient interactions occur when a precipitant agent alters a pharmacokinetic or pharmacodynamics parameter. Their clinical significance may range from negligible to life-threatening, so thorough assessment of a patient's diet and micronutrient use is important. Some drug-nutrient interactions may be negated or mitigated by separating the interacting agents (e.g., agents that undergo a chelation interaction), although this is not true of all interactions (e.g., "cheese reaction"). Drug-nutrient interactions are especially prevalent in critically ill patients receiving continuous enteral nutrition, although

Table 9.1 Drug-nutrient interactions [43]

Pathway	Effects	Herbal/nutrient	Drug/medications
CYP3A4 p-glycoprotein	*Inducers*	St John's wort	Cyclosporine, tacrolimus, digoxin, protease inhibitors, NNRTIs
CYP3A4 CYP2D6	*Inhibition*	Goldenseal Berberine	Cyclosporine, tacrolimus, amitriptyline, clozapine, donepezil, tramadol, methadone
CYP3A4	Inhibition	Grapefruit juice Seville orange juice aka bitter orange	Benzodiazepines, atorvastatin, oxycodone, cyclosporine, tacrolimus, sertraline
CYP2E1	Inhibition	Allyl sulfides Garlic Watercress	Acetaminophen
CYP2E1 CYP1A2	Inhibition	Cruciferous vegetables Sulfur-containing supplements	Acetaminophen, haloperidol, theophylline
CYP2C19	Induction	Ginkgo biloba	Omeprazole
CYP3A4 CYP2C9	Inhibition	Ginseng	Warfarin
CYP3A4	Inhibition	Echinacea	Midazolam
CYP3A4 CYP1A2	Inhibition	Resveratrol	Cyclosporine, tacrolimus, cisapride, testosterone

their significance may be reduced with the holding of tube feeding around the administration of the interaction medication; however, this introduces complications associated with underfeeding and issues related to tolerance of enteral nutrition. Patients who have undergone a renal transplantation are also prone to many drug-nutrient interactions associated with the use of the calcineurin inhibitors tacrolimus and cyclosporine. To prevent potential complications associated with drug-nutrient interactions, it is important to conduct a thorough reconciliation of the patient's diet and medication use including herbal supplements.

References

1. Chan L-N. Drug nutrient interactions. J Parenter Enter Nutr. 2013;37:450–9.
2. Chan L-N. Drug-nutrient interactions. In: Shils ME, Shike M, Olson JA, editors. Modern nutrition in health and disease. 10th ed. Philadelphia: Lippincott Williams & Wilkins; 2006. p. 1539–53.
3. Brown R, Quercia RA, Sigman R. Total nutrient admixture: a review. J Parenter Enter Nutr. 1986;10:650–8.
4. Slattery E, Rumore MM, Douglas JS, Seres DS. 3-in-1 vs 2-in-1 parenteral nutrition in adults: a review. J Parenter Enter Nutr. 2014;29:631–5.
5. Malatani RT. Enteral feeding and fluoroquinolones. Int J Pharm. 2014;4(4):74–7.
6. Neuvonen PJ. Interactions with the absorption of tetracyclines. Drugs. 1976;11(1):45–54.
7. Sridharan K, Sivaramakrishnan G. Interaction of citrus juices with cyclosporine: systematic review and meta-analysis. Eur J Drug Metab Pharmacokinet. 2016;41(6):665–73.
8. An G, Mukker JK, Derendorf H, Frye RF. Enzyme- and transporter-mediated beverage-drug interactions: an update on fruit juices and green tea. J Clin Pharmacol. 2015;55(12):1313–31.
9. Bailey DG, Spence JD, Munoz C, Arnold JM. Interaction of fruit juices with felodipine and nifedipine. Lancet. 1991;337(8736):268–9.
10. Estudante M, Morais JG, Soveral G, Benet LZ. Intestinal drug transporters: an overview. Adv Drug Deliv Rev. 2013;65(10):1340–56.
11. Roth M, Obaidat A, Hagenbuch B. OATPs, OATs and OCTs: the organic anion and cation transporters of the SLCO and SLC22A gene superfamilies. Br J Pharmacol. 2012;165(5):1260–87.
12. Verrotti A, Trotta D, Morgese G, Chiarelli F. Valproate-induced hyperammonemic encephalopathy. Metab Brain Dis. 2002;17(4):367–73.
13. Chopra A, Kolla BP, Mansukhani MP, Netzel P, Frye MA. Valproate-induced hyperammonemic encephalopathy: an update on risk factors, clinical correlates and management. Gen Hosp Psychiatry. 2012;34(3):290–8.
14. Coppola G, Epifanio G, Auricchio G, Federico RR, Resicato G, Pascotto A. Plasma free carnitine in epilepsy children, adolescents and young adults treated with old and new antiepileptic drugs with or without ketogenic diet. Brain and Development. 2006;28(6):358–65.
15. Moreno FA, Macey H, Schreiber B. Carnitine levels in valproic acid-treated psychiatric patients: a cross-sectional study. J Clin Psychiatry. 2005;66(5):555–8.
16. Okamura M, Terada T, Katsura T, Saito H, Inui K. Inhibitory effect of zinc on PEPT1-mediated transport of glycyl-sarcosine and beta-lactam antibiotics in human intestinal cell line Caco-2. Pharm Res. 2003;20(9):1389–93.
17. Okamura M, Terada T, Katsura T, Inui K. Inhibitory effect of zinc on the absorption of beta-lactam antibiotic ceftibuten via the peptide transporters in rats. Drug Metab Pharmacokinet. 2008;23(6):464–8.
18. Ogawa R, Echizen H. Clinically significant drug interactions with antacids: an update. Drugs. 2011;71(14):1839–64.
19. Rodríguez Cruz MS, González Alonso I, Sánchez-Navarro A, SayaleroMarinero ML. In vitro study of the interaction between quinolones and polyvalent cations. Pharm Acta Helv. 1999;73(5):237–45.
20. Mueller BA, Brierton DG, Abel SR, Bowman L. Effect of enteral feeding with ensure on ensure on oral bioavailabilities of ofloxacin and ciprofloxacin. Antimicrob Agents Chemother. 1994;38(9):2101–5.
21. Cohn SM, Sawyer MD, Burns GA, Tolomeo C, Milner KA. Enteric absorption of ciprofloxacin during tube feeding in the critically ill. J Antimicrob Chemother. 1996;38(5):871–6.
22. Mimoz O, Binter V, Jacolot A, Edouard A, Tod M, Petitjean O, et al. Pharmacokinetics and absolute bioavailability of ciprofloxacin administered through a nasogastric tube with continuous enteral feeding to critically ill patients. Intensive Care Med. 1998;24(10):1047–51.
23. Wright DH, Pietz SL, Konstantinides FN, Rotschafer JC. Decreased in vitro fluoroquinolone concentrations after admixture with an enteral feeding formulation. JPEN J Parenter Enteral Nutr. 2000;24(1):42–8.
24. Berlin I, Zimmer R, Cournot A, Payan C, Pedarriosse AM, Puech AJ. Determination and comparison of the pressor effect of tyramine during long-term moclobemide and tranylcypromine treatment in healthy volunteers. Clin Pharmacol Ther. 1989;46:344–51.

25. Bieck PR, Antonin KH. Tyramine potentiation during treatment with MAO inhibitors: brofaromine and moclobemidevs irreversible inhibitors. J Neural Transm. 1989;Suppl 28:21–31.

26. Blackwell B, Mabbitt LA. Tyramine in cheese related to hypertensive crises after monoamine-oxidase inhibition. Lancet. 1965;1(7392):938–40.

27. Gillman PK. A reassessment of the safety profile of monoamine oxidase inhibitors: elucidating tired old tyramine myths. J Neural Transm. 2018;125(11):1707–17.

28. Linezolid. Lexi-Drugs. Lexicomp. Wolters Kluwer Health, Inc. Riverwoods. Available at: http://online.lexi.com. Accessed 27 Feb 2019.

29. Isoniazid. Lexi-Drugs. Lexicomp. Wolters Kluwer Health, Inc. Riverwoods. Available at: http://online.lexi.com. Accessed 27 Feb 2019.

30. Bennett WM. Drug interactions and consequences of sodium restriction. Am J Clin Nutr. 1997;62(2 Suppl): 678S–81S.

31. Yeh DD, Fuentes E, Quraishi SA, Cropano C, Kaafarani H, Lee J, et al. Adequate nutrition may get you home: effect of caloric/protein deficits on discharge destination of critically ill surgical patients. J Parenter Enter Nutr. 2016;40(1):37–44.

32. Wohlt PD, Zheng L, Gunderson S, Balzar SA, Johnson BD, Fish JT. Recommendations for the use of medications with continuous enteral nutrition. Am J Health Syst Pharm. 2009;66:1458–67.

33. Au Yeung SC, Ensom MH. Phenytoin and enteral feedings: does evidence support an interaction? Ann Pharmacother. 2000;34:896–905.

34. Bauer LA. Interference of oral phenytoin absorption by continuous nasogastric feedings. Neurology. 1982;32:570–2.

35. Penrod LE, Allen JB, Cabacungan LR. Warfarin resistance and enteral feedings: 2 case reports and a supporting in vitro study. Arch Phys Med Rehabil. 2001;82:1270–3.

36. Martin JE, Lutomski DM. Warfarin resistance and enteral feedings. J Parenter Enter Nutr. 1989;13:206–8.

37. Kuhn TA, Garnett WR, Wells BK, Karnes HT. Recovery of warfarin from an enteral nutrient formula. Am J Hosp Pharm. 1989;46:1395–9.

38. Dickerson RN, Garmon WM, Kuhl DA, Minard G, Brown RO. Vitamin K-independent warfarin resistance after concurrent administration of warfarin and continuous enteral nutrition. Pharmacotherapy. 2008;28:308–13.

39. Dickerson RN. Warfarin resistance and enteral tube feeding: a vitamin K-independent interaction. Nutrition. 2008;24(10):1048–52.

40. Dickerson RN, Maish GO 3rd, Minard G, Brown RO. Clinical relevancy of the levothyroxine-continuous enteral nutrition interaction. Nutr Clin Pract. 2010;25(6):646–52.

41. Rollins CJ. Drug-nutrient interactions. In: Mueller CM, editor. The a.S.P.E.N. adult nutrition support core curriculum. 2nd ed. Silver Spring: American Society of Parenteral and Enteral Nutrition; 2012. p. 298–312.

42. Coreg (carvedilol) package insert. Research Triangle Park: GlaxoSmithKline; 2017.

43. JoyM. 2019. ASN Kidney News Online. Retrieved from https://www.kidneynews.org.

44. Abuhelwa AY, Williams DB, Upton RN, Foster DJ. Food, gastrointestinal PH, and models of oral drug absorption. Eur J Pharm Biopharm. 2017;112:234–48.

Part III
Preventative Strategies for Chronic Kidney Disease Among Adults

Diet has a profound impact on numerous disease states, and nutritional interventions are at the core of therapeutic and preventative strategies aimed at several common disease states. Hypertension affects a large proportion of the general population and is almost universally found among patients with chronic kidney disease (CKD) and end-stage renal disease (ESRD). Because of its strong link to cardiovascular morbidity and mortality, prevention and treatment of hypertension is one of the most important public health priorities. Diabetes mellitus represents another disease state with alarming impact on CKD development and progression, which represents the number one cause of kidney disease in the developed world. Obesity has taken epidemic proportions in developed countries and is a cause of the rising incidence of diabetes and hypertension, while also having a direct impact on the development and progression of chronic kidney disease. Finally, cardiovascular disease is both a cause and a consequence of CKD, and its therapy is intricately intertwined with the management of CKD.

The chapters in this section discuss how dietary interventions can be used to prevent or treat these disease states. The chapter by Biruete and Kistler summarizes the nutritional interventions that effectively lower blood pressure in patients with and without CKD, including weight loss interventions, restricting salt intake and diets such as the Dietary Approaches to Stop Hypertension (DASH) diet and the Mediterranean diet. Elger et al. describe the role of diabetes mellitus in the genesis of kidney disease and provide a summary of how dietary interventions can be integrated with pharmacologic management of diabetes and other concomitant comorbidities. Friedman provides a detailed description of the roles obesity plays in the development of kidney disease and how weight loss interventions could impact the incidence and progression of CKD. Finally, Beto et al. summarize relevant guidelines for cardiovascular disease management and synthesize the role of nutritional strategies in interventions targeting cardiovascular diseases in patients with CKD. Given the high prevalence and profound impact of these disease states on the health and well-being of the general population and of patients with CKD, the chapters in this section represent a summary of critical importance to a wide range of practitioners.

Chapter 10
Hypertension

Annabel Biruete and Brandon Kistler

Keywords Blood pressure · Weight loss · Sodium · Potassium · Magnesium · Omega-3 · DASH diet Mediterranean diet · Lifestyle · Chronic kidney disease

Key Points
- Diet is a main part of the treatment of hypertension in individuals with and without chronic kidney disease.
- Weight loss in those with overweight and obesity is an effective strategy to reduce blood pressure.
- Among nutrients, sodium and potassium are the ones with the most consistent data showing reductions in blood pressure.
- Among dietary patterns, the DASH diet with and without sodium reduction and the Mediterranean diet have been shown to reduce blood pressure.

Introduction

According to the American Heart Association (AHA) and the American College of Cardiology (ACC), hypertension is defined as systolic blood pressure (SBP) $\geq$130 mmHg and/or diastolic blood pressure (DBP) $\geq$80 mmHg [1]. In the United States, among people $\geq$18 years of age, the prevalence of hypertension was 29% in 2015–2016, with the highest prevalence among those $\geq$60 years of age (63%) and the non-Hispanic Black population (40%) [2]. However, these numbers could be expected to increase with recent changes in BP classifications. A reduction of blood pressure toward normal levels is important, as prolonged hypertension and diabetes mellitus are the leading causes of chronic kidney disease (CKD), and prolonged uncontrolled hypertension may lead to end-stage kidney disease [3].

Lifestyle interventions are vital for the management of hypertension. Among interventions that may reduce blood pressure, weight loss in those with overweight and obesity, increases in physical activity, and dietary interventions have been shown to be effective [1]. Several studies (observational,

The editors acknowledge Kristie J. Lancaster's contribution to this chapter in *Nutrition in Kidney Disease*, *Second Edition*, Nutrition and Health, DOI 10.1007/978-1-62703-685-6_1, © Springer Science+Business Media New York 2014

A. Biruete (✉)
Division of Nephrology, Department of Medicine, Indiana University School of Medicine, Indianapolis, IN, USA
e-mail: abiruete@iu.edu

B. Kistler
Department of Nutrition and Health Science, Ball State University, Muncie, IN, USA

cross-sectional, and randomized controlled trials) have assessed the effects of single nutrients, individual foods, and dietary patterns on blood pressure in individuals with hypertension. Within nutrients, a decrease in dietary sodium intake [4], while an increase in potassium [5], magnesium [6], calcium [7], and omega-3 fatty acids [8], either from food or supplements, has been associated with reductions in blood pressure. Within individual food groups, fruits and vegetables [9], and dairy [10], among others have also been assessed. However, nutrients are not consumed in isolation; therefore, dietary patterns may provide a better overall indication of the effect of diet on blood pressure. Dietary patterns, such as the Dietary Approaches to Stop Hypertension (DASH) diet and the Mediterranean diet, have been shown to be effective in reducing blood pressure [11]. The DASH diet has been recommended by the Joint National Committee (JNC) and the AHA Nutrition Committee of the Council on Lifestyle and Cardiometabolic Health, while the European Renal Nutrition Working Group from the European Renal Association-European Dialysis and Transplantation Association has suggested the Mediterranean diet as the diet of choice for patients with CKD [12, 13]. This chapter will cover the evidence on the effect of these nutrients and dietary patterns on the management of hypertension, with a particular interest in slowing the progression of CKD.

Current Dietary Recommendations For Hypertension and Chronic Kidney Disease

The Joint National Committee (JNC) and American Heart Association (AHA)/ American College of Cardiology (ACC) Recommendations

Lifestyle interventions are a vital part of the management of hypertension. Current recommendations for the management of hypertension are included in Table 10.1 [14].These recommendations were established by the 7th JNC [15] and endorsed again by the 8th JNC [16], in addition to the latest AHA/ACC guidelines [14]. Furthermore, these were recently endorsed by the Kidney Disease Outcomes Quality Initiative (KDOQI) [17]. These recommendations include weight loss in those with overweight and obesity or maintenance of weight in those with a body mass index (BMI) < 25 kg/m^2, adopting a DASH-type diet with the reduction of dietary sodium, increase in physical activity, and reduction or moderate consumption of alcohol. These modifications are recommended to happen in combination, and not in isolation, as an additive effect on blood pressure may be obtained.

Table 10.1 Lifestyle modifications to manage hypertension

Modification	Dose	Approximate SBP	
		Hypertension	Normotension
Weight reduction	Maintain normal body weight. If BMI is ≥25 kg/m^2, work toward ideal body weight. In general, for every 1-kg weight loss, expect a reduction of ~1 mmHg in SBP.	−5 mmHg	−2/3 mmHg
DASH dietary pattern	Dietary pattern rich in fruits, vegetables, and low-fat dairy products with a reduced content of saturated and total fat (see Table 10.2)	−11 mmHg	−3 mmHg
Dietary sodium	Aim for less than 1500 mg/d, but as intake is usually high, aim for a 1000 mg/d reduction.	−5/6 mmHg	−2/3 mmHg
Dietary potassium	Aim for 3500–5000 mg/d, preferably by consumption of a diet rich in potassium versus supplements.	−4/5 mmHg	−2 mmHg

Abbreviations: *SBP* systolic blood pressure, *BMI* body mass index, *DASH* Dietary Approaches to Stop Hypertension
Modified from Ref. [14]

Weight Loss

Weight loss in individuals with overweight and obesity is one of the most effective interventions in reducing blood pressure. In a randomized controlled trial by the Trials of Hypertension Prevention Collaborative Group, participants were assigned to one of four groups: (1) sodium reduction + weight loss (of at least 10 lb/4.5 kg), (2) no sodium reduction + weight loss, (3) sodium reduction (≤1840 mg/day (80 mmol/day)) with no weight loss, or (4) no sodium reduction and no weight loss [18]. At 6 months, those in the weight loss group had a reduction of 6.0 ± 8.1 mmHg and 5.5 ± 6.9 mmHg in SBP and DPB, respectively [18]. Furthermore, those in the combined group of weight loss and sodium reduction had a reduction of 6.2 ± 8.6 mmHg and 5.6 ± 6.9 mmHg in SBP and DBP, respectively.

In a meta-analysis of 25 randomized controlled trials by Neter et al. [19], reductions in SBP and DBP per kilogram of weight loss were estimated to be −1.05 mmHg (95% CI −1.43,−0.66) and −0.92 mmHg (95% CI −1.28,−0.55), respectively. Moreover, in those studies where there was a weight loss of ≥5 kg, as expected, there were larger drops in SBP (−6.63 mmHg vs. −2.70 mmHg) and DBP (−5.12 mmHg vs. −2.01 mmHg) [19]. Due to the marked effect of weight loss on blood pressure in individuals with hypertension, the 7th and 8th Reports of the JNC [15, 16] recommend weight reduction or maintenance of normal body weight, as it may lead to a significant reduction of blood pressure, with a higher effect in those with hypertension versus those with normal blood pressure. However, as observed in the meta-analysis by Neter et al. [19], any weight loss in those with overweight and obesity may result in a beneficial effect on blood pressure.

The evidence on the effect of weight loss on blood pressure in patients with CKD, however, is scarce. MacLaughlin et al. [20] reported the effects of a nine-session structured weight loss program (reduced-energy renal diet, physical activity, and gastrointestinal lipase inhibitor) in patients with CKD (non-dialysis and dialysis-dependent) with a BMI of >30 or >28 kg/m^2 if there was a diagnoses of hypertension, diabetes, and/or dyslipidemia. They found that at 6 months, there was a mean weight loss of 4.5 ± 0.4 kg, which was maintained for up to 24 months. Even though there was a modest, but significant decrease in SBP of 3 ± 2 mmHg only at 18 months, when they stratified by compliance to the weight loss program, those who were compliant (attended seven to nine sessions) had a SBP decrease of 8 mmHg (95% CI −2,−14) [20].

Dietary Interventions

Sodium

Sodium is the most researched nutrient for its effect on blood pressure. Observational studies have shown a relationship between dietary sodium intake and blood pressure. The INTERSALT study, which was an epidemiological study of 10,079 men and women, aged 20 to 59 y, from 32 countries, showed that in individuals with and without hypertension, a sodium intake >2300 mg/day was associated with an increase of 3–6 mmHg and 0–3 mmHg of SBP and DBP, respectively [21]. In subgroup analyses, the relationship remained consistent regardless of sex, age, and individuals without a diagnosis of hypertension [21]. The INTERMAP study, an epidemiological study of 4680 men and women 40 to 59 y from China, Japan, the UK, and the United States showed that an intake of ~2700 mg of sodium/day (measured as urinary sodium) was associated with an increase of 3.7 mmHg in SBP [22]. Furthermore, in a sub-analysis of the Trials of Hypertension Prevention, Cook et al. [23] showed that per 1000 mg increase in dietary sodium intake, there was an increase of 13% in all-cause mortality (95% CI 1.03, 1.24). Due to these consistent associations between dietary sodium intake and blood pressure, and the relationship between high blood pressure and morbidity and mortality, several organizations including the World Health Organization (WHO) [24] and the AHA/ACC have recommended to lower dietary sodium intake in individuals with and without hypertension.

Epidemiological Versus Individual Sodium Assessment: Limitations of Urinary Sodium

Self-reported dietary sodium intake through dietary recalls and food frequency questionnaires may be biased as individuals may underreport due to memory or conscious or unconscious misreporting due to social desirability bias [25]. Additionally, due to the large amount of manufactured foods, the accuracy of the dietary recalls may be compromised. Because of these and other reasons, urinary sodium has been used as a surrogate marker of intake with the premise of sodium intake equals sodium excretion [26]. However, recent evidence suggests that, at the individual level, single-day urinary collections (spot-urine and 24-hour) may not be an accurate measure of dietary sodium intake [27]. Strikingly, in a tightly controlled environment (Mars simulation flight), Lerchl et al. [28] were only able to differentiate between 2400 mg, 3600 mg, and 4800 mg of sodium intake about 50% of the time by single 24-hour urine specimens [28]. However, with 3-day and 7-day collections, accuracy improved but was not perfect [28]. Therefore, using individual urinary sodium measurements as a proxy for dietary intake to assess adherence to interventions may not be the best way of estimating dietary sodium intake.

Dietary Sodium Sources in the Typical American Diet

Sodium intake around the world is well above the recommendation of less than 2300 mg/day, with intakes of ~3400 mg/day in the United States and as high as ~5900 mg/day in China [21]. Contrary to popular belief, dietary sodium intake comes mostly from foods with sodium added as a preservative (mostly ultra-processed foods), followed by the sodium naturally contained in foods, and lastly from added table salt. In a CDC report of What We Eat In America (WWEIA), 65% of dietary sodium came from foods obtained at a store (either supermarket or convenience) and ~25% from restaurants. Specifically, the top ten sources of dietary sodium were bread and rolls, cold cuts/cured meats, pizza, poultry, soups, sandwiches, cheese (naturally and processed), pasta-mixed dishes, meat-mixed dishes, and savory snacks. In total, these foods contributed ~40% of the total sodium intake [29].

Dietary Sodium Intake Recommendations

For adults, the 2019 US Dietary Reference Guidelines (DRIs) recommend an Adequate Intake (AI) of 1500 mg of sodium/day and an upper limit (UL) or now termed Chronic Disease Risk Reduction (CDDR) intake of 2300 mg/day, with no difference between males and females [30]. Similarly, the 2015–2020 Dietary Guidelines for Americans recommend consuming less than 2300 mg sodium/day [31]. However, both the DRIs and the Dietary Guidelines for Americans are intended for healthy individuals and not for the treatment of disease.

The AHA/ACC recommend for individuals with prehypertension and hypertension a sodium intake of less than 2400 mg/day initially and even lowering to 1500 mg/day as it may result in additional reduction in blood pressure [32]. However, the guideline also mentions that when dietary sodium intake is high, even a decrease of 1000 mg/day may help in lowering blood pressure [32]. For individuals with CKD and hypertension, the Kidney Disease Improving Global Outcomes (KDIGO) guidelines for the management of blood pressure in CKD recommend a dietary sodium intake of less than 2000 mg/day [33].

Translation of the recommendations by nutrition professionals and adoption by individuals is challenging. Population-level education and awareness have been shown to be successful in reducing dietary sodium intake [34]. At the individual level, focusing on the location where food is consumed (i.e., at home vs. outside of home), the top sources of dietary sodium and food preparation may help to reduce dietary sodium intake.

Dietary Sodium Restriction in CKD

The reduction of dietary sodium is one of the main nutritional recommendations for patients with CKD. In a systematic review and meta-analysis by McMahon et al. [35], reducing sodium intake decreased SBP by 8.75 mmHg (95% CI $-11.33, -6.16$) and DBP by -3.70 mmHg (95% CI $-5.09, -2.30$ mmHg). Although a reduction in sodium intake may be advised to limit the progression of CKD (to control blood pressure), a small number of long-term studies have assessed changes in estimated glomerular filtration rate (eGFR), time to dialysis, or even mortality [35]. Campbell et al. [36] assessed the acute (2 weeks) effects of a low (aim of 1380–1840 mg of sodium/day) versus high (supplementation of 2760 mg of sodium/day) sodium intake on blood pressure in a randomized, controlled, crossover study in individuals with eGFR of 15–59 ml/min/1.73m^2. During the low-sodium period, SBP was reduced by 10 mmHg (95% CI $-20, -1$) and DBP by 6 mmHg (95% CI $-10, -1$) [36].

Potassium

Benefits of Potassium

Both observational and experimental data have suggested that increasing potassium intake can lower blood pressure by increasing natriuresis and possibly reducing vascular resistance. One of the original observational studies to demonstrate the negative relationship between potassium intake and both SBP and DBP was the previously mentioned INTERSALT study [37]. This negative relationship between potassium intake and blood pressure may also influence the risk of developing hypertension. In an analysis of the PREVEND trial, the lowest sex-specific tertile of potassium excretion (which equated to <68 mmol/24 hour in men and < 58 mmol/24 hour in females) was associated with a modest increase in the likelihood of developing hypertension (SBP ≥140 mmHg, DBP ≥90 mmHg, or antihypertensive medication; adjusted HR 1.20 [95%CI 1.05, 1.37]) [38]. Furthermore, a meta-analysis of prospective cohort studies also demonstrated a reduction in blood pressure-related cardiovascular endpoints including stroke (RR = 0.79 [95%CI 0.68, 0.90]), coronary heart disease (RR = 0.93 [95%CI 0.87, 0.99]), and combined cardiovascular diseases (RR = 0.74 [95%CI 0.60, 0.91]) with increasing potassium intake[39].

Meta-analyses of trials examining the influence of potassium intake on blood pressure have fairly consistently found a reduction in SBP and DBP with increasing potassium intake [40–42]. However, more detailed analyses have found that certain groups such as those with greater age, hypertension, increased body weight, and higher sodium intake may experience a greater benefit [40]. In addition to dietary sources of potassium, studies have also found that potassium supplements may be used to lower BP [43].

A major motivation for lowering blood pressure in patients with CKD is to slow the decline in kidney function. It is worth noting that analyses of large cohorts have produced mixed results on the relationship between higher potassium intake and CKD progression [44–46]. In the CRIC study (the Chronic Renal Insufficiency Cohort), patients with the highest quartile of potassium excretion (≥67.1 mmol/day [2617 mg/day]) experienced more rapid decline in kidney function (halving of eGFR or incident end-stage kidney disease) than the lowest quartile (<39.4 mmol/day [1537 mg/day]; HR 1.59 [95%CI 1.25, 2.03]) [44]. On the other hand, a posthoc analysis of participants in the ONTARGET and TRANSCEND trials found that patients with higher potassium excretion had slower CKD progression (OR 0.74 [95%CI 0.67, 0.82]) [45]. Finally, in a comparison of quartiles of potassium excretion from participants in the MDRD study (Modification of Diet in Renal Disease), there was no relationship between potassium and developing kidney failure (HR 0.95 [95%CI 0.87, 1.04]). However, this same analysis did find a reduction in all-cause mortality with higher potassium excretion (HR 0.83 [95%CI 0.74, 0.94]) [46].

Current Intake

Dietary potassium intake is consistently observed to be below dietary recommendations [37]. Much like the tendency for underreporting sodium, potassium is often overreported in self-reported data [47, 48]. Therefore, 24-hour urinary potassium, although not a perfect measure, may be a better indication of intake. Using 24-hour urinary analysis, Jackson and colleagues reported daily excretions of those with hypertension (1993.7 ± 42.8 mg/day), prehypertension (2080.6 ± 50.2), and optimal blood pressure (2154.2 ± 53.4) [49]. Despite the frequent focus on fruits and vegetables as a source of potassium, it has been estimated that processed foods contribute 40% of dietary potassium intake compared to just 30% from minimally processed foods [50].

Recently, the Food and Drug Administration (FDA) approved several changes to the nutrition facts label that may influence potassium intake. Among these label changes are the mandatory addition of potassium to the label and the changing of the daily value of potassium from 3500 to 4700 mg/day. The objective of these changes is to increase dietary potassium intake at the population level. However, contrary to other nutrients (e.g., phosphorus), data on potassium bioavailability is scarce. Naismith and Braschi [51] showed that there is a lower bioavailability of potassium from fruits and vegetables as compared to animal foods and juices. However, other studies have shown that there was no difference in serum potassium following the consumption of similar amounts of potassium in the form of potatoes or potassium gluconate [52]. Presumably, the addition of potassium to the food label will provide many food manufacturers with motivation to further increase potassium in processed foods. This approach has played out in other countries, where sodium chloride has been substituted with potassium chloride [53] and sodium benzoate by potassium sorbate in soft drinks [54], in an attempt to increase dietary potassium. These changes may be of particular concern to clinicians working with patients with CKD, especially those with other risk factors for developing hyperkalemia.

Dietary Potassium Recommendations

For adults, the 2019 US DRIs recommend a dietary potassium AI of 3400 mg/d and 2600 mg/day for males and females, respectively [30]. The AI decreased from the 2005 DRI report as it was solely based on dietary intake and not taking supplements into consideration. The panel chose not to set an upper limit for potassium due to the lack of reported adverse events associated with potassium intake from food in healthy adults [55]. The ACC/AHA guidelines recommend that patients with elevated blood pressure, including hypertension, should increase potassium intake unless contraindicated by the presence of CKD or drugs that may increase serum potassium [56].

Concerns About Hyperkalemia in CKD

Despite the potential benefits associated with increasing potassium intake, higher intakes are a challenge to patients with late stages of CKD who cannot adequately excrete excess potassium [57]. Potassium challenges (>2 g/day) have been associated with increased serum potassium in patients with CKD [58, 59], but the relationship between dietary potassium intake and serum potassium has been shown to be weak [60] or nonsignificant [61] in patients on hemodialysis. This may be due to a multitude of other factors that can influence serum potassium or hyperkalemia risk including factors that influence potassium distribution (acidosis, insulin, and medications), excretion (CKD stage, medications), and other factors (diabetes, male gender, BMI, muscle catabolism) [61, 62].

Due to the potential consequences of hyperkalemia, the KDOQI recommends that patients in CKD stages 1 and 2 aim for an intake greater than 4000 mg/day while limiting potassium in patients with stages 3 and 4 to no more than 2000 mg to 4000 mg/day [63].

Magnesium

The role of magnesium on the regulation of blood pressure seems to be related to the direct effects on vascular tone and reactivity [64]. Additionally, magnesium deficiency has been shown to lead to hypertension in experimental models. However, results from observational studies and randomized controlled trials in humans have been inconsistent in showing a positive effect on blood pressure. In a meta-analysis of 38 trials by Zhang et al. [6], a modest effect was observed with the supplementation of magnesium. It was reported that with a median supplementation of 368 mg/d and duration of 3 months, SBP was reduced by 2 mmHg (95% CI −3.58,−0.43) and DBP by 1.78 mmHg (95% CI −2.82,−0.73) [6]. As it seems that there is a minor effect on blood pressure, focus on sodium, potassium, sodium-to-potassium ratio, and dietary patterns has been preferred, and no recommendations have been given by the JNC or AHA/ACC. However, by following a DASH diet and Mediterranean-style diet, magnesium intake is likely to increase for many adults.

Calcium

The relationship between calcium intake (from foods and/or supplements) and blood pressure has been reported in several observational studies. There are multiple ways by which calcium may affect blood pressure, including effect on vascular reactivity, central and peripheral sympathetic nervous system, changes in hormones regulated by calcium, and natriuresis [65]. A meta-analysis of 42 studies by Griffith et al. [66] showed that interventions that aimed to increase dietary calcium intake, either through diet or supplementation, led to a modest decrease in SBP of 1.44 mmHg (95% CI −2.20, −0.68) and DBP of 0.84 mmHg (95% CI −1.44, −0.24). Moreover, when studies of dietary interventions were compared to supplementation studies, they found that the drop in SBP was bigger in the dietary interventions (−2.10 mmHg [95% CI −2.93, −1.26] vs. −1.09 [95% CI −2.12, −0.06]) [66]. The effect was similar in DBP (−1.09 mmHg [95% CI −1.67, −0.52] vs. −0.87 mmHg [95% CI −1.71, −0.03]) [66].

Dairy is the main calcium-containing food category. Lana et al. [67] recently assessed the effects of low-fat versus full-fat dairy on blood pressure in an observational study of 715 community-living hypertensive adults >60 years old. Those who consumed ≥7 servings/week of whole-fat dairy had DBP 1.40 mmHg higher (95% CI 0.01, 2.81) than those who consumed <1 serving/week. Conversely, if there was an intake of ≥7 servings/week of low-fat dairy compared to <1 serving/week, DBP was 1.74 mmHg lower (95% CI −3.26, −0.23) [67]. In a meta-analysis of five cohort studies, Ralston et al. [10] showed that total dairy food intake (RR 0.87 [95% CI 0.81, 0.94]) and low-fat dairy intake (RR 0.84 [95% CI 0.74–0.95]) were associated with lower risk for high blood pressure. However, full-fat dairy and cheese intakes were not associated with lower risk for elevated blood pressure [10]. Of note, two to three servings of dairy (low-fat) are recommended in the DASH diet. Thus, the additive effect on blood pressure through a dietary pattern rather than just the increase of calcium/dairy may be more relevant for individuals with hypertension.

Other Nutrients [68]

Nutrients such as protein, omega-3 fatty acids, and vitamin C have also been associated with reductions in blood pressure. In the case of protein, a secondary analysis of the INTERSALT study by Stamler et al. [69] showed that when protein intake was 30% above the mean (~84 g/day) compared with 30% below the mean (44 g/day), SBP and DBP were lower by 3 and 2.5 mmHg, respectively. Moreover, in the INTERMAP study, the protein source was more relevant than total protein intake. Elliott et al. [70] showed that after adjustment for height and weight, there was an inverse association of plant-based protein, but not animal protein, and blood pressure, where SBP and DBP were reduced by −1.95 and −1.22, respectively.

For omega-3 fatty acids, the INTERMAP study showed that omega-3 fatty acids (total, linolenic acid, and long-chain) were associated with very modest reductions in blood pressure. However, in a meta-analysis where omega-3 fatty acids were supplemented as eicosapentanoic (EPA) and/or docosahexanoic (DHA) acids, Miller et al. [71] reported a reduction in SBP of 1.52 mmHg (95% CI −2.25,−0.079) and DBP of 0.99 mmHg (95% CI −1.54,−0.44). However, there are limited studies directly assessing the effect of omega-3 fatty acids and blood pressure, and therefore, more studies are needed to conclusively recommend the supplementation of omega-3 fatty acids.

Finally, high intake of vitamin C has also been associated with lower blood pressure, but this effect may be related to the consumption of fruits and vegetables. However, in a meta-analysis of 29 randomized controlled trials, Juraschek et al. [72] reported that the supplementation of vitamin C (mostly short-term with a median duration of 8 weeks) was associated with a reduction in SBP of 3.84 mmHg (95% CI −5.29,−2.38) and DBP of 1.48 (95% CI −2.86,−0.10).

Dietary Patterns

As nutrients are not consumed in isolation and the addition or restriction of individual food groups may not reflect consistent and sustainable effects, the study and application of dietary patterns in individuals with hypertension and those with CKD have been advocated. Among dietary patterns, the DASH diet and the Mediterranean diet have been shown to be effective in reducing blood pressure in individuals with hypertension.

DASH Diet

The Dietary Approaches to Stop Hypertension or DASH diet trial was designed to test the effect of a complete dietary pattern rather than single nutrients or foods [73] (Table 10.2). This trial had three groups: (1) typical American diet, (2) typical American diet + fruits and vegetables, and (3) combination diet ("ideal" diet that was later called DASH diet) [74]. The DASH trial investigators formulated this "ideal" diet from previous studies investigating the effects of single nutrients and food groups on blood pressure [73]. After 8 weeks, the DASH diet reduced SBP by 5.5 mmHg (95% CI −7.4,−3.7) and DBP by 3.0 mmHg (95% CI −4.3,−1.6) [74]. Among individuals with hypertension, SBP was reduced by 11.4 mmHg (95% CI −15.9.−6.9) and DBP by 5.5 mmHg (95% CI −8.2,−2.7) [74]. Importantly, reductions in blood pressure were more pronounced in individuals with hypertension, minority populations (i.e., African Americans), and females [75] and were observed with a sustained dietary sodium intake of 3000 mg/day. Further research (the DASH-sodium trial) found that the DASH diet pattern with the lowest amount of sodium (1500 mg/day) had the biggest reduction in blood pressure compared to a high-sodium DASH diet (3300 mg/day) [76]. Since these initial

Table 10.2 Food groups servings in the DASH diet

Food group	Servings per day			Significance of food group
	1600 kcal	2000 kcal	2600 kcal	
Grains	6	6–8	10–11	Major sources of energy and fiber
Vegetables	3–4	4–5	5–6	Rich sources of potassium, magnesium, and fiber
Fruits	4	4–5	5–6	Important sources of potassium, magnesium, and fiber
Fat-free or low-fat milk and milk products	2–3	2–3	3	Major sources of calcium and protein
Lean meats, poultry, and fish	3–6	≤6	6	Rich sources of protein and magnesium
Nuts, seeds, and legumes	3/wk	4–5/wk	1	Rich sources of energy, magnesium, protein, and fiber
Fats and oils	2	2–3	3	The DASH study had 27% of calories as fat, including fat in or added to foods
Sweets and added sugars	0	≤5/wk	≤2	Sweets should be low in fat.

Reprinted from "Your Guide to Lowering Your Blood Pressure with DASH." National Heart, Lung, and Blood Institute, National Institutes of Health. NIH Publication No. 06-5834. Originally printed December 2006, Revised August 2015

trials, several researchers have tested the effect of the DASH diet on blood pressure. A systematic review and meta-analysis of a total of 11 randomized controlled trials by Ndanuko et al. [11] yielded similar results, where they observed a reduction in SBP of 4.90 mmHg (95% CI −6.22,−3.58) and DBP of 2.63 mmHg (95% CI −3.34,−1.92). Importantly, 8 out of the 11 studies analyzed had a positive effect on SBP and 10 out of 11 on DBP [11].

Similarly, the PREMIER trial [77] tested the effects of behavioral interventions (18 face-to-face meetings) that included weight loss (at least 15 lb/6.8 kg), at least 180 minute/week of moderate-intensity physical activity, dietary sodium intake of ≤2300 mg/day, and alcohol intake of ≤1oz for men or <0.5 oz for women, with or without a DASH-type diet, compared to a group that received advice only, where participants were provided a 30-minute session with information about weight, sodium intake, physical activity, and the DASH diet. After 6 months, the groups randomized to the behavioral therapies had a similar drop in SBP (without DASH diet −3.7 mmHg (95% CI −5.3,−2.1) and with DASH diet −4.3 mmHg (95% CI −5.9,−2.8)) and DBP (without DASH diet −1.7 mmHg (95% CI −2.8, −0.6) and with DASH diet −2.6 mmHg (95% CI −3.7, −1.5))[77]. Importantly, some of the lifestyle modifications were maintained after 18 months [78].

In addition to reduced blood pressure, a follow-up question could be if the DASH diet reduces the risk of CKD or progression of CKD. In a prospective analysis of the Atherosclerosis Risk in Communities (ARIC) study, those participants who had the lowest DASH-style diet score (calculated from food-frequency questionnaires) had a 16% higher risk of developing kidney disease (95% CI, 1.07–1.26). Similarly, in a secondary analysis of the Tehran Lipid and Glucose Study, Yuzbashian et al. [79] showed that those with a hypertension diagnosis consuming a diet with the highest DASH-style diet score had a 38% lower risk of incident CKD (95% CI 0.44, 0.87). Finally, in the NIH-American Association of Retired Persons (AARP) Diet and Health Study, those with the highest DASH diet score had a 15% lower risk for death due to a renal cause and/or dialysis (95% CI 0.77, 0.94) [80]. However, these studies were prospective observational studies and not randomized controlled trials testing the effect of a DASH diet on the progression of CKD. Moreover, a common fear of recommending a diet high in fruits and vegetables in moderate to advanced CKD, such as the DASH diet, is the risk of hyperkalemia. In a pilot controlled-feeding study, Tyson et al. [81] showed that a 2-week reduced-sodium DASH diet had no effects on serum potassium. However, no further randomized controlled trials have assessed the effects of the DASH diet on serum potassium.

Mediterranean Diet

The Mediterranean diet can be difficult to define due to the differing political and cultural influences that make up the Mediterranean region. However, common components of the diet include fruits and vegetables, whole grains, seafood, nuts, legumes, extra virgin olive oil, small amounts of red wine, and limited amounts of red and processed meats.

Observational trials, primarily using Mediterranean diet scores, have found negative associations between the Mediterranean diet and blood pressure [82] and the incidence of hypertension [83]. The most notable intervention looking at the Mediterranean diet and cardiovascular outcomes is the PREDIMED (Prevención con Dieta Mediterranea) Trial [84]. PREDIMED included a cohort of more than 7000 participants in Spain who were allocated to groups that added either olive oil or mixed nuts to participant's diets. It was initially questioned whether the addition of olive oil and mixed nuts actually tested the effects of the full Mediterranean diet [85]. A secondary analysis of PREDIMED initially found a reduction in DBP in each of the intervention groups [84]. It is worth noting that the original PREDIMED trial was recently republished due to protocol deviations [86]. Outside the Mediterranean region, a randomized trial of 166 Australian adults over the age of 64 compared a Mediterranean diet with habitual intake [87]. Compared to the habitual intake group, there was a significant reduction in SBP at 3 (−1.3 mmHg, 95% CI −2.2, −0.3) and at 6 months (−1.1 mmHg, 95% CI −2.0, −0.1).

There are multiple meta-analyses looking at the influence of the Mediterranean diet on blood pressure. In a systematic review and meta-analysis by Ndanuko et al. [11], prescription of a Mediterranean diet led to a reduction in SBP of 3.02 (95% CI −3.47, −2.58 mmHg). In a separate analysis looking at trials at least a year in duration, a small influence of the Mediterranean diet was found in both SBP (−1.44 mm Hg) and DBP (−0.70 mmHg) [88]. However, the authors recommended that the results be interpreted with caution due to the small number of studies and heterogeneity of results.

The Mediterranean lifestyle, which also includes high amounts of physical activity, represents a major lifestyle change for cultures outside the region [89]. Reviewing studies that have been successful in achieving high compliance with the Mediterranean diet outside of this region, a number of factors were identified that may improve compliance. These included dietitian involvement, written resources, recipes, regular contact, and provision of the primary foods included in a Mediterranean diet.

In terms of the CKD population, the European Renal Nutrition Group from the European Renal Association and European Dialysis and Transplantation Association recommended the Mediterranean diet as the diet of choice for patients with CKD [13]. The main benefits of the Mediterranean diet in CKD include the intake of protein mostly from plant-based sources, intake of monounsaturated and polyunsaturated fats, nutrient-dense food intake from non-processed foods, and high dietary fiber intake (30–50 g/day) [13]. There have been observational studies looking at the effect of a Mediterranean diet and changes in kidney function. Particularly, the NIH-AARP Diet and Health Study reported that those individuals who adhere to a Mediterranean diet had a reduced risk of end-stage kidney disease (HR = 0.84, 95% CI 0.74–0.95) [80].

Ongoing Research

The Gut Microbiota and Blood Pressure

Recent evidence suggests that the gut microbiota may be related to blood pressure control [90]. Li et al. [91] assessed the fecal microbiota of healthy individuals and individuals with prehypertension and hypertension. They observed that the bacterial richness was lower in those with prehypertension and hypertension. Interestingly, when they grouped together bacterial genera common in prehypertension and hypertension versus healthy, as well as metabolites that differed between these groups, they were able to identify individuals with pre- or hypertension with almost 90% accuracy. Finally, when they transplanted the fecal microbiota to germ-free mice (without any gastrointestinal bacteria), the mice transplanted with the fecal microbiota of an individual with hypertension, the mice had higher SBP and DBP, as well as lower bacterial diversity, compared to mice that were transplanted the microbiota of a healthy individual. A combination of this and other studies supports the relationship between the gut microbiota and regulation of blood pressure. Currently, studies are assessing the effects of modulating the gut microbiota through dietary interventions and short- and long-term effects on blood pressure.

Central Blood Pressure

While almost all of the evidence to date has looked at the effect of diet on peripheral blood pressures measured at the brachial artery, central blood pressure measured at the aorta may be a better indication of the pressure experienced by end organs such as the kidneys and a better measure of the risk for CKD progression [92]. Technology to noninvasively estimate aortic blood pressure from peripheral blood pressure waveforms is becoming increasingly available, and dietitians may wish to also consider the effect of diet on central blood pressure in patients with a goal of limiting CKD progression.

Conclusion

Nutrition is a vital component of the treatment of hypertension in those with and without CKD. Among the variety of interventions, weight loss, dietary sodium reduction while increasing dietary potassium, and a DASH or a Mediterranean diet have been shown to be effective in reducing blood pressure and have been associated with improved renal outcomes (i.e., kidney function and rate of kidney function decline).

References

1. Whelton PK, Carey RM, Aronow WS, Casey DE Jr, Collins KJ, Dennison Himmelfarb C, et al. 2017 ACC/AHA/AAPA/ABC/ACPM/AGS/APhA/ASH/ASPC/NMA/PCNA Guideline for the prevention, detection, evaluation, and management of high blood pressure in adults: a report of the American College of Cardiology/American Heart Association Task Force on Clinical Practice Guidelines. Circulation. 2018;138(17):e484–594.
2. Fryar CD, Ostchega Y, Hales CM, Zhang G, Kruszon-Moran D. Hypertension prevalence and control among adults: United States, 2015–2016. NCHS Data Brief. 2017;(289):1–8.
3. Collins AJ, Foley RN, Gilbertson DT, Chen SC. United States Renal Data System public health surveillance of chronic kidney disease and end-stage renal disease. Kidney Int Suppl. 2015;5(1):2–7.
4. He FJ, Li J, Macgregor GA. Effect of longer-term modest salt reduction on blood pressure. Cochrane Database Syst Rev. 2013;4:CD004937.
5. Whelton PK, He J, Cutler JA, Brancati FL, Appel LJ, Follmann D, et al. Effects of oral potassium on blood pressure. Meta-analysis of randomized controlled clinical trials. JAMA. 1997;277(20):1624–32.
6. Zhang X, Li Y, Del Gobbo LC, Rosanoff A, Wang J, Zhang W, et al. Effects of magnesium supplementation on blood pressure: a meta-analysis of randomized double-blind placebo-controlled trials. Hypertension. 2016;68(2):324–33.
7. Dickinson HO, Nicolson DJ, Cook JV, Campbell F, Beyer FR, Ford GA, et al. Calcium supplementation for the management of primary hypertension in adults. Cochrane Database Syst Rev. 2006;2:CD004639.
8. Morris MC, Sacks F, Rosner B. Does fish oil lower blood pressure? A meta-analysis of controlled trials. Circulation. 1993;88(2):523–33.

9. Shin JY, Kim JY, Kang HT, Han KH, Shim JY. Effect of fruits and vegetables on metabolic syndrome: a systematic review and meta-analysis of randomized controlled trials. Int J Food Sci Nutr. 2015;66(4):416–25.

10. Ralston RA, Lee JH, Truby H, Palermo CE, Walker KZ. A systematic review and meta-analysis of elevated blood pressure and consumption of dairy foods. J Hum Hypertens. 2012;26(1):3–13.

11. Ndanuko RN, Tapsell LC, Charlton KE, Neale EP, Batterham MJ. Dietary patterns and blood pressure in adults: a systematic review and meta-analysis of randomized controlled trials. Adv Nutr. 2016;7(1):76–89.

12. Van Horn L, Carson JA, Appel LJ, Burke LE, Economos C, Karmally W, et al. Recommended dietary pattern to achieve adherence to the American Heart Association/American College of Cardiology (AHA/ACC) guidelines: a scientific statement from the American Heart Association. Circulation. 2016;134(22):e505–e29.

13. Chauveau P, Aparicio M, Bellizzi V, Campbell K, Hong X, Johansson L, et al. Mediterranean diet as the diet of choice for patients with chronic kidney disease. Nephrol Dial Transplant. 2018;33(5):725–35.

14. Whelton PK, Carey RM, Aronow WS, Casey DE Jr, Collins KJ, Dennison Himmelfarb C, et al. 2017 ACC/AHA/AAPA/ABC/ACPM/AGS/APhA/ASH/ASPC/NMA/PCNA guideline for the prevention, detection, evaluation, and management of high blood pressure in adults: executive summary: a report of the American College of Cardiology/American Heart Association Task Force on Clinical Practice Guidelines. Hypertension. 2018;71(6):1269–324.

15. Chobanian AV, Bakris GL, Black HR, Cushman WC, Green LA, Izzo JL Jr, et al. The seventh report of the joint national committee on prevention, detection, evaluation, and treatment of high blood pressure: the JNC 7 report. JAMA. 2003;289(19):2560–72.

16. James PA, Oparil S, Carter BL, Cushman WC, Dennison-Himmelfarb C, Handler J, et al. 2014 evidence-based guideline for the management of high blood pressure in adults: report from the panel members appointed to the Eighth Joint National Committee (JNC 8). JAMA. 2014;311(5):507–20.

17. Kramer HJ, Townsend RR, Griffin K, Flynn JT, Weiner DE, Rocco MV, et al. KDOQI US commentary on the 2017 ACC/AHA hypertension guideline. Am J Kidney Dis. 2019;73(4):437–58.

18. The Trials of Hypertension Prevention Collaborative Research Group. Effects of weight loss and sodium reduction intervention on blood pressure and hypertension incidence in overweight people with high-normal blood pressure. The Trials of Hypertension Prevention, phase II. Arch Intern Med. 1997;157(6):657–67.

19. Neter JE, Stam BE, Kok FJ, Grobbee DE, Geleijnse JM. Influence of weight reduction on blood pressure: a meta-analysis of randomized controlled trials. Hypertension. 2003;42(5):878–84.

20. MacLaughlin HL, Sarafidis PA, Greenwood SA, Campbell KL, Hall WL, Macdougall IC. Compliance with a structured weight loss program is associated with reduced systolic blood pressure in obese patients with chronic kidney disease. Am J Hypertens. 2012;25(9):1024–9.

21. Stamler J. The INTERSALT Study: background, methods, findings, and implications. Am J Clin Nutr. 1997;65(2 Suppl):626S–42S.

22. Stamler J, Chan Q, Daviglus ML, Dyer AR, Van Horn L, Garside DB, et al. Relation of dietary sodium (salt) to blood pressure and its possible modulation by other dietary factors: the INTERMAP study. Hypertension. 2018;71(4):631–7.

23. Cook NR, Appel LJ, Whelton PK. Sodium intake and all-cause mortality over 20 years in the trials of hypertension prevention. J Am Coll Cardiol. 2016;68(15):1609–17.

24. WHO. Sodium intake for adults and children. Geneva: World Health Organization (WHO); 2012.

25. Hebert JR, Clemow L, Pbert L, Ockene IS, Ockene JK. Social desirability bias in dietary self-report may compromise the validity of dietary intake measures. Int J Epidemiol. 1995;24(2):389–98.

26. McLean RM. Measuring population sodium intake: a review of methods. Nutrients. 2014;6(11):4651–62.

27. Titze J, Rakova N, Kopp C, Dahlmann A, Jantsch J, Luft FC. Balancing wobbles in the body sodium. Nephrol Dial Transplant. 2016;31(7):1078–81.

28. Lerchl K, Rakova N, Dahlmann A, Rauh M, Goller U, Basner M, et al. Agreement between 24-hour salt ingestion and sodium excretion in a controlled environment. Hypertension. 2015;66(4):850–7.

29. Hoy MK, Goldman JD, Murayi T, Rhodes DG, Moshfegh AJ. Sodium intake of the U.S. population: what we eat in America, NHANES 2007–2008. In: Group FSR, editor. 2011.

30. Stallings VA, Harrison M, Oria M, Committee to Review the Dietary Reference Intakes for Sodium and Potassium, Food and Nutrition Board, Health and Medicine Division, National Academies of Sciences, Engineering, and Medicine. Dietary Reference Intakes for Sodium and Potassium. Washington, DC: National Academies Press (US); 2019.

31. U.S. Department of Health and Human Services and U.S. Department of Agriculture. 2015–2020 dietary guidelines for Americans. 8th ed. December 2015. Available at https://health.gov/dietaryguidelines/2015/guidelines/.

32. Eckel RH, Jakicic JM, Ard JD, de Jesus JM, Houston Miller N, Hubbard VS, et al. 2013 AHA/ACC guideline on lifestyle management to reduce cardiovascular risk: a report of the American College of Cardiology/American Heart Association Task Force on Practice Guidelines. Circulation. 2014;129(25 Suppl 2):S76–99.

33. Kidney Disease: Improving Global Outcomes (KDIGO) Blood Pressure Work Group. KDIGO clinical practice guideline for the management of blood pressure in chronic kidney disease. Kidney Int. 2012;2:337–414.

34. Trieu K, McMahon E, Santos JA, Bauman A, Jolly KA, Bolam B, et al. Review of behaviour change interventions to reduce population salt intake. Int J Behav Nutr Phys Act. 2017;14(1):17.
35. McMahon EJ, Campbell KL, Bauer JD, Mudge DW. Altered dietary salt intake for people with chronic kidney disease. Cochrane Database Syst Rev. 2015;2:CD010070.
36. Campbell KL, Johnson DW, Bauer JD, Hawley CM, Isbel NM, Stowasser M, et al. A randomized trial of sodium-restriction on kidney function, fluid volume and adipokines in CKD patients. BMC Nephrol. 2014;15:57.
37. Intersalt Cooperative Research Group. Intersalt: an international study of electrolyte excretion and blood pressure. Results for 24 hour urinary sodium and potassium excretion. BMJ. 1988;297(6644):319–28.
38. Kieneker LM, Gansevoort RT, Mukamal KJ, de Boer RA, Navis G, Bakker SJ, et al. Urinary potassium excretion and risk of developing hypertension: the prevention of renal and vascular end-stage disease study. Hypertension. 2014;64(4):769–76.
39. D'Elia L, Barba G, Cappuccio FP, Strazzullo P. Potassium intake, stroke, and cardiovascular disease a meta-analysis of prospective studies. J Am Coll Cardiol. 2011;57(10):1210–9.
40. Geleijnse JM, Kok FJ, Grobbee DE. Blood pressure response to changes in sodium and potassium intake: a metaregression analysis of randomised trials. J Hum Hypertens. 2003;17(7):471–80.
41. Cappuccio FP, MacGregor GA. Does potassium supplementation lower blood pressure? A meta-analysis of published trials. J Hypertens. 1991;9(5):465–73.
42. Aburto NJ, Hanson S, Gutierrez H, Hooper L, Elliott P, Cappuccio FP. Effect of increased potassium intake on cardiovascular risk factors and disease: systematic review and meta-analyses. BMJ. 2013;346:f1378.
43. Vongpatanasin W, Peri-Okonny P, Velasco A, Arbique D, Wang Z, Ravikumar P, et al. Effects of potassium magnesium citrate supplementation on 24-hour ambulatory blood pressure and oxidative stress marker in prehypertensive and hypertensive subjects. Am J Cardiol. 2016;118(6):849–53.
44. He J, Mills KT, Appel LJ, Yang W, Chen J, Lee BT, et al. Urinary sodium and potassium excretion and CKD progression. J Am Soc Nephrol. 2016;27(4):1202–12.
45. Smyth A, Dunkler D, Gao P, Teo KK, Yusuf S, O'Donnell MJ, et al. The relationship between estimated sodium and potassium excretion and subsequent renal outcomes. Kidney Int. 2014;86(6):1205–12.
46. Leonberg-Yoo AK, Tighiouart H, Levey AS, Beck GJ, Sarnak MJ. Urine potassium excretion, kidney failure, and mortality in CKD. Am J Kidney Dis. 2017;69(3):341–9.
47. Whelton PK. Sodium and potassium intake in US adults. Circulation. 2018;137(3):247–9.
48. Mercado CI, Cogswell ME, Valderrama AL, Wang CY, Loria CM, Moshfegh AJ, et al. Difference between 24-h diet recall and urine excretion for assessing population sodium and potassium intake in adults aged 18-39 y. Am J Clin Nutr. 2015;101(2):376–86.
49. Jackson SL, Cogswell ME, Zhao L, Terry AL, Wang CY, Wright J, et al. Association between urinary sodium and potassium excretion and blood pressure among adults in the United States: National Health and nutrition examination survey, 2014. Circulation. 2018;137(3):237–46.
50. Weaver CM, Dwyer J, Fulgoni VL 3rd, King JC, Leveille GA, MacDonald RS, et al. Processed foods: contributions to nutrition. Am J Clin Nutr. 2014;99(6):1525–42.
51. Naismith DJ, Braschi A. An investigation into the bioaccessibility of potassium in unprocessed fruits and vegetables. Int J Food Sci Nutr. 2009;59(5):438–50.
52. Macdonald-Clarke CJ, Martin BR, McCabe LD, McCabe GP, Lachcik PJ, Wastney M, et al. Bioavailability of potassium from potatoes and potassium gluconate: a randomized dose response trial. Am J Clin Nutr. 2016;104(2):346–53.
53. van Buren L, Dotsch-Klerk M, Seewi G, Newson RS. Dietary impact of adding potassium chloride to foods as a sodium reduction technique. Nutrients. 2016;8(4):235.
54. Saltmarsh M. Recent trends in the use of food additives in the United Kingdom. J Sci Food Agric. 2015;95(4):649–52.
55. Institute of Medicine (U.S.). Panel on dietary reference intakes for electrolytes and water. In: Dietary reference intakes for water, potassium, sodium, chloride, and sulfate, vol. xviii. Washington, DC: National Academies Press; 2005. p. 617.
56. Whelton PK, Carey RM, Aronow WS, Casey DE Jr, Collins KJ, Dennison Himmelfarb C, et al. 2017 ACC/AHA/AAPA/ABC/ACPM/AGS/APhA/ASH/ASPC/NMA/PCNA guideline for the prevention, detection, evaluation, and management of high blood pressure in adults: a report of the American College of Cardiology/American Heart Association Task Force on Clinical Practice Guidelines. J Am Coll Cardiol. 2018;71(19):e127–248.
57. Ueda Y, Ookawara S, Ito K, Miyazawa H, Kaku Y, Hoshino T, et al. Changes in urinary potassium excretion in patients with chronic kidney disease. Kidney Res Clin Pract. 2016;35(2):78–83.
58. Keith NM, Osterberg AE. The tolerance for potassium in severe renal in-sufficiency: a study of ten cases. J Clin Invest. 1947;26(4):773–83.
59. Winkler AW, Hoff HE, Smith PK. The toxicity of orally administered potassium salts in renal insufficiency. J Clin Invest. 1941;20(2):119–26.
60. Noori N, Kalantar-Zadeh K, Kovesdy CP, Murali SB, Bross R, Nissenson AR, et al. Dietary potassium intake and mortality in long-term hemodialysis patients. Am J Kidney Dis. 2010;56(2):338–47.

61. St-Jules DE, Goldfarb DS, Sevick MA. Nutrient non-equivalence: does restricting high-potassium plant foods help to prevent hyperkalemia in hemodialysis patients? J Ren Nutr. 2016;26(5):282–7.
62. Yeung SMH, Vogt L, Rotmans JI, Hoorn EJ, de Borst MH. Potassium: poison or panacea in chronic kidney disease? Nephrol Dial Transplant. 2019;34(2):175–80.
63. Beto JA, Ramirez WE, Bansal VK. Medical nutrition therapy in adults with chronic kidney disease: integrating evidence and consensus into practice for the generalist registered dietitian nutritionist. J Acad Nutr Diet. 2014;114(7):1077–87.
64. Romani AMP. Beneficial role of Mg(2+) in prevention and treatment of hypertension. Int J Hypertens. 2018;2018:9013721.
65. McCarron DA, Morris CD. The calcium deficiency hypothesis of hypertension. Ann Intern Med. 1987;107(6):919–22.
66. Griffith LE, Guyatt GH, Cook RJ, Bucher HC, Cook DJ. The influence of dietary and nondietary calcium supplementation on blood pressure: an updated metaanalysis of randomized controlled trials. Am J Hypertens. 1999;12(1 Pt 1):84–92.
67. Lana A, Banegas JR, Guallar-Castillon P, Rodriguez-Artalejo F, Lopez-Garcia E. Association of dairy consumption and 24-hour blood pressure in older adults with hypertension. Am J Med. 2018;131(10):1238–49.
68. Lancaster KJ. Hypertension. In: Nutrition in kidney disease. 2nd ed; 2014. p. 93–101.
69. Stamler J, Elliott P, Kesteloot H, Nichols R, Claeys G, Dyer AR, et al. Inverse relation of dietary protein markers with blood pressure. Findings for 10,020 men and women in the INTERSALT study. INTERSALT Cooperative Research Group. INTERnational study of SALT and blood pressure. Circulation. 1996;94(7):1629–34.
70. Elliott P, Stamler J, Dyer AR, Appel L, Dennis B, Kesteloot H, et al. Association between protein intake and blood pressure: the INTERMAP Study. Arch Intern Med. 2006;166(1):79–87.
71. Miller PE, Van Elswyk M, Alexander DD. Long-chain omega-3 fatty acids eicosapentaenoic acid and docosahexaenoic acid and blood pressure: a meta-analysis of randomized controlled trials. Am J Hypertens. 2014;27(7):885–96.
72. Juraschek SP, Guallar E, Appel LJ, Miller ER 3rd. Effects of vitamin C supplementation on blood pressure: a meta-analysis of randomized controlled trials. Am J Clin Nutr. 2012;95(5):1079–88.
73. Sacks FM, Obarzanek E, Windhauser MM, Svetkey LP, Vollmer WM, McCullough M, et al. Rationale and design of the Dietary Approaches to Stop Hypertension (DASH). A multicenter controlled-feeding study of dietary patterns to lower blood pressure. Ann Epidemiol. 1995;5(2):108–18.
74. Appel LJ, Moore TJ, Obarzanek E, Vollmer WM, Svetkey LP, Sacks FM, et al. A clinical trial of the effects of dietary patterns on blood pressure. DASH Collaborative Research Group. N Engl J Med. 1997;336(16):1117–24.
75. Champagne CM. Dietary interventions on blood pressure: the Dietary Approaches to Stop Hypertension (DASH) trials. Nutr Rev. 2006;64(2 Pt 2):S53–6.
76. Sacks FM, Svetkey LP, Vollmer WM, Appel LJ, Bray GA, Harsha D, et al. Effects on blood pressure of reduced dietary sodium and the Dietary Approaches to Stop Hypertension (DASH) diet. DASH-Sodium Collaborative Research Group. N Engl J Med. 2001;344(1):3–10.
77. Appel LJ, Champagne CM, Harsha DW, Cooper LS, Obarzanek E, Elmer PJ, et al. Effects of comprehensive lifestyle modification on blood pressure control: main results of the PREMIER clinical trial. JAMA. 2003;289(16):2083–93.
78. Elmer PJ, Obarzanek E, Vollmer WM, Simons-Morton D, Stevens VJ, Young DR, et al. Effects of comprehensive lifestyle modification on diet, weight, physical fitness, and blood pressure control: 18-month results of a randomized trial. Ann Intern Med. 2006;144(7):485–95.
79. Yuzbashian E, Asghari G, Mirmiran P, Amouzegar-Bahambari P, Azizi F. Adherence to low-sodium Dietary Approaches to Stop Hypertension-style diet may decrease the risk of incident chronic kidney disease among high-risk patients: a secondary prevention in prospective cohort study. Nephrol Dial Transplant. 2018;33(7):1159–68.
80. Smyth A, Griffin M, Yusuf S, Mann JF, Reddan D, Canavan M, et al. Diet and major renal outcomes: a prospective cohort study. The NIH-AARP Diet and Health Study. J Ren Nutr. 2016;26(5):288–98.
81. Tyson CC, Lin PH, Corsino L, Batch BC, Allen J, Sapp S, et al. Short-term effects of the DASH diet in adults with moderate chronic kidney disease: a pilot feeding study. Clin Kidney J. 2016;9(4):592–8.
82. Psaltopoulou T, Naska A, Orfanos P, Trichopoulos D, Mountokalakis T, Trichopoulou A. Olive oil, the Mediterranean diet, and arterial blood pressure: the Greek European Prospective Investigation into Cancer and Nutrition (EPIC) study. Am J Clin Nutr. 2004;80(4):1012–8.
83. Nunez-Cordoba JM, Valencia-Serrano F, Toledo E, Alonso A, Martinez-Gonzalez MA. The Mediterranean diet and incidence of hypertension: the Seguimiento Universidad de Navarra (SUN) Study. Am J Epidemiol. 2009;169(3):339–46.
84. Toledo E, Hu FB, Estruch R, Buil-Cosiales P, Corella D, Salas-Salvado J, et al. Effect of the Mediterranean diet on blood pressure in the PREDIMED trial: results from a randomized controlled trial. BMC Med. 2013;11:207.
85. Appel LJ, Van Horn L. Did the PREDIMED trial test a Mediterranean diet? N Engl J Med. 2013;368(14):1353–4.
86. Estruch R, Ros E, Salas-Salvado J, Covas MI, Corella D, Aros F, et al. Primary prevention of cardiovascular disease with a mediterranean diet supplemented with extra-virgin olive oil or nuts. N Engl J Med. 2018;378(25):e34.

87. Davis CR, Hodgson JM, Woodman R, Bryan J, Wilson C, Murphy KJ. A Mediterranean diet lowers blood pressure and improves endothelial function: results from the MedLey randomized intervention trial. Am J Clin Nutr. 2017;105(6):1305–13.
88. Nissensohn M, Roman-Vinas B, Sanchez-Villegas A, Piscopo S, Serra-Majem L. The effect of the mediterranean diet on hypertension: a systematic review and meta-analysis. J Nutr Educ Behav. 2016;48(1):42–53. e1
89. Murphy KJ, Parletta N. Implementing a mediterranean-style diet outside the mediterranean region. Curr Atheroscler Rep. 2018;20(6):28.
90. Marques FZ, Mackay CR, Kaye DM. Beyond gut feelings: how the gut microbiota regulates blood pressure. Nat Rev Cardiol. 2018;15(1):20–32.
91. Li J, Zhao F, Wang Y, Chen J, Tao J, Tian G, et al. Gut microbiota dysbiosis contributes to the development of hypertension. Microbiome. 2017;5(1):14.
92. Cohen DL, Townsend RR. Central blood pressure and chronic kidney disease progression. Int J Nephrol. 2011;2011:407801.

Chapter 11
Diabetes Mellitus and Chronic Kidney Disease (Stages 1–5)

Meaghan Elger, Arti Sharma Parpia, and Dana Whitham

Keywords Nephropathy · Diabetes · Hypoglycemia · Dialysis · Insulin · Hyperglycemia · Blood glucose

Key Points
- To describe screening procedures and identification of diabetic nephropathy
- To integrate the goals of diabetes therapy with the progressive dietary restrictions necessary with declining kidney function
- To clearly identify the nutrition recommendations for patients with concurrent comorbidities (diabetes mellitus [DM], chronic kidney disease [CKD], hypertension [HTN], cardiovascular disease [CVD]) and to dispel any myths that remain related to the above

Introduction

Diabetic kidney disease (DKD) continues to be the leading cause of end-stage kidney disease (ESKD) in North America, accounting for approximately half of the new cases of kidney failure [1]. DKD has a complex etiology and multiple risk factors that include a long duration of diabetes (DM), hyperglycemia, hypertension, elevated total and low-density lipoprotein (LDL) cholesterol, obesity, and cigarette smoking [2]. The incidence and severity of DKD are increased in Hispanics and Native Americans and are three- to six-fold higher in African Americans compared to Caucasians [3–5], thereby indicating a genetic susceptibility of the disease. Treatment goals include the stabilization of kidney function, the prevention of other microvascular diseases, the prevention of cardiovascular disease (CVD), and the management and prevention of acute complications of poor glycemic control. While cardiovascular death rates have improved over the past decade, heart disease and stroke are still responsible for about 65% of deaths in people with diabetes [2, 6]. The presence of albuminuria doubles the risk of CVD in those with type 2 diabetes mellitus (T2DM) and highlights the need for screening and aggressive interventions aimed at reducing CVD risk [2, 7, 8]. In both type 1 diabetes mellitus (T1DM) and T2DM, the majority of the increased risk of CVD appears to be attributed to those individuals who also have DKD [8]. Albuminuria and estimated glomerular filtration rate (eGFR) are

M. Elger · D. Whitham (✉)
St. Michael's Hospital, Centre for Diabetes & Endocrinology, Toronto, ON, Canada
e-mail: Dana.Whitham@unityhealth.to

A. S. Parpia
St. Michael's Hospital, Toronto, ON, Canada

© Springer Nature Switzerland AG 2020
J. D. Burrowes et al. (eds.), *Nutrition in Kidney Disease*, Nutrition and Health,
https://doi.org/10.1007/978-3-030-44858-5_11

independently and additively associated with increased risk of CVD events, CVD mortality, and all-cause mortality [8]. This chapter will focus on the medical nutrition therapy for the treatment of diabetic kidney disease.

Prevalence and Screening

Persistent albuminuria in the range of 30–300 mg/day is frequently considered the earliest stage of nephropathy and a marker for the development of ESKD in diabetes. Without specific interventions, approximately 20–30% of people with T1DM will develop albuminuria (>300 mg/day) within 15 years of diagnosis, but with tighter glycemic control and intensive blood pressure management, less than half will progress to overt nephropathy [9, 10]. In the Diabetes Control and Complications Trial/Epidemiology of Diabetes Interventions and Complications (DCCT/EDIC) trial, which compared intensive blood glucose control to conventional control, less than 2% of the intensively treated patients developed renal insufficiency (defined as serum creatinine >2.0 mg/dL or renal replacement therapy [RRT]) over an average 30 years of diabetes duration [11]. Evidence is available to support that the renal risk is equivalent in the two types of diabetes and that the lower prevalence of ESKD seen in T2DM is due to a later disease onset and thereby shorter duration of exposure. High rates of comorbidities and other diseases in people with T2DM may also shorten the lifespan and thus impact prevalence [12, 13]. In people with T2DM, 20–40% will progress to overt nephropathy (defined as albuminuria >300 mg/day), but by 20 years duration, only 20% will have progressed to ESKD [14].

The albumin creatinine ratio (ACR) is most commonly used for screening. All patients with T1DM of at least 5 years' duration and all those with T2DM or with comorbid hypertension should be screened annually through both assessment of urinary albumin and eGFR [2]. Monitoring albuminuria annually can also help assess response to drug therapy and lifestyle modification.

Decreased GFR can occur in the absence of albuminuria in adults with diabetes; therefore, serum creatinine should be measured at least annually to estimate GFR and the stage of CKD in all adults with diabetes, regardless of the degree of albuminuria [2]. GFR can be calculated using age, sex, race, and serum creatinine in estimation equations. The Chronic Kidney Disease Epidemiology Collaboration (CKD-EPI) equation is the preferred equation due to its accuracy, especially at higher levels of GFR [15, 16].

Glycemic Control

Evidence from three main trials has guided the development of glycemic targets, namely, the Diabetes Control and Complications Trial (DCCT) in people with T1DM [17], and the United Kingdom Prospective Diabetes Study (UKPDS) [18] and Kumamoto [19] in those with T2DM. These landmark trials demonstrated a significant decrease in microvascular complications with improved glycemic control. Three major subsequent trials examined the impact of glycemic control on people with longer durations of diabetes, namely, the Action to Control Cardiovascular Risk in Diabetes (ACCORD) [20], Action in Diabetes and Vascular Disease: Preterax and Diamicron MR Controlled Evaluation (ADVANCE) [21], and the Veteran Affairs Diabetes Trial (VADT) [22]. Similarly, the importance of glycemic control on the reduction of microvascular complications was confirmed. These later trials and the follow-up observational studies of the DCCT [23] and UKPDS [24, 25] also demonstrated a decrease in macrovascular complications with improved glycemic control. With respect to DKD specifically, intensive glycemic control has been shown to reduce the development of albuminuria and the progression to overt proteinuria [2, 17]. For every percentage decrease in A1C, there is a 25%

reduction in nephropathy [18, 24, 25]. Current American Diabetes Association (ADA) guidelines recommend targeting an A1C of less than 7% [2] with individualization down to a target of 6.5% or up to 8% depending on duration of disease, life expectancy, complications, risk of hypoglycemia, and other comorbidities. The Kidney Disease Outcomes Quality Initiative (KDOQI) guidelines also recommend a target A1C of less than 7%, except in individuals with CKD stages 1–4 who have existing comorbidities, have a limited life expectancy, or are at high risk for hypoglycemia, when a looser A1C is acceptable [26].

Lipids

Cardiovascular risk factors including hypertension, dyslipidemia, increased body weight, smoking, family history, and presence of chronic kidney disease should be assessed at least annually in all patients with diabetes [2]. Lifestyle strategies continue to include a diet low in saturated and trans fat, as saturated fat remains a large driver of LDL cholesterol production. The use of viscous fiber, n-3 fatty acids, plant sterols and stanols, weight loss (if indicated), and physical activity are also recommended [6, 27, 28]. Refer to Chapter 13 for further information and lifestyle strategies aimed at treating dyslipidemia.

Blood Pressure

It is estimated that 65% of patients with T2DM also have hypertension (HTN). The ADA recommends a blood pressure target of <140/90 mmHg for those at lower risk of cardiovascular disease and individualization of targets based on cardiovascular risk. As most individuals with CKD are considered at higher risk of cardiovascular disease, a blood pressure target of <130/80 mmHg is appropriate [1, 27, 29, 30]. Use of either angiotensin-converting enzyme (ACE) inhibitors or angiotensin II receptor blockers (ARBs) is routinely recommended because of their additional reno-protective effects.

Due to the nephrotoxic effects of high dietary sodium intake, such as worsening albuminuria and increased blood pressure, the Kidney Disease: Improving Global Outcomes (KDIGO) guidelines recommend a sodium restriction of <90 mmol/day (<2000 mg) in CKD patients in stages 1–4 [7]. The 2019 position statement of the ADA suggests that people with diabetes limit their sodium intake to less than 2300 mg daily but that reductions should not aim to go below 1500 mg/day [31]. The Dietary Approaches to Stop Hypertension (DASH) diet is generally not recommended for patients with a GFR <60 mL/min, due to its higher protein, phosphorus, and potassium content, but can be used in patients with early stages of CKD, balancing out the risk of hyperkalemia with the expected benefits [29]. Refer to Chapter 10 for more details on lifestyle modifications for the treatment of HTN.

Medical Nutrition Therapy (MNT)

Medical nutrition therapy is an integral component of both diabetes and CKD management. MNT can lower A1C by 1–1.9% for people with T1DM and 0.3–2.0% for people with T2DM [31], which is as effective as many antidiabetic medications. Nutrition therapy for people with diabetes and CKD should balance the general nutrition guidelines for diabetes with the need for dietary restriction of sodium, potassium, and phosphorus. Nutrition recommendations will differ across the stages of DKD based on balancing the risk-to-benefit ratio of the intervention. The goals of medical nutrition therapy for individuals with diabetes and CKD to prevent acute and long-term complications include [31]:

1. Maintenance of target blood glucose levels
2. Achievement of optimal serum lipids and blood pressure
3. Adequate energy and protein intake to attain or maintain an acceptable body weight and nutritional status
4. Achievement of biochemical parameters and fluid status within defined standards

All nutrition goals should be considered within the context of patient-centered care and include lifestyle, personal and cultural preferences, financial situation, and respect for the individual's willingness to make changes. A registered dietitian should be included in the care team to help people balance the nutrition recommendations for DM and CKD.

Weight Management and Energy Needs Estimation

Among patients with diabetes, there is an association between obesity and risk for CKD. The NKF-KDOQI clinical practice guidelines for diabetes and CKD suggest that a normal body mass index (BMI) (18.5–24.9 kg/m^2) may reduce the risk of loss of kidney function and CVD [26]. Factors that may contribute to the relationship between obesity and CKD include physical compression of the kidneys by visceral obesity, renin-angiotensin system activation, hyperinsulinemia, and glomerular hyperfiltration, among others [26]. For overweight individuals with T2DM in stages 1–3 CKD, moderate weight loss of 5–10% improves insulin sensitivity, glycemic and blood pressure control, and proteinuria [32–35].

The primary approach for achieving weight loss is therapeutic lifestyle changes, which include a moderate reduction in energy intake (500–1000 kcal/day) and a moderate increase in physical activity (contributing approximately 200 or more kcal/day). This should result in slow but progressive weight loss (1–2 lb/week) [26, 31]. Women should target between 1200 and 1500 kcals per day and men approximately 1500 and 1800 kcals daily [31]. The goal would be to mitigate loss of lean body or bone mass through use of an energy-controlled, balanced, and slow approach to weight loss. Diets centered on food group exclusion or those that are overly restrictive carry the risk of excessive lean body mass loss, nonadherence, and relapse. Individuals following these types of diets should be carefully monitored by a registered dietitian [31]. Furthermore, individuals with CKD and diabetes should use caution with low-carbohydrate/high-animal protein diets (>20% of total daily calories) as excessive protein intakes are associated with increased albuminuria and a more rapid rate of loss of kidney function [31]. The Institute of Medicine defines a low-carbohydrate diet as a restriction of total carbohydrate (CHO) to <130 g/day [36]. For people on a low-CHO diet who have DKD, there should be careful monitoring of lipids, renal function, and protein intake and attention to adjustment of antihyperglycemic therapy [2]. No one diet has been demonstrated as superior, and in general, all diets that lead to a net caloric deficit and those with greater adherence are associated with greater weight loss and improvements in metabolic markers [37, 38]. The weight loss plan should be selected with consideration for individual preferences, likely adherence, treatment goals, and long-term risk versus benefit.

Weight loss can be achieved through lifestyle changes or through bariatric surgery. Bariatric surgery remains the most effective and sustained weight loss strategy. For those with CKD, bariatric surgery was associated with a 58% lower risk of a greater than 30% decline in eGFR and a 57% lower risk of doubling serum creatinine [39]. With that said, major clinical outcomes such as progression of DKD or the development of ESKD are still unknown, and therefore findings should be interpreted with caution [39].

Recommendations for physical activity should be modest and based on the patient's willingness and ability. The ADA guidelines recommend a goal of at least 150 min/week of moderate intensity activity (50–70% maximum heart rate) over at least 3 days/week. Resistance exercises three times per week are also encouraged [2, 31]. It is important to monitor blood glucose levels before exercising in people with T1DM because vigorous exercise could lead to hypo- or hyperglycemia, depending on the initial blood glucose levels and type of exercise. For planned exercise, a reduction in insulin dosage is the preferred method to prevent hypoglycemia. However, for unplanned exercise, an additional 10–15 g of CHO may be needed for every 60 min of moderate-intensity exercise [31]. A greater amount of carbohydrate is required with more intensive exercise.

At all stages of CKD, a primary goal for MNT is to prevent protein and energy malnutrition, which increases the risk of poor clinical outcomes, morbidity, and mortality [7]. Uremia-associated anorexia is generally not seen until the later stages of CKD [40]; however, other factors such as inflammatory cytokines and depression may also induce anorexia. Energy prediction equations or estimated energy ranges can be used to estimate an individual's caloric requirements. Energy recommendations for individuals with CKD range between 23 and 35 kcal/kg/day [41]. More specifically, KDOQI nutrition guidelines recommend a caloric intake of 25–35 kcal/kg/day for non-dialyzed CKD patients [42]. Estimated energy ranges are used because analysis of the validity of prediction equations in this population is limited. A study by Kamimura et al. [43] concluded that the Harris-Benedict equation accurately predicted resting energy expenditure (REE) in patients with diabetes when compared to indirect calorimetry. Interestingly, in CKD patients without diabetes, the Harris-Benedict equation has been shown to significantly overestimate REE [43, 44]. As a result, the Harris-Benedict equation and the suggested 25–35 kcal/kg/day can be used to determine energy requirements, although both may tend toward overestimation in this patient population.

Dietary Strategies For Carbohydrate (CHO) Management

As carbohydrate (CHO) is the macronutrient with the largest impact on postprandial serum glucose levels, careful management of CHO intake is essential to any diabetes meal-planning approach, and strategies should focus on the quantity and quality of CHO.

Quantity

The ADA guidelines state that there is no ideal percentage of calories from CHO, protein, and fat for managing diabetes and no longer recommend a minimum CHO intake. A "constant carbohydrate" meal plan suits patients who use diet alone to control their blood glucose levels, those on fixed doses of insulin or antihyperglycemic medications, or patients who are not suitable for CHO counting. Emphasis is placed on keeping the amount of CHO relatively constant for each meal and spacing meals throughout the day. Insulin should be adjusted around usual CHO intake, as much as possible, rather than CHO being altered to meet the insulin regimens.

The "carbohydrate counting" method provides the most flexibility and is the preferred meal-planning approach for adjusting insulin around usual dietary intake. Initially, careful record-keeping by reading food labels and measuring portion sizes of CHO foods combined with both pre- and post-meal blood glucose readings is essential until an accurate ratio of insulin to grams of CHO (I/C ratio) is established. Once established, the patient counts the grams of available CHO to be eaten and then matches it with the proper amount of insulin. Ideally, blood glucose readings should be taken before each meal and the insulin dose decided based on the amount of CHO to be consumed, the blood glucose reading at that time, and any recent or upcoming activity. This concept requires motivation, skill in CHO counting, and self-reflection to select and assess insulin doses. Individuals who have pre-meal glucose values within target range but who are not meeting A1C targets should consider monitoring 2-h postprandial glucose (PPG). Treatment should be aimed at reducing PPG values to <180 mg/dL and thereby comparably reducing A1C [2].

Recently, ketogenic diets have been gaining more popularity in the media, and research suggests that this type of dietary pattern may be beneficial for people with type 2 diabetes. There is insufficient data to support the use of ketogenic diets in type 1 diabetes [31]. Ketogenic diets are very low-CHO diets in which people consume less than 50 g of CHO per day. At this level of CHO, the body depletes the glycogen stores in the liver and muscle and begins to metabolize fat to produce ketone bodies, which can be used as an alternative fuel source [45]. The benefits of a ketogenic diet appear to be short-term weight loss [46, 47], improved glycemic control [48–50], reductions in diabetes oral medication and insulin doses [49, 50], and improved lipid profile [45, 46, 48].

Since ketogenic diets are very high in protein [49, 50], caution should be used in people with CKD. The KDIGO guidelines recommend avoiding high-protein diets, defined as >1.3 g/kg/day, for people with CKD [7]. Caution also needs to be used in people taking a sodium-glucose co-transporter 2 (SGLT2) inhibitor due to the risk of ketoacidosis [31, 51].

Quality

Controlling high postprandial blood glucose levels is an ongoing challenge in diabetes management. People spend the majority of their day in a postprandial state, and it is imperative for optimal glycemic control that they achieve target readings post meal [52]. Both the quantity and the quality of CHO found in foods influence PPG levels. Most experts agree, and the ADA's position is, that the quantity of CHO consumed is a more reliable predictor of PPG and that the quality of CHO has a smaller, but still significant, effect [31, 53].

Glycemic Index

The main method used to categorize CHO-containing foods based on their glycemic response is the glycemic index (GI) [31, 53]. Significant improvements in postprandial glucose, total cholesterol, and markers of inflammation have been demonstrated in clinical trials using low-GI diets [54–56]. Low-GI foods such as pasta, parboiled rice, barley, oats, beans, peas, lentils, and pumpernickel, rye, or wholegrains breads are recommended in place of higher GI foods.

The GI of a food varies substantially depending on the CHO makeup of the food, the length of time it was stored, how it was cooked, how it was processed, the acid content of the food, its ripeness, and its variety (e.g., types of potatoes or rice) [53–55]. The International Tables of Glycemic Index [57] can be useful when a potassium or phosphorus restriction is warranted due to declining renal function.

Fiber

High-fiber diets (50 g fiber/day) have been shown to reduce glycemia in subjects with T1DM and T2DM, and to reduce hyperinsulinemia and lipemia in subjects with T2DM through delaying gastric emptying [31, 53]. Potential barriers to achieving such a high-fiber intake include gastrointestinal side effects and the high potassium and phosphorus content of high-fiber grains, fruits, and vegetables. As

Table 11.1 Low potassium sources of fiber

Food item	Serving size	Amount of fiber (g)	Amount of potassium (mg)
Fruits			
Pear (with skin)	1 medium	5.3	206
Raspberries	1/2 cup	4.2	98
Blackberries	1/2 cup	4.0	123
Apple (with skin)	1 medium	3.5	195
Blueberries	1/2 cup	2.0	59
Strawberries (sliced)	1/2 cup	2.0	134
Vegetables			
Green peas, canned, drained	1/2 cup	4.0	93
Mixed vegetables, boiled	1/2 cup	2.8	163
Carrots, boiled	1/2 cup	2.2	194
Asparagus	6 spears	2.0	194
Green and yellow snap beans, boiled	1/2 cup	1.6	96
Cauliflower	1/2 cup	1.0	169
Cabbage, boiled	1/2 cup	1.3	155
Grains			
Popcorn, air-popped	2 cups	2.5	56
Whole wheat pasta, cooked	1/2 cup	2.4	33
Whole-grain bread	1 slice	2.1	71
Instant cream of wheat	1 cup	1.2	36
Barley (cooked)	1 cup	7.4	134

Created by authors. Source: Health Canada. The Canadian nutrient file, 2018 version. Ottawa, ONT. Available from http://food-nutrition.canada.ca/cnf-fce/index-eng.jsp. Accessed February 25, 2019

a first priority, the ADA encourages people with diabetes to aim for the same fiber intake goals set for the general population (14 g/1000 kcal/day) [58]. Diabetes Canada (DC) recommends higher intakes (≥20 g/1000 kcal/day) [51]. For people with CKD, fiber intake should be encouraged within the constraints of the progressing renal diet. Where possible, fiber intake can be sought from increases in low-potassium fruits and vegetables and through the use of fiber supplements (Table 11.1).

Carbohydrate Conclusion and Final Recommendations

Recommendations surrounding CHO intake should be individualized, but for a person with DM and CKD, any reductions in carbohydrate should be moderate and the impact on protein intake needs to be considered. To improve glycemic control, priority can be given to carbohydrate distribution, proper insulin-to-CHO matching, and selecting low-GI, high-fiber foods that are low in potassium and phosphorus. Figure 11.1 provides a stepwise process for modifying carbohydrate intake to accommodate renal dietary restrictions.

Protein Guidelines for Diabetes and CKD

There is no evidence to suggest that protein needs in people with diabetes without diabetic kidney disease are different than that of the general population (1–1.5 g/kg or 15–20% of calories) [31]. Higher protein intakes are said to contribute to satiety when distributed throughout the day and effect

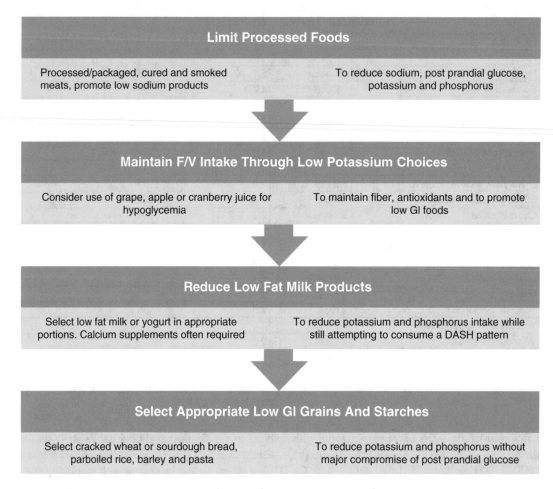

Fig. 11.1 Stepwise restriction protocol for MNT of diabetes complicated by CKD

the clearance of glucose from the blood [41, 51, 59]. As such, for those with DKD, achieving ideal but not excessive protein intake well distributed throughout the day is encouraged. The 2012 KDIGO guidelines for CKD suggest lowering protein intake to 0.8 g/kg/day in adults with diabetes and a GFR <30 ml/min/1.73m^2 and avoiding high protein intakes (>1.3 g/kg/day) in adults with CKD at risk of progression [7].

Prior to the widespread use of renin-angiotensin system blockade agents, protein restrictions were found to significantly reduce proteinuria; however, in a more recent systematic review and meta-analyses, there was no significant improvement in GFR or progression to nephropathy [60, 61]. While malnutrition remains the greatest risk related to restricted protein diets (i.e., <0.7 g/kg/day) [41], the recommendation to avoid restricted protein diets is due to evidence that they do not alter glycemic or cardiovascular outcomes or the rate at which the GFR declines [31, 60, 61] and not simply because of the risk of protein-energy malnutrition.

As was evident with carbohydrate, both amount and type of protein are of importance. Evidence suggests that plant-based protein diets (tofu, legumes, nuts, whole grains) are not associated with CKD progression and that diets that contain more vegetables and fruits are associated with a lower risk of CKD progression [62]. The benefit of including more sources of plant-based proteins should be balanced with potassium and phosphorus restrictions.

In summary, protein intakes should be carefully monitored and maintained at no less than 0.8 g/kg/day. Excessive intakes may accelerate GFR decline, and protein restrictions (below 0.7 g/kg/day) have demonstrated limited benefit and are not recommended.

Dietary Fat Recommendations

Lifestyle modifications should include weight loss as indicated; an increase in physical activity; adoption of healthy diet patterns such as the Mediterranean, Portfolio, or Dietary Approaches to Stop Hypertension (DASH) diets; a reduction in saturated and trans fats; and an increase in viscous fiber, plant sterols, and n-3 fatty acids [31, 51]. Saturated fat and *trans*-fatty acids are the principal dietary determinants of plasma LDL cholesterol, which is the major risk factor for CVD, and as such, limiting their intake is still recommended. The type of fat consumed is considered more important than the amount of fat. In the most recent update to the Canadian and American diabetes guidelines, there is an emphasis on ensuring that reductions in saturated fat occur without replacing those calories with refined carbohydrate. Saturated fat should be substituted with sources of unsaturated fat or with low glycemic index foods [31, 51]. These recommendations state that saturated fat should make up no more than <7–9% of total daily energy intake and that *trans* fat should be eliminated from the diet [31, 51].

Diet Patterns

The KDOQI Diabetes Work Group suggests that the DASH and DASH-sodium diets [63], which emphasize sources of protein other than red meat, may be alternatives to lower total protein intake in persons with HTN, diabetes, and CKD stages 1–2 [26]. Diets that emphasize proteins from plant sources (vegetables, soy, whole grains, legumes, nuts) instead of animal sources (particularly red meat) may be renal-sparing [7, 61, 64–66]. DASH diets have been shown to reduce the risk of developing diabetes and CVD and lead to better blood pressure (BP) control [67]. In a study of 14,882 patients with an eGFR>60, the DASH diet was associated with a decreased risk of developing CKD after follow-up of 23 years. One of the most limiting factors of the DASH diet is its high intake of potassium (~4.5 g/day) and phosphorus (~1.7 g/day) and, as a result, would be best suited to those in the initial stages of DKD [67].

The Mediterranean diet is associated with a decreased incidence of major CV events and the preservation of eGFR [67]. It has general principles similar to that of the DASH diet but with a higher monounsaturated fat profile. In a 15-year observational study, the Mediterranean diet showed a decreased risk of rapid decline in eGFR [67]. There appears to be substantial reno-protective effects; however, further information is required of clinical endpoints [67]. See Chap. 31 for more information on dietary patterns.

Alcohol

General population guidelines recommend moderation in alcohol, and further precautions should be considered within the context of diabetes and CKD. Consideration should be paid to medication interactions, presence of HTN, lipid metabolism, fluid balance, and risk of hypoglycemia. A moderate amount of alcohol is considered to be two or less drinks per day for men and one drink or less per day for women [31]. A standard 15 g portion of alcohol is defined as 12 oz of beer, 5 oz of wine, and 1.5 oz of distilled spirits. Moderate amounts of alcohol can be consumed with food without causing hyperglycemia or hypoglycemia [68, 69]. Beer contains high amounts of phosphorus and should be discouraged for patients requiring a phosphate restriction. Alcohol should also be included in the total daily fluid allowance for patients requiring fluid restriction.

Nutritive and Nonnutritive Sweeteners

Nutritive sweeteners (also known as added sugars) contain carbohydrate and provide energy at appreciable levels (4 kcal/g) [70]. The negative health effects of added sugars are likely related to adding excess calories. Studies looking at isocaloric substitutions of fructose-containing sugars for starches have not shown negative effects on lipoproteins, body weight, blood pressure, and glycemic control [71–73]. Additionally, the impact of fructose-containing sugars on glycemic control may be influenced by the food source, for example, fruit, yogurt, and whole grains versus refined starches and sugar-sweetened beverages [74]. Currently, the ADA and DC recommend that people with diabetes limit their intake of added sugars to ≤10% of total calories and recommend eliminating sugar-sweetened beverages because they often add excess calories and have no added nutritional benefit [31, 51].

Nonnutritive sweeteners (NNS) contain little to no calories and generally have negligible impacts on blood glucose, so they may be a useful substitute for added sugars. The Food and Drug Administration (FDA) is responsible for evaluating the safety of NNS. The ADA recommendations state that sugar alcohols and NNS are safe when consumed within the acceptable daily intakes established by the FDA [31]. Most NNS are excreted unchanged in either the urine or the feces, meaning that they do not influence potassium levels [70]. NNS currently approved for use in the United States include acesulfame K, aspartame, luohanguo, neotame, saccharin, stevia, and sucralose.

ESKD and DM

Diabetes is the most common cause of end-stage kidney disease (ESKD), and dialysis patients with diabetes have a lower survival rate compared to nondiabetics with ESKD [75]. Furthermore, these patients have the poorest rehabilitation potential and the highest incidence of hospitalizations, mostly attributable to cardiovascular events [76, 77].

In addition to a decreased need of insulin and antihyperglycemic agents, there is sometimes a normalization of hyperglycemia and A1C in ESKD [78]. To further complicate the issue of optimizing glycemic control, both hemodialysis and peritoneal dialysis (PD) are comprised of unique aspects that affect the management of DM.

Hemodialysis

Hemodialysis (HD) is the most common form of RRT used to treat people with DM [75, 76]. Poor glycemic control upon initiation of HD indicates worse survival [79, 80]. MNT for patients with diabetes on hemodialysis remains the same as that outlined by KDOQI [26] but with consideration for additional acute complications (e.g., hypoglycemia).

Dietary intake for dialysis patients may be impacted by treatment schedules interfering with a patient's usual mealtime and post-treatment fatigue. Furthermore, hemodialysis patients generally consume fewer calories on dialysis days compared with non-dialysis days [81]. These factors can precipitate hypoglycemia, so a patient may need to eat before coming to treatment and/or bring a snack to consume afterward. Use of glucose-containing dialysates may be indicated to prevent hypoglycemia [82–84]. It is important to encourage regular eating habits to promote consistent blood glucose patterns. In addition, insulin regimens which offer greater flexibility and insulin secretagogues with a shorter half-life may have added benefits for people with variable dietary intakes.

Peritoneal Dialysis

The management of DM in peritoneal dialysis (PD) is especially challenged by the use of hypertonic dialysis solutions. Side effects related to intraperitoneal (IP) exposure to high glucose concentrations may include acute hyperglycemia, an inflammatory state, hyperlipidemia, fibrosis, enhanced protein loss, generalized intra-abdominal fat accumulations, increased risk of CVD, weight gain, and obesity. The underlying diabetic state may compound or exacerbate these problems [85–87]. Carbohydrate-sparing dialytic regimens, such as amino acid-based fluids and icodextrin, may reduce glucose-related toxicity. Icodextrin is a glucose polymer-based solution which may provide better glycemic control, increase ultrafiltration (UF) volume, improve blood pressure control, and be less hyperlipidemic [86, 88, 89].

Glycemic control is complex with PD, and poor control can increase thirst which may lead to fluid retention [90]. Sodium and fluid control are essential to adequate glycemic control in PD to optimize ultrafiltration. The use of lower percent glucose dialysate solutions which may subsequently lead to less IP glucose absorption and could minimize hyperglycemia.

Medical Nutrition Therapy on Dialysis

The nutritional therapy of patients with DM who are receiving maintenance dialysis is similar to those in the later stages of CKD, with the exception of protein requirements and generally stricter restrictions of phosphorus, potassium, and fluid. In the ESKD population, there is a high incidence of protein-energy wasting related to many factors, including, but not limited to, amino acid losses through dialysis, metabolic acidosis, and uremia-associated anorexia. Recommended protein intake is 1.0 to 1.2 g/kg/day for both hemodialysis and peritoneal dialysis patients [42]. Optimizing carbohydrate distribution to achieve euglycemia, minimizing dyslipidemia, and attaining a total energy intake appropriate for weight management should continue to be encouraged. In addition, patients should be educated regarding appropriate hypoglycemia management with consideration of potassium and fluid restrictions.

Malnutrition and Dialysis

Diabetes is the most significant predictor of loss of lean body mass in dialysis patients, independent of inadequate dialysis dose, metabolic acidosis, and insufficient protein intake [77]. Compared to ESKD patients without DM, patients with DM have increased muscle breakdown [91–93]. Since protein-energy wasting is a strong predictor of mortality, ensuring adequate protein and caloric intake is imperative to preventing malnutrition in patients receiving maintenance dialysis. Oral nutrition supplements (ONS) may be useful to increase protein and caloric intake. The choice of an ONS should be based on the overall nutrient profile to meet the individual's metabolic needs, palatability, and affordability. Refer to Chap. 22 for more information about protein-energy wasting.

Fluid Control

Fluid control may be more difficult in patients with DM because hyperglycemia may increase thirst and urination. In those with diabetic neuropathy, symptoms of dry mouth, decreased salivary flow rates, and the effects of xerogenic drugs may worsen fluid control [94–98]. Fluid intake may be higher if dental problems impair chewing or if gastroparesis is severe and solid food is not tolerated. Patients should be educated on tips to control thirst without further exacerbating hyperglycemia. Tips may include brushing or rinsing teeth more often, sucking on lemon or lime wedges, using ice chips in limited quantities, and using sugar-free gum or candies.

Diabetic Gastroparesis

Gastroparesis is defined as nonobstructive delayed gastric emptying with impaired gastric acid secretion and GI motility. It is a common complication in patients with long-standing diabetes due to autonomic neuropathy. Symptoms include early satiety, postprandial fullness, anorexia, nausea, bloating, belching, epigastric discomfort, abdominal pain, and emesis of undigested food. Patients with gastroparesis may be at risk for electrolyte and nutrient deficits, anorexia, and malnutrition [99].

Diets low in fat and fiber may help to prevent early satiety. Patients can also try eating small, frequent meals, chewing food thoroughly, avoiding fluids with meals, and remaining upright for 2 h after meals [2]. If a person struggles to consume solid foods, ONS may be considered as liquid supplements are energy and nutrient dense and empty more easily from the stomach.

People taking insulin or insulin secretagogues should be counseled to consume their carbohydrate-containing foods first at a meal to prevent hypoglycemia. Basal/bolus regimens using a long-/longer-acting and rapid insulin are preferred as they allow for more variability in meal content and timing. People taking mealtime insulin may also benefit from taking their insulin after their meal to ensure they only take insulin for the carbohydrate consumed [99].

MNT Summary

Table 11.2 summarizes the nutrition recommendations for patients with diabetes and CKD. There is no evidence for additional vitamin and mineral supplements in persons with diabetes who do not have underlying deficiencies. Routine supplementation with antioxidants is not advised because of uncertainties related to long-term efficacy and safety [31, 51]. A stepwise MNT protocol for CKD (nondialysis) from the authors is presented in Fig. 11.1.

Monitoring Glycemic Control

Treatment efficacy can be assessed by measuring A1C and using self-monitoring of blood glucose (SMBG). The A1C should be measured quarterly in patients whose therapy has changed or in those who are not meeting blood glucose goals. In patients who are meeting treatment goals and who have

Table 11.2 Daily nutrition recommendations for diabetes and chronic kidney disease

Nutrient	Stages 1–4	Stage 5/end-stage kidney disease
Energy	25–35 kcal/kg/day	25–35 kcal/kg/day
Protein	0.6–0.8 g/kg/day (avoid protein intake >1.3 g/kg/day)	1.0–1.2 g/kg/day
Carbohydrate	Specific recommendation not provided Include whole-grain carbohydrates, sources of fiber, and fresh fruit and vegetables	Specific recommendation not provided Include whole-grain carbohydrates, sources of fiber, and fresh fruit and vegetables but may need to be limited if elevated serum potassium or phosphorus levels
Fat	Specific recommendation not provided May benefit from increased intake of omega-3 and mono- and polyunsaturated fats	Specific recommendation not provided
Potassium	<2400 mg/day, if elevated serum potassium	HD: <2400 mg/day PD: Individualized
Phosphorus	800–1000 mg/day, if elevated serum phosphorus	HD: 800–1200 mg/day PD: 800–1000 mg/day
Sodium	Lower salt intake to less than 2300 mg/day or 2000 mg day if possible but no less than 1500 mg	Lower salt intake to less than 2300 mg/day or 2000 mg day if possible but no less than 1500 mg
Fluid	Usually not restricted	HD: 1 L + urine output PD: Individualized

Adapted from multiple sources [7, 26, 31, 41, 42, 51]

stable blood glucose control, the A1C test should be performed at least twice yearly [2]. Caution should be used when evaluating A1C in people with CKD as it may be reduced due to the shortened lifespan of erythrocytes and the presence of anemia [26]. Estimated average glucose (EAG) levels may be helpful in late-stage CKD to evaluate glycemic control. See http://professional.diabetes.org/diapro/glucose_calc for conversion of EAG to approximate A1C levels.

SMBG is helpful for evaluating and making treatment decisions. For a person on insulin and insulin secretagogues, SMBG is important for safety around hypoglycemia and driving. The optimal frequency and timing of SMBG for patients with T2DM on basal insulin and/or antihyperglycemic agents is unclear. However, the ADA recommends testing fasting blood glucose daily for people on basal insulin to assist with dose titration [2]. For people on multiple daily injections, the recommendation is to test at least three to four times per day, including testing prior to meals and snacks, at bedtime, occasionally after meals, after treatment of hypoglycemia, and prior to driving. A single random test is a poor guide to overall glycemic control, and checking fasting values alone may be insufficient, as PPG reduction may significantly impact glycemic control [100, 102].

Diabetes technology has advanced greatly in recent years, and it is now quite common for individuals with T1DM to use continuous glucose monitoring (CGM). CGM has the most impact when used daily and should be considered for patients with hypoglycemia unawareness or for those who are otherwise unable to meet targets [102]. Flash monitoring use has also grown dramatically in recent years and has the benefit of a lower cost, no calibration, water resistance, and an accuracy that is reasonable for people with T2DM [2]. At this point, there is insufficient data to support the use of CGM and flash monitoring in people on dialysis.

The goals for monitoring glycemic control in people receiving maintenance dialysis are similar to those without RRT, but exact target levels for best outcomes have not been clearly established. Evidence exists to suggest that adequate monitoring of glucose in dialysis patients is uncommon despite the risk of additional diabetes-related complications [103, 104]. It is important to note that glucose polymer-based peritoneal dialysate solutions (icodextrin) may interfere with glucose dehydrogenase-based glucose meters giving false readings, so a compatible glucose meter is needed [98].

Hypoglycemia/Uremia

As kidney function decreases, risk of hypoglycemia increases. Prolonged insulin action and decreased renal gluconeogenesis may be the two physiological mechanisms responsible for the increased propensity toward hypoglycemia in the earlier stages of CKD. As CKD progresses, uremic factors start to play a greater role. Uremic gastroparesis, poor appetite, and taste changes may add to the preexisting risk. When these combine with the risk of depression, fatigue, and a progressively restrictive diet, the risk of hypoglycemia increases sharply. An A1C at or below target may indicate those patients with whom to be more cautious of hypoglycemia, but screening for symptoms of hypoglycemia in all patients is essential. Dose adjustments for antihyperglycemic agents and insulin may be needed.

Due to potassium and fluid restriction in CKD, the usual methods for treating hypoglycemia (e.g., 3/4 cup of orange juice) may need to be adjusted. Better choices that will provide 15 g of CHO are 1 tbsp. of honey, six Life Savers, or commercial glucose tablets. Once the blood glucose returns to normal, if the next regular meal will be more than 1 h, then the patient should eat a snack with an additional 15g of CHO and protein source to stabilize the glucose level [31, 51].

Pharmacological Management of Diabetes Within CKD

Antihyperglycemic Agents

Antihyperglycemic agents now include seven major classes of medications, all targeted at different or multiple metabolic defects of type 2 diabetes or to modify processes related to appetite, nutrient absorption, or excretion. At diagnosis, people with T2DM usually have less than 50% of their normal insulin secretion and, after 6 years, less than 25%. This progressive decline in beta cell function is the reason many fail oral therapy and require insulin [105]. It also highlights the importance of dynamic pharmacological management of the disease.

Metabolic clearance of many medications and their active metabolites is an issue with renal impairment that increases the risk of hypoglycemia. As such, the degree of renal impairment needs to be considered when selecting antihyperglycemic agents for people with CKD. See Table 11.3 for a summary of available therapies and safety considerations in CKD.

Sick Day Medication List

Certain medications commonly taken by people with diabetes need to be held during times of illness with increased risk of dehydration and when there is an acute decline in kidney function [108]. The acronym "SAD MANS," which stands for **S**ulfonylureas, **A**CE inhibitors, **D**iuretics and direct renin inhibitors, **M**etformin, **A**ngiotensin receptor blockers, **N**on-steroidal anti-inflammatory drugs, and SGLT2 inhibitors, can be used to help remember which medications to stop [109].

Table 11.3 Medications

Class	Oral agent	Action	Efficacy (A1C %)	Side effects and CV benefit	CKD cautions (eGFR < 60)
Secretagogues:					
Sulfonylureas	Glimepiride Glipizide Glyburide	↑ insulin secretion	1–2%	Weight gain, minimal to significant hypoglycemia, ↑ risk of CV-related mortality (sulfonylureas)	Glimepiride – initiate at 1 mg Glipizide – initiate at 2.5 mg Glyburide – avoid
Meglitinides	Nateglinide Repaglinide				Nateglinide – 60 mg with meals when eGFR<30 Repaglinide – 2.5 mg with meals when eGFR<30
Biguanides	Metformin	↓ hepatic glucose production	1–2%	GI side effects, vitamin B12 deficiency	Do not initiate if eGFR 30–45 Reduce dose to 500–1000 mg if eGFR 30–45 Discontinue if eGFR<30
TZD	Pioglitazone Rosiglitazone	↑ insulin sensitivity	1–2%	Weight gain, edema, heart failure, bone fractures, bladder cancer (pioglitazone)	No dose adjustments as metabolized in liver, but not recommended due to side effect of fluid retention
Alpha glucosidase inhibitors	Acarbose Miglitol	Inhibits intestinal digestion/absorption	0.5%	GI side effects	Acarbose – avoid if eGFR<30 Miglitol – avoid if eGFR<25
GLP-1 receptor agonists	Albiglutide Exenatide Dulaglutide Liraglutide Lixisenatide Semaglutide	↑ glucose-dependent insulin secretion, slows gastric emptying, enhances satiety	1–2%	Weight loss, GI side effects, ↑ risk of diabetic retinopathy complications (semaglutide), risk of thyroid C-cell cancers (liraglutide, albiglutide, dulaglutide, exenatide) *CV benefit:* Liraglutide Semaglutide	Albiglutide – caution when eGFR<15 Exenatide – avoid when eGFR<30 Dulaglutide – caution when eGFR<15 Liraglutide – cautionwhen eGFR<15 Lixisenatide – caution when eGFR 15–59; avoid if eGFR<15 Semaglutide– no dose adjustments necessary

(continued)

Table 11.3 (Continued)

Class	Oral agent	Action	Efficacy (A1C %)	Side effects and CV benefit	CKD cautions (eGFR < 60)
DPP-4 inhibitors	Alogliptin Linagliptin Saxagliptin Sitagliptin	Prolongs survival of endogenously released incretin hormones	1%	Potential risk of acute pancreatitis, rare joint pain	Alogliptin – 12.5 mg if eGFR 30–60; 6.25 mg if eGFR<30 Linagliptin – no dose adjustment necessary Saxagliptin – 2.5 mg if eGFR ≤50 Sitagliptin – 50 mg if eGFR 30–50; 25 mg if eGFR<30
SGLT2 inhibitors	Canagliflozin Dapagliflozin Empagliflozin	Inhibits glucose reabsorption in the proximal nephron, resulting in glucosuria	0.4–0.7%	Weight loss, genital infections, hypotension, rare diabetic ketoacidosis (sometimes without hyperglycemia), ↑LDL-C, ↑ fractures and amputation (canagliflozin) *CV benefit:* Canagliflozin Empagliflozin	Canagliflozin – 100 mg if eGFR 45–60; avoid if eGFR<45 Dapagliflozin – avoid if eGFR<60 Empagliflozin – avoid if eGFR<30
Insulin	*Basal:* Degludec Detemir Glargine NPH *Bolus:* Aspart Fiasp Glulisine Inhaled Insulin Lispro Regular *Premixed*	↑ glucose disposal	Unlimited	Weight gain, hypoglycemia	Lower doses may be required as eGFR decreases.
Amylin mimetics	Pramlintide	↓ glucagon secretion, slows gastric emptying, ↑ satiety	0.4% (T1DM) 0.6% (T2DM)	Weight loss, GI side effects, ↓ insulin requirements	No dose adjustment necessary

Adapted from multiple sources [106, 107]

Insulin

Insulin therapy with delivery through syringe, pen, or insulin pump technology remains the mainstay of treatment for people with T1DM and is used frequently in patients with T2DM. Basal insulin is classified according to the duration of action as either intermediate, long-acting, or longer-acting insulin. Prandial (mealtime or bolus) insulin is classified in the same manner as either rapid- or short-acting insulin. Basal/bolus regimens using intermediate or long-/longer-acting insulin once or twice daily with short- or rapid-acting insulin to cover the carbohydrate content of each meal are commonly prescribed. Premixed insulins are also available and include a prandial insulin mixed with an intermediate basal insulin.

Hypoglycemia remains the most common side effect and barrier to optimal glycemic control with insulin. As mentioned earlier, the risk of hypoglycemia increases in people with CKD due to decreased renal gluconeogenesis, gastroparesis, and decreased oral intake. The risk of hypoglycemia is further increased by the decreased renal filtration of insulin as kidney disease progresses to its advanced stages. Once the GFR drops below 20 mL/min, the kidneys are unable to adequately metabolize insulin, and there is a related decline in hepatic insulin metabolism [110]. This leads to a high risk of hypoglycemic events [111, 112]. Thus, as kidney function deteriorates further in ESKD, many patients require reduced amounts, or even cessation, of exogenous insulin [113, 114].

Management of blood glucose during times of poor or variable appetite, gastroparesis, and delayed mealtimes can be best accomplished with a more physiological approach to insulin management through a basal/bolus regimen. Premixed insulin regimens, in contrast, require consistent mealtimes, carbohydrate intake, and snacks to reduce the risk of hypoglycemia. Long- and longer-acting basal insulins have demonstrated significant reductions in nocturnal hypoglycemia when used to replace intermediate insulin. Longer-acting insulin, degludec, may provide even more reduction compared to long-acting insulin, glargine. Additionally, rapid-acting insulin analogues have a reduced frequency of hypoglycemia compared to short-acting insulins, and should be considered for use in individuals with diabetic nephropathy [106].

Conclusion

The incidence of both diabetes and CKD is on the rise. Living with either diabetes or CKD is challenging for anyone. Managing diabetes in the presence of CKD requires additional effort on the part of the patient and the health-care team to improve outcomes and decrease morbidity and mortality in this population. Because of the complexity of diabetes and CKD and their comorbidities, multiple drug therapies, in conjunction with MNT, are necessary to achieve the goals of therapy; therefore, patient adherence becomes a serious concern. The nutrition needs of patients with diabetes and CKD change as the progression and treatment of the disease change. Understanding the treatment goals at each stage is crucial to optimize the nutritional status of patients throughout the course of their disease and to individualize their education and meal plans accordingly.

Case Study

P.W. is a 51-year-old man referred for diabetes education and seen for recurrent hypoglycemia. His past medical history reveals T2DM × 19 years, HTN, hyperlipidemia, stage 3 DKD, obesity, and retinopathy.

Current medications include rapid insulin 40 units at breakfast, 30 units at lunch, and 40 units at supper, lantus insulin 90 units once daily at night, atorvastatin 20 mg once daily, chlorthalidone 25 mg once daily, enalapril 40 mg bid, metoprolol 100 mg once daily, and amlodipine 10 mg once daily.

His physical exam presents with Ht 5′7″, Wt 208 lb. (today), BP 150/90 mmHg, and pedal edema 1+. Laboratory data included A1C 6.5, glucose 100 mg/dL (fasting), SCr.2.6 mg/dL, MAC 123 mm, Hgb 10.1 g/dL, TC 201 mg/dL, TG 671 mg/dL, HDL 32 mg/dL, LDL unable to calculate, ACR 7.4 mg/gm, GFR 42 mL/min, and K+4.8 mmol/L. He routinely only checks BG 2× per day at a.m. and before evening Lantus, reports six to eight episodes of hypoglycemia in the past month, did not bring meter or BG log to appointment.

P.W. is not married, works a sedentary job from his home as a computer analyst, quit smoking 18 years ago, and consumes no alcohol. He complains of poor appetite and lack of energy to exercise. Dietary history revealed that he does not have regular mealtimes and may consume only two meals per day (lunch and supper).

Case Questions and Answers

1. What are the patient's possible causes of hypoglycemia?
   Answer: Inconsistent meal timing and frequency, no consistent patterns in eating, mismatch of insulin and carbohydrate amount, poor appetite, and altered pharmacokinetics of insulin with DKD
2. Since the patient did not bring a meter or SMBG records with him, what is his average blood glucose based on his A1C and would you expect this to be a true representation?
   Answer: Mean plasma glucose is 140. This is a one-time snapshot of his A1C. It would be best to longitudinally follow the A1C. With that said, patient is still in stage 3 DKD and may still have an accurate A1C reading.
3. What strategies related to carbohydrate should this patient follow?
   Answer: Based on fixed doses of insulin, the patient should follow a consistent carbohydrate meal pattern with emphasis on whole grains, fruits and low-fat dairy products.
4. Is weight loss appropriate for this patient? If so, what type of patterned diet would you recommend he follow?
   Answer: Yes, the DASH diet with a caloric restriction would be an appropriate choice for the patient at this stage.
5. What dietary protein intake would you recommend?
   Answer: Based on 0.8 g/kg/day if using actual body wt. (94.5 kg) = 76 g/day, encourage to distribute the protein throughout the day for best impact on blood glucose and satiety. Patient is encouraged to not consume more than 1.3 g/kg/day = 123 g. P.W. should be encouraged to choose plant-based protein sources that are lower in potassium.
6. What is the best treatment for P.W.'s hypoglycemia?
   Answer: Encourage 15 grams of carbohydrate from dextrose tablets, 1 tbsp. honey, ½ cup apple juice, or three hard candies.

References

1. Diabetes Canada Clinical Practice Guidelines Expert Committee. Diabetes Canada 2018 clinical practice guidelines for the prevention and management of diabetes in Canada. Can J Diabetes. 2018;42(Suppl 1):S1–S325.
2. American Diabetes Association. Standards of medical care in diabetes—2019. Diabetes Care. 2019;42(Suppl 1):S1–183.

3. Nelson RG, Knowler WC, Pettitt DJ, Saad MF, Bennett PH. Diabetic kidney disease in Pima Indians. Diabetes Care. 1993;16:335.
4. Brancati FL, Whittle JC, Whelton PK, Seidler AJ, Klag MJ. The excess incidence of diabetic end stage renal disease among blacks. A population based study of potential explanatory factors. JAMA. 1992;268:3079.
5. Smith SR, Svetky LP, Dennis VW. Racial differences in the incidence and progression of renal diseases. Kidney Int. 1991;40:815.
6. Expert Panel on Detection, Evaluation, and Treatment of High Blood Cholesterol in Adults. Executive summary of the third report of the National Cholesterol Education Program (NCEP) expert panel on detection, evaluation, and treatment of high blood cholesterol in adults (Adult Treatment Panel III). JAMA. 2001;285:2486–97.
7. Kidney Disease: Improving Global Outcomes (KDIGO) Chronic Kidney Disease Work Group. KDIGO Clinical practice guideline for the evaluation and management of chronic kidney disease. Kidney Inter. 2013;3:5–14.
8. Tuttle KR, Barkris GL, Bilous RW, Chiang JL, de Boer IH, Goldstein-Fuchs J, et al. Diabetic kidney disease: a report from the ADA consensus conference. Diabetes Care. 2014;37:2864–83.
9. Orchard TJ, Dorman JS, Maser RE, Becker DJ, Drash AL, Ellis D, et al. Prevalence and complications of IDDM by sex and duration. Pittsburg Epidemiology of Diabetes Complications Study II. Diabetes. 1990;39:116.
10. Newman DJ, Mattock MB, Dawnay AB, Kerry S, McGuire A, Yagoob M, et al. Systematic review on early albumin testing for early detection of diabetic complications. Health Technol Assess. 2005;9:iii.
11. DCCT/EDIC Research Group, Nathan DM, Zinman B, et al. Modern day clinical course of type 1 diabetes after 30 years duration: the DCCT/EDIC and Pittsburg Epidemiology of Diabetes Complications Experience (1983–2005). Arch Intern Med. 2009;169:1307.
12. Schering D, Kasten S. The link between diabetes and cardiovascular disease. J Pharm Pract. 2004;17(1):61–5.
13. Ritz E, Stefanski A. Diabetic nephropathy in type 2 diabetes. Am J Kidney Dis. 1996;27:167.
14. Adler S. Diabetic nephropathy: linking histology, cell biology and genetics. Kidney Int. 2004;66:2095.
15. Levey AS, Stevens LA, Schmid CH, Zhang YL, Castro AF III, Feldman HI, et al. CKD-EPI (Chronic Kidney disease Epidemiology Collaboration) A new equation to estimate glomerular filtration rate. Ann Intern Med. 2009;150(9):604.
16. Stevens LA, Schmid CH, Greene T, Zhang YL, Beck GJ, Froissart M, et al. Comparative performance of the CKD Epidemiology Collaboration (CKD-EPI) and the Modification of Diet in Renal Disease (MDRD) study equations for estimating GFR levels above 60 mL/min/1.73 m^2. Am J Kidney Dis. 2010;56(3):486.
17. Diabetes Control and Complications Trial Research Group. The effect of intensive treatment of diabetes on the development and progression of long-term complications in insulin-dependent diabetes mellitus. N Engl J Med. 1993;329:977–86.
18. UK Prospective Diabetes Study Group. Intensive blood-glucose control with sulphonylureas or insulin compared with conventional treatment and risk of complications in patients with type 2 diabetes (UKPDS 33). Lancet. 1998;352:837–53.
19. Ohkubo Y, Kishikawa H, Araki E, Miyata T, Isami S, Motoyoshi S, et al. Intensive insulin therapy prevents the progression of diabetic microvascular complications in Japanese patients with non-insulin-dependent diabetes mellitus: a randomized prospective 6-year study. Diabetes Res Clin Pract. 1995;28:103–17.
20. Action to Control Cardiovascular Risk in Diabetes Study Group, Gerstein HC, Miller ME, et al. Effects of intensive glucose lowering in type 2 diabetes. N Engl J Med. 2008;358:2545–59.
21. ADVANCE Collaborative Group, Patel A, MacMahon S, et al. Intensive blood glucose control and vascular outcomes in patients with type 2 diabetes. N Engl J Med. 2008;358:2560–72.
22. Duckworth W, Abraira C, Moritz T, et al. Glucose control and vascular complications in veterans with type 2 diabetes. N Engl J Med. 2009;360:129–39.
23. Diabetes Control and Complications Trial (DCCT)/Epidemiology of Diabetes Interventions and Complications (EDIC) Study Research Group. Intensive diabetes treatment and cardiovascular outcomes in type 1 diabetes: The DCCT/EDIC study 30-year follow-up. Diabetes Care. 2016;39:686–93.
24. Holman RR, Paul SK, Bethel MA, et al. 10-year follow-up of intensive glucose control in type 2 diabetes. New Engl J Med. 2008;359:1577–89.
25. UK Prospective Diabetes Study Group. Effect of intensive blood-glucose control with metformin on complications in overweight patients with type 2 diabetes (UKPDS 34). Lancet. 1998;352:854–65.
26. National Kidney Foundation. KDOQI clinical practice guideline for diabetes and CKD: 2012 update. Am J Kidney Dis. 2012;60(5):850–86.
27. American Diabetes Association. 9. Cadiovascular disease and risk management: Standards of Medical Care in diabetes – 2019. Diabetes Care. 2019;42:S103–23.
28. KDIGO Kidney Disease: Improving Global Outcomes (KDIGO) Lipid Work Group. KDIGO clinical practice guideline for lipid management in chronic kidney disease. Kidney Inter. 2013;3:259–305.
29. Kidney Disease: Improving Global Outcomes (KDIGO) Blood Pressure Work Group. KDIGO Clinical practice guideline for the management of blood pressure in chronic kidney disease. Kidney Inter. 2012;2:337–414.

30. 2017 ACC/AHA/AAPA/ABC/ACPM/AGS/APhA/ASH/ASPC/NMA/PCNA Guideline for the prevention, detection, evaluation, and management of high blood pressure in adults. J Am Coll Cardiol. 2018;71(19):e127–248. https://doi.org/10.1016/j.jacc.2017.11.006.
31. American Diabetes Association. Lifestyle Management: Standards of Medical Care in Diabetes - 2019. Diabetes Care. 2019;42 Suppl 1:S46–60.
32. Morales E, Valero MA, León M, Hernández E, Praga M. Beneficial effects of weight loss in overweight patients with chronic proteinuric nephropathies. Am J Kidney Dis. 2003;41(2):319.
33. Ross TA, Boucher JL, O'Connell BS, editors. American dietetic association guide to diabetes medical nutrition therapy and education by the Diabetes Care and Education Dietetic Practice Group. Chicago: American Dietetic Association; 2005.
34. Maggio CA, Pi-Sunyer FX. Obesity and type 2 diabetes. Endocrinol Metab Clin N Am. 2003;32:805–22.
35. Saiki A, Nagayama D, Ohhira M, Endoh K, Ohtsuka M, Koide N, et al. Effect of weight loss using formula diet on renal function in obese patients with diabetic nephropathy. Int J Obes. 2005;29(9):1115.
36. National Academy of Sciences, Institute of Medicine. Dietary reference intakes: energy, carbohydrate, fiber, fat, fatty acids cholesterol, protein, and amino acids. Washington, DC: National Academy Press; 2002.
37. Dansinger ML, Gleason JA, Griffith JL, Selker HP, Schaefer EJ. Comparison of the Atkins, Ornish, Weight Watchers and Zone diets for weight loss and heart disease risk reduction: a randomized trial. JAMA. 2005;293:43–53.
38. Unick JL, Beavers D, Jakicic JM, Kitabchi AE, Knowler WC, Wadden TA, et al. Effectiveness of lifestyle interventions for individuals with severe obesity and type 2 diabetes: results from the Look AHEAD trial. Diabetes Care [Internet]. 2011 [cited 2019 Feb 19];34(10):2152.
39. Friedman AN, Wolfe B. Is bariatric surgery an effective treatment for type ii diabetic kidney disease? Clin J Am Soc Nephrol CJASN [Internet]. 2016 [cited 2019 Feb 19];11(3):528–35.
40. Kopple JD, Chumlea W, Gassman J. Relationship between nutritional status and the glomerular filtration rate: results from the MDRD study. Kidney Int. 2000;57:1688–703.
41. Evidence-Based Nutrition Practice Guideline on Chronic Kidney Disease. July 2010. http://andevidencelibrary.com. Copyrighted by the Academy of Nutrition and Dietetics. Accessed 10 Dec 2018.
42. Ikizler TA, Burrowes J, Byham-Gray L, Campbell K, Carrero JJ, Chan W, et al. KDOQI Nutrition in CKD Guideline Work Group. KDOQI clinical practice guideline for nutrition in CKD: 2020 update. Am J Kidney Dis. 2020; in press.
43. Kamimura MA, Avesani CM, Bazanelli AP, Baria F, Draibe SA, Cuppari L. Are prediction equations reliable for estimating resting energy expenditure in chronic kidney disease patients. Nephrol Dial Transplant. 2011;26(2):544–50.
44. Byham-Gray LD, Parott JS, Peters EN, Fogerite SG, Hand RK, Ahrens S, et al. Modeling a predictive energy equation specific for maintenance hemodialysis. JPEN. 2018;42(3):587–96.
45. Kosinski C, Jornayvaz FR. Effects of ketogenic diets on cardiovascular risk factors: evidence from animal and human studies. Nutrients. 2017;9:517.
46. Hamdy O, Tasabehji MW, Elseaidy T, Tomah S, Ashrafsadeh S, Mottalib A. Fat versus carbohydrate-based energy-restricted diets for weight loss in patients with type 2 diabetes. Curr Diab Rep. 2018;18:128.
47. Feinman RD, Pogozelski WK, Astrup A, Bernstein RK, Fine EJ, Westman EC, et al. Dietary carbohydrate restriction as the first approach in diabetes management: critical review and evidence base. Nutrition. 2015;31:1–13.
48. Sainsbury E, Kizirian NV, Patridge SR, Gill T, Colagiuri S, Gibson AA. Effect of dietary carbohydrate restriction on glycemic control in adults: a systematic review and meta-analysis. Diabetes Res Clin Pract. 2018;139:239–52.
49. Westman EC, Yancy WS, Mavropoulos JC, Marquart M, McDuffie JR. The effect fo low-carbohydrate, ketogenic diet versus a low-glycemic index diet on glycemic control in type 2 diabetes mellitus. Nutr Metab. 2008;5:36.
50. Tay J, Luscombe-Marsh ND, Thompson CH, Noakes M, Buckley JD, Wittert GA, et al. A very low-carbohydrate, low-saturated fat diet for type 2 diabetes management: a randomized trial. Diabetes Care. 2014;37:2909–18.
51. Sievenpiper JL, Chan CB, Dworatzek PD, Freeze C, Williams SL. Diabetes Canada 2018 clinical practice guidelines for the prevention and management of diabetes in Canada: nutrition therapy. Can J Diabetes. 2018;42:S64–79.
52. Monnier L, Colette C. Targeting prandial hyperglycemia: how important is it and how best to do this? Curr Diab Rep. 2008;8(5):368–74.
53. Sheard NF, Clark NG, Brand-Miller JC, Franz MJ, Pi-Sunyer FX, Mayer-Davis E, Kulkarni K, Geil P. Dietary carbohydrate (amount and type) in the prevention and management of diabetes: a statement of the American Diabetes Association. Diabetes Care. 2004;27:2226–71.
54. Brand-Miller J, Hayne S, Petocz P, Colagiuri S. Low glycemic index diets in the management of diabetes: a meta-analysis of randomized controlled trials. Diabetes Care. 2003;26:2261–7.
55. Thomas DE, Elliott EJ. The use of low-glycaemic index diets in diabetes control. Br J Nutr. 2010;104:797–802.
56. Wolever TM, Gibbs AL, Mehling C, Chiasson JL, Connelly PW, Josse RG, et al. The Canadian Trial of Carbohydrates in Diabetes (CCD), a 1-y controlled trial of low-glycemic-index dietary carbohydrate in type 2 diabetes: no effect on glycated hemoglobin but reduction in C-reactive protein. Am J Clin Nutr. 2008;87:114–25.
57. Atkinson FS, Foster-Powell K, Brand-Miller JC. International tables of glycemic index and glycemic load values. Diabetes Care. 2008;31:2281–3.

58. Evert AB, Boucher JL, Cypress M, Dunbar SA, Franz MJ, Mayer-Davis EJ, et al. Nutrition therapy recommendations for management of adults with diabetes. Diabetes Care. 2014;37(Supplement 1):S120–43.
59. Nuttall FQ, Gannon MC. Metabolic response of people with type 2 diabetes to a high protein diet. Nutr Metab. 2004;1(1):6.
60. Robertson LM, Waugh N, Robertson A. Protein restriction for diabetic renal disease. Cochrane Database Syst Rev. 2007;4:CD002181.
61. Pan Y, Guo LL, Jin HM. Low-protein diet for diabetic nephropathy: a meta-analysis of randomized controlled trials. Am J Clin Nutr. 2008;88:660–6.
62. Dunkler D, Dehghan M, Teo KK, Heinze G, Gao P, Kohl M, et al. Diet and kidney disease in high risk individuals with type 2 diabetes. JAMA Intern Med. 2013;173(18):1682–92.
63. Azadbakht L, Atabak S, Esmaillzadeh A. Soy protein intake, cardio-renal indices and C-reactive protein indices, and C-reactive protein in type 2 diabetes with nephropathy: a longitudinal randomized clinical trial. Diabetes Care. 2008;31(4):648–54.
64. Sacks FM, Svetkey LP, Vollmer WM, Appel LJ, Bray GA, Harsha D, et al. Effects on blood pressure of reduced dietary sodium and the Dietary Approaches to Stop Hypertension (DASH) diet. DASH-Sodium Collaborative Research Group. N Engl J Med. 2001;344:3–10.
65. Aabadakht L, Esmaillzadeh A. Soy protein consumption and kidney related biomarkers among type 2 diabetics: a crossover randomized clinical trial. J Ren Nutr. 2009;19(6):479–86.
66. Teixeira SR, Tappenden KA, Carson L, Jones R, Prabhudesai M, Marshall WP, et al. Isolated soy protein consumption reduces urinary albumin excretion and improves the serum lipid profile n men with type 2 diabetes mellitus and nephropathy. J Nutr. 2004;134(8):1874–80.
67. Ko GJ, Kalantar-Zadeh K, Goldstein-Fuchs J, Rhee CM. Dietary approaches in the management of Diabetic patients with Kidney Disease. Nutrients. 2017;9:824. https://doi.org/10.3390/nu9080824.
68. Howard AA, Arnsten JH, Gourevitch MN. Effect of alcohol consumption on diabetes mellitus: a systematic review. Ann Intern Med. 2004;140:211–9.
69. Bantle AE, Thomas W, Bantle JP. Metabolic effects of alcohol in the form of wine in persons with type 2 diabetes mellitus. Metabolism. 2008;57:241–5.
70. Fitch C, Keim KS, Academy of Nutrition and Dietetics. Position of the academy of nutrition and dietetics: use of nutritive and nonnutritive sweeteners. J Acad Nutr Diet. 2012;112:739–58.
71. Te Morenga LA, Howatson AJ, Jones RM, Mann J. Dietary sugars and cardiometabolis risk: systematic review and meta-analysis of randomized controlled trials of the effects on blood pressure and lipids. Am J Clin Nutr. 2014;100:65–79.
72. Morenga T, Mallard S, Mann J. Dietary sugars and body weight: systematic review and meta-analyses of randomized controlled trials and cohort studies. BMJ. 2013;346:e7492.
73. Choo VL, Cozma AI, Viguiliouk E, Blanco Mejia S, Kendall CWC, de Souza RJ, et al. The effect of fructose-containing sugar on glycemic control: a systematic review and meta-analysis of controlled trisl. FASEB J. 2016;30:685.5.
74. Choo VL, Viguiliouk E, Blanco Mejia S, Cozma AI, Khan TA, Ha V, et al. Food sources of fructose-containing sugars and glycaemic control: systematic review and meta-analysis of controlled intervention studies. BMJ. 2018;363:k4644.
75. Centres for Disease Control and Prevention (CDC). Incidence of end-stage renal disease attributed to disease among persons with diagnosed diabetes – United States and Puerto Rico. 1996–2007. MMWR Morb Mortal Wkly Rep. 2010;59(42):1361.
76. Locatelli F, Pozzoni P, DelVecchio L. Renal replacement therapy in patients with diabetes and ESRD. J Am Soc Nephrol. 2004;15:S25–9.
77. Lok CE, Oliver MJ, Rothwell DM, Hux JE. The growing volume of diabetes related dialysis: a population based study. Nephrol Dial Transplant. 2004;19:3098–103.
78. Kalantar-Zadeh K, Kopple JD, Regidor DL, Jing J, Shinaberger CS, Aronovitz J, et al. A1C and survival in maintenance hemodialysis patients. Diabetes Care. 2007;30(5):1049–55.
79. Akmal M. Hemodialysis in diabetic patients. Am J Kidney Dis. 2001;38:S195–9.
80. Morioka T, Emoto M, Tabata T, Shoji T, Tahara H, Kishimoto H, et al. Glycemic control is a predictor of survival for diabetic patients on hemodialysis. Diabetes Care. 2001;24:909–13.
81. Burrowes JD, Larive B, Cockram DB, Dwyer J, Kusek JW, McLeroy S, et al. Effects of dietary intake, appetite, and eating habits on dialysis and non-dialysis treatment days in hemodialysis patients: cross-sectional results from the HEMO study. J Ren Nutr. 2003;13(3):191–8.
82. Burmeister JE, Scapini A, da Rosa MD, da Costa MG, Campos BM. Glucose added dialysis fluid prevents asymptomatic hypoglycaemia in regular hemodialysis. Nephrol Dial Transplant. 2007;22:1184–9.
83. Jackson MA, Holland MR, Nicholas J, Lodwick R, Forster D, Macdonald IA, et al. Hemodialysis-induced hypoglycemia in diabetic patients. Clin Nephrol. 2000;54:30–4.

84. Jackson MA, Holland MR, Nicholas J, Talbot M, Spencer H, Lodwick R, et al. Occult hypoglycaemia caused by hemodialysis. Clin Nephrol. 1999;51:242–7.

85. Sitter T, Sauter M. Impact of glucose in PD: saint or sinner? Perit Dial Int. 2005;25:415–25.

86. Torun D, Ogurzkurt L, Sezer S, Zumrutdal A, Singan M, Adam FU, et al. Hepatic subcapsular steatosis as a complication associated with intraperitoneal insulin treatment in diabetic peritoneal dialysis patients. Perit Dial Int. 2005;25:595–600.

87. Strid H, Simren M, Johansson A, Svedlund J, Samuelsson O, Björnsson ES. The prevalence of gastrointestinal symptoms in patients with chronic renal failure is increased and associated with impaired psychological well-being. Nephrol Dial Transplant. 2002;17:1434.

88. Yao Q, Lindholm B, Heimburger O. Peritoneal dialysis prescription for diabetic patients. Perit Dial Int. 2005;25:S76–9.

89. Liu J, Rosner MH. Lipid abnormalities associated with end-stage renal disease. Semin Dial. 2006;19:32–40.

90. Wong Y-H, Szeto C-C, Chow K-M, Leung C, Lam CW, Li PK. Rosiglitazone reduces insulin requirements and c-reactive protein levels in type 2 diabetes patients receiving peritoneal dialysis. Am J Kidney Dis. 2005;46:713–9.

91. Siew ED, Ikizler TA. Insulin resistance and protein energy metabolism in patients with advanced chronic kidney disease. Semin Dial. 2010;23(4):378–82.

92. Pupim LB, Flakoll PJ, Majchrzak KM, Aftab Guy DL, Stenvinkel P, Ikizler TA. Increased muscle protein breakdown in chronic hemodialysis patients with type 2 diabetes mellitus. Kidney Int. 2005;68:1857–65.

93. Noori N, Kopple JD. Effect of diabetes mellitus on protein-energy wasting and protein wasting in end-stage renal disease. Semin Dial. 2010;23(2):178–84.

94. Chavez EM, Taylor GW, Borrel LN, Ship JA. A longitudinal analysis of salivary flow in control subjects and older adults with type 2 diabetes. Oral Surg Oral Med Oral Pathol Oral Radiol Endod. 2000;92:281–91.

95. Moore PA, Guggenheimer J, Etzel KR, Weyant RJ, Orchard T. Type 1 diabetes mellitus, xerostomia and salivary flow rates. Oral Surg Oral Med Oral Pathol Oral Radiol Endod. 2001;92:281–91.

96. Meurman JH, Collin HL, Niskanen L, Töyry J, Alakuijala P, Keinänen S, et al. Saliva in non-insulin-dependent diabetic patients and control subjects. Oral Surg Oral Med Oral Pathol Oral Radiol Endod. 1998;86:69–76.

97. Chavez EM, Borrell LN, Taylor GW, Ship JA. A longitudinal analysis of salivary flow in control subjects and older adults with type 2 diabetes. Oral Surg Oral Med Oral Pathol Oral Radiol Endod. 2001;91:166–73.

98. Sreebny LM, Yu A, Green A, Valdini A. Xerostomia in diabetes mellitus. Diabetes Care. 1992;15:900–4.

99. Krishnasamy S, Abell TL. Diabetic gastroparesis: principles and current trends in management. Diabetes Ther. 2018;9(Suppl. 1):S1–S42.

100. Gerich JE. The importance of controlling postprandial hyperglycemia. Pract Diabetol. 2005;24:22–6.

101. Hirsch IB, Bergenstal RM, Parkin CG, Wright E Jr, Buse JB. A real-world approach to insulin therapy in primary care practice. Clin Diabetes. 2005;23:78–86.

102. Klonoff DC. Continuous glucose monitoring. Diabetes Care. 2005;28:1231–9.

103. Uhlig K, Levey AS, Sarnak MJ. Traditional cardiac risk factors in individuals and chronic kidney disease. Semin Dial. 2003;16:116–27.

104. Ansari A, Thomas S, Goldsmith D. Assessing glycemic control with diabetes and end-stage renal disease. Am J Kidney Dis. 2004;41:523–31.

105. Daugherty KK. Review of insulin therapy. J Pharm Pract. 2004;17(1):10–9.

106. American Diabetes Association. Pharmacologic approaches to glycemic treatment: standards of medical care in diabetes—2018. Diabetes Care. 2018;41(Suppl 1):S73–85.

107. Lipscombe L, Booth G, Butalia S, Dasgupta K, Eurich DT, Goldenberg R, et al. Diabetes Canada 2018 clinical practice guidelines for the prevention and management of diabetes in canada: pharmacologic management of type 2 diabetes in adults. Can J Diabetes. 2018;42:S88–S103.

108. McFarlane P, Cherney D, Gilbert R, Senior P. Diabetes Canada 2018 clinical practice guidelines for the prevention and management of diabetes in Canada: chronic kidney disease. Can J Diabetes. 2018;42:S201–9.

109. Diabetes Canada Clinical Practice Guidelines Expert Committee. Diabetes Canada 2018 clinical practice guidelines for the prevention and management of diabetes in Canada: Appendix 8 – Sick day medication list. Can J Diabetes. 2018;42(Suppl 1):S316.

110. Mak RH, DeFronzo RA. Glucose and insulin metabolism in uremia. Nephron. 1993;61:377.

111. Mak RH. Impact of end-stage renal disease and dialysis on glycemic control. Semin Dial. 2000;13:4–8.

112. Shrishrimal K, Hart P, Michota F. Managing diabetes in hemodialysis patients: observations and recommendations. Cleve Clin J Med. 2009;76(11):649–55.

113. Biesenback G, Raml A, Schmekal B, Eichbauer-Sturm G. Decreased insulin requirement in relation to GFR in nephropathy in type 1 and insulin-treated type 2 diabetic patients. Diabet Med. 2003;20:642–5.

114. Kovesdy CP, Park JC, Kalantar-Zadeh K. Glycemic control and burnt-out diabetes in ESRD. Semin Dial. 2010;23:148–56.

Chapter 12
Implications and Management of Obesity in Kidney Disease

Allon N. Friedman

Keywords Obesity · Kidney · Proteinuria · Glomerular filtration rate · Dialysis · Transplant · Bariatric surgery · Diet · Weight loss · Lifestyle intervention · Nutrition

Key Points
- A variety of anthropometric measurements can be used to estimate body fat in the kidney disease population.
- Glomerular filtration rate-estimating equations should be used cautiously in obese individuals.
- Obesity rates in patients with kidney disease and failure and kidney transplantation are increasing at least as rapidly as in the general population.
- Obesity is linked to structural, functional, hemodynamic, and molecular changes in the kidney that frequently can be reversed with weight loss.
- The pathophysiology of obesity-related kidney disease is complex and likely multifactorial.
- Reduced nephron mass may explain why only certain individuals are likely to develop obesity-related kidney disease.
- Preliminary evidence suggests that intentional weight reduction is renoprotective in people with and without preexisting kidney disease.

Introduction

The obesity crisis sweeping the globe in recent decades has not spared the chronic kidney disease (CKD) population. Of all the problems facing this ill and complex population, few have risen to the forefront with such rapidity, have the capacity to adversely influence health, and are as modifiable as obesity.

This chapter is designed to give the reader a broad familiarity with the epidemiology, basic science, and clinical aspects of obesity throughout the spectrum of CKD. Various controversies will also be addressed. In doing so, this chapter will equip the reader with a comprehensive understanding of this important and rapidly evolving area.

A. N. Friedman (✉)
Department of Medicine, Indiana University School of Medicine, Indianapolis, IN, USA
e-mail: allfried@iu.edu

© Springer Nature Switzerland AG 2020
J. D. Burrowes et al. (eds.), *Nutrition in Kidney Disease*, Nutrition and Health,
https://doi.org/10.1007/978-3-030-44858-5_12

Table 12.1 Classifying overweight and obesity according to BMI, waist circumference, and associated disease risk

Classification	BMI (kg/m²)	Obesity Class	Disease risk[a] relative to normal weight and waist circumference	
			Men ≤ 102 cm Women ≤ 88 cm	Men > 102 cm Women > 88 cm
Underweight	<18.5		–	–
Normal weight[b]	18.5–24.9		–	–
Overweight	25.0–29.9		Increased	High
Obesity	30.0–34.9	I	High	Very high
	35.0–39.9	II	Very high	Very high
Extreme obesity	≥ 40	III	Extremely high	Extremely high

Adapted from [1]

[a]Disease risk for type 2 diabetes, hypertension, and cardiovascular disease

[b]Increased waist circumference can increase risk even in persons of normal weight

Defining Obesity

The definition of "excess" body fat is somewhat arbitrary and lacks a validated threshold. While a number of techniques can be used to accurately measure body fat content and/or patterns of unhealthy fat deposition—among them neutron activation analysis, dual-energy x-ray absorptiometry (DEXA), bioelectrical impedance, air displacement plethysmography, and computed tomography—their use is typically limited to the research environment.

In clinical practice and in medical epidemiology, obesity is determined by simple measurements that "define" excess body fat in a manner that is partly derived from their associations with clinical risk (Table 12.1). Perhaps the most commonly used obesity marker in patients with CKD is the body mass index (BMI), which is defined as a ratio of weight to height (i.e., weight [kg]) divided by height [m²]). Simple to calculate and easy to employ, the BMI is a reasonably good indicator of the total body fat content in the general population as well as in chronic kidney disease and dialysis patients [1–3]. One study of 77 patients with an estimated glomerular filtration rate (eGFR) of 40 ml/min/1.73 m² found that a BMI greater than 30 kg/m² had a 100% positive predictive value for detecting obesity compared with a reference body composition method, while its negative predictive value was only 30% [2]. That is, a high BMI confirmed obesity while a lower BMI did not exclude obesity. This study highlights some of the limitations of using BMI including that it cannot distinguish lean from fat mass, peripheral from central/visceral fat, or fluid excess from fat excess. These limitations have spurred interest in alternative anthropometric measurements such as waist circumference and waist-to-hip ratio that detect excess visceral fat in a manner that the BMI does not. Visceral fat is currently considered an important causal risk factor for insulin resistance, the metabolic syndrome, and cardiovascular disease [4]. Studies suggest that these alternative metrics can add additional prognostic information in the CKD population [5–7].

In summary, commonly used anthropometric measurements have been demonstrated to provide useful information about adiposity status in kidney disease patients. However, their limitations should be kept in mind.

Measuring Kidney Parameters in Obese Individuals

The two most important clinical indicators of kidney function and health are the glomerular filtration rate (GFR) and proteinuria [8]. The GFR can be directly measured using various techniques such as plasma or urinary clearance of inulin or other exogenous markers [9]. Because direct measurement is usually too cumbersome, time consuming, and costly for routine use, most clinicians and many researchers rely on creatinine-based formulas such as the Cockroft-Gault [10], Modification of Diet in Renal Disease (MDRD) [11], and Chronic Kidney Disease Epidemiology Collaboration (CKD-EPI) [12, 13] equations to estimate GFR. However, such equations should be used with caution in individuals who are obese or whose weights are fluctuating for the following reasons: First, estimating equations work reasonably well in the populations they were derived in, but none of the equations were derived in primarily obese populations, which explains why their accuracy is reduced in that setting [14–17] or that of fluctuating weight. Second, estimating equations rely heavily on serum creatinine as an endogenous filtration marker. Serum creatinine is generated directly from muscle so the greater the muscle mass, the greater the creatinine generated. Therefore, any change in muscle mass as a result of weight gain or loss will also influence serum creatinine generation and make it difficult to differentiate changes in glomerular filtration from changes in muscle mass. An alternative endogenous filtration marker to serum creatinine in obese patients is serum cystatin C. Cystatin C is more closely associated with measured GFR than creatinine in very obese individuals [18]. However, even cystatin C may be influenced by body mass [19, 20]. Third, GFR estimating equations usually include an adjustment for body surface area in order to equalize differences in body size between individuals. This indexing strategy is based upon the observed relationship in mammals that GFR is proportional to body size [21] which is itself premised upon the fact that the kidney modifies its excretory (e.g., filtration) capabilities based upon the amount of metabolic byproducts generated by the body [22, 23]. The use of such adjustments in obese individuals presents challenges because it is lean and not fat mass that primarily generates metabolic waste so adjusting for lean *and* fat mass introduces systemic bias and error [24]. Because of these pitfalls clinical trials should ideally directly measure rather than estimate GFR or index it for body size in individuals who are gaining or losing weight [18, 25].

Proteinuria can be measured from a 24-hour urine collection or estimated from a spot urine protein to creatinine ratio. Either method is acceptable in obese individuals. However, the latter is susceptible to bias when used for serial measurements during weight change because urine creatinine is dependent upon muscle mass and will change with weight gain or loss. It will therefore be difficult to distinguish if a rise in the urine protein to creatinine ratio in an obese individual after weight loss represents a true increase in proteinuria or alternatively a reduction in urinary creatinine. In the setting of weight changes a 24-hour urine collection is therefore the preferred method of measurement.

Epidemiology and Trends in Obesity

Obesity is undoubtedly a scourge of modern society. According to the World Health Organization, in 2016, over 1.9 billion adults were overweight and 650 million of these were obese [26]. Though traditionally a problem limited to affluent Western societies, obesity is also increasingly common in underdeveloped regions of the world as they experience economic progress.

The obesity problem has also affected individuals with CKD. The prevalence of obesity in the United States adult CKD population was 44.1% during 2011–2014 [27] as compared to 37.9% in the general populace [28]. This represents a 5% increase in obesity in CKD patients compared to the preceding 12 years. Moreover, over 25% of CKD patients in this time period had class II obesity or higher.

A similar phenomenon has been observed in individuals at the time of initiating dialysis. The mean BMI of incident US dialysis patients increased steadily between 1995 and 2002 at a rate twice as steep as what was seen in the greater US population (8% vs. 4%) [29]. By 2002, nearly one-third of incident dialysis patients were obese with the fastest rate of growth occurring in patients with class II obesity

Table 12.2 Risk factors for weight gain postkidney transplant

Traditional risk factors
Younger age
Female sex
Black ethnicity
Low socioeconomic status
Preexisting obesity
Mental health
Dietary intake
Physical activity
Nontraditional risk factors
Steroid use
Number of rejection episodes
Living donor kidney transplant
Other immunosuppressive medications

Reprinted and modified with permission from [32]

or higher. Limited available data suggest that hemodialysis and peritoneal dialysis patients are equally at risk for obesity [30].

The increased prevalence of obesity extends as well to kidney transplant recipients. The prevalence of obesity as measured by BMI among kidney transplant recipients grew by 44% from 1999 to 2009 to include 33% of all patients [31]. Further major weight gain after transplantation (e.g., greater than 10 kg) is not uncommon [32].

One plausible explanation for the increase in obesity is that the growing abundance of inexpensive, calorie-dense foodstuffs combined with an increasingly sedentary lifestyle affect individuals with CKD at least as much as they do the general populace. The fact that CKD patients are limited in their physical activity may further reduce their ability to live healthier lifestyles.

It is therefore perhaps no coincidence that 47% of patients starting dialysis who also have diabetes [33] are more obese and have a steeper obesity trajectory rate than their nondiabetic peers [29]. Specific renal-related factors may also play a role. One retrospective study of weight gain in peritoneal dialysis patients suggested that absorption of glucose in the dialysate may be a predisposing factor in certain patients [34]. A number of risk factors for weight gain after kidney transplantation have been identified [32] and are shown in Table 12.2.

Of particular interest is steroid use, long known to stimulate the appetite. In fact, the influence of steroid use in weight gain is unclear [35]. While increasingly common steroid-free immunosuppressive regimens have been associated with reduced weight gain, patients still gain weight over time [36, 37].

Obesity and Clinical Risk

Normal Kidney Function and CKD Stages 1–4

The relationship between obesity and the development or progression of CKD has been intensely studied. A consensus is emerging that obesity is responsible for a large proportion of CKD in the population. Population attributable risk analyses estimate that approximately one-fifth to one-fourth of kidney disease cases could be prevented by eliminating overweight and obesity [38]. The true number is invariably higher when accounting for obesity-associated diabetes and hypertension. A population-based analysis reports that the lifetime risk of CKD is 32.5%, 37.6%, and 41% in persons who are normal weight, overweight, or obese, respectively [39].

Weight gain and/or obesity is an independent predictor for the development of proteinuria, kidney stones, acute kidney injury, and chronic kidney disease in the general population [40–46] and in higher risk groups like prehypertensive individuals [47]. These observations extend beyond ethnic or racial lines to include a variety of groups and age ranges. The risk that obesity confers is heightened by the presence of additional risk factors like elevated blood pressure, lipid, or glucose levels that in combination are known as "the metabolic syndrome" [48–50]. A high body mass index has also been linked to the progression of preexisting glomerulonephritis (i.e., IgA nephropathy) and inherited illnesses like polycystic kidney disease and nondiabetic kidney disease [51–53]. Limitations to this body of literature include residual confounding and the estimation rather than direct measurement of GFR.

Obesity is also a risk factor for progression to end-stage renal disease (ESRD), an outcome independent of biases related to estimating GFR. In a population of over 300,000 adults, a higher BMI independently predicted the development of ESRD even after adjusting for baseline blood pressure, the presence of diabetes, and other risk factors [54]. Compared to individuals with normal BMI the adjusted relative risk for ESRD was 1.87 for overweight individuals, 3.57 for individuals with a BMI of 30–34.9 kg/m², 6.12 for those with a BMI of 35–39.9 kg/m², and 7.07 for those with a BMI $\geq$40 kg/m². This relationship applies to younger individuals as well. A study of 1.2 million Israeli adolescents found that overweight and obesity were independently associated with the development of nondiabetic and especially diabetic ESRD over a 25-year mean follow-up period [55]. Interestingly, the presence of obesity at the time of initiation of dialysis has also been linked to a more rapid decline in the residual kidney function [56] as well as a family history of end-stage renal disease [57]. Whether this is due to environmental or genetic factors is not known. Finally, obesity as measured by waist-to-hip ratio independently predicts a higher risk of cardiovascular events in persons with chronic kidney disease [6] though a meta-analysis that included 510,785 patients with CKD stages 3–5 found an increasing BMI to be linked to lower risk of all-cause mortality [58].

CKD Stage 5D (ESRD)

The observation that obesity is associated with improved survival in dialysis patients is well documented. This phenomenon, sometimes known as "reverse epidemiology" or "the obesity paradox," is controversial [59–61]. A more nuanced understanding of this topic requires familiarity with the relationship between adiposity and mortality [62].

In the general populace the relationship between adiposity (as measured by BMI) and mortality is influenced by several factors including demographics, concurrent illnesses, and cause of death. For example, the risk of death from excess fat is higher in whites (vs. blacks), lower at extreme ages, and different between men and women [63]. In analyses that adjust for multiple factors, the death rates of healthy nonsmokers usually increase at either extreme of BMI although the risk is greater at higher BMI. Thus a "J-shaped" relationship between BMI and risk of death is formed [64]. In contrast, in persons who smoke or are ill, mortality risk increases equally at both ends of the spectrum (a "U-shaped" curve) with absolute risk being attenuated overall [63]. In light of these observations it should be expected that for the ESRD population, with all its complexities and multiple competing risks, the relationship between BMI and mortality may not necessarily be straightforward.

The first study analyzing the relationship between adiposity and outcomes in dialysis patients reported that a BMI of 23.3 kg/m² was associated with a 29% reduction in overall, cardiovascular, and noncardiovascular mortality when compared to a BMI of 20.4–23.3 kg/m² [65]. Since then, dozens of studies evaluating obesity risk have been performed in varied populations of hemo- and peritoneal dialysis patients using disparate markers of adiposity, though BMI remains by far the most commonly used. A meta-analysis including several hundred thousand hemodialysis patients found a protective association between a higher BMI and all-cause and cardiovascular mortality though the quality of evidence was rated as low to moderate [58]. Similar analyses in peritoneal dialysis patients are less common, tend to be smaller, and report mixed results. The largest such study included over 40,000 patients and concluded that excess adiposity did not confer an increased mortality risk, whereas having a BMI less than 18.5 kg/m² did [66]. A recent meta-analysis concurred with this finding though the evidence was considered of very low quality [58]. The largest studies of the relationship between adiposity and mortality involve mixed populations of hemodialysis and peritoneal dialysis patients. In general, they support a neutral or protective relationship between excess adiposity and death in the hemodialysis population, with less convincing results in peritoneal dialysis patients [62]. Numerous studies also find that just like in the general populace, age, sex, race, and comorbid risk factors modify the relationship between adiposity and mortality [63, 67–72].

A number of potential concerns about this literature and its conclusions should be addressed. The fact that many of the studies include patients who have already started dialysis (i.e., prevalent patients) introduces the possibility of survival bias because of the possibility that heavier subjects may have died earlier on dialysis. However, survival bias cannot explain why large studies of incident patients also find a protective effect of obesity [30, 66, 68–70, 73]. Obesity was associated with a higher risk for death on peritoneal dialysis over time in at least one study, though the hazard of death was still not especially high [66]. Incompletely accounting for known mortality risk factors such as smoking, blood pressure, and medications due to database limitations could also be a problem. Censoring patients who are transplanted or switch dialysis modalities does not always occur. Yet generally consistent results across studies make it unlikely that these factors explain why adiposity is associated with a protective effect.

Another major limitation is that BMI does not distinguish between different body compartments (e.g., fat mass and lean body mass). This important issue has been tackled in a series of epidemiological experiments. When urine creatinine excretion was used as a surrogate for muscle mass, the predominant predictor of survival was found to be increased muscle mass rather than fat mass [74] (Fig. 12.1). This finding was soon challenged by a study of over 400,000 incident dialysis patients that found no influential effect of lean mass when using equations to estimate body mass compartments [73]. Additional studies using other proxies for muscle and fat mass including serum creatinine [75], mid-arm muscle circumference [76], and triceps skin-fold thickness [76] indicate that greater muscle mass (and perhaps fat mass) has a protective effect on mortality.

Perhaps the greatest concern is that the supportive evidence for the protective effect of obesity is entirely associative in nature. No prospective studies have been performed in this field to demonstrate that weight gain is beneficial for dialysis patients or that weight loss is unhealthy. Observations that weight loss in dialysis patients is associated with higher death rates do not distinguish between intentional and unintentional weight loss [77]. Interventional studies on this topic are therefore sorely needed.

If the assumption is true that increased fat mass is healthier for dialysis patients, what could account for this? One possible explanation is that dialysis patients are unique in that they have survived years of CKD and oftentimes multiple comorbid illnesses, and may be genotypically or phenotypically different from otherwise healthy obese individuals. Additionally, obese dialysis patients have lower rates of certain risk factors such as smoking or hypertension compared to their peers with lower BMI [70, 78]. An abundance of stored fat may also serve as a well-needed reservoir of energy during acute illnesses or the wasting effects of dialysis though it is difficult to explain why severe obesity——with all its associated risks——would be more protective than being overweight or modestly obese (i.e., 28–31 kg/m²) since these states still offer plenty of energy storage [73]. A more speculative mechanism may be the influence of biologically active molecules secreted by adipocytes such as adiponectin or leptin [79].

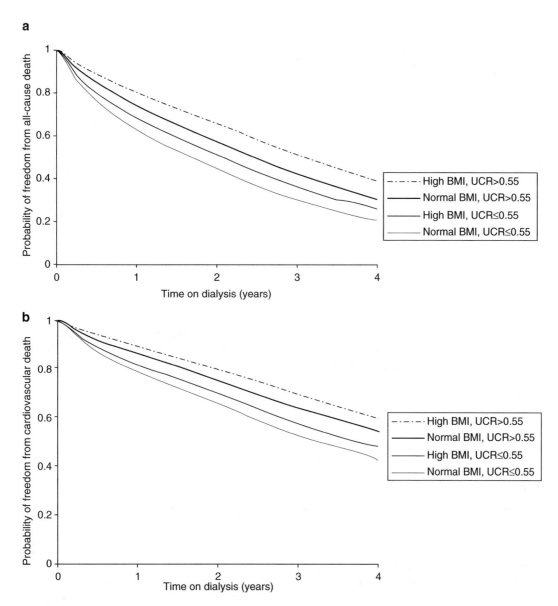

Fig. 12.1 Kaplan-Meier curves for (**a**) all-cause death and (**b**) cardiovascular death by body composition groups. BMI is categorized as normal (18.5–24.9 kg/m^2) and high (≥25 kg/m^2). UCr, 24 hr urine creatinine (g/day). (Reprinted with permission from [74])

While much attention has been focused on how obesity influences mortality in dialysis patients, there is less attention paid to how obesity could affect other important patient outcomes. This is especially true in light of the poor long-term survival in this population [33], making preservation of quality of life and avoidance of hospitalization important alternative goals. Investigators have, however, begun to study how obesity affects dialysis access. Successfully functioning dialysis accesses (e.g., arteriovenous fistulas and peritoneal dialysis catheters) are critical to the well-being of both hemodialysis and peritoneal patients. Accesses that fail to work well typically require great expenditure of resources and expose the patient to discomfort, inconvenience and risk. Whether obesity limits the successful placement and/or function of arteriovenous fistulas, which are usually formed surgically in a subcutaneous fashion in either arm, is controversial [80–82]. It is possible that only the severely obese are at risk for hemodialysis access failure because the adipose tissue physically compresses the access and impedes maturation of normal blood flow [80, 83].

Peritoneal dialysis catheters are inserted by tunneling through the abdominal wall to place the catheter tip in the peritoneal cavity. One concern is that obese individuals may suffer complications with catheter insertion or function due to excessive abdominal wall adiposity or be more predisposed to catheter tunnel infections or infectious peritonitis from an inability to perform aseptic techniques when connecting or disconnecting from the peritoneal dialysate tubing. The preponderance of data suggests that obesity confers an increased risk of catheter infections and peritonitis that could lead to catheter loss [68, 84–86]. For obese individuals in whom traditional abdominal peritoneal dialysis catheter use is not an option, alternative strategies like the use of presternal dialysis catheters exist [87].

Aside from dialysis access issues, future topics ripe for research include whether obesity adversely affects quality of life indicators, arthritis, ambulation, comfort during dialysis, mood, and hospitalization rates, among others.

Kidney Transplant Recipients

The presence of obesity in transplant candidates and recipients has important implications. Because of the concern that obesity predisposes to higher perioperative complications like wound dehiscence or infections [88–90], many transplant centers exclude individuals with BMI greater than 30 or 35 kg/m^2. In fact, the existence of obesity in a potential recipient reduces the likelihood of their receiving a kidney transplant [91]. Concern about using obese living kidney donors has also been raised because of their higher risk of developing end-stage renal disease [92].

Whether obesity at the time of transplantation negatively influences patient or allograft outcomes is hotly debated. Reports in kidney transplant recipients describe an association between a higher body mass index and a greater risk of delayed graft function, long-term renal allograft, and patient survival [89, 93–95] although others have challenged these findings [88, 90, 96–98].

Influence of Obesity on Kidney Function, Structure, and Health

The idea that obesity influences kidney health and function has existed for at least a century. In 1923, Boston practitioner William Preble published his observations that high rates of albuminuria and kidney impairment were frequent in his obese patients [99]. Subsequent reports from the 1970s onward reported an association between obesity and nephrotic syndrome that disappeared with weight loss [100–105]. Kidney biopsies in many but not all of these patients demonstrated focal segmental glomerulosclerosis but other findings include glomerular enlargement (i.e., glomerulomegaly), intraglomerular fibrin deposition, and mesangial glomerulopathy. A number of patients manifested venous hypertension likely as a result of the sleep apnea syndrome [100, 105]. From these early descriptive reports, our understanding of how obesity influences the kidney has grown to encompass a much broader variety of functional, anatomic, and molecular effects.

Kidney Mass

Kidney mass has been demonstrated to grow with weight gain and high protein diet consumption as described in animal models (see below), cross-sectional studies in children and adults, and weight loss trials [106–110]. This is generally believed to occur because the kidney adapts to growing metabolic demand.

Renal Hemodynamics

Data obtained from cross-sectional analyses and studies of (primarily) bariatric surgery-related weight loss report significant effects on renal hemodynamics. Most studies find that obesity is associated with an elevated GFR (and increase in single nephron GFR [111]), renal plasma/blood flow, and filtration fraction (i.e., glomerular filtration rate divided by renal plasma flow) when compared to controls [15, 112–118]. The idea that kidney hemodynamics, similar to kidney mass, is influenced by metabolic requirements is supported by the observation that even in the BMI range of less than 30 kg/m^2, there is a strong association between BMI and filtration fraction [119]. One research group concluded that increased glomerular filtration rate was most likely a result of greater intraglomerular hydraulic pressure caused by dilated glomerular afferent arterioles [112] from deactivation of tubuloglomerular feedback [120, 121]. Weight loss after bariatric surgery appears to reverse these renal hemodynamic changes [18, 113, 122].

Proteinuria

Along with the glomerular filtration rate, proteinuria is one of the strongest clinical markers of kidney disease with a higher level of proteinuria (or albuminuria, the most common measured fraction of proteinuria) commonly indicating kidney damage [8, 123]. A positive relationship has been demonstrated between obesity and the likelihood of urinary protein or albumin excretion that is consistent across race, sex, and ethnicity and that exists in healthy individuals as well as in patients with and without diabetes [124–128]. As with hemodynamic indices, weight loss reverses the effect on proteinuria [129].

Histologic Changes

Analyses of kidney tissue obtained under various circumstances (e.g., during gastric bypass surgery, at the time of kidney transplant implantation, or for medical diagnostic reasons) and patient populations (e.g., kidney donors, bariatric surgery patients, IgA nephropathy, or other kidney diseases) reveal common findings such as glomerulomegaly and a thickened glomerular basement membrane [130–135]. A variety of other findings, including increased glomerular planar surface area, podocyte hypertrophy, expanded mesangial matrix with or without paramesangial deposits, decreased slit diaphragm frequency, tubular atrophy, and arterial hyperplasia and sclerosis have also been observed. Focal segmental glomerular sclerosis is a rare finding, if seen at all. However, the literature in this field is limited by heterogeneity in the populations studied, selection bias in how the biopsies were obtained, the quality of biopsy samples, and the analyses performed.

Molecular Findings

RNA gene expression profiles have been measured in kidney biopsy samples from obese patients with proteinuria and glomerulomegaly with or without focal segmental glomerulosclerosis. Compared to controls, expression of a variety of key genes involved in lipid metabolism, the inflammatory cascade, and insulin homeostasis/resistance were upregulated in obese patients [136].

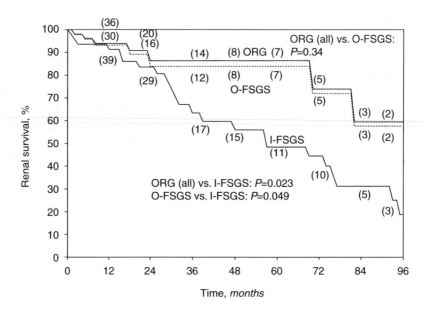

Fig. 12.2 Renal survival (endpoints defined as doubling of serum creatinine or ESRD) over time in ORG (obesity-related glomerulopathy, O-FSGS (obesity-focal segemental glomerulosclerosis), and control I-FSGS (idiopathic-focal segmental glomerulosclerosis). Analysis by the method of Kaplan and Meier with comparison by the log rank test. Symbols are as follows: (bottom solid line) I-FSGS; (top solid line) ORG (all); (dotted line) O-FSGS. ORG (all) vs. O-FSGS, $P = 0.34$; ORG (all) vs. I-FSGS, $P = 0.023$; O-FSGS vs. I-FSGS, $P = 0.049$. (Reprinted with permission from [137])

Obesity-Related Glomerulopathy and Glomerulosclerosis

First described in 2001 [137], obesity-related glomerulopathy (ORG)is a distinct entity and diagnosis of exclusion in obese individuals characterized by proteinuria, glomerulomegaly with or without glomerulosclerosis and, in some cases, a progressive decline in the kidney function [137, 138]. The precise incidence of ORG is unknown and complicated by the fact that it may be superimposed on other disease processes [138]. One center reported the prevalence of ORG to have increased ten-fold between the years 1986 and 2000 [137]. Several studies have tracked long-term outcomes of ORG [137, 139, 140]. While not as aggressive as primary focal segmental glomerulosclerosis, up to one-third of patients developed kidney failure over several years (Fig. 12.2) with the rate varying by geographic location. Of note, all studies of ORG were of limited sample size.

Animal Models of Weight Gain and Loss

The effects of obesity have been examined in several rodent models, many of which have specific genetic mutations that make them susceptible to obesity and diabetes [141–149]. The consensus is that obesity leads to increases in kidney size, blood pressure, circulating insulin and glucose, low density-lipoproteins and triglycerides, albuminuria, and an initial elevation and subsequent decline in the glomerular filtration rate. Histological changes include enlargement of the glomerular tuft area with mesangial expansion, thickening of the glomerular basement membrane, progressive glomerulosclerosis, and tubulointerstitial damage. In addition, type IV collagen and lipid deposition in the glomerulus and macrophage infiltration in the medulla are also seen. All these changes can be prevented or stopped by restricting caloric intake.

Because rodent models may have limited applicability to humans, other animal models offer additional insight. In one such model, dogs in whom obesity was induced over 24 weeks [150] developed relative hypertension, tachycardia and elevations in the glomerular filtration rate, renal plasma flow, kidney weight, and plasma glucose and insulin levels compared to controls. Similar to the rodent models the obese dogs exhibited a marked expansion of the mesangium, glomerular tuft area and Bowman's capsule space and thickening of the glomerular basement membrane. There was also upregulation of Transforming Growth Factor-β1 (TGF- β1), a marker for fibrosis. However, unlike in rodents there was no increase in glomerulosclerosis, a key indicator of irreversible kidney damage. This may represent a fundamental difference between models. A separate study reported that obese dogs had upregulation of a host of intrarenal genes related to sympathetic activation, the inflammatory response, matrix formation, angiogenesis, and endothelial dysfunction, with downregulation of genes associated with the leptin receptor and attenuation of cell survival [151].

Pathogenesis of Obesity-Related Kidney Disease

Apart from its role in promoting diabetes and hypertension, the two most common causes of end-stage renal disease [33], obesity directly damages the kidneys through several putative mechanisms that are reviewed below and shown in Fig. 12.3.

Intraglomerular Hypertension

Intraglomerular hypertension is a result of several factors. Obese individuals have increased proximal tubular sodium uptake perhaps from increased sympathetic activity [153], greater circulating angiotensin II [120], or other mechanisms. The reduced sodium load downstream deactivates tubuloglomerular feedback [121] leading to afferent arteriolar dilation, an increased filtration fraction, and direct transmission of higher (and ultimately detrimental) systemic blood pressures to the glomerulus [154]. Compounding this is a volume expanded state induced by increased proximal tubular sodium uptake [120, 154–156]. A higher glomerular filtration rate and filtration fraction increases oncotic pressure in

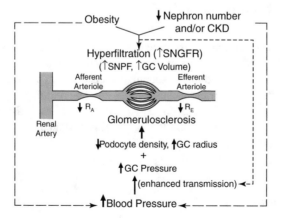

Fig. 12.3 Proposed pathogenesis of glomerulosclerosis in obesity. GC glomerular capillary, SNGFR single-nephron glomerular filtration rate, SNPF single-nephron plasma flow, RA afferent arteriolar resistance, RE efferent arteriolar resistance, CKD chronic kidney disease. (Reprinted with permission from [152])

the peritubular capillaries which in turn also promotes proximal sodium absorption [120]. Taken together, the process involves a vicious cycle that promotes structural damage within the glomerulus.

Podocyte Depletion

Podocytes help maintain the glomerular basement membrane filtration mechanism and have limited capacity for cell division and replacement [157]. Increased caloric intake stimulates glomerular hypertrophy likely through the mammalian target of rapamycin (mTOR) pathway [158, 159]. This causes a maladaptive response in which podocytes attempt but are ultimately unable to sufficiently hypertrophy to maintain the filtration barrier leading to denuded areas on the capillary loops that are a trigger for segmental glomerulosclerosis. This theory is supported by evidence showing that in humans increased glomerular volume associates with reduced podocyte density and greater foot-process width, each of which are risk factors for proteinuria [160]. Angiotension II, aldosterone, plasminogen activator inhibitor-1 (PAI-1), hyperlipidemia, and adiponectin are all upregulated in obesity and have been hypothesized to also contribute to podocyte depletion [161–165].

Nephron Endowment

The reason why only certain obese individuals develop ORG may involve nephron endowment. Individuals born with reduced nephron mass and relatively low nephron numbers, such as in the case of small-for-gestational age or preterm births, are susceptible to developing hypertension and in certain circumstances kidney disease [166]. Similarly, the presence of obesity in persons with reduced nephron mass may lead to kidney damage [167]. One line of evidence that reduced nephron endowment or mass is the key factor in the development of ORG are histological studies showing that patients with ORG have lower glomerular density, lower podocyte density and number, and increased glomerular size compared with controls [160, 168]. However, whether fewer glomeruli are a cause or consequence of ORG has not yet been definitively established.

Renin-Angiotensin-Aldosterone Axis

The deleterious renal effects of renin-aldosterone axis upregulation such as seen in obesity [169] are well established and explain why inhibitors of this axis may be effective treatments for kidney disease in overweight patients [170, 171], though not all evidence is supportive of this strategy [172]. Experimental data in animals and observational data in humans find that angiotensin II and aldosterone play an important role in obesity-related hypertension and kidney disease [173–175]. Possible mechanisms include sympathetic nerve stimulation, insulin resistance, and hemodynamic alterations that promote renal cellular toxicity and fibrosis [175, 176].

Sympathetic Activation

Obstructive sleep apnea, elevated circulating leptin levels, and hyperinsulinemia have all been postulated to cause increase sympathetic nerve activity in obesity with resultant sodium retention [153,

177]. In a dog model, kidney denervation prevented a rise in blood pressure and greatly lowered sodium retention though renal hemodynamics remain unchanged [177].

Obstructive Sleep Apnea

In addition to increased sympathetic activity, obstructive sleep apnea has been linked to obesity-related focal segmental glomerulosclerosis [100] and proteinuria [105, 178, 179], though the association is controversial [180]. One report described how initiation of BiPAP ventilation preceded the disappearance of nephrotic-range proteinuria in a patient with obesity-hypoventilation syndrome and biopsy-proven focal segmental glomerulosclerosis. A postulated mechanism involves regression of pulmonary hypertension-associated abnormalities in renal blood flow and sympathetic nerve activity.

Insulin Resistance and the Metabolic Syndrome

The importance of insulin sensitivity to proper glomerular function was highlighted using a murine model in which insulin receptors were deleted from podocytes [181]. Over time, the mice developed albuminuria and glomerulosclerosis. In humans, the link between insulin resistance, a hallmark of obesity and the metabolic syndrome, and kidney disease is primarily based on associative data [182, 183]. Indeed, it is difficult to tease out the specific effects of insulin resistance from other abnormalities that cluster in patients with the metabolic syndrome.

Lipotoxicity

Excess lipids accumulating in mesangial cells, podocytes, and tubular cells can damage cellular structural integrity and lead to maladaptive metabolic changes that contribute to kidney disease [184]. Targeting pathways involved in lipid metabolism have been shown in animal studies to limit lipid-related injury [138].

Fatty Kidney

Fat accumulation in renal sinuses has been linked to kidney disease [185, 186] perhaps through direct compression of renal parenchyma resulting in increased renal interstitial pressure, sodium reabsorption, and other adverse effects. Of note, weight loss has been shown to reduce renal sinus fat in persons without CKD [187].

Adipocyte Secretory Products

Fat cells are now understood to secrete a range of biologically active molecules some of which have been investigated for possible deleterious effects on the kidney [188]. Two of the most prominent are leptin and adiponectin. Leptin was first studied for its role in appetite and metabolic regulation but is now also understood to mediate the obesity-associated increase in blood pressure [189]. In addition, cell and animal models exposed to leptin develop glomerular endothelial cell proliferation, increased TGF-β1 secretion and glomerulosclerosis and collagen deposition within the glomerulus [190]. Adiponectin has insulin sensitizing effects and its levels are inversely associated with adipose mass [191]. Mice that cannot express adiponectin manifest increased levels of albuminuria and podocyte foot process fusion while treatment with adiponectin reverses these effects [165]. In observational studies, adiponectin is inversely correlated with proteinuria [165, 192]. A direct effect of adiponectin on podocytes is postulated to occur at least in part through stimulation of the AMP-activated protein kinase (AMPK) pathway that inhibits reactive oxygen species [193]. Whether adipokines truly mediate kidney disease or are simply an epiphenomenon remains open to debate as the available evidence is primarily based on in vitro or animal models that may not reflect human physiology. In addition, the fact that some adipokines are filtered and reabsorbed in the nephron makes it challenging to differentiate their biologic effects from those related to changes in GFR.

Strategies and Benefits of Weight Reduction

Patients with CKD who are overweight and obese have an active interest in losing weight [194]. This section will review studies that have expanded our understanding of whether weight reduction strategies offer protection against kidney disease.

Chronic Kidney Disease Stages 1–5

Strategies to lower weight include lifestyle interventions (i.e., diet and exercise), pharmacologic treatment, and bariatric surgery. Interestingly, any renoprotection provided by weight loss appears to be in large part a function of the amount of weight lost and not necessarily how weight is lost [195]. Weight loss medications are limited by dosing and other toxicities in persons with CKD as described in Table 12.3. However, certain medications that may provide kidney protection or are commonly used in patients with CKD also have weight-lowering effects such as the sodium-glucose co-transporter 2 inhibitors and the glucagon-like peptide-1 agonists [198].

Sustained weight loss is typically difficult to attain so a combination of strategies may be necessary. Several studies of lifestyle intervention with or without the use of medications in patients with moderate to advanced CKD have suggested renal and other benefits [199–201]. There are also preliminary data from secondary analyses of anorectic medications that suggest renoprotection [202, 203]. One study performed in patients mostly free of CKD stands out for its design, size and length of follow-up [201]. The Action for Health in Diabetes (Look AHEAD) randomized 5145 individuals with overweight or obesity and type 2 diabetes to an intensive lifestyle intervention or standard support and monitored weight loss over time. A secondary analysis reported that after a median of 8 years, the intensive lifestyle intervention arm had an average 4 kg greater weight loss and a 31% lower likelihood of developing very high risk CKD as compared to controls. Limitations of this study included the small proportion of patients with preexisting kidney disease and a lack of statistical power to detect hard endpoints such as development of ESRD.

Bariatric surgery, which offers more profound and sustained weight reduction than nonsurgical approaches, has also been studied for its effects on kidney health. The consensus based on several

Table 12.3 Long-term pharmacologic treatment for weight loss approved in the United States

Drug (brand name)	Mechanism of action	Common adverse effects	Kidney-related precautions	Dosing adjustment Stages 3–5 CKD	ESRD
Orlistat (Xenical, Alli)	Lipase inhibitor thus inhibiting absorption	Fecal incontinence, oily spotting, fat soluble vitamin deficiency	Reports of acute kidney injury possibly from oxalate nephropathy [196]	None	None
Phentermine/ Topiramate (Qsymia)	Sympathomimetic, anorexic	Dry mouth, constipation, parasthesias, proximal (type 2) renal tubular acidosis, calcium kidney stones	Excreted primarily via the urine	Stage 3: Lower maximum dose Stages 4–5: Avoid use	Avoid use
Buproprion-Naltrexone (Contrave)	Inhibits norepinephrine/ dopamine uptake, opioid antagonist	Nausea, constipation, dry mouth, dizziness, transient increase in blood pressure, contraindicated in uncontrolled hypertension	Excreted primarily via the urine	Low maximum dose	Avoid use
Liraglutide (Saxenda)	Glucagon-like peptide-1 agonist	Nausea/vomiting, diarrhea, anorexia	None	None (limited data – Use with caution)	None (limited data – Use with caution)

Adapted with permission from [197]
Abbreviations: *CKD* chronic kidney disease, *ESRD* end stage renal disease

observational studies is that bariatric surgery reduces the risk of a decline in eGFR and/or progression to a worse prognostic risk CKD category [204–207] (Fig. 12.4). These findings were also observed in susceptible patients with type 2 diabetes [207–209]. However, none of the studies were prospective or randomized in nature and, with only one exception, were mostly free of CKD at baseline [204]. In addition, none of the studies were adequately powered to detect differences in ESRD or mortality. Thus, while bariatric surgery looks promising as a treatment for CKD, additional information is needed to strengthen the clinical evidence, particularly when considering the potential risks. While the risks of 3-month readmission or reoperation are elevated in patients with CKD and ESRD (as is mortality in the latter group) compared to patients without kidney disease, the overall rates are low [210]. Longer-term risks including the development of hyperoxaluria, kidney stones, renal oxalosis, and irreversible kidney failure that can be observed with certain types of bariatric surgery are less well defined though appear to be uncommon [211].

End-Stage Renal Disease (Stage 5D)

Perhaps because of the "obesity paradox" there has been a reluctance to perform weight reduction trials in dialysis patients despite the demonstrated desire of such patients to lose weight [212]. Unfortunately, all weight loss medications are contraindicated in ESRD (see Table 12.3). Preliminary

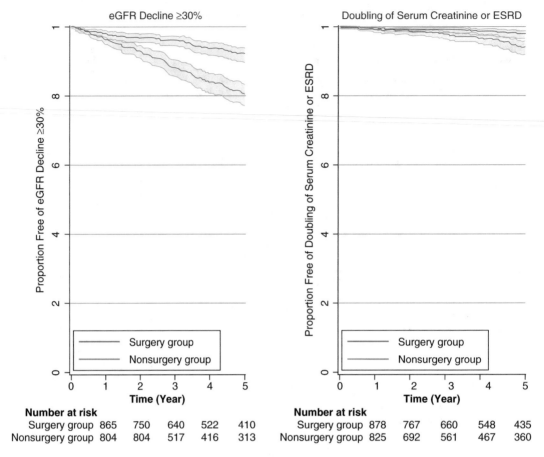

Fig. 12.4 Kaplan-Meier curves estimating time to kidney outcomes by surgery group and control group. The estimated glomerular filtration rate (eGFR) decline ≥30% outcome was defined as having a follow-up outpatient eGFR ≥30% lower than the baseline eGFR value. ESRD was defined as eGFR <15 ml/min/1.73 m^2 or treated ESRD per US Renal Data System registry. Shaded areas represent 95% confidence interval bounds. (Reprinted with permission from [205])

evidence suggests that bariatric surgery in dialysis patients offers comparable weight loss to nondialysis patients with a slightly higher risk of perioperative mortality [213]. Bariatric surgery also increases transplant eligibility in obese patients on dialysis [214, 215].

Kidney Transplant Recipients

Small uncontrolled dietary interventions in incident or prevalent transplant patients reduced weight gain postsurgery [216, 217], though a recent randomized trial was unsuccessful in doing so [218]. Weight-loss medications in kidney transplant recipients should be used cautiously due to drug-drug interactions (see Table 12.3). Pharmacokinetic analyses suggest that immunosuppressive dosing adjustment may be required after Roux-en-Y gastric bypass [219]. Bariatric surgery appears to be effective and fairly safe in inducing weight loss in transplant recipients, though the literature is limited by short follow-up, heterogeneity in the surgical interventions, and a lack of suitable comparison groups [220].

Conclusion

Evidence from laboratory research, human studies, and epidemiologic analyses confirm that the obesity crisis is arguably the largest contributor to the ongoing rise in CKD and ESRD worldwide. Future advances in this field will require further elucidation of the underlying pathophysiologic links between obesity and kidney disease and clinical trials to determine whether weight loss offers renoprotection and how best to tailor available weight loss strategies to fit the needs of individual patients.

References

1. Clinical guidelines on the identification, evaluation, and treatment of overweight and obesity in adults. Bethesda: National Institutes of Health: National Heart, Lung, and Blood Institute; 1998.
2. Agarwal R, Bills JE, Light RP. Diagnosing obesity by body mass index in chronic kidney disease: an explanation for the "obesity paradox?". Hypertension. 2010;56(5):893–900.
3. Leinig C, Pecoits-Filho R, Nascimento MM, Goncalves S, Riella MC, Martins C. Association between body mass index and body fat in chronic kidney disease stages 3 to 5, hemodialysis, and peritoneal dialysis patients. J Ren Nutr. 2008;18(5):424–9.
4. Bergman RN, Kim SP, Catalano KJ, Hsu IR, Chiu JD, Kabir M, et al. Why visceral fat is bad: mechanisms of the metabolic syndrome. Obesity (Silver Spring). 2006;14(1):16S–9S.
5. Kramer H, Shoham D, McClure LA, Durazo-Arvizu R, Howard G, Judd S, et al. Association of waist circumference and body mass index with all-cause mortality in CKD: the REGARDS (reasons for geographic and racial differences in stroke) study. Am J Kidney Dis. 2011;58(2):177–85.
6. Elsayed EF, Tighiouart H, Weiner DE, Griffith J, Salem D, Levey AS, et al. Waist-to-hip ratio and body mass index as risk factors for cardiovascular events in CKD. Am J Kidney Dis. 2008;52(1):49–57.
7. Postorino M, Marino C, Tripepi G, Zoccali C. Abdominal obesity and all-cause and cardiovascular mortality in end-stage renal disease. J Am Coll Cardiol. 2009;53(15):1265–72.
8. National Kidney Foundation. KDOQI clinical practice guidelines for chronic kidney disease: evaluation, classification and stratification. Am J Kidney Dis. 2002;39:S1–S000.
9. Jesudason DR, Clifton P. Interpreting different measures of glomerular filtration rate in obesity and weight loss: pitfalls for the clinician. Int J Obes. 2012;36(11):1421–7.
10. Cockroft D, Gault M. Prediction of creatinine clearance from serum creatinine. Nephron. 1976;16:31–41.
11. Levey AS, Bosch JP, Lewis JB, Greene T, Rogers N, Roth D. A more accurate method to estimate glomerular filtration rate from serum creatinine: a new prediction equation. Modification of diet in renal disease study group. Ann Intern Med. 1999;130(6):461–70.
12. Levey AS, Stevens LA, Schmid CH, Zhang YL, Castro AF, Feldman HI, et al. A new equation to estimate glomerular filtration rate. Ann Intern Med. 2009;150(9):604–12.
13. Inker LA, Schmid CH, Tighiouart H, Eckfeldt JH, Feldman HI, Greene T, et al. Estimating glomerular filtration rate from serum creatinine and cystatin C. N Engl J Med. 2012;367(1):20–9.
14. Verhave JC, Fesler P, Ribstein J, du Cailar G, Mimran A. Estimation of renal function in subjects with normal serum creatinine levels: influence of age and body mass index. Am J Kidney Dis. 2005;46(2):233–41.
15. Friedman AN, Strother M, Quinney SK, Hall S, Perkins SM, Brizendine EJ, et al. Measuring the glomerular filtration rate in obese individuals without overt kidney disease. Nephron Clin Pract. 2010;116(3):c224–c34.
16. Wuerzner G, Bochud M, Giusti V, Burnier M. Measurement of glomerular filtration rate in obese patients: pitfalls and potential consequences on drug therapy. Obes Facts. 2011;4(3):238–43.
17. Nair S, Mishra V, Hayden K, Lisboa PJ, Pandya B, Vinjamuri S, et al. The four-variable modification of diet in renal disease formula underestimates glomerular filtration rate in obese type 2 diabetic individuals with chronic kidney disease. Diabetologia. 2011;54(6):1304–7.
18. Friedman AN, Moe S, Fadel WF, Inman M, Mattar SG, Shihabi Z, et al. Predicting the glomerular filtration rate in bariatric surgery patients. Am J Nephrol. 2014;39(1):8–15.
19. Macdonald J, Marcora S, Jibani M, Roberts G, Kumwenda M, Glover R, et al. GFR estimation using cystatin C is not independent of body composition. Am J Kidney Dis. 2006;48(5):712–9.
20. Vupputuri S, Fox CS, Coresh J, Woodward M, Muntner P. Differential estimation of CKD using creatinine- versus cystatin C-based estimating equations by category of body mass index. Am J Kidney Dis. 2009;53(6):993–1001.
21. Edwards NA. Scaling of renal functions in mammals. Comp Biochem Physiol A Comp Physiol. 1975;52(1):63–6.

22. Friedman A. The importance of considering metabolism when indexing the glomerular filtration rate. Am J Kidney Dis. 2010;56:1218.
23. Singer MA. Of mice and men and elephants: metabolic rate sets glomerular filtration rate. Am J Kidney Dis. 2001;37(1):164–78.
24. Delanaye P, Radermecker RP, Rorive M, Depas G, Krzesinski JM. Indexing glomerular filtration rate for body surface area in obese patients is misleading: concept and example. Nephrol Dial Transplant. 2005;20(10):2024–8.
25. Chang A, Greene TH, Wang X, Kendrick C, Kramer H, Wright J, et al. The effects of weight change on glomerular filtration rate. Nephrol Dial Transplant. 2015;30(11):1870–7.
26. World Health Organization. Obesity and overweight fact sheet 2018 Available from: http://www.who.int/news-room/fact-sheets/detail/obesity-and-overweight.
27. Chang AR, Grams ME, Navaneethan SD. Bariatric surgery and kidney-related outcomes. Kidney Int Rep. 2017;2(2):261–70.
28. Flegal KM, Kruszon-Moran D, Carroll MD, Fryar CD, Ogden CL. Trends in obesity among adults in the United States, 2005 to 2014. JAMA. 2016;315(21):2284–91.
29. Kramer HJ, Saranathan A, Luke A, Durazo-Arvizu RA, Guichan C, Hou S, et al. Increasing body mass index and obesity in the incident ESRD population. J Am Soc Nephrol. 2006;17(5):1453–9.
30. Abbott KC, Glanton CW, Trespalacios FC, Oliver DK, Ortiz MI, Agodoa LY, et al. Body mass index, dialysis modality, and survival: analysis of the United States renal data system Dialysis morbidity and mortality wave II study. Kidney Int. 2004;65(2):597–605.
31. Lentine KL, Axelrod D, Abbott KC. Interpreting body composition in kidney transplantation: weighing candidate selection, prognostication, and interventional strategies to optimize health. Clin J Am Soc Nephrol. 2011;6(6):1238–40.
32. Potluri K, Hou S. Obesity in kidney transplant recipients and candidates. Am J Kidney Dis. 2010;56(1):143–56.
33. U.S. Renal Data System, USRDS 2018 Annual data report: Atlas of End-stage renal disease in the United States. Bethesda: National Institutes of Health, National Institute of Diabetes and Digestive and Kidney Diseases; 2018.
34. Jolly S, Chatatalsingh C, Bargman J, Vas S, Chu M, Oreopoulos DG. Excessive weight gain during peritoneal dialysis. Int J Artif Organs. 2001;24(4):197–202.
35. Elster EA, Leeser DB, Morrissette C, Pepek JM, Quiko A, Hale DA, et al. Obesity following kidney transplantation and steroid avoidance immunosuppression. Clin Transpl. 2008;22(3):354–9.
36. Rogers CC, Alloway RR, Buell JF, Boardman R, Alexander JW, Cardi M, et al. Body weight alterations under early corticosteroid withdrawal and chronic corticosteroid therapy with modern immunosuppression. Transplantation. 2005;80(1):26–33.
37. de Oliveira CM, Moura AE, Goncalves L, Pinheiro LS, Pinheiro FM, Esmeraldo RM. Post-transplantation weight gain: prevalence and the impact of steroid-free therapy. Transplant Proc. 2014;46(6):1735–40.
38. Wang Y, Chen X, Song Y, Caballero B, Cheskin LJ. Association between obesity and kidney disease: a systematic review and meta-analysis. Kidney Int. 2008;73(1):19–33.
39. Yarnoff BO, Hoerger TJ, Shrestha SS, Simpson SK, Burrows NR, Anderson AH, et al. Modeling the impact of obesity on the lifetime risk of chronic kidney disease in the United States using updated estimates of GFR progression from the CRIC study. PLoS One. 2018;13(10):e0205530.
40. Druml W, Metnitz B, Schaden E, Bauer P, Metnitz PG. Impact of body mass on incidence and prognosis of acute kidney injury requiring renal replacement therapy. Intensive Care Med. 2010;36(7):1221–8.
41. Ryu S, Chang Y, Woo HY, Kim SG, Kim DI, Kim WS, et al. Changes in body weight predict CKD in healthy men. J Am Soc Nephrol. 2008;19(9):1798–805.
42. Fox CS, Larson MG, Leip EP, Culleton B, Wilson PW, Levy D. Predictors of new-onset kidney disease in a community-based population. JAMA. 2004;291(7):844–50.
43. de Boer IH, Katz R, Fried LF, Ix JH, Luchsinger J, Sarnak MJ, et al. Obesity and change in estimated GFR among older adults. Am J Kidney Dis. 2009;54(6):1043–51.
44. Ejerblad E, Fored CM, Lindblad P, Fryzek J, McLaughlin JK, Nyren O. Obesity and risk for chronic renal failure. J Am Soc Nephrol. 2006;17(6):1695–702.
45. Bello AK, de Zeeuw D, El Nahas M, Brantsma AH, Bakker SJ, de Jong PE, et al. Impact of weight change on albuminuria in the general population. Nephrol Dial Transplant. 2007;22(6):1619–27.
46. Taylor EN, Stampfer MJ, Curhan GC. Obesity, weight gain, and the risk of kidney stones. JAMA. 2005;293(4):455–62.
47. Munkhaugen J, Lydersen S, Wideroe TE, Hallan S. Prehypertension, obesity, and risk of kidney disease: 20-year follow-up of the HUNT I study in Norway. Am J Kidney Dis. 2009;54(4):638–46.
48. Thomas G, Sehgal AR, Kashyap SR, Srinivas TR, Kirwan JP, Navaneethan SD. Metabolic syndrome and kidney disease: a systematic review and meta-analysis. Clin J Am Soc Nephrol. 2011;6(10):2364–73.
49. Chen J, Muntner P, Hamm LL, Jones DW, Batuman V, Fonseca V, et al. The metabolic syndrome and chronic kidney disease in U.S. adults. Ann Intern Med. 2004;140(3):167–74.

50. Yun HR, Kim H, Park JT, Chang TI, Yoo TH, Kang SW, et al. Obesity, metabolic abnormality, and progression of CKD. Am J Kidney Dis. 2018;72(3):400–10.
51. Bonnet F, Deprele C, Sassolas A, Moulin P, Alamartine E, Berthezene F, et al. Excessive body weight as a new independent risk factor for clinical and pathological progression in primary IgA nephritis. Am J Kidney Dis. 2001;37(4):720–7.
52. Othman M, Kawar B, El Nahas AM. Influence of obesity on progression of non-diabetic chronic kidney disease: a retrospective cohort study. Nephron Clin Pract. 2009;113(1):c16–23.
53. Nowak KL, You Z, Gitomer B, Brosnahan G, Torres VE, Chapman AB, et al. Overweight and obesity are predictors of progression in early autosomal dominant polycystic kidney disease. J Am Soc Nephrol. 2018;29(2):571–8.
54. Hsu CY, McCulloch CE, Iribarren C, Darbinian J, Go AS. Body mass index and risk for end-stage renal disease. Ann Intern Med. 2006;144(1):21–8.
55. Vivante A, Golan E, Tzur D, Leiba A, Tirosh A, Skorecki K, et al. Body mass index in 1.2 million adolescents and risk for end-stage renal disease. Arch Intern Med. 2012;172(21):1644–50.
56. Drechsler C, de Mutsert R, Grootendorst DC, Boeschoten EW, Krediet RT, le Cessie S, et al. Association of body mass index with decline in residual kidney function after initiation of dialysis. Am J Kidney Dis. 2009;53(6):1014–23.
57. Speckman RA, McClellan WM, Volkova NV, Jurkovitz CT, Satko SG, Schoolwerth AC, et al. Obesity is associated with family history of ESRD in incident dialysis patients. Am J Kidney Dis. 2006;48(1):50–8.
58. Ladhani M, Craig JC, Irving M, Clayton PA, Wong G. Obesity and the risk of cardiovascular and all-cause mortality in chronic kidney disease: a systematic review and meta-analysis. Nephrol Dial Transplant. 2017 Mar 1;32(3):439–49.
59. Ikizler TA. Resolved: being fat is good for dialysis patients: the Godzilla effect: pro. J Am Soc Nephrol. 2008;19(6):1059–62.
60. Stenvinkel P, Lindholm B. Resolved: being fat is good for dialysis patients: the Godzilla effect: con. J Am Soc Nephrol. 2008;19(6):1062–4.
61. Levin NW, Handelman GJ, Coresh J, Port FK, Kaysen GA. Reverse epidemiology: a confusing, confounding, and inaccurate term. Semin Dial. 2007;20(6):586–92.
62. Friedman AN. Adiposity in dialysis: good or bad? Semin Dial. 2006;19(2):136–40.
63. Calle EE, Thun MJ, Petrelli JM, Rodriguez C, Heath CW. Body-mass index and mortality in a prospective cohort of U.S. adults. N Engl J Med. 1999;341(15):1097–105.
64. Bhaskaran K, Dos-Santos-Silva I, Leon DA, Douglas IJ, Smeeth L. Association of BMI with overall and cause-specific mortality: a population-based cohort study of 3.6 million adults in the UK. Lancet Diabetes Endocrinol. 2018;6(12):944–53.
65. Degoulet P, Legrain M, Reach I, Aime F, Devries C, Rojas P, et al. Mortality risk factors in patients treated by chronic hemodialysis. Report of the diaphane collaborative study. Nephron. 1982;31(2):103–10.
66. Snyder JJ, Foley RN, Gilbertson DT, Vonesh EF, Collins AJ. Body size and outcomes on peritoneal dialysis in the United States. Kidney Int. 2003;64(5):1838–44.
67. Fleischmann E, Teal N, Dudley J, May W, Bower JD, Salahudeen AK. Influence of excess weight on mortality and hospital stay in 1346 hemodialysis patients. Kidney Int. 1999;55(4):1560–7.
68. McDonald SP, Collins JF, Johnson DW. Obesity is associated with worse peritoneal dialysis outcomes in the Australia and New Zealand patient populations. J Am Soc Nephrol. 2003;14(11):2894–901.
69. Wong JS, Port FK, Hulbert-Shearon TE, Carroll CE, Wolfe RA, Agodoa LY, et al. Survival advantage in Asian American end-stage renal disease patients. Kidney Int. 1999;55(6):2515–23.
70. Stack AG, Murthy BV, Molony DA. Survival differences between peritoneal dialysis and hemodialysis among "large" ESRD patients in the United States. Kidney Int. 2004;65(6):2398–408.
71. Ricks J, Molnar MZ, Kovesdy CP, Kopple JD, Norris KC, Mehrotra R, et al. Racial and ethnic differences in the association of body mass index and survival in maintenance hemodialysis patients. Am J Kidney Dis. 2011;58(4):574–82.
72. Hoogeveen EK, Halbesma N, Rothman KJ, Stijnen T, van Dijk S, Dekker FW, et al. Obesity and mortality risk among younger dialysis patients. Clin J Am Soc Nephrol. 2012;7(2):280–8.
73. Johansen KL, Young B, Kaysen GA, Chertow GM. Association of body size with outcomes among patients beginning dialysis. Am J Clin Nutr. 2004;80(2):324–32.
74. Beddhu S, Pappas LM, Ramkumar N, Samore M. Effects of body size and body composition on survival in hemodialysis patients. J Am Soc Nephrol. 2003;14(9):2366–72.
75. Kalantar-Zadeh K, Streja E, Kovesdy CP, Oreopoulos A, Noori N, Jing J, et al. The obesity paradox and mortality associated with surrogates of body size and muscle mass in patients receiving hemodialysis. Mayo Clin Proc. 2010;85(11):991–1001.
76. Huang CX, Tighiouart H, Beddhu S, Cheung AK, Dwyer JT, Eknoyan G, et al. Both low muscle mass and low fat are associated with higher all-cause mortality in hemodialysis patients. Kidney Int. 2010;77(7):624–9.

77. Ku E, Kopple JD, Johansen KL, McCulloch CE, Go AS, Xie D, et al. Longitudinal weight change during CKD progression and its association with subsequent mortality. Am J Kidney Dis. 2018;71(5):657–65.

78. Gregg EW, Cheng YJ, Cadwell BL, Imperatore G, Williams DE, Flegal KM, et al. Secular trends in cardiovascular disease risk factors according to body mass index in US adults. JAMA. 2005;293(15):1868–74.

79. Zoccali C, Postorino M, Marino C, Pizzini P, Cutrupi S, Tripepi G. Waist circumference modifies the relationship between the adipose tissue cytokines leptin and adiponectin and all-cause and cardiovascular mortality in haemodialysis patients. J Intern Med. 2011;269(2):172–81.

80. Chan MR, Young HN, Becker YT, Yevzlin AS. Obesity as a predictor of vascular access outcomes: analysis of the USRDS DMMS Wave II study. Semin Dial. 2008;21(3):274–9.

81. Kats M, Hawxby AM, Barker J, Allon M. Impact of obesity on arteriovenous fistula outcomes in dialysis patients. Kidney Int. 2007;71(1):39–43.

82. Weyde W, Krajewska M, Letachowicz W, Porazko T, Watorek E, Kusztal M, et al. Obesity is not an obstacle for successful autogenous arteriovenous fistula creation in haemodialysis. Nephrol Dial Transplant. 2008;23(4):1318–22.

83. Plumb TJ, Adelson AB, Groggel GC, Johanning JM, Lynch TG, Lund B. Obesity and hemodialysis vascular access failure. Am J Kidney Dis. 2007;50(3):450–4.

84. Aslam N, Bernardini J, Fried L, Piraino B. Large body mass index does not predict short-term survival in peritoneal dialysis patients. Perit Dial Int. 2002;22(2):191–6.

85. Piraino B, Bernardini J, Centa PK, Johnston JR, Sorkin MI. The effect of body weight on CAPD related infections and catheter loss. Perit Dial Int. 1991;11(1):64–8.

86. McDonald SP, Collins JF, Rumpsfeld M, Johnson DW. Obesity is a risk factor for peritonitis in the Australian and New Zealand peritoneal dialysis patient populations. Perit Dial Int. 2004;24(4):340–6.

87. Twardowski ZJ. Presternal peritoneal catheter. Adv Ren Replace Ther. 2002;9(2):125–32.

88. Johnson DW, Isbel NM, Brown AM, Kay TD, Franzen K, Hawley CM, et al. The effect of obesity on renal transplant outcomes. Transplantation. 2002;74(5):675–81.

89. Kwan JM, Hajjiri Z, Metwally A, Finn PW, Perkins DL. Effect of the obesity epidemic on kidney transplantation: obesity is independent of diabetes as a risk factor for adverse renal transplant outcomes. PLoS One. 2016;11(11):e0165712.

90. Nicoletto BB, Fonseca NK, Manfro RC, Goncalves LF, Leitao CB, Souza GC. Effects of obesity on kidney transplantation outcomes: a systematic review and meta-analysis. Transplantation. 2014;98(2):167–76.

91. Segev DL, Simpkins CE, Thompson RE, Locke JE, Warren DS, Montgomery RA. Obesity impacts access to kidney transplantation. J Am Soc Nephrol. 2008;19(2):349–55.

92. Locke JE, Reed RD, Massie A, MacLennan PA, Sawinski D, Kumar V, et al. Obesity increases the risk of end-stage renal disease among living kidney donors. Kidney Int. 2017;91(3):699–703.

93. Meier-Kriesche HU, Arndorfer JA, Kaplan B. The impact of body mass index on renal transplant outcomes: a significant independent risk factor for graft failure and patient death. Transplantation. 2002;73(1):70–4.

94. Meier-Kriesche HU, Vaghela M, Thambuganipalle R, Friedman G, Jacobs M, Kaplan B. The effect of body mass index on long-term renal allograft survival. Transplantation. 1999;68(9):1294–7.

95. Molnar MZ, Kovesdy CP, Mucsi I, Bunnapradist S, Streja E, Krishnan M, et al. Higher recipient body mass index is associated with post-transplant delayed kidney graft function. Kidney Int. 2011;80(2):218–24.

96. Glanton CW, Kao TC, Cruess D, Agodoa LY, Abbott KC. Impact of renal transplantation on survival in end-stage renal disease patients with elevated body mass index. Kidney Int. 2003;63(2):647–53.

97. Howard RJ, Thai VB, Patton PR, Hemming AW, Reed AI, Van der Werf WJ, et al. Obesity does not portend a bad outcome for kidney transplant recipients. Transplantation. 2002;73(1):53–5.

98. Kovesdy CP, Czira ME, Rudas A, Ujszaszi A, Rosivall L, Novak M, et al. Body mass index, waist circumference and mortality in kidney transplant recipients. Am J Transplant. 2010;10(12):2644–51.

99. Preble W. Obesity: observations on one thousand cases. Boston Med Surg J. 1923;188:617–21.

100. Jennette JC, Charles L, Grubb W. Glomerulomegaly and focal segmental glomerulosclerosis associated with obesity and sleep-apnea syndrome. Am J Kidney Dis. 1987;10(6):470–2.

101. Verani RR. Obesity-associated focal segmental glomerulosclerosis: pathological features of the lesion and relationship with cardiomegaly and hyperlipidemia. Am J Kidney Dis. 1992;20(6):629–34.

102. Kasiske BL, Crosson JT. Renal disease in patients with massive obesity. Arch Intern Med. 1986;146(6):1105–9.

103. Wesson DE, Kurtzman NA, Frommer JP. Massive obesity and nephrotic proteinuria with a normal renal biopsy. Nephron. 1985;40(2):235–7.

104. Warnke RA, Kempson RL. The nephrotic syndrome in massive obesity: a study by light, immunofluorescence, and electron microscopy. Arch Pathol Lab Med. 1978;102(8):431–8.

105. Weisinger JR, Kempson RL, Eldridge FL, Swenson RS. The nephrotic syndrome: a complication of massive obesity. Ann Intern Med. 1974;81(4):440–7.

106. Peters A, Bosy-Westphal A, Kubera B, Langemann D, Goele K, Later W, et al. Why doesn't the brain lose weight, when obese people diet? Obes Facts. 2011;4(2):151–7.

107. Skov AR, Toubro S, Bulow J, Krabbe K, Parving HH, Astrup A. Changes in renal function during weight loss induced by high vs low-protein low-fat diets in overweight subjects. Int J Obes Relat Metab Disord. 1999;23(11):1170–7.
108. Pantoja Zuzuarregui JR, Mallios R, Murphy J. The effect of obesity on kidney length in a healthy pediatric population. Pediatr Nephrol. 2009;24(10):2023–7.
109. Paivansalo MJ, Merikanto J, Savolainen MJ, Lilja M, Rantala AO, Kauma H, et al. Effect of hypertension, diabetes and other cardiovascular risk factors on kidney size in middle-aged adults. Clin Nephrol. 1998;50(3):161–8.
110. Johnson S, Rishi R, Andone A, Khawandi W, Al-Said J, Gletsu-Miller N, et al. Determinants and functional significance of renal parenchymal volume in adults. Clin J Am Soc Nephrol. 2011;6(1):70–6.
111. Denic A, Glassock RJ, Rule AD. Single-Nephron glomerular filtration rate in healthy adults. N Engl J Med. 2017;377(12):1203–4.
112. Chagnac A, Weinstein T, Korzets A, Ramadan E, Hirsch J, Gafter U. Glomerular hemodynamics in severe obesity. Am J Physiol Renal Physiol. 2000;278(5):F817–22.
113. Chagnac A, Weinstein T, Herman M, Hirsh J, Gafter U, Ori Y. The effects of weight loss on renal function in patients with severe obesity. J Am Soc Nephrol. 2003;14(6):1480–6.
114. Anastasio P, Spitali L, Frangiosa A, Molino D, Stellato D, Cirillo E, et al. Glomerular filtration rate in severely overweight normotensive humans. Am J Kidney Dis. 2000;35(6):1144–8.
115. Ribstein J, du Cailar G, Mimran A. Combined renal effects of overweight and hypertension. Hypertension. 1995;26(4):610–5.
116. Scaglione R, Ganguzza A, Corrao S, Parrinello G, Merlino G, Dichiara MA, et al. Central obesity and hypertension: pathophysiologic role of renal haemodynamics and function. Int J Obes Relat Metab Disord. 1995;19(6):403–9.
117. Wuerzner G, Pruijm M, Maillard M, Bovet P, Renaud C, Burnier M, et al. Marked association between obesity and glomerular hyperfiltration: a cross-sectional study in an African population. Am J Kidney Dis. 2010;56(2):303–12.
118. Janmahasatian S, Duffull SB, Chagnac A, Kirkpatrick CM, Green B. Lean body mass normalizes the effect of obesity on renal function. Br J Clin Pharmacol. 2008;65(6):964–5.
119. Bosma RJ, van der Heide JJ, Oosterop EJ, de Jong PE, Navis G. Body mass index is associated with altered renal hemodynamics in non-obese healthy subjects. Kidney Int. 2004;65(1):259–65.
120. Chagnac A, Herman M, Zingerman B, Erman A, Rozen-Zvi B, Hirsh J, et al. Obesity-induced glomerular hyperfiltration: its involvement in the pathogenesis of tubular sodium reabsorption. Nephrol Dial Transplant. 2008;23(12):3946–52.
121. Zingerman B, Herman-Edelstein M, Erman A, Bar Sheshet Itach S, Ori Y, Rozen-Zvi B, et al. Effect of acetazolamide on obesity-induced glomerular hyperfiltration: a randomized controlled trial. PLoS One. 2015;10(9):e0137163.
122. Brochner-Mortensen J, Rickers H, Balslev I. Renal function and body composition before and after intestinal bypass operation in obese patients. Scand J Clin Lab Invest. 1980;40(8):695–702.
123. Vassalotti JA, Stevens LA, Levey AS. Testing for chronic kidney disease: a position statement from the National Kidney Foundation. Am J Kidney Dis. 2007;50(2):169–80.
124. Tozawa M, Iseki K, Iseki C, Oshiro S, Ikemiya Y, Takishita S. Influence of smoking and obesity on the development of proteinuria. Kidney Int. 2002;62(3):956–62.
125. de Jong PE, Verhave JC, Pinto-Sietsma SJ, Hillege HL. Obesity and target organ damage: the kidney. Int J Obes Relat Metab Disord. 2002;26(4):S21–4.
126. Cirillo M, Senigalliesi L, Laurenzi M, Alfieri R, Stamler J, Stamler R, et al. Microalbuminuria in nondiabetic adults: relation of blood pressure, body mass index, plasma cholesterol levels, and smoking: the Gubbio population study. Arch Intern Med. 1998;158(17):1933–9.
127. Toto RD, Greene T, Hebert LA, Hiremath L, Lea JP, Lewis JB, et al. Relationship between body mass index and proteinuria in hypertensive nephrosclerosis: results from the African American study of kidney disease and hypertension (AASK) cohort. Am J Kidney Dis. 2010;56(5):896–906.
128. Kramer H, Reboussin D, Bertoni AG, Marcovina S, Lipkin E, Greenway FL, et al. Obesity and albuminuria among adults with type 2 diabetes: the look AHEAD (action for health in diabetes) study. Diabetes Care. 2009;32(5):851–3.
129. Afshinnia F, Wilt TJ, Duval S, Esmaeili A, Ibrahim HN. Weight loss and proteinuria: systematic review of clinical trials and comparative cohorts. Nephrol Dial Transplant. 2010;25(4):1173–83.
130. Tanaka M, Yamada S, Iwasaki Y, Sugishita T, Yonemoto S, Tsukamoto T, et al. Impact of obesity on IgA nephropathy: comparative ultrastructural study between obese and non-obese patients. Nephron Clin Pract. 2009;112(2):c71–8.
131. Goumenos DS, Kawar B, El Nahas M, Conti S, Wagner B, Spyropoulos C, et al. Early histological changes in the kidney of people with morbid obesity. Nephrol Dial Transplant. 2009;24(12):3732–8.
132. Serra A, Romero R, Lopez D, Navarro M, Esteve A, Perez N, et al. Renal injury in the extremely obese patients with normal renal function. Kidney Int. 2008;73(8):947–55.
133. Rea DJ, Heimbach JK, Grande JP, Textor SC, Taler SJ, Prieto M, et al. Glomerular volume and renal histology in obese and non-obese living kidney donors. Kidney Int. 2006;70(9):1636–41.

134. Alexander MP, Patel TV, Farag YM, Florez A, Rennke HG, Singh AK. Kidney pathological changes in metabolic syndrome: a cross-sectional study. Am J Kidney Dis. 2009;53(5):751–9.

135. Kato S, Nazneen A, Nakashima Y, Razzaque MS, Nishino T, Furusu A, et al. Pathological influence of obesity on renal structural changes in chronic kidney disease. Clin Exp Nephrol. 2009;13(4):332–40.

136. Wu Y, Liu Z, Xiang Z, Zeng C, Chen Z, Ma X, et al. Obesity-related glomerulopathy: insights from gene expression profiles of the glomeruli derived from renal biopsy samples. Endocrinology. 2006;147(1):44–50.

137. Kambham N, Markowitz GS, Valeri AM, Lin J, D'Agati VD. Obesity-related glomerulopathy: an emerging epidemic. Kidney Int. 2001;59(4):1498–509.

138. D'Agati VD, Chagnac A, de Vries AP, Levi M, Porrini E, Herman-Edelstein M, et al. Obesity-related glomerulopathy: clinical and pathologic characteristics and pathogenesis. Nat Rev Nephrol. 2016;12(8):453–71.

139. Praga M, Hernandez E, Morales E, Campos AP, Valero MA, Martinez MA, et al. Clinical features and long-term outcome of obesity-associated focal segmental glomerulosclerosis. Nephrol Dial Transplant. 2001;16(9):1790–8.

140. Tsuboi N, Koike K, Hirano K, Utsunomiya Y, Kawamura T, Hosoya T. Clinical features and long-term renal outcomes of Japanese patients with obesity-related glomerulopathy. Clin Exp Nephrol. 2013;17(3):379–85.

141. Maddox DA, Alavi FK, Santella RN, Zawada ET Jr. Prevention of obesity-linked renal disease: age-dependent effects of dietary food restriction. Kidney Int. 2002;62(1):208–19.

142. Gades MD, Van Goor H, Kaysen GA, Johnson PR, Horwitz BA, Stern JS. Brief periods of hyperphagia cause renal injury in the obese Zucker rat. Kidney Int. 1999;56(5):1779–87.

143. Kasiske BL, Cleary MP, O'Donnell MP, Keane WF. Effects of carbohydrate restriction on renal injury in the obese Zucker rat. Am J Clin Nutr. 1986;44(1):56–65.

144. Alavi FK, Zawada ET, Hoff KK. Renal hemodynamic effects of chronic ketorolac tromethamine treatment in aged lean and obese Zucker rats. Clin Nephrol. 1995;43(5):318–23.

145. Kasiske BL, Cleary MP, O'Donnell MP, Keane WF. Effects of genetic obesity on renal structure and function in the Zucker rat. J Lab Clin Med. 1985;106(5):598–604.

146. Coimbra TM, Janssen U, Grone HJ, Ostendorf T, Kunter U, Schmidt H, et al. Early events leading to renal injury in obese Zucker (fatty) rats with type II diabetes. Kidney Int. 2000;57(1):167–82.

147. Johnson PR, Stern JS, Horwitz BA, Harris RE, Greene SF. Longevity in obese and lean male and female rats of the Zucker strain: prevention of hyperphagia. Am J Clin Nutr. 1997;66(4):890–903.

148. Stern JS, Gades MD, Wheeldon CM, Borchers AT. Calorie restriction in obesity: prevention of kidney disease in rodents. J Nutr. 2001;131(3):913S–7S.

149. Keenan KP, Coleman JB, McCoy CL, Hoe CM, Soper KA, Laroque P. Chronic nephropathy in ad libitum over-fed Sprague-Dawley rats and its early attenuation by increasing degrees of dietary (caloric) restriction to control growth. Toxicol Pathol. 2000;28(6):788–98.

150. Henegar JR, Bigler SA, Henegar LK, Tyagi SC, Hall JE. Functional and structural changes in the kidney in the early stages of obesity. J Am Soc Nephrol. 2001;12(6):1211–7.

151. Gu JW, Wang J, Stockton A, Lokitz B, Henegar L, Hall JE. Cytokine gene expression profiles in kidney medulla and cortex of obese hypertensive dogs. Kidney Int. 2004;66(2):713–21.

152. Karen A, Griffin HK, Bidani AK. Adverse renal consequences of obesity. Am J Physiol Renal Physiol. 2008;294(4) https://doi.org/10.1152/ajprenal.00324.2007.

153. Esler M, Straznicky N, Eikelis N, Masuo K, Lambert G, Lambert E. Mechanisms of sympathetic activation in obesity-related hypertension. Hypertension. 2006;48(5):787–96.

154. Griffin KA, Kramer H, Bidani AK. Adverse renal consequences of obesity. Am J Physiol Renal Physiol. 2008;294(4):F685–96.

155. Fu Y, Hall JE, Lu D, Lin L, Manning RD Jr, Cheng L, et al. Aldosterone blunts Tubuloglomerular feedback by activating Macula Densa mineralocorticoid receptors. Hypertension. 2012 Mar;59(3):599–606.

156. Shah S, Hussain T. Enhanced angiotensin II-induced activation of Na+, K+-ATPase in the proximal tubules of obese Zucker rats. Clin Exp Hypertens. 2006;28(1):29–40.

157. Shankland SJ. The podocyte's response to injury: role in proteinuria and glomerulosclerosis. Kidney Int. 2006;69(12):2131–47.

158. Wiggins JE, Goyal M, Sanden SK, Wharram BL, Shedden KA, Misek DE, et al. Podocyte hypertrophy, "adaptation," and "decompensation" associated with glomerular enlargement and glomerulosclerosis in the aging rat: prevention by calorie restriction. J Am Soc Nephrol. 2005;16(10):2953–66.

159. Fukuda A, Chowdhury MA, Venkatareddy MP, Wang SQ, Nishizono R, Suzuki T, et al. Growth-dependent podocyte failure causes glomerulosclerosis. J Am Soc Nephrol. 2012;23(8):1351–63.

160. Chen HM, Liu ZH, Zeng CH, Li SJ, Wang QW, Li LS. Podocyte lesions in patients with obesity-related glomerulopathy. Am J Kidney Dis. 2006;48(5):772–9.

161. Nagase M, Shibata S, Yoshida S, Nagase T, Gotoda T, Fujita T. Podocyte injury underlies the glomerulopathy of Dahl salt-hypertensive rats and is reversed by aldosterone blocker. Hypertension. 2006;47(6):1084–93.

162. Liang X, Kanjanabuch T, Mao SL, Hao CM, Tang YW, Declerck PJ, et al. Plasminogen activator inhibitor-1 modulates adipocyte differentiation. Am J Physiol Endocrinol Metab. 2006;290(1):E103–E13.
163. Deji N, Kume S, Araki S, Soumura M, Sugimoto T, Isshiki K, et al. Structural and functional changes in the kidneys of high-fat diet-induced obese mice. Am J Physiol Renal Physiol. 2009;296(1):F118–26.
164. Gloy J, Henger A, Fischer KG, Nitschke R, Mundel P, Bleich M, et al. Angiotensin II depolarizes podocytes in the intact glomerulus of the rat. J Clin Invest. 1997;99(11):2772–81.
165. Sharma K, Ramachandrarao S, Qiu G, Usui HK, Zhu Y, Dunn SR, et al. Adiponectin regulates albuminuria and podocyte function in mice. J Clin Invest. 2008;118(5):1645–56.
166. Abitbol CL, Ingelfinger JR. Nephron mass and cardiovascular and renal disease risks. Semin Nephrol. 2009;29(4):445–54.
167. Praga M. Synergy of low nephron number and obesity: a new focus on hyperfiltration nephropathy. Nephrol Dial Transplant. 2005;20(12):2594–7.
168. Tsuboi N, Utsunomiya Y, Kanzaki G, Koike K, Ikegami M, Kawamura T, et al. Low glomerular density with glomerulomegaly in obesity-related glomerulopathy. Clin J Am Soc Nephrol. 2012;7(5):735–41.
169. Tuck ML, Sowers J, Dornfeld L, Kledzik G, Maxwell M. The effect of weight reduction on blood pressure, plasma renin activity, and plasma aldosterone levels in obese patients. N Engl J Med. 1981;304(16):930–3.
170. Praga M, Hernandez E, Andres A, Leon M, Ruilope LM, Rodicio JL. Effects of body-weight loss and captopril treatment on proteinuria associated with obesity. Nephron. 1995;70(1):35–41.
171. Mallamaci F, Ruggenenti P, Perna A, Leonardis D, Tripepi R, Tripepi G, et al. ACE inhibition is renoprotective among obese patients with proteinuria. J Am Soc Nephrol. 2011;22(6):1122–8.
172. Cohen JB, Stephens-Shields AJ, Denburg MR, Anderson AH, Townsend RR, Reese PP. Obesity, renin-angiotensin system blockade and risk of adverse renal outcomes: a population-based cohort study. Am J Nephrol. 2016;43(6):431–40.
173. de Paula RB, da Silva AA, Hall JE. Aldosterone antagonism attenuates obesity-induced hypertension and glomerular hyperfiltration. Hypertension. 2004;43(1):41–7.
174. Ahmed SB, Fisher ND, Stevanovic R, Hollenberg NK. Body mass index and angiotensin-dependent control of the renal circulation in healthy humans. Hypertension. 2005;46(6):1316–20.
175. Ruster C, Wolf G. Renin-angiotensin-aldosterone system and progression of renal disease. J Am Soc Nephrol. 2006;17(11):2985–91.
176. Cohen JB. Hypertension in obesity and the impact of weight loss. Curr Cardiol Rep. 2017;19(10):98.
177. Kassab S, Kato T, Wilkins FC, Chen R, Hall JE, Granger JP. Renal denervation attenuates the sodium retention and hypertension associated with obesity. Hypertension. 1995;25(4 Pt 2):893–7.
178. Sklar AH, Chaudhary BA. Reversible proteinuria in obstructive sleep apnea syndrome. Arch Intern Med. 1988;148(1):87–9.
179. Hall IE, Kashgarian M, Moeckel GW, Dahl NK. Resolution of proteinuria in a patient with focal segmental glomerulosclerosis following BiPAP initiation for obesity hypoventilation syndrome. Clin Nephrol. 2012;77(1):62–5.
180. Casserly LF, Chow N, Ali S, Gottlieb DJ, Epstein LJ, Kaufman JS. Proteinuria in obstructive sleep apnea. Kidney Int. 2001;60(4):1484–9.
181. Welsh GI, Hale LJ, Eremina V, Jeansson M, Maezawa Y, Lennon R, et al. Insulin signaling to the glomerular podocyte is critical for normal kidney function. Cell Metab. 2010;12(4):329–40.
182. Kincaid-Smith P. Hypothesis: obesity and the insulin resistance syndrome play a major role in end-stage renal failure attributed to hypertension and labelled 'hypertensive nephrosclerosis'. J Hypertens. 2004;22(6):1051–5.
183. Dengel DR, Goldberg AP, Mayuga RS, Kairis GM, Weir MR. Insulin resistance, elevated glomerular filtration fraction, and renal injury. Hypertension. 1996;28(1):127–32.
184. de Vries AP, Ruggenenti P, Ruan XZ, Praga M, Cruzado JM, Bajema IM, et al. Fatty kidney: emerging role of ectopic lipid in obesity-related renal disease. Lancet Diabetes Endocrinol. 2014;2(5):417–26.
185. Dwyer TM, Mizelle HL, Cockrell K, Buhner P. Renal sinus lipomatosis and body composition in hypertensive, obese rabbits. Int J Obes Relat Metab Disord. 1995;19(12):869–74.
186. Foster MC, Hwang SJ, Porter SA, Massaro JM, Hoffmann U, Fox CS. Fatty kidney, hypertension, and chronic kidney disease: the Framingham heart study. Hypertension. 2011;58(5):784–90.
187. Zelicha H, Schwarzfuchs D, Shelef I, Gepner Y, Tsaban G, Tene L, et al. Changes of renal sinus fat and renal parenchymal fat during an 18-month randomized weight loss trial. Clin Nutr. 2018;37(4):1145–53.
188. Briffa JF, McAinch AJ, Poronnik P, Hryciw DH. Adipokines as a link between obesity and chronic kidney disease. Am J Physiol Renal Physiol. 2013;305(12):F1629–36.
189. Simonds SE, Pryor JT, Ravussin E, Greenway FL, Dileone R, Allen AM, et al. Leptin mediates the increase in blood pressure associated with obesity. Cell. 2014;159(6):1404–16.
190. Wolf G, Chen S, Han DC, Ziyadeh FN. Leptin and renal disease. Am J Kidney Dis. 2002;39(1):1–11.
191. Goldstein BJ, Scalia R. Adiponectin: a novel adipokine linking adipocytes and vascular function. J Clin Endocrinol Metab. 2004;89(6):2563–8.

192. Tsioufis C, Dimitriadis K, Chatzis D, Vasiliadou C, Tousoulis D, Papademetriou V, et al. Relation of microalbuminuria to adiponectin and augmented C-reactive protein levels in men with essential hypertension. Am J Cardiol. 2005;96(7):946–51.

193. Ix J, Sharma K. Mechanisms linking obesity, chornic kidney disease, and fatty liver disease: the roles of fetuin-a, adiponectin, and AMPK. J Am Soc Nephrol. 2010;21:406–12.

194. Navaneethan S, Kirwan J, Arrigain S, Schreiber M, Sehgal A, Schold S. Overweight, obesity and intentional weight loss in chronic kidney disease: NHANES. Int J Obes. 1999-2006;2012:1–6.

195. Neff KJ, Elliott JA, Corteville C, Abegg K, Boza C, Lutz TA, et al. Effect of roux-en-Y gastric bypass and diet-induced weight loss on diabetic kidney disease in the Zucker diabetic fatty rat. Surg Obes Relat Dis. 2017;13(1):21–7.

196. Weir MA, Beyea MM, Gomes T, Juurlink DN, Mamdani M, Blake PG, et al. Orlistat and acute kidney injury: an analysis of 953 patients. Arch Intern Med. 2011;171(7):703–4.

197. Kramer H, Tuttle KR, Leehey D, Luke A, Durazo-Arvizu R, Shoham D, et al. Obesity management in adults with CKD. Am J Kidney Dis. 2009;53(1):151–65.

198. Apovian CM, Okemah J, O'Neil PM. Body weight considerations in the management of type 2 diabetes. Adv Ther. 2018;36:44–58.

199. MacLaughlin HL, Cook SA, Kariyawasam D, Roseke M, van Niekerk M, Macdougall IC. Nonrandomized trial of weight loss with orlistat, nutrition education, diet, and exercise in obese patients with CKD: 2-year follow-up. Am J Kidney Dis. 2010;55(1):69–76.

200. Friedman A, Chambers M, Kamendulis L, Temmerman J. Short-term changes following a weight reduction intervention in advanced diabetic nephropathy. Clin J Am Soc Nephrol. 2013;8:1892–8.

201. Look AHEAD Research Group. Effect of a long-term behavioural weight loss intervention on nephropathy in overweight or obese adults with type 2 diabetes: a secondary analysis of the look AHEAD randomised clinical trial. Lancet Diabetes Endocrinol. 2014;2(10):801–9.

202. Scirica BM, Bohula EA, Dwyer JP, Qamar A, Inzucchi SE, McGuire DK, et al. Lorcaserin and renal outcomes in obese and overweight patients in the CAMELLIA-TIMI 61 trial. Circulation. 2019;139(3):366–75.

203. Mann JFE, Orsted DD, Brown-Frandsen K, Marso SP, Poulter NR, Rasmussen S, et al. Liraglutide and renal outcomes in type 2 diabetes. N Engl J Med. 2017;377(9):839–48.

204. Imam TH, Fischer H, Jing B, Burchette R, Henry S, DeRose SF, et al. Estimated GFR before and after bariatric surgery in CKD. Am J Kidney Dis. 2017;69(3):380–8.

205. Chang AR, Chen Y, Still C, Wood GC, Kirchner HL, Lewis M, et al. Bariatric surgery is associated with improvement in kidney outcomes. Kidney Int. 2016;90(1):164–71.

206. Friedman AN, Wahed AS, Wang J, Courcoulas AP, Dakin G, Hinojosa MW, et al. Effect of bariatric surgery on CKD risk. J Am Soc Nephrol. 2018;29(4):1289–300.

207. Shulman A, Peltonen M, Sjostrom CD, Andersson-Assarsson JC, Taube M, Sjoholm K, et al. Incidence of end-stage renal disease following bariatric surgery in the Swedish Obese Subjects Study. Int J Obes. 2018;42(5):964–73.

208. Friedman AN, Wolfe B. Is bariatric surgery an effective treatment for type II diabetic kidney disease? Clin J Am Soc Nephrol. 2016;11(3):528–35.

209. O'Brien R, Johnson E, Haneuse S, Coleman KJ, O'Connor PJ, Fisher DP, et al. Microvascular outcomes in patients with diabetes after bariatric surgery versus usual care: a matched Cohort Study. Ann Intern Med. 2018;169(5):300–10.

210. Cohen JB, Tewksbury CM, Torres Landa S, Williams NN, Dumon KR. National postoperative bariatric surgery outcomes in patients with chronic kidney disease and end-stage kidney disease. Obes Surg. 2019 Mar;29(3):975–82.

211. Nasr SH, D'Agati VD, Said SM, Stokes MB, Largoza MV, Radhakrishnan J, et al. Oxalate nephropathy complicating roux-en-Y gastric bypass: an underrecognized cause of irreversible renal failure. Clin J Am Soc Nephrol. 2008;3(6):1676–83.

212. Saeed Z, Janda KM, Tucker BM, Dudley L, Cutter P, Friedman AN. Personal attitudes toward weight in overweight and obese us hemodialysis patients. J Ren Nutr. 2017;27(5):340–5.

213. Modanlou KA, Muthyala U, Xiao H, Schnitzler MA, Salvalaggio PR, Brennan DC, et al. Bariatric surgery among kidney transplant candidates and recipients: analysis of the United States renal data system and literature review. Transplantation. 2009;87(8):1167–73.

214. Takata MC, Campos GM, Ciovica R, Rabl C, Rogers SJ, Cello JP, et al. Laparoscopic bariatric surgery improves candidacy in morbidly obese patients awaiting transplantation. Surg Obes Relat Dis. 2008;4(2):159–64; discussion 64-5

215. Al-Bahri S, Fakhry TK, Gonzalvo JP, Murr MM. Bariatric surgery as a bridge to renal transplantation in patients with end-stage renal disease. Obes Surg. 2017;27(11):2951–5.

216. Jezior D, Krajewska M, Madziarska K, Regulska-Ilow B, Ilow R, Janczak D, et al. Weight reduction in renal transplant recipients program: the first successes. Transplant Proc. 2007;39(9):2769–71.

217. Patel MG. The effect of dietary intervention on weight gains after renal transplantation. J Ren Nutr. 1998;8(3):137–41.
218. Henggeler CK, Plank LD, Ryan KJ, Gilchrist EL, Casas JM, Lloyd LE, et al. A randomized controlled trial of an intensive nutrition intervention versus standard nutrition care to avoid excess weight gain after kidney transplantation: the intent trial. J Ren Nutr. 2018;28(5):340–51.
219. Rogers CC, Alloway RR, Alexander JW, Cardi M, Trofe J, Vinks AA. Pharmacokinetics of mycophenolic acid, tacrolimus and sirolimus after gastric bypass surgery in end-stage renal disease and transplant patients: a pilot study. Clin Transpl. 2008;22(3):281–91.
220. Hadjievangelou N, Kulendran M, McGlone ER, Reddy M, Khan OA. Is bariatric surgery in patients following renal transplantation safe and effective? A best evidence topic. Int J Surg. 2016;28:191–5.

Chapter 13
Nutritional Management of Cardiovascular Disease

Judith A. Beto, Vinod K. Bansal, and Wendy E. Ramirez

Keywords Cardiovascular disease · Chronic kidney disease · Dyslipidemia · Diet · Exercise · Lifestyle modifications · Medical nutrition therapy · Nutrition · Pharmacological intervention · Physical activity Statin therapy

---

Key Points
- Define cardiovascular disease (CVD) in chronic kidney disease (CKD) from a pathophysiological and metabolic perspective
- Review current clinical practice guidelines, evidence-based literature, and peer-reviewed recommendations
- Identify key assessment and intervention strategies in the nutritional management of CVD in CKD
- Outline parameters of lifestyle adaptations, dietary modifications, and pharmacological strategies to achieve CVD risk reduction in CKD

Introduction

The National Kidney Foundation's Kidney Disease Outcome Quality Initiative (KDOQI) and Kidney Disease: Improving Global Outcomes (KDIGO) have produced a cohort of clinical practice guidelines directed toward improving the quality and breadth of care given to patients with chronic kidney disease (CKD) [1]. The 2012 Update of KDOQI Clinical Practice Guideline for Evaluation and Management of CKD continues the definition and stratification of stages 1–5 of kidney disease using estimated glomerular filtration rate (GFR) [2]. This classification system reinforces clinical focus from patients near or at kidney failure (stage 5 requiring renal replacement therapy such as hemodialysis or transplantation) to earlier clinical intervention during stages 1–4 which might delay or retard progression. By applying this classification system to existing population surveys, it is now

J. A. Beto (✉)
Division of Nephrology and Hypertension, Department of Medicine, Loyola University Healthcare, Maywood, IL, USA
e-mail: judithbeto@comcast.net

V. K. Bansal
Division of Nephrology and Hypertension, Department of Medicine, Loyola University Healthcare, Maywood, IL, USA

W. E. Ramirez
Evergreen Health Medical Center, Pharmacy, Kirkland, WA, USA

© Springer Nature Switzerland AG 2020
J. D. Burrowes et al. (eds.), *Nutrition in Kidney Disease*, Nutrition and Health, https://doi.org/10.1007/978-3-030-44858-5_13

conservatively estimated that more than 30 million Americans (one out of seven adults) have some risk factors for CKD [3].

Both CKD and cardiovascular disease (CVD) share common risk factors including obesity, dyslipidemia, sedentary lifestyle, inadequate blood pressure and diabetes control, and multiple dietary factors [4]. Recent analyses have suggested more than a 100% increase in CVD prevalence compared to the general population (65.8% in CKD vs. 31.9% in non-CKD), even when matching for gender, race, age, and other confounding risk factors. Stroke risk is estimated to be more than 3x greater compared to the non-CKD population. Atrial fibrillation also continues to rise in CKD stage 5 particularly among older patients and those on dialysis longer. Heart failure continues to rise as well in conjunction with the aging population [5]. The Healthy People Initiative 2020, coordinated by the United States Department of Health and Human Services, stated a key priority to reduce new cases of CKD and its complications (disability, death, economic costs) using screening, education, and management activities [6].

Population screening for CKD risk factors continues on a nationwide basis in the United States. The screening also addresses CVD risk factors such as hypertension, elevated blood glucose, and obesity. These initiatives include the National Kidney Foundation's Kidney Early Evaluation Program (KEEP), the American Kidney Fund's Know Your Kidneys program, and the National Institute of Diabetes and Digestive and Kidney Disease's National Kidney Disease Education Program (NKDEP) [7–9]. This chapter will focus on the nutritional management of CVD in adults with stages 1–5 CKD with emphasis on dietary composition.

Pathophysiology

The pathophysiological scope of CVD is broad. These include any change in cardiovascular health that would increase the risk for CVD events such as stroke (cerebrovascular disease), coronary heart disease, heart failure, disorders of heart rhythm, atherosclerotic cardiovascular disease, acute coronary syndrome, angina, myocardial infarction, transient ischemic attack, peripheral artery disease, and/or angina. Promoting and achieving optimal cardiovascular health will lower the prevalence and improve prognosis of CVD events. The American Heart Association has focused on seven core health behaviors/factors to reduce the CVD risk, many of which are discussed in greater detail in other chapters: smoking, physical activity (see Chap. 30), diet, weight (see Chap. 12), cholesterol, blood pressure (see Chap. 10), and glucose control (see Chap. 11) [4, 10]. Nutritional management of CVD integrates all of these factors.

Lipid Metabolism

Although elevated serum cholesterol has received the most attention over time in public education programs, an understanding of lipid metabolism is important. Dyslipidemia is defined as elevated serum levels of lipid components in the blood: total cholesterol (TC), high-density lipoproteins (HDL), low-density lipoproteins (LDL), and other lipid particles such as triglycerides [11]. Abnormal lipid profiles are seen in kidney function impairment and particularly in protein-losing nephropathies such as nephrotic syndrome [12].

Lipid metabolism, specifically cholesterol synthesis, takes place in the liver. The liver produces bile which is the primary lipid-reducing agent stored in the gallbladder. Cholesterol can be synthesized in the liver; it can be removed from circulating lipoproteins, and it can also be directly absorbed from the small intestine from cholesterol secreted in the bile or from dietary cholesterol. Excess circulating cholesterol results in hyperlipidemia. Individual variation in lipid response comprises differences in absorption or biosynthesis of primary and receptor-mediated lipid products that may or may not be CKD related. Chronic elevation may lead to deposits on inner arterial walls (fatty plaque) resulting in accumulation and atherosclerosis.

The process of reverse cholesterol transport also exists whereby cholesterol may be removed from areas of lipid accumulation and returned to circulation. The exact mechanisms responsible, however, are still being understood. HDL, as the primary carrier, transports cholesterol back to the liver where it is either reused or excreted. This metabolic process uses a cohort of enzymes and protein pathways to decrease monocyte penetration of wall sites. Macrophages attract oxidized LDL, which appears to increase inflammatory effects [11].

Serum triglycerides, represented primarily as chylomicrons, move into the lymphatic system. From this point, they enter directly into blood circulation at the internal jugular and subclavian vein junction. The exact role of triglycerides in the CVD process is still evolving [13].

Other Metabolic Factors

There are several additional CVD contributing factors in CKD including vascular calcification, homocysteine metabolism abnormalities, and inflammation. These factors often develop early in CKD and are known to be present in the general population as well. The independent and interdependent relationships remain under clinical investigation.

The role of calcification and development of atherosclerotic lesions within the context of bone and mineral metabolism in CKD is discussed in detail in Chap. 23. Homocysteinemia is another risk factor present in CKD. Serum levels increase as much as 30–50% in later stages of CKD and may respond to oral folic acid supplementation of 5–10 mg/d. However, no evidence exists for long term cardioprotective effect with supplementation. Chronic inflammation is a known CVD risk factor but the specific role in reducing CKD has not been defined. Numerous mathermatical formulas have been developed to grade risk (i.e., malnutrition-inflammation index) but there is lack of clinical intervention evidence to support CVD abatement [14, 15].

Existing Clinical Practice Guidelines and Peer-Reviewed Recommendations

The National Cholesterol Education Program has published recommended parameters for fasting serum lipids for non-CKD adults [16]. The American Heart Association, in their most recent updated cholesterol guidelines, assigns a GFR of >60 ml/min/1.73 m^2 as normal risk category, and GFR of 15–59 ml/min/1.73 m^2 as high-risk category, regardless of fasting serum values. The emphasis is now on more customized CVD risk assessments and interventions based on individual characteristics such as age, gender, dialysis vintage, and presence of comorbidities (e.g., hypertension and diabetes), and motivation. Algorithms can be downloaded to guide clinical practice choices based on published guidelines [10].

The 2016 updated KDOQI lipid commentary suggests that all CKD patients should be managed as high CVD risk using existing lipid guidelines for non-CKD high-risk patients [17]. Currently, there are no long-term studies of lipid management in CKD patients that provide any additional information to direct care. Two systematic reviews and meta-analyses supported the beneficial, low-risk effect of dietary and pharmaceutical modifications to reduce the level of serum lipids in CKD stages 1–4, but reported no clear benefit in stage 5 [18, 19]. The role of lowering serum lipids in stage 5 patients currently on hemodialysis remains unclear. Two major randomized clinical trials in the dialysis population showed mixed results with cardiovascular outcome. The use of the statin rosuvastatin did lower LDL significantly, but did not have any benefit in the combined primary endpoint of death from cardiovascular cases, nonfatal myocardial infarct, or nonfatal strokes in a cohort of over 3000 hemodialysis patients [20]. In the SHARP trial (Study of Heart and Renal Protection), a combination therapy of simvastatin plus ezetimibe was used. The overall conclusion was that this therapy was effective in reducing atherosclerotic events by 17% in moderate to advanced CKD patients, but the effect on patients already on dialysis was hard to determine [21]. In two recent retrospective observational database analyses of dialysis populations, some mortality reduction was seen with statin use but findings cannot be applied prospectively [22, 23]. Nevertheless, these studies demonstrate evidence of no harm from continuing statin use after initiation of dialysis.

Assessment

Biochemical

Serum lipids should be assessed if the GFR is >60 ml/min/1.73 m^2 [12, 14]. Patients may have been screened for TC with a nonfasting sample as part of general risk assessment. Ideally, a fasting lipid profile should be obtained. The lipid profile should include TC, HDL, LDL, and triglycerides. Goal ranges as shown in Table 13.1 are the same as the general population. Values reported outside of reasonable laboratory parameters should be repeated for reliability. Instructions for at least a 12-h fast should be reinforced with the patient prior to blood draws for highest accuracy [16].

Serum lipids should be drawn annually or whenever a treatment change warrants reassessment of effect. Serum lipid patterns may change during CKD stages. The ramifications of the duration of lipid abnormalities and their relationship to later CVD risk are unknown. When hyperlipidemia is particularly resistant to standard treatment, the clinician may consider additional biochemical testing for contributory inflammatory markers such as high sensitivity C-reactive protein (CRP) [10, 16]. Hidden sources of infection should be investigated (i.e., foot and nail infection particularly in diabetics) and advanced periodontal disease.

If the GFR is 15–59 ml/min/1.73 m^2, patients should be treated as high risk regardless of serum values. No lipid screening is recommended and no follow-up blood draw is indicated. Rather, the patient is treated as high risk and interventions are initiated [12, 17]. For a more detailed discussion of CKD biochemical assessments, refer to Chap. 5.

Table 13.1 Goals for fasting serum profiles from the National Institutes of Health's National Cholesterol Education program for non-chronic kidney disease

Fasting parameter	Optimal
Total cholesterol	<200 mg/dl (5.2 mmol/L)
LDL cholesterol	<130 mg/dl (3.4 mmol/L)
HDL cholesterol	>60 mg/dl (1.5 mmol/L)
Triglycerides	<150 mg/dl (1.7 mmol/L)

Adapted from [16]
Note: American Heart Association and the Kidney Disease Outcome Quality Initiative designates any patient with chronic kidney disease (GFR <60) as high risk regardless of fasting serum profile [10, 12]

Physical

Measured, rather than self-reported, height and weight should be recorded. The body mass index should be calculated and compared to standardized tables for baseline assessment. Patients with fluid accumulation such as edema, amputees, or other body composition imbalances need special adaptations to standardized formulas [15]. Newer emphasis has been placed on waist-hip circumference as a more predictive measure of body composition. General adult guidelines are a maximum waist circumference of 102 cm (40 in.) for men and 88 cm (35 in.) for women. Physical assessment should include an evaluation of recommended cardiac activity level and intensity based on the 2018 Physical Activity Guidelines for Americans in preparation for lifestyle intervention [25]. For a more detailed discussion of physical activity assessment, refer to Chap. 30.

Patterns of body composition have received some attention in the literature. Ideally, individuals should have optimal lean muscle mass in proper proportion to adipose tissue to achieve a body mass index comparable to a healthy body weight. Serum triglycerides are often elevated in conjunction with obesity and metabolic syndrome [11, 15]. There are several handheld instruments that can be used to estimate lean body mass with individual strengths and weaknesses on reliability and validity of data over time. Employing a single instrument to track changes of an individual over time using their own baseline to measure progress may be more consistent and reliable rather than comparing to a heterogeneous group mean or trend. Adipose tissue location, particularly abdominal fat stores estimated by waist circumference, has also been used in cardiovascular risk factor evaluation. For more detailed discussion of anthropometric assessments, refer to Chap. 4.

A detailed medical history should be taken including but not limited to prior laboratory values, family history of associated lipid or vascular disorders, comorbid conditions, and current medications [26]. If possible, a nutrition-focused physical exam should be performed to provide more detailed information on other risk factors (see Chap. 6).

Nutritional

A registered dietitian will be most able to evaluate the dietary intake and recommend specific food changes to promote CVD risk reduction. Dietary intake patterns can be assessed by one of the many methods. Specific attention should be given to the type of fat consumed by saturation level, pattern of fat consumption throughout the day, and the use of fat in food preparation. Detailed information from a computer analysis of nutrient content from a food record or food frequency questionnaire may be difficult to obtain [26]. Many patients prefer to complete a picture food log of all foods consumed in a single day using their smartphones as a more interactive assessment method. Patterns in food intake will provide a higher degree of dietary understanding and assessment than a single day of intake (see Chap. 7).

Intervention

Lifestyle

The 2018 Physical Activity Guidelines for Americans recommends establishing a consistent daily physical activity pattern for all adults. Sustained cardiac activity will promote the use of circulating lipids for energy, rather than storage as atherosclerotic deposits. Also regular exercise to achieve a sustained cardiovascular benefit heart rate level may reduce serum fat particle size [5]. Patients can visually understand this exercise principle if a bottle of salad oil combined with red vinegar is shown first in a resting state of separated layers and then shaken (as in exercise) to distribute and reduce the fat particle size.

The increased cardiac output and corresponding muscle strength generally have a minimal risk when undertaken within the context of daily activities found in the home (climbing stairs, walking, vacuuming, carrying groceries). CKD patients should be evaluated for anemia and potential deficiencies (i.e., iron, folic acid, vitamin B_{12}) that can reduce the oxygen-carrying capacity of the blood and exhibit symptoms of fatigue. The use of erythropoietin, the kidney hormone decreased in CKD, should be administered and monitored using updated KDIGO guidelines [7].

The 2018 Physical Activity Guidelines for Americans encourages moderate intensity daily activities while discouraging "sitting time," even for individuals with chronic disease. Further recommendations include varying the intensity of the activity such as 10-min or more faster increments of speed as well as a longer duration of lower intensity [25]. Any physicial activity needs to be individualized for adherence and compliance over time. Most physical behaviors require a period of adaptation and variety in order to become sustainable.

A simple pedometer can be used to record steps taken per day. Steps can be used as a simple method of distance but not intensity of activity. For sedentary patients, this may be a good first effort to assess baseline activity. Steps can also be tabulated using smartphone apps or other mobile devices worn on the wrist. Complicated models monitoring stride distances are not necessary. Although the accuracy between pedometers/measures has been shown to be variable, the use of the same method by the same patient on a daily basis minimizes variability and provides a consistent baseline measurement upon which to monitor physical activity. Physical activity can be increased by small increments of as few as 100–250 steps per day until the minimal goal has been reached or as higher goals are attained. The use of any measuring device should become routine over time. The placement of the measuring device in relation to the hip flex movement is important to obtain accurate and consistent results.

To sustain motivation, many individuals benefit from pairing with a "walking buddy" or walking/activity group or class to provide continuous support and motion opportunities. For example, individuals who own dogs often increase their daily walking frequency and distance when compared to individuals who do not. Social support generally has been shown to decrease relative risks of death in both the general and chronic disease populations. Refer to Chap. 30 (Physical Activity and Exercise in Chronic Kidney Disease) for more detailed information.

Other lifestyle changes to reduce CVD risk include cessation of smoking, control of blood glucose and diabetic control (see Chap. 11), and weight maintenance (see Chap. 12).

Dietary

The Dietary Approaches to Stop Hypertension (DASH) study provided evidence to support weight reduction as an evidence-based strategy to aid in blood pressure control (see Chap. 10). As part of this plan, emphasis is placed on choosing sources of unsaturated dietary fat to support reduction of serum lipids as well [8]. Adaptations may be required in CKD stages 1–3 but the reduction in protein portions may aid in slowing CKD progression. Feasibility in CKD 4–5 (predialysis) may be more difficult and not applicable for stage 5 adults on hemodialysis. The increase in dairy products may increase serum phosphorus. The increase in fruits and vegetables may decrease serum triglycerides by reducing simple sugars but may increase dietary potassium. Serum electrolytes should be monitored in later stages of CKD.

A single educational session will not be sufficient to enact a dietary change. Routinely scheduled long-term monitoring is required. The services of a registered dietitian delivered to Medicare-eligible patients diagnosed with diabetes and kidney disease prior to dialysis are reimbursable with a referral from their treating physician [26]. Patients undergoing dialysis therapy are covered for nutritional services within the center where they receive treatment. This professional assessment and ongoing monitoring are essential to attain the dietary goals.

The general dietary principles to treat CVD risk by diet in CKD stages 1–5 are shown in Table 13.2. The key component of dietary intervention is the type and amount of fat consumed with emphasis on reducing saturated and *trans*-fatty acid content. The type and amount of simple carbohydrate is also important when treating elevated serum triglycerides. Adequate protein is needed to maintain protein stores yet balance the amount and type of protein to the level of kidney function. These general population goals are appropriate for both healthy and CKD individuals [10, 26, 28]. As such, the integration of diet modifications can be beneficial to both the individual as well as other individuals living within that household, potentially maximizing the benefit and compliance to everyone.

Table 13.2 Summary of dietary recommendations to reduce CVD risk in CKD stages 1–5

Dietary modification	Intervention method	Anticipated change
Match energy intake to energy output	Calculate and implement amount of calories required using goal body weight	Attain and maintain healthy body weight
Match caloric distribution among diet components	Provide adequate dietary protein while providing sufficient total calories	Maintain normal serum albumin
	Emphasize quality of protein when quantity is limited to potentially retard progression	Decrease risk of protein-calorie malnutrition
Decrease total fat calories to ≤30% of total calories	Decrease total fat calories consumed from all dietary sources	Normalize serum lipids
Decrease total cholesterol intake to <300 mg/day	Reduce intake of dietary cholesterol (i.e., egg yolks, animal fats); substitute whole milk dairy products with skim and low-fat alternatives; replace egg yolks with egg substitute products	Normalize serum cholesterol
Decrease saturated fat calories to <7% of total calories	Decrease intake or avoid saturated fats (i.e., animal fats, butter, full fat dairy products, mayonnaise, avocado, tropical oils such as palm and coconut)	Decrease LDL
Change the type of fats used in food preparation	Promote intake of nonhydrogenated vegetable oils (peanut, canola, olive) or nut oils (walnut, flaxseed)	Decrease LDL
Increase the use of monounsaturated fats within total fat intake amount	Promote use of olive oil, sunflower oil, canola oil	Increase HDL
Increase the use of omega-3 fatty acids within total fat intake amount	Increase consumption of green leafy vegetables, flaxseed, nuts (almonds, walnuts), and use of fatty fish 1–2 servings/week	Increase HDL
Avoid use of *trans*-unsaturated fatty acids	Avoid commercially fried foods, hydrogenated fats, partially hydrogenated vegetable oils and margarines, and processed foods containing these fats	Decrease LDL
		Increase HDL
Decrease total calories to achieve weight loss	Calculate and implement amount of calories required to achieve reduction in current body weight to goal body weight	Decrease in body weight
		Decrease in serum triglycerides
Decrease intake of simple sugars and alcohol consumption	Promote consumption of low glycemic intake foods; reduce or eliminate alcohol consumption	Decrease in serum triglycerides

Adapted from [10, 12, 15, 29]

Determination of Nutrition Prescription

General guidelines suggest reducing total fat calories but also assume individuals will not consume more calories per day than they need to attain or sustain a healthy weight. The estimation of the amount of daily dietary fat to be consumed should be based on a reasonable body weight. Obesity will be promoted or sustained using the current body weight if presently at obese or overweight levels. Body mass index of 25–29.9 kg/m^2 is considered overweight by government guidelines. The consumption of "empty" calories will contribute to overall non-lean body mass. The definition of "healthy" weight in many patients within the context of chronic disease has challenges of its own, and the use of formulas contained in the KDOQI guidelines have been shown to be used inconsistently in practice [24].

Recent literature from the chronic dialysis population (CKD stage 5) has shown a trend toward greater survival at higher body weight levels compared to normal and underweight levels. Although the exact mechanism is not fully understood, this "J-curve" observation may be related to the cushion of additional body fat stores available for energy during concurrent hospitalization or stress periods. It is important to maintain a reasonable body weight during CKD stages 1–4 and avoid malnutrition when progressing to CKD stage 5. The exact benefit or need for a "cushion" of fat stores and muscle mass, however, has yet to be determined [30].

Amount and Type of Dietary Fat

The balance of diet composition between fat, carbohydrate, and protein should be individualized by a registered dietitian, customized to level of kidney function and patient direct interaction. A typical 2000 kcal per day diet focused towards CVD risk reduction should contain ≤30% total fat. This is calculated as 600 kcal (30% of 2000 kcal and 600/9 kcal/g of fat) which equals approximately 66 g or less of total fat per day. Guidelines suggest no more than 7% of total calories (140 kcal or 16 g of fat) should come from saturated fat [10, 12, 16].

Saturated fat has more hydrogen bonds than polyunsaturated and monounsaturated fat. Typically, saturated fat remains solid at room temperature (such as animal fat from meat, lard, butter), whereas unsaturated fat is softer or liquid at room temperature (such as vegetable oils or tub compared to stick margarine). These hydrogen bonds are more difficult to break down and metabolize, thus circulating as larger fat particles in the serum. The composition of the diet should be changed to encourage the intake of predominantly polyunsaturated and monounsaturated sources within the total daily fat intake.

Trans-fatty acids have been altered during processing to change the natural *cis* configuration (the most unsaturated version) to the *trans* configuration (primarily to increase shelf life). *Trans*-fatty acids function as saturated fatty acids during metabolism and have been implicated in reducing HDL and increasing LDL cholesterol [11]. They are found predominantly in processed foods to promote shelf life (cookies, crackers, baked goods). A general trend has been to increase public awareness of and to reduce the amount of *trans*-fatty acids in the food supply.

Monosaturated and polyunsaturated fats should comprise the majority of diet intake. Omega-3, n-6, and n-9 fatty acids should be emphasized. Simple choices such as the use of canola oil and olive oil can be practical diet choices. Fish oil dietary supplementation does not replace healthy fat choices in the overall diet [10, 15].

Nutrition labels allow for rounding of fat grams on a label to 0.5 or 0 g if that food contains less than 5 g of fat per portion, and rounding to the nearest 1 g if the food contains more than 5 g of fat per portion. If a consumer uses the nutrition label as the general guide to counting fat grams per day, the accuracy of their estimate can be proportionate to the number of food items they consume each day. Nutrition labels in the United States must now also contain *trans*-fatty acid composition [31]. The

American Heart Association has a Heart-Check Mark Food Certification Program [32] with specific nutritional guidelines that aid consumers in selecting a wide variety of foods that meet the nutrition prescription discussed in this chapter.

Incorporation of the Type of Carbohydrate, Dietary Fiber, and Plant Sterols

Replacement of simple carbohydrates with more complex dietary sources in conjunction with weight reduction has been shown to decrease serum triglycerides [11, 13, 15]. Pending United States food label changes will require "added sugar" to help compare to natural sugar occurring in the food item [31]. The level of dietary fiber has generally decreased in the Western diet pattern with the increased consumption of refined foods, higher animal protein, and lower plant sources. Increasing dietary fiber and including plant sterols in the diet have also been identified as effective dietary interventions to address hyperlipidemia [15, 16, 29].

Increasing the consumption of dietary fiber to levels of 20–30 g/day has been linked to lower LDL levels. Soluble fiber binds to bile acids which may decrease the absorption of cholesterol. Both soluble and insoluble fiber may also decrease the gastrointestinal transit time which may improve insulin sensitivity by slowing carbohydrate absorption. Insoluble fiber is found primarily in wheat products but may be less effective on LDL serum levels than soluble fiber. Soluble fiber is found in a wide variety of foods including barley, bran, raw or partially cooked fruits and vegetables, nuts and seeds, and oats and oatmeal. A wide variety of over-the-counter psyllium capsules and soft fiber equivalents are available as alternatives or supplements to dietary modification. Fiber intake should be increased gradually over time in conjunction with liberal fluid intake to decrease gastrointestinal symptoms until the gut adapts to a higher load [15, 16]. Excess dietary fiber intake by diet or supplements can result in negative effects of gastrointestinal symptoms and potential malabsorption of selected nutrients. Dietary fluid and potassium restrictions will require adaptations when progression to CKD stage 5 is eminent [26–28].

Plant sterols and their stanol esters are naturally present in small quantities in plant sources. Most research has been done in soybean derivatives where they have been chemically concentrated to produce commercial products marketed as butter or margarine substitutes. Plant sterol esters in this new format which exceed what can be consumed by diet alone have been shown to potentially lower LDL in the general population. Clinical trials have included more than 1800 people with doses of up to 25 g/day. No clinical studies have been done in CKD patients, but they are rated as a safe food-grade additive. A daily intake of approximately two tablespoons consumed as part of two separate meals per day (total 2–3 g/day) is the recommended dose with no evidence that higher levels produce a greater effect [29]. Refer to Chap. 31 for detailed discussion of dietary patterns.

Pharmacological

Drug intervention for CVD risk reduction includes anticoagulation and lipid-lowering focus. A recent summary of the controversies on the use of anticoagulant therapies in CKD reviewed the challenges involved to reduce the stroke risk while balancing bleeding issues in the CKD population [33]. Green leafy vegetables (spinach, kale, broccoli) are high in vitamin K which may affect the coagulation profile in warfarin.

There are several classes of drugs used for reducing serum lipids as shown in Table 13.3. The majority of early stage CKD adults (stages 1–3) are typically followed by non-nephrologists. The AHA/ACC(American College of Cardiology) general lipid management guidelines for the non-CKD population are applicable to this population [10]. A recent overview focused on the controversies

Table 13.3 Summary of selected pharmacological agents to address dyslipidemia in CKD stages 1–5

Mechanism of action/drug class	Selected pharmacological agent by generic name	Brand name
Oral agents		
Bile acid sequestrants	Cholestyramine	Questran
	Cholestipol	Colestid
	Colesevelam	Welchol
Fibric acid	Fenofibrate	Tricor
	Gemfibrozil	Lopid
Statins	Atorvastatin	Lipitor
	Fluvastatin	Lescol
	Lovastatin	Mevacor, Altoprev (extend release)
	Pitavastatin[a]	Livalo
	Pravastatin	Pravachol
	Rosuvastatin	Crestor
	Simvastatin	Zocor
Cholesterol inhibitor	Ezetimibe	Zetia
Nicotinic acid	Niacin	Niacor, Slo-niacin (sustained release), Niaspan (extended release)
Combinations	Ezetimibe and simvastatin	Vytorin
	Niaspan and lovastatin	Advicor
Injectable Agents		
Proprotein convertase subtilisin/kexin type 9	Alirocumab+	Praluent
	Evolocumab+	Repatha

Adapted from [10, 12, 17, 34, 35]
[a]Contraindicated in impaired renal function
+Not studied in CKD population

regarding lipid management in CKD [17]. Special considerations may need to be given to older age (>70 years of age), those with known CKD/CVD risk, and post-kidney transplant patients. The 2013 KDIGO clinical practice guidelines for lipid management in CKD recommended adults ≥50 years of age with nondialysis dependent CKD be treated with a statin or statin plus ezetimibe regardless of lipid (LDL-C) levels. The guidelines did not recommend initiation of a statin for adults undergoing renal replacement therapy (CKD stage 5) but suggested that prior statin prescriptions could be continued and monitored as part of standard of care [12, 17].

Each drug has a unique mechanism by which it changes lipid metabolism or absorption. The most common mechanism is metabolically blocking the enzymes that aid in the manufacture of cholesterol. Others use a variety of mechanisms to change the way in which dietary cholesterol is absorbed. All are taken orally and use the gastrointestinal tract as an important metabolic medium. A complete drug interaction analysis should be performed by a registered pharmacist at regular intervals to monitor potential problems. For example, some statins interfere with the absorption of drugs such as immunosuppressive agents such as cyclosporine. Refer to Chap. 9 for detailed discussion of drug-nutrient interactions.

The strongest evidence for the use of statins (HMG CoA reductase inhibitors) is in CKD stages 1–4 [18, 19]. All agents should be evaluated and monitored for drug–nutrient interactions, side effects, and tolerance in CKD stages 1–5. As noted earlier, retrospective analyses of patients undergoing dialysis showed no harm in continuing a prescribed statin [22, 23].

Regular bowel habits will promote the efficacy of many of these oral drugs. The gastrointestinal tract can increase absorption of specific dietary components such as potassium in CKD as a compensatory mechanism to decrease absorption–reabsorption by the kidneys. Constipation may be a problem due to lower fluid intake and binding features of concurrent drugs such as phosphate binders in later stages of CKD.

A new class of injectable proprotein convertase subtilisin/kexin type 9 agents have recently been introduced for biweekly administration. Their development focused on heterozygous familiar hypercholesterolemia, an inherited disorder of elevated LDL increasing the risk of atherosclerotic lesions [34, 35]. The clinical trials did not include CKD patients. One of the drugs (alirocumab) did not affect serum creatinine but the half-life of the drug was reduced when administered with a statin [34].

The type of pharmacological intervention used is not as important as the attainment of the overall goal of lipid reduction. Each drug has specific potency effects, doses, and safety data. A variety of options may be necessary to achieve compliance within financial and administration issues while avoiding side effects and potential complications. Dietary and pharmacological intervention should be used together to maximize lipid reduction effect as their mechanisms of action are complementary, not competitive [10, 12, 17].

Conclusion

The diagnosis of CKD implies a high CVD risk. The reduction of CVD risk in CKD stages 1–5 requires a multifactorial healthcare team approach. Practitioners need to use comprehensive assessment techniques to evaluate and individualize treatment at every step to the unique needs of the patient. Intervention strategies that include physical activity, dietary changes, and pharmacological options need to be continually monitored to achieve goals. The skills of a registered dietitian nutritionist are necessary to provide the support and continuous balance of nutritional components to modify existing habits and promote new patterns. A strong integrated health team approach is necessary to diagnose, evaluate, and treat CVD risk throughout the CKD stages. Evidence-based clinical practice guidelines provide templates upon which to plan and coordinate quality care.

Case Questions and Answers

Learners are encouraged to adapt the case study outline to reflect their own practice experience to individualize to their professional setting.

Visit 1:
Mr. Jones, age 45, arrives as a new patient in the general medicine clinic. He has no specific complaints or symptoms. He is coming at the insistence of his adult son who was recently diagnosed with high blood pressure. Height 68 inches, weight 260 lbs (118 kg), sitting blood pressure 155/90 mmHg. A follow-up appointment is scheduled in two weeks.

1. What biochemical tests should be ordered before the next visit?
   Answer:

   - Metabolic screening panel to assess diabetes, liver, and renal function status
   - Lipid profile
   - Urine screening for proteinuria

2. Identify additional information needed to evaluate CKD and CVD risk factors.
   Answer:

   - Calculation of eGFR
   - A detailed medical history including but not limited to prior laboratory values, family history of CVD/CKD
   - An initial evaluation and current understanding of blood pressure as a risk factor

3. What initial nutritional management might be planned for this visit or in preparation for the next visit?
   Answer:

   - Initial discussion of Table 13.2 parameters
   - Perform nutrition-focused physical examination, if time allows
   - Assign diet assessment by written or picture food log (daily camera/phone record of food consumed for 1–2 days) for completion by the next visit
   - Invite involvement of other family members who have health/food support role to come to the next visit

4. What pharmacological interventions might be considered?
   Answer:

   - Consideration of diuretic as first-line agent for blood pressure control

Visit 2:
During the next visit two weeks later, the following fasting laboratory values are reported: serum glucose (100 mg/dl; 5.5 mmol/L), HbA1c (5.0%), fasting lipids (TC 226 mg/dl/5.85 mmol/l; LDL 132 mg/dl/3.4 mmol/l; HDL 32 mg/dl/0.82 mmol/l; triglycerides 310 mmol/l;3.5 mmol/l); estimated GFR 75 ml/min/1.73 m². Blood pressure is 140/80. Mrs. Jones, who does most of the food preparation, is present.

1. Identify key nutritional management activities that might be applicable.
   Answer:

   - 2016 updated KDOQI commentary suggests that all CKD patients should be managed as high CVD risk
   - Nutrition-focused physical examination if not completed on first visit
   - Focus can begin by review of picture food log, if available, with education on relationship of type of fat to CVD disease using Table 13.2
   - Discussion on weight management principles to reduce BMI and correlation to disease reduction risk
   - Referral to individual nutritional counseling plan and awareness of group support activities/classes
   - Incorporation of digital/social/electronic app and education resources

2. Identify the stage of CKD for Mr. Jones.
   Answer:

   - Estimated GFR of 75 ml/min/1.73m² is Stage 2 (mild CKD GFR 60–89 ml/min)

3. Identify key CVD risk factors with appropriate actions/goals.
   Answer:

   - Comparison of lipid levels to Table 13.1 for CVD risk along with BMI
   - Diet composition, weight reduction, and pharmacological interventions should be considered as action and goal key points

4. Evaluate the pharmacological intervention(s).
   Answer:

   - Evaluation of compliance, tolerance of diuretic prescription
   - Adding statin prescription should be considered using Table 13.3

Visit 3:
The follow-up visit in three months documents a blood pressure of 130/70 and a weight of 240 lbs (109 kg). Mr. Jones reports he is going to "start" walking when the weather gets better.

1. Plan a set of individualized goals for Mr. Jones including follow-up and monitoring.
   Answer:

   - Continue diet awareness and weight loss progress using Table 13.2. (20 lbs lost in past 3 months)
   - Discuss new weight loss target for the next 3 months
   - Discuss activity and relation to CKD and CVD risks
   - Reinforce blood pressure correlation to weight loss and activity
   - Reinforce diet composition changes and blood pressure to CVD and CKD risks

2. Postulate the results of a dietary assessment and actions to reduce CVD risk based on your assessment.
   Answer:

   - Reinforce diet composition changes, particularly the type of dietary fat
   - Review the efficacy of diet/activity resources and provide new options to encourage sustained or new approaches to current action goals

3. Identify the strengths and barriers to achieve your planned goals for Mr. Jones.
   Answer:

   - Strengths: Family support; stated action plan to "start walking"; initial weight loss; blood pressure control; medication compliance in relation to blood pressure and statin
   - Barriers: Not currently walking; comparison of self in relation to family actions; the presence or absence of family members at follow-up visits; sustaining motivation factors; availability of pedometer or phone app for steps/day awareness of daily lifestyle patterns

4. Evaluate the pharmacological intervention(s).
   Answer:

   - Assessment of tolerance and compliance to current pharmacy strategies based on Table 13.3
   - Plan for repeat lipid profiles to assess the efficacy of statin prescription to Table 13.1
   - Reinforce diuretic or current medication for blood pressure control

References

1. National Kidney Foundation. Guidelines development process. [cited 2019 Feb 26]. Available from: https://www.kidney.org/professionals/guidelines/content/guideline-development-process.
2. Kidney Disease: Improving Global Outcomes (KDIGO) CKD Work Group. KDIGO 2012 Clinical practice guideline for the evaluation and management of chronic kidney disease. Kidney Int Suppl. 2013;3:1–150.
3. Centers for Disease Control and Prevention. National chronic kidney disease fact sheet, 2017. [cited 2019 Feb 26]. Available from: https://www.cdc.gov/diabetes/pubs/pdf/kidney_factsheet.pdf.
4. Benjamin EJ, Muntner P, Alonso A, Bittencourt MC, Callaway CW, Carson AP, Chamberlain AM, et al. AHA statistical update: heart disease and stroke statistics 2019 update: a report from the American Heart Association. Circulation. 2019;139:e56–e528. https://www.ncbi.nlm.nih.gov/pubmed/30700139.
5. Bansal N, Katz R, Robinson-Cohen C, Odden MC, Dalrymple L, Shlipak MG, et al. Absolute rates of HF, CHD, and stroke in CKD: an analysis of three community-based cohort studies. JAMA Cardiol. 2017;2:314–8.
6. United States Department of Health and Human Services. Healthy People Initiative 2020, Chronic Kidney Disease. [cited 2019 Feb 26]. Available from: https://www.healthypeople.gov/2020/topics-objectives/topic/chronic-kidney-disease.
7. National Kidney Foundation. Kidney Early Evaluation Program (KEEP). [cited 2019 Feb 26]. Available from: https://www.kidney.org/keephealthy.
8. American Kidney Fund. Know Your Kidneys Program. [cited 2019 Feb 26]. Available from: https://www.kidney-fund.org/prevention/free-kidney-health-screenings
9. National Institutes of Health. National Kidney Disease Education Program. [cited 2019 Feb 26]. Available from: https://niddk.nih.gov/health-information/communication-programs/nkdep/identify-manage-patients

10. Grundy SM, Stone NJ, Bailey AL, Beam C, Birtcher KK, Blumenthal RS, et al. 2018 AHA/ACC/AACVPR/AAPA/ ABC/ACPM/ADA/AGS/A[jA/ASPC/NLA/PCNA guideline on the management of blood cholesterol: a report of the American College of Cardiology/American Heart Association Task Force on Clinical Practice Guidelines. Circulation. 2018. https://doi.org/10.1161/CIR.0000000000000625.
11. Gropper SS, Smith JL, Carr TP. Advanced nutrition and human metabolism. 7th ed. Boston: Cengage Learning; 2013. p. 138–74.
12. Kidney Disease Improving Global Outcomes (KDIGO) Lipid Work Group. KDIGO clinical practice guidelines for lipid management in chronic kidney disease. Kidney Int Suppl. 2013;3:259–305.
13. Miller M, Stone NJ, Ballantyne C, Bittner V, Criqui M, Ginsberg HN, Goldberg AC, Howard WJ, Jacobson MS, Kris-Etherton PM, Lennie TA, Levi M, Mazzone T, Pennathur S. Triglycerides and cardiovascular disease: a scientific statement from the American Heart Association. Circulation. 2011;123:2252–332.
14. Mahei S, Ocrici E, Popescu I, Enciu AM, Albulescu L, et al. Inflammation-related mechanisms in chronic kidney disease prediction, progression, and outcome. J Immunol Res. 2018;2018:1. https://doi.org/10.1155/2018/2180373.
15. Byham-Gray L, Stover J, Wiesen K, editors. A clinical guide to nutrition care in kidney disease. 2nd ed. Chicago: Academy of Nutrition and Dietetics; 2013.
16. Expert Panel on Detection, Evaluation, and Treatment of High Blood Cholesterol in Adults. Executive summary of the third report of the National Cholesterol Education Program [NCEP]. [cited 2019 Feb 26]. Available from: www. ncbi.nlm.nih.gov/nlmcatalog/101160954.
17. Markossian T, Burge N, Ling B, Schneider J, Pacold I, Bansal V, et al. Controversies regarding lipid management and statin use for cardiovascular risk reducation in patients with CKD. Am J Kidney Dis. 2016;67:965–77.
18. Upadhyay A, Earley A, Lamont JL, Haynes S, Wanner C, Balk EM. Lipid-lowering therapy in persons with chronic kidney disease. Ann Intern Med. 2012;157:251–62.
19. Palmer SC, Craig JC, Navaneethan SD, Tonelli M, Pellegrinin F, Strippoli GF. Benefits and harms of statin therapy for persons with chronic kidney disease. Ann Intern Med. 2012;157:263–75.
20. Fellstrom BC, Jardine AG, Schmieder RE, Holdaas H, Bannister K, Beutler J, et al. Rosuvastatin and cardiovascular events in patients undergoing hemodialysis. N Engl J Med. 2009;360:1395–407.
21. Barigent C, Landray MJ, Reith C, Emberson J, Wheeler DC, Tomson C, et al. The effects of lowering LDL cholesterol with simvastatin plus ezetimibe in patients with chronic kidney disease: study of heart and renal protection: a randomised placebo-controlled trial. Lancet. 2001;377:2181–92.
22. Chan KE, Thadhani R, Lazarus JM, Hakim RM. Modeling the 4D study: statins and cardiovascular outcomes in long-term hemodialysis patients with diabetes. Clin J Am Soc Nephrol. 2010;5:856–66.
23. Streja E, Gosmanova EO, Molnar MZ, Soahoa M, Morcidi H, Potukuchi PE, et al. Association of continuation of statin therapy initiated before transition to chronic dialysis therapy with mortality after dialysis initiation. JAMA Netw Open. 2018;1(6):e182311.
24. Harvey KS. Methods for determining health body weight in end stage renal disease. J Ren Nutr. 2006;16:269–76.
25. 2018 Physical Activity Guidelines Advisory Committee. Physical activity guidelines for Americans scientific report. 2nd ed. Washington, DC: United States Department of Health; 2018.
26. Kent PS, McCarthy MP, Burrowes JD, McCann L, Pavlinac J, Goeddeke-Merickel MS, et al. Academy of Nutrition and Dietetics and the National Kidney Foundation revised 2014 standards of practice and standards of professional performance for registered dietitian nutritionists (competent, proficient, and expert) in nephrology nutrition. J Acad Nutr Diet. 2014;24(5):275–285.e45.
27. National Kidney Foundation. KDIGO clinical practice guideline for anemia in chronic kidney disease. Kidney Int Suppl. 2012;2(4):279–335.
28. National Heart Lung Blood Institute. Your guide to lowering you blood pressure with DASH. [cited 2019 Feb 26]. Available from: https://www.nhlbi.nih.gov/files/docs/public/heart/new_dash.pdf
29. Rysz L, Franczyk B, Olszewski R, Banach M, Gluba-Brzozka A. The use of plant sterols and stanols as lipid-lowering agents in cardiovascular disease. Curr Pharm Des. 2017;23(17):2488–95.
30. Kalantar-Zadeh K, Kopple JD, Kilpatrick RD, McAllister CJ, Shinaberger CS, Gjertson DW, Greenland S. Association of morbid obesity and weight change over time with cardiovascular survival in hemodialysis population. Am J Kidney Dis. 2005;46(3):489–500.
31. Food and Drug Administration. Food labeling guide. [cited 2019 Feb 26]. Available from: https://www.fda.gov/ Food/GuidanceRegulation//GuidanceDocumentsRegulatoryInformation/labelingnutrition/ucm2006828.htm.
32. American Heart Association. Heart-check mark nutritional guidelines. [cited 2019 Feb 26]. https://www.heart.org/ en/healthy-living/company-collaboration/heart-check-certification.
33. Bansal V, Herzog C, Sarnak M, Choi M, Methta R, Jaar B, et al. Oral anticoagulants to prevent stroke in nonvalvular atrial fibrillation in patients with CKD stage 5: an NKF-KDOQI controversies report. Am J Kidney Dis. 2017;70(6):859–68.
34. Product Insert: Alirocumab (Pralvent). [cited 2019 Mar 10]. Available from: https://www.praluent.com.
35. Product Insert: Evolocumab (Repatha). [cited 2019 Mar 10]. Available from: https://www.repatha.com.

Part IV
Chronic Kidney Disease in Adults Treated by Renal Replacement Therapies

Medical nutrition therapy (MNT) for patients with varying stages of chronic kidney disease (CKD) is at the forefront of nutritional management of the disease. These patients are a heterogeneous group who require different treatment strategies including nutrition support, depending on the stage of the disease (i.e., 1–5D), the concurrent comorbidities, and treatment modalities (i.e., maintenance hemodialysis, peritoneal dialysis, and kidney transplantation). During the early stages of CKD (1–3), the goals of MNT are to prevent protein-energy wasting (PEW) and/or protein-calorie malnutrition (PCM), to maintain an optimal nutritional status, to prevent cardiovascular disease and bone disease, and to retard progression of the disease. A moderate- to low-protein diet with an adequate energy intake is recommended for patients during the early stages of CKD. As the stage of the disease progresses to 4–5 (non-dialysis), a low-protein diet is recommended and the goals of MNT are the same as the earlier stages with the addition of reducing or controlling symptoms of uremia. An optimal nutritional status during this stage is critical since a poor nutritional status at the start of dialysis is a predictor of poor outcome. Once dialysis begins (stage 5D), the purpose of MNT is to prevent or treat PEW and/or PCM; to reduce accumulation of fluid, waste products, potassium, and phosphorus; and to prevent cardiovascular and bone disease.

The chapters in this section include the updated KDOQI/Academy evidence-based clinical practice guidelines for nutrition in chronic kidney disease. In addition, a case study is included at the end of each chapter to evoke critical thinking in the reader and to foster further learning about the nutritional management of the specific stage of kidney disease and renal replacement therapy.

Harvey discusses medical nutrition therapies for patients with non-dialysis-dependent CKD (i.e., stages 1–5) including healthy eating patterns such as plant-based diets and the Mediterranean and DASH diets. Furthermore, topics such as anemia management and a low-antigen diet for treating IgA nephropathy are addressed. Nutritional management of patients receiving renal replacement therapies (i.e., hemodialysis, peritoneal dialysis, and transplantation) are presented in chapters by Blair, Patel and Burrowes, and Pieloch, respectively. Lastly, because of the importance of nutritional management in preventing and treating PEW and/or PCM in maintenance dialysis patients, a chapter is dedicated to nutrition support in this population. Chan presents an in-depth review of oral and enteral nutrition supplements, intra-dialytic parenteral nutrition (IDPN), intraperitoneal nutrition (IPN), enteral tube feedings, and total parenteral nutrition (TPN).

Chapter 14
CKD Stages 1–5 (Nondialysis)

Katherine Schiro Harvey

Keywords Diet quality · Malnutrition · Protein restriction · Energy needs · IgA nephropathy · Anemia
Diabetes · Comorbid conditions

Key Points
- Describe nutrition risks associated with chronic kidney disease, including protein-energy malnutrition, diabetes, cardiovascular disease, mineral bone disease, and anemia.
- Identify appropriate nutrition interventions to prevent and/or treat nutrition risks associated with chronic kidney disease, including healthy eating patterns, and estimating protein calorie needs.
- Discuss nutrition therapies to treat chronic kidney disease complications such as diabetes, cardiovascular disease, hypertension, hyperlipidemia, and anemia.
- Describe nutrition strategies that may be appropriate for treating IgA nephropathy.
- Describe how self-management techniques can be used to enhance nutrition knowledge and promote behavior changes in people with chronic kidney disease.

Introduction

Chronic kidney disease (CKD) is a worldwide public health problem and a progressive, debilitating condition. In the United States, it is estimated that 15% of the population have CKD, equivalent to 37 million Americans or one in seven adults [1]. Most individuals with CKD are unaware that they have the disease, as the symptoms are "hidden" until it has progressed to later stages and complications become apparent. The National Kidney Foundation Kidney Disease Outcomes Quality Initiative (NKF KDOQI) defines CKD as abnormalities of the kidney structure or function lasting longer than 3 months, with implications on health [2]. Additionally, a greater than 3-month reduction in kidney function as estimated by the glomerular filtration rate (GFR) and the presence of proteinuria are included in the definition (Table 14.1) [3]. The stages and prevalence of CKD are detailed in Chap.1.

Approximately 750,000 people in the United States have Stage 5 CKD and are receiving maintenance dialysis or received a transplant [4]. Most people with CKD (>29 million) are at stages 1 through 4, at the risk of progressing to stage 5. But the risk is even greater that they will develop comorbid conditions associated with CKD and die prematurely. The NKF recommends that all individuals at high risk of CKD should be screened regularly through assessment of markers of kidney damage and GFR [5]. Appropriate interventions should be initiated to prevent development

K. S. Harvey (✉)
Renal Nutrition Services, Puget Sound Kidney Centers, Mountlake Terrace, WA, USA
e-mail: kathyh@pskc.net

© Springer Nature Switzerland AG 2020 239
J. D. Burrowes et al. (eds.), *Nutrition in Kidney Disease*, Nutrition and Health,
https://doi.org/10.1007/978-3-030-44858-5_14

Table 14.1 Chronic kidney disease prognosis and stages[a]

Prognosis of CKD by GFR and Albuminuria Categories: KDIGO 2012				Persistent albuminuria categories Description and range		
				A1	**A2**	**A3**
				Normal to mildly increased	Moderately increased	Severely increased
				<30 mg/g <3 mg/mmol	30–300 mg/g 3–30 mg/mmol	>300 mg/g >30 mg/mmol
GFR categories (ml/min/ 1.73 m²) Description and range	G1	Normal or high	≥90			
	G2	Mildly decreased	60–89			
	G3a	Mildly to moderately decreased	45–59			
	G3b	Moderately to severely decreased	30–44			
	G4	Severely decreased	15–29			
	G5	Kidney failure	<15			

Green, low risk (if no other markers of kidney disease, no CKD); yellow, moderately increased risk; orange, high risk; red, very high risk.
[a]Reprinted with permission from Inker et al. [3]

Table 14.2 Risk factors for chronic kidney disease[a]

Primary risk factors for chronic kidney disease	Secondary risk factors for chronic kidney disease
Diabetes	Obesity
High blood pressure	Autoimmune diseases
Family history of chronic kidney disease	Urinary tract and/or systemic infections
Age 60 years or older	Overuse of over-the-counter painkillers or exposure to toxic chemicals
Ethnic groups	Kidney loss, damage, injury, or infection

[a]Created with data from [5]

and/or progression of CKD, and treat complications. Primary and secondary risk factors for CKD are listed in Table 14.2.

Certain ethnic populations that have high rates of diabetes or high blood pressure are at an increased risk of CKD, such as African Americans, Hispanics, Asians, Pacific Islanders, and Native Americans. The prevalence of CKD is 1.5–3 times higher in these groups compared to whites [5].

CKD involves complex, comorbid conditions, including malnutrition, diabetes, cardiovascular disease (CVD), hypertension, dyslipidemias, and bone and mineral metabolism disorders (BMD).

Nutrition plays a significant role in CKD treatment as CVD, hypertension, obesity, and diabetes are related to a sedentary lifestyle and a high processed food diet. Therefore, Medical Nutrition Therapy (MNT) is the cornerstone treatment for managing CKD and its complications. People with CKD who receive MNT provided by an expert renal dietitian show less decline in GFR compared to those who do not receive MNT; they have better markers of nutrition health, improved survival, and decreased health care costs [6–8]. Clinical guidelines recommend that all individuals with CKD receive expert dietary advice and information tailored to their specific individual situations [3, 9]. This chapter discusses nutrition therapies appropriate for CKD stages 1–5 (nondialysis) which can reduce comorbid complications, and slow the progression to stage 5 dialysis. Additional information for treating those with hypertension, diabetes, obesity, and CVD is discussed in Chaps.10, 11, 12, and 13.

Quantity vs. Quality

Traditional diet therapies for CKD focus on adjusting specific nutrients (protein, sodium, phosphorus, potassium) in the diet to help manage and balance blood chemistries and prevent buildup of toxic wastes. Diets typically include small amounts of animal protein foods, along with limited amounts of fruits and vegetables, and avoidance of whole grains and dairy foods. Extra fats and sugars may be added to maintain calorie intake and satiety. Although these diets provide the appropriate mix of protein, calories, sodium, potassium, and phosphorus, they are generally not considered "healthy" by current nutrition standards. Over the past several years, research has emerged demonstrating that the total diet quality may be more important and effective in treating CKD compared to limited specific nutrition quantities [10–13]. Healthy diets based on a variety of whole grains, vegetables, fruits, plant proteins including legumes and nuts, fish, poultry, low fat dairy foods, and plant-based oils are showing promise both in preventing CKD, reducing its complications, and slowing progression to dialysis. Large population studies have evaluated vegetarian diets, Mediterranean diets and the Dietary Approaches to Stop Hypertension (DASH) diet, all showing effectiveness in treating and preventing CKD [10–13]. Studies focusing on increased intake of fruits and vegetables in CKD show improved acid/base balance and decreased uremic toxins [14–16]. Therefore, current CKD diet recommendations include emphasis on eating patterns consistent with the overall diet quality rather than just limiting nutrients. Within food groups, specific food choices may be required to balance sodium, potassium and phosphorus levels, but there is little evidence that avoiding total food groups such as whole grains, legumes, or dairy foods is warranted. Nutrition therapies must be monitored to provide adequate calories and protein, but also a variety of whole foods consistent with overall healthy diets.

Malnutrition in CKD

Improving and/or maintaining nutrition health in people with CKD is a priority of MNT. Protein energy malnutrition (PEM – malnutrition due to the lack of calories and nutrients) or protein-energy wasting (PEW – decreased body lean and fat tissue stores related to inadequate nutrient intake and also metabolic conditions such as acidosis, inflammation, and anemias) at the start of dialysis therapy is associated with increased mortality, as evidenced by a variety of markers of nutritional health. Early studies by Held showed that the relative risk of death more than doubled in subjects who began dialysis with serum albumin less than 2.5 g/dL compared with those who began dialysis with albumin greater than 4.0 g/dL [17]. Kopple reported that both average calorie intake and body mass index (BMI) in people with CKD tend to decrease as GFR declines [18]. Ikizler has shown that protein intake also declines with GFR [19]. More recent studies report that low energy and/or protein intake are associated with a significant decline of nutritional parameters and an increased risk of morbidity and mortality [20]. Studies by Fried and O'Sullivan report that reduced lean body mass is an important measure for protein deficit and is also predictive of increased mortality in this patient population [21, 22].

Metabolic acidosis is common in CKD and is associated with increased protein catabolism. The degradation of essential branched chain amino acids and muscle protein is stimulated during metabolic acidosis, resulting in muscle catabolism and suppression of albumin synthesis [23]. Evidence strongly suggests a chronic inflammatory state in CKD, especially as the GFR drops below 60 ml/min/1.73 m². Inflammation is associated with anorexia, increased skeletal muscle protein breakdown, increased whole body protein catabolism, cytokine mediated hypermetabolism, and disruption of growth hormone and insulin-like growth factor-1(IGF-1) axis leading to decreased anabolism [24].

Overall, as the GFR drops below 60 mL/min/1.73 m² (stage 3), both calorie and protein intake spontaneously decrease [18, 19]. Even though there is a lack of data regarding optimal dietary and energy patterns in order to slow the progression of CKD and maintain proper nutritional status, it is critical that nutrient intake be assessed and appropriate recommendations made in the earlier stages of CKD to prevent and treat PEM and PEW. Although obesity is a major risk factor for CKD, once CKD is established, higher BMI becomes linked with greater survival [25–28]. This "obesity paradox" is evident in the more advanced stages of CKD (stages 4 and 5) and has been substantiated by a large number of observational studies with large sample sizes [25–28]. However, in the earlier stages of CKD (stages 1–3), obesity is associated with more rapid loss of kidney function and progression of CKD [25–28]. Better outcomes occur in those with BMI < 30 kg/m² [25–28]. Therefore, it is acceptable to promote gradual weight loss in obese subjects with CKD, especially in stages 1–3. Weight loss should be achieved through a combination of increased physical activity to promote lean tissue and a high-quality diet, including a wide variety of foods, balanced in all essential nutrients. Rapid weight loss results in the loss of lean rather than fat tissue but slow weight loss while following a healthy eating plan, in combination with resistance exercise, can help prevent muscle catabolism in CKD [29, 30].

Protein Needs

Consuming a traditional Western diet high in animal-based proteins will induce increases in GFR and ultimately lead to glomerular hyperfiltration [31]. High protein intake increases renal blood flow and elevates intraglomerular pressure, resulting in the excretion of protein-derived nitrogenous waste products. Overtime this may lead to an increase in the kidney volume and weight [31].

For over 50 years, researchers have studied the effects of restricting protein intake on kidney function in CKD. The largest study published to date, the Modification of Diet in Renal Disease (MDRD), evaluated more than 800 subjects with CKD [32]. After many years of subject follow-up, data evaluation, and re-evaluation, results remain inconclusive on the benefits of a low protein diet on progression of CKD. However, several prior and subsequent studies and meta-analyses appear to support the role of limiting protein intake on progression of CKD [9, 31, 33–40].

Protein quality may be of more importance than total protein intake, as evidenced by current research on the effect of the vegetarian, Mediterranean and DASH diets in CKD [10, 11].Consuming plant proteins results in less uremic toxins, improved gut microbiome leading to decreased inflammation, and reduced metabolic acidosis and hyperphosphatemia [11, 12]. The large NHANES III study evaluated protein intake and CKD outcomes and found lower mortality is those subjects who consumed more of their protein from plant sources [41].

Table 14.3   High biological value protein foods[a]

For people with chronic kidney disease, at least 50% of protein intake should be from these foods:	
Fish, seafood	Tofu
Poultry	Soy milk, soy cheese, soy yogurt
Eggs	Dried beans and legumes
Milk, cheese, yogurt	Nuts and nut butters

[a]Created with data from [42, 43]

Current protein recommendations for CKD stages 1–5 (nondialysis) range from 0.55 to 0.60 g/kg/day and from 0.60 to 0.80 g/kg/day for those with diabetes [2, 9]. It is generally recommended that at least 50% of the protein should be of high biological value (Table 14.3) [42, 43]. Because these recommendations are less than most typical Western diets, some people may adapt more easily if protein intake is gradually decreased to goal levels, depending on usual intake. It may be advantageous to first alter the protein quality to substitute more plant protein foods, rather than drastically reducing total intake. Additionally, overall health, activities, metabolic condition, and stress must be considered when calculating protein needs. For those clients who require more protein (malnutrition, wound healing, infections, trauma, strenuous activities, etc.), high-quality plant protein foods should be considered as the healthy alternative to eating more animal proteins.

The protein recommendation of 0.55 to 0.60 gm/kg/day is much less than that recommended for healthy adults. Limiting protein to this level can increase the risk of malnutrition and will require intensive education and ongoing counseling by a renal dietitian. The nutritional status must be maintained with adequate calorie intake to prevent iatrogenic malnutrition. Increasing the intake of fruits, vegetables, grains, and healthy fats will provide needed nutrients. Depending on individual needs, food choices may need to be adapted to limit intake of sodium, potassium, and phosphorus. The recommended limit of sodium is 2300 mg/day, which is easily tracked as sodium content of food is readily available on nutrition labels. It is recommended that phosphorus intake be limited and that potassium intake be adjusted to maintain normal serum values. However, the phosphorus and potassium content of foods is not easily obtained, and does not necessarily coincide with their effect on serum levels. The phosphorus in many high phosphorus plant foods is minimally absorbed and thus has little impact on serum levels. Moreover, evidence supporting the effect of high potassium-containing foods on serum levels is virtually nonexistent. Therefore, when treating CKD patients with hyperphosphatemia and/or hyperkalemia, the renal nutrition expert will need to critically evaluate not only food intake but medications and overall metabolic and physical health [44, 45].

Energy Needs

There is a lack of data regarding optimal energy requirements to slow the progression of CKD and to maintain a proper nutritional status. Resting energy expenditure (REE) may be low, normal, or elevated in patients with CKD as compared to the general population [22]. Inflammation and prevalence of comorbid conditions such as poorly controlled diabetes and cardiovascular disease may cause an increase in metabolic rate and elevated REE, which is a major risk factor for the development of protein-energy wasting [20, 46].

Indirect calorimetry is considered the best technique for determining energy expenditure but is often laborious and cumbersome to routinely use in the clinical setting [47, 48]. Commonly used equations such as the Harris-Benedict, Schofield, or Mifflin-St Jeor equations have not been extensively studied in the CKD population. Kamimura demonstrated that Harris-Benedict and Schofield overestimated REE when compared with indirect calorimetry in 124 CKD patients not yet on dialy-

Table 14.4 Equation for estimating lean body mass in CKD[a]

LBM-H	(1 if male; 0 if female) × 6.82 + height (cm) × 0.18 + weight (kg) × 0.40 + HGS (n) × 0.01−18.12
LBM-M	(1 if male; 0 if female) × 7.36 + height (cm) × 0.22 + weight (kg) × 0.37 + MAMC (cm) × 0.24−26.43

Abbreviations: *LBM-H* lean body mass estimated from handgrip strength, *HGS* hand grip strength, *LBM-M* lean body mass estimated from mid-arm muscle circumference, *MAMC* mid-arm muscle circumference
[a]Created with data from [47]

sis [49]. Byham-Gray suggested the addition of laboratory data such as albumin, C-reactive protein (CRP), and creatinine in addition to using anthropometric data when estimating REE in CKD patients [48].

Recently, Tian developed and evaluated two new equations for estimating lean body mass (LBM) based on hand-grip strength (HGS) and mid-arm muscle circumference (MAMC) in 300 patients with stages 3–5 CKD (Table 14.4). Results suggested that LBM values estimated using both equations were numerically close to and significantly correlated with those measured using DEXA ($p < 0.01$) [47].

In the absence of a validated REE formula for CKD, KDOQI and the Academy of Nutrition and Dietetics (Academy) recommend calculating energy needs at 25–35 kcal/kg/day for those who are metabolically stable in order to provide adequate calories to drive the use of protein for repair rather than energy [9, 50, 51]. Calorie needs will be affected by age, gender, activity level, body composition, and overall health status.

Calculating Nutrient Needs in Underweight and Obese Conditions

Data from the United States Renal Data System (USRDS) indicate an increase in the prevalence of overweight and obesity in the CKD population [4]. Dietary management of these patients need to address issues of excess energy consumption. As mentioned previously, obesity has complex effects in those with CKD. Patients with low BMI have increased risk of all-cause and cardiovascular mortality, while an elevated BMI results in improved survival [46]. This conflicting data may be a result of limitations of BMI in differentiating adipose tissue from lean mass. Obese patients may have more energy reserves and this may play a role in mitigating the deleterious effects of increased REE in CKD [46]. Prevention and treatment of obesity is complex, and studies on intentional weight loss to slow progression of CKD have not been performed.

The ideal (healthiest) BMI range for CKD is unknown. The KDOQI guidelines suggest a "normal weight" BMI of 18.5–24.9 [9]. When the client's actual BMI is near this range, current body weight is recommended for nutrient calculations [52]. In obese CKD patients (BMI ≥ 30), some clinicians use adjusted body weight for calculating nutrient needs, which aims to capture what is considered to be metabolically active weight rather than excess adiposity [53]. However, adjusted body weight formulas have no scientific validity and evidence-based research does not support their use [52]. Energy recommendations calculated with an adjusted body weight are very different from calculated needs based on indirect calorimetry[54]. The Evidence Analysis Library Chronic Kidney Disease Guideline does not recommend using adjusted body weight formulas and encourages using best clinical judgment in practice [9]. The Academy of Nutrition and Dietetics Evidence Analysis Library Adult Weight Management Guideline recommends using actual body weight and the Mifflin-St Jeor equation when estimating energy needs in overweight noncritically ill patients [55]. Therefore, it is generally recommended that actual body weight be used whenever feasible to determine energy needs in both underweight and overweight individuals, followed by the addition or subtraction of calories for weight gain or loss, depending on the patient's condition and nutrition needs [52–55].

There is no evidence-based research for determining protein needs in underweight or obese CKD patients. The American Society for Parenteral and Enteral Nutrition (A.S.P.E.N) recommends using actual body weight for calculating protein needs in critically ill obese subjects [56]. Studies on non-ill obese subjects without CKD also recommend actual body weight for calculating protein needs [57, 58]. However, in both overweight and underweight CKD patients, calculating 0.55 to 0.60 gm protein/kg/day (0.60 to 0.80 gm/kg/day for those with diabetes) actual body weight could greatly underestimate or overestimate protein needs.

It has been suggested that protein needs could be calculated as a percentage (e.g., 10–12%) of estimated energy requirements once those are determined, but there is no evidence to support this method. The practitioner should exercise good clinical judgment when determining protein requirements and consider encouraging more plant protein when a higher protein intake is indicated. Clinicians must monitor patient outcomes to determine whether protein recommendations are adequate and meeting patient needs. As always, registered dietitian nutritionists (RDN) must be flexible to adjust goals and prescriptions according to their patient's individual conditions. Well-controlled metabolic studies and/or randomized-controlled trials are needed to determine actual energy and protein requirements in obese and underweight CKD patients.

Micronutrients and Supplements

Vitamin supplementation needs in CKD can vary, depending on renal disorders, co-morbid conditions, appetite, and intake. Due to compromised kidney function, some vitamin levels can be higher or lower, depending on excretion and metabolism [59]. Traditional CKD diet recommendations which restrict foods and food groups due to protein, phosphorus, and potassium content could result in suboptimal intakes of several vitamins, although not always [60]. When diet focuses on quality over quantity, it is possible to achieve healthier nutrient intakes. Thus, routine vitamin supplements may not be needed. The clinician will need to assess patients individually to determine needs, considering disease and metabolic states, stage of CKD, appetite, and overall intake.

Multiple-Vitamin-Mineral (MVI) supplements should be avoided as they often contain extra minerals such as phosphorus, potassium, magnesium, etc. Vitamin A supplements are contraindicated as they can lead to high serum and liver levels. Vitamins D and E should be individualized to specific conditions. For those patients with suboptimal intakes, it is generally safe to recommend a water-soluble-vitamin-supplement at dietary reference intake (DRI) levels (Table 14.5) [9, 43, 61]. Biotin needs may be higher due to decreased biotin consumption when protein intake is low. Higher levels of vitamin C should be avoided due to risk of oxalosis [62]. Some clinicians prefer extra folate, pyri-

Table 14.5 Dietary reference intakes for adults.[a] Vitamin supplementation table recommendations in chronic kidney disease stages 1–4. Higher levels may be acceptable based on specific patient needs

Vitamin	US DRI (Adults > 18 years)
Vitamin C	75–90 mg/d
Thiamin (B-1)	1.1–1.2 mg/d
Riboflavin (B-2)	1.1–1.3 mg/d
Niacin	14–16 mg/d
Folate	0.4 mg/d
Pyridoxine (B-6)	1.3–1.7 mg/d
Cobalamin (B-12)	2.4 mcg/d
Biotin	30 mcg/d

[a]Created with data from [61]

doxine (B-6), and cobalamin (B-12) to help prevent hyperhomocysteinemia, although some studies show that treating this condition with high levels of B-vitamins is unwarranted and possibly harmful [63]. Moreover, there is limited evidence that folate supplements along with vitamin B complex can affect markers of nutrition health such as body weight, CRP, and serum albumin. Folic acid supplementation when combined with Enalapril has been shown to help stabilize the kidney function in CKD [9].

Use of alternative, complementary and herbal supplement products is common in CKD populations. Many products are advertised as kidney protective or beneficial for kidney dysfunction. However, few of these products have been adequately studied in humans, and even fewer have been trialed in CKD [64, 65]. Since there is no regulation of the supplement industry in the United States, the purity, safety and effectiveness of these products is unknown. One study testing 44 herbal products for authenticity concluded that most were of poor quality and contained contaminants, non-listed ingredients, and fillers [66]. Patients should be reminded that every product they consume must be filtered by their kidneys, and it can affect kidney health. Clinicians should routinely ask patients about their use of supplements to help identify risks. There are safe herbal products available, and the renal nutrition expert should work with patients to find appropriate items that meet their needs. (See Chaps. 32 and 33 for additional information.)

Comorbidities of CKD

Individuals with CKD often have multiple comorbidities, such as diabetes, CVD, hypertension, dyslipidemia, and BMD. Nutrition plays an important role in the management of these comorbidities and kidney function. As previously mentioned, CKD diet recommendations should emphasize overall diet quality rather than focusing on individual nutrients. Emerging research recommends comprehensive eating patterns such as the Mediterranean and DASH for the management of chronic diseases such as CKD, diabetes, and cardiovascular diseases. These diets emphasize a variety of whole grains, vegetables, fruits, and plant proteins. Evidence suggests that these diets may be helpful in managing comorbidities of CKD, delay progression, and prevent complications in CKD patients [10, 12, 13].

Diabetes

Diabetes is the most common comorbid risk factor for CKD. Roughly, 40% of all individuals with CKD have diabetes [1, 4]. Nutrition management for patients with CKD and diabetes must include intensive treatment of hyperglycemia to help prevent elevated albuminuria and delay kidney disease progression. Treatment of hyperglycemia includes medications, balanced nutrition, and physical activity. Depending on the stage of CKD, each of these approaches should be individualized to patient needs [67, 68].

A recent review of the benefits of the Mediterranean diet shows that this eating pattern can have a protective effect against the development of diabetes and also may improve glycemic control and reduce CVD risk factors in diabetic patients [69]. The DASH diet, which is most well known for reducing hypertension, shows benefits of improved glycemic control, weight loss, and improved insulin sensitivity in diabetic patients [70].

In order to address hyperglycemia in the diabetic CKD population, it is recommended that the amount and type of carbohydrates in the diet be adjusted. Emphasis should be placed on reducing refined carbohydrates and added sugars, focusing on quality carbohydrates from vegetables, legumes, fruits, dairy, and whole grains [71].

Low carbohydrate diets that include higher protein levels should be avoided due to the relationship of high protein diets and progression of kidney disease [72]. Current protein recommendations for CKD range from 0.55 to 0.60 g/kg/day [2, 3, 9]. Expert panels agree that 0.60 to 0.80 g/kg/day is appropriate for diabetic patients with CKD stages 1–5 (nondialysis) [9, 67, 68, 72]. Focusing on the quality of protein (plant vs. animal) may also be beneficial, as studies have shown that plant protein diets may help preserve kidney function in CKD [67, 68, 72]. (See Chap.11 for additional information.)

Cardiovascular Disease

Sixty-five percent of people with CKD have CVD. It is the leading cause of death, and most individuals with CKD will die prematurely of CVD, not surviving to stage 5 dialysis. Nutrition interventions to treat or stabilize CVD conditions include treating traditional risk factors such as hypertension and dyslipidemias, plus the nontraditional risk factor more specific to CKD, abnormal bone mineral metabolism [4].

Hypertension

Hypertension is both a cause and a complication of CKD and the CVD associated with it, with 50–75% of patients having blood pressure greater than 140/90 mm Hg. It is generally recommended that people with kidney disease should maintain blood pressure levels ≤130/80 mm Hg, adjusting for the level of albuminuria and age [73]. The DASH trial showed a comprehensive eating pattern successfully reduced blood pressure in adults [74]. In 2001, the DASH research group showed that adding sodium restriction of 1.5–2.4 g/d to the DASH dietary plan further reduced blood pressure levels [75].

In 2016, the first controlled feeding study of the DASH diet in moderate CKD was done and showed a reduced-sodium DASH diet to be beneficial for blood pressure (BP) control in moderate CKD [76]. The reduced sodium content used in the study was 2.4 gm/day. Additional restriction to 1.5 gm/d may lower blood pressure further; however, this may be difficult to achieve in most Western-type diets due to the prevalence of sodium additives in food production.

Compared to the typical American diet, the DASH plan is lower in fat and sodium and higher in potassium, magnesium, calcium, fiber, and antioxidants. DASH results indicate that a whole foods approach, which may include interactions between nutrients, can be more effective in treating hypertension than simply limiting or increasing one nutrient [74].

The low sodium DASH diet can be a safe and effective treatment for hypertension and preventing progression of CVD. Protein and phosphorus-containing foods may need adjustment to avoid intakes higher than recommended. As CKD progresses, adjusting potassium intake to help manage serum levels may become necessary also. Potassium excretion is usually sufficient to control serum levels in early stages of CKD, but common blood pressure medications (e.g., angiotensin-converting enzyme inhibitors [ACE inhibitors] and angiotensin II receptor blockers [ARBs]) can interfere with potassium excretion even when the urine output is good. These drugs are recommended in CKD as they not only control hypertension but also protect the kidneys and can slow CKD progression. The side effects of increasing serum potassium often occur in stages 4 and 5, when diet restriction becomes necessary. Although there are many common lists of high potassium-containing foods, there is little evidence to support the effect of restricting these foods on serum potassium level. Initial studies done on potassium intake and serum levels used potassium solutions rather than whole foods [44]. Potassium absorption and its effect on intracellular and serum levels from foods is impacted by a person's acid-base balance, glucose and insulin levels, bowel excretion, and

Table 14.6 Causes of high serum potassium in people with CKD[a]

Potential causes of high serum potassium in people with CKD	
Acidosis	Changes in gastric function (vomiting,
Blood glucose/insulin variations	diarrhea, constipation)
Intracellular/extracellular fluid shifts	Medications (ACEs, ARBs, Heparin)
Low urine output	Tissue breakdown (infection, injury, catabolism)
Variations in thyroid function	Blood transfusions
Changes in aldosterone/renin activity	Bleeding
Variations in total volume status	

[a]Created with data from [77, 78]

medications. One study showed that reported potassium intake only accounted for 2% of the variance in serum potassium levels [77]. Therefore, the renal nutrition expert will need to consider all potential causes of hyperkalemia rather than just focusing on limiting high potassium foods [78] (Table 14.6).

Additional lifestyle changes that can impact hypertension include weight loss in obese subjects. The beneficial effects of weight loss and exercise on hypertension and the progression of CKD are unknown [73]. Weight loss to obtain and maintain appropriate body weight for height (BMI < 25.5 kg/m^2) is most likely beneficial in early CKD stages, along with fitness programs to improve muscle mass, flexibility, and strength. But considering the high risk of malnutrition as kidney function declines, weight loss programs should be approached with caution when CKD progresses. Maintaining adequate calorie and protein intake is the first priority. In obese subjects, controlled and gradual weight loss might be appropriate if patients are monitored closely to ensure that they are able to consume adequate protein and that they are not losing muscle mass. This becomes especially critical as appetite and food intake spontaneously decline with decreasing kidney function [18, 19]. Exercise programs that include resistance training can help reduce catabolism and help maintain muscle mass in people with stage 4 CKD [29, 30] (See Chap. 30).

Dyslipidemias

Abnormal lipid levels are common in people with CKD and can contribute to the progression of CKD and CVD. It is recommended that all people with CKD should be evaluated for lipid disorders. Hyperlipidemia treatment recommendations include the use of statin drugs plus lifestyle interventions [79, 80].

Therapeutic lifestyle changes (TLC) for treating dyslipidemia are similar to those for treating hypertension, including diet modifications, exercise, moderate alcohol intake, and smoking cessation. As with hypertension, a few studies have evaluated the effect of exercise and weight loss on abnormal lipid profiles in CKD, and the effect of weight reduction on dyslipidemia in obese subjects with CKD is unknown. Regarding diet modifications, current research suggests that eating patterns similar to the DASH and Mediterranean diets are most beneficial in treating lipid disorders [81]. (See Chap.13 for additional information.)

Mineral and Bone Disorders

Bone disorders and abnormalities in calcium, phosphorus, vitamin D, parathyroid hormone (PTH) metabolism, and fibroblast growth factor-23 (FGF-23) begin in the early stages of CKD. Reduction in the kidney function even at stages 2 and 3 will result in phosphate retention, hyperphosphatemia, elevated PTH, decreased 1,25 vitamin D, and increased levels of FGF-23 [82–84]. Conversion of

25(OH)D to 1,25 (OH)D is reduced, lowering intestinal calcium absorption and increasing PTH. FGF-23 and PTH normally enhance phosphate excretion in the kidneys, but as CKD advances, the kidneys no longer respond efficiently to either of it. Down regulation of vitamin D and PTH resistance at the tissue level is also evident. As the GFR falls below 60 mL/min/1.73 m^2, serum levels of phosphorus, calcium, PTH, and vitamin D will begin to show abnormalities [82, 83].

The pathogenesis and progression of abnormal bone metabolism in CKD is complex, involving a combination of minerals and hormones that act on multiple organ systems throughout the body. The consequences of PTH, vitamin D, and FGF-23 abnormalities include high turnover bone disease, bone resorption, osteomalacia, adynamic bone disease, overt fractures, microfractures, and bone pain [82]. More importantly, the high mortality of patients with CKD may be directly related to soft tissue calcification resulting from hyperphosphatemia, hypercalcemia, or high PTH. Vascular calcification has been implicated in the high rate of atherosclerosis and cardiac dysfunction seen in the CKD population [82–86].

Biochemical monitoring of bone health should begin in CKD stage 3, with baseline measurements of serum PTH, calcium, phosphorus, and alkaline phosphatase. Frequency of testing should be determined by baseline levels and progression of kidney disease, generally every 6–12 months. As CKD progresses to stage 4, frequency of testing could increase up to every 3–6 months, and up to monthly by stage 5, depending on serum levels and the presence of biochemical abnormalities [82, 83]. 25(OH)D should be assessed beginning at stage 3. Repeat testing is dependent on baseline values and therapeutic interventions. Vitamin D deficiency should be treated as in the general population.

For all biochemical measurements of mineral and bone disorders, therapeutic treatments should be based on serial measurements and trends rather than single values. Progressive or persistent high serum phosphorus should be treated to lower levels toward the normal range, beginning with a low phosphorus diet. Secondary treatment for hyperphosphatemia includes phosphate binders, but calcium-based binders should be avoided when possible to prevent hypercalcemia.

Specific goal levels for PTH are not known. It is recommended that when PTH is progressively rising or persistently above the upper normal limit, patients should first be evaluated and treated for hyperphosphatemia, high phosphorus intake, hypocalcemia, and vitamin D deficiency. Treatment with calcitriol and vitamin D analogs is not routinely recommended for high PTH levels except in those with severe and progressive hyperparathyroidism at CKD stages 4 and 5 [82, 83].

The restriction of dietary phosphorus in conjunction with a low-protein diet can have a direct effect on lowering serum phosphorus and PTH and is associated with a significant increase in blood levels of 1,25(OH)$_2$D$_3$ [84, 87]. The average phosphate intake in the typical American diet varies from 1000 to 1600 mg/d, based on naturally occurring phosphorus in foods, which tends to be concentrated in high-protein foods such as meats, dairy products, and eggs. Although legumes, whole grains, and nuts contain significant amounts of phosphorus, they are poorly absorbed, and thus contribute much less to the total dietary phosphorus load [45]. Phosphorus-containing food additives used in processed, convenience, and fast foods make a significant contribution to phosphorus consumption. It is estimated that a typical American diet that includes the regular use of processed foods can add an additional 500–1000 mg phosphorus; this increases the daily consumption to 1500–2600 mg/d. Phosphorus consumed in the form of food additives is readily absorbed compared to naturally occurring phosphorus, thus representing a large phosphorus burden [88–90].

It has been advised that phosphorus intake be restricted to maintain normal serum phosphorus levels, or 10–12 mg phosphorus per gram of protein [9]. But tracking the amount of phosphorus in foods is difficult as it is not included on food labels and it is frequently missing from nutrient database tables. Because naturally occurring phosphorus is found in high-protein foods, a protein-controlled diet, as is recommended with CKD, tends to be lower in phosphorus than the typical American diet. CKD patients following a vegetarian low-protein diet have lower serum phosphorus levels compared to those on an animal-based low-protein diet [45, 91]. The phosphorus content of convenience, processed, and fast foods must also be considered in planning a low-phosphorus intake. Because ingredients in processed foods change often, frequent consultation with food manufacturers is needed in order to obtain accurate nutrient amounts.

Even with a dietary phosphorus restriction, phosphate binders may be required in stage 3 or 4 CKD to help control serum phosphorus. When taken with meals and snacks, these compounds bind phosphate in the intestine before it can be absorbed. See Chap. 23 for additional information on bone and mineral disorders in CKD.

Anemia

Anemia develops during the course of CKD and the incidence of anemia increases as GFR declines, primarily due to insufficient production of erythropoietin (EPO) by the diseased kidneys [3]. Additional causes of anemia may be blood loss from repeated laboratory testing, gastrointestinal bleeding, acute and chronic inflammation, or deficiency of iron, folate, or vitamin B12. It is recommended that all patients with CKD be evaluated for anemia. If hemoglobin (Hgb) falls below 13 g/dL in males or 12 g/dL in females, an anemia workup is warranted. This workup should include assessment of complete blood count (CBC), reticulocyte count, percent transferrin saturation (TSAT), serum ferritin, serum B12, and folate [92, 93].

Anemia in CKD is generally normocytic and normochromic. Microcytosis may reflect iron deficiency; macrocytosis may indicate B12 or folate deficiency. Elevated reticulocyte count may suggest active hemolysis, such as hemolytic uremic syndrome. An abnormal white blood cell count and/or platelet count may reflect a more generalized bone marrow dysfunction such as malignancy or vasculitis. Low levels of serum iron, percent TSAT, or ferritin may indicate iron deficiency [94]. If iron deficiency is present, a stool occult blood test may be recommended to test for gastrointestinal bleeding. If a reversible cause of anemia is not present or has been corrected, then erythropoietin (EPO) deficiency is the most likely primary cause of anemia and erythropoietin stimulating agents (ESA) may be necessary.

Iron Deficiency

In CKD stages 3–5, iron deficiency is indicated if TSAT is <30% and/or serum ferritin level is <500 ng/mL [91, 92]. Due to the quantity of iron required, increasing iron intake from foods will not adequately replenish iron stores. Depending on severity of iron deficiency and previous responses to iron therapy, oral or IV iron supplementation will be needed. Oral iron is often prescribed to provide 200 mg elemental iron daily. Ferrous sulfate is commonly used although there are other oral iron preparations available. There is no evidence to suggest that one is better utilized than another. Intestinal iron absorption is inversely related to iron stores. If iron supplementation goals are not met within 3 months of oral iron supplements, IV iron therapy may be considered.

ESA Therapy

Once iron deficiency and other causes of anemia have been resolved, ESA therapy may be warranted if Hgb falls below 10 mg/dL. The decision to treat with ESA therapy should be individualized based on symptoms and previous responses to therapy. During ESA therapy, Hgb and iron status should be monitored at least every 3 months. In general, it is not recommended that ESA therapy be used to maintain Hgb > 11.5 mg/dL.

The most common cause of an inadequate response to EPO therapy for the treatment of anemia is iron deficiency. If iron-replete patients are not achieving their Hgb goal, they should be evaluated for conditions such as B12/folate deficiencies, hypothyroidism, infection or inflammation, blood loss, malignancy, bone marrow disorders, or hemoglobinopathies. Additionally, malnutrition can result in the unavailability of the needed substrate for protein synthesis in hematopoietic cells [92, 93]. It is unclear whether the presence of anemia in CKD directly worsens prognosis or progression to stage 5 CKD; however, low Hgb levels in CKD are associated with higher rates of hospitalizations, CVD, cognitive impairment, and mortality [92, 93].

IgA Nephropathy

IgA nephropathy (IgAN) is one of the most common kidney diseases in the world, after diabetes and high blood pressure. It is believed to be an autoimmune disease, due to immune complex-mediated glomerulonephritis characterized by the deposition of IgA within the mesangial regions of the glomeruli. Many patients develop a chronic, slowly progressive decline in kidney function over 10–20 years, leading to stage 5 CKD in 20–40% of cases [95–97]. Treatment often includes medications to suppress the immune system, control blood pressure, and lower cholesterol. Specific diet therapies involving nutrition interventions have also been examined.

Omega-3 (n-3) Polyunsaturated Fatty Acids

The omega-3 polyunsaturated fatty acids (PUFA) eicosapentanoic acid (EPA) and docosahexanoic acid (DHA) (found in cold water fish, flaxseed oil, and canola oil) have anti-inflammatory effects in humans. EPA and DHA undergo biologic transformation into trienoic eicosanoids, which lead to decreased production of proinflammatory mediators, resulting in vasodilatory rather than vasoconstriction properties. In the kidney, EPA is used as substrate which results in reduced manifestations of mesangial cell activation [98]. Prospective studies have evaluated the effect of EPA and DHA supplements on the progression of IgAN and found that in long-range follow-up, the rate of loss of kidney function can be lowered with doses of 1.9 g EPA and 1.4 g DHA [99]. As a person would need to consume approximately two servings of salmon per day to obtain that amount of EPA and DHA, supplements provide a convenient way to increase noninflammatory polyunsaturated fatty acids (PUFA). An additional benefit may come from reducing the intake of pro-inflammatory PUFAs, which are found in vegetable oils such as safflower, sunflower, and corn oils.

Low Antigen Content Diet

The rationale for use of a low antigen content diet for the treatment of IgAN involves the pathogenesis of IgA renal lesions. IgA is secreted by β-cells as part of the mucosal immune system in the intestinal tract, as triggered by viral and dietary antigens crossing the intestinal mucosal barrier [98]. Animal studies have shown IgA that is produced in response to dietary antigens can form glomerular deposits [100]. Studies in humans have shown that a low antigen content diet was able to reduce nephritogenic dietary antigens [101]. More recent studies have investigated the relation of IgAN to celiac disease and treatments with a gluten free diet [102]. Besides gluten, the low antigen content diet includes avoidance of foods containing common allergens such as nuts, dairy foods, citrus foods such as oranges and grapefruit, cantaloupe, honeydew, berries, chocolate, shellfish, eggs, and sulfites. Although the diet is complicated and restrictive in many foods and nutrients, a qualified renal dietitian could combine the low antigen components with an appropriate renal diet in those patients with IgAN. Regular nutrition assessments would be necessary to assure that the patient was consuming adequate nutrients.

Self-Management Behavior and Medical Nutrition Therapy

Nutrition management in CKD involves complex diet therapies; patients must learn to balance protein, calories, sodium, phosphorus, and possibly potassium. Additionally, if patients are diagnosed with diabetes, they must also incorporate methods to control carbohydrate intake and appropriate blood glucose levels. Emphasis should be placed on eating patterns consistent with overall diet quality rather than just limiting nutrients. The plate method has been recommended as a teaching tool to emphasize healthy eating patterns, and simplify meal planning (Fig. 14.1, kidney-healthy plate) [103].This tool can be utilized with CKD patients and adjusted depending on individual needs. Using a healthy plate method to teach diabetic kidney disease meals would include: ½ of plate nonstarchy vegetables, ¼ of plate healthy protein, and ¼ of plate grains, starchy vegetables, or fruit. Individuals limiting phosphorus and potassium can adjust the plate method to include fruits and vegetables lower in potassium, less processed foods, and a reduced amount of dairy and animal products. CKD patients concerned about heart health could adjust the plate to emphasize healthy fats such as fish, nuts, seeds and healthy oils. When following a vegetarian diet, the plate method can be adjusted to include vegetarian protein sources such as beans, lentils, tofu, nuts, and seeds. See Table 14.7 for examples of these meals.

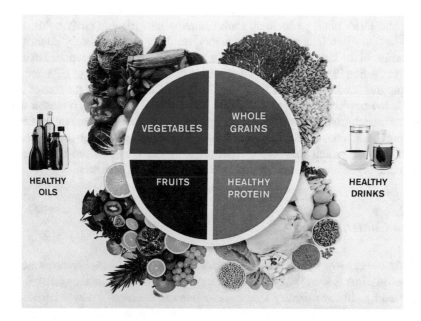

Fig. 14.1 Kidney-healthy plate. The plate method can be used to plan high-quality, kidney-healthy meals that provide adequate calories and protein, appropriate for treating diabetes and CVD. (Reprinted with permission from Puget Sound Kidney Centers, Everett WA)

Table 14.7 Sample kidney-healthy meals, based on kidney-healthy plate

Diabetes meal	Low-potassium, low-phosphorus meal	Heart-healthy meal	Vegetarian meal
Fresh eggs scrambled with chopped onion, peppers, spinach, and zucchini. Whole grain toast	Chicken stir-fry with green beans, onions, peppers, carrots, and mushrooms. Couscous Apple slices	Grilled salmon Whole grain pasta tossed with olive oil and herbs Sautéed bell peppers, mushrooms, spinach, onions, and garlic	Mixed bean chili with chopped tomatoes and cilantro Corn bread Green salad with balsamic vinaigrette

Depending on the patient's overall health, clinicians may additionally advise lifestyle changes such as quitting smoking, increasing levels of physical activity and exercise. These are not behavioral changes that patients can learn in brief office visits with clinicians but involve intense education in new lifestyles. Partnership and collaboration between healthcare providers and patients is crucial in promoting self-management in CKD patients [104].

Studies have shown that MNT provided by a RDN is effective in preventing and treating malnutrition and mineral and electrolyte disorders, and in minimizing the impact of other comorbid conditions such as hypertension and diabetes [6, 7, 9]. Referrals for MNT should begin during stage 3 CKD when GFR is less than 50 mL/min/1.73 m². The RDN should monitor the nutritional status every 1–3 months, or more frequently depending on the risk of malnutrition or mineral and electrolyte disorders. Nutrition therapies must be adjusted to help maintain nutritional health and improve outcomes, depending on patient conditions. RDNs providing MNT teach self-management skills to their clients in order to promote lifestyle changes that will result in the most successful outcomes for the CKD patient.

Conclusion

Effective nutrition care for people with CKD stages 1 through 5 (nondialysis) involves complex therapeutic interventions. Patients must be assessed for individual nutrition risks and needs to prevent malnutrition, electrolyte imbalances, and bone and mineral metabolism disorders. Many patients presenting with CKD are also diagnosed with comorbid conditions such as diabetes, cardiovascular disease, hypertension, and dyslipidemia. MNT must include treatment of these conditions and must be coordinated with CKD nutrition therapies. The ultimate goal is to slow the progression of CKD and comorbid conditions and prevent complications of bone mineral metabolism while maintaining overall nutritional health. This can be accomplished through effective MNT provided by the RDN.

Case Study

B.H. has been referred to a nephrologist by the local Community Health Center. Last month, B.H. went to the Health Center complaining of "flu symptoms" like fatigue, chronic cough, nausea, headaches, and fever. B.H. is 66 years old male, height 182 cm, body weight 83 kg, with a previous diagnosis of diabetes. He quit smoking last year but drinks alcohol occasionally. BH eats two meals per day at restaurants, plus an afternoon snack at work. Meals are frequently eggs and hash browns or pancakes, and meat and potatoes with a small salad, or deli sandwich. Snacks include chips, crackers, popcorn. Exercise includes housework and light yard work. Medications included Glyburide 2.5 mg every day. His blood pressure was 163/89 mm Hg with trace peripheral edema in his lower extremities. His lungs were clear. Laboratory test results showed: creatinine 2.3 mg/dL, BUN 51 mg/dL, HbA1C 6.1%, potassium 4.6 meq/L, bicarbonate 26 meq/L, TC 219 mg/dL. The Health Center prescribed Lasix 20 mg once daily, Lisinopril 5 mg once daily, and referred B.H. to the nephrologist. When the nephrologist sees B.H. a month later his blood pressure is 150/80 mm Hg. Trace edema is still present below the knees. Cough, headache, and fever have resolved, but he complains of ongoing fatigue and low energy. Current laboratory tests show creatinine 1.8 mg/dL, BUN 52 mg/dL, Hgb 9.6 gm/dL, potassium 5.3 meq/L, calcium 9.2 meq/L, phosphorus 5.0 mg/dL, Intact PTH 79 pg/mL, albumin 4.9 g/dL, glucose 95 mg/dL. Calculated GFR is 40 ml/min/1.73 m^2, CKD Stage 3. The nephrologist orders an anemia workup including iron studies. Ferritin is 83 ng/mL and TSAT is 18%. The nephrologist discusses CKD with him, the importance of achieving a lower blood pressure, and good blood glucose control. B.H. is told to add Norvasc 5 mg and FeSO4 325 mg (four tablets daily) to his medications and is referred to a dietitian for nutrition assessment and therapy.

Case Questions and Answers

1. Why is EPO therapy not prescribed, considering B.H.'s low Hgb?
   Answer: Ferritin and TSAT levels indicate iron deficiency. EPO therapy is not appropriate until iron stores are adequate. Therefore, B.H. is first prescribed iron therapy to replenish iron stores.
   Additional Follow-Up
   One month later, B.H. and his wife meet with the dietitian. She questions B.H. about lifestyle and usual eating patterns. He eats two meals per day at restaurants, plus an afternoon snack at work. Meals are frequently eggs and hash browns or pancakes, and meat and potatoes (steak, burger, fries) with a small salad. B.H. may occasionally have a deli style sandwich. Snacks are chips, crackers, or popcorn. Exercise includes housework and light yard work on weekends.
2. What are nutrition priorities for B.H.?
   Answer: Priorities include adjusting meals/snacks to include balanced servings of healthy proteins, whole grains, fruits, and vegetables. Since B.H. eats most of his meals in restaurants, education should include choosing healthier protein portions and other foods from menus, how to add fruits/vegetables to each meal, planning for healthy snack foods. The RDN should consider discussion on planning a few home-prepared meals if B.H. is receptive. His current exercise should be encouraged, and consider increasing physical activities as appropriate.
   Additional Follow-Up
   One month later B.H. and his wife return for follow-up, after seeing the nephrologist. Body weight is 81 kg with no signs of edema. Current laboratory values include serum phosphorus 4.8 mg/dL, potassium 4.6 meq/L, Hgb 10.1 gm/dL, ferritin 110 ng/dL, TSAT 23% and blood pressure 132/79. Evening blood glucose levels have been 180–200 mg/dL. B.H. reviews his food records with the dietitian, showing the changes he has made over the past several weeks, including eating 2 meals at home each week. He has reduced his meat portions and added fruit to his meals and afternoon snacks.
3. What additional nutrition therapy should be presented to B.H. at this clinic visit?
   Answer: By substituting fruit for meats, B.H. could significantly increase his carbohydrate intake resulting in higher blood glucose levels. Nutrition therapy should include a review of usual meal/snack patterns, focus on reducing fruits that affect blood glucose and substituting more low glycemic fruits and vegetables. Carbohydrate content of meals should be reviewed, including how to choose and plan appropriate amounts to balance carbs.
   Additional Follow-Up
   Two months later, B.H. returns for follow-up. Current laboratory values (from his nephrology visit) include serum phosphorus 4.3 mg/dL, Hgb 11.7 gm/dL, blood pressure 129/80, random blood glucose range from 90 to 130 mg/dL, and body weight has decreased to 78 kg. No medication changes are noted. B.H. reports that with his smaller protein, starch (potato, bread) and snack food portions, he often feels like he is not getting enough to eat.

4. Is B.H.'s recent weight loss a benefit or risk, considering his usual weight, diabetes, hypertension, and CKD?

   Answer: Although B.H. is within healthy weight range for his height (BMI 23.6), ongoing weight loss may be a concern. B.H. reports that he often feels hungry. He is probably not eating enough food as he has been focusing on limiting protein and carbohydrates. Nutrition therapy should include review of meal plans, suggestions for increasing quantities and or ways to add calories so that he feels more satisfied and limits further weight loss.

References

1. Centers for Disease Control and Prevention. Chronic Kidney Disease in the United States, 2019. Atlanta, GA: US Department of Health and Human Services, Centers for Disease Control and Prevention; 2019. https://www.cdc.gov/kidneydisease/publications-resources/2019-national-facts.html. Access 5/1/20.
2. National Kidney Foundation. KDOQI 2012 clinical practice guidelines for the evaluation and management of chronic kidney disease. Kidney Int. 2013;3(1):1–150.
3. Inker LA, Astor BC, Fox CH, Isakova T, Lash JP, Peralta CA, et al. KDOQI US commentary on the 2012 KDIGO clinical practice guideline for the evaluation and management of CKD. Am J Kidney Dis. 2014;63(5):713–35.
4. Saran R, Robinson B, Abbott KC, Bragg-Gresham J, Chen X, Gipson D, et al. US Renal Data System 2019 Annual Data Report: epidemiology of kidney disease in the United States. Am J Kidney Dis. 2020;75(1)(suppl 1):Svi–Svii.
5. About chronic kidney disease. National Kidney Foundation. https://www.kidney.org/atoz/content/about-chronic-kidney-disease. Access 10/6/18.
6. de Waal D, Heaslip E, Callas P. Medical nutrition therapy for chronic kidney disease improves biomarkers and slows time to dialysis. J Ren Nutr. 2015;26(1):1–9.
7. Kramer H, Yakes Jimenez E, Brommage D, Vassalotti J, Montgomery E, Steiber A, et al. Medical nutrition therapy for patients with non-dialysis-dependent chronic kidney disease: barriers and solutions. J Acad Nutr Diet. 2018;118(10):1958–65.
8. Kopple JD, Fouque D. Pro: the rationale for dietary therapy for patients with advanced chronic kidney disease. Nephrol Dial Transplant. 2018;33(3):373–8.
9. Ikizler TA, Burrowes J, Byham-Gray L, Campbell K, Carrero JJ, Chan W, et al. KDOQI Nutrition in CKD Guideline Work Group. KDOQI clinical practice guideline for nutrition in CKD: 2020 update. Am J Kidney Dis. 2020; in press.
10. Chauveau P, Aparicio M, Bellizzi V, Campbell K, Hong X, Johansson L, et al. Mediterranean diet as the diet of choice for patients with chronic kidney disease. Nephrol Dial Transplant. 2017;5(33):725–35.
11. Chauveau P, Koppe L, Combe C, Lasseur C, Trolonge S, Aparicio M. Vegetarian diets and chronic kidney disease. Nephrol Dial Transplant. July 5 2018. https://doi.org/10.1093/ndt/gfy164.
12. Rebholz CM, Crews DC, Grams MD, Steffen LM, Levey AS, Miller ER, et al. Dash (dietary approaches to stop hypertension) diet and risk of subsequent kidney disease. Am J Kidney Dis. 2016;68(6):853–61.
13. Smyth A, Griffin M, Yusuf S, Mann JFE, Reddan D, Canavan M, et al. Diet and major renal outcomes: a prospective cohort study. The NIH-AARP diet and health study. J Ren Nutr. 2016;26(5):288–98.
14. Chen W, Bushinsky DA. Addressing racial disparity in the progression of chronic kidney disease: prescribe more fruits and vegetables? Am J Nephrol. 2018;47:171–3.
15. Cupisti A, D'Alessandro CD, Gesualdo L, Cosola C, Gallieni M, Egidi MF, et al. Non-traditional aspects of renal diets: focus on fiber, alkali and vitamin K1 intake. Nutrients. 2017;5(9):444. https://doi.org/10.3390/nu9050444.
16. Goraya N, Simoni J, Jo CH, Wesson D. A comparison of treating metabolic acidosis in CKD stage 4 hypertensive kidney disease with fruits and vegetables or sodium bicarbonate. Clin J Am Soc Nephrol. 2013;8:371–81.
17. Held PJ, Port FK, Gaylin DS, et al. Evaluations of initial predictors of mortality among new ESRD patients: the USRDS case mix study. Abstracts. J Am Soc Nephrol. 1991;2:328.
18. Kopple JD, Greene T, Chumlea WC, Hollinger D, Maroni BJ, Merrill D, et al. Relationship between nutritional status and the glomerular filtration rate: results from the MDRD study. Kidney Int. 2000;57:1688–703.
19. Ikizler TA, Green JH, Wingard RL, Parker RA, Hakim RM. Spontaneous dietary protein intake during progression of chronic renal failure. J Am Soc Nephrol. 1995;6:1386–91.
20. Carrero JJ, Stenvinkel P, Cuppari L, Ikizler TA, Kalantar-Zadeh K, Kaysen G, et al. Etiology of the protein-energy wasting syndrome in chronic kidney disease: a consensus statement from the International Society of Renal Nutrition and Metabolism (ISRNM). J Ren Nutr. 2013;23(2):77–90.
21. Fried LF, Boudreau R, Lee JS, Chertow G, Kurella-Tamura M, Shlipak MG, et al. Kidney function as a predictor of loss of lean mass in older adults: health, aging, and body composition study. J Am Geriatr Soc. 2007;55:1578–84.

22. O'Sullivan AJ, Lawson JA, Chan M, Kelly JJ. Body composition and energy metabolism in chronic renal insufficiency. Am J Kidney Dis. 2002;39(2):369–75.
23. Mitch WE, Maroni BJ. Factors causing malnutrition in patients with chronic uremia. Am J Kidney Dis. 1999;33:176–9.
24. Stenvinkel P, Heimburger O, Paultre F, Diczfalusy U, Wang T, Berglund L, et al. Strong association between malnutrition, inflammation, and atherosclerosis in chronic renal failure. Kidney Int. 1999;55:1899–911.
25. Rhee CM, Ahmadi SF, Kalantar-Zedeh K. The dual roles of obesity in chronic kidney disease: a review of the current literature. Curr Opin Nephrol Hypertens. 2016;25(3):208–16.
26. Stenvinkel P, Zoccoli C, Ikizler TA. Obesity in CKD-what should nephrologists know? J Am Soc Nephrol. 2013;24:1727–36.
27. Mohebi R, Simforoosh A, Tohidi M, Azizi F, Hadaegh F. Obesity paradox and risk of mortality events in chronic kidney disease patients: a decade of follow-up in Tehran lipid and glucose study. J Ren Nutr. 2015;25(4):345–50.
28. Kalantar-Zadeh K, Rhee CM, Chou J, Ahmadi SF, Park J, Chen JLT, et al. The obesity paradox in kidney disease: how to reconcile it with obesity management. Kidney It Rep. 2017;2(2):271–81.
29. Van Huffel L, Tomson CR, Ruige J, Nistor I, Van Biesen W, Bolignano D. Dietary restriction and exercise for diabetic patients with chronic kidney disease: a systematic review. PLoS One. 2014;9(11):e113667.
30. Sah SK, Siddiqui MA, Darain H. Effect of progressive resistive exerise training in improving mobility and functional ability of middle adulthood patients with chronic kidney disease. J Kidney Dis Transpl. 2015;26(5):912–23.
31. Ko GJ, Obi Y, Tortoricci AR, Kalantar-Zadeh K. Dietary protein intake and chronic kidney disease. Curr Opin Clin Nutr Metab Care. 2017;20(1):77–85.
32. Kovesdy CP, Kalantar-Zadeh K. Back to the future: restricted protein intake for conservative management of CKD, triple goals of renoprotection, uremia mitigation, and nutrition health. Int Urol Nephrol. 2016;48(5):725–9.
33. Ihle BU, Becher GJ, Whitworth JA, Charlwood RA, Kincaid-Smith PS. The effect of protein restriction on the progression of renal insufficiency. N Engl J Med. 1989;321:1773–7.
34. Walser M, Hill SB, Ward L, Magder L. A crossover comparison of progression of chronic renal failure: ketoacids versus amino acids. Kidney Int. 1993;43:933–9.
35. Klahr S, Levey AS, Beck GJ, Caggiula AW, Hunsicker L, Kusek JW, et al. The effects of dietary protein restriction and blood-pressure control on the progression of chronic renal disease. N Engl J Med. 1994;330:877–84.
36. Walser M, Hill S. Can renal replacement be deferred by a supplemented very low protein diet? J Am Soc Nephrol. 1999;10:110–6.
37. Levey AS, Green T, Beck GJ, Caggiula AW, Kusek JW, Hunsicker LG, et al. Dietary protein restriction and the progression of chronic renal disease: what have all of the results of the MDRD study shown? J Am Soc Nephrol. 1999;10:2426–39.
38. Levey A, Greene T, Sarnak M, Wang X, Beck GJ, Kusek JW, et al. Effect of dietary protein restriction on the progression of kidney disease: long-term follow-up of the Modification of Diet in Renal Disease (MDRD) study. Am J Kidney Dis. 2006;48:879–88.
39. Menon V, Kopple J, Wang X, Beck GJ, Collins AJ, Kusek JW, et al. Effect of a very low-protein diet on outcomes: long-term follow-up of the Modification of Diet in Renal Disease (MDRD) study. Am J Kidney Dis. 2009;53:208–17.
40. Fouque D, Guebre-Egziabher F. Do low-protein diets work in chronic kidney disease patients? Semin Nephrol. 2009;29:30–8.
41. Chen X, Wei G, Jalili T, Metos J, Giri A, Cho ME, et al. The associations of plant protein intake with all-cause mortality in CKD. Am J Kidney Dis. 2016;67:423–30.
42. Brookhyser Hogan J. The vegetarian diet for kidney disease: preserving kidney function with plant based eating. Laguna Beach: Basic Health Publications; 2010.
43. Wiggins KL. Guideline 2: nutrition care of adult dialysis patients. In: Guidelines for nutrition care of renal patients. 3rd ed. Chicago: American Dietetic Association; 2002. p. 5–18.
44. St-Jules DE, Goldfarb DS, Sevick MA. Nutrient non-equivalence: does restricting high-potassium plant foods help to prevent hyperkalemia in hemodialysis patients? J Ren Nutr. 2016;26(5):282–7.
45. Moe SM, Zidehsarai MP, Chambers MA, Jackman LA, Radcliffe JS, Trevino LL, et al. Vegetarian compared with meat dietary protein source and phosphorus homeostasis in chronic kidney disease. Clin J Am Soc Nephrol. 2011;6(2):257–64.
46. Naderi N, Kleine CE, Park C, Hsiung JT, Soohoo M, Tantisattamo E, et al. Obesity paradox in advanced kidney disease: from bedside to the bench. Prog Cardiovasc Dis. 2018;61(2):168–81.
47. Tian X, Chen Y, Yang ZK, Ou Z, Dong J. Novel equations for estimating lean body mass in patients with chronic kidney disease. J Ren Nutr. 2018;28(3):156–64.
48. Byham-Gray L, Parrott JS, Peters EN, Fogerite SG, Hand RK, Ahrens S, et al. Modeling a predictive energy equation specific for maintenance hemodialysis. J Parenter Enteral Nutr. 2017;42(3):587–96.
49. Kamimura MA, Avesani CM, Bazanelli AP, Baria F, Draibe SA, Cuppari L. Are prediction equations reliable for estimating energy expenditure in chronic kidney disease patients? Nephrol Dial Transplant. 2011;26:544–50.
50. Byham-Gray LD. Weighing the evidence: energy determinations across the spectrum of kidney disease. J Ren Nutr. 2006;16:17–26.

51. Beto JA, Ramirez WE, Bansal VK. Medical nutrition therapy in adults with chronic kidney disease: integrating evidence and consensus into practice for the generalist registered dietitian nutritionist. J Acad Nutr Diet. 2014;114(7):1077–87.
52. Schiro Harvey K. Methods for determining healthy body weight in end stage renal disease. J Ren Nutr. 2006;16(3):269–76.
53. Ash S, Campbell KL, Bogard J, Millichamp A. Nutrition prescription to achieve positive outcomes in chronic kidney disease. Nutrients. 2014;6:416–51.
54. Ireton-Jones C. Adjusted body weight, con: why adjust body weight in energy expenditure calculations? Nutr Clin Pract. 2005;20:474–9.
55. Academy of Nutrition and Dietetics Evidence Analysis Library Adult Weight Management. https://www.andeal.org/template.cfm?template=guide_summary&key=621&highlight=Adult%20Weight%20management&home=1. Accessed 10/7/18.
56. McClave SA, Taylor BE, Martindale RG, Warren MM, Johnson DR, Braunschweig C, et al. Guidelines for the provision and assessment of nutrition support therapy in the adult critically ill patient: Society of Critical Care Medicine (SCCM) and American Society for Parenteral and Enteral Nutrition (A.S.P.E.N.). J Parenter Enteral Nutr. 2016;40(2):159–211.
57. Dutheil F, Lac G, Courteix D, Dore E, Chapier R, Roszyk L, et al. Treatment of metabolic syndrome by combination of physical activity and diet needs an optimal protein intake: a randomized controlled trial. Nutr J. 2012;11:72. https://doi.org/10.1186/1475-2891-11-72.
58. Weijs PJM, Wolfe RR. Exploration of the protein requirement during weight loss in obese older adults. Clin Nutr. 2016;35(2):394–8.
59. Handelman GJ, Levin NW. Guidelines for vitamin supplements in chronic kidney disease patients: what is the evidence? J Ren Nutr. 2011;21(1):117–9.
60. Jankowska M, Szupryczynska N, Debska-Slizien A, Borek P, Kaczkan M, Rutkowski B, et al. Dietary intake of vitamins in different options of treatment in chronic kidney disease: is there a deficiency? Transplant Proc. 2016;48(5):1427–30.
61. National Institute of Health. Office of dietary supplements. https://ods.od.nih.gov/Health_Information/Dietary_Reference_Intakes.aspx. Accessed 10/8/2018.
62. Handelman GJ. New insight on vitamin C in patients with chronic kidney disease. J Ren Nutr. 2011;21(1):110–2.
63. Rafeq Z, Roh JD, Guarina P, Kaufman J, Joseph J. Adverse myocardial effects of B-vitamin therapy in subjects with chronic kidney disease and hyperhomocysteinaemia. Nutr Metab Cardiovasc Dis. 2013;23(9):836–42.
64. Vamenta-Morris H, Dreisbach A, Shoemaker-Moyle M, Abdel-Rahman EM. Internet claims on dietary and herbal supplements in advanced nephropathy: truth or myth. Am J Nephrol. 2014;40(5):393–8.
65. Osman NA, Nassanein SM, Leil MM, NasrAllah MM. Complementary and alternative medicine use among patients with chronic kidney disease and kidney transplant recipients. J Ren Nutr. 2015;25(6):466–71.
66. Newmaster SG, Grguric M, Shanmughanandhan D, Ramalingam S, Ragupathy S. DNA barcoding detects contamination and substitution in North American herbal products. BMC Med. 2013;11:222.
67. National Kidney Foundation. KDOQI clinical practice guidelines and clinical practice recommendations for diabetes and chronic kidney disease. Am J Kidney Dis. 2007;49(suppl 2):S1–S180.
68. National Kidney Foundation. KDOQI clinical practice guideline for diabetes and CKD: 2012 update. Am J Kidney Dis. 2012;60(5):850–86.
69. Boucher JL. Mediterranean eating pattern. Diabetes Spectr. 2017;30(2):72–6.
70. Campbell AP. DASH eating plan: an eating pattern for diabetes management. Diabetes Spectr. 2017;30(2):76–81.
71. American Diabetes Association. 4. Lifestyle management: standards of medical care in diabetes-2018. Diabetes Care. 2018;41(Suppl.1):S38–50.
72. Ko GJ, Kalantar-Zadeh K, Goldstein-Fuchs J, Rhee CM. Dietary approaches in the management of diabetic patients with kidney disease. Nutrients. 2017;9(8). https://doi.org/10.3390/nu9080824.
73. Taler SJ, Agarwal R, Bakris GL, Flynn JT, Nilsson PM, Rahman M, et al. KDOQI US commentary on the 2012 KDIGO clinical practice guideline for management of blood pressure in CKD. Am J Kidney Dis. 2013;62(2):201–13.
74. Conlin PR, Chow D, Miller ER, Svetkey LP, Lin PH, Harsha DW, et al. The effect of dietary patterns on blood pressure control in hypertensive patients: results from the Dietary Approaches to Stop Hypertension (DASH) trial. Am J Hypertens. 2000;13:949–55.
75. Sacks FM, Svetkey LP, Vollmer WM, Appel LJ, Bray BA, Harsha D, et al. Effects on blood pressure of reduced dietary sodium and the Dietary Approaches to Stop Hypertension (DASH) diet. N Engl J Med. 2001;344:3–10.
76. Tyson CC, Lin PH, Corsino L, Batch BC, Allen J, Sapp S, et al. Short-term effects of the DASH diet in adults with moderate chronic kidney disease: a pilot feeding study. Clin Kidney J. 2016;9(4):592–8.
77. Noori N, Kalantar-Zadeh K, Kovesdy CP, Murali SB, Bross R, Nissenson AR, et al. Dietary potassium intake and mortality in long-term hemodialysis patients. Am J Kidney Dis. 2010;56:338–47.
78. Nissenson AR, Fine RN, Gentile DE. Clinical dialysis. 3rd ed. Norwalk: Appleton & Lange; 1995. p. 258, 730.

79. Sarnak MJ, Bloom R, Mutner P, Rahman M, Saland JM, Wilson PWF, et al. KDOQI US commentary on the 2013 KDIGO clinical practice guideline for lipid management in CKD. Am J Kidney Dis. 2015;65(3):354–66.

80. Marino A, Tannock LR. Role of dyslipidemia in patients with chronic kidney disease. J Postgrad Med. 2013;125(4):28–37.

81. KDIGO clinical practice guideline for lipid management in chronic kidney disease. Kidney Int. 2013;Supplement 3(3):284–85.

82. KDIGO 2017 clinical practice guideline update for the diagnosis, evaluation, prevention, and treatment of chronic kidney disease-mineral and bone disorder (CKD-MBD). Kidney Int. 2017;Supplement 7(1):1–60.

83. Isakova T, Nickolas TL, Denburg M, Yarlagadda S, Weiner DE, Gutierrez OM, et al. KDOQI US commentary on the 2017 KDIGO clinical practice guideline update for the diagnosis, evaluation, prevention, and treatment of chronic kidney disease-mineral and bone disorder (CKD-MBD). Am J Kidney Dis. 2017;70(6):737–51.

84. Martinez I, Saracho R, Montenegro J, Llach F. The importance of dietary calcium and phosphorous in the secondary hyperparathyroidism of patients with early renal failure. Am J Kidney Dis. 1997;29:496–502.

85. Andress DL. Vitamin D in chronic kidney disease: a systemic role for selective vitamin D receptor activation. Kidney Int. 2006;69:33–43.

86. Kramer H, Toto R, Peshock R, Cooper R, Victor R. Association between chronic kidney disease and coronary artery calcification: the Dallas Heart Study. J Am Soc Nephrol. 2005;16:507–13.

87. Barsotti G, Cupisti A. The role of dietary phosphorus restriction in the conservative management of chronic renal disease. J Ren Nutr. 2005;15:189–92.

88. Uribarri J, Calvo MS. Hidden sources of phosphorus in the typical American diet: does it matter in nephrology? Semin Dial. 2003;16:186–8.

89. Sullivan C, Sayre SS, Leon JB, Machekano R, Love TE, Porter D, et al. Effect of food additives on hyperphosphatemia among patients with end-stage renal disease, a randomized controlled trial. JAMA. 2009;301:629–35.

90. Carrigan A, Klinger A, Choquette SS, Luzuriaga-McPherson A, Bell EK, Darnell B, et al. Contribution of food additives to sodium and phosphorus content of diets rich in processed foods. J Ren Nutr. 2014;24(1):13–9.

91. Saloma L, Rix M, Kamper AL, Thomassen JQ, Sloth JJ, Astrup A. Short-term effect of the New Nordic Renal Diet on phosphorus homeostatsis in chronic kidney disease stages 3 and 4. Nephrol Dial Transplant. 2018;34:1691. https://doi.org/10.1093/ndt/gfy366.

92. KDIGO Anemia Work Group. KDIGO clinical practice guideline for anemia in chronic kidney disease. Kidney Int Suppl. 2012;2:279–335.

93. Kliger AS, Foley RN, Goldfarb DS, Goldstein SL, Johansen K, Singh A, et al. KDOQI US commentary on the 2012 KDIGO clinical practice guideline for anemia in CKD. Am J Kidney Dis. 2013;62(5):849–59.

94. Pocket guide to nutrition assessment of the patient with kidney disease. 5th ed. McCann L, editor. New York, National Kidney Foundation; 2015.

95. National Institute of Diabetes and Digestive and Kidney Diseases, National Institutes of Health. IgA Nephropathy. November 2015. https://www.niddk.nih.gov/health-information/kidney-disease/iga-nephropathy. Accessed 7 Feb 2019.

96. Donadio JV. The emerging role of omega-3 polyunsaturated fatty acids in the management of patients with IgA nephropathy. J Ren Nutr. 2001;11:122–8.

97. Pettersson EE, Rekola S, Berglund L, Sundqvist KG, Angelin B, Diczfalusy U, et al. Treatment of IgA nephropathy with omega-3-polyunsaturated fatty acids: a prospective, double-blind, randomized study. Clin Nephrol. 1994;41:183–90.

98. Souba WW, Wilmore DW. Diet and nutrition in the care of the patient with surgery, trauma, and sepsis. In: Shils ME, Olson JA, Shike M, Ross AC, editors. Modern nutrition in health and disease. 9th ed. Philadelphia: Lippincott Williams & Wilkins; 1999. p. 1609.

99. Donadio JV, Larson TS, Bergstralh EJ, Grande JP. A randomized trial of high dose compared with low-dose omega-3 fatty acids in severe IgA nephropathy. J Am Soc Nephrol. 2001;12:791–9.

100. Genin G, Laurent B, Sabatier JC, Colon S, Berthoux FC. IgA mesangial deposits in C3H/He mice after oral immunization with ferritin or bovine serum albumin. Clin Exp Immunol. 1986;63:385–91.

101. Ferri C, Puccini R, Longombardo G, Paleologo G, Migliorini P, Moriconi L, et al. Low-antigen-content diet in the treatment of patients with IgA nephropathy. Nephrol Dial Transplant. 1993;8:1193–8.

102. Cheung CK, Barratt J. Gluten and IgA nephropathy: you are what you eat? Kidney Int. 2016;88(2):215–8.

103. Maryniuk MD. From pyramids to plates to patterns: perspectives on meal planning. Spectr Diabetes J. 2017;30(2):67–70.

104. Chiou CP, Lu YC, Hung SY. Self-management in patients with chronic kidney disease. Hu Li Za Zhi-Chin J Nurs. 2016;63(2):5–11.

Chapter 15
Maintenance Hemodialysis

Debra Blair

Keywords Protein-energy wasting · Medical nutrition therapy · Renal replacement therapy · Maintenance hemodialysis · Conventional hemodialysis · Nocturnal hemodialysis · Short daily hemodialysis · Frequent hemodialysis · Long hemodialysis · Home hemodialysis · Stage 5 chronic kidney disease

> **Key Points**
> - Describe the goals of medical nutrition therapy for patients receiving conventional hemodialysis, nocturnal hemodialysis, and short daily hemodialysis.
> - Describe the differences in nutrition therapy between the different types of maintenance hemodialysis.
> - Identify factors that may impact the nutritional status of patients receiving maintenance hemodialysis.

Introduction

Medical nutrition therapy (MNT) is an essential component to achieving improved health outcomes for stage 5 chronic kidney disease (CKD) patients on dialysis. Recent data indicate that more than 700,000 adults in the United States have stage 5 CKD with prevalent cases increasing by about 20,000 annually [1]. Almost nine in ten patients who choose a renal replacement therapy (RRT) start on maintenance hemodialysis (HD), and approximately 60% stay with this modality over time. Recognizing that more than a third of new Stage 5 CKD patients have had minimal or no kidney care prior to starting RRT highlights the need for prompt and ongoing nutrition assessment and intervention [1]. Most patients present to dialysis with comorbid conditions that may have already negatively impacted their nutritional status. Protein-energy wasting (PEW) is common and is associated with increased morbidity and mortality for dialysis patients, and MNT is essential to improve health outcomes [2, 3]. Nutritional management should include ongoing nutrition education, nutrition assessment, individualized interventions, and routine monitoring of nutritional status.

The editors acknowledge Karen Wiesen's contribution to this chapter in *Nutrition in Kidney Disease*, *Second Edition*, Nutrition and Health, DOI 10.1007/978-1-62703-685-6_1, © Springer Science+Business Media New York 2014

D. Blair (✉)
Rutgers, The State University of New Jersey, Clinical and Preventive Nutrition Sciences, School of Health Professions, Newark, NJ, USA
e-mail: blairda@shp.rutgers.edu

Table 15.1 Types of hemodialysis modalities

Type of hemodialysis	Location	Typical duration	Frequency
Conventional hemodialysis	Home	3–5 h	3–4×/week
	In-center	3–5 h	3×/week
Nocturnal hemodialysis	Home	>5 h	3–7×/week
	In-center	6–8 h	3×/week
Short daily hemodialysis	Home	2–3 h	5–7×/week
	In-center	2–3 h	5–6×/week

Regardless of the RRT modality, MNT goals remain the same:

1. Achieve or maintain neutral or positive nitrogen balance.
2. Achieve and maintain good nutritional status.
3. Prevent excessive accumulation of electrolytes, minerals, and fluid between treatments.
4. Minimize the effects of metabolic disorders which are associated with stage 5 CKD.

When a patient is ready to start RRT, there are now more choices both in-center and at home that are demonstrating some positive benefits. In addition to conventional HD, alternatives include nocturnal hemodialysis (NHD) and short daily hemodialysis (SDHD) (also known as long HD and frequent HD) (Table 15.1). To meet the individual's needs and preferences, flexibility exists within these HD types in regards to treatment location, time of day, and duration [4]. Peritoneal dialysis (PD) and renal transplantation treatment options are discussed in Chaps. 16 and 18, respectively. This chapter will review the MNT for hemodialysis modalities and discuss factors that may impact nutrition assessment and the overall nutritional status.

Factors Influencing Nutritional Status

Malnutrition in the maintenance HD population is prevalent and is associated with poor health outcomes including increased morbidity and mortality [5–10]. Between 28% and 54% of dialysis patients worldwide have some degree of protein-energy wasting (PEW) according to recent estimates by the International Society of Renal Nutrition and Metabolism (ISRNM)[2]. Recognizing the importance of early detection, prevention, and treatment of PEW in dialysis patients, the National Kidney Foundation (NKF) Kidney Disease Outcomes Quality Initiative (KDOQI) and the Academy of Nutrition and Dietetics Clinical Practice Guidelines for Nutrition in Chronic Kidney Disease: 2020 Update recommends that a panel of measures be taken to routinely assess the nutritional status [11]. These include the use of anthropometric measures, physical assessment, biochemical parameters, and diet histories and interviews. (For an in-depth review of specific parameters utilized in the nutrition assessment, refer to Chaps. 4, 5, 6 and 7). Composite nutritional indices commonly used to assess the nutritional status or malnutrition risk in hemodialysis patients include subjective global assessment (SGA), which incorporates medical history and physical assessment, and the malnutrition inflammation score (MIS), which additionally considers laboratory data and body mass index (BMI) [9]. Since many factors contribute to the nutritional risk of hemodialysis patients (e.g., inflammation, anorexia, acidosis, fluid volume, dialysis-related losses, and dialysis adequacy), it is important to consider how each may affect the nutrition assessment.

Inflammation

Serum albumin strongly correlates with poor outcomes in hemodialysis patients [6–8, 12]. A serum albumin level between 3.5 and 4.0 g/dL is associated with a two-fold increased risk of death, and a low albumin at the initiation of dialysis increases the risk of hospitalization as well as the length of stay in the first year of dialysis [6, 13]. Although long used as an indicator of malnutrition, serum albumin is a negative acute phase reactant and it is more often a marker of inflammation which can impact albumin synthesis [14, 15]. An estimated 30% to 50% of hemodialysis patients have high levels of inflammatory markers (e.g., C-reactive protein, interleukin-6) [16]. Causes of inflammation specific to hemodialysis include the type of dialysis access (more inflammation with central venous catheter vs. fistula or graft), dialyzer membrane (biocompatible is recommended), and dialysate solution [4, 16]. Additional factors like comorbidities, periodontal disease, infection, cardiovascular disease, changes in gut microbiota, and obesity may also contribute to inflammation [16–18]. Recognizing inflammation as a major driving force of low albumin in hemodialysis patients assists the practitioner in developing strategies to improve outcomes. In 2008, the ISRNM proposed a definition and diagnostic criteria for PEW that better reflect the type of wasting that occurs in CKD, characterized by very low albumin levels, the presence of inflammation and oxidative stress, and higher levels of protein breakdown vs. protein synthesis [19, 20]. See Chap. 22 for further information on PEW in CKD.

Anorexia

Reduced appetite is common in hemodialysis patients affecting an estimated 35%–50%, especially on dialysis treatment days [20–22]. Although initiation of RRT ameliorates some of the uremia present by stage 5 CKD, other factors contributing to anorexia may persist and include taste and olfactory changes, dental issues and dry mouth, inflammation, infection, gastroparesis and early satiety, constipation, comorbidities, pill burden, psychosocial and socioeconomic factors, and age [22–24]. Since poor appetite is associated with a decreased quality of life and an increased risk of hospitalization and death for dialysis patients, appetite assessment is important in developing strategies to promote adequate nutritional intake [25, 26].

Acidosis

Metabolic acidosis (serum bicarbonate <22 mEq/L) in stage 5 CKD is a consequence of a decreased ability of the kidneys to maintain acid-base balance. Results of a large cohort study revealed an estimated 40% of hemodialysis patients exhibit acidosis, and low serum bicarbonate is associated with a 25% increased risk of all-cause and cardiovascular mortality [27]. Hemodialysis attempts to correct this acid-base imbalance through a delivered dose of bicarbonate in the dialysate. Potential nutrition-related effects of low serum bicarbonate in dialysis patients include increased protein degradation, decreased muscle mass, and increased bone mineral loss [27–31]. Since correction of acidosis has been shown to correct the protein catabolism [32], the updated KDOQI guidelines recommend that predialysis serum bicarbonate levels be maintained at 24–26 mmol/L[11].

Fluid Volume

High interdialytic fluid weight gain (IDWG), defined as >4% of the body weight between dialysis treatments, contributes to inflammation and is associated with increased hospitalizations and mortality [33–37]. Excessive IDWG may also be a factor in low serum albumin test results due to dilutional hypoalbuminemia. It has been hypothesized that this correlation may explain some of the mortality associated with low albumin [36]. Fluid overload also increases the risk of cardiovascular disease, hypertension, and heart failure in dialysis patients [37]. Sodium limits, both dietary and in the dialysate, along with fluid restriction can help to maintain the fluid balance.

Dialysis-Related Losses

HD has long been considered a catabolic procedure. Approximately 4–9 g net amino acids and 1–2 g protein are lost during HD compared to 5–15 g protein during PD [38–41]. The use of high-flux membranes, bio-incompatible membranes, and reuse of high-flux dialyzers have been shown to increase amino acid losses [42–44]. Dialysate protein losses are also higher with polysulfone dialyzers processed with bleach and losses significantly increase after the sixteenth use [27]. HD has been shown to induce a protein catabolic state that can stimulate muscle and whole-body protein loss, decrease protein synthesis, and increase energy expenditure with the effects lasting up to 2 hours postdialysis [45–47].

Hemodialysis Adequacy

Conventional hemodialysis, initiated in the 1960s, was initially used once weekly. However, since uremic symptoms returned and became more severe 24–36 hours before the next dialysis, along with increased extravascular volume, hypertension, and the development of peripheral neuropathy, HD was increased to twice weekly. Further improvement in the progression of uremic peripheral neuropathy occurred with thrice weekly dialysis and this was "accepted as standard" since the early 1970s [48].

Adequate dialysis is important because underdialysis impacts appetite and dietary intake. Assessment of dialysis adequacy is based on Kt/V (a marker for dialysis adequacy where K = clearance, t = time, and V = volume). According to a recent KDOQI update on dialysis adequacy, recommendations are for "a target single pool Kt/V (spKt/V) of 1.4 per hemodialysis session for patients treated thrice weekly, with a minimum delivered spKt/V of 1.2"and "for hemodialysis schedules other than thrice weekly… a target standard Kt/V of 2.3 volumes per week with a minimum delivered dose of 2.1 using a method of calculation that includes the contributions of ultrafiltration and residual kidney function"[4].

In numerous observational studies, the use of short daily HD and NHD has been shown to reduce anorexia, improve protein intake, and have a positive impact on a number of nutritional markers [39, 43, 49, 50]. Results from the Frequent HD Study, however, did not show any significant effect on nutritional parameters with either NHD or SDHD [51]. Both of these treatment modalities may not be widely available to all dialysis patients because of reimbursement obstacles and limited experience by dialysis providers. Research is ongoing.

KDOQI highlights the importance of presenting the benefits and risks of HD options to patients, "considering individual patient preferences, the potential quality of life and physiological benefits," along with some of the potential risks of more frequent HD ("possible increase in vascular access procedures, and potential for hypotension during dialysis") and longer HD at home ("possible increase in vascular access complications, potential for increased caregiver burden, and possible accelerated decline in residual kidney function") [4].

Nutrient Recommendations

Energy

Conventional Hemodialysis

Current KDOQI recommendations for energy intake in metabolically stable adults are the same regardless of dialysis modality (i.e., 25–35 kcal/kg body weight per day) [11]. Energy intakes may need to be adjusted according to age, gender, activity level, weight goals, body composition, comorbidities or inflammation to maintain normal nutritional status [11, 52].

Many HD patients are unable to consume the recommended energy intake, resulting in a low body weight and body mass index (BMI), both of which are associated with increased mortality in the HD patient [11, 39]. The average energy intake has been reported at 24–27 kcal/kg/day [21, 52]. In the Hemodialysis (HEMO) Study, patients averaged 23 kcal/kg/day, which is significantly less than the KDOQI guidelines for calories and less than the HEMO target of 28 kcal/kg/day [53]. Energy intake was less and patient reported appetite was suboptimal on dialysis days when compared to nondialysis days [54].Restricting food during in-center hemodialysis, a common policy at many dialysis clinics in the United States, is thought to be a missed opportunity for nutrition. A recent consensus statement from the ISRNM recommends that "meals and supplements during hemodialysis should be considered as a part of the standard-of-care practice for patients without contraindications"[55].

Other factors contributing to poor intake in HD patients include fatigue after dialysis or the catabolic, physiologic, and metabolic effects of dialysis on the body, taste disturbances, medications, the overly restricted renal diet, delayed gastric emptying, repeated hospitalizations, and psychosocial concerns [24, 54, 56]. A standard dialysate solution containing 200 mg/dL glucose contributes only a small amount of calories during thrice weekly dialysis and does not significantly contribute to energy intake [39]. Assessment and counseling by the dietitian is important in helping the patient achieve an adequate intake. The use of nutritional supplements may need to be considered.

Nocturnal Hemodialysis/Short Daily Hemodialysis

There have been limited studies examining the nutritional needs of patients receiving NHD and SDHD. The current recommendations are extrapolated from the needs of the conventional HD patient (i.e., thrice weekly dialysis). The diet should be individualized to the patient based on lab data, interdialytic fluid weight gains, and duration of dialysis. Because of the frequency and duration of dialysis, the diet for NHD tends to be more liberal than conventional HD. There are no established energy guidelines for NHD or SDHD so current recommendations follow the KDOQI nutrition guidelines for conventional HD, and energy needs can be adjusted as needed to maintain the weight (Table 15.2). With both NHD and SDHD, appetite has been reported to improve leading to an increase in both protein and calorie intake [39, 57, 58]. Weight gain may occur so energy needs should be adjusted and exercise encouraged if the patient is physically able to participate [39, 58].

Table 15.2 Daily nutrient recommendations for adult hemodialysis patients

Nutrient	Conventional hemodialysis	Nocturnal/ short daily hemodialysis
Energy (kcal/kg BW)	25–35	None established. Use KDOQI
Protein (g/kg BW/ day)	1.0–1.2	Use KDOQI
Sodium	<2.3 g/day	NHD: 2.4–4 g/day
		SDHD: 2–3 g
		Monitor BP control, fluid balance.
Potassium	2–3 g/day	Dependent on serum levels.
Calcium	800–1000 mg total elemental	Same
Phosphorus	800–1000 mg or 10–12 mg/g protein	NHD: Mild to unrestricted
		SDHD: Suggest HD restriction; adjust to control serum levels.
Fluid	750–1000 mL + UO	Individualize for BP, UO, and fluid balance.
Thiamine	1.2–1.5 mg/day	Same
Riboflavin	1.1–1.3 mg/day	Same
Niacin	20 mg/day	Same
Biotin	30 μ/day	Same
Pantothenic acid	5–10 mg/day	Same
Cobalamin	2–3 μ/day	Same
Pyridoxine	10 mg/day	Same
Folate	1–10 mg/day[a]	Same[a]
Vitamin C	75–90 mg/day	Same
Vitamin A	None	None
Vitamin D	Individualize	Individualize
Vitamin E	None	None
Vitamin K	None[b]	None[b]
Zinc	If needed[c]	If needed[c]
Copper	None	None
Iron	Individualize[d]	Individualize[d]
Selenium	None	None
Magnesium	None	None
Aluminum	None	None

Source: Data from [11, 33, 39, 58, 93–97]

Abbreviations: BW body weight, HD hemodialysis, NHD nocturnal hemodialysis, SDHD short daily hemodialysis, KDOQI Kidney Disease Outcomes Quality Initiative, BP blood pressure, UO urine output

[a]1 mg is the standard recommendation but higher amounts may be needed. See text

[b]May need supplements if on antibiotics and have poor oral intake

[c]May be supplemented up to 15 mg elemental zinc

[d]Varies based on serum ferritin, transferrin saturation

Protein

Conventional Hemodialysis

Adequate protein intake is important to ensure that the patient maintains positive or neutral nitrogen balance. The KDOQI nutrition guidelines recommend a dietary protein intake of 1.0–1.2 g/kg body weight for the metabolically stable adult dialysis patient [11]. Protein recommendations are the same for dialysis patients with diabetes; however, higher levels of protein may be considered for those at risk of hyper- and/or hypoglycemia [11]. Vegetarian patients will require ongoing counseling by the dietitian to help ensure they consume adequate protein from legumes or soy products without excess mineral load. Protein recommendations are based on a small number of nitrogen balance studies and do not differentiate for age. While it is possible that protein needs of the elderly patient receiving maintenance HD may be slightly reduced, the catabolic effects of dialysis along with other comorbid conditions may outweigh this reduction. A small number of studies have shown that the risk level for malnutrition in elderly HD patients is higher than that in younger patients [49, 50, 59, 60].

Protein intake is often inadequate in HD patients and contributes to PEW. In the HEMO Study, less than 20% of the patients at baseline met the current KDOQI Nutrition Guidelines for protein with an average intake of 0.93 g/kg/day [53]. Protein needs are also influenced by metabolic acidosis, infection, inflammation, or surgical procedures associated with increased catabolism. Current protein recommendations are based on older metabolic studies and do not take into account the newer, highly permeable dialyzer membranes that have been shown to increase amino acid losses and lower serum albumin levels [44]. Further research on the effect of new dialyzer membranes and dialysis techniques on nutritional requirements is needed. There is limited data on the protein needs of the acutely ill maintenance HD patient, and KDOQI recommends that these patients receive at least 1.2 g protein/kg/day with needs individualized based on concurrent illness and inflammation [11]. Hospitalized HD patients generally consume less than the recommended amount of protein and may need intensive nutrition counseling, monitoring, and possibly nutritional support to provide adequate protein to meet their needs.

Protein Nitrogen Appearance (PNA) or Protein Catabolic Rate (PCR)

In stable dialysis patients (i.e., no catabolic or anabolic processes), protein nitrogen appearance (PNA), or protein catabolic rate (PCR) is used to estimate protein intake (normalized as grams per kg per day) [41]. The KDOQI nutrition guidelines note that nPCR has been shown to be a predictor of albumin and mortality in HD patients [11]. In catabolic patients, PNA will overestimate protein intake; the reverse is true for anabolic patients [41]. Urea nitrogen appearance rate is estimated from the interdialytic changes in serum urea nitrogen in the HD patient. After PNA is calculated, it can be normalized (nPNA) to body size or actual edema free body weight [41]. Normalizing to body weight may be more appropriate for underweight or overweight individuals, since nPNA may otherwise overestimate or underestimate protein intake respectively [41].

Nocturnal Hemodialysis/Short Daily Hemodialysis

There are no established guidelines for protein requirements in NHD or SDHD, so current recommendations are to implement the KDOQI guidelines for protein, and adjust to maintain adequate serum albumin levels (see Table 15.2) [11, 58]. Patients receiving NHD usually have adequate protein intakes possibly due to an increased clearance of middle- and larger-molecular weight substances during the longer dialysis procedure [58]. Patients on SDHD have been shown to also have increased protein intakes possibly due to the increased frequency of dialysis [61, 62].

Sodium and Fluid

Conventional Hemodialysis

Sodium and fluid control are very important in patients receiving maintenance HD. When the glomerular filtration rate (GFR) falls below 15 mL/min/1.73 m^2, the kidneys' ability to compensate and excrete sodium declines leading to sodium retention. Since a patient's GFR declines within the first few months on HD to 1–2 mL/min/1.73 m^2 and the patient becomes oliguric or anuric, diet and dialysis become the two controlling factors in sodium and fluid balance [39]. Excessive fluid and sodium intake between treatments can result in sodium and fluid overload leading to hypertension and cardiac problems such as congestive heart failure (CHF) [63, 64]. In addition, removal of large interdialytic fluid weight gains to achieve a dry weight may not be possible during one treatment and may cause intradialytic hypotension, cramping, angina, arrhythmias, and malaise [39, 65]. The recommended sodium intake for HD patients is <2.3 g/day while the recommended fluid intake is 750–1000 mL plus urine output, and in general should not exceed 1500 mL/day [11, 38, 39, 65]. The goal is to minimize interdialytic fluid weight gains and control blood pressure. Ideally, interdialytic fluid weight gains between treatments should not exceed 2–3 kg or 3% to 4% of the patient's dry weight [33, 65]. Some nephrology specialists think that lower sodium intakes of 1–1.5 g/day would be beneficial, but this may impact the nutritional status of the patient by limiting intake of important nutrients, especially if poor food choices are made. The accessibility of high sodium convenience and fast foods makes patient adherence difficult. Reduced or low sodium convenience foods in the grocery store may have potassium chloride added to replace sodium making them potentially dangerous for the HD patient. Patients should be counseled on avoiding high sodium foods, label reading, making appropriate choices when eating out, and ways to help control thirst. While high interdialytic fluid weight gains can indicate excessive consumption of sodium and fluid, very low interdialytic weight gains, especially in the elderly, may be an early indicator of poor oral intake [66]. The elderly dialysis patient, already at risk for malnutrition, may over restrict both food and fluid intake. A thorough diet history, along with a review of other nutritional parameters, should be obtained to assess the nutritional adequacy of the diet.

Nocturnal Hemodialysis/Short Daily Hemodialysis

Sodium and fluid restriction in the NHD and SDHD patient is dependent on fluid balance, blood pressure control, and the type of dialysis machine used. The current Dietary Reference Intake (DRI) for sodium is 1500 mg/day for adults. Decreasing sodium intakes if above 2300 mg/day is recommended and is a good starting point for the stable patient, but no formal guidelines for these cohorts have been published. The hypotensive NHD patient may require a more liberal sodium prescription. Fluid intake should be individualized based on interdialytic weight gain. A fluid restriction may not be required for the NHD patient as long as the patient does not gain more than he/she can safely remove while maintaining hemodynamic stability. This may vary slightly from patient to patient based on the dialysis prescription, but it is approximately 2–4 L/night [58].

Patients on SDHD dialyze 2–3 h/day so they are limited in the amount of fluid they can safely remove in one treatment. Patients may dialyze on a conventional HD machine or the NxStage System

One™ machine. There are no formal guidelines, but clinical experience suggests that 1–1.5 L/h can be removed safely depending on the type of dialysis machine used for treatment.

Potassium

Conventional Hemodialysis

As the GFR falls, the kidneys lose their ability to filter potassium, and fecal potassium excretion increases [39, 67]. Potassium removal during HD averages between 70 and 150 mEq per treatment [68]. This will vary depending on the dialyzer clearance and the potassium concentration of the dialysate, i.e., the higher the dialysate concentration, the less the removal of potassium. Most patients receiving maintenance HD are placed on a dialysate bath of 2–3 mEq/L, with the standard being 2 mEq/L [39, 68]. Low-potassium dialysate (0–1 mEq/L) is rarely used in the outpatient dialysis setting because of the increased risk of cardiac arrest due to hypokalemia [39]. Patients with a low predialysis serum potassium (<3.5 mEq/L) will generally require an upper range of the dialysate bath (3 mEq/L) especially if oral intake is poor. Hyperkalemia may be categorized as either mild (serum potassium 5.5–6.5 mEq/L) or moderate (>6.5 mEq/L) and may result in cardiac arrhythmias and cardiac arrest [39].

The recommended dietary potassium restriction is 2–3 g/day and should be individualized based on serum lab values [38, 39, 52]. Nutritional counseling regarding food sources of potassium and patient education about the complications of hyperkalemia are important to help the patient avoid elevated potassium levels during the interdialytic period. The primary sources of potassium are fruits, vegetables, and dairy along with nuts, seeds, nut butters, and dried beans and peas. Patients should also avoid salt substitutes, which contain potassium chloride, and check with their doctor or dietitian before using any herbal products or dietary supplements. Patients should also be counseled to check the nutrition facts label on packaged foods for the potassium content, and to be aware that the ingredients of reduced or low sodium products may include potassium chloride. For patients who are chronically nonadherent and whose dialysate bath cannot be lowered, a short-term oral suspension dose of Kayexalate® (sodium polystyrene) or Veltassa® (patiromer) may be given [39, 52, 69]. While the primary cause of hyperkalemia may be dietary intake, nondietary factors such as medications, hyperglycemia, metabolic acidosis, pica behaviors, and inadequate dialysis may also lead to elevated serum potassium levels and should be investigated if dietary causes can be ruled out (Table 15.3) [67, 68, 70, 71].

Nocturnal Hemodialysis/Short Daily Hemodialysis

A potassium restriction in NHD is normally not required unless mid-week serum levels are high [58, 72]. If a patient skips one night of treatment and has a high interdialytic potassium level, then that patient should be placed on a potassium restriction over the longest skip period [58]. Although no specific recommendations are available, clinical experience suggests that a 2.5–3 g/day potassium diet may be appropriate depending on the degree of hyperkalemia. Patients who are hypokalemic will need to increase their dietary potassium intake; however, if they are unable to maintain normal serum levels by diet alone, they should receive a potassium supplement or have the potassium concentrate of the dialysate adjusted [58].

There have been limited studies on potassium removal in SDHD. One study using the NxStage™ System showed an average of 73 mmol of potassium cleared per treatment [73]. Kohn demonstrated an average of 55 mEq is removed with a range of 35–80 mEq [74]. Potassium

Table 15.3 Dietary and nondietary causes of hyperkalemia in hemodialysis patients

Dietary causes
Use of salt substitutes
Pica behavior
Use of herbal or over-the-counter vitamin/mineral supplements
Excessive consumption of high-potassium foods
Excessive consumption of liquid nutritional supplements
Nondietary causes
Severe, chronic constipation
Loss of remaining residual renal function
High dialysate potassium concentration
Frequent use of chewing tobacco
Metabolic acidosis
Inadequate dialysis
Blood transfusions
Hemolysis of blood sample due to error in blood draw or specimen handling
Hyperglycemia: Potassium shifts from cell into serum
Conditions causing release of potassium through tissue destruction such as catabolism, starvation, infection, burns, surgical stress, chemotherapy
Drug interactions: Beta blocking agents, spironolactone, angiotensin-converting enzyme inhibitors, cyclosporine, digoxin
Comorbid conditions such as Addison's disease, sickle-cell anemia, hypoaldosteronism

Data from [33, 39, 67, 68]

clearance on SDHD is not as good as on PD, but slightly better than conventional HD when one compares weekly potassium removal. There are no formal guidelines on dietary potassium intake in SDHD and more research is needed. Since most patients on SDHD transition from conventional HD, clinical experience suggests patients continue with their conventional HD dietary recommendations and then adjust the diet during the initial training period to control serum levels.

Calcium, Phosphorus, Parathyroid Hormone, and Calcitriol/Vitamin D Analogs

Conventional Hemodialysis

The kidneys play a crucial role in mineral homeostasis [75–77]. Features of abnormal mineral metabolism in stage 5 CKD include hypocalcemia/hyperphosphatemia, defective intestinal absorption of calcium, altered vitamin D metabolism, and altered handling of phosphate, calcium, and magnesium [75]. Dialysis patients frequently develop metabolic bone disease or renal osteodystrophy, but abnormal mineral metabolism also has systemic effects such as cardiovascular, arterial, and valvular calcification along with metastatic calcification of soft tissue (calciphylaxis), erythropoietin stimulating agent (ESA) resistant anemia, and increased morbidity and mortality [78]. Several studies have shown coronary calcification in 83%–92% of dialysis patients [79–81]. Factors that may predispose to soft-tissue calcification include hyperphosphatemia, secondary hyperparathyroidism, local tissue injury, the rise in pH of tissue, removal of calcification inhibitors by dialysis, and excessive calcium intake.

Calcium Balance

The primary route of calcium excretion is the kidney, and in maintenance hemodialysis patients the normal deposition into the bone reservoir may be limited due to low turnover bone disease. Serum calcium is not a good indicator of calcium because excesses are not retained in plasma but rather deposited in soft and vascular tissue. Contributing to the risk of hypercalcemia in maintenance hemodialysis patients is the prevalence of calcium enhanced foods, calcium supplements or calcium-based phosphate binders, the use of calcitriol and vitamin D analogs, and dialysate calcium concentration [82]. The KDOQI nutrition guidelines suggest limiting the total elemental calcium intake to 800–1000 mg/day [11]. The use of calcium-based binders is discouraged when at all possible [83]. Interventions to prevent hypercalcemia in maintenance hemodialysis include evaluating calcium load, recommending changes as needed (i.e., adjusting the dose of calcitriol and vitamin D analogs, modifying dialysate calcium concentration, using noncalcium-based phosphate binders), and educating patients regarding limiting calcium-fortified foods.

Parathyroid Hormone (PTH) and Calcitriol/Vitamin D Analogs

Parathyroid hormone (PTH) is secreted in response to hypocalcemia to conserve calcium in the renal tubules. PTH acts on the kidneys to trigger calcitriol production (activation of vitamin D) and to enhance urinary excretion of phosphorus. Calcitriol, stimulated by PTH, increases phosphorus and calcium absorption from the gut and increases bone remodeling by stimulating the release of calcium and phosphorus from bone. By Stage 5 CKD, the kidneys are no longer able to activate vitamin D, so the active form of vitamin D (calcitriol) or a vitamin D analog (doxercalciferol, paricalcitol, or other) may be prescribed. Active vitamin D therapy is initiated and adjusted based on PTH, serum calcium, and phosphorus levels. Over suppression of PTH is avoided to prevent adynamic bone disease. More recently, oral or IV calcimimetic medications, Sensipar® or Parsabiv®, respectively, have been used to regulate PTH secretion via the calcium sensing receptors.

Phosphorus

Regulation of phosphorus homeostasis is complex, and preventing hyperphosphatemia is a challenge for maintenance hemodialysis patients. Prolonged elevated serum phosphorus leads to soft tissue and vascular calcification, and is associated with increased morbidity and mortality for maintenance hemodialysis patients. An analysis of United States Renal Data System (USRDS) data of more than 6400 hemodialysis patients demonstrated that serum phosphorus >6.5 mg/dL was associated with a 27% higher mortality risk [78]. Phosphorus management focuses on receiving adequate dialysis, reducing phosphorus intake, evaluating the phosphorus content of meals and snacks, and matching the amount of phosphate binding medication accordingly.

The KDOQI guidelines for bone disease recommends no more than 800–1000 mg phosphorus per day [76]; however, in some cases this may be difficult to achieve since many high phosphorus foods are also high in protein. The phosphorus restriction needs to be adjusted to dietary protein requirements to prevent protein malnutrition. For patients with higher protein needs, calculating phosphorus based on protein requirements (using 10–12 mg phosphorus/gram protein) should provide a reasonable phosphorus goal [76]. Phosphorus is not currently required to be listed on food labels, and the use of phosphate-based food additives has contributed to hidden sources of phosphorus outside the traditionally known high-phosphorus foods. The inorganic phosphates used as food additives are also

100% absorbable as compared to the 50%–60% absorption rate from naturally occurring phosphorus [84]. Refer to Chap. 23 for a review of bone and mineral disorders in CKD.

Nocturnal Hemodialysis/Short Daily Hemodialysis

With NHD, weekly phosphate removal is twice that of conventional HD, so phosphate levels are generally normal or low and calcium-phosphorus balance is normal [72, 85, 86]. Phosphorus restriction is not needed in the majority of NHD patients, but it is dependent on the patients' appetite, oral intake, and serum phosphorus levels. A large percentage of patients may be able to decrease or discontinue use of phosphate binders. Phosphorus levels should be monitored and the diet individualized. In patients who are hypophosphatemic and unable to increase dietary phosphorus intake, phosphate may be added to the bicarbonate bath [85].

Phosphorus control is not as effective with SDHD compared to NHD. Weekly phosphorus removal has been shown to be 606– 694 mg per treatment and is dependent on predialysis levels of phosphorus as well as the time on dialysis [73, 74]. Phosphorus removal is increased when levels are greater than 5 mg/dL [73, 74]. Phosphorus binder dose has been shown to either increase or decrease slightly depending on the HD duration and frequency and dietary protein and phosphorus intake [62, 73, 74]. Phosphorus intake may be higher due to improved appetite and higher protein intakes. There are no formal evidence-based guidelines for dietary phosphorus restrictions in SDHD. However, based on current studies, it is prudent to restrict phosphorus intake to control serum levels.

Lipids

Conventional Hemodialysis

There is a high prevalence of lipid abnormalities in the dialysis population, which is a risk factor for cardiovascular disease (CVD). The mortality rate from CVD in patients undergoing maintenance HD is almost 50% [39]. HD patients generally have normal or high total cholesterol, low-density lipoproteins (LDL) and triglycerides (TG), and normal or low high-density lipoproteins (HDL) [39, 87]. According to the Dialysis Morbidity and Mortality Study (DMMS), only 20% of patients receiving maintenance HD meet the recommended normal lipid parameters outlined by the National Cholesterol Education Program (NCEP) Adult Treatment Panel (ATP III) [70]. The KDOQI recommended therapeutic lifestyle changes (TLC) are covered in detail in Chap. 13. Briefly, it recommends: (a) a reduction in saturated fat to <7% of total calories; (b) a reduction in total fat to 25%–35% of total calories with monounsaturated fat providing up to 20% of calories and polyunsaturated fat up to 10%; (c) total dietary cholesterol <200 mg/day; (d) increased dietary fiber; and (e) modifications in calories to attain or maintain a desired weight along with exercise and smoking cessation [88].

Before beginning any dietary modifications, the dietitian should assess the patient for signs of PEW since addition of a fat restricted diet may compromise caloric intake and further affect nutritional status [89]. Patients also encounter difficulty trying to comply with the fat recommendations in addition to a complex renal diet. Dietary modification may be undertaken if the patient is well-nourished; however, pharmacological intervention with lipid-lowering medication may be the only intervention used if the patient is unable or unwilling to further modify their diet. Encouraging general recommendations for modifying saturated fat along with smoking cessation and promoting exercise should be emphasized.

Nocturnal Hemodialysis/Short Daily Hemodialysis

While there are no specific recommendations for NHD and SDHD, it would be prudent to encourage patients to follow general therapeutic lifestyle recommendations suggested by the KDOQI guidelines for dyslipidemias [88] due to the high risk of CVD in the dialysis population.

Vitamins, Minerals, and Trace Elements

Maintenance Hemodialysis (Conventional, Nocturnal, Short Daily Hemodialysis)

The importance of adequate intakes of vitamins, minerals, and trace elements is well known including their roles in metabolic processes, cell function, growth, and anemia management. Although the Food and Nutrition Board of the National Research Council/National Academy of Sciences has determined a recommended daily allowance (RDA) of vitamins and minerals sufficient for most healthy people, the RDAs for conventional hemodialysis patients, NHD, and SDHD have not been established. Intake of essential vitamins, minerals and trace elements in maintenance HD patients is complicated by factors like dietary restrictions, appetite issues, losses during the dialysis process, comorbidities, and medication interactions. It has been estimated that less than 50% of maintenance HD patients achieve sufficient intake of most vitamins through diet, though intakes of minerals like sodium, phosphorus, and potassium may exceed recommendations [90]. The use of renal-specific vitamin and mineral supplementation for maintenance HD patients, though widely accepted, has been a topic of debate due to concerns regarding cost, pill burden, and other potential downsides [91].

The current recommendations for vitamins and minerals in NHD and SDHD are the same as those for conventional HD. There is some concern that there may be an increased loss of water-soluble vitamins, especially vitamin C, because patients are dialyzing twice as many days. In the few studies that have been done, lower levels of vitamin C and thiamine have been found [58, 72, 92, 93]. Further research is needed regarding vitamin/mineral requirements in stage 5 CKD patients and how these needs may be affected by hemodialysis modalities (i.e., conventional HD, NHD, SDHD).

Water-Soluble Vitamins

Water-soluble vitamins are small, nonprotein bound substances which are removed by dialysis and may be lost at a rate greater than normal urinary excretion [94]. Dialysis membrane pore size, surface area, and increased flow rates can adversely affect water-soluble vitamin retention [95, 96]. Some drugs such as immunosuppressants, anticonvulsants, and chemotherapy drugs used to treat comorbid conditions can also interfere with vitamin absorption [97]. The water-soluble vitamins most likely to be deficient in maintenance hemodialysis patients are pyridoxine (B-6), folic acid, and vitamin C [38, 94–96]. See Chap. 33 for an in-depth review of micronutrient requirements in CKD.

Vitamin B-6

Adequate stores of vitamin B-6 (pyridoxamine) are necessary for erythropoietin to be effective in promoting red blood cell (RBC) formation, and deficiency symptoms also include peripheral neuropathy [95, 97]. Levels of B-6 are low to normal in patients receiving conventional HD, with higher losses for patients on high-flux/high-efficiency dialyzers, and increased needs for those receiving erythropoietin stimulating therapy (ESA) [52, 95, 96]. Vitamin B-6, along with folic acid and vitamin B-12, is a cofactor in homocysteine metabolism; low levels may result in hyperhomocysteinemia which may contribute to an increased cardiovascular risk in patients receiving maintenance HD [98–101]. Therefore, the requirement for pyridoxamine is 10 mg/day, higher than the RDA of 1.3–1.7 mg/day [102].

Folic Acid

For maintenance HD patients, adequate serum levels of folic acid and vitamin B-12 (cobalamin) are particularly important for their roles in RBC production [39, 95, 97, 103]. Although levels are generally normal, folate losses may be higher in maintenance HD especially with high-flux dialysis [96–98]. Therefore, folic acid needs are estimated as 1 g/day for HD patients, which is higher compared to the RDA (0.4 mg/day).

Vitamin C

Vitamin C has antioxidant properties; it regulates iron distribution and storage, and it may help to promote intestinal iron absorption [52, 95, 104]. Vitamin C levels can be low if not supplemented, since it is removed during dialysis and the patient's dietary intake of vitamin C may be marginal [94, 102]. KDOQI nutrition guidelines suggest a vitamin C intake of 75 mg/day for women and 90 mg/day for men [11]. Higher doses may lead to oxalosis resulting in increased oxalate deposition in soft tissue, and can also increase the risk of kidney stones [38, 94, 95, 97, 104]. Whether or not vitamin C supplementation can help reduce inflammation and oxidative stress and aid in improving ESA response is still unclear and research is ongoing [38, 95].

Vitamin B-12

Vitamin B-12 (cobalamin) plays a role in folic acid metabolism and the formation of RBC. Levels may be normal as vitamin B-12 may not be removed as much as other water-soluble vitamins [39, 97]. There have been reports of B-12 deficiency in patients on high-flux dialyzers, and ESA and high-dose folic acid supplementation may increase requirements [96–98]. Vitamin B-12 levels may decrease as the length of time on dialysis increases [39]. At this time, the RDA for vitamin B-12 (2.4 μg/day) is recommended for maintenance hemodialysis patients.

Other Water-Soluble Vitamins

Little research has been done to determine the exact requirements for vitamin B-1 (thiamine), vitamin B-2 (riboflavin), biotin, niacin, and pantothenic acid in Stage 5 CKD, and serum levels are usually normal [95]. However, thiamine deficiency has been reported in some dialysis patients and several symptoms of thiamine deficiency, such as CHF with fluid overload (wet beriberi), lactic acidosis, and unexplained encephalopathy, can mimic uremic complications making an early diagnosis difficult [95, 105, 106]. Biotin levels have been shown to be normal, but supplementation may help with dialysis-related intractable hiccups [106–108]. A renal vitamin supplement which includes thiamine, niacin, biotin, riboflavin, and pantothenic acid at RDA levels is generally recommended (see Table 15.2).

Fat-Soluble Vitamins

Vitamin A

Vitamin A is not removed by dialysis and can accumulate in kidney failure. Vitamin A levels increase with duration of time on dialysis but not frequency, and levels are generally two to five times higher in dialysis patients than in the general population [39, 95, 109]. Elevated vitamin A levels are thought to be due to the lack of removal of retinol-binding protein (RBP) by the kidney. Toxicity occurs when the amount of retinol exceeds the binding capability of RBP. Symptoms include hypercalcemia, anemia, hypertriglyceridemia, and increased alkaline phosphate levels. These symptoms may mimic uremia and a diagnosis of toxicity cannot be made without assessing serum vitamin levels [39, 95, 109, 110]. Vitamin A supplementation is not recommended.

Nutritional Vitamin D (Cholecalciferol, Ergocalciferol)

Hemodialysis patients are prone to vitamin D deficiency, defined as serum 25-hydroxyvitamin D [25(OH)D] < 30 ng/mL, due to less outdoor activity and therefore sunlight exposure, decreased intake of dietary sources of vitamin D, and decreased synthesis of vitamin D observed with low glomerular filtration rate (GFR) [65]. Although by Stage 5 CKD the kidneys can no longer convert vitamin D to the active form needed for bone mineral metabolism, adequate nutritional vitamin D is important for many nonbone functions (immune function, insulin sensitivity and secretion, cell growth, gene transcription, muscle strength) [111]. Recommendations for the frequency of serum 25(OH)D testing and daily supplementation with nutritional vitamin D vary. Both vitamin D2 (ergocalciferol) and D3 (cholecalciferol) have been successfully used for repletion in maintenance HD patients. The Kidney Disease: Improving Global Outcomes (KDIGO) CKD mineral and bone disorder (CKD-MBD) guidelines suggest that "25(OH)D (calcidiol) levels might be measured, and repeated testing determined by baseline values and therapeutic interventions" and "that vitamin D deficiency and insufficiency be corrected using treatment strategies recommended for the general population"[77]. Use of a renal vitamin with D may be a strategy in preventing vitamin D deficiency.

Vitamin E

Vitamin E is not removed by dialysis and levels have been reported to be low, normal, or high [39, 94, 110]. Low serum levels of vitamin E are thought to be associated with the development of atherosclerosis and cardiovascular events in the dialysis population, but research into the role of vitamin E in decreasing oxidative stress, inflammation, and mortality has not demonstrated any appreciable benefit [106, 110]. Vitamin E may cause an increased risk of deep vein thrombosis and a vitamin K-like responsive hemorrhagic condition in patients taking an anticoagulant [39, 95]. Research indicates that supplementation ≥400 IU may increase all-cause mortality in the general population; 15 IU/day is the recommended amount for HD patients [33, 112], though current KDOQI nutrition guidelines suggest that vitamin E should not be routinely supplemented [11].

Vitamin K

Vitamin K was thought not to be deficient in patients receiving maintenance dialysis; however, recent research indicates that 30% or more of maintenance HD patients demonstrate subclinical vitamin K deficiency [113–115]. Adequate levels of Vitamin K may play a role in bone health by decreasing the frequency of bone fractures [116]. Further clinical trials are needed to look at the benefits or potential side effects of vitamin K supplementation; therefore, at this time there is still not enough evidence to recommend routine supplementation. Patients at possible risk for vitamin K deficiency are those receiving long-term antibiotic therapy, those eating poorly over an extended period of time, or those patients on unsupplemented total parenteral nutrition [39, 98]. Excessive vitamin K can interfere with anticoagulant therapy; therefore, patients receiving vitamin K supplements should be closely monitored [39, 94, 97].

Minerals and Trace Elements

Minerals and trace elements are mainly supplied by diet; however, serum levels can also be affected by environmental exposure, length of dialysis, concentrations of the dialysate, poor nutrition, impaired absorption, or age [95, 98, 117]. Many minerals and trace elements are protein bound so uremia itself may alter levels; however, losses during dialysis are probably minimal [95, 117]. Levels of some minerals and trace elements will be affected by the concentration gradient between the dialysate fluid and the serum. This section will provide an overview of select minerals in maintenance HD. See Chap. 33 for further information.

Aluminum

There is no known need for aluminum supplementation in humans, though it is pervasive in small amounts in many substances including water. Since it is excreted by the kidney, there is a risk for toxic levels in stage 5 CKD and patients on maintenance hemodialysis [95]. Age, PTH, citrate, vitamin D, and fluorine may increase aluminum absorption in the gut, and the length of time on dialysis may increase aluminum levels in bone [39, 95]. Aluminum toxicity in dialysis patients is due to increased uptake and storage and is associated with dialysis encephalopathy syndrome, refractory anemia, and a reduction in bone formation leading to aluminum-induced adynamic bone disease (ABD) or osteomalacia [39, 95]. A primary source of aluminum is aluminum-containing antacids and patients should avoid long-term use of these medications. However, as stated in the KDOQI Clinical Practice Guidelines: Bone Metabolism and Disease in Chronic Renal Failure [76], aluminum-based binders may be used on a short-term basis for patients with chronic hyperphosphatemia (refer to Chap. 23).

Copper

Copper levels in maintenance hemodialysis patients are typically normal, and deficiency is rarely seen unless the patient has a malabsorptive condition or is receiving long-term parenteral nutrition with inadequate supplementation [95]. Serum copper levels can be affected by excessive intake and inflammation (ceruloplasmin is an acute phase reactant); high zinc intakes can interfere with copper absorption [95, 98]. Copper supplementation is not recommended for hemodialysis patients.

Iron

Iron deficiency is common in patients receiving maintenance HD because of frequent blood sampling, dialysis associated losses, decreased availability of ferritin, losses during surgery, and gastrointestinal losses [95]. ESA therapy increases RBC production thereby increasing iron utilization

[95, 118]. Monitoring iron balance using transferrin saturation and serum ferritin is important to correct deficiency and prevent iron overload. Patients with CKD are unable to obtain adequate iron from diet alone, and oral iron supplementation may not be effective since absorption can be decreased by the presence of an inflammatory state, iron stores, age, sex, timing of supplement administration, and simultaneous use of iron inhibiting medications such as calcium [119, 120]. The need for iron supplementation in maintenance HD patients should be individualized and is typically based on serum ferritin and transferrin saturation levels. Intravenous (IV) iron is usually administered during HD when deficient. IV iron therapy has fewer gastrointestinal side effects and is more efficient.

Magnesium

Magnesium levels in patients receiving maintenance HD are generally normal to mildly elevated due to a decrease in gastrointestinal absorption and the fact that high magnesium-containing foods such as green leafy vegetables and legumes, are generally restricted [39, 52]. Hypermagnesemia occurs primarily from excessive intake of over-the-counter medications such as antacids or laxatives, alcoholism, or magnesium-based phosphorus binders. Magnesium can be removed using a lower magnesium dialysate (0.75–1.5 mEq/L) [39]. Hypermagnesemia can cause hypertension, weakness, and arrhythmias. Long-term hypermagnesemia may cause adynamic bone disease by suppressing PTH secretion [52, 121]. Deficiency can result in muscle weakness, seizures, and arrhythmias and may interfere with the release of PTH leading to hypocalcemia [39, 121]. Supplementation is not routinely prescribed unless the patient develops a magnesium deficiency.

Selenium

Selenium levels have been found to be low in patients receiving maintenance HD and may be associated with low protein intakes [95, 122]. Selenium supplementation may help improve immune function by decreasing oxidative stress [38, 117]. Toxicity is rare but until more clinical evidence is established, regular supplementation is not recommended.

Zinc

The prevalence of zinc deficiency in patients receiving maintenance HD is not known but can occur, and toxicity is rare [39, 95, 123]. Zinc is protein bound so levels may be falsely low when serum albumin levels are low. Calcium and iron supplements as well as fiber and alcohol intake can interfere with zinc absorption [95, 98]. These factors decrease the reliability of using serum zinc alone as a diagnostic tool for zinc deficiency, or for monitoring patients receiving zinc supplements [95, 98]. Assessment of patient response to supplementation should use a combination of laboratory levels and changes in clinical symptoms. Chronic uremia can impair taste acuity; however, controversy exists as to whether or not zinc supplementation will improve taste perception [124, 125]. Short-term zinc supplementation may be beneficial for wound healing though optimal dose levels have not been determined [98]. Therefore, until more definitive outcomes are determined, the zinc recommendation for maintenance HD is the same as the RDA (15 mg/ day).

Conclusion

Maintaining adequate nutritional status is a challenge for maintenance HD patients regardless of the modality chosen. Understanding the different types of hemodialysis and their nutritional implications is important in maintaining the nutritional status and improving outcomes. Tailoring diet recommendations according to individual needs for protein, sodium, potassium, phosphorus, and fluid is the cornerstone of successful MNT, and keeping the diet as liberal as possible helps to promote optimal intake and quality of life in this patient population. Recognizing the prevalence of PEW in maintenance HD patients highlights the importance of ongoing nutrition assessment and intervention. Bone disease, anemia, and dyslipidemia management are all areas for the dietitian to attain competence and initiate into practice. A variety of assessment and educational tools are available via the National Kidney Foundation and the Academy of Nutrition and Dietetics, which are also sources of evidence-based guidelines for health professionals working with hemodialysis patients.

Acknowledgments Although Karen Weisen and Graeme Mendel did not contribute to the maintenance hemodialysis chapter in this edition, their previous contributions are invaluable and have provided the foundation for this revision.

Case Study

R.G. is a 67-year-old female, recently retired elementary school teacher who presents as a new HD patient. She has a history of resistant hypertension and lives with her son and daughter-in-law. Her appetite has been poor for the past month, and she complains that "foods don't taste right" and of feeling fatigued. She has had a 10-lb weight gain over the past month with signs of edema prior to starting HD. Height 5′2″, weight 127 lb. (57.7 kg); initial estimated dry weight (EDW) has been ordered at 122 lb. (55.4 kg); usual body weight (UBW) 117 lb. (53.2 kg). Medications include: cholecalciferol 1000 mg/day and an over-the-counter multivitamin with minerals; she was recently prescribed sevelamer carbonate (Renvela®) 800 mg as a phosphorus binder three times a day with meals. Initial predialysis labs: Ca 7.8 mg/dL, P 6.5 mg/dL, PTH 300 pg/mL, Na 127 mEq/L, K$^+$4.7 mEq/L, Cholesterol 102 mg/dL, BUN 39 mg/dL, Cr 5.4 mg/dL, Alb 3.2 g/dL, CO$_2$ 19 mEq/L, spKt/V 1.2, urine output = ~500 mL. HD prescription: Tuesday, Thursday, Saturday, 4 hour treatment; access: catheter. A 24-hour diet recall indicates the patient consumes an estimated 1000 kcal and 30 g protein over three meals and an occasional snack. R.G. avoids salt and salty foods; she followed a low protein, DASH-style diet prior to starting dialysis. Estimated sodium intake is 1500–2000 mg, potassium 3000 mg, and phosphorus 1100 mg.

After 1 week of HD, her appetite begins to improve and predialysis labs are Ca 8.0 mg/dL, P 6.0 mg/dL, PTH 375 pg/mL, Na 132 mEq/L, K$^+$5.8 mEq/L, BUN 44 mg/dL, Creatinine 5.0 mg/dL, Alb 3.3 g/dL, CO$_2$ 22 mEq/L, Cholesterol 150 mg/dL; EDW has been adjusted to 118 lb. (53.6 kg). Sevelamer (Renvela®) was increased to 1600 mg at each meal and patient was also instructed to take 800 mg with snacks which she had not been doing.

Case Questions and Answers

1. What are the diet recommendations for R.G. on conventional HD based on her weight and initial labs?
   Answer: The recommended diet is 64 g protein (UBW × 1.2 g/kg), 2 g sodium, 2 g potassium, 800–1000 mg phosphorus. Fluid intake should be kept to 1500 mL (urine output plus 1000 mL)

and adjusted according to IDWG. Based on R.G.'s initial intake of 1000 kcal and 30 g protein, she will have to add a minimum ~600 kcal and ~35 g of protein to her diet. Sodium intake is acceptable but she will need to decrease her intake of higher potassium fruit/juice and vegetables (as recommended on the DASH diet) to bring the potassium content of the diet within guidelines.

2. Are R.G.s' medications at the start of HD appropriate? Any recommendations for changes?
   Answer: The multivitamin with minerals should be changed to a renal B- and C-complex with folic acid. Serum 25-hydroxyvitamin D [25(OH)D] should be checked and current nutritional vitamin D supplement assessed. A renal vitamin containing cholecalciferol (D3) should be considered. PTH is above the KDOQI recommended range, and active vitamin D (calcitriol) or analog should be initiated. She is currently on a small dose of a phosphorus binder (sevelamer), and with the increased protein in the diet and elevated phosphorus, an increase in binders will be needed.

3. By the third month, R.G.'s appetite and energy level have improved. EDW has stabilized at 53.2 kg and IDWGs are 2–3 kg; current labs include: serum albumin 3.9 g/dL, K+3.6 mEq/L, P 5.5 mg/dL, Ca 9.8 mg/dL, PTH 390 pg/mL; fistula as access. She decides to resume teaching on a substitute basis and switches to in-center nocturnal hemodialysis (NHD). What diet and/or medication changes are indicated?
   Answer: A more liberal K+ intake should be considered since current serum K+ is at the lower end of the recommended range. PTH is still above the KDOQI recommended range; the addition of a calcimimetic (Sensipar® or Parsabiv®) could be considered and/or calcitriol adjusted, and serum calcium monitored (current corrected calcium = 9.9 mg/dL). Since NHD is associated with improved phosphorus control, intake may need to be liberalized and the binder dose adjusted.

4. As summer approaches, R.G. expresses an interest in trying short daily hemodialysis (SDHD) at home. After her training has been completed and she transitions to SDHD, what improvements/changes might be anticipated?
   Answer: Anticipated improvements include increased appetite and protein/calorie intake, increased serum albumin, increased dry weight (may need to adjust EDW); serum phosphorus levels may be slightly higher and diet and/or the phosphate binder dose adjusted as needed.

References

1. United States Renal Data System. 2018 USRDS annual data report: epidemiology of kidney disease in the United States. National Institutes of Health, National Institute of Diabetes and Digestive and Kidney Diseases. Bethesda;2018. www.usrds.org . Accessed 13 Jan 2019.
2. Carrero JJ, Thomas F, Nagy K, Arogundade F, Avesani CM, Chan M, et al. Global prevalence of protein-energy wasting in kidney disease: a meta-analysis of contemporary observational studies from the International Society of Renal Nutrition and Metabolism. J Ren Nutr. 2018;28(6):380–92.
3. Lodebo BT, Shah A, Kopple JD. Is it important to prevent and treat protein-energy wasting in chronic kidney disease and chronic dialysis patients? J Renal Nutr. 2018;28(6):369–79.
4. National Kidney Foundation. KDOQI clinical practice guideline for hemodialysis adequacy: 2015 update. Am J Kidney Dis. 2015;66(5):884–930.
5. Hakim RM, Levin N. Malnutrition in hemodialysis patients. Am J Kidney Dis. 1993;21:125–37.
6. Zeir M. Risk of mortality in patients with end-stage renal disease: the role of malnutrition and possible therapeutic implications. Horm Res. 2002;56:30–4.
7. Pupim LB, Caglar K, Hakim RM, Shyr Y, Ikizler TA. Uremic malnutrition is a predictor of death independent of inflammatory status. Kidney Int. 2004;66:2054–60.
8. Kopple JD. Effect of nutrition on morbidity and mortality in maintenance dialysis patients. Am J Kidney Dis. 1994;24:1002–9.
9. Sabatino A, Regolisti G, Karupaiah T, Sahathevan S, Sadu Singh BK, Khor BH, et al. Protein-energy wasting and nutritional supplementation in patients with end-stage renal disease on hemodialysis. Clin Nutr. 2017;36(3): 663–71.

10. Ikizler TA, Cano NJ, Franch H, Fouque D, Himmelfarb J, Kalantar-Zadeh K, et al. Prevention and treatment of protein energy wasting in chronic kidney disease patients: a consensus statement by the International Society of Renal Nutrition and Metabolism. Kidney Int. 2013;84:1096–107.

11. Ikizler TA, Burrowes J, Byham-Gray L, Campbell K, Carrero JJ, Chan W, et al. KDOQI Nutrition in CKD Guideline Work Group. KDOQI clinical practice guideline for nutrition in CKD: 2020 update. Am J Kidney Dis. 2020; in press.

12. Lowrie EG, Lew NL. Death risk in hemodialysis patients: the predictive value of commonly measured variables and an evaluation between facilities. Am J Kidney Dis. 1990;15(5):458–82.

13. Pupim LB, Evanson JA, Hakim RM, Ikizler TA. The extent of uremic malnutrition at the time of initation of maintenance dialysis is associated with the subsequent hospitalization. J Ren Nutr. 2003;13:259–6.

14. Friedman AN, Fadem SZ. Reassessment of albumin as a nutritional marker in kidney disease. J Am Soc Nephrol. 2010;21:223–30.

15. Kaysen GA, Dubin JA, Muller HG, Rosales L, Levin NW, Mitch WE. Inflammation and reduced albumin synthesis associated with stable decline in serum albumin in hemodialysis patients. Kidney Int. 2004;65:1408–15.

16. Jofré R, Rodriguez-Benitez P, López-Gómez JM, Peŕez-Garcia R. Inflammatory syndrome in patients on hemodialysis. Am Soc Nephrol. 2006;17:S274–80.

17. Sabatino A, Piotti G, Cosola C, Gandolfini I, Kooman JP, Fiaccadori E. Dietary protein and nutritional supplements in conventional hemodialysis. Semin Dial. 2018;31:583–91.

18. Stenvinkel P, Alvestrand A. Inflammation in end-stage renal disease: sources, consequences, and therapy. Semin Dial. 2002;15(5):329–37.

19. Fouque D, Kalantar-Zadeh K, Kopple J, Cano N, Chauveau P, Cuppari L, et al. A proposed nomenclature and diagnostic criteria for protein-energy wasting in acute and chronic kidney disease. Kidney Int. 2008;73:391–8.

20. Mak RH, Ikizler TA, Kovesdy CP, Raj DS, Stenvinkel P, Kalantar-Zadeh K. Wasting in chronic kidney disease. J Cachexia Sarcopenia Muscle. 2011;2:9–25.

21. Bossola M, Muscaritoli M, Tazza L, Panocchia N, Liberatori M, Giungi S, et al. Variables associated with reduced dietary intake in hemodialysis patients. J Ren Nutr. 2005;15:244–52.

22. Carrero JJ. Identification of patients with eating disorders: clinical and biochemical signs of appetite loss in dialysis patients. J Ren Nutr. 2009;19(1):10–5.

23. Kalantar-Zadeh K, Block G, McAllister J, Humphreys MH, Kopple JD. Appetite and inflammation, nutrition, anemia and clinical outcomes in hemodialysis patients. Am J Clin Nutr. 2004;80:299–307.

24. Mehrotra R, Kopple JD. Nutritional management of maintenance dialysis patients: why aren't we doing better? Ann Rev Nutr. 2001;21:343–79.

25. Molfino A, Kaysen GA, Chertow GM, Doyle J, Delgado C, Dwyer T, et al. Validating appetite assessment tools among patients receiving hemodialysis. J Ren Nutr. 2016;26(2):103–10.

26. Lopes AA, Elder SJ, Ginsberg N, Andreucci VE, Cruz JM, Fukuhara S, et al. Lack of appetite in haemodialysis patients—associations with patient characteristics, indicators of nutritional status and outcomes in the international DOPPS. Nephrol Dial Transplant. 2007;22:3538–46.

27. Kopple JD, Kalantar-Zadeh K, Mehrotra R. Risks of chronic metabolic acidosis in patients with chronic kidney disease. Kidney Int. 2005;67:S21–7.

28. Walls J. Effect of correction of acidosis on nutritional status in dialysis patients. Miner Electrolyte Metab. 1997;23:234–6.

29. Kalantar-Zadeh K, Mehrotra R, Fouque D, Kopple JD. Metabolic acidosis and malnutrition inflammation complex syndrome in chronic renal failure. Semin Dial. 2004;17:455–65.

30. Blair D, Bigelow C, Sweet SJ. Nutritional effects of delivered bicarbonate dose in maintenance hemodialysis patients. J Ren Nutr. 2003;13(3):205–11.

31. Vashistha T, Kalantar-Zadeh K, Molnar MZ, Torle'n K, Mehrotra R. Dialysis modality and correction of uremic metabolic acidosis: relationship with all-cause and cause-specific mortality. Clin J Am Soc Nephrol. 2013;8:254–64.

32. Papadoyannakis NJ, Stefanidis CJ, McGeown M. The effect of the correction of metabolic acidosis on nitrogen and potassium balance of patients with chronic renal failure. Am J Clin Nutr. 1984;40:623–7.

33. McCann L. Pocket guide to nutrition assessment of the patient with chronic kidney disease. 5th ed. New York: National Kidney Foundation; 2015.

34. Ohashi Y, Sakai K, Hase H, Joki N. Dry weight targeting: the art and science of conventional hemodialysis. Semin Dial. 2018;31:551–6.

35. Bossola M, Pepe G, Vulpio C. The frustrating attempt to limit the interdialytic weight gain in patients on chronic hemodialysis: new insights into an old problem. J Ren Nutr. 2018;28(5):293–301.

36. Dekker MJE, Konings C, Canaud B, van der Sande FM, Stuard S, Raimann JG, et al. Interactions between malnutrition, inflammation, and fluid overload and their associations with survival in prevalent hemodialysis patients. J Ren Nutr. 2018;28(6):435–44.

37. Wong MMY, McCullough, Bieber BA, Bommer J, Hecking M, Levin NW, et al. Interdialytic weight gain: trends, predictors, and associated outcomes in the international Dialysis outcomes and practice patterns study (DOPPS). Am J Kidney Dis. 2017;69(3):367–79.
38. Kopple JD, Kalantar-Zadeh K. Malnutrition and IDPN in patients with ESRD. In: Principles and practices of dialysis. 4th ed. Philadelphia: Lippincott Williams & Wilkins; 2009. p. 473–88.
39. Kalantar-Zadeh K, Kopple JD. Nutritional management of patients undergoing maintenance hemodialysis. In: Kopple JD, Massry SG, editors. Kopple and Massry's nutritional management of renal disease. 2nd ed. Philadelphia: Lippincott Williams & Wilkins; 2004. p. 433–58.
40. Bossola M, Muscaritoli M, Tazza L, Giungi S, Tortorelli A, Rossi Fanelli F, et al. Malnutrition in hemodialysis patients: what therapy? Am J Kidney Dis. 2005;46:371–86.
41. Ikizler TA. Nutrition and peritoneal dialysis. In: Handbook of nutrition and the kidney. 5th ed. Philadelphia: Lippincott Williams & Wilkins; 2005. p. 228–44.
42. Gutierrez A, Bergstrom J, Alvestrand A. Protein catabolism in sham-hemodialysis: the effect of different membranes. Clin Nephrol. 1992;38:20–9.
43. Ikizler TA, Flakoll PJ, Parker RA, Hakim RM. Amino acid and albumin losses during hemodialysis. Kidney Int. 1994;46:830–7.
44. Fouque D, Pelletier S, Guebre-Egziabher F. Have recommended protein and phosphate intake recently changed in maintenance hemodialysis? J Ren Nutr. 2011;1:35–8.
45. Kaplan AA, Halley SE, Lapkin RA, Graeber CW. Dialysate protein losses with bleach processed polysulphone dialyzers. Kidney Int. 1995;47:573–8.
46. Ikizler TA, Pupim LA, Brouillette JR, Levenhagen DK, Farmer K, Hakim RM, et al. Hemodialysis stimulates muscle and whole body protein loss and alters substrate oxidation. Am J Physiol Endocrinol Metab. 2002;282:E107–16.
47. Pupim LB, Flakoll PJ, Ikizler TA. Protein homeostasis in chronic hemodialysis patients. CurrOpin Clin NutrMetab Care. 2004;7:890–5.
48. Blagg CR. The early history of dialysis for chronic renal failure in the United States: a view from Seattle. Am J Kidney Dis. 2007;49(3):482–96.
49. Cianciaruso B, Brunori G, Traverso G, Paanarello G, Enia G, Strippoli P, et al. Nutritional status in the elderly patient with uraemia. Nephrol Dial Transplant. 1995;10:65–8.
50. Chauveau P, Combe C, Laville M, Fouque D, Azar R, Cano N, et al. Factors influencing survival in hemodialysis patients aged older than 75 years: 2.5 year outcome study. Am J Kidney Dis. 2001;37:997–1003.
51. Kaysen GA, Greene T, Larive B, Mehta RL, Lindsay RM, Depner TA, et al. The effect of frequent hemodialysis on nutrition and body composition: frequent hemodialysis network trial. Kidney Int. 2012;82:90–9.
52. Hutson B, Stuart N. Nutrition management of the adult hemodialysis patient. In: a clinical guide to nutrition care in kidney disease. 2nd ed. Chicago: American Dietetic Association; 2013.
53. Rocco MV, Paranandi L, Burrowes JD, Cockram DB, Dwyer JT, Kusek JW, et al. Nutritional status in the HEMO study cohort at baseline. Am J Kidney Dis. 2002;39:245–56.
54. Burrowes JD, Larive B, Cockram DB, Dwyer J, Kusek JW, McLeroy S, et al. Effects of dietary intake, appetite and eating habits on dialysis and non-dialysis treatment days in hemodialysis patients: cross sectional results from the HEMO study. J Ren Nutr. 2003;13:191–8.
55. Kistler BM, Benner D, Burrowes JD, Campbell KL, Fouque D, Garibotto G, et al. Eating during hemodialysis treatment: a consensus statement from the International Society of Renal Nutrition and Metabolism. J Ren Nutr. 2018;28(1):4–12.
56. Boxall MC, Goodship THJ. Nutritional requirements in hemodialysis. In: Mitch WE, Klahr S, editors. Handbook of nutrition and the kidney. 4th ed. Philadelphia: Lippincott Williams & Wilkins; 2005. p. 218–27.
57. Punal J, Lema LV, Sanhez-Guisande D, Ruano-Ravina A. Clinical effectiveness and quality of life of conventional haemodialysis versus short daily haemodialysis: a systematic review. Nephrol Dial Transplant. 2008;10:1–13.
58. McPhatter LL. Nocturnal home hemodialysis. In: a clinical guide to nutrition care in kidney disease. 2nd ed. Chicago: American Dietetic Association; 2013.
59. Wolfson M. Nutrition in elderly dialysis patients. Semin Dial. 2002;15:113–5.
60. Burrowes JD, Dalton S, Backstrand J, Levin NW. Patients receiving maintenance hemodialysis with low vs high levels of nutritional risk have decreased morbidity. J Am Diet Assoc. 2005;105:563–71.
61. Galland R, Traeger J. Short daily hemodialysis and nutritional status in patients with chronic renal failure. Semin Dial. 2004;2:104–8.
62. Ayus JC, Achinger SG, Mizani MR, Chertow GM, Furmaga W, Lee S, et al. Phosphorus balance and mineral metabolism with 3 h daily dialysis. Kidney Int. 2007;71:336–42.
63. Ahmad S. Dietary sodium restriction for hypertension in dialysis patients. Semin Dial. 2004;17:284–7.
64. Wilson J, Shah T, Nissenson AR. Role of sodium and volume in the pathogenesis of hypertension in hemodialysis. Semin Dial. 2004;17:260–4.

65. Goldstein-Fuchs J. Nutrition intervention for chronic renal diseases. In: Mitch WE, Klahr S, editors. Handbook of nutrition and the kidney. 5th ed. Philadelphia: Lippincott Williams & Wilkins; 2005. p. 267–301.
66. Testa A, Plou A. Clinical determinants of interdialytic weight gain. J Ren Nutr. 2001;11:155–60.
67. Beto J, Bansai VK. Hyperkalemia: evaluating dietary and non-dietary etiology. J Ren Nutr. 1992;2:28–9.
68. Musso CG. Potassium metabolism in patients with chronic kidney disease. Part II: patients on dialysis (stage 5). Int UrolNephrol. 2004;36:469–72.
69. Veltassa prescribing information. www.veltassa.com. 2 Feb 2019.
70. Constantino J, Roberts C. Life-threatening hyperkalemia from chewing tobacco in a hemodialysis patient. J Ren Nutr. 1997;7:106–8.
71. Ifudu O, Reydel K, Vlacich V, Delosreyes G, et al. Dietary potassium is not the sole determinant of serum potassium concentration in hemodialysis patients. Dial Transplant. 2004;33:684–8.
72. Pierratos A, Ouwendyk M, Francoeur R, Vas S, Raj DS, Ecclestone AM, et al. Nocturnal hemodialysis: three year experience. J Am Soc Nephrol. 1998;9:859–68.
73. Argoudelis A, McCarty C, Re R, et al.. Phosphorus and potassium removal with short daily hemodialysis. In: Poster presentation. Annual Dialysis Conference. 2009.
74. Kohn OF, Coe FL, Ing TS. Solute kinetics with short-daily home hemodialysis using slow dialysate rate flow. Hemodial Int. 2010;14:39–46.
75. Goodman WG. Calcium, phosphorus and vitamin D. In: Handbook of nutrition & the kidney. 5th ed. Philadelphia: Lippincott Williams & Wilkins; 2004. p. 47–69.
76. National Kidney Foundation. Clinical practice guidelines: bone metabolism and disease in chronic renal failure. Am J Kidney Dis. 2003;42:S12–143.
77. Kidney Disease: Improving Global Outcomes (KDIGO) CKD–MBD work group. KDIGO clinical practice guideline for the diagnosis, evaluation, prevention, and treatment of chronic kidney disease–mineral and bone disorder (CKD–MBD). Kidney Int. 2009;76(113):S1–S130.
78. Block GA, Klassen PS, Lazarus M, Ofsthun N, Lowrie EG, Chertow GM. Mineral metabolism, mortality and morbidity in maintenance hemodialysis. J Am Soc Nephrol. 2004;15:2208–18.
79. Goodman W, Goldin J, Kuizon B, Yoon C, Gales B, Sider D, et al. Coronary-artery calcification in young adults with end-stage renal disease who are undergoing dialysis. N Engl J Med. 2000;342:1478–83.
80. Goodman W, London G, Amann K, Block G, Giachelli C, Hruska KA, et al. Vascular calcification in chronic kidney disease. Am J Kidney Dis. 2004;43:572–9.
81. Schwarz U, Buzello M, Ritz E, Stein G, Raabe G, Wiest G, et al. Morphology of coronary atherosclerotic lesions in patients with end-stage renal failure. Nephrol Dial Transplant. 2000;15:218–23.
82. Beto J, Bhatt N, Gerbeling T, Patel C, Drayer D. Overview of the 2017 KDIGO CKD-MBD update: practice implications for adult hemodialysis patients. J Ren Nutr. 2019;29(1):2–15.
83. Kidney Disease: Improving Global Outcomes (KDIGO) CKD-MBD update work group. KDIGO 2017 clinical practice guideline update for the diagnosis, evaluation, prevention, and treatment of chronic kidney disease–mineral and bone disorder (CKD-MBD). Kidney Int Suppl. 2017;7:1–59.
84. Murphy-Gutekunst L. Hidden phosphorus in popular beverages: part I. J Ren Nutr. 2005;15:e1–6.
85. Lockridge RS, Spencer M, Craft V, Pipkin M, Campbell D, McPhatter L, et al. Nightly home hemodialysis: five and one-half years of experience in Lynchburg, Virginia. Hemodial Int. 2004;8:61–9.
86. Schulman G. Nutrition in daily dialysis. Am J Kidney Dis. 2003;41:S112–5.
87. Goldstein-Fuchs J. Dyslipidemias in chronic kidney disease. In: A clinical guide to nutrition care in kidney disease. 2nd ed. Chicago: American Dietetic Association; 2013.
88. National Kidney Foundation. KDOQI clinical practice guidelines for managing dyslipidemia in chronic kidney disease patients. Am J Kidney Dis. 2003;41:S1–91.
89. Saltissi D, Morgan C, Knight B, Chang W, Rigby R, Westhuyzen J. Effect of lipid-lowering dietary recommendations on the nutritional intake and lipid profiles of chronic peritoneal dialysis patients and hemodialysis patients. Am J Kidney Dis. 2001;37:1209–15.
90. Luis D, Zlatkis K, Comenge B, Garcia Z, Navarro JF, Lorenzo V, et al. Dietary quality and adherence to dietary recommendations in patients undergoing hemodialysis. J Ren Nutr. 2016;26(3):190–5.
91. Tucker BM, Safadi S, Friedman AN. Is routine multivitamin supplementation necessary in US chronic adult hemodialysis patients? A systematic review. J Ren Nutr. 2015;25(3):257–64.
92. Coveney N, Polkinghorne KR, Linehan L, Corradini A, Kerr PG. Water-soluble vitamin levels in extended hours hemodialysis. Hemodial Int. 2010;15:30–8.
93. Kannampuzha J, Donnelly SM, McFarlane PA, Chan CT, House JD, Pencharz PB, et al. Glutathione and riboflavin status in supplemented patients undergoing home nocturnal hemodialysis versus standard hemodialysis. J Ren Nutr. 2010;20:199–208.

94. Makoff R, Gonick H. Renal failure and the concomitant derangement of micronutrient metabolism. Nutr Clin Pract. 1999;14:238–46.
95. Masud T. Trace elements and vitamins in renal disease. In: Handbook of nutrition and the kidney. 5th ed. Philadelphia: Lippincott Williams & Wilkins; 2004. p. 196–217.
96. Kasama R, Koch T, Canals-Navas C, Pitone JM. Vitamin B6 and hemodialysis: the impact of high-flux/high efficiency dialysis and review of the literature. Am J Kidney Dis. 1996;27:680–6.
97. Rocco MV, Makoff R. Appropriate vitamin therapy for dialysis patients. Semin Dial. 1997;10:272–7.
98. Wiggins KL. Renal care: resources and practical applications. Chicago: American Dietetic Association; 2004. p. 39–60.
99. Shemin D, Bostom AG, Selhub J. Treatment of hyperhomocysteinemia in end-stage renal disease. Am J Kidney Dis. 2001;38:S91–4.
100. Obeid R, Kuhlmann MK, Kohler H, Herrmann W. Response of homocysteine cystathionine, and methylmalonic acid to vitamin treatment in dialysis patients. Clin Chem. 2005;51:196–201.
101. Clement L. Homocysteine: the newest uremic toxin? Renal Nutr Forum. 2003;23:1–4.
102. Fletcher RH, Fairfield KM. Vitamins for chronic disease prevention in adults. JAMA. 2002;287:3127–9.
103. Schaefer RM, Tschner M, Kosch M. Folate metabolism in renal failure. Nephrol Dial Transplant. 2002;17:24–7.
104. Handelman GJ. New insight on vitamin C in patients with chronic kidney disease. J Ren Nutr. 2011;21:110–2.
105. Hung SC, Hung SH, Tarng DC, Yang WC, Chen TW, Huang TP. Thiamine deficiency and unexplained encephalopathy in hemodialysis and peritoneal dialysis patients. Am J Kidney Dis. 2001;38:941–7.
106. Handleman GJ, Levin NW. Guidelines for vitamin supplements in chronic kidney disease patients: what is the evidence? J Ren Nutr. 2011;21:117–9.
107. Jung U, Helbich-Endermann M, Bitsch R, Schenider BR, Stein G. Are patients with chronic renal failure (CRF) deficient in biotin and is regular biotin supplementation required? Z Ernahrungswiss. 1998;37:363–7.
108. Jones WO, Nidus BD. Biotin and hiccups in chronic dialysis patients. J Ren Nutr. 1991;1:80–3.
109. Muth I. Implications of hypervitaminosis a in chronic renal failure. J Ren Nutr. 1991;1:2–8.
110. Holden RM, Ki V, Morton AR, Clase C. Fat-soluble vitamins in advanced CKD/ESRD: a review. Semin Dial. 2012;25:334–43.
111. Blair D, Byham-Gray L, Lewis E, McCaffrey S. Prevalence of vitamin D [25(OH)D] deficiency and effects of supplementation with ergocalciferol (vitamin D2) in stage 5 chronic kidney disease patients. J Ren Nutr. 2008;18(4):375–82.
112. Miller ER, Pastor-Barriuso R, Dalal D, Riemersma RA, Appel LJ, Guallar E. Meta-analysis: high dose vitamin E supplementation may increase all-cause mortality. Ann Intern Med. 2005;142:37–46.
113. Pilkey RM, Morton AR, Boffa MB, Noordhof C, et al. Subclinical vitamin K deficiency in hemodialysis patients. Am J Kidney Dis. 2007;49:432–9.
114. Cranenburg ECM, Schurgers LJ, Uiterwijk HH, Beulens JWJ, et al. Vitamin K intake and status are low in hemodialysis patients. Kidney Int. 2012;82:605–10.
115. Elliott MJ, Booth SL, Hopman WM, Holden RM. Assessment of potential biomarkers of subclinical vitamin K deficiency in patients with end-stage kidney disease. Can JKidney Health Dis. 2014;1:13. http://www.cjkhd.org/content/1/1/13. Accessed 13 April 2019
116. Kohlmeier M, Saupe J, Shearer MJ, Schaefer K, Asmus G. Bone health of adult hemodialysis patients is related to vitamin K status. Kidney Int. 1997;51:1218–21.
117. Rucker D, Thadhani R, Tonelli M. Trace elements status in hemodialysis patients. Semin Dial. 2010;23:389–95.
118. Skikine BS, Ahluwalia B, Fergusson B, Chonko A, Cook JD. Effects of erythropoietin therapy on iron absorption in chronic renal failure. J Lab Clin Med. 2000;135:452–8.
119. Cook JD, Dassenko SA, Whittaker P. Calcium supplementation: effect on iron absorption. Am J Clin Nutr. 1991;53:106–11.
120. Hallberg I, Hulten L, Gramatkovski E. Iron absorption from the whole diet in men: how effective is the regulation of iron absorption? Am J Clin Nutr. 1997;66:347–56.
121. Ng AHM, Hercz G, Kandel R, Grynpas MD. Association between fluoride, magnesium, aluminum and bone quality in renal osteodystrophy. Bone. 2003;34:216–24.
122. Smith AM, Temple K. Selenium metabolism and renal disease. J Ren Nutr. 1997;7:69–72.
123. Erten Y, Kayata M, Sezer S, Ozdemir FN. Zinc deficiency: prevalence and causes in hemodialysis patients and effect on cellular immune response. Transplant Proc. 1998;30:850–1.
124. Matson A, Wright M, Oliver A, Woodrow G, King N, Dye L, et al. Zinc supplementation at conventional doses does not improve the disturbance of taste perception in hemodialysis patients. J Ren Nutr. 2003;13:224–8.
125. van der Eijk I, Allman Farinelli MA. Taste testing in renal patients. J Ren Nutr. 1997;7:3–9.

Chapter 16
Peritoneal Dialysis

Chhaya Patel and Jerrilynn D. Burrowes

Keywords Peritoneal dialysis · Protein-energy wasting · Medical nutrition therapy

Key Points
- Describe the goals of medical nutrition therapy for patients receiving peritoneal dialysis.
- Describe the differences in nutrition therapy between the different types of renal replacement therapies.
- Identify factors that may impact the nutritional status of patients receiving peritoneal dialysis.

Introduction

Medical nutrition therapy (MNT) plays an integral role in the health of the patient with stage 5 chronic kidney disease (CKD) receiving maintenance dialysis. The health professional must understand the role of nutrition in stage 5 CKD, the factors affecting assessment and maintenance of adequate nutritional status, and the nutritional implications associated with the different types of renal replacement therapies (RRTs). Studies have shown that older age, diabetes mellitus (DM), hypertension (HTN), cardiovascular disease (CVD), and a higher body mass index (BMI) ($\geq$30 kg/m^2) are associated with CKD [1–3]. Based on the data from four cohorts of the National Health and Nutrition Examination Survey (NHANES) (2001–2004; 2005–2008; 2009–2012; 2013–2016), overall CKD prevalence in the general U.S. adult population has remained relatively stable from 2001 to 2016: stages 1–5 CKD--4.2% to 4.8%; stages 3–5 CKD--6.6% to 6.9%, respectively) [4]. However, the prevalence of CKD among people with DM decreased over time (from 43.6% in 2001–2004 to 36.0% in 2013–2016). A similar decrease was not seen among individuals with HTN, whose CKD prevalence remains at about 31% [4].

The editors acknowledge Karen Wiesen's contribution to this chapter in *Nutrition in Kidney Disease, Second Edition*, Nutrition and Health, DOI https://doi.org/10.1007/978-1-62703-685-6_1, © Springer Science+Business Media New York 2014.

C. Patel (✉)
DaVita Dialysis, Program Manager Nutrition Services, Divisional Lead Dietitian for ORCA Division, Dietitian Council and EPIC Mentor, Walnut Creek, CA, USA
e-mail: cpatel@davita.com

J. D. Burrowes
Department of Biomedical, Health and Nutritional Sciences, School of Health Professions and Nursing, Long Island University-Post, Brookville, NY, USA

© Springer Nature Switzerland AG 2020
J. D. Burrowes et al. (eds.), *Nutrition in Kidney Disease*, Nutrition and Health,
https://doi.org/10.1007/978-3-030-44858-5_16

Table 16.1 Types of dialysis modalities

Type of dialysis	Location	Duration	Frequency
Conventional hemodialysis	In-center	3–5 hours	3×/week
Peritoneal dialysis			
CAPD	Home	Varies with type of PD	Daily
CCPD	Home	4–6 exchanges	4–6×/daily
Home hemodialysis	Home	3–5 hours	3×/week
Home nocturnal hemodialysis	Home	7–10 hours	5–7×/week
In-center nocturnal hemodialysis	In-center	7–8 hours	3×/week
Home short daily hemodialysis	Home	2–3 hours	5–7×/week
In-center short daily hemodialysis	In-center	2–3 hours	5–6×/week

CAPD continuous ambulatory peritoneal dialysis, *CCPD* continuous cyclic peritoneal dialysis, *PD* peritoneal dialysis

In 2016, there were 124,675 newly reported cases of end-stage renal disease (ESRD), with 9.7% starting peritoneal dialysis (PD). By the end of 2016, there were 726,331 prevalent cases of ESRD with 7% of these cases treated with PD [5]. Moreover, since 2000, the number of incident and prevalent PD patients has increased by 60.2% and 87.9%, respectively [5].

The nutritional status of the patient at the initiation of RRT is an important risk factor for future outcomes, since malnutrition is associated with increased morbidity and mortality in patients receiving maintenance dialysis [6–8]. Therefore, nutritional management should include a comprehensive nutrition assessment, individualized interventions, ongoing diet education, and continuous monitoring of nutritional status. The goals of MNT in stage 5 CKD are (1) to achieve and maintain a neutral or positive nitrogen balance; (2) to achieve and maintain an adequate nutritional status; (3) to prevent the accumulation of electrolytes and minimize fluid imbalance; and (4) to minimize the effect of metabolic disorders associated with stage 5 CKD.

Patients beginning RRT now have a choice of modalities that include hemodialysis (HD), PD, nocturnal home hemodialysis (NHD), short daily hemodialysis (SDHD), and renal transplantation (Table 16.1). This chapter will review the MNT for PD and discuss factors that may impact nutrition assessment and the overall nutritional status.

Factors Influencing Nutritional Status

Malnutrition in patients receiving maintenance dialysis is associated with increased morbidity and mortality, and they are more susceptible to infections and fatigue [6–9]. Studies have shown that about one-third of PD patients have some degree of malnutrition [10]. A recent study found that 20% of PD patients had some degree of malnutrition based on the malnutrition-inflammation score (MIS) [11]. Factors that influence nutritional status include anorexia associated with chronic disease, the dialysis procedure itself, impaired nutrient absorption, poor dietary intake, acidosis, increased protein catabolism, and inflammation. Routine monitoring of nutritional status is important in the early detection and prevention of malnutrition. A variety of assessment tools is important since there is limited evidence to suggest the use of one tool over the other [12]. Moreover, some of the traditional anthropometric and biochemical measures used to assess the nutritional status may be influenced by other factors that affect nutritional status in dialysis patients. The recent clinical practice guidelines on nutrition in CKD patients from the Academy of Nutrition and Dietetics Evidence Analysis Library (Academy EAL)/Kidney Disease Outcomes Quality Initiative (KDOQI) Guidelines recommends that registered dietitian nutritionists (RDNs) (or international equivalents) conduct a comprehensive nutrition assessment which includes, but is not limited to, an assessment of appetite, a history of dietary intake, biochemical data, anthropometric measurements and a nutrition-focused physical exam [12]. This section will provide a brief overview of some of these factors. However, refer to Chaps. 4, 5, 6, and 7 for more information on individual parameters used in the nutrition assessment.

Serum albumin concentration has long been used as a marker of nutritional status in the maintenance dialysis population, although there are several factors that can influence this biochemical marker such as hydration status, inflammation, and liver disease. Regardless of its limitations, serum albumin has been shown to independently correlate with an increased risk of mortality in dialysis patients [13–15]. In PD patients, the baseline serum albumin concentration <3.0 g/dL had a more than 3-fold higher adjusted risk of all-cause and cardiovascular mortality and a 3.4-fold higher risk of infection-related mortality compared to serum albumin 4.0–4.19 g/dL [14].

The terminology defining malnutrition in the dialysis patient has evolved. Historically, it was divided into two types. Classic or type 1 malnutrition, which was defined by a loss of lean body mass, inadequate oral intake, normal to mildly depleted serum albumin, and normal C-reactive protein (CRP) levels, is responsive to nutrition interventions [16, 17]. Type 2 malnutrition, which is caused by inflammation and characterized by markedly low serum albumin despite adequate oral intake, increased oxidative stress, elevated CRP and other proinflammatory markers, is not reversible with nutrition intervention alone [18]. Type 2 is now referred to as the malnutrition-inflammation complex syndrome (MICS) because of the interrelationship between malnutrition and inflammation. The challenge for the clinician when identifying the type of malnutrition present is difficult, and emerging evidence has indicated that these definitions are not necessarily accurate for the CKD patient. In 2008, the International Society of Renal Nutrition and Metabolism (ISRNM) proposed the definition and specific diagnostic criteria for protein-energy wasting (PEW) which better reflects the type of wasting that occurs in CKD [18]. PEW is defined as the "state of decreased body stores of protein and energy fuels (body protein and fat masses)" [18, 19].

An assessment of anorexia or poor appetite is a subjective factor in the nutrition assessment; however, recent studies have shown that it is predictive of poor clinical outcomes as well as being associated with inflammation [20]. Anorexia is estimated to be present in one-third of patients receiving maintenance dialysis [21, 22]. In a recent study, anorexia was a key risk factor for inadequate protein intake and malnutrition in patients undergoing PD, which highlights the need to closely monitor patients with appetite disturbances [23].

The etiology of anorexia is multifactorial and includes uremia, inflammation, infection, delayed gastric emptying, comorbid conditions, medications, psychosocial and socioeconomic factors, absorption of glucose in PD, early satiety, and age [22–24]. An assessment of appetite is a key contributor in the evaluation of the nutritional status, since it is associated with reduced protein and energy intakes and inflammation. The Appetite and Diet Assessment Tool (ADAT) has been used to assess appetite in dialysis patients [25]. The predictive value of appetite in the clinical management of dialysis patients has been validated in several studies [22, 26, 27]. See Chap. 22 for further information on PEW in CKD.

Metabolic acidosis impacts nutritional status by increasing protein catabolism and possibly decreasing protein synthesis, which leads to negative nitrogen balance and loss of lean body mass [28]. Correction of acidosis with sodium bicarbonate has been shown to correct protein catabolism [29]. Metabolic acidosis may induce insulin resistance and chronic inflammation, both of which may also increase protein catabolism; however, more research is needed in this area [29, 30]. The Academy EAL/KDOQI guidelines recommend that in adults with CKD stages 3–5D, serum bicarbonate levels should be maintained at 24–26 mEq/L [12].

The dialysis procedure has long been considered a catabolic procedure. Approximately 4–9 g net amino acids and 1–2 g protein are lost during the HD procedure and 2–4 g net amino acids and 5–15 g protein during PD [31–34]. PD is not as catabolic as HD unless the patient has peritonitis. A mild inflammatory response may be triggered by bioincompatability of the peritoneal dialysate, endotoxin transfer from the dialysate, or the PD catheter itself that can lead to protein catabolism [35]. Patients receiving PD who are classified as high transporters by the peritoneal equilibration test (PET) have a higher incidence of poor nutrition due to the loss of larger amounts of protein into the dialysate [33, 36]. Serum albumin levels are usually low in these patients and they may require nutritional supplementation.

PD Adequacy

Assessment of dialysis adequacy [37] should be part of the routine evaluation of nutritional status in patients receiving PD. The relationship between Kt/V (a marker for dialysis adequacy where K = clearance, t = time, and V = volume) and the protein equivalent of nitrogen appearance (PNA) may be confounded by mathematical coupling. Using Kt alone, the non-normalized dose of dialysis may be more closely associated with serum albumin levels [38].

The relationship between the nutritional intake and the dose of dialysis in patients receiving continuous PD was evaluated as part of the CANUSA (Canada-USA) peritoneal dialysis study [35]. A number of different nutritional markers were evaluated and, in the first 6 months, there was a positive correlation between the PD dose and all of the nutritional markers except serum albumin level. After 6 months, reduction in overall clearance because of loss of residual renal function was associated with a trend toward declining nutritional parameters [35]. The current minimum recommendation for continuous PD is a weekly total Kt/V of 1.7 [39]. Project data from a large dialysis corporation in 2018 showed that inadequate dialysis was associated with PD loss. Patients with $Kt/V < 1.7$ had 2.5 times higher drop or loss rate than patients with $Kt/V \geq 1.7$. It is also important to note that patients with serum albumin <3.0 mg/dL had two times higher loss rate than patients with serum albumin $\geq$3.6 mg/dL [39].

Nutrient Recommendations in Peritoneal Dialysis

Energy

The Academy EAL/KDOQI guidelines recommend that in adults receiving maintenance dialysis who are metabolically stable, an energy intake of 25–35 kcal/kg body weight (BW) per day should be prescribed [12]. Energy intakes should be adjusted for age, gender, the level of physical activity, body composition, weight status goals, and concurrent illness or the presence of inflammation to maintain normal nutritional status. These recommendations are based on metabolic studies which showed that 35 kcal/kg IBW/day was necessary to maintain neutral nitrogen balance and stable body composition. Since patients 60 years or older may be more sedentary and have less lean body mass, a lower energy intake of 30 kcal/kg BW/day is thought to be acceptable. Energy intake should include calories from both the diet and the dialysate since calories absorbed during dialysis can be significant and lead to weight gain. Several formulas have been published for determining caloric load from the dialysate (Table 16.2) [40–43].The most accurate method for estimating calories absorbed from the dialysate is to compare the grams of glucose infused with the grams of glucose in the effluent [40]. Glucose absorption differs between therapies with patients on continuous cyclic peritoneal dialysis (CCPD) absorbing approximately 40% of calories due to shorter dwell times, while patients on continuous ambulatory peritoneal dialysis (CAPD) absorb approximately 60% of calories [40, 41]. Dextrose absorption may help older patients with inadequate energy intake. The clinician needs to be reminded that patients are taught to adjust their usual dextrose prescription for incidences of fluid overload or dehydration and low blood pressure, so caloric contribution from dextrose may vary. It may be difficult to restrict calories in PD patients for weight reduction without compromising protein intake and

Table 16.2 Suggested methods to estimate calories absorbed from peritoneal dialysis

Formula	Comments
$(11.3X - 10.0) \times$ L inflow $\times 3.4$ = kcal absorbed from glucose X = average glucose concentration infused [44]	Does not account for differences in membranes
Glucose absorbed (kcal) = $(1 - D/Do)x_1$ D/Do is the fraction of glucose remaining and the x_1 is the initial glucose infused [35]	Considers dialysis modality and membrane transport type

Simple estimate:
    G glucose infused (based on total vol of exchanges) $\times$ %
    absorption (per modality) = G glucose absorbed
    G glucose absorbed $\times 3.4$ = glucose kcal absorbed
% Absorption:
    APD: 40%
    CAPD: 60%
    Icodextrin: 20–35%
G glucose/L:
    1.5% = 15 g
    2.5% = 25 g
    4.25% = 42.5 g
    7.5% icodextrin = 75 g
	Does not consider membrane transport type or type of PD modality
	Provides a rough estimate

Data from [40–44]. Adapted with permission from Academy of Nutrition & Dietetics: A Clinical Guide to Nutrition Care in Kidney Disease, 2004
APD automated peritoneal dialysis, *CAPD* continuous ambulatory peritoneal dialysis, *PD* peritoneal dialysis, *vol* volume

nutritional status. Patients should be encouraged to limit excessive sugars and fats and to exercise, if possible, to help with weight control. Assessment and counseling by the dietitian are important to help the patient achieve an adequate intake.

Icodextrin is an alternative polyglucose PD solution produced from the hydrolysis of cornstarch. Because it is a macromolecule, icodextrin is absorbed more slowly by the peritoneal membrane resulting in a sustained ultrafiltration (UF) and lower glucose absorption [43–46]. Icodextrin provides a caloric load similar to a 2.5% dextrose dialysate solution over the longer dwell. One of the metabolites of icodextrin is maltose, which can interfere with certain blood glucose monitors and strips that may cause a falsely elevated reading [43, 45–47].

Protein

Protein requirements in PD are higher than in HD because of increased losses during the dialysis procedure [31–33, 47]. As stated previously, PD patients lose between 5 and 15 g protein/day through the peritoneum with the average being 9 g. Approximately half of the protein lost is in the form of albumin [48, 49]. During episodes of peritonitis, this loss can increase by 50% or more and may remain elevated for 2–3 weeks after resolution of the infection [50, 51].

Metabolic balance studies in clinically stable PD patients showed that 1.2–1.3 g protein/kg/day is required to maintain neutral or positive nitrogen balance [52]. Based on these studies, the Academy EAL/KDOQI guidelines recommend prescribing a dietary protein intake of 1.0–1.2 g/kg BW/day in PD patients who are metabolically stable to maintain adequate nutritional status [12]. At least 50% of the protein should come from high biological value (HBV) sources.

Achieving this amount of protein is sometimes difficult for some PD patients and the dietitian needs to assess actual protein intake for adequacy. Older patients may need higher protein intakes and protein supplements because of protein losses and non-nutritional causes including psychosocial issues. PD patients who follow a vegetarian eating pattern will require ongoing counseling by the dietitian to help ensure they consume adequate protein from legumes or soy products without an excess mineral load.

Protein Nitrogen Appearance in Peritoneal Dialysis

Protein nitrogen appearance (PNA) or protein catabolic rate (PCR) is used to estimate protein intake in the clinically stable dialysis patient. Protein is metabolized to nitrogenous waste products and, in the stable patient, the waste products removed (in grams/day) are equal to protein intake. PNA is calculated from the urea nitrogen appearance (UNA) rate, which is calculated from 24-h collections of urea dialysate and urine concentrations in the PD patient. Mandolfo et al. evaluated several equations used to calculate PNA in CAPD patients to determine which formula provides the most appropriate estimate of protein intake and nitrogen appearance [53]. After PNA is calculated, it can be normalized to the body weight (nPNA). PNA may also be normalized to the actual edema-free body weight; however, this method will give a higher nPNA in malnourished patients with low body weights than in overweight patients with a good nutritional status [50]. In these cases, normalizing to IBW may be more appropriate. If the patient is catabolic, the PNA will be high in proportion to the actual dietary protein intake and, if the patient is anabolic, then the reverse will occur.

Nutrition Support

PD patients who are malnourished at the initiation of dialysis or those who develop malnutrition or peritonitis later will have increased dietary protein and energy needs [50]. Achieving adequate intake may be difficult since oral intake may have spontaneously declined. It may be necessary to liberalize the diet and encourage the patient to use oral nutrition supplements (ONS) in the form of modular protein powders or nutritionally complete liquid products [54, 55].The use of amino acids in intraperitoneal nutrition (IPN) has been shown to improve the nutritional status in malnourished PD patients [56, 57]. IPN is an option for the patient who has failed to achieve/maintain an adequate protein intake [56–58]. The use of IPN is limited by cost and insurance reimbursement. Refer to Chap. 17 on nutrition support in hemodialysis and peritoneal dialysis.

Sodium and Fluid

The recommended sodium restriction for patients receiving PD is 2–3 g/day, which should be individualized depending on the cardiac status, blood pressure control, residual renal function, and fluid balance. Sodium is usually cleared easily in PD, with the majority of patients clearing 3–4 g of sodium daily depending on the dialysis prescription [59]. Excess dietary sodium intake will affect volume retention and blood pressure control [60–62]. Patients receiving PD who are volume-overloaded, hypertensive, and unresponsive to management by medication may require a stricter sodium and fluid restriction [61].

Data suggests there is a strong association between the volume status and nutritional status in PD patients [63]. Cheng et al. assessed fluid status in 28 PD patients using repeated bioimpedance analysis (BIA), and the nutritional status was assessed by handgrip strength and subjective global assessment. After a follow-up of 9 months, patients were divided into groups based on changes in BIA (continuous and steadily improved fluid status vs. consistent fluid overload). Patients in the former group showed an improved nutritional status (prevalence of malnutrition decreased significantly, $p < 0.01$) compared to the latter group where the nutritional status deteriorated significantly ($p < 0.05$). The researchers concluded that the improved fluid status was associated with improvement in the nutritional status, whereas deterioration in fluid status was associated with the prevalence of malnutrition [63].

To correct volume overload, it may be necessary to use a hypertonic dialysate solution. The frequent use of high dextrose concentrations can damage the peritoneum leading to alterations in and possible loss of UF by the peritoneal membrane [46, 64, 65]. Hypertonic dextrose solutions can also aggravate hypertriglyceridemia, hyperglycemia, and hyperinsulinemia and promote weight gain [40]. Patients may initially start out with a liberal sodium intake (e.g., 3 g/day) but it may become necessary to reassess the patient for declining residual renal function and uncontrolled blood pressure to determine whether a reduction in sodium intake is indicated.

Fluid removal in PD is regulated by the strength of the dialysate concentration used (i.e., the higher the concentration, the more fluid removed) [42, 46]. Patients are taught to monitor their blood pressure, weight, and drain volumes to identify if and when any change in their normal dialysis prescription may be needed. Ultrafiltration using glucose occurs quickly and early in the PD exchange, which can present a problem for the volume overloaded patient who requires a higher UF during the long overnight CAPD dwell or the daytime CCPD dwell [46]. In these circumstances, icodextrin can be used as an alternative dialysate [44].

The recommended fluid allowance for patients receiving PD should be individualized for each patient with the goal of minimizing the use of hypertonic exchanges. The typical daily fluid allowance should be 1 L and not exceed 2 L; however, patients with a high urine output may need to have additional fluid [33, 43]. A daily fluid allowance may be less depending on the cardiac status, blood pressure control, rate of UF, and amount of remaining residual renal function.

Potassium

Hyperkalemia is less common in patients receiving PD due to the continuous nature of the dialysis. Some patients may not require a potassium restriction. However, in patients who need to restrict dietary potassium, 3–4 g/day is recommended and this amount should be adjusted based on laboratory values to maintain serum potassium levels within the normal range [43]. It is advisable to have patients spread their high potassium food choices throughout the day. Patients with diabetes should be cautioned not to treat low blood glucose levels with only high potassium fruit juices such as orange juice, as this may cause hyperkalemia. While the primary cause of hyperkalemia may be dietary intake, nondietary factors such as medications, hyperglycemia, metabolic acidosis, pica behaviors, and inadequate dialysis can also lead to elevated serum potassium levels and should be investigated if dietary causes can be ruled out (Table 16.3) [66–70]. In addition, some patients may become hypokalemic due to nausea, vomiting, diarrhea, or inadequate dietary intake and may require liberalization of the diet and potassium supplements [66, 67].

Table 16.3 Dietary and nondietary causes of hyperkalemia in hemodialysis patients

Dietary causes
Use of salt substitutes
Pica behavior
Use of herbal or over-the-counter vitamin/mineral supplements
Excessive consumption of high-potassium foods
Excessive consumption of liquid nutritional supplements
Nondietary causes
Severe, chronic constipation
Loss of remaining residual renal function
High dialysate potassium concentration
Frequent use of chewing tobacco
Metabolic acidosis
Inadequate dialysis
Blood transfusions
Hemolysis of blood sample due to error in blood draw or specimen handling
Hyperglycemia: potassium shifts from cell into serum
Conditions causing release of potassium through tissue destruction such as catabolism, starvation, infection, burns, surgical stress, and chemotherapy
Drug interactions: beta-blocking agents, spironolactone, angiotensin-converting enzyme inhibitors, cyclosporine, digoxin
Comorbid conditions such as Addison's disease, sickle-cell anemia, hypoaldosteronism

Data from [31, 60, 66, 68]. Adapted from Beto and Bansai [68]

Calcium/Phosphorus/Vitamin D

Calcium and phosphorus balance in healthy individuals is maintained through interactions between the kidneys, parathyroid glands, bones, and intestines. In CKD, the decline in the glomerular filtration rate (GFR) results in increased phosphorus retention and decreased production of 1,25-dihydroxycholecalciferol ($1,25(OH)_2$ Vit D) or calcitriol, the active form of vitamin D. Decreases in calcitriol can result in reduced intestinal calcium absorption, decreased mineral reabsorption/excretion by the kidneys, increased bone turnover, and increased parathyroid hormone (PTH) production [71]. These metabolic changes, along with hyperphosphatemia, can lead to secondary hyperparathyroidism, renal osteodystrophy, and elevated PTH levels [72]. Active vitamin D can be given orally to correct vitamin D deficiency and suppress PTH production and secretion; however, calcitriol supplementation can also increase intestinal absorption of calcium and phosphorus and increase calcium mobilization from the bone leading to further mineral imbalance [71]. Vitamin D analogs are available to suppress PTH with less impact on calcium and phosphorus. Cinacalcet has been shown to consistently reduce serum of PTH, calcium, and phosphate levels and to increase the proportion of patients within recommended ranges for each of these parameters. Management of secondary hyperparathyroidism (SHPT) with cinacalcet has been associated with reductions in the relative risk of parathyroidectomy, bone fractures, and cardiovascular hospitalization, and with an improvement in quality of life parameters [72]. Regardless of therapy, all patients should be closely monitored to keep calcium, phosphorus, and PTH levels within recommended guidelines. Refer to Chap. 23 for a review of bone disease management and mineral disorders in CKD.

Both excessive calcium load and hyperphosphatemia are associated with bone disease, vascular and soft tissue calcification, and increased cardiovascular mortality because they contribute to an elevated Ca × P product [73–75]. Research indicates that a Ca × P product >55 is related to an increase in mortality in CKD patients [76]. Calcium load is affected by the amount of dialysate calcium, dietary calcium intake, and use of calcium-based medications, specifically phosphorus binders, while serum phosphorus is controlled by dialysis adequacy, diet restrictions, and the use of phosphorus binders [77].

The Academy EAL/KDOQI guidelines recommend adjusting dietary phosphorus intake to maintain serum phosphate levels in the normal range [12]. Traditionally, CKD-specific recommendations suggested maintaining the phosphorus intake between 800 and 1000 mg/day in patients receiving maintenance dialysis in order to maintain serum phosphate in the normal range [78–80]. The Academy EAL/KDOQI workgroup noted that the efficacy of this recommendation has not been established. Furthermore, this dietary phosphorus intake range is higher than the current recommended dietary allowance (RDA) for phosphorus in the general adult population (i.e., 700 mg/day) [81]. In some cases, the dietary phosphorus intake may be difficult to achieve since many high phosphorus foods are also high in protein. Therefore, the phosphorus restriction needs to be adjusted to dietary protein requirements to prevent protein malnutrition.

Phosphorus is not currently required to be listed on food labels, and the use of phosphate-based food additives has contributed to hidden sources of phosphorus outside the traditionally known high phosphorus foods. The inorganic phosphates used as food additives are also 100% absorbable as compared to the 50–60% absorption rate from naturally occurring phosphorus [72, 82]. Refer to Chap. 23 for a review of bone disease management and mineral disorders in CKD.

Lipids

There is a high prevalence of lipid abnormalities in the dialysis population, which is a contributing risk factor to CVD. Briefly, KDOQI recommends (1) a reduction in saturated fat to <7% of total calories; (2) a reduction in the total fat to 25–35% of total calories with monounsaturated fat providing up to 20% of calories and polyunsaturated fat up to 10%; (3) total dietary cholesterol intake of <200 mg/day; (4) increased dietary fiber; and (5) modifications in calories to attain or maintain a desired weight along with exercise and smoking cessation [83, 84]. Before beginning any dietary modification, the dietitian should assess the patient for any signs of PEW, as addition of a low-fat modified diet can compromise caloric intake, which can further compromise nutritional status [85]. Patients may also encounter difficulty when adhering to the recommendations for dietary fat intake in addition to a complex renal diet. Dietary modification may be undertaken if the patient is well-nourished; however, pharmacological intervention with lipid-lowering medication(s) may be the only intervention used if the patient is unable or unwilling to further modify his/her diet. Encouraging general recommendations for modifying saturated fat intake along with smoking cessation and promoting exercise should be encouraged.

Patients receiving PD often have elevated low-density lipoprotein (LDL) cholesterol, serum total cholesterol, and triglyceride (TG) levels along with abnormalities in serum apoproteins, which are thought to be related to glucose uptake from the dialysate and increased protein losses during dialysis [33, 46, 86]. There is little data on the effectiveness of diet modification on lipid levels in PD patients with the exception of maintaining good glycemic control in those with diabetes [85]. Strict fat-restricted diets may also compromise protein and energy intake, and lipid-lowering medications are generally the first line of treatment along with encouraging general therapeutic lifestyle changes (TLC) such as smoking cessation and exercise. Maintaining adequate protein intake is the primary goal. Minimizing saturated fat, trans fat, and sugar intake should be recommended, but strict dyslipidemia diets may not be appropriate for patients receiving PD if the nutritional status is compromised [83–85]. Refer to Chap. 13 on nutritional management of cardiovascular disease in CKD.

Fiber

Constipation is an important cause of technique failure and poor dialysis efficacy in patients on PD, often manifesting as an abrupt reduction in drainage of PD fluid [87, 88]. Dietary fiber improves constipation by increasing fecal mass, which stimulates increased bowel activity and transit time [89]. In the nonrenal population, a clear dose response relationship has been found between the fiber intake and the fecal output [90]. A high fiber intake is also associated with a number of clinical and health benefits, including improved glucose tolerance, improved lipid levels and early satiety [91]. A similar response may be expected in patients on PD, but it is complicated by the dietary restrictions imposed by the renal diet [92].

Vitamins, Minerals, and Trace Elements

The dietary reference intakes (DRIs) for the patient receiving maintenance dialysis have not been established, and the vitamin and mineral recommendations are the same for HD and PD. Kidney failure can cause impaired or excessive excretion of micronutrients due to the loss of glomerular filtration or impaired tubular function leading to either a deficiency or toxicity of certain micronutrients [93]. Further research is needed in this area.

Water-Soluble and Fat-Soluble Vitamins

There are numerous causes of water-soluble vitamin deficiencies in dialysis patients which include anorexia, alterations in metabolism caused by renal failure, the dialysis procedure, drugs which may affect absorption, and the renal diet restrictions [33, 94]. Water-soluble vitamins are small, nonprotein bound substances that are removed by dialysis and may be lost at a rate greater than normal urinary excretion [94]. Dialysis membrane pore size, surface area, and increased flow rates can adversely affect water-soluble vitamin retention [95, 96]. Some drugs such as immunosuppressants, anticonvulsants, and chemotherapy drugs used to treat comorbid conditions can also interfere with vitamin absorption [97, 98]. A water-soluble renal vitamin supplement is generally recommended at levels to meet the DRIs for the general healthy population to help maintain normal levels (Table 16.4). The fat-soluble vitamins are not removed by dialysis and can accumulate in patients with kidney failure.

Minerals and Trace Elements

Minerals and trace elements are mainly supplied by the diet; however, serum levels can also be affected by environmental exposure, concentration of the dialysate, poor nutrition, impaired absorption, or age [95, 99, 100]. Many minerals and trace elements are protein bound, so uremia itself may alter levels; however, losses during dialysis are probably minimal [95, 100]. Refer to Chap. 33 for further information on micronutrient and trace elements requirements in CKD.

Table 16.4 Daily nutrient recommendations for adult dialysis patients

Nutrient	Peritoneal dialysis
Energy (kcal/kg BW) (Includes dialysate kcal)	25–35
Protein (g/kg BW)	1.0–1.2 (≥50% HBV)
Sodium (g/day)	2–3 (Monitor BP control, fluid balance)
Potassium (g/day)	3–4-unrestricted (Monitor serum levels)
Calcium (mg total elemental)	≤2000
Phosphorus (mg or mg/g protein)	Individualize
Fluid (mL)	1000 + UOP (Individualize for fluid balance)
Thiamine (mg/day)	1.2–1.5 mg/day
Riboflavin (mg/day)	1.1–1.3 mg/day
Niacin (mg/day)	20 mg/day
Biotin (µg/day)	30
Pantothenic acid (mg/day)	5–10
Cobalamin (µg/day)	2–3
Pyridoxine (mg/day)	10
Folate (mg/day)	1–10
Vitamin C (mg/day)	60–100
Vitamin A	None
Vitamin D	Individualize
Vitamin E	Optional[a]
Vitamin K	None[b]
Zinc	If needed[c]
Copper	None
Iron	Individualize[d]
Selenium	None
Magnesium	None
Aluminum	None

Data from [31, 60, 76, 94, 95, 97]

Abbreviations: *BW* body weight, *HBV* high biological value, *BP* blood pressure, *UOP* urine output

[a]400 IU may be indicated. See text

[b]May need supplements if on antibiotics and have poor oral intake

[c]May be supplemented up to 15 mg elemental zinc

[d]Varies based on the EPO dose

Conclusion

Diet is an essential component in the treatment of patients receiving maintenance dialysis. The diet for stage 5 CKD presents many challenges for the patient receiving maintenance dialysis that include lifestyle changes in food choices and preparation, adjusting to new medication regimens such as phosphorus binders with meals, and possibly having to combine the renal diet with other dietary modifications (e.g., diabetes or lipidemia). The diet must be individualized for each patient to help promote adherence and to maintain an optimal intake while balancing protein, sodium, potassium, phosphorus, and fluid requirements.

There are a variety of educational materials available to help educate both the patient and the professional. The National Kidney Foundation and the Academy of Nutrition and Dietetics provide both patient and professional educational material in the area of kidney disease that can be accessed online or by contacting the organizations. Understanding the different types of RRTs and their nutritional implications are important in maintaining the nutritional status and improving outcomes.

Case Study

C.T. is a 34-year-old male, self-employed graphic designer who presents for training on CAPD after transferring from HD at another unit following failure of his 13-year-old kidney transplant. He has a history of esophageal reflux and hypertension. C.T. lives alone and his reported appetite is fair. He notes an 8-lb weight loss prior to starting HD and now complains of occasional indigestion stating food occasionally feels like it is lodged in his throat producing a feeling of choking. Height 6′2″, weight 182 lb (82.7 kg), target weight 182 lb (82.7 kg), usual weight 190 lb (86.4 kg). Medications: prenatal vitamin, Tums (as needed), 10 mg prednisone, 1 (800 mg) sevelamer carbonate as phosphorus binder three times a day with meals. Initial labs: Ca 9.0 mg/dL, P 6.3 mg/dL, Na 141 mEq/L, K^+ 4.7 mEq/L, Chol 102 mg/dL, BUN 39 mg/dL, SCr 7.8 mg/dL, SAlb 3.4 g/dL, CO_2 22 mEq/L, Kt/V 2.0, urine output = 1500 mL. CAPD prescription: 3 (2.5 L) 1.5% dextrose plus 1 (2.5 L) 2.5% dextrose. Twenty-four hour diet recall indicates that the patient consumes an estimated 1800–2000 kcal and 70–80 g protein over three meals with an occasional snack. C.T. does not use the salt shaker at the table and has had difficulty decreasing his dairy intake. Estimated sodium intake is 2000–2500 mg, potassium 3000 mg, and phosphorus 1800 mg.

After 3 months on PD, C.T. complains of increased dysphagia and decreased oral intake. There has been no change in the CAPD prescription. Target weight 180 lb (81.8 kg). Labs: Ca 8.6 mg/dL, P 3.0 mg/dL, Na 142 mEq/L, K^+ 2.8 mEq/L, BUN 28 mg/dL, SAlb 3.1 g/dL, TP 6.1 g/dL, Chol 110 mg/dL, Kt/V 2.1, urine output 1400 mL. C.T. is referred for a barium swallow that indicates a severe hiatal hernia and Schatzki's ring. He had an esophageal dilation and dysphagia resolved. After 1 year on PD, C.T.'s UF declines leading to poor clearance and fluid retention. He complains of early satiety, nausea, and severe anorexia and develops 3+ edema to the knee. Use of diuretics and 4.25% dextrose is unsuccessful. A repeat Kt/V has dropped to 1.4. His PD prescription was changed to 4 (2.5 L) 2.5% dextrose plus 1 (2.5 L) 1.5% dextrose. One week after changing the PD prescription, C.T.'s appetite begins to improve and his labs and clinical parameters are: Ca 9.5 mg/dL, P 6.0 mg/dL, Na 128 mEq/L, K^+ 5.8 mEq/L, BUN 44 mg/dL, SCr 8.0 mg/dL, SAlb 3.3 g/dL, CO_2 24 mEqQ/L, Chol 150 mg/dL, urine output 500 mL, 1+ edema, weight 184 lb (83.6 kg), and the estimated target weight 182 lb (82.7 kg).

Case Questions and Answers

1. What are C.T.'s estimated calorie and protein needs for CAPD? Using the simple formula for estimating glucose, how many calories is C.T. getting from his dialysis prescription (3 (2.5 L) 1.5% dextrose plus 1 (2.5 L) 2.5% dextrose)?
   Answer: C.T. has no edema so using 35 kcal/kg/day of his current body weight puts estimated kcal needs at 2894 kcal. Based on 1.3 g protein/kg body weight, his protein needs are 107.5 g. Based on a 60% absorption rate for CAPD, C.T. receives approximately 357 kcal from his dialysate.

2. What are the diet recommendations for C.T. for CAPD based on his weight and initial labs?
   Answer: The recommended diet is 107 g protein, 3 g sodium (since he has no overt cardiac issues or problems with fluid retention), 3–4 g potassium, and 1070–1284 mg phosphorus (using 10–12 mg/g protein). Fluid intake should be kept to 2000–2500 mL (urine output plus 1000 mL) and adjusted based on UF. Based on C.T.'s initial intake of 1800–2000 kcal and 70–80 g protein and allowing for the 357 kcal absorbed from the dialysate, he will have to add a minimum 500–700 kcal and 27–37 g of protein to his diet. Sodium and potassium intake is acceptable but he will need to decrease his intake of dairy foods to bring the phosphorus content of the diet within guidelines.

3. Are C.T.'s medications at the start of CAPD appropriate? What is his corrected calcium? Any recommendations for changes in his medications?
   Answer: The prenatal vitamin should be changed to a renal B- and C-complex with folic acid. His corrected calcium is 9.5 mg/dL and, to avoid any elevation in calcium, his Tums was discontinued and he was placed on Velphoro, a noncalcium containing binder. He is currently on a small dose of phosphorus binders (sevelamer) and with the increased protein in the diet and elevated phosphorus, an increase in binders will be needed. Sevelamer carbonate was increased to 1600 mg at each meal and C.T. was also instructed to take 800 mg with snacks, which he had not been doing.

4. At 3 months what diet and/or medication changes are indicated for C.T.?
   Answer: At 3 months, C.T. presents with low serum potassium, low serum phosphorus, declining serum albumin, and BUN secondary to poor oral intake due to dysphagia. His binders should be decreased by one-third and potassium intake liberalized along with a prescription for an oral potassium supplement until his labs indicate normal levels and oral intake has improved. It should be suggested that he use a liquid nutritional calorie and protein supplement until after his dilation since his oral intake is limited.

5. When C.T. changes his exchanges as per the new PD prescription, what dietary modifications are necessary based on the weight and laboratory data? (Calculate corrected calcium and evaluate.)
   Answer: Due to edema, his target weight should be used to calculate his daily protein needs at 1.2 g/kg body weight. His protein needs will now change to 99 g/day. Because of edema, C.T.'s sodium intake should be decreased to 2–2.5 g/day. His phosphorus is elevated so his binders should be increased to at least 1600 mg with each meal and 800 mg with snacks and a dietary phosphorus restriction restarted. Corrected calcium is high so his Ca intake should be lowered. Fluid restriction should be limited to 1500 mL/day or less (urine output plus 1000 mL) and his weight should be monitored. His serum albumin level should be monitored for changes. C.T. should be encouraged to consume 107 gm protein per day.

References

1. Herrington WG, Smith M, Bankhead C, Matsushita K, Stevens S, Holt T, et al. Body mass index and risk of advanced chronic kidney disease: prospective analysis from a primary cohort of 1.4 million adults in England. PLoS One. 2017;12(3):e0173515.
2. Garofalo C, Borrelli S, Minutolo R, Chiodini P, De Nicola L, Conte G. A systematic review and meta-analysis suggests obesity predicts onset of chronic kidney disease in the general population. Kidney Int. 2017;91(5):1224–35.
3. Centers for Disease Control and Prevention. Chronic kidney disease in the United States, 2019. Atlanta: U.S. Department of Health and Human Services, Centers for Disease Control and Prevention; 2019.
4. United States Renal Data System. (USRDS). Chapter I: CKD in the general population. 2018 USRDS annual data report: epidemiology of kidney disease in the United States. Bethesda: National Institutes of Health, National Institute of Diabetes and Digestive and Kidney Diseases; 2018. Accessed from: https://www.usrds.org/2018/view/v1_01.aspx.
5. United States Renal Data System. (USRDS). Chapter 1: Incidence, prevalence, patient characteristics, and treatment modalities. 2018 USRDS annual data report: Epidemiology of kidney disease in the United States. Bethesda:

National Institutes of Health, National Institute of Diabetes and Digestive and Kidney Diseases; 2018. Accessed from: https://www.usrds.org/2018/view/v2_01.aspx.

6. Pupim LB, Evanson JA, Hakim RM, Ikizler TA. The extent of uremic malnutrition at the time of initiation of maintenance hemodialysis is associated with subsequent hospitalization. J Ren Nutr. 2003;13:259–66.

7. Zha Y, Qian Q. Protein nutrition and malnutrition in CKD and ESRD. Nutrients. 2017;9(3):E208.

8. Kang SS, Chang JW, Park Y. Nutritional status predicts 10-year mortality in patients with end-stage renal disease on hemodialysis. Nutrients. 2017;9:399.

9. Davies SJ, Phillips L, Naish PF, Russell GI. Quantifying comorbidity in peritoneal dialysis patients and its relationship to other predictors of survival. Nephrol Dial Transplant. 2002;17(6):1085–92.

10. Naeeni AE, Poostiyan N, Teimouri Z, Mortazavi M, Soghrati M, Poostiyan E, et al. Assessment of severity of malnutrition in peritoneal dialysis patients via malnutrition inflammatory score. Adv Biomed Res. 2017;6:128.

11. Naini AE, Karbalaie A, Abedini M, Askari G, Moeinzadeh F. Comparison of malnutrition in hemodialysis and peritoneal dialysis patients and its relationship with echocardiographic findings. J Res Med Sci. 2016;21:78.

12. Ikizler TA, Burrowes J, Byham-Gray L, Campbell K, Carrero JJ, Chan W, et al. KDOQI Nutrition in CKD Guideline Work Group. KDOQI clinical practice guideline for nutrition in CKD: 2020 update. Am J Kidney Dis. 2020; in press.

13. Pupim LB, Caglar K, Hakim RM, Shyr Y, Ikizler TA. Uremic malnutrition is a predictor of death independent of inflammatory status. Kidney Int. 2004;66:2054–60.

14. Mehrotra R, Duong U, Jiwakanon S, Kovesdy CP, Moran J, Kopple JD, et al. Serum albumin as a predictor of mortality in peritoneal dialysis: comparisons with hemodialysis. Am J Kidney Dis. 2011;58(3):418–28.

15. de Mutsert R, Grootendorst DC, Indemans F, Boeschoten EW, Krediet RT, Dekker FW, Netherlands Cooperative Study on the Adequacy of dialysis-II Study Group. Association between serum albumin and mortality in dialysis patients is partly explained by inflammation, and not by malnutrition. J Ren Nutr. 2009;19(2):127–35.

16. Ikizler TA, Burrowes J, Byham-Gray L, Campbell K, Carrero JJ, Chan W, et al. KDOQI Nutrition in CKD Guideline Work Group. KDOQI clinical practice guideline for nutrition in CKD: 2020 update. Am J Kidney Dis. 2020; in press.

17. Stenvinkel P, Heimburger O, Lindholm B, Kaysen GA, Bergström J. Are there two types of malnutrition in chronic renal failure? Evidence for relationships between malnutrition, inflammation and atherosclerosis (MIA syndrome). Nephrol Dial Transplant. 2000;15:953–60.

18. Fouque D, Kalantar-Zadeh K, Kopple J, Cano N, Chauveau P, Cuppari L, et al. A proposed nomenclature and diagnostic criteria for protein-energy wasting in acute and chronic kidney disease. Kidney Int. 2008;73:391–8.

19. Mak RH, Ikizler TA, Kovesdy CP, Raj DS, Stenvinkel P, Kalantar-Zadeh K. Wasting in chronic kidney disease. J Cachexia Sarcopenia Muscle. 2011;2:9–25.

20. Bossola M, Muscaritoli M, Tazza L, Panocchia N, Liberatori M, Giungi S, et al. Variables associated with reduced dietary intake in hemodialysis patients. J Ren Nutr. 2005;15:244–52.

21. Kalantar-Zadeh K, Block G, McAllister CJ, Humphreys MH, Kopple JD. Appetite and inflammation, nutrition, anemia and clinical outcome in hemodialysis patients. Am J Clin Nutr. 2004;80:299–307.

22. Bergstrom J. Appetite in CAPD patients. Perit Dial Int. 1995;16:8–21.

23. Young V, Balaam S, Orazio L, Bates A, Badve SV, Johnson DW, et al. Appetite predicts intake and nutritional status in patients receiving peritoneal dialysis. J Ren Care. 2016;42(20):123–31.

24. Mehrotra R, Kopple JD. Nutritional management of maintenance dialysis patients: why aren't we doing better? Annu Rev Nutr. 2001;21:343–79.

25. Burrowes JD, Powers SN, Cockram DB, McLeroy SL, Dwyer JT, Cunniff PJ, et al. From the hemodialysis study. Use of an appetite and diet assessment tool in a hemodialysis clinical trial: the hemodialysis (HEMO) study. J Ren Nutr. 1996;6:229–32.

26. Molfino A, Kaysen GA, Chertow GM, Doyle J, Delgado C, Dwyer T, et al. Validating appetite assessment tools among patients receiving hemodialysis. J Ren Nutr. 2016;26(2):103–10.

27. Oliveria CM, Kubrusly M, Lima AT, Torres DM, Cavalcante NM, Jeronimo AL, et al. Correlation between nutritional markers and appetite self-assessments in hemodialysis patients. J Ren Nutr. 2015;25(3):301–7.

28. Kraut JA, Madias NE. Metabolic acidosis of CKD: an update. Am J Kidney Dis. 2016;67(2):307–17.

29. Kovesdy CP. Metabolic acidosis and kidney disease: does bicarbonate therapy slow the progression of CKD? Nephrol Dial Transplant. 2012;27:3056–62.

30. Kalantar-Zadeh K, Mehrotra R, Fouque D, Kopple JD. Metabolic acidosis and malnutrition inflammation complex syndrome in chronic renal failure. Semin Dial. 2004;17:455–65.

31. Kalantar-Zadeh K, Kopple JD. Nutritional management of patients undergoing maintenance hemodialysis. In: Kopple JD, Massry SG, editors. Kopple and Massry's nutritional management of renal disease. 2nd ed. Philadelphia: Lippincott Williams & Wilkins; 2004. p. 433–58.

32. Bossola M, Muscaritoli M, Tazza L, Giungi S, Tortorelli A, Rossi Fanelli F, et al. Malnutrition in hemodialysis patients: what therapy? Am J Kidney Dis. 2005;46:371–86.

33. Ikizler TA. Nutrition and peritoneal dialysis. In: Handbook of nutrition and the kidney. 5th ed. Philadelphia: Lippincott Williams & Wilkins; 2005. p. 228–44.
34. Tijong HL, Zijlstra FJ, Rietveld T, Wattimena JL, Huijmans JG, Swart GR, et al. Peritoneal dialysis losses and cytokine generation in automated peritoneal dialysis with combined amino acids and glucose solutions. Mediators Inflamm. 2007;2007:97272.
35. McCusker FX, Teehan BP, Thorpe KE, Keshaviah PR, Churchill DN. How much peritoneal dialysis is required for the maintenance of a good nutritional state? Canada-USA (CANUSA) Peritoneal Dialysis Study Group. Kidney Int Suppl. 1996;56:S56–61.
36. Bergstrom J. Why are dialysis patients malnourished? Am J Kidney Dis. 1995;26:229–41.
37. National Kidney Foundation. Clinical practice guidelines for peritoneal dialysis adequacy. Am J Kidney Dis. 2006;48:S98–129.
38. Jager KJ, Merkus MP, Husiman RM, Boeschoten EW, et al. NECOSAD Study Group. Nutritional status over time in hemodialysis and peritoneal dialysis. J Am Soc Nephrol. 2001;12:1272–9.
39. Brunelli SM, Cohen DE, Gray KS, Cassin M, Van Hout B, Rodriguez J, et al. Identification of factors that are associated with risk of modality failure among patients treated with peritoneal dialysis. DaVita Clinical Research. Poster presentation at the American Society of Nephology Kidney Week, October 23–28, 2018.
40. Grodstein GP, Blumenkrantz MJ, Kopple JD, Moran JK, Coburn JW. Glucose absorption during continuous ambulatory peritoneal dialysis. Kidney Int. 1981;19:564–7.
41. Bodnar DM, Busch S, Fuchs J, Piedmonte M, Schreiber M. Estimating glucose absorption in peritoneal equilibration tests. Adv Perit Dial. 1993;9:114–8.
42. Burkart J. Metabolic consequences of peritoneal dialysis. Semin Dial. 2004;17:498–504.
43. McCann L. Nutrition management of the adult peritoneal dialysis patient. In: A clinical guide to nutrition care in kidney disease. 2nd ed. Chicago: American Dietetic Association; 2013.
44. Chhabra D, Nash K. Icodextrin: an alternative peritoneal dialysis fluid. Expert Opin Drug Metab Toxicol. 2008;4:1455–64.
45. Hamburger RJ, Iknaus MA. Icodextrin fulfills unmet clinical need of PD patients: improved ultrafiltration. Dial Transplant. 2003;32:675–84.
46. Teitelbaum I, Burkart J. Peritoneal dialysis. Am J Kidney Dis. 2003;42:1082–96.
47. Heimburger O, Stenvinkel P, Lindholm B. Nutritional effects and nutritional management of chronic peritoneal dialysis. In: Kopple JD, Massry SG, editors. Kopple and Massry's nutritional management of renal disease. 2nd ed. Philadelphia: Lippincott Williams & Wilkins; 2004. p. 477–510.
48. Krediet RT, Zuyderhoudt FM, Boeschoten EW, Arisz L. Peritoneal permeability to proteins in diabetic and non-diabetic continuous ambulatory peritoneal dialysis patients. Nephron. 1986;42(2):133–40.
49. Balafa O, Halbesma N, Struijk DG, Dekker FW, Krediet RT. Peritoneal albumin and protein losses do not predict outcome in peritoneal dialysis patients. Clin J Am Soc Nephrol. 2011;6(3):561–6.
50. Lindholm B, Bergstrom J. Protein and amino acid metabolism in patients undergoing continuous ambulatory peritoneal dialysis (CAPD). Clin Nephrol. 1988;30:S59–63.
51. Blumenkrantz MJ, Kopple JD, Moran JK, Coburn JW. Metabolic balance studies and dietary protein requirements in patients undergoing continuous ambulatory peritoneal dialysis. Kidney Int. 1982;21:849–61.
52. Kopple JD, Blumenkrantz MJ. Nutritional requirements for patients undergoing continuous ambulatory peritoneal dialysis. Kidney Int Suppl. 1983;16:S295–302.
53. Mandolfo S, Zucchi A, Cavalieri DL, Corradi B, Imbasciati E. Protein nitrogen appearance in CAPD patients: what is the best formula? Nephrol Dial Transplant. 1996;11(8):1592–6.
54. Liu PJ, Ma F, Wang QY, He SL. The effects of oral nutritional supplements in patients with maintenance dialysis therapy: a systematic review and meta-analysis of randomized clinical trials. PLoS One. 2018;13(9):e0203706.
55. Satirapoj B, Limwannata P, Kleebchaiyaphum C, Prapakorn J, Yatinan U, Chotsriluecha S, et al. Nutritional status among peritoneal dialysis patients after oral supplement with ONCE dialyze formula. Int J Nephrol Renovasc Dis. 2017;10:145–51.
56. Tijong HL, van den Berg JW, Wattimena JL, Rietveld T, van Dijk LJ, van der Wiel AM, et al. Dialysate as food: combined amino acid and glucose dialysate improves protein anabolism in renal failure patients on automated peritoneal dialysis. J Am Soc Nephrol. 2005;16:1486–93.
57. Tijong HL, Swart R, Van den Berg JW, Fieren MW. Dialysate as food as an option for automated peritoneal dialysis. NDT Plus. 2008;1(Suppl 4):iv36–40.
58. Lindholm B, Bergstrom J. Nutritional aspects on peritoneal dialysis. Kidney Int. 1992;42:S165–71.
59. Nolph KD, Sorkin MI, Moore H. Autoregulation of sodium and potassium removal during continuous ambulatory peritoneal dialysis. Trans Am Soc Artif Intern Organs. 1980;26:334–8.
60. McCann L. Pocket guide to nutrition assessment of the patient with chronic kidney disease. 4th ed. New York: National Kidney Foundation; 2009.
61. Lameire N, Van Biesen W. Hypervolemia in peritoneal dialysis patients. J Nephrol. 2004;17:58–66.

62. Wang X, Axelsson J, Lindholm B, Wang T. Volume status and blood pressure in continuous ambulatory peritoneal dialysis patients. Blood Purif. 2005;23:373–8.
63. Cheng L, Tang W, Wang T. Strong association between volume status and nutritional status in peritoneal dialysis patients. Am J Kidney Dis. 2005;45(5):891–902.
64. Krediet RT, van Westrhenen R, Zweers MM, Struijk DG. Clinical advantages of new peritoneal dialysis solutions. Nephrol Dial Transplant. 2002;17:16–8.
65. Davies SJ, Phillips L, Naish PF, Russel GI. Peritoneal glucose exposure and changes in membrane solute transport with time on peritoneal dialysis. J Am Soc Nephrol. 2001;12:1046–51.
66. Musso CG. Potassium metabolism in patients with chronic kidney disease. Part II: patients on dialysis (stage 5). Int Urol Nephrol. 2004;36:469–72.
67. Rostand SG. Profound hypokalemia in continuous ambulatory peritoneal dialysis. Arch Intern Med. 1983;143:377–8.
68. Beto J, Bansai VK. Hyperkalemia: evaluating dietary and non-dietary etiology. J Ren Nutr. 1992;2:28–9.
69. Ifudu O, Reydel K, Vlacich V, Delosreyes G, Friedman EA. Dietary potassium is not the sole determinant of serum potassium concentration in hemodialysis patients. Dial Transplant. 2004;33:684–93.
70. Constantino J, Roberts C. Life-threatening hyperkalemia from chewing tobacco in a hemodialysis patient. J Ren Nutr. 1997;7:106–8.
71. Goodman WG. Calcium, phosphorus and vitamin D. In: Handbook of nutrition & the kidney. 5th ed. Philadelphia: Lippincott Williams & Wilkins; 2004. p. 47–69.
72. Beto J, Bhatt N, Gerbeling T, Patel C, Drayer D. Overview of the 2017 KDIGO CKD-MBD update: practice implications for adult hemodialysis patients. J Ren Nutr. 2019;29(1):2–15.
73. Qunibi WY. Consequences of hyperphosphatemia in patients with end-stage renal disease (ESRD). Kidney Int Suppl. 2004;66:S8–12.
74. Coladonato JA. Control of hyperphosphatemia among patients with ESRD. J Am Soc Nephrol. 2005;16:S107–14.
75. Rodriguez-Benot A, Martin-Malo A, Alvarez-Lara MA, Rodriguez M, Aljama P. Mild hyperphosphatemia and mortality in hemodialysis patients. Am J Kidney Dis. 2005;46:68–77.
76. Block GA, Klassen PS, Lazarus M, Ofsthun N, Lowrie EG, Chertow GM. Mineral metabolism, mortality and morbidity in maintenance hemodialysis. J Am Soc Nephrol. 2004;15:2208–18.
77. McCann L. Total calcium load in dialysis patients: an issue of concern for dietitians. Dial Transplant. 2004;33:282–9.
78. Clinical practice guidelines for nutrition in chronic renal failure. K/DOQI, National Kidney Foundation. Am J Kidney Dis. 2000;35(6 Suppl 2):S1–140.
79. K/DOQI clinical practice guidelines for bone metabolism and disease in chronic kidney disease. Am J Kidney Dis. 2003;42(4 Suppl 3):S1–201.
80. Ketteler M, Block GA, Evenepoel P, Fukagawa M, Herzog CA, McCann L, et al. Executive summary of the 2017 KDIGO chronic kidney disease-mineral and bone disorder (CKD-MBD) guideline update: what's changed and why it matters. Kidney Int. 2017;92(1):26–36.
81. Institute of Medicine. Dietary reference intakes for calcium, phosphorus, magnesium, vitamin D, and fluoride. Washington, DC: National Academies Press; 1997.
82. Murphy-Gutekunst L. Hidden phosphorus in popular beverages: part I. J Ren Nutr. 2005;15:e1–6.
83. Goldstein-Fuchs J. Dyslipidemias in chronic kidney disease. In: A clinical guide to nutrition care in kidney disease. 2nd ed. Chicago: American Dietetic Association; 2013.
84. National Kidney Foundation. KDOQI clinical practice guidelines for managing dyslipidemia in chronic kidney disease patients. Am J Kidney Dis. 2003;41:S1–91.
85. Saltissi D, Morgan C, Knight B, Chang W, Rigby R, Westhuyzen J. Effect of lipid-lowering dietary recommendations on the nutritional intake and lipid profiles of chronic peritoneal dialysis patients and hemodialysis patients. Am J Kidney Dis. 2001;37:1209–15.
86. Kadiroglu AK, Ustundag S, Kayabasi H, Yilmaz Z, Yildirim Y, Sen S, et al. A comparative sudy of the effect of icodextrin based peritoneal dialysis and hemodialysis on lipid metabolism. Indian J Nephrol. 2013;23(5):358–61.
87. Setyapranata S, Holt SG. The gut in older patients on peritoneal dialysis. Perit Dial Int. 2015;35(6):650–4.
88. Kosmadakis G, Albaret J, Da Costa Correia E, Somda F, Aguilera D. Constipation in peritoneal dialysis patients. Perit Dial Int. 2019;39(5):399–404.
89. Yang J, Wang H-P, Zhou L, Xu C-F. Effect of dietary fiber on constipation: a meta analysis. World J Gastroenterol. 2012;18(48):7378–83.
90. DeVries J, Miller PE, Verbeke K. Effects of cereal fiber on bowel function: a systematic review of intervention trials. World J Gastroenterol. 2015;21(29):8952–63.
91. Ludwig DS, Pereira MA, Kroenke CH, Hilner JE, Van Horn L, Slattery ML, et al. Dietary fiber, weight gain, and cardiovascular disease risk factors in young aduls. JAMA. 1999;282:1539–46.

92. Sutton D, Ovington S, Engel B. A multi-centre, randomised trial to assess whether increased dietary fibre intake (using a fibre supplement or high-fibre foods) produces healthy bowel performance and reduces laxative requirement in free living patients on peritoneal dialysis. J Ren Care. 2014;40(3):157–63.
93. Jankowska M, Rutkowski B, Debska-Slizien A. Vitamins and microelement bioavailability in different stages of chronic kidney disease. Nutrients. 2017;9(3):282.
94. Makoff R, Gonick H. Renal failure and the concomitant derangement of micronutrient metabolism. Nutr Clin Pract. 1999;14:238–46.
95. Masud T. Trace elements and vitamins in renal disease. In: Handbook of nutrition & the kidney. 5th ed. Philadelphia: Lippincott Williams & Wilkins; 2004. p. 196–217.
96. Jankowska M, Lichodziejewska-Niemierko M, Rutkowski B, Debska-Slizien A, Malgorzewicz S. Water soluble vitamins and peritoneal dialysis—state of the art. Clin Nutr. 2017;36(6):1483–9.
97. Rocco MV, Makoff R. Appropriate vitamin therapy for dialysis patients. Semin Dial. 1997;10:272–7.
98. Kosmadakis G, Da Costa Correia E, Carceles O, Somda F, Aguilera D. Vitamins in dialysis: who, when and how much? Ren Fail. 2014;35(4):638–50.
99. Wiggins KL. Renal care: resources and practical applications. Chicago: American Dietetic Association; 2004. p. 39–60.
100. Rucker D, Thadhani R, Tonelli M. Trace elements status in hemodialysis patients. Semin Dial. 2010;23:389–95.

Chapter 17
Nutrition Support in Hemodialysis and Peritoneal Dialysis

Winnie Chan

Keywords Protein-energy wasting · Hemodialysis · Peritoneal dialysis · Nutrition support · Nutrition counseling · Oral nutritional supplements · Intradialytic feeding · Enteral tube feeding · Intradialytic parenteral nutrition · Intraperitoneal parenteral nutrition · Intraperitoneal amino acid · Total parenteral nutrition

Key Points
- Protein-energy wasting (PEW) is common among patients undergoing maintenance dialysis, and many signs of PEW can be improved with nutrition support therapy.
- Early and regular nutrition counseling by registered dietitian (or international equivalent) is essential for the prevention and treatment of PEW in maintenance dialysis patients.
- When nutrition counseling alone is unable to bridge the gap between protein-energy intake and the target requirements, oral nutritional supplements (ONS) should be prescribed to improve nutritional status.
- Intradialytic feeding through monitored in-center provision of ONS or high-protein meals may be a cost-effective strategy to improve dietary intake in hemodialysis patients.
- ONS should be prescribed taking into account of important success factors including patient's requirements, preference, compliance, and tolerance.
- Renal-specific ONS may be prescribed to increase protein and energy intakes without inducing excess levels of fluid and electrolytes.
- When maintenance dialysis patients with PEW are unable to meet protein and energy requirements with nutrition counseling and ONS, enteral tube feeding should be considered.
- Intradialytic parenteral nutrition (IDPN) should only be used as supplemental nutrition in hemodialysis patients with PEW, and adequate spontaneous protein and energy intakes are required to compensate for the difference between those provided by IDPN and the target requirements.
- Intradialytic amino acid therapy remains a viable option for protein-energy wasted peritoneal dialysis patients with insufficient dietary intake, as well as those with tolerance, compliance, and suitability issues of oral intake and other forms of enteral supplementation.

W. Chan (✉)
University of Birmingham, School of Sport, Exercise and Rehabilitation Sciences, Birmingham, UK

© Springer Nature Switzerland AG 2020
J. D. Burrowes et al. (eds.), *Nutrition in Kidney Disease*, Nutrition and Health,
https://doi.org/10.1007/978-3-030-44858-5_17

Introduction

One of the most frequently encountered issues for patients with chronic kidney disease (CKD), especially those reaching end-stage renal disease undergoing maintenance dialysis, is a progressive deterioration of nutritional status, characterized by a unique state of nutritional and metabolic derangements [1], including simultaneous loss of body protein and energy stores, ultimately leading to muscle and fat wasting, as well as visceral protein pool contraction [2–4]. This condition, termed as protein-energy wasting (PEW), has a reported global prevalence of 28–54% among dialysis patients [5] and progresses with dialysis vintage [6–8]. Importantly, PEW substantially increases morbidity and mortality, and exerts deleterious effects on quality of life [1, 9].

The mechanisms causing PEW in maintenance dialysis patients are complex and multifactorial. A conceptual model for the etiology of PEW has been proposed by the International Society of Renal Nutrition and Metabolism (ISRNM) and is summarized in Fig. 17.1 [1]. A common and important cause of PEW in maintenance dialysis patients is inadequate dietary protein and energy intakes due to anorexia, resulting from retention of uremic toxins, the dialysis procedure, intercurrent illnesses, inflammation, and metabolic acidosis [1, 10]. Of relevance, these conditions also contribute to the development of PEW independently. Additionally, inadequate protein and energy intakes can occur secondary to dietary restrictions, comorbidities that affect gastrointestinal function, poor socioeconomic status, depression, physical impairment that limits patient's ability to obtain and prepare food, and peritoneal dialysis-specific factors (i.e., abdominal discomfort, early satiety with peritoneal dialysate infusion, peritoneal glucose absorption) [1, 10, 11]. Along with a spontaneous reduction in dietary protein and energy intakes, the pathophysiology of PEW is attributable to other highly prevalent factors, including physical inactivity, metabolic derangements, endocrine disturbances, and dialysis-related factors such as nutrient losses and catabolism [1, 10–13]. In particular, losses of protein, amino acids, and water-soluble vitamins are evident in both hemodialysis and peritoneal dialysis procedures [12, 13], whereas loss of glucose is most apparent in the hemodialysis procedure, because glucose is provided continuously by the peritoneal route [12, 13]. Of note, increased protein catabolism and

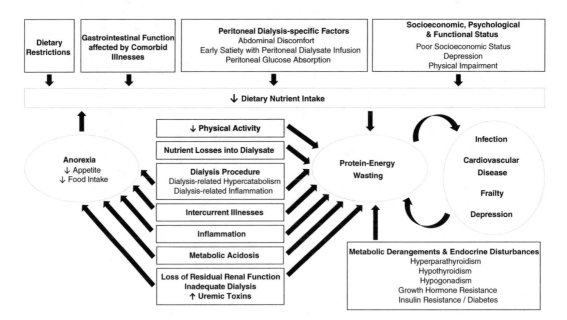

Fig. 17.1 Etiology and direct clinical implications of protein-energy wasting in maintenance hemodialysis and peritoneal dialysis

dialysis-induced inflammation were observed in both hemodialysis and peritoneal dialysis patients [12–14], though the catabolic effect is higher in the former except when peritonitis occurs [12]. Ultimately, PEW may cause infection, cardiovascular disease, frailty, and depression, with these complications in turn exacerbating PEW [1, 10].

Although PEW is caused by a multitude of factors, it is recognized that many of these causes are associated with reduced nutrient intake [3], as shown in Fig. 17.1. Indeed, many signs of PEW can be improved with nutrition support therapy. This chapter focuses specifically on the targets for nutrition support and the types of nutrition support strategies in the management of PEW in maintenance dialysis patients, including nutrition counseling, oral and enteral nutritional supplementation, intradialytic parenteral nutrition (IDPN), and intraperitoneal parenteral nutrition (IPPN) therapies.

Targets for Nutrition Support in Hemodialysis and Peritoneal Dialysis Patients

For maintenance dialysis patients, recommendations for dietary protein and energy intakes from current evidence-based clinical practice guidelines and expert consensus statement are broadly similar. Accordingly, at least 1.0 g protein/kg body weight (BW)/day should be recommended for stable patients on hemodialysis and peritoneal dialysis (Table 17.1) [10, 15–18]. Compared with nondialysis-dependent stages 3–5 CKD patients, higher protein intakes are recommended due to inevitable losses of protein and amino acids into the dialysate and the inflammatory stimulus associated with the dialysis procedure. Protein requirements may be marginally higher in peritoneal dialysis [15, 18] as losses of proteins into the dialysate are 5–15 g/day greater in peritoneal dialysis compared to hemodialysis [15, 19], and protein losses increase with episodes of peritonitis [15, 19]. At least 50% of the protein intake should be of high biological value, that is, food sources containing a full spectrum of essential amino acids [10, 15, 16].

An energy intake of 25–35 kcal/kg BW/day is usually recommended for patients on maintenance hemodialysis and peritoneal dialysis (see Table 17.1) [10, 15, 16, 18], although the European Best Practice Guidelines (EBPG) on Nutrition recommends a higher upper limit for energy intake,

Table 17.1 Recommended protein and energy intakes for maintenance dialysis patients

	Hemodialysis	Peritoneal dialysis
National Kidney Foundation Kidney Disease Outcomes Quality Initiative and the Academy of Nutrition and Dietetics (KDOQI/ Academy) [16]	1.0–1.2 g protein/kg BW/day 25–35 kcal/kg BW/ day	1.0–1.2 g protein/kg BW/ day 25–35 kcal/kg BW/day
European Society for Clinical Nutrition and Metabolism (ESPEN) [15]	1.2–1.4 g protein/kg IBW/day 35 kcal/kg IBW/day	1.2–1.5 g protein/kg IBW/ day 35 kcal/kg IBW/day
European Best Practice Guidelines (EBPG) [17, 18]	>1.1 g protein/kg IBW/day 30–40 kcal/kg IBW/day	≥1.2 g protein/kg IBW/day 35 kcal/kg IBW/day
International Society of Renal Nutrition &Metabolism (ISRNM) [10]	>1.2 g protein/kg IBW/day 30–35 kcal/kg IBW/day	>1.2 g protein/kg IBW/day Peritonitis: >1.5 g protein/kg IBW/day 30–35 kcal/kg IBW/day including kcal from dialysate

Abbreviations: BW body weight, *IBW* ideal body weight

that is, 30–40 kcal/kg BW/day for hemodialysis patients [17]. These recommendations should be based on age, gender, physical activity level, body composition, goals for weight status, and concurrent illness or presence of inflammation to maintain normal nutritional status [16]. Of relevance, a recent metabolic study showed that measured dietary energy requirements are lower than many current recommendations in patients undergoing maintenance hemodialysis [20]. In view of the highly variable dietary energy requirements, careful monitoring of the nutritional status of individual patients is crucial. In addition, it should be noted that patients undergoing peritoneal dialysis absorb calories from the glucose in the dialysate and as such, this should be incorporated into the calculation of dietary energy intake, that is, 25–35 kcal/kg BW/day including kcal from dialysate.

Nutrition Counseling

Although the spontaneous decline in dietary protein and energy intakes that occurs in nondialysis-dependent CKD patients usually improves after the initiation of dialysis, anorexia may persist in a considerable proportion of maintenance dialysis patients due to the factors outlined in Fig. 17.1. These include the loss of residual renal function, inadequate dialysis with resultant retention of uremic toxins, intercurrent illnesses, systemic inflammation, the dialysis procedure, and other physiological, physical, and psychological factors that directly limit dietary protein and energy intakes. Notably, it is highly probable that some of the dietary restrictions are continued to prevent hyperphosphatemia, hyperkalemia, and metabolic acidosis. In addition to identifying and treating the potential underlying causes, early and regular nutrition counseling by registered dietitians (or international equivalents) represents an integral component for the prevention and treatment of PEW in maintenance dialysis patients. The ISRNM proposed an algorithm for the nutritional management and support in CKD patients, with continuous nutrition counseling and sufficient nutrient intake being indicated as important preventive measures for PEW, alongside the optimization of the renal replacement therapy prescription, and management of metabolic acidosis, inflammation, as well as comorbidities including type 2 diabetes mellitus, congestive heart failure, and depression [10]. Pertinently, nutrition counseling was shown to improve nutritional status in both hemodialysis and peritoneal dialysis patients [21, 22].

Transitioning from nutrition management of nondialysis-dependent CKD to maintenance dialysis therapy requires a thorough revision of nutrition support therapy. Priority should be given to the identification of deficiencies in dietary protein and energy intakes, and the provision of appropriate dietary advice for patients at increased risk of PEW, for example, protein and energy intakes <1.0 g/kg BW/day and <25 kcal/kg BW/day, respectively, for both maintenance hemodialysis and peritoneal dialysis patients [10, 15–17].

Attention should be given to increasing protein-rich foods, yet avoiding excessive consumption of dietary phosphorus, potassium, and sodium. Of relevance, higher protein intakes are subjected to a higher dietary phosphorus load. Survival benefit was observed in maintenance dialysis patients with a combination of increased protein intake and decreased serum phosphorus [23]; therefore, nutrition counseling of these patients should aim to reduce the load of dietary phosphorus without compromising protein intake. Such an approach should consist of educating patients to minimize the consumption of highly absorbable phosphorus foods (e.g., processed foods such as cheese) and foods containing phosphorus-based additives (e.g., soft drinks), as the phosphorus content in both is almost completely absorbed by the gastrointestinal tract [24]. (See Chap. 23.) Simultaneously, the consumption of plant-based proteins relative to animal-based proteins should be increased, as plant-based phosphorus is less readily absorbed by the human gastrointestinal tract compared with animal-based phosphorus, that is, gastrointestinal absorption of 20–40% of plant-based phosphorus versus 40–60% of animal-based phosphorus [24]. Of importance, the consumption of plant-based proteins was found to be associated with lower serum phosphorus levels [25] and lower mortality [26]. Moreover, boiling should be the preferred cooking method for protein-rich foods compared to other common cooking methods [24], as boiling reduces phosphorus content along with lowering the content of sodium, potassium, and other minerals in both plant-based and animal-based protein foods [24, 27]. Recently, a novel, visual, and user-friendly tool of "phosphorus pyramid" was developed for nutrition counseling in CKD patients [27]. The pyramid consists of six levels with foods arranged based on their phosphorus content, phosphorus to protein ratio, and phosphorus bioavailability. It also provides guidance on recommended frequency of consumption, ranging from "unrestricted" to "avoid as much as possible."

Finally, prolonged and often unnecessary periods of fasting should be avoided, such as protracted laboratory testing, missed meals due to the dialysis schedule, and inadequate dietary intake during acute illness and hospitalization. Consequently, periodic re-evaluation and ongoing nutrition counseling are essential dietetic practices for all maintenance dialysis patients. Nutrition counseling should be intensive upon initiation of dialysis, and provided on a monthly or bimonthly basis thereafter [16]. In the presence of inadequate nutritional intake, PEW, and illnesses that can cause deterioration in nutritional status, a more intensive monitoring schedule should be implemented [16].

Oral and Enteral Nutritional Supplementation

When nutrition counseling alone proves insufficient to bridge the gap between protein-energy intake and the target requirements in maintenance dialysis patients, oral nutritional supplementation should be the next appropriate step of nutrition support to restore and prevent further losses of protein and energy stores. In particular, the Kidney Disease Outcomes Quality Initiative and the Academy of Nutrition and Dietetics (KDOQI/Academy) suggests a minimum of a 3-month trial of oral nutritional supplements (ONS) to improve nutritional status if dietary counseling alone does not achieve sufficient energy and protein intakes to meet nutritional requirements [16]. Specific indications for initiating ONS have been proposed by the ISRNM [10] and are shown in Table 17.2. ONS can typically provide an additional 7–10 kcal/kg/day and 0.3–0.4 g protein/kg/day, and the utilization of ONS requires the complement of a spontaneous dietary intake of >20 kcal/kg/day and 0.4–0.8 g protein/kg/day in order to attain the recommended dietary energy and protein requirements [9, 10]. Oral nutritional supplementation is frequently considered as a highly feasible means of nutrition support in mild to moderate protein-energy wasted dialysis patients, as usual intakes in many of these patients often exceed the required minimum spontaneous intake (i.e., 20–24 kcal/kg/day for hemodialysis patients, 30 kcal/kg/day inclusive of glucose absorption from dialysate for peritoneal dialysis patients, and 0.8–1.0 g protein/kg/day for both dialysis modalities) [28].

Indeed, the effectiveness of oral nutritional supplementation has been investigated in different research settings. In metabolic studies, the use of ONS during hemodialysis led to positive whole-body protein

Table 17.2 Indications for initiating oral nutritional supplementation in maintenance dialysis patients proposed by the International Society of Renal Nutrition and Metabolism (ISRNM)

Suggested criteria for initiating oral nutritional supplementation [10]
Poor appetite and/or poor oral intake
Dietary protein intake <1.2 g/kg/day and dietary energy intake <30 kcal/kg/day
Serum albumin <3.8 g/dL or serum prealbumin[a] <28 mg/dL
Unintentional weight loss >5% of ideal body weight or estimated dry weight over 3 months
Worsening nutritional markers over time
Subjective global assessment score within PEW range

Abbreviation: PEW protein-energy wasting

[a]Only for maintenance dialysis patients without residual renal function

balance [29, 30], with the anabolic effects sustained in the postdialytic period [30]. In clinical trials, the use of ONS has demonstrated efficacy in improving nutritional status in maintenance dialysis patients. Table 17.3 provides a list of studies, including both randomized controlled trials (RCTs) and nonrandomized controlled trials (NRCTs), along with the nutritional and clinical outcomes in these studies.

In general, the effect of ONS has been investigated predominately in hemodialysis patients [31–43], and far less attention has been received by peritoneal dialysis patients [40, 44, 45]. The type of ONS evaluated in the current literature were food-based supplements [31] and commercial products [32–45] taken at home or during dialysis, comprising of protein-energy [31–35, 41–44], protein-based [36–38, 40, 45], energy-based [39], and renal-specific [33, 34, 42, 43] formulations. A major drawback throughout the literature was the limited use of a placebo group [38], although most studies included a comparative group where maintenance dialysis patients were either not supplemented [34, 37, 41, 42, 44], received nutrition counseling only [31–33, 36, 39, 40, 43, 45], or treated with a combination of ONS and IDPN [35]. The duration of supplementation ranged from 3 months to over a year. The nutritional benefits of these supple-

Table 17.3 Studies examining the effects of oral nutritional supplements (ONS) on nutritional outcomes in maintenance dialysis patients

Study	Dialysis modality	Study type and duration	Sample size	Nutritional entry criteria	Type of ONS	Nutritional and other relevant parameters significantly improved by ONS
Calegari et al. [31]	Hemodialysis	RCT: ONS vs. nutritional guidance 3 months	$n = 18$	SGA >9, and TST <90%, or AC/AMC <90%, or serum albumin <3.5 g/dL, or BMI <18.5 kg/m^2	Protein-energy supplement (food-based supplement)	↑ SGA ↑ QoL
Wilson et al. [32]	Hemodialysis	RCT: ONS vs. dietary counseling 9 months	$n = 46$	↓ Serum albumin	Protein-energy supplement (commercial formula)	↑ Serum albumin
Fouque et al. [33]	Hemodialysis	RCT: ONS vs. dietary advice 3 months	$n = 86$	Serum albumin <40 g/L and BMI <30 kg/m^2	Protein-energy supplement (renal-specific commercial formula)	↑ DPI ↑ DEI ↑ SGA ↑ QoL
Hung et al. [34]	Hemodialysis	RCT: ONS vs. no supplementation 3 months	$n = 55$	No nutritional entry criteria specified	Protein-energy supplement (renal-specific commercial formula)	↑ DEI ↑ Body fat mass
Cano et al. [35]	Hemodialysis	RCT: ONS vs. IDPN 12 months	$n = 186$	Two out of four malnutrition markers: BMI <20 kg/m^2, >10% weight loss within 6 months, serum albumin <35 g/dL, and serum prealbumin <300 mg/L	Protein-energy supplement (commercial formula)	↑ nPNA ↑ Serum albumin ↑ Serum prealbumin ↑ BMI

Table 17.3 (continued)

Hiroshige et al. [36]	Hemodialysis	RCT (CO): ONS vs. dietary advice 12 months	$n = 44$	Serum albumin <3.5 g/dL and complain of anorexia	Protein supplement (BCAA commercial formula)	↑ DPI ↑ DEI ↑ Plasma albumin ↑ Dry body weight ↑ Body fat % ↑ Lean body mass
Bolasco et al. [37]	Hemodialysis	RCT: ONS vs. no supplementation 3 months	$n = 30$	Serum albumin <3.5 g/dL, nPNA <1.1 g/kg/day, and BMI >20 kg/m^2	Protein supplement (AA commercial formula)	↑ ePCR ↑ Serum albumin ↑ Total proteins ↑ Body weight ↑ Hb ↓ CRP
Tomayko et al. [38]	Hemodialysis	RCT: Two ONS groups vs. placebo 6 months	$n = 38$	No nutritional entry criteria specified	Protein supplement (whey and soy commercial formulae)	↓ IL-6 (whey and soy) ↑ Gait speed and walking distance (whey and soy)
Allman et al. [39]	Hemodialysis	RCT: ONS vs. dietary advice 6 months	$n = 21$	BMI <27 kg/m^2	Energy supplement (glucose polymer commercial formula)	↑ DEI ↑ Body weight ↑ Body fat ↑ Lean body mass
Moretti et al. [40]	Hemodialysis and peritoneal dialysis	RCT (CO): ONS vs. dietary advice 6 months	$n = 49$	No nutritional entry criteria specified	Protein supplement (liquid hydrolyzed collagen commercial formula)	↑ nPCR ↑ Albumin
Teixido-Planas et al. [44]	Peritoneal Dialysis	RCT: ONS vs. no supplementation 6 months	$n = 65$	No nutritional entry criteria specified	Protein-energy supplement (commercial formula)	↑ Body weight ↑ TST ↑ MAMC ↑ LBM ↑ Creatinine LBM related to body surface area ↑ Creatinine generation rate ↑ Lymphocytes
Gonzalez-Espinoza et al. [45]	Peritoneal dialysis	RCT: ONS vs. nutritional counseling 6 months	$n = 28$	Moderate or severe malnutrition rated by SGA	Protein supplement (egg-albumin commercial formula)	↑ DPI ↑ DEI ↑ nPNA ↑ Serum albumin ↑ TST ↑ MAMA ↑ SGA
Cheu et al. [41]	Hemodialysis	NRCT: ONS vs. no supplementation 13.5 months	$n = 470$	Serum albumin <3.8 g/dL	Protein-energy supplement (commercial formula)	↑ Serum albumin ↓ Hospitalization

(continued)

Table 17.3 (continued)

Scott et al. [42]	Hemodialysis	NRCT: ONS vs. no supplementation/standard care 3 months	$n = 88$	No nutritional entry criteria specified	Protein-energy supplement (renal-specific commercial formula)	↑ Serum albumin ↑ QoL
Sezer et al. [43]	Hemodialysis	NRCT: ONS vs. dietary advice 6 months	$n = 62$	Serum albumin <4 g/dL, and/or ≥5% loss of dry weight over the past 3 months	Protein-energy supplement (renal-specific commercial formula)	↑ Serum albumin ↑ Dry weight ↑ TST

Abbreviations: *AA* amino acid, *AC* arm circumference, *AMC* arm muscle circumference, *BCAA* branched chain amino acids, *BMI* body mass index, *CO* cross-over, *CRP* c-reactive protein, *DEI* dietary energy intake, *DPI* dietary protein intake, *ePCR* equilibrated protein catabolic rate, *Hb* hemoglobin, *IL-6* interleukin-6, *LBM* lean body mass, *MAMA* mid arm muscle area, *MAMC* mid arm muscle circumference, *nPCR* normalized protein catabolic rate, *nPNA* normalized protein nitrogen appearance, *NRCT* nonrandomized controlled trial, *ONS* oral nutritional supplements, *QoL* quality of life, *RCT* randomized controlled trial, *SGA* subjective global assessment, *TST* triceps skinfold thickness

ments were improvements in dietary intakes of protein [33, 35–37, 40, 45] and energy [33, 34, 36, 39, 45]; nutritional biomarkers including levels of serum albumin [32, 35–37, 40–43, 45], prealbumin [35], and total proteins [37]; subjective global assessment (SGA) composite nutritional score [31, 33, 45]; body weight [36, 37, 39, 43, 44]; BMI [35]; and anthropometric estimates of muscle mass [36, 39, 44, 45] and fat mass [34, 36, 39, 43–45]. The beneficial effects were evident as early as 1 month [36, 39], and were found to be sustainable [32, 35, 36, 39, 41, 45]. Improvements in inflammation [37, 38], physical functioning [38], and quality of life [31, 33, 42] were also observed. Although hospitalization and mortality were often reported [32, 35, 40], most studies did not possess the statistical power to adequately assess the efficacy of ONS on these outcomes. However, findings from large observational studies indicated lower rates of hospitalization [41] and mortality [46] in maintenance hemodialysis patients who received ONS.

In order to maximize the benefits of nutritional supplementation, ONS should not be used as a nutritional substitution; it should be taken separately from regular meals once to thrice daily, preferably 1–3 hours after main meals [10, 15]. Findings from metabolic studies support the consumption of a late evening supplement as it may decrease the length of overnight starvation and the sequential catabolism [15, 47, 48]. ONS may also be consumed during hemodialysis to prevent dialysis-associated alterations of protein metabolism [10, 15]. In particular, intradialytic feeding through monitored in-center provision of ONS and high-protein meals has been proposed as a feasible, economical, and patient-friendly approach to improve dietary protein and energy intakes in hemodialysis patients [49]. Many of the perceived negative effects such as postprandial hypotension and other hemodynamic instabilities, gastrointestinal symptoms, inadequate dialysis, risks of aspiration, and contamination are not commonly observed [49–51], and can be prevented with judicious selection of patients coupled with continuous monitoring. Nevertheless, definitive RCTs that balance the potential benefits against the risks of intradialytic feeding are currently missing. Further large-scale RCTs should be performed to provide clear guidance of intradialytic feeding.

Furthermore, ONS should be prescribed based on patient's requirements, preference, compliance, and tolerance, as these are important success factors. The acceptability of ONS in terms of appearance, smell, taste, texture, and type of preparation (e.g., milkshake, juice, pudding, bar, or fortification powder) should be considered. Among the standard ONS that have been formulated for the general diseased populations, the preferred choice of supplement should be high in protein and energy without excessive amounts of potassium and phosphorus. Of relevance, protein-energy dense, low-electrolytes, renal-specific ONS are currently available, and these may be prescribed as an alternative to increase protein and energy intakes without inducing excess levels of fluid and electrolytes [33]. Gastrointestinal side effects can affect the outcome of oral nutrition support, and an extended period of monotonous supplementation may lead to flavor and taste fatigue, as well as noncompliance with the prescribed supplement. Consequently, frequent monitoring and evaluation by the registered dietitian (or international equivalent) during the supplementation period is crucial, and implementation of the necessary changes to the supplement prescription is an important measure to improve patient's adherence and hence the overall effectiveness of oral nutritional supplementation. Both the KDOQI/Academy [16] and EBPG [17, 18] provided recommendations for nutritional monitoring in maintenance hemodialysis and peritoneal dialysis patients, shown in Table 17.4. Unstable or protein-energy wasted maintenance dialysis patients may require intensive monitoring [52].

Table 17.4 Recommendations for nutritional monitoring in maintenance hemodialysis and peritoneal dialysis patients

Guidelines	Nutritional assessment parameters (dialysis modality)	Frequency of monitoring	Recommended levels
National Kidney Foundation Kidney Disease Outcomes Quality Initiative and the Academy of Nutrition and Dietetics (KDOQI/Academy) [16]	Dietary interview and/or diary (HD and PD)	≤12 months	–
	nPCR (HD and PD)	≤12 months	–
	Body weight (HD and PD)	≤1 month	–
	BMI (HD and PD)	≤1 month	–
	Skinfold thickness (HD and PD)	≤12 months	–
	Waist circumference (HD and PD)	≤12 months	–
	Handgrip strength (HD and PD)	≤12 months	–
	7-point SGA (HD and PD)	≤12 months	–
	MIS (HD)	≤12 months	–
	Creatinine kinetics (HD and PD)	≤12 months	–
	Serum albumin (HD and PD)[a]	≤12 months	–
	Serum prealbumin (HD and PD)	≤12 months	–
European Best Practice Guidelines (EBPG) [17, 18]	Dietary interview (HD and PD)	3–12 months	–
	nPNA (HD and PD)	1 month	>1 g/kg BW/day
	Body weight (HD and PD)	Every dialysis	–
	BMI (HD and PD)	1 month	>23 kg/m²
	SGA (PD)	3 months	–
	Midweek predialysis creatinine (HD)	1 month	–
	Serum albumin (HD and PD)[a]	1–3 months	≥40 g/L
	Serum prealbumin (HD)	1–3 months	≥300 mg/L
	Serum cholesterol (HD)	3 months	>Minimum laboratory threshold

Abbreviations: BMI body mass index, *BW* body weight, *HD* hemodialysis, *MIS* malnutrition inflammation score, *nPCR* normalized protein catabolic rate, *nPNA* normalized protein nitrogen appearance, *PD* peritoneal dialysis, *SGA* subjective global assessment
[a]By bromocresol green method

When maintenance hemodialysis and peritoneal dialysis patients are failing to reach the recommended dietary protein and energy intakes with ONS and nutrition counseling, exhibiting severe PEW, presenting with spontaneous intakes of <20 kcal/kg/day, or in stress conditions, enteral feeding by nasogastric or nasojejunal tubes should be considered [10, 15, 16, 28]. The latter should be reserved for patients with gastroparesis unresponsive to prokinetic treatment [15]. Daily nutrition support is important in these patients, and enteral nutrition should always be preferable to parenteral nutrition because feeding through the gastrointestinal tract helps maintain its normal structure and function [15]. Parenteral nutrition is an invasive and expensive feeding method with a higher risk of metabolic and septic complications.

Percutaneous endoscopic gastroscopy (PEG) and jejunostomy may also be considered for hemodialysis patients, especially for long-term enteral tube feeding[15], but these methods of feeding delivery have been contraindicated in peritoneal dialysis patients due to the increased risk of peritonitis [15]. Nevertheless, the use of a PEG in peritoneal dialysis patients has shown to be an effective nutrition support strategy in selected cases [53–55]. In patients with diagnosed peritonitis, early initiation of parenteral nutrition has been shown to maintain a positive nitrogen balance [56]. In cases of encapsulating peritoneal sclerosis, parenteral nutrition support may confer nutritional benefits and improved tolerance compared to enteral tube feeding [57].

Although enteral tube feeding is often considered an important nutrition support option in maintenance dialysis patients with PEW, the effectiveness and the associated complications have not been well investigated. Limited evidence from a small-scale clinical trial [58] and a cohort study [59] showed that nasogastric and gastrostomy feedings using a variety of standard and renal-specific formulas are effective in improving biochemical and anthropometric measures of nutritional status in hemodialysis patients, including increases in serum albumin [58, 59], dry weight [58], as well as muscle mass and fat mass [58]. Of note, hypophosphatemia may occur in enteral tube feeding through a renal-specific formula [59], highlighting the need for phosphorus monitoring during feeding. Formulas with high-protein, low-carbohydrate content should be the preferred choice for peritoneal dialysis patients [15]. Further large-scale RCTs should be performed to examine the efficacy of enteral tube feeding on nutritional parameters, clinical outcomes, and quality of life in maintenance dialysis patients.

Intradialytic Parenteral Nutrition

Intradialytic parenteral nutrition is a form of partial parenteral nutrition involving the administration of nutrients, usually a mixture of amino acids, dextrose, and lipid emulsions, during regularly scheduled hemodialysis sessions. IDPN is delivered via intravenous infusion through the venous drip chamber of the extracorporeal circulation lines. It has been proposed as a safe and convenient approach of nutritional supplementation in maintenance hemodialysis patients. However, the indications for IDPN therapy vary among clinical practice guidelines. The consensus is that IDPN should not be the initial choice of nutrition support in maintenance hemodialysis patients with PEW. Dietary counseling and oral nutritional supplementation are crucial, and both should be attempted as initial steps for nutrition support in this patient group [16, 17, 28, 60]. When nutrition counseling and the use of ONS are unable to reach the target protein and energy requirements, both enteral tube feeding and IDPN have been proposed as the next appropriate steps [16, 17, 28, 60].

In particular, both the KDOQI/Academy and EBPG suggest the use of IDPN only under two conditions: (1) when dietary counseling, use of ONS, and enteral tube feeding have all failed to achieve the requirements for protein and energy, and (2) when the spontaneous protein and energy intakes in conjunction with IDPN are able to attain the required targets [16, 17], for example, spontaneous intake >20 kcal/kg and >0.8 g protein/kg daily [17]. Otherwise, daily total or partial parenteral nutrition should be considered [16, 17]. On the other hand, the ESPEN guidelines suggest the use of IDPN even before attempting enteral tube feeding, because of the risk associated with feeding tube placement [28]. In contrast, the American Society for Parenteral and Enteral Nutrition only recommends enteral tube feeding, and does not recommend IDPN due to the lack of evidence supporting its application in clinical practice [60]. In view of the contrasting recommendations among the existing clinical practice guidelines, the decision to prescribe IDPN should be based on clinical judgment of an individual's benefit–risk balance.

The types of IDPN available were a compounded admixture-based IDPN and a commercial admixture-based IDPN [61]. While the former are all-in-one bags specifically prepared by pharmacy for individual patients, the latter are commercially premixed all-in-one bags designed to cover the needs of most maintenance hemodialysis patients. Electrolyte-free admixtures are also commercially available [61]. The commercial mixture remains a common option in clinical practice, because the process of compounding an individualized mixture is time-consuming and costly. From a practical perspective, the most concentrated solutions are frequently used in maintenance hemodialysis patients due to the risk of volume overload and the time constraint of accommodating IPDN within the standard dialysis session [61].

IDPN suffers from time limitations due to hemodialysis frequency and duration, usually 4 hours thrice weekly [9]. The maximum concentration of calories of all-in-one admixtures is 1 kcal/ml, and the suggested maximum fluid, calories, and amino acids for safe delivery through IDPN are 1000 ml, 1000 kcal, and 50 g, respectively [61]. Taking into account the nondialysis days and the loss of 4–8 g amino acids per dialysis session, the provision of calories and amino acids for a 70 kg patient are marginally less than 3000 kcal and 150 g per week, respectively, or approximately 6 kcal/kg/day and 0.30 g protein/kg/day [61, 62]. For IDPN to satisfy the protein and energy requirements of a maintenance hemodialysis patient, the patient's spontaneous dietary intakes are required to meet the actual difference between those provided by IDPN and the target requirements. In this case, with protein and energy targets being 1.0–1.2 g/kg/day and 25–35 kcal/kg/day, respectively, a spontaneous intake of at least 0.7 g protein/kg/day and 19 kcal/kg/day is required. These are broadly corroborated by the recommendations from the EBPG, that is, a spontaneous intake of >0.8 g protein/kg/day and >20 kcal/kg/day [17]. Given the limited provision of protein and energy, IDPN is likely to be most effective in maintenance hemodialysis patients at risk of PEW or with mild to moderate PEW, rather than with severe PEW [9]. The presence of severe PEW is often accompanied with spontaneous intakes of <0.8 g protein/kg/day and <20 kcal/kg/day. Under these conditions, both IDPN and oral intake are generally unable to meet the nutritional targets. Hence, IDPN is not recommended for maintenance hemodialysis patients with severe PEW. Instead, a more aggressive nutrition support approach should be prompted for these patients, such as enteral tube feeding or total parenteral nutrition [61].

The efficacy of IDPN has been investigated in multiple research settings. In metabolic studies, the use of IDPN led to increased whole-body protein synthesis and fractional albumin synthesis, as well as decreased whole-body proteolysis [63–65]. These metabolisms mitigated the negative effects of hemodialysis on protein synthesis and degradation, leading to positive net protein balance [66]. However, the anabolic effect of IDPN was found to dissipate in the postdialytic period [30]. Of interest, performing brief exercise at the beginning of the dialysis session was shown to improve the anabolic effect of IDPN therapy markedly [65].

In clinical trials, the use of IDPN has demonstrated efficacy in improving nutritional status in maintenance dialysis patients. Table 17.5 provides a list of studies, including both RCTs and NRCTs, along with the nutritional and clinical outcomes in these studies. In general, the effect of IDPN has been evaluated using both individually compounded and commercial mixtures [35, 67–73], with varying nutritional composition. While some studies enrolled maintenance hemodialysis patients with some degree of PEW [35, 67, 68, 70, 71], others did not specify the application of nutritional entry criteria [69, 72, 73]. The use of IDPN was compared to a variety of control treatments including dietary counseling [71, 72], ONS [35], isocaloric glucose solution [67], another IDPN admixture

Table 17.5 Studies examining the effects of intradialytic parenteral nutrition (IDPN) on nutritional outcomes in maintenance hemodialysis patients

Study	Study type and duration	Sample size	Nutritional entry criteria	IDPN formula	Nutritional and other relevant parameters significantly improved by IDPN
Guarnieri et al. [67]	RCT: Two IDPN groups vs. isocaloric 5% glucose solution 2 months	$n = 18$	Unable to improve oral energy intake, and negative nitrogen balance	Two IDPN groups: Group 1- EAAs with added histidine Group 2- EAAs and non-EAAs	↑ Body weight (in EAAs with added histidine group)
Cano et al. [68]	RCT: IDPN vs. no IDPN 3 months	$n = 26$	Serum transthyretin <300 mg/L	EAAs and non-EAAs with added glycyl-tyrosine	↑ DEI ↑ DPI ↑ Serum pre-albumin ↑ Serum albumin ↑ Interdialytic creatinine appearance ↑ Skin-test reactivity ↑ Plasma leucine ↑ Plasma apolipoprotein A-1 ↑ Body weight ↑ AMC
Navarro et al. [69]	RCT: IDPN vs. no IDPN 3 months	$n = 17$	No nutritional entry criteria specified	EAAs and non-EAAs	↑ PCR ↑ Serum albumin ↑ Serum transferrin
Cano et al. [70]	RCT: Two IDPN groups (differed by fat emulsions: olive oil or soybean oil) 5 weeks	$n = 35$	Three of the five criteria: BMI <20 kg/m², >10% weight loss within 6 months, serum albumin <35 g/L, serum transthyretin (prealbumin) <300 mg/L, and nPCR <1 g/kg/day	Two IDPN groups: Group 1- AAs, glucose, olive oil Group 2 - AAs, glucose, soybean oil	Both olive oil and soybean oil groups: ↑ nPCR ↑ Serum albumin Soybean oil group only: ↑ Serum pre-albumin ↑ Creatinine Comparison between olive oil and soybean oil groups: ↑ BMI (olive oil group)
Cano et al. [35]	RCT: IDPN+ONS vs. ONS only 1 year	$n = 186$	Two of the four criteria: BMI <20 kg/m², >10% weight loss within 6 months, serum albumin <35 g/L, and serum prealbumin <300 mg/L	Standard lipid emulsion of 50%, glucose 50% of nonprotein energy supply, and standard AA	Both IDPN+ONS and ONS only groups: ↑ nPNA ↑ DEI ↑ DPI ↑ Body weight ↑ BMI ↑ Serum albumin ↑ Serum pre-albumin

Table 17.5 (continued)

Marsen et al. [71]	RCT: IDPN + nutritional counseling vs. nutritional counseling only 16 weeks	n = 107	SGA score = B or C (moderate to severe malnutrition), and two of the three criteria: albumin <35 g/L, prealbumin <250 mg/L, and phase angle alpha <4.5° assessed by BIA	Individualized compounded solution containing glucose, AAs, fat, vitamins, trace elements, and L-carnitine	↑ Serum pre-albumin
Hiroshige et al. [72]	NRCT: IDPN vs. dietary counseling 1 year	n = 28	Malnutrition was ascertained at the start of the study, but nutritional entry criteria were undefined	200 ml 50% dextrose, 200 ml 7.1% EAAs, 200 ml 20% lipid emulsion	↑ Serum albumin ↑ Serum transferrin ↑ Total lymphocyte count ↑ DEI ↑ DPI ↑ Dry body weight ↑ BMI ↑ TSF ↑ MAMC ↑ MAC
Toigo et al. [73]	RCT: Two IDPN groups 6 months	n = 21	No nutritional entry criteria specified	Two IDPN groups: Group 1 - EAAs Group 2 - Isonitrogenous EAAs plus non-EAAs	Both EAAs and Isonitrogenous EAAs plus non-EAAs groups: ↑ PCR EAAs group: ↑ NCV

Abbreviations: AA amino acids, *AMC* arm muscle circumference, *BIA* bioelectrical impedance analysis, *BMI* body mass index, *DEI* dietary energy intake, *DPI* dietary protein intake, *EAAs* essential amino acids, *IDPN* intradialytic parenteral nutrition, *MAC* midarm circumference, *MAMC* midarm muscle circumference, *non-EAAs* nonessential amino acids, *NCV* nerve conduction velocity, *nPCR* normalized protein catabolic rates, *nPNA* normalized protein nitrogen appearance, *NRCT* nonrandomized controlled trial, *ONS* oral nutritional supplements, *PCR* protein catabolic rate, *RCT* randomized controlled trial, *SGA* subjective global assessment, *TSF* tricep skinfold thickness

[70, 73], or no IDPN supplementation [68, 69]. However, the characteristics of the control groups, particularly the latter group where patients received no IDPN supplementation, were often ill-defined with limited information on the patients' diet. Also, it remains unclear whether nutrition counseling was provided as part of the control treatment. Moreover, no studies have compared IDPN to enteral tube feeding.

Among the available literature, the duration of IDPN supplementation ranged from 2 months to 1 year. The nutritional benefits of IDPN were improvements in dietary intakes of protein [35, 68–70, 72] and energy [35, 68, 72], nutritional biomarkers including levels of serum albumin [35, 68–70, 72], prealbumin [35, 68, 70, 71, 73], and transferrin [69, 72]; body weight [35, 67, 68, 72] and BMI [35, 70, 72]; as well as anthropometric measurements of muscle mass [68, 72] and fat mass [72].

Although the use of IDPN was associated with improvements in nutritional status, the landmark study by the French Intradialytic Nutrition Evaluation (FINE) study group showed that IDPN conferred no further nutritional benefit than the use of ONS [35]. The investigators of the FINE study randomly assigned 186 maintenance hemodialysis patients with PEW to receive 1-year of IDPN and ONS or ONS alone [35]. The nutritional supplementation goal for both groups was to increase dietary protein and energy intakes to the recommended targets of 1.2 g/kg/day and 30–35 kcal/kg/day, respectively [35]. In addition to exhibiting similar improvements in markers of nutritional status in both groups [35], the primary outcome, 2-year mortality rate, was not different between the two groups (43% in IDPN and ONS group; and 39% in ONS alone group) [35]. Similarly, hospitalization rate and functional status were not influenced by the addition of IDPN in the supplementation regimen [35]. These observations suggest that the route of nutrient administration (i.e., combined parenteral-oral or oral) has no influence on markers of nutritional status and survival as long as equal and adequate amounts of protein and calories are provided to attain the target nutritional requirements. The FINE study also demonstrated that increased serum prealbumin, as a result of either parenteral-oral or oral feeding, was associated with decreased 2-year mortality and hospitalization rates [35] independently of a chronic inflammatory status, hence providing the first prospective association between response to nutritional therapy and improved clinical outcomes [35]. These findings further strengthen the rationale for nutrition support in maintenance hemodialysis patients with PEW.

Notably, the high cost of IDPN and the regulatory concerns are substantial barriers to regular utilization of IDPN. Also, the cost-effectiveness of IDPN has not been adequately examined, with only one study reporting significant reductions in number of hospitalizations, cost of hospitalizations, and length of hospital stay after 6 months of IDPN therapy, but no overall cost savings were achieved when the cost of IDPN was taken into account [74]. However, this study lacked comparison to a concurrent non-IDPN control group, hence limiting the interpretation of its findings [74].

Thus far, IDPN displayed no major adverse effects compared to oral nutritional supplementation [35]. The most frequently reported adverse effects were digestive symptoms, hypotension, and muscle cramps, but these issues occurred at a similar rate compared to patients receiving ONS [35]. Other possible adverse events include deranged liver function and vascular access–related symptoms, although the former has not been reported in the literature [35].

In addition, disorders of glucose metabolism, lipid intolerance, as well as mineral and electrolyte imbalances may occur, but these abnormalities can be minimized by frequent laboratory monitoring and seeking appropriate clinical intervention. Specifically, the development of hyperglycemia during IDPN infusion may be treated with either subcutaneous or intravenous insulin, or with insulin added to the IDPN solution [75]. In cases of rebound hypoglycemia, oral consumption of carbohydrate within the last 30 minutes of IDPN infusion may be necessary [76]. Additionally, IDPN is contraindicated if triglyceride levels are >300 mg/dL because lipids in the IDPN formula may exacerbate hypertriglyceridemia, although elevations of lipids have not been reported and were not observed by the FINE study group [35]. Nevertheless, it is important to monitor serum cholesterol and triglyceride concentrations because improvement in these parameters may signal an improvement in oral intake, potentially rendering a decision to discontinue IDPN therapy. Furthermore, mineral and electrolyte imbalances, such as hypokalemia and hypophosphatemia, may be relieved by adding potassium and phosphorus to the IDPN solution. The former may also be managed by increasing the potassium concentration in the dialysate. On the other hand, hyperkalemia and hyperphosphatemia may occur. These may be important signs for improvement in the patient's oral diet. It is therefore crucial to monitor blood biochemistry profile and oral diet simultaneously. Due to the risk of electrolyte abnormalities, stringent monitoring of electrolytes is highly recommended, particularly during the first week of IDPN therapy [28]. Of note, to prevent volume overload, the ultrafiltration rate should be adjusted to remove the additional fluid provided by IDPN.

Overall, IDPN has been demonstrated to be safe with a very low complication rate. In the unlikely event of adverse consequences, IDPN should be terminated. Also, IDPN should not be implemented as a long-term nutrition support strategy [9]. It should be discontinued as soon as sustained improvements in nutritional status and spontaneous dietary intakes are observed, thus making IDPN unnecessary [77]. Most patients undergoing maintenance hemodialysis respond to IDPN after 3–6 months of therapy; hence, nutritional status should be evaluated after this time period [35]. Lack of improvement after 3–6 months of IDPN therapy should render a decision to discontinue [77]. When oral intake combined with IDPN is unable to attain the target nutritional requirements, or in cases of a malfunctioned gastrointestinal tract, total parenteral nutrition should be considered [16, 17].

Intraperitoneal Parenteral Nutrition

IPPN is a form of parenteral nutrition unique to maintenance peritoneal dialysis patients [28]. It occurs intermittently as part of the regular peritoneal dialysis regimen via intraperitoneal administration. IPPN replaces a portion of the regular peritoneal dialysate, that is, dextrose-based dialysate, with an amino acid–containing dialysate. Specifically, IPPN utilizes either an amino acid–based peritoneal dialysate containing no glucose [28, 78–81], or a combined amino acid and glucose peritoneal dialysate [82–85], both of which substitute for one to two exchanges of the conventional dextrose-based peritoneal dialysate. Since IPPN involves the administration of an amino acid–containing dialysate, it is also termed as intraperitoneal amino acid (IPAA) therapy. The purpose of IPAA therapy is to maintain ultrafiltration and small solute clearance while compensating for deceased dietary protein intake, obligatory peritoneal losses of amino acids and proteins, and normalizing plasma amino acid concentrations [79]. It has long been established that the quantity of amino acids provided by an amino acid–based dialysate during one exchange exceeds the daily losses of amino acids induced by the dialysis procedure [16, 86].

The efficacy of IPAA administration has been investigated in multiple settings. In metabolic studies, an early investigation showed that the use of an amino acid–based dialysate led to positive nitrogen balance, net protein anabolism, and normalized fasting plasma amino acid pattern [78], as well as elevated serum total protein and transferrin concentrations [78]. Another study confirmed its utility in promoting protein synthesis with no effect on protein breakdown [87]. Despite these positive findings from metabolic studies, clinical trials ranging from 3 months to 3 years showed an inconclusive effect on nutritional improvement using amino acid–based dialysate. These studies include both RCTs and NRCTs [79–81] and are summarized in Table 17.6. Such discrepancies may be explained by inadequate sample size to detect a significant difference, and the presence of comorbid conditions such as peritonitis, heart failure, and infectious illnesses during the study period that may confound the outcome [79, 88]. Also, long-term study may be further hampered by a high dropout rate, as well as inconsistency in dietary control and monitoring [79, 88]. Notably, the most remarkable nutritional improvement was observed in hypoalbuminemic peritoneal dialysis patients [80, 81]. Thus far, only one RCT examined the effect of amino acid–based dialysate on hospitalization and survival [79], with negative results among peritoneal dialysis patients with PEW.

While amino acid–based dialysate received the most attention in IPAA therapy, the utilization of combined amino acid and glucose peritoneal dialysate remains a potential option. Hitherto, the evaluation of this approach is limited to the metabolic settings. An early study demonstrated a cumulative effect of the combined use of dextrose and amino acids [85], whereby glucose-induced insulin secretion suppressed endogenous muscle breakdown [85], and the availability of amino acid enhanced muscle synthesis [85]. Hence, muscle mass could be preserved with the utilization of a combined amino acid and glucose peritoneal dialysate [85]. Additionally, two further studies showed that peritoneal dialysate containing both amino acids and glucose improves protein kinetics including protein synthesis [84] and net protein balance [83], thereby promoting protein anabolism [83]. These preliminary findings suggest that the use of combined amino acid and glucose dialysate

Table 17.6 Studies examining the effects of intraperitoneal parenteral nutrition (IPPN) on nutritional outcomes in maintenance peritoneal dialysis patients

Study	Study type & duration	Sample size	Nutritional entry criteria	IPPN treatment protocol	Nutritional & other relevant outcomes with IPPN therapy
Misra et al. [81]	NRCT (CO): Treatment group (1.1% amino acid dialysate) vs. control group (dextrose-based dialysate) 12 months	n = 18	Serum cholesterol ≥5.5 mmol/L	Treatment phase (6 months): A dextrose exchange was replaced with a 2 L amino acid dialysate Control phase (6 months): Usual PD regimen with dextrose dialysate exclusively	↑ Serum albumin (only in patients with baseline albumin <30 g/L) No effect on: Transferrin Lipid profile (total cholesterol, LDL, HDL, triglycerides, Lp-a, Apo-B, Apo-A₁) Dialysis adequacy Ultrafiltration Dialysate protein excretion
Jones et al. [80]	RCT: Treatment group (1.1% amino acid dialysate with no glucose) vs. control group (1.5% dextrose dialysate) 3 months	n = 134	At least two of the three criteria: Dietary protein intake ≤1.0 g/kg, serum albumin ≤3.7 g/dL for men or ≤3.5 g/dL for women, and evidence of malnutrition on SGA	Treatment group: One or two 2 L amino acid–based dialysate in place of the same number of dextrose-based exchanges Control group: Usual PD regimen using dextrose-based dialysate only	↑ Insulin-like growth factor-1 ↓ Serum potassium ↓ Serum phosphorus ↑ Serum prealbumin ↑ Serum transferrin ↑ Serum albumin (only in patients with baseline albumin <3.5 g/dL) ↑ MAMC No changes in peritoneal membrane transport characteristic
Li et al. [79]	RCT: Treatment group (1.1% amino acid dialysate with no glucose) vs. control group (1.5% dextrose dialysate) 3 years	n = 60	At least two of the three criteria: Protein nitrogen intake ≤0.9 g/kg, serum albumin ≤3.5 g/dL, and evidence of malnutrition on SGA	Treatment group: One 2 L bag of amino acid–based dialysate in place of one exchange of dextrose-based dialysate Control group: Usual PD regimen with dextrose-based dialysate exclusively	↑ nPNA ↑ DPI ↓ Serum prealbumin ↓ Serum transferrin ↓ Serum triglyceride ↑ LBM (only in women) ↑ BMI (only in women) ↑ MTAC of creatinine No effect on: Mortality Hospitalization CRP Serum albumin Composite nutritional index Serum cholesterol Dialysis adequacy Ultrafiltration MTAC of urea

Abbreviations: Apo-A₁ apoprotein A₁, *Apo-B* apolipoprotein B, *BMI* body mass index, *CO* cross-over, *CRP* c-reactive protein, *DPI* dietary protein intake, *HDL* high-density lipoprotein cholesterol, *LBM* lean body mass, *LDL* low-density lipoprotein cholesterol, *Lp-a* lipoprotein a, *MAMC* midarm muscle circumference, *MTAC* mass transfer area coefficient, *nPNA* normalized protein equivalent of nitrogen appearance, *NRCT* nonrandomized controlled trial, *PD* peritoneal dialysis, *RCT* randomized controlled trial, *SGA* subjective global assessment may improve nutritional status of peritoneal dialysis patients with inadequate dietary intake. However, large-scale clinical trials are required to evaluate the long-term clinical relevance of this strategy.

It should be recognized that increased serum urea concentration associated with exacerbated uremic symptoms, as well as metabolic acidosis, is a potential complication of IPAA therapy that requires close monitoring with appropriate intervention [10, 78]. This may include the administration of oral alkalinizing agents, and the prevention of excessive amino acids and protein load from the combined peritoneal and oral intakes. Generally, limiting the use of amino acid–based dialysate to one exchange daily lowers the risk of such complications [80, 89, 90]. On the other hand, IPAA therapy may reduce the infused daily glucose load, thereby reducing the risk and the tendency of hyperglycemia, hypercholesterolemia, and hypertriglyceridemia [16]. In addition to exerting beneficial effects on lipid profile, substituting amino acids for glucose in peritoneal dialysate may serve as an immediate strategy for glycemic control in diabetic patients with uncontrolled hyperglycemia.

Both the KDOQI/Academy and ESPEN guidelines suggest the use of IPAA therapy when protein and energy requirements cannot be met by ONS and enteral tube feeding [16, 28]. The KDOQI/Academy guideline specified that IPAA should only be used if spontaneous protein and energy intakes in conjunction with IPAA are able to meet the required protein and energy targets [16]. Otherwise, daily total or partial parenteral nutrition should be considered [16, 28]. Overall, IPAA therapy remains a viable option for protein-energy wasted peritoneal dialysis patients with insufficient dietary intake, as well as those with tolerance, compliance, and suitability issues of oral intake and other forms of enteral supplementation [10, 16, 28].

Conclusion

PEW is highly common among patients undergoing maintenance dialysis. Although the etiology of PEW is complex and multifactorial, many of these causes are associated with reduced protein and energy intakes. Indeed, many signs of PEW can be ameliorated with nutrition support therapy. Regular nutrition counseling should be provided for all maintenance dialysis patients to prevent PEW. When nutrition counseling alone is insufficient to meet protein and energy requirements, oral nutritional supplementation should be the next appropriate step of nutrition support for maintenance dialysis patients to restore and prevent further losses of protein and energy stores. Only when these initial attempts fail to maintain optimal nutritional status, enteral tube feeding, total parenteral nutrition, and partial parenteral nutrition such as IDPN and IPPN may be considered for protein-energy wasted maintenance dialysis patients.

Case Study

A 51-year-old Caucasian man (Mr. Smith) with a medical history of stage 5 CKD secondary to hypertension and glomerulonephritis presents with progressive decline of kidney function, poor appetite, nausea, lethargy, and decreased urine output. His nutritional assessment parameters are as follows: height = 170 cm; weight = 75.6 kg; BMI = 26.2 kg/m^2; 5% unintentional weight loss over the past 3 months; SGA score = 4; serum albumin = 3.4 g/dL; and pedal edema. Peritoneal dialysis is started with the aim of removing excess fluid and uremic toxins, as well as improving nutritional status.

At 3 months after initiating peritoneal dialysis, Mr. Smith is feeling better. His pedal edema is resolving. His uremic symptoms, appetite, and oral intake are improving. His nutritional assessment parameters are as follows: dry body weight = 73.6 kg; BMI = 25.5 kg/m^2; serum albumin = 4.0 g/dL; and SGA score = 6. Upon physical examination, Mr. Smith is euvolemic. His total intakes of protein and energy including the calories provided by the peritoneal dialysate are 1.3 g protein/kg/day and 33 kcal/kg/day, respectively.

Having been treated with peritoneal dialysis for 3 years, Mr. Smith is admitted to hospital due to turbid peritoneal effluent accompanied by constant abdominal pain. He had two prior episodes of peritonitis in the past few years. The laboratory findings and bacterial culture of the peritoneal dialysate confirm PD-associated peritonitis. At the same time, Mr. Smith experiences nausea, poor appetite, and reduced food intake. His food record chart indicates an ingestion of approximately 0.6 g protein/kg/day and 24 kcal/kg/day on the first few days of hospital admission.

Mr. Smith is given a 2-week course of intraperitoneal antibiotics upon diagnosis of peritonitis. He is also prescribed a trial of renal-specific ONS, providing an additional 25 g protein and 500 kcal daily. With the completion of the antibiotic therapy and the resolution of the peritonitis, improvements in appetite and oral intake are observed. He is subsequently discharged from the hospital. Upon hospital discharge, his estimated total protein and energy intakes including the use of ONS are 1.2 g/kg/day and 32 kcal/kg/day, respectively. His nutritional assessment parameters are as follows: dry weight = 71.5 kg; BMI = 24.7 kg/m^2; 6% unintentional weight loss over the past 3 months; serum albumin = 3.4 g/dL; and SGA score = 4. In view of recurrent peritonitis, his renal replacement therapy is changed from peritoneal dialysis to hemodialysis.

At 2–3 months after transition to hemodialysis, his nutritional parameters are as follows: dry weight = 76.1 kg; BMI = 26.3 kg/m^2; serum albumin = 4.1 g/dL; and SGA score = 6. Upon physical examination, he is euvolemic. His food diary shows an estimated consumption of 1.2 g protein/kg/day and 33 kcal/kg/day excluding the use of ONS.

Over the course of the next few years, he is relatively stable, and receives regular nutrition counseling from a registered dietitian. He is compliant with his hemodialysis regimen and manages to maintain nutritional assessment parameters within acceptable ranges. After 3–4 years on hemodialysis, Mr. Smith is admitted to hospital for 3 weeks with pneumonia. His nutritional assessment parameters immediately post-discharge are as follows: dry weight = 68.8 kg; BMI = 23.8 kg/m^2; 9% unintentional weight loss over the past 2 months; temporal wasting indicated by physical examination; serum albumin = 3.2 g/dL; and SGA score = 4. His diet history indicates a spontaneous dietary intake of 0.9 g protein/kg/day and 25 kcal/kg/day.

Over the course of the next 3 months, there is no improvement in Mr. Smith's nutritional assessment parameters. His nutritional status continues to decline despite liberalization of his diet and the use of ONS. His nutritional assessment parameters are as follows: dry weight = 64.2 kg; BMI = 22.2 kg/m^2; unintentional weight loss of 7% over the past 3 months; muscle and fat wasting upon physical examination; serum albumin = 3.1 g/dL; and SGA score = 2. His diet history shows a consumption of 0.7 g protein/kg/day and 19 kcal/kg/day.

Although enteral tube feeding is proposed to Mr. Smith, he is very reluctant to attempt the suggested feeding methods including nasogastric tube feeding and percutaneous endoscopic gastrostomy feeding. With Mr. Smith's agreement, the multidisciplinary team decides to commence IDPN. At 5 months after starting IDPN, there is only marginal improvement in Mr. Smith's nutritional assessment parameters, and no improvement is observed for spontaneous dietary protein and energy intakes. IDPN is subsequently discontinued. After further discussion with Mr. Smith, he eventually consents to initiate enteral nutrition via nasogastric tube feeding. Subsequently, there are progressive improvements in spontaneous dietary protein and energy intakes, as well as various nutritional assessment parameters.

Case Questions and Answers

1. Is Mr. Smith presented with PEW upon initiation of peritoneal dialysis?
   Answer: Yes, PEW can emerge in early CKD, and the risk of PEW increases as CKD progresses. Mr. Smith displays signs of PEW including poor appetite, nausea, 5% weight loss over the past 3 months, moderate PEW on SGA, and mild hypoalbuminemia.

2. Compared to nondialysis-dependent CKD, what are the specific concerns with the recommendations for dietary protein and energy intakes in maintenance peritoneal dialysis?
   Answer: Compared to nondialysis-dependent CKD, higher protein and energy intakes are recommended by current evidence-based practice guidelines and expert consensus statement, that is, 1.0–1.5 g protein/kg BW/day and 25–35 kcal/kg BW/day. Every effort should be made to remove any unnecessary dietary restrictions. Education on calorie-dense foods and high biological value protein is necessary, as well as ways to improve oral intake.

3. After initiating peritoneal dialysis, should Mr. Smith aim for a dietary energy intake of 25–35 kcal/kg BW/day?
   Answer: No, Mr. Smith absorbs calories from glucose in the dialysate, and the calories provided by the peritoneal dialysate should be subtracted from 25 to 35 kcal/kg BW/day to derive the target dietary energy intake.

4. Is Mr. Smith presented with PEW at 3 months after the initiation of peritoneal dialysis?
   Answer: Mr. Smith has no obvious signs of PEW at 3 months after the initiation of peritoneal dialysis. His total protein and energy intakes are within the target requirement ranges, alongside improvements in appetite and oral intake. Although a reduction in body weight is observed, it is likely a resolution of volume overload reflected by euvolemia upon physical examination. Mr. Smith is no longer hypoalbuminemic, and his SGA score is not suggestive of PEW.

5. On the first day of his peritonitis-associated hospital admission, he was prescribed a renal menu (i.e., a menu that is protein-energy dense and low in electrolytes). Is this menu adequate as a form of nutrition support therapy? If not, what should be the next appropriate step of nutrition support and how would you optimize the outcome?
   Answer: No, the prescription of a renal menu is insufficient to meet both protein and energy requirements. This is indicated by low protein and energy intakes on the food record chart, alongside reported symptoms of nausea, poor appetite, and reduced food intake. A full nutritional assessment is required, and the use of ONS should be considered as the next appropriate step. ONS should be prescribed based on the patient's requirements, preference, compliance, and tolerance, as these are important success factors.

6. After his recovery from peritonitis, should he be discharged from the hospital with an ONS prescription?
   Answer: Yes, although Mr. Smith is meeting both protein and energy requirements, it is derived from both oral diet and the use of ONS. An oral diet alone remains insufficient to attain the requirements. Mr. Smith is displaying signs of PEW including 6% unintentional weight loss over the past 3 months, hypoalbuminemia, and moderate PEW on SGA. Regular nutritional assessment and continuous dietary counseling are essential after the initiation of hemodialysis.

7. Should the use of ONS be discontinued at 2–3 months after transition to hemodialysis?
   Answer: Yes, the use of ONS should be discontinued, because his nutritional status has improved with no obvious signs of PEW. He is attaining both protein and energy targets without the use of ONS.

8. Mr. Smith was prescribed a trial of renal-specific ONS during the episode of pneumonia-associated hospitalization. Should he continue to take the ONS after hospital discharge?

   Answer: Yes, ONS should be continued upon hospital discharge, because Mr. Smith is displaying signs of PEW including unintentional weight loss, temporal wasting on physical examination, moderate PEW on SGA, and hypoalbuminemia. His spontaneous dietary protein and energy intakes are insufficient to meet protein and energy requirements, but both intakes are higher than the required minimum for ONS to be effective (e.g., 20–24 kcal/kg/day and 0.8–1.0 g protein/kg/day). Regular monitoring and intensive nutrition counseling are critical during the supplementation period. Implementing changes to the ONS prescription may be necessary to improve Mr. Smith's adherence and hence the overall effectiveness of ONS.

9. Despite liberalization of his diet and the use of ONS, his nutritional status continues to decline. Is Mr. Smith an ideal candidate for enteral tube feeding?

   Answer: Yes, Mr. Smith is an ideal candidate for enteral tube feeding. He is exhibiting severe PEW on SGA, hypoalbuminemia, and unintentional weight loss of 7% over the past 3 months. His spontaneous dietary protein and energy intakes are <0.8 g/kg/day and <20 kcal/kg/day. Continuation of ONS and nutrition counseling are unlikely to achieve the recommended dietary protein and energy requirements. Daily nutrition support is important for Mr. Smith, and enteral nutrition should always be preferable to parenteral nutrition as feeding through the gastrointestinal tract helps to maintain its normal structure and function.

10. Should IDPN be discontinued after a trial period of 5 months?

    Answer: Yes, most maintenance hemodialysis patients respond to IDPN after 3–6 months of therapy. Lack of improvement after 3–6 months should render a decision to discontinue.

References

1. Carrero JJ, Stenvinkel P, Cuppari L, Ikizler TA, Kalantar-Zadeh K, Kaysen G, et al. Etiology of the protein-energy wasting syndrome in chronic kidney disease: a consensus statement from the International Society of Renal Nutrition and Metabolism (ISRNM). J Ren Nutr. 2013;23(2):77–90.
2. Kovesdy CP, Kopple JD, Kalantar-Zadeh K. Management of protein-energy wasting in non-dialysis-dependent chronic kidney disease: reconciling low protein intake with nutritional therapy. Am J Clin Nutr. 2013;97(6):1163–77.
3. Lodebo BT, Shah A, Kopple JD. Is it important to prevent and treat protein-energy wasting in chronic kidney disease and chronic dialysis patients? J Ren Nutr. 2018;28(6):369–79.
4. Fouque D, Kalantar-Zadeh K, Kopple J, Cano N, Chauveau P, Cuppari L, et al. A proposed nomenclature and diagnostic criteria for protein-energy wasting in acute and chronic kidney disease. Kidney Int. 2008;73(4):391–8.
5. Carrero JJ, Thomas F, Nagy K, Arogundade F, Avesani CM, Chan M, et al. Global prevalence of protein-energy wasting in kidney disease: ameta-analysis of contemporary observational studies from the International Society of Renal Nutrition and Metabolism. J Ren Nutr. 2018;28(6):380–92.
6. Chertow GM, Johansen KL, Lew N, Lazarus JM, Lowrie EG. Vintage, nutritional status, and survival in hemodialysis patients. Kidney Int. 2000;57(3):1176–81.
7. den Hoedt CH, Bots ML, Grooteman MP, van der Weerd NC, Penne EL, Mazairac AH, et al. Clinical predictors of decline in nutritional parameters over time in ESRD. Clin J Am Soc Nephrol. 2014;9(2):318–25.
8. Avram MM, Mittman N, Fein PA, Agahiu S, Hartman W, Chattopadhyay N, et al. Dialysis vintage, body composition, and survival in peritoneal dialysis patients. Adv Perit Dial. 2012;28:144–7.
9. Sabatino A, Regolisti G, Karupaiah T, Sahathevan S, Sadu Singh BK, Khor BH, et al. Protein-energy wasting and nutritional supplementation in patients with end-stage renal disease on hemodialysis. Clin Nutr. 2017;36(3):663–71.
10. Ikizler TA, Cano NJ, Franch H, Fouque D, Himmelfarb J, Kalantar-Zadeh K, et al. Prevention and treatment of protein energy wasting in chronic kidney disease patients: a consensus statement by the International Society of Renal Nutrition and Metabolism. Kidney Int. 2013;84(6):1096–107.
11. Cano NJ. Chapter 39: Oral and enteral supplements in kidney disease and kidney failure. In: Nutritional management of renal disease. Amsterdam: Elsevier; 2013. p. 659–72.
12. Lindholm B, Wang T, Heimburger O, Bergstrom J. Influence of different treatments and schedules on the factors conditioning the nutritional status in dialysis patients. Nephrol Dial Transplant. 1998;13(Suppl 6):66–73.

13. Laville M, Fouque D. Nutritional aspects in hemodialysis. Kidney Int. 2000;58:S133–S9.
14. Velloso MS, Otoni A, de Paula SA, de Castro WV, Pinto SW, Marinho MA, et al. Peritoneal dialysis and inflammation. Clinica chimica acta. Int JClin Chem. 2014;430:109–14.
15. Cano N, Fiaccadori E, Tesinsky P, Toigo G, Druml W, Kuhlmann M, et al. ESPEN guidelines on enteral nutrition: adult renal failure. Clin Nutr. 2006;25(2):295–310.
16. Ikizler TA, Burrowes J, Byham-Gray L, Campbell K, Carrero JJ, Chan W, et al. KDOQI Nutrition in CKD Guideline Work Group. KDOQI clinical practice guideline for nutrition in CKD: 2020 update. Am J Kidney Dis. 2020; in press.
17. Fouque D, Vennegoor M, ter Wee P, Wanner C, Basci A, Canaud B, et al. EBPG guideline on nutrition. Nephrol Dial Transplant. 2007;22(Suppl 2):ii45–87.
18. Dombros N, Dratwa M, Feriani M, Gokal R, Heimburger O, Krediet R, et al. European best practice guidelines for peritoneal dialysis. 8 Nutrition in peritoneal dialysis. Nephrol Dial Transplant. 2005;20(Suppl 9):ix28–33.
19. Blumenkrantz MJ, Gahl GM, Kopple JD, Kamdar AV, Jones MR, Kessel M, et al. Protein losses during peritoneal dialysis. Kidney Int. 1981;19(4):593–602.
20. Shah A, Bross R, Shapiro BB, Morrison G, Kopple JD. Dietary energy requirements in relatively healthy maintenance hemodialysis patients estimated from long-term metabolic studies. Am J Clin Nutr. 2016;103(3):757–65.
21. Leon JB, Majerle AD, Soinski JA, Kushner I, Ohri-Vachaspati P, Sehgal AR. Can a nutrition intervention improve albumin levels among hemodialysis patients? A pilot study. J Ren Nutr. 2001;11(1):9–15.
22. Prasad N, Gupta A, Sinha A, Sharma RK, Kumar A, Kumar R. Changes in nutritional status on follow-up of an incident cohort of continuous ambulatory peritoneal dialysis patients. J Ren Nutr. 2008;18(2):195–201.
23. Shinaberger CS, Greenland S, Kopple JD, Van Wyck D, Mehrotra R, Kovesdy CP, et al. Is controlling phosphorus by decreasing dietary protein intake beneficial or harmful in persons with chronic kidney disease? Am J Clin Nutr. 2008;88(6):1511–8.
24. Cupisti A, Kalantar-Zadeh K. Management of natural and added dietary phosphorus burden in kidney disease. Semin Nephrol. 2013;33(2):180–90.
25. Moe SM, Zidehsarai MP, Chambers MA, Jackman LA, Radcliffe JS, Trevino LL, et al. Vegetarian compared with meat dietary protein source and phosphorus homeostasis in chronic kidney disease. Clin J Am Soc Nephrol. 2011;6(2):257–64.
26. Chen X, Wei G, Jalili T, Metos J, Giri A, Cho ME, et al. The associations of plant protein intake with all-cause mortality in CKD. Am J Kidney Dis. 2016;67(3):423–30.
27. D'Alessandro C, Piccoli GB, Cupisti A. The "phosphorus pyramid": a visual tool for dietary phosphate management in dialysis and CKD patients. BMC Nephrol. 2015;16:9.
28. Cano NJ, Aparicio M, Brunori G, Carrero JJ, Cianciaruso B, Fiaccadori E, et al. ESPEN guidelines on parenteral nutrition: adult renal failure. Clin Nutr. 2009;28(4):401–14.
29. Veeneman JM, Kingma HA, Boer TS, Stellaard F, De Jong PE, Reijngoud DJ, et al. Protein intake during hemodialysis maintains a positive whole body protein balance in chronic hemodialysis patients. Am J Physiol Endocrinol Metab. 2003;284(5):E954–65.
30. Pupim LB, Majchrzak KM, Flakoll PJ, Ikizler TA. Intradialytic oral nutrition improves protein homeostasis in chronic hemodialysis patients with deranged nutritional status. J Am Soc Nephrol. 2006;17(11):3149–57.
31. Calegari A, Barros EG, Veronese FV, Thome FS. Malnourished patients on hemodialysis improve after receiving a nutritional intervention. J Bras Nefrol. 2011;33(4):394–401.
32. Wilson B, Fernandez-Madrid A, Hayes A, Hermann K, Smith J, Wassell A. Comparison of the effects of two early intervention strategies on the health outcomes of malnourished hemodialysis patients. J Ren Nutr. 2001;11(3):166–71.
33. Fouque D, McKenzie J, de Mutsert R, Azar R, Teta D, Plauth M, et al. Use of a renal-specific oral supplement by haemodialysis patients with low protein intake does not increase the need for phosphate binders and may prevent a decline in nutritional status and quality of life. Nephrol Dial Transplant. 2008;23(9):2902–10.
34. Hung SC, Tarng DC. Adiposity and insulin resistance in nondiabetic hemodialysis patients: effects of high energy supplementation. Am J Clin Nutr. 2009;90(1):64–9.
35. Cano NJ, Fouque D, Roth H, Aparicio M, Azar R, Canaud B, et al. Intradialytic parenteral nutrition does not improve survival in malnourished hemodialysis patients: a 2-year multicenter, prospective, randomized study. J Am Soc Nephrol. 2007;18(9):2583–91.
36. Hiroshige K, Sonta T, Suda T, Kanegae K, Ohtani A. Oral supplementation of branched-chain amino acid improves nutritional status in elderly patients on chronic haemodialysis. Nephrol Dial Transplant. 2001;16(9):1856–62.
37. Bolasco P, Caria S, Cupisti A, Secci R, Saverio DF. A novel amino acids oral supplementation in hemodialysis patients: a pilot study. Ren Fail. 2011;33(1):1–5.
38. Tomayko EJ, Kistler BM, Fitschen PJ, Wilund KR. Intradialytic protein supplementation reduces inflammation and improves physical function in maintenance hemodialysis patients. J Ren Nutr. 2015;25(3):276–83.
39. Allman MA, Stewart PM, Tiller DJ, Horvath JS, Duggin GG, Truswell AS. Energy supplementation and the nutritional status of hemodialysis patients. Am J Clin Nutr. 1990;51(4):558–62.

40. Moretti HD, Johnson AM, Keeling-Hathaway TJ. Effects of protein supplementation in chronic hemodialysis and peritoneal dialysis patients. J Ren Nutr. 2009;19(4):298–303.
41. Cheu C, Pearson J, Dahlerus C, Lantz B, Chowdhury T, Sauer PF, et al. Association between oral nutritional supplementation and clinical outcomes among patients with ESRD. Clin J Am Soc Nephrol. 2013;8(1):100–7.
42. Scott MK, Shah NA, Vilay AM, Thomas J 3rd, Kraus MA, Mueller BA. Effects of peridialytic oral supplements on nutritional status and quality of life in chronic hemodialysis patients. J Ren Nutr. 2009;19(2):145–52.
43. Sezer S, Bal Z, Tutal E, Uyar ME, Acar NO. Long-term oral nutrition supplementation improves outcomes in malnourished patients with chronic kidney disease on hemodialysis. JPEN J Parenter Enteral Nutr. 2014;38(8):960–5.
44. Teixido-Planas J, Ortiz A, Coronel F, Montenegro J, Lopez-Menchero R, Ortiz R, et al. Oral protein-energy supplements in peritoneal dialysis: a multicenter study. Perit Dial Int. 2005;25(2):163–72.
45. Gonzalez-Espinoza L, Gutierrez-Chavez J, del Campo FM, Martinez-Ramirez HR, Cortes-Sanabria L, Rojas-Campos E, et al. Randomized, open label, controlled clinical trial of oral administration of an egg albumin-based protein supplement to patients on continuous ambulatory peritoneal dialysis. Perit Dial Int. 2005;25(2):173–80.
46. Lacson E Jr, Wang W, Zebrowski B, Wingard R, Hakim RM. Outcomes associated with intradialytic oral nutritional supplements in patients undergoing maintenance hemodialysis: a quality improvement report. Am J Kidney Dis. 2012;60(4):591–600.
47. Ricanati ES, Tserng KY, Kalhan SC. Glucose metabolism in chronic renal failure: adaptive responses to continuous glucose infusion. Kidney Int Suppl. 1983;16:S121–7.
48. Schneeweiss B, Graninger W, Stockenhuber F, Druml W, Ferenci P, Eichinger S, et al. Energy metabolism in acute and chronic renal failure. Am J Clin Nutr. 1990;52(4):596–601.
49. Kalantar-Zadeh K, Ikizler TA. Let them eat during dialysis: an overlooked opportunity to improve outcomes in maintenance hemodialysis patients. J Ren Nutr. 2013;23(3):157–63.
50. Kistler BM, Benner D, Burrowes JD, Campbell KL, Fouque D, Garibotto G, et al. Eating during hemodialysis treatment: aconsensus statement from the International Society of Renal Nutrition and Metabolism. J Ren Nutr. 2018;28(1):4–12.
51. Choi MS, Kistler B, Wiese GN, Stremke ER, Wright AJ, Moorthi RN, et al. Pilot study of the effects of high-protein meals during hemodialysis on intradialytic hypotension in patients undergoing maintenance hemodialysis. J Ren Nutr. 2019;29(2):102–11.
52. Cano NJM, Heng A-E. Nutritional problems in adult patients with stage 5 chronic kidney disease on dialysis (both haemodialysis and peritoneal dialysis). NDT Plus. 2009;3(2):109–17.
53. Patel MG, Raftery MJ. Successful percutaneous endoscopic gastrostomy feeding in continuous ambulatory peritoneal dialysis. J Ren Nutr. 1997;7(4):208–11.
54. Fein PA, Madane SJ, Jorden A, Babu K, Mushnick R, Avram MM, et al. Outcome of percutaneous endoscopic gastrostomy feeding in patients on peritoneal dialysis. Adv Perit Dial. 2001;17:148–52.
55. Paudel K, Fan SL. Successful use of continuous ambulatory peritoneal dialysis in 2 adults with a gastrostomy. Am J Kidney Dis. 2014;64(2):316–7.
56. Rubin J. Nutritional support during peritoneal dialysis-related peritonitis. Am J Kidney Dis. 1990;15(6):551–5.
57. de Freitas D, Jordaan A, Williams R, Alderdice J, Curwell J, Hurst H, et al. Nutritional management of patients undergoing surgery following diagnosis with encapsulating peritoneal sclerosis. Perit Dial Int. 2008;28(3):271–6.
58. Sayce HA, Rowe PA, McGonigle RJS. Percutaneous endoscopic gastrostomy feeding in haemodialysis out-patients. J Hum Nutr Diet. 2000;13(5):333–41.
59. Holley JL, Kirk J. Enteral tube feeding in a cohort of chronic hemodialysis patients. J Ren Nutr. 2002;12(3):177–82.
60. Brown RO, Compher C. A.S.P.E.N. clinical guidelines: nutrition support in adult acute and chronic renal failure. JPEN J Parenter Enteral Nutr. 2010;34(4):366–77.
61. Sabatino A, Regolisti G, Antonucci E, Cabassi A, Morabito S, Fiaccadori E. Intradialytic parenteral nutrition in end-stage renal disease: practical aspects, indications and limits. J Nephrol. 2014;27(4):377–83.
62. Hoffer LJ. How much protein do parenteral amino acid mixtures provide? Am J Clin Nutr. 2011;94(6):1396–8.
63. Pupim LB, Flakoll PJ, Brouillette JR, Levenhagen DK, Hakim RM, Ikizler TA. Intradialytic parenteral nutrition improves protein and energy homeostasis in chronic hemodialysis patients. J Clin Invest. 2002;110(4):483–92.
64. Pupim LB, Flakoll PJ, Ikizler TA. Nutritional supplementation acutely increases albumin fractional synthetic rate in chronic hemodialysis patients. J Am Soc Nephrol. 2004;15(7):1920–6.
65. Pupim LB, Flakoll PJ, Levenhagen DK, Ikizler TA. Exercise augments the acute anabolic effects of intradialytic parenteral nutrition in chronic hemodialysis patients. Am J Physiol Endocrinol Metab. 2004;286(4):E589–97.

66. Ikizler TA, Pupim LB, Brouillette JR, Levenhagen DK, Farmer K, Hakim RM, et al. Hemodialysis stimulates muscle and whole body protein loss and alters substrate oxidation. Am J Physiol Endocrinol Metab. 2002;282(1):E107–16.
67. Guarnieri G, Faccini L, Lipartiti T, Ranieri F, Spangaro F, Giuntini D, et al. Simple methods for nutritional assessment in hemodialyzed patients. Am J Clin Nutr. 1980;33(7):1598–607.
68. Cano N, Labastie-Coeyrehourq J, Lacombe P, Stroumza P, di Costanzo-Dufetel J, Durbec JP, et al. Perdialytic parenteral nutrition with lipids and amino acids in malnourished hemodialysis patients. Am J Clin Nutr. 1990;52(4):726–30.
69. Navarro JF, Mora C, Leon C, Martin-Del Rio R, Macia ML, Gallego E, et al. Amino acid losses during hemodialysis with polyacrylonitrile membranes: effect of intradialytic amino acid supplementation on plasma amino acid concentrations and nutritional variables in nondiabetic patients. Am J Clin Nutr. 2000;71(3):765–73.
70. Cano NJ, Saingra Y, Dupuy AM, Lorec-Penet AM, Portugal H, Lairon D, et al. Intradialytic parenteral nutrition: comparison of olive oil versus soybean oil-based lipid emulsions. Br J Nutr. 2006;95(1):152–9.
71. Marsen TA, Beer J, Mann H. Intradialytic parenteral nutrition in maintenance hemodialysis patients suffering from protein-energy wasting. Results of a multicenter, open, prospective, randomized trial. Clin Nutr. 2017;36(1):107–17.
72. Hiroshige K, Iwamoto M, Kabashima N, Mutoh Y, Yuu K, Ohtani A. Prolonged use of intradialysis parenteral nutrition in elderly malnourished chronic haemodialysis patients. Nephrol Dial Transplant. 1998;13(8):2081–7.
73. Toigo G, Situlin R, Tamaro G, Del Bianco A, Giuliani V, Dardi F, et al. Effect of intravenous supplementation of a new essential amino acid formulation in hemodialysis patients. Kidney Int Suppl. 1989;27:S278–81.
74. Cranford W. Cost effectiveness of IDPN therapy measured by hospitalizations and length of stay. Nephrol News Issues. 1998;12(9):33–5, 7–9.
75. Gosmanov AR, Umpierrez GE. Management of hyperglycemia during enteral and parenteral nutrition therapy. Curr Diab Rep. 2013;13(1):155–62.
76. Moore E. Challenges of nutrition intervention for malnourished dialysis patients. J Infus Nurs. 2008;31(6):361–6.
77. Sarav M, Friedman AN. Use of intradialytic parenteral nutrition in patients undergoing hemodialysis. Nutr Clin Pract. 2018;33(6):767–71.
78. Kopple JD, Bernard D, Messana J, Swartz R, Bergstrom J, Lindholm B, et al. Treatment of malnourished CAPD patients with an amino acid based dialysate. Kidney Int. 1995;47(4):1148–57.
79. Li FK, Chan LY, Woo JC, Ho SK, Lo WK, Lai KN, et al. A 3-year, prospective, randomized, controlled study on amino acid dialysate in patients on CAPD. Am J Kidney Dis. 2003;42(1):173–83.
80. Jones M, Hagen T, Boyle CA, Vonesh E, Hamburger R, Charytan C, et al. Treatment of malnutrition with 1.1% amino acid peritoneal dialysis solution: results of a multicenter outpatient study. Am J Kidney Dis. 1998;32(5):761–9.
81. Misra M, Reaveley DA, Ashworth J, Muller B, Seed M, Brown EA. Six-month prospective cross-over study to determine the effects of 1.1% amino acid dialysate on lipid metabolism in patients on continuous ambulatory peritoneal dialysis. Perit Dial Int. 1997;17(3):279–86.
82. Tjiong HL, Swart R, Van den Berg JW, Fieren MW. Dialysate as food as an option for automated peritoneal dialysis. NDT Plus. 2008;1(Suppl 4):iv36–40.
83. Tjiong HL, van den Berg JW, Wattimena JL, Rietveld T, van Dijk LJ, van der Wiel AM, et al. Dialysate as food: combined amino acid and glucose dialysate improves protein anabolism in renal failure patients on automated peritoneal dialysis. J Am Soc Nephrol. 2005;16(5):1486.
84. Tjiong HL, Rietveld T, Wattimena JL, van den Berg JW, Kahriman D, van der Steen J, et al. Peritoneal dialysis with solutions containing amino acids plus glucose promotes protein synthesis during oral feeding. Clin J Am Soc Nephrol. 2007;2(1):74.
85. Garibotto G, Sofia A, Canepa A, Saffioti S, Sacco P, Sala M, et al. Acute effects of peritoneal dialysis with dialysates containing dextrose or dextrose and amino acids on muscle protein turnover in patients with chronic renal failure. J Am Soc Nephrol. 2001;12(3):557–67.
86. Wolfson M, Jones M. Intraperitoneal nutrition. Am J Kidney Dis. 1999;33(1):203–4.
87. Delarue J, Maingourd C, Objois M, Pinault M, Cohen R, Couet C, et al. Effects of an amino acid dialysate on leucine metabolism in continuous ambulatory peritoneal dialysis patients. Kidney Int. 1999;56(5):1934–43.
88. Park MS, Choi SR, Song YS, Yoon SY, Lee SY, Han DS. New insight of amino acid-based dialysis solutions. Kidney Int. 2006;70:S110–S4.
89. Tjiong HL, Swart R, van den Berg JW, Fieren MW. Amino acid-based peritoneal dialysis solutions for malnutrition: new perspectives. Perit Dial Int. 2009;29(4):384–93.
90. Dombros N, Dratwa M, Feriani M, Gokal R, Heimburger O, Krediet R, et al. European best practice guidelines for peritoneal dialysis. 5 Peritoneal dialysis solutions. Nephrol Dial Transplant. 2005;20(Suppl 9):ix16–20.

Chapter 18
Kidney Transplantation

Daniel Pieloch

Keywords Kidney · Transplant · Transplantation · Nutrition · Dietitian · Medical nutrition therapy Immunosuppression · Obesity · Education · Diabetes · Protein · Energy

---

Key Points
- Nutritional management of kidney transplant candidates and recipients continues to evolve with advancements in immunosuppression, revised transplant regulations, standardization of practice, and further research in transplant nutrition.
- Transplant regulations now mandate that a registered dietitian be part of the multidisciplinary transplant team in all phases of transplant (pre-, peri-, and post).
- Competencies for dietitians practicing in kidney transplantation have been recently established and further define the scope and role that nutrition plays in all three phases of transplant.

  - Pretransplant: To provide medical nutrition therapy (MNT) for candidates with nutrition risk factors that impact transplant outcomes and to provide nutrition clearance or risk stratification for transplant listing.
  - Peritransplant: To perform nutrition assessments, manage postsurgical nutrition needs, and provide posttransplant diet education.
  - Posttransplant: To provide MNT to optimize kidney allograft function and improve patient survival. Hyperglycemia and hypophosphatemia are common findings early posttransplantation (1–8 weeks). Weight gain, new-onset diabetes, bone disease, diarrhea, and progression of CKD are often found late posttransplantation (>8 weeks).

Introduction

The kidney was the first human organ to be transplanted successfully in 1954. With advances in immunosuppressive therapy and surgical techniques that lead to better long-term survival and improved quality of life, kidney transplantation is now considered the preferred treatment option for most patients with advanced chronic kidney disease (CKD).

The editors acknowledge Maureen P. McCarthy's contribution to this chapter in *Nutrition in Kidney Disease, Second Edition*, Nutrition and Health, DOI 10.1007/978-1-62703-685-6_1, © Springer Science+Business Media New York 2014

D. Pieloch (✉)
Robert Wood Johnson University Hospital, Transplant Center, RWJ Barnabas Health, New Brunswick, NJ, USA
e-mail: Daniel.pieloch@rwjbh.org

There are roughly 96,000 candidates waiting to receive a kidney transplant on the United Network for Organ Sharing (UNOS) waiting list [1]. Over 30,000 patients were added to the waiting list in 2016, while approximately 19,000 received a kidney transplant [1]. Every year, thousands of kidney transplant candidates die on the waiting list or are removed for no longer being an acceptable transplant candidate. In 2016, close to 14,000 kidney transplant candidates were removed from the UNOS waitlist for these reasons [1].

Living donation is considered the best transplant option as it portends higher patient and graft survival rates compared to deceased donation. Unfortunately, while the number of patients requiring a kidney transplant continues to climb, the rate of kidney transplantation from living donation remains flat [1]. Less than 30% of all kidney transplants come from living donors [1]. Because of the overall shortage in donor organs, waiting times for deceased donor kidneys continues to be long. Waiting times drastically vary by geographic region with an estimated 5-year wait-time ranging between 15.7% and 90.9% of recipients, depending on the donation service area [1].

The purpose of this chapter is to provide an up-to-date and practical resource for clinicians providing nutritional care to kidney transplant candidates and recipients. This includes information on nutrition assessment, the nutritional impact of induction and maintenance immunosuppressive medications, transplant-specific nutrition education, macro- and micronutrient recommendations, and common nutritional findings in all three phases of transplantation (pre, peri, and post).

Kidney Transplant Nutrition

The role that nutrition plays in kidney transplant candidates and recipients significantly expanded with the conditions set forth by the Centers for Medicare and Medicaid Services (CMS) in 2007. CMS mandated that nutrition services be an essential component of the transplant process. These regulations now require that a registered dietitian be part of a multidisciplinary transplant team in all phases of transplant including the pretransplant evaluation, the transplant surgery admission, and posttransplant after discharge [2].

Prior to the establishment of these regulations, it is estimated that only 59% of transplant programs involved dietitians in the care of their kidney transplant recipients and often only during the transplant surgery admission [3]. Although CMS sets forth minimum nutrition requirements, they do not prescribe specific nutrition practice [3]. Over the last decade, kidney transplant programs and dietitians established varying practices in the nutritional management of transplant candidates and recipients in part due to limited research and lack of formal established guidelines in transplant nutrition.

In 2017, a *Framework for Standardized Transplant Specific Competencies* was published for dietitians practicing in all solid organ transplants [3]. These competencies were developed based on the revised transplant regulations, transplant dietitian survey research, and agreement from experts in the field of transplant nutrition. The competencies highlight several key areas including transplant-specific MNT, the role of the transplant dietitian in each phase of transplant, quality and performance improvement, training including orientation and continuing education requirements for transplant dietitians, and general knowledge of transplant principles and regulations [3]. This framework helps set the benchmark for the role nutrition plays in the management of kidney transplant candidates and recipients.

Pretransplant Phase

According to the Organ Procurement and Transplantation Network (OPTN), adult kidney transplant candidates can only be registered on the waiting list if they have a calculated creatinine clearance or glomerular filtration rate (GFR) less than or equal to 20 mL/min [4]. Therefore, candidates initiating a kidney transplant evaluation present with advanced CKD, most already on dialysis. A kidney transplant evaluation is required to be multidisciplinary and the decision regarding transplant candidacy requires input from the transplant program's nephrologist, surgeon, nurse coordinator, social worker, and dietitian [2].

It is important to note that kidney transplant programs have become more conservative in their selection of transplant candidates since 2007, as they are held more accountable for graft and patient survival outcomes for the patients they transplant. An example of this impact was the sudden use of conservative obesity cut-offs by transplant programs nationally, which considered those who were morbidly obese too high risk for transplant [5].

Because of the rigorous process of the pretransplant evaluation, most kidney transplant candidates selected for the waiting list are generally well-nourished with relatively low nutritional risk. Since candidates can wait for years on the waiting list, programs often evaluate these candidates periodically. Yearly transplant re-evaluations are common and identify changes in medical condition and reaffirms transplant candidacy.

Since 80% of candidates are on dialysis at the time of transplant, many of these patients also have an established relationship with a dietitian at their dialysis center and receive ongoing MNT [1]. Therefore, the primary goal during the pretransplant phase is as follows [3]:

- To identify and provide MNT for those modifiable nutrition risk factors that significantly affect short- and long-term transplant outcomes
- To provide nutrition clearance or nutrition risk assessment for transplant listing
- To educate the potential recipient on the nutritional requirements for transplantation
- To introduce the posttransplant diet

Pretransplant Obesity

Obesity is the most common nutritional risk/barrier identified in the kidney transplant candidate. Most transplant programs have implemented an absolute obesity criterion for kidney transplantation, typically using body mass index (BMI) as a cutoff and can range from >32 to >42 kg/m^2. Many older studies link obesity to poor graft and patient survival [6, 7]. More recent studies show that pretransplant obesity does not impact graft or patient survival particularly for those who have been transplanted after the year 2000 [8–10]. This is true even in morbidly obese recipients [8, 10]. Some data even suggests that certain morbidly obese populations have better outcomes than many commonly transplanted normal weight recipients [8]. While higher rates of short-term complications such as delayed graft function (DGF), acute rejection, and delayed wound healing can still be linked to pretransplant obesity, long-term outcomes are unaffected [7]. Pretransplant morbid obesity does impact length of stay during the transplant admission, but no greater than many other prevalent risk factors found for transplant recipients; for example, African-American, history of coronary artery disease or diabetes, being dialysis dependent, or over the age of 50 years [11].

Improvement of outcomes seen in the obese kidney population may be due to better surgical techniques and less reliance on older immunosuppressive agents known to impact wound healing. More recently, because of this trend, obesity criterion has been relaxed with less reliance on BMI as a tool to measure that criterion by many kidney transplant programs.

Pretransplant Malnutrition

Malnutrition is common in patients with end-stage renal disease (ESRD), but acceptable transplant candidates are often healthier than that of the average ESRD patient. Not surprisingly, kidney transplant candidates with a BMI < 22 kg/m^2 have higher rates of malnutrition and portend the worse outcomes compared to all other weight groups [12]. Weight loss is inversely correlated with death on the waiting list, even in those with a BMI above 30 kg/m^2 [13]. Differentiation of intentional versus unintentional weight loss on outcomes has not been well established but unintentional weight loss is likely more concerning. Similar to the dialysis population, pretransplant serum albumin is a strong predictor of posttransplant mortality [14].

Pretransplant Diabetes

Diabetic nephropathy is the leading cause of ESRD in the United States and, therefore, it is no surprise that 46% of all kidney candidates on the waiting list have diabetes [1, 15]. While genetic predisposition, age, gender, and ethnicity play a role, uncontrolled blood glucose levels can lead to rapid recurrence of diabetic nephropathy in the allograft [16]. According to the findings of a 2019 transplant dietitian survey presented at NATCO's 8th Annual Transplant Nutrition Conference, poor glycemic control identified in the pretransplant phase is often considered an absolute contraindication to transplant with many programs utilizing a hemoglobin A1c (HbA1c) level of 8–10% or greater as an absolute cutoff (unpublished data). Glycemic control tends to worsen after transplantation in part due to the "burnt-out diabetes" effect. Although the physiology is not fully understood, it is believed that insulin renal degradation and clearance is impaired with advancing CKD [17]. Once transplanted, the new kidney can normally excrete insulin, which may be the reason why many patients with normal or prediabetic glucose levels prior to transplant develop type 2 diabetes after transplantation. Therefore, it is important to assess a patient's full understanding and compliance of their diabetes management rather than solely relying on lab values during the pretransplant evaluation, particularly if they are prediabetic or if their diabetes has improved with no intervention or poor adherence to treatment.

Peritransplant Phase

The intended transplant recipient is typically admitted to the hospital the day of surgery where the average hospital length of stay (LOS) is between 2 and 7 days [15]. The transplant surgery is performed under general anesthesia and can last between 2 and 4 hours. The kidney allograft is placed in the pelvis and the native kidneys are not typically removed unless they are the source of uncontrollable hypertension, frequent infections, or pain due to polycystic transformation.

Because kidney transplant surgery does not usually violate the abdominal cavity, diet advancement after surgery proceeds quickly. Liquid intake is often initiated within 24 hours and solid foods within 48 hours after surgery. Recipients are often adequately nourished entering surgery with any nutrition-related issues having been addressed and resolved prior to surgery. Barring any unexpected nutritional deficits or postoperative complications impacting nutrition, focus of the remaining hospital stay should be on the management of postsurgical nutrition needs and posttransplant discharge nutrition education.

Transplant regulatory requirements of the dietitian during the transplant surgery admission include, at a minimum, a nutrition assessment of the transplant recipient, documented participation in the transplant multidisciplinary care planning process, and a transplant discharge nutrition education plan [3].

Induction Therapy

Induction therapy provides a high degree of immunosuppression at the time of surgery that persists through the early-posttransplant period. Nearly all kidney transplant recipients receive induction therapy to reduce the risk of early allograft rejection [1, 18]. Many of these induction agents are biological, either monoclonal (muromonab-CD3, daclizumab, basiliximab, alemtuzumab) or polyclonal (antithymocyte globulin) antibodies. Most undergo induction with a polyclonal anti-T cell depleting antibody [1]. Nondepleting monoclonal antibodies are used in 20% of recipients, making it the second most common induction agent [1].

Inducing immunosuppression is generally associated with a slightly higher risk of infectious complications and malignancy beyond that of standard immunosuppression. Short-term adverse effects, such as fever, chills, and gastrointestinal distress, are more frequent with polyclonal antibody therapy than with other induction agents [19, 20]. However, premedication with antihistamines and acetaminophen is often given to reduce the frequency and severity of these reactions.

High-dose corticosteroid use in the early-posttransplant period, specifically methylprednisolone, remains a cornerstone of most immunosuppression regimens [15]. A commonly prescribed regimen includes 6 intravenous doses of 125 mg methylprednisolone after surgery followed by conversion to oral prednisone at a dose of 30 mg daily with a gradual taper to a maintenance dose [15].

Maintenance Therapy

Maintenance immunosuppression is essential to prevent rejection and to preserve long-term function of the allograft. Maintenance immunosuppression is a delicate balance with too much increasing the risk of infection or malignancy and too little leading to rejection and loss of graft. Most recipients receive triple therapy for maintenance immunosuppression, which includes a calcineurin inhibitor (CNI), a corticosteroid, and an antimetabolite [15].

Calcineurin Inhibitors

Calcineurin inhibitors inhibit the action of calcineurin, an enzyme that activates T-cells of the immune system, which play a key role in cell-mediated immunity. Tacrolimus remains the CNI of choice over cyclosporine as it is superior in improving graft survival and preventing acute rejection [1, 21]. Ironically, these drugs are nephrotoxic and can cause hypertension and hyperkalemia especially with high levels [22]. Hypophosphatemia and hypomagnesemia are also common findings after kidney transplantation due to CNI-induced urinary excretion of phosphate and magnesium [23]. Increased intake of foods high in phosphorous and magnesium may not be sufficient for repletion and often necessitates use of supplementation [23]. Both CNIs can cause hyperglycemia and gastrointestinal distress, but tacrolimus is associated with a higher incidence of posttransplant diabetes and gastrointestinal side effects [24, 25] .

Antiproliferative Agents

Mycophenolate is currently utilized in 95.2% of all kidney transplant recipients either in the form of mycophenolate mofetil (Cellcept®) or mycophenolate sodium (Myfortic®) [1]. Azathioprine (Imuran®) is an older agent, but it is still used in select patient populations. These antimetabolites work by inhibiting purine synthesis and T-cell proliferation with mycophenolate, additionally inhibiting B-cell proliferation [19]. The most common and well-known nutritional side effect of mycophenolate is gastrointestinal distress including nausea, vomiting, and diarrhea. Splitting the dosage into two to four intervals throughout the day has been shown to improve symptoms [19]. Azathioprine can exhibit similar side effects.

Corticosteroids

Corticosteroids have immunosuppressive, anti-inflammatory, and lympholytic effects. While some transplant programs still believe in a steroid-free approach, corticosteroid use in kidney transplantation has increased from 63.8% to 71.8% over the last decade [1]. Prednisone is the most commonly prescribed maintenance corticosteroid at a dosage of 5–10 mg daily [17]. While steroids are notorious for having negative nutritional side effects such as sodium retention, impaired wound healing, increased appetite, weight gain, hyperglycemia, and osteoporosis, among others, it is important to note that these adverse effects are believed to be dose-dependent and occur more frequently at higher dosages [19]. The side effects of long-term corticosteroid use at maintenance dose levels are not well studied and remain unclear.

m-TOR Inhibitors

The m-TOR inhibitors, sirolimus and everolimus, have declined in use over the last 15 years and are currently used in fewer than 2% of all new recipients [1]. This is likely due to concerns about increased mortality and adverse events, some nutrition-related including hyperlipidemia, anemia, mouth ulcers, and impaired wound healing [26].

Common Transplant Admission Findings

Hypophosphatemia

Several reasons exist why hypophosphatemia is common after kidney transplantation. CNI and corticosteroid use can increase renal excretion and inhibit the reabsorption of phosphate [27]. Parathyroid hormone (PTH) levels should fall after transplantation but can remain elevated in some recipients, leading to additional increases in urinary phosphate excretion [28]. Vitamin D levels may also remain low after transplantation, leading to impaired phosphate absorption from the intestine [27]. Phosphate supplements are commonly prescribed but can lead to diarrhea. K-Phos Neutral is the most palatable supplement that provides the largest dose of phosphate with the least amount of potassium [29]. The nadir in observed serum phosphate measurements is generally found 1 month after transplantation [30].

Hyperglycemia

Hyperglycemia occurs and is often sustained in most recipients during their transplant admission even in those with no history of pretransplant diabetes. The stresses of surgery and exposure to immunosuppression medications have metabolic effects that exacerbate hyperglycemia [31]. A myriad of factors, including daily immunosuppression changes, high-dose corticosteroid tapering, the diminishing metabolic effect of surgery, increasing PO intake, and improving renal function, makes optimal glycemic control difficult during this period and often requires daily adjustments to the management plan [31]. Aggressive glycemic control in the early period is not common. Perhaps the risk of hypoglycemic complications outweighs the detrimental effects of short-term hyperglycemia during this critical phase. It can take weeks to months to identify the recipient's maintenance diabetes medication regimen after transplant.

Delayed Graft Function

Once the kidney allograft is anastomosed and reperfused, urine production may rapidly commence. Immediate graft function is accompanied by a high urine output and a gradual decrease in serum blood urea nitrogen and creatinine levels over a period of days. However, slow or delayed graft function (requiring acute dialysis) may occur. This can be the result of acute tubular necrosis (ATN), an ischemic injury sustained by the kidney during organ procurement, preservation, or reperfusion [32]. ATN can be oliguric or anuric and may last for several days to weeks before recovery of renal function is observed [15]. Hypotension and hypovolemia can also cause ATN posttransplantation [32]. Other reasons for delayed graft function can include ureteral obstruction, thrombosis, early rejection or recurrent diseases such as focal segmental glomerulosclerosis (FSGS) [32].

Nutrition Requirements

Nutrition requirement recommendations for adult kidney transplant recipients are shown in Table 18.1. A paucity of research exists regarding the nutritional requirements for kidney transplant recipients. Over the years, recommendations have emerged for all solid organ transplant recipients often citing references to nontransplant patient populations [35, 36]. These recommendations are primarily based on critical care guidelines, which make them more relevant to the other types of organ recipients including heart, liver, intestine, and lung. Specific kidney transplant recommendations have been proposed but should be considered in context when incorporating into practice, as they are also similar to recommendations for critical care patients and utilize research from a different era of transplantation [29, 37–39].

Table 18.1 Daily nutrient recommendations for adult kidney transplant recipients

Nutrient	Transplant admission (first week)	Early posttransplantation (weeks 2–8)	Late posttransplantation (>8 weeks)
Protein	1.3 g/kg	1.0–1.1 g/kg	0.8 g/kg[a]
Calories	30–33 kcal/kg	25–30 kcal/kg	20–25 kcal/kg[a]
Carbohydrate calories	45–65% of total calories with emphasis on complex carbohydrates; limit from added sugars[b]		
Fat	20–35% of daily calories from fat with less than 10% from saturated fat[b]		
Sodium	2–4 g	2–4 g	2–4 g
Potassium	2–4 g if hyperkalemic[c]	2–4 g if hyperkalemic[c]	unrestricted[c]
Phosphorus	DRI[c] (may need supplementation to normalize serum levels)	DRI[c] (may need supplementation to normalize serum levels)	DRI[c]
Calcium	1200–1500 mg[c]	1200–1500 mg[c]	1200–1500 mg[c]
Other vitamins	DRI[c]	DRI[c]	DRI[c]
Other minerals	DRI[c]	DRI[c]	DRI[c]
Trace elements	DRI[c]	DRI[c]	DRI[c]
Fluid	2–4 L (may be less with slow or delayed graft function)	2–4 L (may be less with slow or delayed graft function)	2–4 L

Abbreviation: *DRI* dietary reference intake
[a]Considered approximate energy/protein requirements for most adults. Source: References [33, 34]
[b]Source: Adapted from the USDA 2015–2020 Dietary Guidelines
[c]Source: Adapted from Ref.[29]

Calories and Protein

Transplant Admission (First Week)

In the early stages, after kidney transplantation, metabolic stress and immunosuppressive drugs are believed to cause higher protein catabolism rates and increased energy expenditure, but this is not well studied. Previously accepted energy and protein recommendations for kidney transplant recipients during the first week after surgery have ranged from 30 to 35 kcal/kg/day and 1.3–2.0 g/kg protein/day, similar to that of other solid organ recipients who require more extensive surgery, longer recovery periods, and where pretransplant malnutrition is more prevalent [29, 35–39].

In contrast, kidney transplant recipients are generally well nourished entering surgery, spend less than 24 hours in the intensive care unit, and are discharged within a few days. This may make energy and protein requirements in the first few days after kidney transplantation more similar to that of patients undergoing elective surgery rather than critical care patients undergoing surgery, particularly as surgical techniques and immunosuppression management has evolved over the years.

A study by Tannus et al. using indirect calorimetry showed that a 2- to 3-hour elective surgery does not result in increased energy expenditure 24 hours postoperatively [40]. However, a direct correlation between elective surgery and kidney transplantation is inappropriate as induction corticosteroid therapy alone is believed to impact energy and protein needs, although as to what degree has not been carefully studied.

A precyclosporine era study of eight kidney transplant recipients experiencing DGF requiring hemodialysis for at least a week showed that intake of 33 kcal/kg and 1.3 g pro/kg daily achieved neutral nitrogen balance after 10–14 days of high-dose corticosteroids (starting at 120 mg/day and tapered to 70–90 mg/day) during the hospital admission [41].

It is also important to note that the high calorie and protein requirements of dialysis patients decreases almost immediately upon the recovery of renal function and is quickly followed by a general improvement in overall nutritional status [42]. Therefore, protein and energy needs during the transplant admission should decline fairly quickly as renal function improves, corticosteroids are weaned, and surgical stress abates.

To date, there is insufficient information to validate energy and protein recommendations for kidney transplant recipients in the modern age of transplantation. Therefore, based on available data, it is this author's opinion that calorie and protein needs during the transplant admission may be more appropriately estimated at 30–33 kcal/kg/day and 1.3 g protein/kg/day for an uncomplicated kidney transplant recipient. This equates to 30–50% higher energy needs and 60% higher protein needs compared to a normal healthy adult. It is important to note that few kidney transplant recipients will be able to reach these moderate calorie and protein levels in the first few days after surgery when nutritional needs are likely the highest.

Early Posttransplantation (Weeks 2–8)

Kidney transplant recipients are usually discharged 2–7 days after surgery when renal function improves enough whereby serum creatinine starts to plateau or decline, fluid and electrolyte balance is controlled, and the recipient is clinically stable [19]. Energy and protein recommendations for kidney transplant recipients during the early posttransplantation period have ranged from 30 to 35 kcal/kg and from 1.3 to 2.0 g pro/kg daily [29, 35–39]. However, at the time of discharge, it is estimated that resting energy expenditure (REE) is only 7% higher in kidney transplant recipients compared to that of a normal healthy adult [43].

Protein needs remain higher in the early posttransplantation period as intake less than 1 g/kg/day in the first 28 days after kidney transplantation (i.e., when high-dose corticosteroids are progressively reduced) can lead to negative nitrogen balance and muscle mass loss [44, 45]. However, protein intakes of 1.3–2.0 g pro/kg/day may be excessive in the early posttransplantation period.

Upon discharge, the surgical wound may take 4–8 weeks to heal and renal function usually optimizes within 3 months after transplantation. Based on the information above, this author believes that after discharge, a 20–25% increase in energy and 25–40% increase in protein needs seem appropriate to remain in positive nitrogen balance until the surgical wound has healed and corticosteroids are minimized. This also appears to be more in line with current practice. Therefore, calorie and protein needs during this time can be estimated at 25–30 kcal/kg/day and 1.0–1.1 g protein/kg/day, respectively.

Late Posttransplantation (>8 Weeks)

Once the surgical wound has healed and the effects of induction corticosteroids have weaned, a kidney transplant recipient without other complication factors has an REE very similar to that of a normal healthy adult [43, 46]. Therefore, calorie and protein needs can be estimated at 20–25 kcal/kg/day and 0.8 g protein/kg/day in the late posttransplantation phase but should be adjusted so the recipient achieves or maintains a healthy weight [33, 34].

Carbohydrate and Fat

Limited research to date has been performed on carbohydrate and fat intake in the kidney transplant population. Therefore, it is recommended that adult kidney transplant recipients follow the 2015–2020 Dietary Guidelines for Americans by consuming between 20% and 35% of daily calories from fat with less than 10% from saturated fat and a carbohydrate intake of 45–65% of total calories [47]. Higher than recommended fat intake is associated with dyslipidemia, hypertension, and cardiovascular disease, while excessive carbohydrate intake is linked to hyperglycemia and impaired wound healing [48, 49].

Sodium

A sodium restriction has not been shown to improve graft function or reduce mortality in stable kidney transplant recipients; therefore, it has been suggested that a sodium restriction be instituted only in the presence of hypertension, allograft dysfunction, or fluid retention [50]. Still a conservative daily sodium intake of 2–4 g per day should be considered for all kidney transplant recipients as hypertension is the most common posttransplant complication occurring in 90% of recipients [51]. Maintenance-dose corticosteroids may cause fluid retention. As such, sodium restriction of 3 g/day with a normal amount of protein intake has been shown to stabilize kidney function in transplant recipients [52].

Vitamins, Minerals, and Trace Elements

Hypophosphatemia and hypomagnesemia are well-known complications in the early transplant period, and they are monitored frequently and often require supplementation. Other micronutrients have not been well studied in the kidney transplant population, but it is believed that most recipients take in adequate amounts. Supporting this theory is a recent study of 584 kidney recipients transplanted in North America showing that nearly all recipients are sufficient in folate and vitamin B12 [53]. Also, many programs continue to recommend a general multivitamin after transplant. Vitamin and mineral recommendations for kidney transplant recipients should generally comply with Dietary Reference Intake (DRI) guidelines.

Common Posttransplant Findings

Posttransplant Weight Gain

Much emphasis is placed on pretransplant obesity, but posttransplant weight gain is significantly more influential on graft and patient survival outcomes [54]. Weight gain after kidney transplant is epidemic. In fact, the average kidney transplant recipients start out overweight and gains greater than 10% of their body weight in the first year after transplantation [55]. Kidney recipients who gain weight after transplantation simultaneously show measurable reductions in lean body mass [56].

After successful transplantation, a feeling of well-being, improved physical and psychological quality of life, and long-term corticosteroid use are often anecdotally cited as the cause for weight gain. Recipients often blame their weight gain on steroid induced hyperphagia; however, low-dose corticosteroid does not cause weight gain in the modern era of kidney transplantation [57, 58].

Weight gain caused by reduced metabolic needs after transplantation tend to be underreported. Compared to receiving maintenance dialysis, kidney transplant recipients require roughly a third less daily calories. Reduction in one's typical caloric intake is difficult; therefore, it should be a major focus of posttransplant diet education.

Interestingly, recipients who gain weight compared to those with stable weight after transplant have similar energy and macronutrient intakes but lower daily physical activity [56]. This suggests physical activity plays an important role in successful weight loss after transplantation. However, a false perception exists among recipients that exercise may harm their transplant [57]. In one study, a dietary regimen of a 25 kcal/kg/day and 0.8 g pro/kg/day, low sodium, low cholesterol, and increased physical activity resulted in a 4–11% reduction in body weight 1 year after kidney transplantation [59].

Weight loss is challenging after kidney transplantation even with intensive nutrition intervention [55]. Therefore, the importance of weight management and physical activity should be addressed early during the pretransplant phase, particularly stressing the impact both have on transplant outcomes.

Posttransplant Diabetes

Diabetes is a major concern posttransplant and its incidence is reported to be as high as 46% in candidates prior to transplantation with an additional 20% developing new-onset diabetes mellitus after transplantation (NODAT) [1, 56]. In the early transplant period, high-dose corticosteroids and the stress response from surgery are well-known causes of hyperglycemia, but the impact of low-dose maintenance corticosteroids on diabetes is controversial. While large retrospective studies have found that a steroid-free program reduces the odds of developing NODAT, the only prospective, double-blind, randomized, placebo-controlled study showed that early withdrawal of corticosteroids also has little impact on NODAT [60, 61].

Calcineurin inhibitors, utilized in most immunosuppression regimens, are linked to insulin resistance and reduced glucose delivery and thus associated with impaired fasting glucose and the development of NODAT [54, 62, 63]. An underreported cause of worsening blood glucose levels and NODAT may be the normalization of insulin degradation and excretion with the return of renal function after transplant.

Physical activity has been shown to improve blood glucose levels in the kidney transplant population and should be strongly encouraged [64]. Posttransplant weight gain is also linked to the development of diabetes and other comorbidities; therefore, weight management strategies should be made a priority [65]. Lastly, until evidence emerges specific to the kidney transplant population, recipients should be advised to follow guidelines for the management of type 2 diabetes in the general population [65].

Bone Disease

Bone disease is common in kidney transplant recipients and may progress rapidly within the first 2 years [54]. The pathophysiology is multifactorial including preexisting renal osteodystrophy, bone loss related to immunosuppression, alterations in vitamin D and parathyroid levels, and changes in mineral metabolism [66, 67]. Contemporary immunosuppression regimens have lowered fracture rates in kidney transplant recipients and are less than that of comparable patients who remain on dialysis, but the overall risk remains high [68, 69]. Calcium, phosphorus, and 1,25-dihydroxy vitamin D levels improve with normalizing renal function; however, a deficiency in 25-hydroxy vitamin D and elevated PTH levels often persist [67, 70]. Supplementation with both active and inactive vitamin D shows beneficial effects on bone mineral density in kidney transplant recipients with daily supplementation of 0.25–0.5 μg calcitriol (1,25-dihydroxyvitamin D) being a common recommendation [65, 67]. More effective therapy is dual supplementation with calcium and vitamin D compared to vitamin D supplementation alone [65].

Acute Kidney Injury

Acute kidney injury (AKI) is common in kidney transplant recipients, and it is associated with an increase in graft loss and mortality [71]. Transplant recipients can develop AKI for all the usual reasons, but risk factors such as having a single functioning kidney, underlying CKD, and immunosuppression are unique causes in this population. These include acute rejection, drug toxicity, infections, urinary tract obstruction, and vascular thrombosis [72].

Acute rejection occurs in up to 10% of kidney transplant recipients annually [72]. Cell-mediated rejection is treated with corticosteroids or antithymocyte globulin, while antibody-mediated rejection is mostly treated with some combination of plasmapheresis, intravenous immunoglobins (IVIG), rituximab, proteasome inhibitors, and corticosteroids [72]. Excessive CNI exposure can also cause AKI but typically resolves when holding or reducing the dosage [72].

Incidence of urinary tract infections is significantly higher in the kidney transplant population and reported to be as high as 75% in the first 2 years after kidney transplantation [73]. Pyelonephritis will develop in 19% of transplant recipients within the same time frame [73]. Contributing to this high incidence are immunosuppression, neurogenic bladder in diabetics, or small noncompliant bladders in long-standing anuric patients as well as the increased risk of reflux nephropathy from a shorter ureter [72]. Significant consequences of BK virus are often only found in the immunocompromised and the immunosuppressed patient, occurring in up to 10% of transplanted recipients and can cause nephropathy or ureteral stricture [72]. Generally, standard nutritional guidelines should be followed in the management of AKI in the kidney transplant population.

Dehydration

Adequate hydration after kidney transplant is vital to the success of the allograft. AKI caused by dehydration is often reversed with adequate hydration in normal healthy kidneys. However, kidney allografts are believed to be less resilient. Preventing volume depletion early after transplant is particularly important when maximum concentrating ability has not been achieved and CNI levels are kept higher [74].

Liberal fluid intake of 2–4 L/day is routinely recommended to kidney transplant recipients to maintain adequate renal perfusion. Although high fluid intake is thought to have a protective effect on kidney function, the benefit of fluid intake >4L in kidney transplant recipients is unproven [75].

CKD Progression

The average life-span of a transplanted kidney is 8–12 years for a deceased donor kidney and 12–20 years for a living-related transplant. The majority of these patients will have progression of CKD in their allograft after transplantation [76]. The progression of CKD is typically slower than that of nontransplant CKD patients [77]. Recurrence of primary native kidney disease after transplantation can occur, and it is the third most common cause of allograft loss after rejection and patient death [72]. Nutritional management of CKD in the transplant recipient and the general population should be similar. Thus, kidney transplant recipients should follow standard nutritional guidelines for management of CKD progression.

Diarrhea

The frequency of posttransplant diarrhea can be as high as 33%, and it is most often infectious or drug-induced [78]. The primary infectious causes are *Clostridium difficile* infection, norovirus infection, and cytomegalovirus (CMV) gastrointestinal infection [79]. Posttransplant diarrhea related to immunosuppressive therapy is most notably due to mycophenolate mofetil, mycophenolate sodium, and to a lesser extent tacrolimus. When this occurs, a change in immunosuppressive dosing or medication often leads to remission in roughly two-thirds of these cases [80].

Dyslipidemia

Dyslipidemia is seen in about 60% of patients after kidney transplantation [65]. A contributor is the immunosuppressive drugs, in particular mTORs, where hyperlipidemia is a common side effect [54]. Although mTOR use has rapidly declined over the last few years, CNIs, which are widely used, can also cause drug-induced hyperlipidemia [81]. Suggestions for diet modification include a high-fiber, low glycemic index, low saturated fat diet rich in sources of vitamin E and monosaturated fat [65]. In cases where diet intervention is unsuccessful for 3 months, drug therapy may be indicated.

Cardiovascular Disease

Cardiovascular disease (CVD) is still the primary cause of death in the kidney transplant population [82]. In addition to conventional CVD risk factors (e.g., obesity, diabetes, hypertension, or dyslipidemia), transplant-specific risk factors such as delayed graft function, rejection episodes, and use of immunosuppressant medications can influence the development of CVD in kidney transplant recipients [83, 84]. Although most risk factors are nonmodifiable, diet and obesity are two factors that can be modified.

Few studies have investigated the benefits of dietary modification in the kidney transplant population. Adherence to a Dietary Approaches to Stop Hypertension (DASH) diet has been shown to lower the risk of kidney function decline and all-cause mortality [50]. A Mediterranean-style diet has been linked with a lower risk of NODAT and better survival rates after kidney transplantation [85].

Other Important Posttransplant Education Topics

Alcohol Consumption

Recommendations on alcohol consumption after kidney transplant are mixed and vary by program. Some programs believe total abstinence is best as alcohol is thought to interfere with transplant immunosuppression. Others do not advise a restriction as moderate alcohol consumption has been linked to a lower prevalence to NODAT and reduced risk of kidney transplant mortality [86].

Food Safety

Kidney transplant recipients are considered high risk for foodborne illnesses because of the immunosuppressive medications; it is estimated that they are 15–20% more susceptible than the general population [87]. In the early transplant period, this risk is thought to be higher due to induction immunosuppression.

It is common practice for transplant programs to distribute food safety information to recipients although delivery, content, and format often vary. A 2010 study of transplant recipients found that information regarding safe food-handling practices is often missing, limited in scope, or misperceived by transplant recipients [88]. Transplant recipients are generally aware of the importance of food safety after transplantation but prefer information provided to them by someone knowledgeable on the topic, such as a transplant dietitian [89]. The United States Department of Agriculture (USDA) guidelines for preventing foodborne illness should be followed by all transplant recipients. The USDA has recently developed a comprehensive booklet that addresses food safety specifically for organ transplant recipients [90]. Strict enforcement should be encouraged particularly in the early transplant period.

Herbals

The use of herbal products is generally contraindicated in the kidney transplant population due to the lack of efficacy, safety, and quality control standards. Numerous herbals are known to be nephrotoxic and others such as St. John's wort have been shown to interact with the absorption or metabolism of immunosuppression medication [37].

Food–Drug Interactions

Grapefruit is the most recognized food to avoid after kidney transplant due to its well-documented food–drug interactions with multiple medications including the immunosuppressing CNIs. Pomegranate-containing products are also commonly being avoided following a 2013 case report identifying a tacrolimus–pomegranate interaction [91]. Potential new food-immunosuppressant drug interactions have emerged with pomelo, tangerine, ginger, and turmeric, but further research is needed to substantiate these claims [92, 93]. Immunosuppression medications have a narrow therapeutic window; therefore, all foods known to interact with these medications should be avoided.

Conclusion

Nutritional management in the field of kidney transplantation continues to keep pace with advancements in surgical technique, immunosuppression, and evidenced-based practice. The scope and role that nutrition services play as part of the multidisciplinary transplant team is now defined in all three phases of transplant (pre-, peri-, and post). Pretransplant nutrition evaluations are meant to identify and improve nutritional risk factors that can negatively impact outcomes after transplant and help determine transplant candidacy. Performing nutritional assessments, managing postsurgical nutrition needs, and providing posttransplant diet education are essential components during the peritransplant phase. The goal after transplantation is to provide MNT to optimize kidney allograft function and improve recipient survival. Common findings in early posttransplant period include hyperglycemia and hypophosphatemia. Weight gain, new-onset diabetes, bone disease, diarrhea, and progression of CKD are nutritional concerns often found late post transplantation period. In order to provide appropriate nutritional care for transplant recipients, it is critical to understand their unique physiology, complications, and management.

Case Study

Pretransplant

L.L. is a sedentary 55-year-old black female presenting for transplant evaluation with advanced CKD (GFR 16 mL/min) presumed due to longstanding type 2 diabetes. Past medical history includes placement of a coronary artery stent and gout. Physical exam shows large abdominal obesity but is otherwise unremarkable. BMI is 36 kg/m². A 15-pound weight gain over the last 3 months was identified. Her glycemic control improved almost spontaneously last year, and she is now off insulin. HbA1c is 6.6. Blood glucose monitoring happens when "she remembers." Avoiding salt and sugary beverages is her primary diet strategy. L.L. works as an office supervisor, but she is now on disability due to worsening symptoms associated with advanced CKD. L.L. sees her nephrologist monthly.

Case Questions and Answers – Pretransplant

1. What are the primary objectives of the pretransplant nutrition evaluation for L.L.?
   Answer: The primary objectives of the pretransplant nutrition evaluation are to identify and provide MNT for modifiable nutrition risk factors that negatively affect transplant outcomes, to provide nutrition clearance or nutrition risk assessment for transplant listing, and to educate on the nutritional requirements for transplantation.

2. Which of the following is most likely to prevent L.L. from receiving a kidney transplant? Explain your response.

   (a) BMI of 36 kg/m²
   (b) 15-pound weight gain in the last 3 months

(c) Large abdominal obesity

(d) All the above

Answer: c. Large abdominal obesity. Kidney transplantation may be an absolute contraindication for some candidates with large abdominal obesity due to greater surgical risks and potential wound complications from a large pannus. A BMI of 36 kg/m^2 alone does not increase graft failure or patient mortality. Also, potential recipients may see significant fluid gains when approaching the need for dialysis.

3. L.L. no longer requires insulin and has a HbA1c of 6.6. Do you believe she requires MNT for her diabetes prior to receiving a kidney transplant? Explain your response.

Answer: Yes. The improvement in her glycemic control occurred spontaneously suggesting a "burnt-out diabetes" effect from advancing CKD. In addition, her current approach to diet and blood glucose monitoring suggests noncompliance and/or further education is required.

Peritransplant

Five years after the transplant evaluation L.L. received a deceased kidney donor transplant. The course was complicated by delayed graft function likely from ATN caused by ischemic injury sustained during organ procurement. No nutritional deficits were identified prior to surgery which lasted 2.5 hours. The diet was quickly advanced post-op day 1 and tolerated well throughout the hospital course. Induction immunosuppression therapy included rabbit antithymocyte globulin (rATG) and 6 intravenous doses of 125 mg methylprednisolone, and was later introduced to tacrolimus, myfortic, and prednisone. Mild hyperglycemia was prevalent throughout, and hypophosphatemia was identified later in the admission. Serum creatinine plateaued at 6.0 mg/dL. L.L. was discharged 12 days after surgery with declining serum creatinine.

Case Questions and Answers – Peritransplant

1. Which of the following could be causing L.L.'s hypophosphatemia? Explain your response.

(a) Tacrolimus

(b) Corticosteroids

(c) Elevated PTH

(d) Low vitamin D levels

(e) All the above

Answer: e. All the above. CNI and corticosteroid use can increase renal excretion and inhibit the reabsorption of phosphate. PTH levels should fall after transplantation but can remain elevated, leading to increased urinary phosphate excretion. Vitamin D levels can remain low after transplantation, leading to impaired phosphate absorption from the intestine.

2. What are common causes of delayed graft function after kidney transplantation?

(a) ATN

(b) Ureteral obstruction

(c) Thrombosis

(d) Early rejection

(e) All the above

Answer: e. All the above

3. Why do you think L.L. was mildly hyperglycemic throughout her admission?
   Answer: Aggressive glycemic control during the transplant admission is not common. Optimal control is often difficult for a myriad of reasons (e.g., metabolic effect of surgery, immunosuppression changes, improving renal function, and varied PO intake) and the risk of hypoglycemic complications often outweighs any detrimental effects of short-term mild hyperglycemia during this critical phase.

Posttransplant

During a routine posttransplant clinic visit, L.L. presents with a BMI of 33 kg/m^2 and 8% weight gain since receiving her transplant 1 year ago. She believes the 5 mg of daily prednisone is causing her weight gain, because she has been consuming the same amount of calories that successfully led her to lose weight prior to transplant while on maintenance dialysis. She expressed concerns about being more physically active for fear of hurting the allograft. Her diarrhea has resolved with an adjustment of her myfortic dosing last visit. Baseline serum creatinine is 0.9 mg/dL, but this visit, it was found to be 1.2 mg/dL. She also inquired about taking a vitamin supplement containing pomegranate extract.

Case Questions and Answers– Posttransplant

1. Do you think the 5-mg dose of daily prednisone is causing L.L. to gain weight? Explain your response.
   Answer: No. Kidney transplant recipients often blame their weight gain on steroid-induced hyperphagia, but low-dose corticosteroid is not linked to weight gain in the modern era of transplantation.

2. Why do you think L.L. is gaining weight on the same diet that successfully helped her lose weight prior to transplant? Explain your response.
   Answer: Energy needs are considerably higher on maintenance dialysis compared to after kidney transplantation. Therefore, small to moderate reductions in pretransplant caloric intake can still lead to weight gain after transplant. The hesitation to being more physically activity may also be contributing to her weight gain. Increasing physical activity levels after kidney transplantation is encouraged and important to prevent weight gain.

3. Which of the following can cause an acute rise in serum creatinine from 0.9 to 1.2 mg/dL in L.L?

   (a) Dehydration
   (b) Tacrolimus toxicity
   (c) Acute rejection
   (d) a and c only
   (e) All the above

   Answer: All the above

4. Would you recommend that L.L. take a vitamin supplement that contains pomegranate extract? Explain your response.
   Answer: No. Products containing pomegranate should be avoided due to a potential tacrolimus–pomegranate interaction.

References

1. Hart A, Smith JM, Skeans MA, Gustafson SK, Wilk AR, Robinson A, et al. OPTN/SRTR 2016 annual data report: kidney. Am J Transplant. 2018;18(1):18–113.
2. Centers for Medicare & Medicaid Services (CMS), HHS. Medicare program; hospital conditions of participation: requirements for approval and re-approval of transplant centers to perform organ transplant. Final rule. Fed Regist. 2007;72(61):15197–280.
3. Pieloch D, Friedman GG, DiCecco S, Ulerich L, Beer S, Hasse J. A standardized framework for transplant-specific competencies for dietitians. Prog Transplant. 2017;27(3):281–5.
4. Waiting time for candidates registered at age. Organ procurement and transplantation network policies. https://optn.transplant.hrsa.gov/governance/policies/. Accessed Jan 2019.
5. Pondrum S. The AJT report: news and issues that affect organ and tissue transplantation. Am J Transplant. 2012;12:1663–4.
6. Potluri K, Hou S. Obesity in kidney transplant recipients and candidates. Am J Kidney Dis. 2010;56:143–56.
7. Gore JL, Pham PT, Danovitch GM, Wilkinson AH, Rosenthal JT, Lipshutz GS, et al. Obesity and outcome following renal transplantation. Am J Transplant. 2006;6(2):357–63.
8. Pieloch D, Dombrovskiy V, Osband AJ, Lebowitz J, Laskow DA. Morbid obesity is not an independent predictor of graft failure or patient mortality after kidney transplantation. J Ren Nutr. 2014;24(1):50–7.
9. Hill CJ, Courtney AE, Cardwell CR, Maxwell AP, Lucarelli G, Veroux M, et al. Recipient obesity and outcomes after kidney transplantation: a systematic review and meta-analysis. Nephrol Dial Transplant. 2015;30(8):1403–11.
10. Krishnan N, Higgins R, Short A, Zehnder D, Pitcher D, Hudson A, et al. Kidney transplantation significantly improves patient and graft survival irrespective of BMI: acohort study. Am J Transplant. 2015;15(9):2378–86.
11. Pieloch D, Mann R, Dombrovskiy V, DebRoy M, Osband AJ, Mondal Z, et al. The impact of morbid obesity on hospital length of stay in kidney transplant recipients. J Ren Nutr. 2014;24(6):411–6.
12. Molnar MZ, Keszei A, Czira ME, Rudas A, Ujszaszi A, Haromszeki B, et al. Evaluation of the malnutrition-inflammation score in kidney transplant recipients. Am J Kidney Dis. 2010;56(1):102–11.
13. Molnar MZ, Streja E, Kovesdy CP, Bunnapradist S, Sampaio MS, Jing J, et al. Associations of body mass index and weight loss with mortality in transplant-waitlisted maintenance hemodialysis patients. Am J Transplant. 2011;11(4):725–36.
14. Molnar MZ, Kovesdy CP, Bunnapradist S, Streja E, Mehrotra R, Krishnan M, et al. Associations of pretransplant serum albumin with post-transplant outcomes in kidney transplant recipients. Am J Transplant. 2011;11(5):1006–15.
15. Holechek MJ, Paredes M. Kidney transplantation. In: Ohler L, Cupples SA, editors. Transplantation nursing secrets. Philadelphia: Hanley & Belfus; 2003.
16. Bhalla V, Nast CC, Stollenwerk N, Tran S, Barba L, Kamil ES, et al. Recurrent and de novo diabetic nephropathy in renal allografts. Transplantation. 2003;75(1):66–71.
17. Kalantar-Zadeh K, Derose SF, Nicholas S, Benner D, Sharma K, Kovesdy CP. Burnt-out diabetes: impact of chronic kidney disease progression on the natural course of diabetes mellitus. J Ren Nutr. 2009;19(1):33–7.
18. KDIGO clinical practice guideline for the care of kidney transplant recipients. Am J Transplant. 2009;9(3):1–155.
19. Kalluri HV, Hardinger KL. Current state of renal transplant immunosuppression: present and future. World J Transplant. 2012;2(4):51–68.
20. Hill P, Cross NB, Barnett AN, Palmer SC, Webster AC. Polyclonal and monoclonal antibodies for induction therapy in kidney transplant recipients. Cochrane Database Syst Rev. 2017;1:CD004759.
21. Karpe KM, Talaulikar GS, Walters GD. Calcineurin inhibitor withdrawal or tapering for kidney transplant recipients. Cochrane Database Syst Rev. 2017;7:CD006750.
22. Muntean A, Lucan M. Immunosuppression in kidney transplantation. Clujul Med. 2013;86(3):177–80.
23. Pochineni V, Rondon-Berrios H. Electrolyte and acid-base disorders in the renal transplant recipient. Front Med (Lausanne). 2018;5:261.
24. Shivaswamy V, Boerner B, Larsen J. Post-transplant diabetes mellitus: causes, treatment, and impact on outcomes. Endocr Rev. 2016;37(1):37–61.
25. Helderman JH, Goral S. Gastrointestinal complications of transplant immunosuppression. J Am Soc Nephrol. 2002;13(1):277–87.
26. Andrade LG, Tedesco-Silva H. Critical analysis of graft loss and death in kidney transplant recipients treated with mTOR inhibitors. J Bras Nefrol. 2017;39(1):70–8.
27. Sakhaee K. Post-renal transplantation hypophosphatemia. Pediatr Nephrol. 2010;25(2):213–20.
28. Ghanekar H, Welch BJ, Moe OW, Sakhaee K. Post-renal transplantation hypophosphatemia: a review and novel insights. Curr Opin Nephrol Hypertens. 2006;15(2):97–104.
29. Cochran CC, Kent PS. Nutrition management of the adult renal transplant patient. In: Byham-Gray L, Weissen K, editors. A clinical guide to nutrition in kidney disease. Chicago: American Dietetic Association; 2004.

30. van Londen M, Aarts BM, Deetman PE, van der Weijden J, Eisenga MF, Navis G, et al. Post-transplant hypophosphatemia and the risk of death-censored graft failure and mortality after kidney transplantation. Clin J Am Soc Nephrol. 2017;12:1301–10.

31. Crutchlow MF, Bloom RD. Transplant-associated hyperglycemia: a new look at an old problem. Clin J Am Soc Nephrol. 2007;2(2):343–55.

32. Siedlecki A, Irish W, Brennan DC. Delayed graft function in the kidney transplant. Am J Transplant. 2011;11(11):2279–96.

33. Comparative standards: estimating approximate energy requirements for adults. Academy of Nutrition and Dietetics Nutrition Care manual. http://nutritioncaremanual.org/topic.cfm?ncm_toc_id=268183&showtbar=1&showbar=1. Accessed Jan 2019.

34. Dietary reference intakes for energy, carbohydrate, fiber, fat, fatty acids, cholesterol, protein, and amino acids. Food and Nutrition Board of the Institute of Medicine, National Academy of Sciences. 2005. https://ods.od.nih.gov/Health_Information/Dietary_Reference_Intakes.aspx. Accessed Jan 2019.

35. Hasse JM. Nutrition assessment and support of organ transplant recipients. J Parenter Enter Nutr. 2001;25(3):120–31.

36. Hasse JM, Linda SB. Comprehensive guide to transplant nutrition. Chicago: American Dietetic Association; 2002.

37. McCarthy MP. Transplantation. In: Byham-Gray L, Stover J, Weissen K, editors. A clinical guide to nutrition in kidney disease. 2nd ed. Chicago: Academy of Nutrition and Dietetics; 2013.

38. Guichard SW. Nutrition in the kidney transplant recipient. In: Danovitch GM, editor. Handbook of kidney transplantation. 4th ed. Philadelphia: Lippincott Williams & Wilkins; 2005.

39. Goral S, Bleicher MB. Handbook of nutrition and the kidney. Philadelphia: Lippincott Williams & Wilkins; 2010.

40. Tannus AF, Valença de Carvalho RL, Suen VM, Cardoso JB, Okano N, Marchini JS. Energy expenditure after 2- to 3-hour elective surgical operations. Rev Hosp Clin Fac Med Sao Paulo. 2001;56(2):37–40.

41. Cogan MG, Sargent JA, Yarbrough SG, Vincenti F, Amend WJ Jr. Prevention of prednisone-induced negative nitrogen balance. Effect of dietary modification on urea generation rate in patients on hemodialysis receiving high-dose glucocorticoids. Ann Intern Med. 1981;95(2):158–61.

42. Martins C, Pecoits-Filho R, Riella MC. Nutrition for the post-renal transplant recipients. Transplant Proc. 2004;36(6):1650–4.

43. Marino LV, Romão EA, Chiarello PG. Nutritional status, energy expenditure, and protein oxidative stress after kidney transplantation. Redox Rep. 2017;22(6):439–44.

44. Whittier FC, Evans DH, Dutton S, Ross G Jr, Luger A, Nolph KD, et al. Nutrition in renal transplantation. Am J Kidney Dis. 1985;6(6):405–11.

45. Chadban S, Chan M, Fry K, Patwardhan A, Ryan C, Trevillian P, Westgarth F, The CARI guidelines. Protein requirement in adult kidney transplant recipients. Nephrology (Carlton). 2010;15(1):68–71.

46. Schütz T, Hudjetz H, Roske AE, Katzorke C, Kreymann G, Budde K, et al. Weight gain in long-term survivors of kidney or liver transplantation--another paradigm of sarcopenic obesity? Nutrition. 2012;28(4):378–83.

47. Nolte Fong JV, Moore LW. Nutrition trends in kidney transplant recipients: the importance of dietary monitoring and need for evidence-based recommendations. Front Med. 2018;31(5):302.

48. Mottillo S, Filion KB, Genest J, Joseph L, Pilote L. Poirier P the metabolic syndrome and cardiovascular risk a systematic review and meta-analysis. J Am Coll Cardiol. 2010;56(14):1113–32.

49. Terranova A. The effects of diabetes mellitus on wound healing. Plast Surg Nurs. 1991;11(1):20–5.

50. Osté MCJ, Gomes-Neto AW, Corpeleijn E, Gans ROB, de Borst MH, van den Berg E, et al. Dietary approach to stop hypertension (DASH) diet and risk of renal function decline and all-cause mortality in renal transplant recipients. Am J Transplant. 2018;18(10):2523–33.

51. Schwenger V, Zeier M, Ritz E. Hypertension after renal transplantation. Curr Hypertens Rep. 2001;3(5):434–9.

52. Bernardi A, Biasia F, Pati T, Piva M, D'Angelo A, Bucciante G. Long-term protein intake control in kidney transplant recipients: effect in kidney graft function and in nutritional status. Am J Kidney Dis. 2003;41(3):146–52.

53. Scott TM, Rogers G, Weiner DE, Livingston K, Selhub J, Jacques PF, et al. B-vitamin therapy for kidney transplant recipients lowers homocysteine and improves selective cognitive outcomes in the randomized FAVORIT ancillary cognitive trial. J Prev Alzheimers Dis. 2017;4(3):174–82.

54. Veroux M, Corona D, Sinagra N, Tallarita T, Ekser B, Giaquinta A, et al. Nutrition in kidney transplantation. Int J Artif Organs. 2013;36(10):677–86.

55. Henggeler CK, Plank LD, Ryan KJ, Gilchrist EL, Casas JM, Lloyd LE, et al. A randomized controlled trial of an intensive nutrition intervention versus standard nutrition care to avoid excess weight gain after kidney transplantation: the INTENT trial. J Ren Nutr. 2018;28(5):340–51.

56. Zelle DM, Kok T, Dontje ML, Danchell EI, Navis G, van Son WJ, et al. The role of diet and physical activity in post-transplant weight gain after renal transplantation. Clin Transpl. 2013;27(4):484–90.

57. Stanfill A, Bloodworth R, Cashion A. Lessons learned: experiences of gaining weight by kidney transplant recipients. Prog Transplant. 2012;22(1):71–8.

58. Woodle ES, First MR, Pirsch J, Shihab F, Gaber AO, Van Veldhuisen P. A prospective, randomized, double-blind, placebo-controlled multicenter trial comparing early (7 day) corticosteroid cessation versus long-term, low-dose corticosteroid therapy. Ann Surg. 2008;248(4):564–77.

59. Guida B, Trio R, Laccetti R, Nastasi A, Salvi E, Perrino NR, et al. Role of dietary intervention on metabolic abnormalities and nutritional status after renal transplantation. Nephrol Dial Transplant. 2007;22(11):3304–10.

60. Luan FL, Steffick DE, Ojo AO. New-onset diabetes mellitus in kidney transplant recipients discharged on steroid-free immunosuppression. Transplantation. 2011;91(3):334–41.

61. Pirsch JD, Henning AK, First MR, Fitzsimmons W, Gaber AO, Reisfield R, Shihab F, Woodle ES. New-onset diabetes after transplantation: results from a double-blind early corticosteroid withdrawal trial. Am J Transplant. 2015;15(7):1982–90.

62. Hjelmesaeth J, Hagen LT, Asberg A, Midtvedt K, Størset O, Halvorsen CE, et al. The impact of short-term ciclosporin A treatment on insulin secretion and insulin sensitivity in man. Nephrol Dial Transplant. 2007;22(6):1743–9.

63. Burroughs TE, Lentine KL, Takemoto SK, Swindle J, Machnicki G, Hardinger K, et al. Influence of early post-transplantation prednisone and calcineurin inhibitor dosages on the incidence of new-onset diabetes. Clin J Am Soc Nephrol. 2007;2(3):517–23.

64. Orazio L, Hickman I, Armstrong K, Johnson D, Banks M, Isbel N. Higher levels of physical activity are associated with a lower risk of abnormal glucose tolerance in renal transplant recipients. J Ren Nutr. 2009;19(4):304–13.

65. Chan M, Patwardhan A, Ryan C, Trevillian P, Chadban S, Westgarth F, et al. Evidence-based guidelines for the nutritional management of adult kidney transplant recipients. J Ren Nutr. 2011;21(1):47–51.

66. Miles AM, Markell MS, Sumrani N, Hong J, Friedman EA. Severe hyperparathyroidism associated with prolonged hungry bone syndrome in a renal transplant recipient. J Am Soc Nephrol. 1997;8(10):1626–31.

67. Bouquegneau A, Salam S, Delanaye P, Eastell R, Khwaja A. Bone disease after kidney transplantation. Clin J Am Soc Nephrol. 2016;11(7):1282–96.

68. Weisinger JR, Carlini RG, Rojas E, Bellorin-Font E. Bone disease after renal transplantation. Clin J Am Soc Nephrol. 2006 Nov;1(6):1300–13.

69. Ball AM, Gillen DL, Sherrard D, Weiss NS, Emerson SS, Seliger SL, et al. Risk of hip fracture among dialysis and renal transplant recipients. JAMA. 2002;288(23):3014–8.

70. Lou I, Foley D, Odorico SK, Leverson G, Schneider DF, Sippel R, et al. How well does renal transplantation cure hyperparathyroidism? Ann Surg. 2015;262(4):653–9.

71. Mehrotra A, Rose C, Pannu N, Gill J, Tonelli M, Gill JS. Incidence and consequences of acute kidney injury in kidney transplant recipients. Am J Kidney Dis. 2012;59(4):558–65.

72. Abu Jawdeh BG, Govil A. Acute kidney injury in transplant setting: differential diagnosis and impact on health and health care. Adv Chronic Kidney Dis. 2017;24(4):228–32.

73. Pellé G, Vimont S, Levy PP, Hertig A, Ouali N, Chassin C, et al. Acute pyelonephritis represents a risk factor impairing long-term kidney graft function. Am J Transplant. 2007;7(4):899–907.

74. Weber M, Berglund D, Reule S, Jackson S, Matas AJ, Ibrahim HN. Daily fluid intake and outcomes in kidney recipients: post hoc analysis from the randomized ABCAN trial. Clin Transpl. 2015;29(3):261–7.

75. Magpantay L, Ziai F, Oberbauer R, Haas M. The effect of fluid intake on chronic kidney transplant failure: a pilot study. J Ren Nutr. 2011;21(6):499–505.

76. Parajuli S, Clark DF, Djamali A. Is kidney transplantation a better state of CKD? Impact on diagnosis and management. Adv Chronic Kidney Dis. 2016;23(5):287–94.

77. Marcén R, Pascual J, Tenorio M, Ocaña EJ, Teruel JL, Villafruela JJ, et al. Chronic kidney disease in renal transplant recipients. Transplant Proc. 2005;37(9):3718–20.

78. Ekberg H, Tedesco-Silva H, Demirbas A, Vítko S, Nashan B, Gürkan A, et al. Reduced exposure to calcineurin inhibitors in renal transplantation. N Engl J Med. 2007;357(25):2562–75.

79. Echenique IA, Penugonda S, Stosor V, Ison MG, Angarone MP. Diagnostic yields in solid organ transplant recipients admitted with diarrhea. Clin Infect Dis. 2015;60(5):729–37.

80. Shin HS, Chandraker A. Causes and management of postrenal transplant diarrhea; an underappreciated cause of transplant-associated morbidity. Curr Opin Nephrol Hypertens. 2017;26:484–93.

81. Holdaas H, Potena L, Saliba F. mTOR inhibitors and dyslipidemia in transplant recipients: a cause for concern? Transplant Rev. 2015;29(2):93–102.

82. Rao NN, Coates PT. Cardiovascular disease after kidney transplant. Semin Nephrol. 2018;38(3):291–7.

83. Meier-Kriesche HU, Baliga R, Kaplan B. Decreased renal function is a strong risk factor for cardiovascular death after renal transplantation. Transplantation. 2003;75(8):1291–5.

84. Neale J, Smith AC. Cardiovascular risk factors following renal transplant. World J Transplant. 2015;5(4):183–95.

85. Osté MC, Corpeleijn E, Navis GJ, Keyzer CA, Soedamah-Muthu SS, van den Berg E, et al. Mediterranean style diet is associated with low risk of new-onset diabetes after renal transplantation. BMJ Open Diabetes Res Care. 2017;5(1):283.

86. Zelle DM, Agarwal PK, Ramirez JL, van der Heide JJ, Corpeleijn E, Gans RO, et al. Alcohol consumption, new onset of diabetes after transplantation, and all-cause mortality in renal transplant recipients. Transplantation. 2011;92(2):203–9.
87. Obayashi PA. Food safety for the solid organ transplant patient: preventing foodborne illness while on chronic immunosuppressive drugs. Nutr Clin Pract. 2012;27(6):758–66.
88. Kosa KM, Cates SC, Adams-King J, O'Brien B. Improving foodborne illness prevention among transplant recipients. Health Promot Pract. 2011;12(2):235–43.
89. Medeiros LC, Chen G, Kendall P, Hillers VN. Food safety issues for cancer and organ transplant patients. Nutr Clin Care. 2004;7(4):141–8.
90. United States Department of Agriculture. Food safety and inspection service. Food safety for transplant recipientswww.fsis.usda.gov/shared/PDF/Food_Safety_for_Transplant_Recipients.pdf. Accessed Feb 2019.
91. Khuu T, Hickey A, Deng MC. Pomegranate-containing products and tacrolimus: a potential interaction. J Heart Lung Transplant. 2013;32(2):272–4.
92. Moore LW. Food, food components, and botanicals affecting drug metabolism in transplantation. J Ren Nutr. 2013;23(3):71–3.
93. Egashira K, Sasaki H, Higuchi S, Ieiri I. Food-drug interaction of tacrolimus with pomelo, ginger, and turmeric juice in rats. Drug Metab Pharmacokinet. 2012;27(2):242–7.

Part V
Nutrition in Chronic Kidney Disease Among Special Needs Populations

Chronic kidney disease (CKD) is not discriminatory; it affects individuals of all races, ethnicities, socioeconomic statuses, and age groups. The nutritional management of CKD is similar for these demographic characteristics with the exception of age. The types and risks of kidney disease are different for each group in the life cycle. The incidence of CKD in infancy, childhood, and adolescence differs from that in adults and the elderly, in that the incidence in the former group results primarily from congenital anomalies and inherited disorders. To the contrary, the aging process stresses the kidney and impacts progression of the disease. Furthermore, vascular disease appears to be the primary cause of CKD in the elderly. The nutritional concerns of individuals with CKD throughout the life cycle (i.e., pregnancy, infancy, childhood, adolescence, and the elderly) are presented in this section. Case studies are also included at the end of each chapter.

Stover and Trolinger discuss nutrition management during pregnancy throughout the stages of CKD (non-dialysis), while on dialysis, and post kidney transplantation. The authors also address breastfeeding in this population. Infancy, childhood, and adolescence are a critical time in the life cycle because significant growth and development takes place during these stages. Nelms and Warady address the special needs of the pediatric patient with chronic kidney disease which includes nutrient requirements, assessment of nutritional status, and age-related monitoring interventions that take place during the life stage. This chapter also addresses the transition from pediatric to adult care. Lastly, Goldstein-Fuchs ends this section with a discussion about the aging adult with chronic kidney disease.

Chapter 19
Pregnancy

Jean Stover and Mandy Trolinger

Keywords Pregnancy · Intensive dialysis · Medications · Vitamins · Minerals · Nutrition · CKD Kidney transplant

Key Points
- Discuss medical and nutritional management of pregnant CKD patients prior to dialysis therapy.
- Identify modifications in dialysis therapy and nutritional management for the pregnant CKD patient.
- Discuss medical and nutritional management of pregnant CKD patients post-kidney transplant.

Introduction

Pregnancy is possible for women with chronic kidney disease (CKD) either prior to or while undergoing dialysis or after renal transplantation. However, the outcomes are different compared to the overall population and its management may be complicated [1]. Women who become pregnant in later stages of CKD are at a significant greater risk for worsening kidney function. One recent study has shown, however, that women with stages 3–4 CKD, although they had more adverse events during pregnancy, did not experience worsening kidney function [2]. Another retrospective study in women who became pregnant after a kidney transplant did not show a significantly increased risk for loss of kidney function or graft loss compared to nonpregnant recipients with similar clinical characteristics [3]. Immunosuppressive medications (especially cyclosporine), however, have been known to contribute to infants born small for gestational age. These medications have not been shown to increase abnormalities in the fetus, except for mycophenolate mofetil, which is now believed to be teratogenic. The incidence of premature birth also does remain high for women during all stages of CKD [4].

Fertility generally returns for women who have a good functioning kidney transplant [3]. Otherwise, women with CKD tend to become pregnant less frequently than those with normal kidney function. There is also a significant decrease in conception for women undergoing dialysis. Although it has been reported that the occurrence of pregnancy in the dialysis population has increased, pregnancy is

J. Stover
DaVita Kidney Care, Philadelphia, PA, USA

M. Trolinger (✉)
Colorado Kidney Care, Lone Tree, CO, USA
e-mail: mtrolinger@cokidneycare.com

© Springer Nature Switzerland AG 2020
J. D. Burrowes et al. (eds.), *Nutrition in Kidney Disease*, Nutrition and Health,
https://doi.org/10.1007/978-3-030-44858-5_19

still considered relatively uncommon [4]. This chapter will discuss special considerations and management for women during all stages of CKD, while on dialysis and after kidney transplantation.

Confirmation of Pregnancy

The confirmation of pregnancy in women in the later stages of CKD and those undergoing dialysis generally requires a pelvic ultrasound in addition to the blood test that measures levels of the β subunit of human gonadotropin (hCG). The rationale for the additional testing is that the kidney excretes small amounts of hCG produced by somatic cells, and in renal failure, this test can appear positive by usual standards [5]. Once pregnancy is confirmed, and the woman wishes to proceed, she should be referred to a high-risk obstetrics practice.

CKD (Prior to Dialysis)

There is an increased risk of comorbid conditions such as preeclampsia, and babies who are born preterm in pregnant women with later stages of CKD [5]. Nutritional modifications needed based on energy and protein needs for CKD without dialysis combined with nutritional recommendations for pregnancy are speculative. Vitamin and mineral needs are discussed later in this chapter and presented in Table 19.1. Also, some medications may need to be changed or added once pregnancy is suspected and definitely when it is confirmed (see section on "Medications").

Table 19.1 Nutrient recommendations for the pregnant patient with CKD [9, 10, 12–17]

Energy	35 kcal/kg pregravida SBW + 350–450 kcal/day in second and third trimester for all stages of CKD, while undergoing dialysis and post-kidney transplant; she may need a nutritional supplement to meet needs.
Protein	*CKD, stages 1 to 5:* 0.6–0.8 g/kg pregravida SBW + 10–25 g/day; plant-based protein restricted diets may be appropriate as well. *HD:* 1.2 g/kg pregravida SBW (and maybe more with intensive HD) + 10–25 g/day. *PD:* 1.2–1.3 g/kg pregravida SBW + 10–25 g/day. *Post-kidney transplant:* 0.8 g/kg + 10–25 g/day. May need a nutritional supplement to meet needs.
Vitamins	*CKD stages 1 to 3: prenatal* *CKD stages 4 and 5: renal vitamin or prenatal* *HD/PD: renal vitamin and total daily intake of 2–4 mg folic acid = d*oubling a standard renal vitamin is generally advised *Post-kidney transplant:* prenatal vitamins, which include vitamin and mineral recommendations for pregnancy in general; 600 mcg daily of folate
	Vitamin D—analogs have been given, but not enough information on safety during pregnancy; 25(OH)D may be beneficial; should meet general pregnancy needs of 15 mcg/day post-kidney transplant.
	Vitamin A—not usually given; thus, renal vitamins are generally given instead of prenatal vitamins in later stages of CKD; OK in early stages of CKD and post-transplant.
Minerals	*Iron*—30 mg daily; usually given in oral form for CKD without dialysis and post-kidney transplant to meet needs for pregnancy, and IV during dialysis (generally iron sucrose or gluconate) to achieve iron studies in goal range for general dialysis population.
	Calcium—given as calcium acetate or carbonate to bind phosphorus or as calcium carbonate for a calcium supplement; keep in mind that there is increased absorption of calcium from dialysate with more frequent dialysis.
	Sodium, potassium, and phosphorus—can often be liberalized in the diet with more dialysis; phosphate binders may not be needed.
	Zinc—11 mg/day for CKD and post-kidney transplant; at least 15 mg/day recommended for dialysis patients.

Abbreviations: *SBW* standard body weight, *HD* hemodialysis, *PD* peritoneal dialysis, *IV* intravenously

Dialysis

Intensive dialysis is a key component to successful pregnancy outcome for women undergoing dialysis. The amount of dialysis is increased in efforts to create a less uremic environment and mimic more normal kidney function during fetal development. Improved infant survival has resulted when the mother receives at least 24 hours of hemodialysis per week [5]. The greater time commitment for intensive dialysis is an important message to convey to women in this population as soon as pregnancy is confirmed, as it involves an alteration in lifestyle.

Nocturnal hemodialysis (NHD) performed at home, in which individuals receive 3–4 times as much dialysis as conventional in-center hemodialysis, may be the ideal modality for pregnant dialysis patients. This dialysis regimen has been associated with increased fertility, longer gestation periods with higher birth weights, and fewer complications for the mother and fetus [6]. Thus, women with advanced CKD contemplating pregnancy may be encouraged to seek a program offering this modality, if feasible.

Hypertension can be a serious complication of pregnancy for women with CKD [1]. Severe hypotension, on the other hand, may promote fetal distress [7]. More frequent dialysis will improve efforts to avoid potential hypertension due to volume overload and potential hypotension with the need to remove large volumes of fluid during the treatment.

The content of the dialysate used for hemodialysis during pregnancy will vary depending on the amount of dialysis given as well as the mother's dietary intake and levels of serum electrolytes, calcium, and bicarbonate. Frequent monitoring of all of these levels should be completed during the pregnancy. With more dialysis, a higher potassium dialysate concentration (generally 3.0 mEq/L) may be required to maintain normal serum potassium levels. The bicarbonate concentration of the dialysate may also need to be decreased due to the higher bicarbonate concentrations currently used. With more frequent dialysis and/or nausea and vomiting during pregnancy, the possibility of developing metabolic alkalosis exists [8, 9].

Even though the fetus requires adequate calcium for proper skeletal development, it is usually not necessary to increase the dialysate calcium content when calcium-containing medications are taken and more frequent dialysis is given [9]. A standard 2.5 mEq/L calcium dialysate concentration is frequently used. There is also some production of calcitriol by the placenta, which makes it important to frequently monitor serum calcium levels to avoid hypercalcemia [8, 9].

There are older case reports in the literature that discuss successful pregnancy outcomes for women undergoing peritoneal dialysis. More frequent exchanges with lesser volumes of instilled peritoneal fluid are necessary as the pregnancy progresses to allow more intense dialysis with less abdominal discomfort [10]. One report utilizes tidal dialysis with the automated cycler machine to promote both comfort and increased dialysis clearance [11].

Energy and Protein Needs

Initial and ongoing nutrition assessment and counseling of the pregnant patient with CKD is very important due to modified energy, protein, vitamin, and mineral needs for this population. The dietitian should meet with the patient to discuss an overview of nutritional needs as soon as possible after the pregnancy is confirmed and she has agreed to follow through with it. Regular follow-up using dietary recalls and/or food intake records to evaluate nutrition adequacy is suggested when feasible.

Generally, 35 kcal/kg/day of pregravida standard body weight (SBW) or adjusted SBW is prescribed in the first trimester, and 350–450 kcal/day is added to this value for the second and third trimesters for all stages and modalities of treatment for CKD [12]. Daily protein needs for the pregnant patient with stages 1–5 CKD prior to initiating dialysis are speculated to be: 0.6–0.8 g/kg + 10–25 g/day. Plant-based protein restricted diets with keto acid or amino acid supplementation may be appropriate and more effective as well [13]. Generally, at least 1.2 g/kg SBW plus 10–25 g/day for women undergoing hemodialysis and 1.2–1.3 g/kg SBW plus 10–25 g/day for those receiving peritoneal dialysis is recommended [14–17]. It may be easier to meet these needs with liberalization of sodium, potassium, and phosphorus content due to the increased amount of solute removal with more dialysis. At times though, the patient may even require protein or calorie/protein supplements to attain her estimated energy and protein requirements. Generally, a regular commercial supplement may be used with increased dialysis time and more solute removal.

Vitamins and Minerals

Prenatal vitamins are generally given in the earlier stages of CKD and post-kidney transplant, but some have also prescribed these in later CKD stages. Water-soluble vitamins are usually preferred over prenatal vitamins due to the need to avoid excess vitamin A for all individuals with CKD undergoing dialysis. With increased requirements for water-soluble vitamins during pregnancy, as well as increased losses anticipated with more intensive dialysis, a standard renal vitamin containing 1 mg folic acid is often doubled. Folate deficiency has been linked to neural tube defects in infants born to women without CKD; therefore, at least 2–4 mg of folic acid per day is recommended for pregnant women undergoing dialysis [9, 16]. Presently, there are renal vitamin preparations already containing greater than 1 mg folic acid and even added zinc, and these may also be used as long as they contain recommended amounts of other water-soluble vitamins during pregnancy.

Vitamin D analogs have been given intravenously during dialysis to pregnant women needing suppression of the parathyroid hormone (PTH) and to maintain normal serum levels of calcium. There still does not seem to be definitive information available concerning whether these forms of vitamin D cross the placental barrier and, if so, whether they are safe relative to fetal development [18–20]. It may be beneficial to provide supplements of 25(OH)D, as it does cross the placental barrier and can be utilized by the fetus [21, 22]. Low levels of 25(OH)D have been associated with preeclampsia for pregnant women without CKD [23]. Moreover, although not a vitamin, cinacalcet, a calcimimetic medication used for PTH suppression, is generally avoided due to lack of knowledge about its safety during pregnancy.

There are increased iron needs due to worsening anemia for all women during pregnancy. At least 30 mg iron per day is recommended during pregnancy, so women with CKD who are not receiving dialysis should receive this as an oral preparation [17]. Intravenous iron in the form of iron sucrose has been given safely and effectively to pregnant patients during hemodialysis [19], based on goal ranges for serum levels of transferrin saturation and ferritin used in the general dialysis population. Ferric gluconate is also considered a category B drug in pregnancy, which means that animal studies have not shown adverse effects when this drug is given during pregnancy and there are no adequate human studies available [5]. Although not as well absorbed, oral iron preparations have also been used for pregnant dialysis patients instead of intravenous iron, either alone or in combination with a vitamin.

Zinc supplements are prescribed in the amount of at least 15 mg/day to prevent increased risks of fetal malformation, preterm delivery, low birth weight, and pregnancy-induced hypertension [9, 17]. Zinc is included in prenatal vitamins and in some renal vitamins, or it is provided as an added supplement.

Calcium-containing phosphate binders are generally given to the pregnant dialysis patient if needed. Sometimes serum phosphorus levels are less than goal range. In these instances, calcium supplements in the form of calcium carbonate are given between meals and phosphate supplements are prescribed if needed. It has been recommended that a daily intake of at least 1500 mg calcium be provided [24]. This is usually achieved easily for hemodialysis patients undergoing frequent dialysis with a 2.5 mEq/L dialysate content (see Chap. 15).

Weight Gain and Serum Albumin

Due to fluid retention with CKD, it is difficult to determine actual solid body weight gain during pregnancy. For women undergoing dialysis, it has been suggested that the pregnant dialysis patient's estimated dry weight (EDW) or target weight (TW) be increased by 0.5 kg/week during the second and third trimesters, when most weight gain occurs [10]. More frequent treatments with gentle fluid removal may help with this assessment, but a team approach involving regular collaboration with the dialysis technicians, nurses, physicians, dietitian, and patient is very important when determining true weight gain.

The evaluation of adequate protein intake is also difficult, as the expected decrease of serum albumin during pregnancy is about 1 g/dL for women without CKD [25]. Recommendations are to continue weekly dietary recalls or records to assess daily protein/calorie intake.

Medications

Since blood pressure control is very important for the pregnant dialysis patient, the goal is to keep measurements less than or equal to 140/90 mmHg [5]. If there is no apparent fluid overload but hypertension exists, medications are utilized. There are several antihypertensive agents considered safe during pregnancy including methyldopa, β-blockers, and labetalol. There is less experience using calcium channel blockers and clonidine, but these are likely to be safe as well. Angiotensin-converting enzyme inhibitors (ACEIs) and angiotensin receptor blockers (ARBs), on the other hand, are contraindicated during pregnancy. When given late in the second trimester and during the third trimester, they have been linked to oligohydramnios, an ossification defect in the fetal skull, dysplastic kidneys, neonatal anuria, and death from hypoplastic lungs [5].

Anemia becomes worse during pregnancy due to increased plasma volume without an increase in red blood cell mass. Erythropoiesis usually increases in the first trimester, but this process is limited or absent for individuals with CKD (27). Epoetin alfa given during dialysis has been used safely for this population, with no known congenital anomalies reported. The dose frequently needs to be increased as the pregnancy progresses to maintain a hemoglobin greater than or equal to 10–11 g/dL [24]. It has also been noted in the literature that darbepoetin has been given successfully during pregnancy to women with CKD prior to initiating dialysis, when undergoing dialysis and following kidney transplantation [26, 27].

Breastfeeding

There is little in the literature regarding the safety of breastfeeding an infant born to a mother with CKD. The theoretical question is always whether the content of the breast milk will be high in urea and cause a diuresis in the infant that must be supplemented with extra water. Most women who plan to breastfeed, especially those undergoing dialysis, decide not to once the infant is born, as the pregnancy has been difficult.

Transplant recipients have generally been advised against breastfeeding due to the antirejection medications they are taking. Other than mycophenolate mofetil, sirolimus, everolimus, and belatacept, which are contraindicated for breastfeeding, data are limited for the safety of many immunosuppressants, while glucocorticoids and azathioprine are considered relatively safe [28]. Newer data as mentioned in The National Transplant Pregnancy Registry, now suggests that there is minimal fetal exposure via breast milk to tacrolimus and cyclosporine [5, 28]. Counseling practices, however, still differ among transplant centers. Women who choose to breast feed require an extra 500 kcal daily [12, 28]. Furthermore, antihypertensives believed to be safe for women with CKD during pregnancy are still appropriate during breastfeeding; this includes some ACE inhibitors [5].

Conclusion

Pregnancy for women with CKD is a complex medical condition. Those who are not yet receiving dialysis will hopefully have some access to a dietitian for counseling on appropriate nutrient needs. The dietitian must realize the importance of ensuring that the patient is counseled and evaluated regularly to provide adequate energy and protein in her diet to meet the needs of the developing fetus. The patient must also be guided to include adequate amounts of folate and other vitamins that have significance during pregnancy. The management of calcium, phosphorus, and vitamin D required may need to be modified for the patient's safety, and zinc will need to be supplemented as well.

As mentioned previously, fertility usually returns for women who have had a successful kidney transplant. It has been suggested, however, that these women plan pregnancy for at least 1–2 years after the transplant. Those who have a serum creatinine less than or equal to 1.4 mg/dL and have minimal proteinuria (<500 g/24 hours) seem to have the best outcomes [29].

The management of a pregnant patient with CKD, especially if she is undergoing dialysis, requires a team approach involving nephrology and high-risk obstetrics healthcare professionals. Regular follow-up and communication are important to promote positive outcomes.

Case Study

L.T. is a 34-year-old Caucasian female with a history of hypertension and reflux nephropathy. When she was 29 years old, she underwent a living kidney donor transplant and has not had any episodes of rejection. She recently found out she is 6 weeks pregnant. She presents to your office today for counseling and education. She just saw her OB/GYN for an initial visit and ultrasound, which was normal. She has been referred to high-risk OB and will see them next week. At this time, she is also interested in breastfeeding.

Her current medications are tacrolimus 2 mg twice a day, mycophenylate mofetil 1000 mg twice a day, prednisone 5 mg daily, lisinopril 20 mg every morning, labetalol 200 mg twice a day, multivitamin one time a day, calcium carbonate 1000 mg daily, and vitamin D3 2000 units twice a day.

Her current vital signs are as follows:

- Ht: 66 inches tall (medium frame)
- Wt: 165 pounds
- BP: 141/82
- HR: 70
- Temp: 97.8 °F
- Her physical exam is normal.

Most recent lab results are as follows:

- Hgb 14.2 g/dL
- BUN 14 mg/dL
- SCr 1 mg/dL
- Urine protein level: 100 mg/24 hours urine
- Albumin 3.9 g/dL
- Tacrolimus 12-hour trough level 7 ng/mL
- The rest of her electrolyte and mineral levels were normal.

Case Questions and Answers

1. What are the recommendations for getting pregnant after a renal transplant?
   Answer: There is not an increased risk of loss of kidney function if the post-transplant SCr is <1.5 mg/dL and protein excretion is <500 mg/24 hours. It is also recommended to wait at least 1 year after transplant and have no kidney rejection episodes in the last year.
2. What concerns are there for her current immunosuppressant regimen?
   Answer: First, mycophenolate mofetil is contraindicated in pregnancy due to its teratogenic effects. The patient should meet with her transplant provider and discuss changing to another immunosuppressant immediately. Monthly serum tacrolimus levels should be monitored as the dose usually increases during pregnancy to maintain an adequate 12-hour trough level.
3. What are your recommendations for her blood pressure medications?
   Answer: Lisinopril is contraindicated in pregnancy, but labetalol is appropriate for pregnancy. She would need to stop her lisinopril immediately and then she could increase her labetalol to get her blood pressure to goal as long as her heart rate remains at goal as well. Otherwise, she would need to add another blood pressure medication that is not contraindicated in pregnancy.
4. L.T. states that she would like to breastfeed after delivery. What are her caloric needs during breastfeeding and are there any concerns regarding her medications?
   Answer: The National Transplant Pregnancy registry has not seen a significant increase in adverse effects in infants in the presence of tacrolimus, azathioprine, or cyclosporine while breastfeeding. The drug levels in breast milk are lower than what the fetus is exposed to in utero. She would also need to remain on an antihypertensive regimen that is considered safe during breastfeeding. L.T. would still need to consider the benefits versus the risks with breastfeeding while on certain medications and decide if she would be comfortable with this decision as well.
5. What are her caloric and protein recommendations during pregnancy and during breastfeeding?
   Answer: Caloric intake during pregnancy depends on the prepregnancy BMI, SBW, and activity level. During the second and third trimesters, the caloric intake recommendations per day range from an additional amount of 350 to 450 kcal/day. Weekly weights should be monitored throughout the pregnancy, so an adjustment in kcal intake can be made if necessary, to maintain an appropriate weight gain during pregnancy.

   Protein: 1.1 g/kg/day pregravida SBW based on 0.8 g/day for nonpregnant women plus 25 g/day for pregnancy. Recommended folate requirements for pregnancy are 600 mcg/day, calcium 1000 mg/day, and vitamin D3 starting at 15 mcg daily. This patient is already taking adequate calcium and vitamin D3. Not sure what her current multivitamin contains, but could substitute a prenatal vitamin for this, and decrease her current calcium and vitamin D3 supplements, if needed.

   During breastfeeding, she should increase her daily caloric intake by 500 kcal.

6. Are vegetarian protein-restricted diets for pregnant patients with CKD prior to undergoing dialysis proven to be safe and effective?

   Answer: Yes, a few case reports with keto/amino acid supplemented protein-restricted vegetarian have been shown to be safe and effective.

7. What lifestyle changes must be considered when counseling women with CKD undergoing dialysis once pregnancy is confirmed?

   Answer: Commitment to increased and more frequent dialysis time.

8. What are energy needs calculated for the pregnant CKD patient?

   Answer: 35 kcal/kg pregravida SBW + 350–450/day in second and third trimesters.

9. What are protein needs calculated for the pregnant hemodialysis patient?

   Answer: 1.2 g/kg pregravida SBW + 10–25 g/day, and even higher with more intensive dialysis.

10. Which vitamin is supplemented in the diet of pregnant patients with CKD to prevent neural tube defects?

    Answer: Folic acid.

11. What is the minimum amount of dialysis per week recommended for a pregnant dialysis patient and why?

    Answer: At least 24 hours/week to create a less uremic environment for the fetus to promote positive outcomes. Also, this allows the patient more liberal dietary intakes to meet nutrient needs during pregnancy.

12. How is anemia treated for pregnant women with CKD undergoing dialysis?

    Answer: Intravenous epoetin alfa or darbepoetin and iron given during dialysis.

References

1. Piccoli GB, Zakharova E, Attini R, Ibarra Hernandez M, Orozco Guillien A, Alrukhaimi M, et al. Pregnancy in chronic kidney disease; need for higher awareness. A pragmatic review focused on what could be improved in the different CKD stages and phases. J Clin Med. 2018;7(11):415.
2. He Y, Liu J, Cai Q, Lv J, Yu F, Chen Q, Zhao M. The pregnancy outcomes in patients with stage 3-4 chronic kidney disease and the effects of pregnancy in the long-term kidney function. J Nephrol. 2018;31(6):953–60.
3. Sevitsky S, Baruch R, Schwartz IF, Schwartz D, Nakache R, Goykhman Y, Katz P, Grupper A. Long-term effects of pregnancy on renal graft function in women after kidney transplantation compared with matched controls. Transplant Proc. 2018;50(5):1461–5.
4. Cabiddu G, Spotti D, Genone G, Maroni G, Gregorini G, Santoro D. A best-practice position statement on pregnancy after kidney transplantation: focusing on the unsolved questions. The Kidney and Pregnancy Study Group of the Italian Society of Nephrology. J Nephrol. 2018;31(5):665–81.
5. Fitzpatrick A, Mohammedi F, Jesudason S. Managing pregnancy in chronic kidney disease: improving outcomes for mother and baby. Int J Women's Health. 2016;8:273–85.
6. Chang JY, Jang H, Chung BH, Youn YA, Sung IK, Kim YS, Yang CW. The successful clinical outcomes of pregnant women with advanced chronic kidney disease. Kidney Res Clin Pract. 2016;35(2):84–9.
7. Haase M, Morgera S, Bamberg C, Halle H, Martini S, Hocher B, et al. A systematic approach to managing pregnant dialysis patients—the importance of an intensified haemodiafiltration protocol. Nephrol Dial Transplant. 2005;20(11):2537–42.
8. Manisco G, Poti M, Maggiulli G, Di Tullio M, Losappio V, Vernaglione L. Pregnancy in end-stage renal disease patients on dialysis: how to achieve a successful delivery. Clin Kidney J. 2015;8(3):293–9.
9. Hou S. Pregnancy and renal disease. In: Educational review manual in nephrology. 2nd ed. New York: Castle Connolly Graduate Medical Publishing; 2008. p. 251–78.
10. Hou S. Pregnancy in women treated with dialysis: lessons from a large series over 20 years. Am J Kidney Dis. 2010;56(1):5–6.
11. Chang H, Miller MA, Bruns FJ. Tidal peritoneal dialysis during pregnancy improves clearance and abdominal symptoms. Perit Dial Int. 2002;22(2):272–4.
12. Kominiarek MA. Nutrition recommendations in pregnancy and lactation. Med Clin North Am. 2016;100:1199.

13. Rossella A, et al. Pregnancy, proteinuria, plant-based supplemented diets and focal segmental gomerulosclerosis: a report on there cases and critical appraisal of the literature. Nutrients. 2017;9(7):770.
14. Clinical practice guidelines for nutrition in chronic renal failure. K/DOQI, National Kidney Foundation. Am J Kidney Dis. 2000;35(6 Suppl 2):S1–S140.
15. Institute of Medicine. Dietary reference intake tables. https://ods.od.nih.gov/Health_Information/Dietary_Reference_Intakes.aspx. Accessed May 6, 2020.
16. Stover J. Nutritional management of pregnancy in chronic kidney disease. Adv Chronic Kidney Dis. 2007;14(2):212–4.
17. Wiggins KL. Nutrition care of adult pregnant ESRD patients. In: Guidelines for nutrition care of renal patients. 3rd ed. Chicago: American Dietetic Association; 2002. p. 105–7.
18. Fredericksen MC. Physiologic changes in pregnancy and their effect on drug disposition. Semin Perinatol. 2001;25(3):120–3.
19. Vidal LV, Ursu M, Martinez A, Roland SS, Wibmer E, Pereira D, et al. Nutritional control of pregnant women on chronic hemodialysis. J Ren Nutr. 1998;8(3):150–6.
20. Stover J. Pregnancy in chronic kidney disease (CKD). In: Byham-Gray L, Stover J, Wiesen K, editors. A clinical guide to nutrition care in kidney disease. Chicago: American Dietetic Association; 2013. p. 151–6.
21. Hollis BW, Wagner CL. Nutritional vitamin D status during pregnancy: reasons for concern. CMAJ. 2006;174(9):1287–90.
22. Schroth RJ, Lavelle CL, Moffatt ME. Review of vitamin D deficiency during pregnancy: who is affected? Int J Circumpolar Health. 2005;64(2):112–20.
23. Baker AM, Haeri S, Camargo CA Jr, Espinola JA, Stuebe AM. A nested case-control study of midgestation vitamin D deficiency and risk of severe preeclampsia. J Clin Endocrinol Metab. 2010;95(11):5105–9.
24. Reddy SS, Holley J. Management of the pregnant dialysis patient. Adv Chronic Kidney Dis. 2007;14(2):146–55.
25. Hyten FE. Nutrition and metabolism. In: Hyten F, editor. Clinical physiology in obstetrics. Oxford: Blackwell Scientific Publications; 1988. p. 177.
26. Sobiło-Jarek L, Popowska-Drojecka J, Muszytowski M, Wanic-Kossowska M, Kobelski M, Czekalski S. Anemia treatment with darbepoetin alpha in pregnant female with chronic renal failure: report of two cases. Adv Med Sci. 2006;51:309–11.
27. Goshorn J, Youell TD. Darbepoetinalfa treatment for post-renal transplantation anemia during pregnancy. Am J Kidney Dis. 2005;46(5):e81–6.
28. Transplant Pregnancy Registry International. https://www.transplantpregnancyregistry.org/.
29. Shah S, Verma P. Overview of pregnancy in renal transplant patients. Int J Nephrol. 2016;2016:4539342.

Chapter 20
Infancy, Childhood, and Adolescence

Christina L. Nelms and Bradley A. Warady

Keywords Children · Pediatric · Chronic kidney disease · Nutritional management · Growth · Dietary modification · Enteral nutrition · Parenteral nutrition

Key Points
- Children typically have different causes of kidney failure than adults.
- The preferred treatment of pediatric end-stage kidney disease is transplantation; peritoneal dialysis (PD) is the preferred dialysis modality for children <9 years.
- Adequacy of linear growth is a unique challenge with pediatric chronic kidney disease (CKD).
- Normal growth and weight gain are clinical targets for children with CKD and thus make adequacy of dietary intake and prevention of protein-energy wasting (PEW) critical.
- Multiple tools are required for an accurate nutrition assessment and include use of standardized growth charts.
- Calorie and individual macronutrient needs should be in accordance with the KDOQI nutrition guidelines for protein, as well as the acceptable macronutrient distribution ranges (AMDRs) and recommended energy intake for healthy children.
- The intake of most individual micronutrients should be 100% of the DRI for age, taking into account dialysis losses.
- Sodium and potassium intake should be regularly monitored, keeping in mind that young children may have sodium-wasting disorders that mandate salt supplementation.
- Phosphorus management is important for prevention of cardiovascular disease (CVD), but phosphorus intake should not be overly restricted such that low phosphorus levels result. Calcium intake should be between 100% and 200% of the DRI for age.
- Fluid needs vary greatly in pediatric patients and are dependent on the level of residual kidney function in those patients with CKD.
- Infants and young children on dialysis require close attention to their nutritional goals to help optimize growth and cognitive development.

C. L. Nelms (✉)
PedsFeeds, LLC – Pediatric Renal Nutrition Consulting and Education, Kearney, NE, USA

University of Nebraska, Kearney, NE, USA

B. A. Warady
University of Missouri-Kansas City School of Medicine, Kansas City, MO, USA

Division of Nephrology, Dialysis and Transplantation, Children's Mercy Kansas City, Kansas City, MO, USA

© Springer Nature Switzerland AG 2020
J. D. Burrowes et al. (eds.), *Nutrition in Kidney Disease*, Nutrition and Health,
https://doi.org/10.1007/978-3-030-44858-5_20

- Children and adolescents may have unique challenges related to family dynamics and social-emotional development, and they require individualization of nutrition instruction with consideration of these factors.
- Enteral nutrition should focus on oral intake, followed by oral and/or tube feeding supplementation if further intake is needed. If enteral nutrition does not meet intake and growth needs, parenteral nutrition, including intradialytic parenteral nutrition (IDPN), may need to be considered.
- The nutrition counseling provided to transplant recipients may be different from that provided to the CKD and dialysis populations.
- Transition of the emerging adult from pediatric-focused to adult-focused care is an educational process designed to prevent negative health outcomes in the CKD population.

Introduction

The *Kidney Disease Outcomes Quality Initiative (KDOQI) Clinical Practice Guideline for Nutrition in Children with CKD: 2008 Update* outlines goals for the nutritional management of children in all stages of chronic kidney disease (CKD) as: (1) "maintenance of an optimal nutritional status," (2) "avoidance of uremic toxicity, metabolic abnormalities and malnutrition," and (3) "reduction of the risk of chronic morbidities and mortality in adulthood" [1]. Although further research has refined knowledge and pediatric renal nutrition care since its publication, the KDOQI pediatric nutrition guidelines remain the foundation for the clinical nutrition management of the pediatric CKD patient.

Although "traditional" issues such as phosphorus and hypertension management remain pivotal in children as well as in adults with kidney disease, additional pediatric specific concerns merit the careful attention of a trained professional, making pediatric renal nutrition a subspecialty within the field of renal dietetics and nutrition care [2]. A pediatric renal dietitian, trained with expertise in childhood nutrition and growth, is best positioned to provide care for this niche population. Heavy emphasis is not only placed upon growth, but neurocognitive development and life-long morbidity and mortality risks are also important considerations. Finally, meeting the differing nutrition priorities of infants and young children, school-aged children, and adolescents, and the unique psychosocial concerns and risks for metabolic and uremic derangements in children of all ages with CKD, are all challenges the clinician must face to provide optimal nutrition care [3].

Etiology of CKD in Children

In patients aged 0–21 years, the definition of "pediatric," the United States Renal Data Systems (USRDS) [4] reports there are 2.7 cases of CKD per 1000 population based on children with single payer insurance. Whereas diabetic kidney disease and hypertensive nephrosclerosis are common disorders in adult patients, these are rare in pediatrics. Structural disorders account for 56–57.6% of CKD cases in children, with congenital anomalies of the kidney and urinary tract (CAKUT) such as posterior urethral valves or renal dysplasia accounting for the largest percentage (49.1%) of those patients, followed by glomerular diseases (6.8–20.5%) with steroid-resistant nephrotic syndrome (e.g., focal segmental glomerulosclerosis) topping that group at 10.4%. The relationship to age is significant as CAKUT predominates as the cause of end-stage kidney disease (ESKD) in young children, while glomerular disease is most prevalent in the adolescent ESKD population [5].

Treatment Modalities

Traditionally, peritoneal dialysis (PD) has been the most common dialysis modality for the pediatric patient who has advanced to ESKD and has the need for renal replacement therapy. However, this preference has been shifting, particularly in the adolescent population [6]. Currently, of all dialysis patients under 19 years of age in the United States, approximately 60% receive hemodialysis (HD) and 40% receive PD [7], with a gradually increasing majority of patients >9 years of age receiving HD. Automated PD is the most common PD modality used in North America and is characterized by multiple dialysis exchanges at night and a long daytime dwell [6]. Standard HD treatments are typically three times weekly for 4–5 hours in a dialysis center. However, a limited number of centers are using some form of intensified dialysis, whether conducted at home or in the dialysis center [8]. Home hemodialysis is used in 1.8% of the overall dialysis population [9], with its use in pediatric patients also very limited at present. However, reports of both nocturnal and short, daily home dialysis have been reported with good outcomes in nutritional management and quality of life measures [8, 10]. As noted previously, transplantation is the preferred treatment option for children with stage 5 CKD as it offers the best opportunities for rehabilitation in terms of educational and psychosocial functioning, as well as better survival rates [7, 11]. In most centers, candidates for transplantation must weigh more than 10 kg [11].

Linear Growth

Growth in children with CKD is often poor, and there are multiple factors in addition to poor nutritional status that may contribute to this outcome. Age at onset of disease, etiology and severity of the primary renal disorder, renal bone disease, fluid and electrolyte imbalance, metabolic acidosis, inflammation, anemia, abnormalities of the growth hormone-insulin growth factor (IGF) axis, and suboptimal levels of sex hormones are additional factors, which influence growth and impact final adult height [1, 12]. According to the 2017 USRDS data report [13], children receiving dialysis have a high prevalence of severe linear stunting, defined as less than the 3rd percentile for length or height, compared to US norms. Children aged 0–4 years had the highest incidence at 52.7%. The prevalence of severe short stature decreases slightly by age group, with it being present in 33% of children with ESKD in the 5- to 9-year age group, 29.4% in ages 10–13 and 23.8% of those patients 14–17 years of age. In contrast to the dialysis population, 12% of North American children who are part of the Chronic Kidney Disease in Children (CKiD) study, with glomerular filtration rate (GFR) values from 30 to 90 ml/min/1.73 m^2, are reported to have had severe short stature upon admission to the study [14]. Linear growth retardation is clearly a challenge for children with CKD of all stages. Linear growth is not only important in this population because of quality of life issues that may develop during childhood or young adulthood, but also because severely reduced height has been associated with increased morbidity and mortality in children with CKD and ESKD [12, 14, 15], with a 14% and 12% increase in mortality risk, respectively, for each standard deviation below average a child is for height and height velocity.

The impact of nutritional intake on growth is most important in the first 2 years of life, during which time half of the final adult height is typically achieved. In a global assessment of children less than 2 years of age and undergoing maintenance PD, the use of gastrostomy feedings, as opposed to nasogastric or solely oral feedings, was associated with improved growth [16]. Gastrostomy feedings may be associated with less frequent emesis, especially when compared to nasogastric tube feedings, which may, in turn, improve total caloric intake. Despite these results and as suggested above, recent research indicates that the achievement of standard nutritional goals for energy and protein may not be enough to ensure adequacy of growth in the pediatric CKD population [17]. Since many children have CKD disorders that are characterized by polyuria and salt depletion, care should be taken to ensure an adequate sodium and fluid intake. Failure to meet the often substantial quantity of sodium needs can compromise linear growth [18]. Serum bicarbonate (CO_2) may provide a portion of the sodium as the serum CO_2 level should be corrected to at least 22 mmol/dL in CKD stages 2–5, which is also important for adequacy of growth [1]. CKiD data have demonstrated that serum CO_2 levels <18 mmol/dL have lower heights and weights, and remarkably, only one-third of children with a low serum CO_2 value in this cohort received alkali supplementation [14]. Appropriate management of anemia and renal osteodystrophy is also mandatory, the latter most often requiring dietary phosphate restriction in addition to the use of phosphate binders and vitamin D in those patients with advanced CKD.

One of the most important interventions is often the provision of recombinant human growth hormone (rhGH) because of the resistance to growth hormone that exists as a result of the presence of an increased concentration of IGF binding proteins [19]. Recent evidence lends support to an early initiation of rhGH therapy to avoid growth delay if metabolic and nutritional issues have been addressed and poor height velocity persists [1, 16, 20, 21]. Currently, the use of rhGH is recommended when the height standard deviation scores (SDSs) or height velocity SDS is <1.88 (<3rd percentile) [1, 14]. Finally, a study by Tom et al. [17], supported by work from Fischbach [22], would also seem to indicate that increased dialysis may be necessary to overcome growth delays, even when nutritional factors have been addressed and growth hormone is utilized [22–24].

Adequacy of Weight Gain and Nutritional Intake

Protein-energy wasting (PEW) has been defined by the International Society of Renal Nutrition and Metabolism (ISRNM) [25] as loss of body protein mass and energy reserves in persons with CKD. PEW differs from classic malnutrition, which typically includes adaptive factors such as an increase in appetite and a decrease in metabolic rate [26, 27]. Unfortunately, poor intake and subsequent growth failure, as seen in children with CKD, are often characterized by maladaptive responses such as a decline in appetite and an increase in energy needs. Additionally, these patients may experience muscle wasting of lean body mass without fat decrease. Uremic failure-to-thrive has been a term used to describe pediatric patients with PEW, as it describes the growth component that is an essential factor to consider in children [28]. Although not yet well studied in children on dialysis, the CKiD study has provided evidence that PEW occurs in 7–20% of children with predialysis CKD [29]. Use of a modified definition, which involves linear growth, with severe stunting indicative of PEW, is consistent with criteria used to define this condition in the general pediatric population. Biochemical parameters (e.g., reduced serum total cholesterol, serum albumin, C-reactive protein (CRP), or serum transthyretin), reduced body mass index (BMI), reduced muscle mass measured by mid-upper arm circumference, and decreased appetite are additional criteria by which a diagnosis of PEW can be made [29]. Recently, a joint position paper by the American Society or Parenteral and Enteral Nutrition (ASPEN) and the Academy of Nutrition and Dietetics (Academy) has classified PEW as a subtype of pediatric malnutrition in an attempt to standardize definitions [30].

In adult and pediatric patients, new evidence is providing some answers as to why poor dietary intake and negative energy balance are frequently seen in the CKD population. Proinflammatory, anti-appetite cytokines, such as tumor necrosis factor alpha (TNF-α) and interleukin (IL)-6, are elevated in this population. Specific appetite modulators are altered as well. Leptin, known to suppress appetite and originating from adipose tissue, has been found to be elevated in the setting of a decreased GFR [31]. Although total ghrelin, which typically increases appetite, is normal in the CKD population, the majority of circulating ghrelin is desacyl ghrelin, which is associated with a decreased appetite [31]. A similar finding was noted in HD patients [32]. In the young PD patient, the increased intraperitoneal pressure that results from the presence of dialysate can also have a negative influence on appetite. Appetite, while not a direct marker of poor anthropometrics, has been associated with increased hospitalizations, emergency room visits, and overall poorer quality of life when rated anything less than "very good" [33].

Successful treatment of nutritional inadequacy in this population is difficult because many factors that are not fully defined or understood likely influence outcome [26]. However, several small studies have suggested possible intervention strategies [23, 34–36]. Options to increase calorie and protein intake include supplemental oral feedings, tube feedings, intradialytic parenteral nutrition (IDPN) for those patients who receive HD, or other routes of parenteral nutrition [34]. Oral appetite stimulants have been shown to enhance intake. One study of 25 pediatric dialysis patients with inadequate weight gain reported that the use of megestrol acetate at a dose of 7 mg/kg/day provided evidence of increasing weight over a limited period of time, with minimal side effects [35]. However, more data are needed before megestrol acetate or any other appetite stimulant is recommended for routine use in children with CKD and a poor nutritional status. Increased dialysis time for patients on HD is another strategy that may not only increase linear growth as previously mentioned, but may improve overall weight gain as well. It is speculated that fewer diet restrictions and reduced inflammation made possible by improved clearance may be the reasons for improved dietary intake and weight gain [23, 36]. Of course, the patients' quality of life needs to be considered when recommendations for increased dialysis time are being considered.

In years past, most pediatric CKD patients were underweight or at risk for being underweight. Whereas this may still be the case in developing countries [37], in western countries the risk of overweight and obesity is comparable with that seen in the general population. Recent International Pediatric PD Network (IPPN) registry [38] data from over 1000 children in 35 countries indicates that overweight and obesity, as measured by BMI, are a global problem in pediatric CKD patients with 19.7% of all children exhibiting overweight (≥85th percentile BMI) or obesity (≥95th percentile BMI) at initiation of PD. South and southeast Asia, central Europe, and Turkey have the highest percentages of underweight patients, while the United States and the Middle East have the highest percentages of overweight and obesity, reflective of a high prevalence in the general population in these areas. India and southeast Asia also reported a surprisingly high rate of obesity compared to their general population, but this may be influenced by the commonality of dialysis being more available to affluent families who can afford the treatment.

Short stature appears to be a risk factor for overweight and obesity, given that CKiD data demonstrates that the average child with CKD is in a healthy centile curve for weight, but short stature results in an increased BMI [14]. This indicates that linear height stunting should be addressed to improve proportionality [38]. Using height age to calculate BMI, as is recommended by the KDOQI guidelines, 17% of children with CKD in North America are overweight and 20% are obese [14]. In addition, 20.8% and 12.5% of children in Europe with CKD younger than 16 were overweight and obese, respectively, when using BMI calculated with height age [39]. In both populations (i.e., North America and Europe), short stature was a risk factor for elevated BMI.

Dietary and lifestyle changes need to be addressed for this population. Overweight children suffer from more chronic conditions and have poorer health than children with weights in an ideal range for age [40]. In fact, the CKiD study found an increased prevalence of dyslipidemia, abnormal glucose synthesis, and hypertension in obese pediatric patients with CKD [41]. If the patient is significantly overweight or the patient has reached his/her final adult height, a gradual loss of weight is recommended. However, if the patient is still growing linearly, weight maintenance may be beneficial, allowing for a gradual increase in height to reduce the BMI.

To prevent excessive, rapid weight loss or inadequate nutrition, the provision of adequate protein and other nutrients are essential. A focus on increased physical activity and limiting simple carbohydrates is an appropriate and moderate approach to slow weight loss or to achieve weight maintenance and minimize risk. It is important to avoid excess weight loss and inadequate intake even in obese populations, since CKD patients are at risk for muscle loss and an inability to utilize adipose stores. Children with CKD tend to have high adiposity, especially centrally, as well as low muscle mass [29, 42, 43]. Obese sarcopenia – the term used for malnourished obese individuals – has been demonstrated in other at-risk pediatric populations [44]. The term may extrapolate to pediatric renal populations given that the prevalence of overweight and obesity is common, but at the same time, many of these patients report poor appetites and have poor musculature.

Assessment

The assessment of nutritional status of children with CKD is complicated by the myriad of factors that may influence stature, body weight, and intake. Consequently, a variety of assessment tools are recommended to provide a more complete picture than any single measure. The frequency of the assessment is recommended to be at least twice as often as the assessment of healthy children. A more frequent assessment may be necessary for children with comorbid conditions, increasing disease severity, changes in residual kidney function or dialysis modality, and for younger age children [1, 45]. Figure 20.1 demonstrates a sample pediatric initial or annual assessment form. The KDOQI pediatric nutrition guideline outlines the recommendations for assessment in the pediatric CKD population. A review of the complete medical picture, including biochemical parameters, dietary and fluid intake, bowel habits, urine output, medications, and physical activity, aids in the nutrition assessment. Details of the KDOQI recommendations regarding the content and frequency of assessment in a given patient's age group are presented in Table 20.1 [1].

Anthropometric values are a key component of assessment. Length is the preferred measurement in children younger than 2 years of age, while height, which is measured standing, should be used in children aged 2 and older. Length should be measured with a length board to ensure accuracy, while height should be measured with a stadiometer. Measurements for children younger than age two should be compared to the World Health Organization (WHO) growth charts or assessed as a standard deviation score (SDS). Poor or declining linear growth as an SDS may be one measure of inadequate nutrition; however, and as noted previously, growth is influenced by many factors in this population. Parental height should be compared with the child's placement on the growth chart. Predicted adult height can be calculated for boys as the mother's height plus 5 inches (34 cm) averaged with the father's height and for girls as the father's height minus 5 inches (34 cm) averaged with the mother's height [1].

Length or height velocity can provide further insight to assessment of linear growth. Assessment of height velocity can be judged as a percentile or a SDS. References data from the Fels Longitudinal Study [46] provides data on expected height velocity for age. Serial measurements provide for the best assessment and data can be compared every 6 months. Shorter intervals may not provide accurate velocity readings [1]. Although many of the same factors that influence height in this population affect height velocity as an assessment metric, trending may provide greater insight regarding the influence of the nutritional status.

Weight is another important anthropometric measure. Weight can also be assessed as a percentile compared to a standard growth chart or as a SDS. Again, the WHO growth charts should be used in children younger than two. It is important that the weight assessed is a euvolemic weight as oliguria and associated fluid retention may increase weight and not give an accurate picture of the actual lean body mass. In contrast, children with polyuria can be fluid-depleted with a measured weight that is below their true dry weight. The use of noninvasive blood volume monitoring which measures hematocrit determines the capacity to refill the vascular space when fluid is removed by HD [1, 47]. This tool may aid in determining if a HD patient has reached his/her dry weight. Signs of edema, blood pressure control, and biochemical markers such as serum albumin or serum sodium may also help determine a patient's dry weight.

When characterized by a percentile, dry weight may need to be compared to a patient's "height age" or the age that aligns with the 50th percentile based on current height. This is important when a patient is very small or short to give a more accurate assessment of the appropriateness of the weight for size. While weight trends may provide important information about adequacy of the nutritional status, a single weight is of limited value without taking other indices (e.g., BMI) into consideration.

Growth:

Age: Gestational Age: or N/A

Weight: kg   Length or Height: cm   BMI: kg/m2   Head Circumference cm or N/A

Weight %ile: Length or Height %ile: BMI or Weight/Length %ile: HC %ile:

Weight SDS: Length or Height SDS: Height Velocity SDS:

Previous Weight SDS: Date: % change in SDS:

Previous Length or Height SDS: Date: % change in SDS:

Previous Height Velocity SDS: Date: % change in SDS:

Previous weight: Date: Weight gain: g/day or kg/month

Laboratory Values: (Range for age and clinical status)

Calcium	Date:	Appropriate? Yes/No	Reference Range:
Phosphorus	Date:	Appropriate? Yes/No	Reference Range:
PTH	Date:	Appropriate? Yes/No	Reference Range:
Albumin	Date:	Appropriate? Yes/No	Reference Range:
BUN	Date:	Appropriate? Yes/No	Reference Range:
nPCR (HD only)	Date:	Appropriate? Yes/No	Reference Range:
Potassium:	Date:	Appropriate? Yes/No	Reference Range:
Sodium:	Date:	Appropriate? Yes/No	Reference Range:
Zinc:	Date:	Appropriate? Yes/No	Reference Range:
Aluminum:	Date:	Appropriate? Yes/No	Reference Range:
Cholesterol:	Date:	Appropriate? Yes/No	Reference Range:
LDL:	Date:	Appropriate? Yes/No	Reference Range:
Triglycerides	Date:	Appropriate? Yes/No	Reference Range:
HDL:	Date:	Appropriate? Yes/No	Reference Range:

Fig. 20.1 Sample pediatric renal nutrition initial or annual assessment form

Medications:

Phosphorus binders: _____

Iron/erythropoietin therapy: _____

Vitamins/supplements: _____

Stool softeners/GI medications: _____

Other pertinent medications: _____

Diet/Intake:

Diet Order: _____

Tube Feeding Prescription: (N/A) _____

Infant Formula Order: (N/A) _____

      Bolus Feeding Regimen: Continuous Feeding Rate:

IDPN: (N/A) _____

Subjective Assessment:

Oral intake reported (specify meals, snacks, amounts):

Primary food preparer:

Primary food purchaser:

Fig. 20.1 (continued)

Additional food resources (WIC, SNAP, etc): _____

Other persons present at meal and/or snack times: _____

_____

Physical appearance:

Evidence of muscle wasting: None   Mild   Moderate   Severe

Evidence of fat wasting: None   Mild   Moderate   Severe

Oral cavity concerns (note issues with teeth, sores or marks on the tongue, etc) _____

Reported Physical Activity:

_____

Appetite Description:

_____

Questions Patient/Family has at this time:

Fig. 20.1 (continued)

Table 20.1 Recommended parameters and frequency of nutritional assessment for children with CKD stages 2–5 and 5D

Minimum interval (mo)

Measure	Age 0–1 year			Age 1–3 years			Age 3 years			
	CKD 2–3	CKD 4–5	CKD 5D	CKD 2–3	CKD 4–5	CKD 5D	CKD 2	CKD 3	CKD 4–5	CKD 5D
Dietary intake	0.5–3	0.5–3	0.5–2	1–3	1–3	1–3	6–12	6	3–4	3–4
Height or length-for-age										
percentile or SDS	0.5–1.5	0.5–1.5	0.5–1	1–3	1–2	1	3–6	3–6	1–3	1–3
Height or length velocity-for-age										
percentile or SDS	0.5–2	0.5–2	0.5–1	1–6	1–3	1–2	6	6	6	6
Estimated dry weight and weight-for-age										
percentile or SDS	0.5–1.5	0.5–1.5	0.25–1	1–3	1–2	0.5–1	3–6	3–6	1–3	1–3
BMI-for-height-age										
percentile or SDS	0.5–1.5	0.5–1.5	0.5–1	1–3	1–2	1	3–6	3–6	1–3	1–3
Head circumference-for-age percentile or SDS	0.5–1.5	0.5–1.5	0.5–1	1–3	1–2	1–2	N/A	N/A	N/A	N/A
nPCR	N/A	N/A	N/A	N/A	N/A	N/A	N/A	N/A	N/A	1[a]

Reprinted with permission from National Kidney Foundation [1]
Abbreviations: *N/A* not applicable, *SDS* standard deviation score, *nPCR* normalized protein catabolic rate
[a]Only applies to adolescents receiving HD

Ideal body weight (IBW) is another clinical tool that can help assess nutritional status. Dry weight can be compared to IBW. Ideal body weight is the weight needed to be at the 50th percentile for BMI for age or height age. This can be calculated by taking the 50th percentile BMI for current height or height age × height (in meters) squared to obtain a weight value in kilograms. Percent IBW can be assessed by dividing the actual dry weight by the IBW and converting to a percentage. The percentage can then help determine if a patient is underweight or overweight, and by what degree [1, 48].

Growth standards based on growth charts should also be used for the assessment of BMI, with a target range of the 3rd to the 85th percentile (with a BMI of >85th percentile defined as overweight and >95th percentile as obese) [1]. This is supported by an international survey defining thinness in pediatric patients. Grades 1, 2, and 3 thinness are similar in assessment to grades of malnutrition, with grade 2 thinness corresponding with the 3rd percentile BMI [49]. The closer a patient is to the 3rd percentile, the more at risk he/she is of an acute illness or decline in appetite, which quickly moves them to below the 3rd percentile. In children and adolescents, BMI should be compared to height age as physical and sexual development is more likely to be consistent with the height age as opposed to chronological age [1]. However, once final height and development have been reached, it is no longer appropriate to use height age. Using chronological age to calculate BMI may also overestimate the appropriate BMI [48]. A landmark study by Wong et al. has indicated that mortality risk increases in a U-shaped curve for BMIs that are very low or high for age in pediatric CKD patients [15]. Since BMI is not an appropriate measure in children under the age of 2, weight for length percentile is the comparable metric in this age group.

Since it has been determined that children with CKD have an abnormally high adipose to lean tissue ratio [42, 43], the measure of waist-to-height ratio (WHr) has recently been evaluated in the CKiD population, as well as in transplant recipients. WHr may aid in the assessment of adiposity in children with borderline BMI values. A WHr of >0.49 indicates adiposity [50, 51].

Head circumference is an anthropometric measure specific to pediatrics. It should be measured and compared to normative curves as provided by the WHO standards in children aged three and younger [1]. A small head, with absence of comorbidities, may indicate nutritional insufficiency. Prematurity may also affect this measurement.

Normalized protein catabolic rate (nPCR) is the only calculation based on biochemical values validated for pediatric dialysis patients, but only in adolescents. nPCR, also known as normalized protein nitrogen appearance (nPNA), indirectly assesses dietary protein intake in dialysis patients with less measurement error than dietary diaries or 24-hour recalls. A child who has a desirably low predialysis urea may be a well-nourished patient who is adequately dialyzed or an individual with an inadequate dietary protein intake. Normalized PCR can help differentiate between the two possibilities.

Recent research indicates that nPCR is a more valid marker of nutritional status than serum albumin in adolescents receiving HD, the latter measure being influenced by inflammation and fluid status [1]. The nPCR is measured in grams of protein per weight in kilograms per day. For adolescents, nPCR values between 1.0 and 1.2 g/kg/d have been associated with positive outcomes for appropriate growth and overall nutritional status [52]. Target values for infants and children have not been clearly delineated, but theoretically, they should be higher than for adolescents as greater rates of weight gain are expected at younger ages. Because nPCR fluctuates on a daily basis depending on what is eaten, a single value does not provide an optimal picture of usual or average protein intake; therefore, monthly measurements are more informative. The nPCR can be calculated as part of the monthly assessment of clearance for the adolescent HD patient using the following formula:

The G must be calculated first:

- **G (mg/min) (urea generation rate) = {(C2 × V2) – (C1 × V1)}/t**
- C2 is the predialysis blood urea nitrogen (BUN) mg/dL
- C1 is the postdialysis BUN
- V2 is the predialysis total body water (dL; V2 = 5.8 dL × predialysis weight in kg)
- V1 is the postdialysis total body water (dL; V1 = 5.8 dL × postdialysis weight in kg)
- t is the time (in minutes) from the end of the dialysis treatment to the beginning of the next treatment

The modified Borah equation is then used to calculate nPCR.

- **nPCR (g/kg/d) = 5.43 × est G/V1 + 0.17**
- V1 is the postdialysis total body water (L; V1 = 0.58 × postdialysis weight in kg)

A goal of at least 1 g/kg/d of dietary protein intake as measured by nPCR is expected for weight maintenance in adolescents, and those who have values lower than this may be experiencing weight loss and inadequate nutritional intake. Additionally, very high values could indicate catabolism and the need for enhanced nutritional supplementation. Values in the 1–1.2 g/kg/d range are ideal for those expected to gain weight [1, 52]. Although PCR has been used to estimate dietary protein intake in children on PD [53–55], outcome measures for interpreting PCR measurements, as well as targets of therapy, are not well established. Therefore, monitoring of PCR is not currently recommended as part of routine practice for the nutritional management of children on PD [56].

Dietary intake is the final assessment parameter. Assessment of intake as it relates to nutritional status is best carried out via a 3-day food record or three, 24-hour recalls. A single 24-hour recall may be inadequate to account for day-to-day variance, but the 24-hour recall may be preferable for some patients or families in whom keeping written dietary records is burdensome. A skilled pediatric dietitian should assess dietary intake with these methods for the determination of the adequacy of intake for energy, protein, and other macro- and micronutrients [1]. Use of technology may aid this process for some patients and families who are savvy with its use. Taking photographs of intake before and after consumption may be sent digitally, and it may increase the accuracy of the intake assessment [57].

In addition to the recommendations pertaining to assessment contained in the KDOQI guidelines, other possible assessment tools have been or are currently being studied in pediatric populations and may be added to the assessment regimen in the future. Subjective global assessment (SGA) was first validated in general pediatric populations as the subjective global nutrition assessment (SGNA) [44] and was consequently validated in the pediatric renal population [58].

Additionally, bioelectrical impedance (BIA) or bioimpedance spectroscopy (BIS) may have a role in better defining dry weight and assisting in the assessment of cardiovascular dynamics in pediatric patients on dialysis [27, 59, 60]. BIA has been reported to be noninvasive, simple, and inexpensive to use, but may be most useful when conducted serially by an experienced clinician. Dual-energy X-ray absorptiometry (DXA) has been used in a limited manner in the pediatric CKD population for body composition measurement because of expense and/or poor predictive value, respectively [1, 48]. Mid-upper arm circumference (MUAC) has been validated in the general pediatric population for tracking overweight and malnutrition. Although it has not been independently validated in pediatric patients with CKD, it has been used in several pediatric renal studies assessing nutritional status [61–65]. A small single study has looked at air displacement plesmography (ADP) in children receiving dialysis, with positive results regarding the assessment of body composition and fluid status [65]. However, more information is needed before standard recommendations regarding its application can be made. Finally, handgrip strength as a surrogate for musculature and nutritional status has also been evaluated in pediatric CKD [66]. However, the data are limited and thus this measure cannot be recommended to be included as part of the routine nutritional assessment until further data are obtained. (Refer to Chap. 4 for further details on anthropometric assessment in the general renal population.)

Nutrient Requirements

The KDOQI guidelines provide recommendations by age group for macro- and micronutrient intake. These recommendations should be used as an initial starting point with subsequent individualization to the patient's needs [1]. Many variables affect these needs, including periods of catabolic stress, comorbid conditions, and genetic variation. Children who are significantly above or below their IBW may need adjustment as well. A child may need to have his/her nutrient needs calculated based on height age when he or she has failed to meet goals for weight gain with nutrient needs based on chronological age, especially if height age and chronological age are very different. Adjustment for prematurity may also need to be considered, using adjusted age for calculated needs. Adjusted age is the age that an infant would be if he/she had reached full term (40 week gestation). It can be used for any child born earlier than 37 weeks. For example, if born at 32 weeks, at 4 months of age the child would have an adjusted age of 2 months, since the child was approximately 2 months early. Nutrient needs for the premature infant who has not yet reached term gestation may be significantly greater, and referral to appropriate sources for preterm nutrition needs is recommended.

Energy

Caloric intake is important for growth and age-appropriate weight gain and prevention of lean tissue loss. A recent study demonstrated that caloric needs for children with CKD stage 3 were comparable to healthy children and that resting energy expenditure (REE) actually declined slightly as CKD progressed [67]. However, other factors such as catabolism and comorbidities may also play a role in the determination of energy needs as CKD progresses. In short, estimated energy requirements (EERs), as recommended for healthy children, is a good starting place to predict energy needs for children with all stages of CKD, with adjustments as needed following a routine nutrition assessment and evaluation [67, 68]. In 2002, guidelines for calculating energy needs in pediatric patients were published by the Institute of Medicine (IOM) Food and Nutrition Board (Tables 20.2 and 20.3) [1]. Body size and response to these recommendations must be considered for CKD patients when adjusting the recommendations to meet the needs of the individual patient [1]. Children with PEW/cachexia may

Table 20.2 Estimated energy requirements calculations

0–3 months: [89 × weight in kg – 100] + 175
4–6 months: [89 × weight in kg – 100] + 56
7–12 months: [89 × weight in kg – 100] + 22
13–35 months: [89 × weight in kg – 100] + 20
3- to 8-year-old male: 88.5 – 61.9 × age in years + PA × [26.7 × weight in kg = 903 × height in meters] + 20
3- to 8-year-old female: 135.3 – 30.8 × age in years + PA × [10 × weight in kg = 934 × height in meters] + 20
9- to 18-year-old male: 88.5 – 61.9 × age in years + PA × [26.7 × weight in kg = 903 × height in meters] + 25
9- to 18-year-old female: 135.3 – 30.8 × age in years + PA × [10 × weight in kg = 934 × height in meters] + 25

Data from Institute of Medicine [178]
Abbreviation: *PA* physical activity factor (see Table 20.3)

Table 20.3 Physical activity factors[a]

	Sedentary	Low active	Active	Very active
	Typical activities of daily living only	30–60 minutes of daily moderate activity	≥60 minutes of daily moderate activity	≥60 minutes of daily moderate activity + additional 60 of vigorous or 120 minutes of moderate activity
Males	1.0	1.13	1.26	1.42
Females	1.0	1.16	1.31	1.56

Data from Institute of Medicine[178]
[a]For use in estimated energy equations

have higher energy needs [26, 68]. CKiD data indicates that children with CKD predialysis consume an average of 100% of the EER [69, 70], but that energy intake and appetite decline when nearing ESKD. Moreover, weight loss is a common indicator of progression toward ESKD [70, 71].

In the case of the child on PD, glucose absorption from the peritoneal dialysis solution provides approximately 9 kcal/kg daily [72]. However, the quantity of glucose that is absorbed varies between children and may be influenced by factors such as the number of cycles for patients receiving automated PD, dwell time, body surface area, and peritoneal membrane transport capacity. Although these calories are typically not considered when calculating energy recommendations, high or high-average transporters may absorb significantly more glucose calories than low or low-average transporters [1]. This variation in glucose absorption is the reason that KDOQI does not recommend including this parameter into the determination of energy intake. However, since oral caloric intake may be quite low for the PD patient [73], calories from dextrose may be considered "bonus" calories. In contrast, if a child is gaining significant weight while receiving PD with the regular use of hypertonic dialysis solutions, calories received from glucose should be considered as a possible source of energy and the dietary intake may require modification.

Protein

A positive nitrogen balance is important to support growth and prevent catabolism in pediatric CKD patients. However, in the patient with advanced CKD, free access to dietary protein must be modified because of the phosphorus load that accompanies the protein. On average, the dietary protein intake for oral eaters, especially for the youngest ages (≤3 years), exceeds Dietary Reference Intakes (DRIs) for healthy children [69]. At the same time, there is no documented benefit of reducing protein intake to slow the progression of CKD in children. In addition, low protein diets may interfere with nutritional status and growth in the pediatric population. Therefore, the aim of nutritional management is to avoid *excessive* protein intake in order to minimize the risk of uremia. Protein of high biological value is encouraged because it minimizes urea production by reusing circulating nonessential amino acids (AAs) for protein maintenance.

For predialysis children and adolescents, the KDOQI guidelines recommend limiting dietary protein intake to no more than 140% of the DRI for age for stage 3 CKD (30–59 ml/min/1.73 m^2), and 120% of the DRI for stage 4 and 5 CKD (<30 ml/min/1.73 m^2). This may aid in the minimization of uremic symptoms and limit excess phosphorus intake. However, to ensure adequate growth and palatability of the diet, at least 100% of the DRI for age should be recommended [1]. Dietary protein recommendations for children on dialysis are 100% of the age-appropriate DRI plus 0.1 g/kg/d for HD patients and 0.2–0.3 g/kg/d for PD patients to account for dialysis-related losses. For patients on PD, protein requirements are highest on a g/kg basis for infants and toddlers, because protein losses are inversely related to body weight and peritoneal surface area [1].

Noteworthy is the fact that the Food and Nutrition Board revised DRI guidelines for protein intake in 2002. These recommendations, which are lower than the previous Recommended Dietary Allowances (RDA), were used to develop the 2008 KDOQI nutrition update [1]. However, and as noted above, the KDOQI references (Table 20.4) should be used as a minimum starting point with individualized recommendations contingent upon patient-specific clinical and biochemical follow-up.

A number of additional issues need to be taken into consideration when addressing the patient's protein requirements. Protein needs may be overestimated using the DRI based on weight in obese patients or underestimated in small or malnourished children and adolescents. Obese children have a higher amount of adipose tissue and thus protein needs based on lean tissue may be less than the patient's actual weight would indicate. Common practice allows for the use of an adjusted body

Table 20.4 Recommended dietary protein intake (DRI) in children with CKD Stages 3–5 and 5D

		Recommended for CKD stage 3	Recommended for CKD stages 4–5		
	DRI	(g/kg/d)	(g/kg/d)	Recommended for HD	Recommended for PD
Age	(g/kg/d)[a]	(100–140% DRI)	(100–120% DRI)	(g/kg/d)[a]	(g/kg/d)[b]
0–6 months	1.5	1.5–2.1	1.5–1.8	1.6	1.8
7–12 months	1.2	1.2–1.7	1.2–1.5	1.3	1.5
1–3 years	1.05	1.05–1.5	1.05–1.25	1.15	1.3
4–13 years	0.95	1.05–1.5	1.05–1.25	1.15	1.3
14–18 years	0.85	0.85–1.2	0.85–1.05	0.95	1

Reprinted with permission from National Kidney Foundation [1]
Abbreviations: *CKD* chronic kidney disease, *HD* hemodialysis, *PD* peritoneal dialysis
[a]DRI 0.1 g/kg/d to compensate for dialytic losses
[b]DRI 0.15–0.3 g/kg/d depending on the patient's age to compensate for peritoneal losses

weight (ABW) as a weight-based number to calculate dietary protein needs in the obese pediatric patient. The formula used to calculate ABW is as follows:

$$\left[\left(\text{actual weight} - \text{ideal weight} \right) \times 25\% + \text{ideal body weight} \right]$$

Likewise, small children may have a higher proportion of lean tissue and clinical judgment should be used in assessing protein needs. Wasted children may need additional protein to account for catabolism [1]. Protein requirements may also be increased in patients with proteinuria, acidosis, peritonitis, high peritoneal membrane transport status and longer dialysis times, or in those patients who are receiving glucocorticoids. It may be useful to trend blood urea nitrogen (BUN) values to determine if protein intake is adequate [72, 74].

Although some children may have inadequate protein intake, such as vegetarians or especially vegans, or children with anorexia and overall poor intake, the majority of children will meet dietary protein needs. Counseling to increase specific sources of protein and/or calorie intake may need to be considered in these cases. Larger and taller children may have difficulty meeting protein needs while limiting dietary phosphorus intake; high-quality proteins should be encouraged in these instances. Young children receiving enteral formulas, especially those receiving peritoneal dialysis, may need protein supplementation in the form of protein modulars added to the formula.

Carbohydrates, Fats, and Lipid Management

The macronutrients that comprise total energy intake should be within the acceptable macronutrient distribution range (AMDR) that is recommended by the IOM [11]. Additionally, the American Academy of Pediatrics (AAP) recommends that children aged four and older with dyslipidemia limit total fat to <30% of calories, saturated fat to 7–10% of calories, and cholesterol to <300 mg/day [75]. These recommendations are especially pertinent for the pediatric patient with CKD, since 39–65% have evidence of dyslipidemia [76]. Dyslipidemia often presents with CKD Stages 3–5 [77, 78] or as an adverse effect of immunosuppressant therapy posttransplant [41]. Hypertriglyceridemia is the most common lipid disorder, and it is often accompanied by abnormalities of very-low-density lipoproteins (VLDL), low-density lipoproteins (LDL), and total cholesterol, and low levels of high-density lipoproteins (HDL). Factors which may contribute to the development of dyslipidemia include a reduced ability of HDL to carry cholesterol to the liver, functional abnormalities of LDL, nephrotic syndrome, and insulin resistance.

Table 20.5 Macronutrient needs for children with CKD

	Stage 3 CKD	Stages 4–5 CKD	Hemodialysis	Peritoneal dialysis
Energy	EER for age or height age			
Protein	100–140% of DRI	100–120% of DRI	g/kg/d 0–6 months: 1.6 71–2 months: 1.3 1–3 years: 1.15 4–13 years: 1.05 4–18 years: 0.95	g/kg/d 0–6 months: 1.8 7–12 months: 1.5 1–3 years: 1.3 4–13 years: 1.1 4–18 years: 1.0
Fat	AMDR: Age 1–3: 30–40% of calories Age 4–18: 25–35% of calories	Stage 5: <30% of calories; <7% of calories from saturated fat, avoid trans fat	<30% of calories; <7% of calories from saturated fat, avoid trans fat	
Carbohydrate	AMDR: 45–65% of calories			AMDR: 45–65% of calories, ensure oral calories + calories from PD do not exceed AMDR

Data from National Kidney Foundation [1]

Abbreviations: *CKD* chronic kidney disease, *EER* estimated energy requirement, *DRI* dietary reference intake, *AMDR* acceptable macronutrient range

In terms of management, glucose calories absorbed from peritoneal dialysis solutions may increase the percentage of caloric intake from carbohydrate sources and should be assessed when counseling patients on total percentage of macronutrient intake. In nonmalnourished/wasted children, an increase in fiber, focusing on complex carbohydrates and limited added sugar intake, is recommended [1, 75]. If carbohydrate and fat modulars are used to increase the caloric content of formulas or supplements, it should be done proportionately to maintain an appropriate ratio within the AMDR. Use of "heart healthy" oils such as canola, olive, or peanut oils can be promoted to replace other saturated or trans fats in the diet and increase monounsaturated fat intake [79].

The Kidney Disease: Improving Global Outcomes (KDIGO) Clinical Practice Guideline for Lipid Management in Chronic Kidney Disease [80] recommends obtaining an initial and annual lipid panel for children with CKD and transplant. The guidelines also recommend the use of lifestyle changes to treat dyslipidemia as opposed to medication, citing concerns about lifetime medication accumulation and unknown effects on growth. Most lipid-reducing medications are not indicated for children younger than 10 years of age [76, 80]. Simple changes can be made to reduce saturated fat intake and increase healthy fats, and replace simple carbohydrates with complex carbohydrates without tightly restricting the diet. Physical activity should also be encouraged for all types of dyslipidemias [75].

See Table 20.5 for a summary of macronutrient needs for pediatric CKD.

Vitamins and Minerals

Adequacy of vitamin and mineral intake is important for growth and overall health. Vitamin and mineral supplementation recommendations in pediatric CKD patients are, however, complicated by the lack of substantial research on the subject. Although one small study [81] that looked at various B vitamin intakes in children on dialysis found the majority of children had adequate intakes and high serum levels, other studies documented water-soluble vitamin intake below recommendations [82, 83]. A more recent study of children receiving dialysis and who were prescribed a standard water-soluble "renal" vitamin found that serum levels of vitamins or minerals could be high, normal, or low

[84]. Fat-soluble vitamins A and E were elevated, which might be expected, but folate and vitamin B12, both typically in a water-soluble supplement, were often elevated. However, in some patients, folate levels and select minerals such as zinc, copper, and selenium were depressed. This exemplifies the fact that there are many variables that influence vitamin and mineral status, and an individual's needs and circumstances must always be taken into consideration. Other factors that may be influential in vitamin and mineral needs include treatment modality or CKD stage (e.g., predialysis, HD, PD, or transplant), the frequency and amount of dialysis, PD membrane transport status, use of certain medications (e.g., increased iron requirements if receiving erythropoietin therapy), and age.

Since the amount or variety of dietary intake may be limited by anorexia or dietary restrictions, the dietitian/clinician must carefully assess a patient's intake for risk of vitamin and mineral deficiencies. The KDOQI pediatric nutrition guidelines recommend a daily vitamin supplement for children on dialysis, emphasizing adequacy of water-soluble vitamin intake as there is likely minimal harm associated with additional or even excess water-soluble vitamins and a greater risk for inadequate intake [1]. A renal-formulated vitamin most likely meets these needs. Although there are no known marketed pediatric renal vitamins in North America, liquid "adult" renal vitamins can be titrated to more closely meet the DRIs of young children. Adolescents typically have similar water-soluble vitamin needs to adult patients and can take similar vitamin supplements. Providing a supplement that delivers a quantity that is at or slightly above the DRI for age should be the aim.

Although there is minimal concern with most of the B vitamins, caution regarding excess vitamin C intake is warranted, given the associated kidney stone risk [85]. Vitamin C is frequently lost through dialysis, and so adequacy of intake should be ensured.

KDOQI recommends meeting the DRI for all vitamins and minerals with the exclusion of phosphorus, potassium, and sodium; however, supplementation of fat-soluble vitamins is generally avoided unless there is a clear need, as blood levels are typically normal or elevated [82]. Children and adults on dialysis have both been found to exhibit elevated levels of serum retinol, retinol-binding protein, and transthyretin [86, 87]. Recently, Manichkavasagar et al. demonstrated that serum retinol levels were elevated in 77% of children with CKD, as early as stage 2 [87]. Levels were elevated even in patients with intakes below national recommendations. Importantly, vitamin A metabolites reduced osteoblastic action and increased osteoclastic action, allowing for the release of calcium from the bones and hypercalcemia. Joyce et al. also found that 94% of dialysis patients had elevated retinol levels [84]. Although little may be able to be done to modify vitamin A intake in oral eaters, children who receive formula can have alterations to reduce vitamin A intake including the addition of formulas low in vitamin A content. As a result of the influence of vitamin A on serum calcium status, it is recommended to assess serum retinol levels in children with hypercalcemia of unknown etiology [87].

There is some question about whether vitamin E has a role in improving the management of anemia in CKD through a reduction in oxidative stress [88]. However, there is insufficient evidence at this time to routinely recommend supplementation, especially since Joyce et al. also found that 87% of dialysis patients have elevated vitamin E levels [84].

Specific attention should be given to the assessment of nutritional vitamin D (25(OH)D3) status. Vitamin D insufficiency is common in the healthy pediatric population [89]. To prevent the risk of rickets and to support the role of vitamin D in a number of physiologic activities, the AAP recommends that all infants, children, and adolescents receive at least 400 IU of vitamin D daily, which is an increase from the previous recommendation of 200 IU daily [89]. Major health organizations in both the United States and Canada recommend vitamin D supplementation for all exclusively breast-fed infants, especially those with dark skin, limited sunlight availability or exposure, and vitamin D-deficient mothers [89–91]. Importantly, children with all stages of CKD [92–94] are at greater risk than the general population for vitamin D insufficiency (<30 ng/mL) and deficiency (<20 ng/mL) [92]. Moreover, low levels of 25 (OH) 3 have been seen in the majority of patients with advanced CKD or on dialysis [92, 94, 95]. It appears that the prevalence of low nutritional vitamin D levels has increased in recent years because children with CKD may be less physically active and more likely to

Table 20.6 Micronutrient needs for children with CKD

	Predialysis CKD	Dialysis
Water-soluble vitamins	Supplement if assessment of intake indicates deficiency	Supplement recommended
Fat-soluble vitamins	Avoid vitamin A supplementation, vitamin E and K at DRI, assess and supplement 1, 25 dihydroxyvitamin D and 25-hydroxyvitamin D as needed	
Trace minerals	Assess and supplement copper, selenium, and zinc as needed; limit heavy metals	
Calcium	100–200% DRI	
Phosphorus	100% DRI if PTH at target, 80% DRI if PTH elevated	80% DRI

Data from National Kidney Foundation[1] and Manichkavasagar et al. [87]
Abbreviations: *CKD* chronic kidney disease, *DRI* dietary reference intake, *PTH* parathyroid hormone

spend time inside, and those children on dialysis may be even further limited. Children with CKD have reduced endogenous synthesis in the skin, reduced production in the liver, and loss of vitamin D-binding proteins in the urine and through PD losses [92, 93].

Children with CKD are frequently prescribed 1,25 dihydroxyvitamin D (calcitriol) because of the reduced capacity of the diseased kidney to convert 25-hydroxyvitamin D (ergocalciferol or cholecalciferol) to the active form. It has been well documented and long known that bone metabolism and growth concerns arise if 1,25 dihydroxyvitamin D is not provided [1, 92]. However, it is important to recognize that not only is the generation of activated vitamin D a substrate-dependent process in patients with CKD that is dependent upon adequate levels of 25(OH)D3, but that 25(OH)D3 itself likely plays an important role. In patients with CKD, research has shown links to immune function, prevention of malignancy, and cardiac function, irrespective of the provision of activated vitamin D [92, 93, 95]. There is now evidence that maintenance of a 25(OH)D3-replete state may have a role in lowering parathyroid hormone (PTH) levels in children with CKD [92, 95]. The recent Clinical Practice Recommendations for Native Vitamin D Therapy in Children with Chronic Kidney Disease Stages 2–5 and on Dialysis recommend monitoring 25(OH)D3 levels every 6–12 months, and if low, intervening and rechecking the level after 3 months of therapy [92]. Intensive therapy is recommended initially, based on the initial serum level and age, with a lower maintenance dose recommended after repletion; this is considered a first-line therapy for secondary hyperparathyroidism.

Recommendations for treatment are based on age and severity of deficiency, and stratified by intensive replacement phase and maintenance phase. Children younger than 1 year of age are to be repleted with 600 IU/day with a maintenance dose of 400 IU daily. Those older than one may be repleted with 2000–8000 IU, depending on severity of depletion and then should continue on a maintenance dose of 1000–2000 IU daily depending on stage of CKD [92]. Refer to Chap. 33 for further discussion of micronutrients in the general CKD population. Table 20.6 summarizes micronutrient needs.

It is well known that anemia is common in CKD, but the role of iron and therapies for the management of anemia in pediatric patients with CKD is beyond the scope of this chapter.

Sodium

The specific approach to be used for sodium management is very much dependent upon the clinical status of the patient. Restriction of dietary sodium is appropriate for children with CKD who experience salt and water retention and associated hypertension. This is particularly important as CVD is the most frequent cause of mortality in children and adults with ESKD. In contrast, it is not appropriate to restrict salt for children with salt-wasting syndromes such as obstructive uropathy, renal dysplasia, or renal tubular disease. In addition, infants receiving PD may require sodium supplementation to prevent sodium depletion, a decrease in extracellular volume, and impaired growth [18, 96]. In fact, failure to provide adequate supplemental salt to young patients receiving PD has been associated with severe cerebrovascular complications [1]. The need for sodium supplementation for patients with a salt-losing disorder typically decreases with age as the common western high sodium diet provides more than adequate intake. These children may actually develop® hypertension that would benefit from sodium restriction.

Newly updated in 2019, the Dietary Reference Intakes for Sodium and Potassium [97] recommend an AI of 800–1500 mg for children age 1 and older, depending on the age of the child or adolescent and a Chronic Disease Risk Reduction (CDRR) intake of no more than 1200–2300 mg, also depending on the age, while the KDOQI nutrition guidelines recommend 1500–2400 mg/day, based on the DRI Upper Tolerable Limit (UL) for age. Restaurant meals and salt added by manufacturers provide 75% of the daily sodium intake of most people living in North America [98]. Data from the CKiD study indicates that children with CKD actually consume significantly more sodium than recommended [69]. Of the 658 children included in the study, all age groups exceeded recommended sodium intake with an average daily intake of 3089 mg; 25% of the adolescent population (age 14–18 years) consumed more than 5150 mg of sodium daily. The largest source of dietary sodium in the CKiD population was fast food. Limiting processed foods and teaching label reading are, in turn, two important issues a clinician/dietitian should address with patients/parents with respect to sodium intake [69].

Significant pressure from social groups, the lack of available lower sodium foods, and palatability may make these sodium goals difficult to achieve, especially for many adolescents. Diet liberalization, within reason and within the constraints of maintaining appropriate blood pressure, may allow for improved nutritional adequacy. Homemade baby foods prepared from fresh ingredients are lower in sodium, and commercial baby foods also do not contain added salt. Lunch ideas should be discussed, especially for children who eat at school. Salt substitutes are contraindicated in children with hyperkalemia, because manufacturers' use potassium chloride to replace some or all of the sodium chloride in some food products.

Potassium

Dietary potassium must be restricted for many children with advanced CKD. The need to restrict potassium usually correlates with the severity of CKD, with many children not requiring a restriction of dietary potassium until they are near or reach the need for renal replacement therapy [1]. Data from the CKiD study has revealed that only 7% of children predialysis had elevated potassium levels and that, on average, the dietary intake of potassium was less than recommended for healthy children [69]. However, infants and toddlers with CKD often have congenital disorders, such as renal dysplasia or obstructive uropathies, that increase the risk for hyperkalemia. Thus, this population may need special care and recommendations for limiting potassium [1]. Infants with these disorders should be provided a low potassium containing formula such as Similac PM 60/40® (Abbott Nutrition, Columbus, Ohio). In addition, the need for potassium restriction may be hastened when certain medications, such as angiotensin-converting enzyme (ACE) inhibitors or angiotensin receptor blockers (ARBs), are prescribed [99].

Persistence of elevated potassium levels may require further intervention. Ion-exchange resins (e.g., sodium polystyrene sulfonate (SPS), calcium polystyrene sulfonate) can be used to reduce potassium content of enteral beverages. Although no official protocol has been established, most centers typically recommend decanting formula or other beverages if appropriate, for a half hour or less [100]. Originally, it was recommended to add 1 g of SPS to the formula per mEq of potassium in the formula. However, in practice, many clinicians start more conservatively at half this amount. The formula is shaken and refrigerated, and after the allotted time, the formula is decanted and a minimal amount of formula containing the bound potassium residue is discarded [101]. The amount of SPS used should be individualized based on the patient's lab values. However, SPS is not a benign medication. Oral and rectal administration has been associated with multiple side effects including gastrointestinal distress, vomiting and diarrhea and, more severely, bowel necrosis. Formulas treated with SPS may also contribute to alterations of other nutrients, including increased iron, sulfur and pH, and lowered calcium, phosphorus, magnesium, zinc, copper, and manganese [102]. As the ion exchange process by which SPS removes potassium replaces it with sodium, a greatly increased sodium content of the formula can be a by-product. It is difficult to know exactly what quantity of nutrients will be present in a formula that has been treated with SPS and it is, in turn, difficult to monitor micronutrient intakes in children receiving treated formula. A recent study also showed severe biochemical derangements in the children who receive treated formula, including severely low serum potassium levels [103]. An alternative to using an exchange resin is the use of formulas that are designed to be especially low in key nutrients such as potassium. These products are not intended for sole source nutrition and can be used as a supplement to an oral diet, or be mixed with another formula to titrate individual nutrient levels [104].

Once the infant starts taking additional oral food, caregivers can be advised to offer low potassium choices and limit high potassium foods, including several fruits and vegetables. Of course, use of a very low potassium formula as a supplement to oral intake may allow for more freedom in oral diet choices for the toddler. These nonsole source products work well for greater solid food variety and allow for some higher potassium items.

While older children with mild-to-moderate CKD may not need a tight dietary potassium restriction, children receiving hemodialysis, irrespective of the primary cause of kidney failure, will typically need to limit high potassium foods including milk, yogurt, bananas, cantaloupe, tomato and potato products, and potassium-fortified foods. Children receiving PD may, on the other hand, not need a restriction or as tight of a restriction and, in some instances, may require supplementation. This is in part dependent upon the peritoneal membrane transport status, with high transporters often losing large amounts of potassium across the peritoneal membrane [1].

There are no clear guidelines on how much dietary potassium is appropriate for pediatric CKD patients. The adult guideline recommendation of 2400 mg/day may be extrapolated to <30–40 mg/kg/d or 0.8–1 mmol/kg/d. For infants and toddlers, 1–3 mmol/kg/d may be a reasonable starting place [1]. It is important to remember that there may be nondietary causes of hyperkalemia, including constipation, acidosis, inflammation, catabolism/starvation, elevated glucose levels, suboptimal dialysis adequacy, increased HD potassium bath, increased activity, and medications [99]. All of these issues, including dietary intake, should be considered when addressing/correcting hyperkalemia.

Table 20.7 summarizes electrolyte and fluid needs.

Table 20.7 Electrolyte and fluid needs for children with CKD

	Predialysis CKD	Hemodialysis	Peritoneal dialysis
Sodium	Limit to DRI (upper tolerable limit) if hypertensive; if polyuric, consider supplementation		Supplementation to be considered for all infants Limit to DRI (upper tolerable limit) if hypertensive; if polyuric, consider supplementation
Potassium	If at risk for hyperkalemia: Infants and young children: 1–3 mmol/kg/d Older children: 0.8–1 mmol/kg/d		High transporters may need supplement; low transporters' needs similar to HD patients
Fluid	Typically unrestricted unless edematous; supplement if polyuric	Supplement if polyuric If oliguric: fluid restriction = insensible fluid losses + urine output + additional losses (i.e., vomiting, diarrhea) – amount to be deficited	

Data from National Kidney Foundation [1]

Abbreviations: *CKD* chronic kidney disease, *DRI* dietary reference intake, *HD* hemodialysis

Phosphorus and Calcium

The incidence of renal bone disease is higher in children compared to adults due to high bone turnover in the growing skeleton. To prevent growth failure as well as CVD associated with poor calcium-phosphorus balance, so-called CKD-mineral bone disorder (CKD-MBD), the achievement of target values for calcium (Ca++), phosphorus (PO4), and PTH is extremely important.

The KDOQI Bone Guidelines for Children with CKD [105] previously made recommendations for the strict control of serum PTH levels and the Ca × PO4 product, including a PTH goal of 200–300 pg/mL for patients receiving dialysis. The KDIGO bone guidelines allow greater variance with PTH targets, recommending 2–9 times normal values in pediatric ESKD, although there is virtually no evidence supporting the use of values on the high end of the recommended range [21]. Data from the IPPN suggested that a iPTH value of 1.7–3 times normal range (approximately 100–200 pg/mL) may be a better target [106]. However, the latest KDIGO update stressed the importance of including calcium and alkaline phosphatase in the evaluation of bone metabolism, as well as trending PTH values since a single value may be spurious. It also recommends evaluation as early as CKD stage 2 [107].

Maximum dietary phosphorus intake and intake of calcium from calcium-containing phosphorus binders and diet are also outlined in the KDOQI bone guidelines because of their importance in bone management [105]. It is recommended to limit dietary phosphorus intake to the DRI if iPTH values are elevated and to 80% of the DRI if serum phosphorus levels are elevated in patients with CKD. Eighty percent of the DRI for age is appropriate for all pediatric dialysis patients [21]. An intake below 500 mg of phosphorus in any age group, however, may not be compatible with adequate oral intake for those who consume all their calories from food as opposed to tube feedings or formulas. Current recommendations from the KDOQI nutrition guidelines indicate that serum phosphorus levels should ideally be normal for age. However, some evidence discourages overrestriction of dietary phosphorus [108], given the associated possibility for PEW. This would support the previously published KDOQI bone guidelines allowing for serum phosphorus in the range of 3.5–5.5 mg/dL for adolescents and 4–6 mg/dL for younger children on dialysis, which is slightly higher than normal values. Normal serum phosphorus levels for age for patients with CKD stages 1–4 are also recommended by the KDOQI pediatric bone guidelines [105]. A lower serum phosphorus level may be more attainable in those with residual renal output as opposed to children who are anuric or severely oliguric. The 2017 KDIGO guidelines recommend "lowering phosphorus toward a normal range," which acknowledges that it may be more realistic for some patients to achieve a normal serum phosphorus value than others [107].

Many factors such as urine output, amount of dialysis, type of dialysis, and membrane transport characteristics influence phosphorus management. Traditional peritoneal dialysis or thrice weekly hemodialysis provides limited phosphorus removal. Patients with residual kidney function and patients on PD who are high transporters also tend to have lower serum phosphorus levels [109]. Children receiving more frequent dialysis, especially nocturnal dialysis, may require little or no binders and in some cases may actually have to supplement phosphorus [17, 22].

Recommendations for dietary counseling to control phosphorus intake are moving away from the traditional food lists of "good" and "bad" food choices and focusing more on the limitation of processed foods and phosphate additives. It is prudent to limit dairy and meat intake within the bounds of adequate protein intake, as these are naturally rich sources of phosphorus as well. In a typical mixed-food diet comprised of natural foods, about 60% of phosphorus is absorbed. However, nearly 100% of phosphorus is absorbed from processed foods in which phosphate additives have been used in the manufacturing process. Without changing protein or calcium content, it may be possible for the adolescent to consume an extra 1000 mg of phosphorus in the diet, by only including more processed versus natural foods [110]. One of the most challenging aspects of phosphorus-related counseling for children and families with CKD is that phosphorus may be difficult to detect. Phosphorus is abbreviated in many different additive forms and many standard nutrient databases underestimate the phosphorus content of food due to an increased use of these additives in the last decade [111]. This is of particular concern as the typical adolescent diet may be comprised of many of these items such as colas, fast food, and convenience quick-cooking products.

Because children on formula often have controlled phosphorus intake and are typically placed on a low phosphate formula, or optimally are breastfed, hyperphosphatemia is most often not a concern in these children. Similac PM 60/40® is the only infant formula designed specifically for pediatric CKD patients that is currently available in the United States. Renastart® (Vitaflo, Alexandria VA) in the United States and Nephea Kid® in Canada (Meta X, Hamburg, Germany) are pediatric renal formulas designed to be mixed with other formulas to lower select nutrients such as phosphorus and potassium. However, if electrolyte balance allows, a general infant formula that has a lower phosphorus content may work as well, especially in earlier stages of CKD. Other formulas designed for older children may also be an option (see discussion in *Infants* section). Typically, the choice of a low phosphorus formula is continued beyond 1 year of age to delay introducing phosphorus-rich cow's milk.

The provision of adequate dietary protein within the constraints of a phosphorus limitation can be difficult given that protein-rich foods are typically good sources of phosphorus. Because of the increased use of phosphate additives, especially in many animal products, the "typical American" diet today is higher in phosphorus than it was in past decades. In the case of a nondialysis patient with CKD, who does not need additional high-biological value protein to cover dialysis losses, there is new evidence that a vegetarian diet may be appropriate [112]. Although this study included adults, many pediatric clinicians have reported improved phosphorus values with a more plant-based diet. As a result of the phytate content of legumes and nuts, which binds some phosphorus, a well-planned, natural-food-based vegetarian diet may actually be lower in phosphorus than the traditionally prescribed diet that limits high-phosphorus legumes and nuts. Additionally, a natural-based vegetarian diet may provide other benefits such as increased fiber and reduced saturated fat that may be important in modifying the cardiovascular milieu associated with CKD.

Education of the pediatric patient and his/her family about the reasons and methods for dietary phosphorus restriction and the impact on patient outcome is important. The "renal diet" is not easy to comply with and may be particularly challenging for the pediatric patient whose normal diet is exceedingly high in phosphorus. In some cases, a patient's family may have social or cultural barriers that also influence the ability to achieve the necessary dietary management. The experiences of one center suggests that intensified diet education, using many different learning styles and tools, may be important for understanding the diet and improved phosphorus levels [113].

Successful individualization of the low phosphorus diet also requires attention to adherence. Preferences of the child should be considered when attempting to increase intake and include as many favorite foods as possible: within dietary limits to manage electrolyte and other laboratory values. At the same time, the calorie to phosphorus ratio should be considered to maximize total nutrient intake, especially for those who struggle with weight gain or adequate rate of weight gain. Timing of meals and amount consumed at mealtimes should also be assessed, especially when prescribing a binder regimen. Popular phosphorus binders available include calcium carbonate, calcium acetate (Phoslo® or Phoslyra®), sevelamer carbonate (Renvela®), and sevelamer acetate (Renagel®). Sevelamer carbonate and acetate are noncalcium options for pediatric patients, and there is limited experience on the use of pretreated beverages (such as formula) with sevelamer to lower the phosphorus content [114]. The KDOQI guidelines [1] indicate that calcium-based binders should be the first choice for infants and young children; however, noncalcium-based binders may be used if hypercalcemia is a concern [105, 107].

There is evidence that self-monitoring in the pediatric population is beneficial to phosphorus control. Teaching patients to adjust the phosphorus binder dose to the amount of phosphorus consumed at a meal or snack has also been shown to not only empower the pediatric patient, but to also lead to improved phosphorus levels [115].

When considering calcium needs, a clinician must balance the need for adequacy of intake for bone mineralization and growth versus the concern for excess intake and the subsequent development of adynamic bone disease or cardiac calcification. High doses of active vitamin D may contribute to increased intestinal calcium absorption [1]. The KDOQI guidelines recommend that calcium intake for children and adolescents should be between 100% and 200% of the DRI for age from dietary intake and calcium binders or supplements combined [1]. However, calcium intake may need to be further adjusted if the patient is hypo- or hypercalcemic. A calcium supplement, given away from meals and not more than 500 mg at a time for best absorption, may be appropriate if the patient is not meeting the DRI for age or is hypocalcemic [105]. Calcium intake may also be low due to dietary restrictions, reduced intestinal absorption due to low levels of 1,25-(OH)2 D, or poor appetite and intake [1].

Fluid

Fluid needs can vary for the child with CKD and who is receiving dialysis. Children whose primary kidney disorder is characterized by polyuria will often require a substantial fluid intake to prevent dehydration in the setting of mild-to-moderate CKD [1]. Supplementation of fluid via enteral formula or as free water may be necessary, with careful monitoring of electrolyte needs. Regular assessment of hydration via laboratory assessment or physical appearance is important. In contrast to the nonoliguric patient, children who have limited urine output or who are anuric often need fluid restriction, especially if they are edematous or have hypertension. An assessment of 24-hour urine output and other losses (such as diarrhea or emesis, insensible losses), as well as ultrafiltration capacity/fluid removal for those patients on dialysis, helps determine the most appropriate fluid allowance [1]. Foods that contain fluid may need to be evaluated or restricted if fluid intake continues to be excessive, even after counseling. When fluid restriction is required, families should be taught that food that is liquid at room temperature contains water and must be counted as part of the daily fluid allotment. Sucking on crushed ice, chewing gum, or enjoying a frozen piece of fruit may aid with the dry mouth that many patients experience. Limiting sodium intake is also very important as ingested sodium increases thirst.

Age-Related Intervention and Monitoring

Infants and Toddlers (Ages 0–3 Years)

Infants and toddlers with CKD may demand much of the clinicians' time and resources. Growth and associated cognitive development are most active during the first few years of life. Consequently, growth, biochemical profiles, and adequacy of intake must be monitored closely during this time. One dialysis center has reported that dietetic contacts were needed twice as frequently for the care of children younger than age 5 compared to those aged 5 and older, indicating that younger children require more close monitoring, intervention, and clinician time than older children [116].

Most infants with CKD are satisfied with small volumes of oral feedings and often have slow or no progression through the normal stages of acquired oral feeding skills, thus often having inadequate intake or intake that is not age-appropriate. Use of gastrostomy feeding tubes is preferred to nasogastric tubes for long-term use, and they are often necessary as most children with advanced CKD are unable to spontaneously take adequate caloric intake [117]. However, growth and weight gain should be carefully monitored to prevent overfeeding and development of obesity, since IPPN data suggest that gastrostomies are a risk factor for obesity [38]. Obesity is also a risk factor for mortality in young children [38]. Advanced stages of CKD are commonly associated with feeding problems. Children with a history of invasive medical procedures (e.g., intubation, tube feeding, suctioning) around their mouth or nose may also have aversions to stimulation around those areas, which may preclude adequate food and fluid intake. Some children may be able to take formula or even pureed baby foods, but they are unable to advance textures. This scenario can be especially common in young children with CKD, since many have spent time in the Neonatal Intensive Care Unit (NICU) soon after birth. Involvement of the speech language pathologist, occupational therapist, or behavioral feeding therapist may aid with the advancement of oral feeding [118, 119]. In the absence of these specialists, the clinician should still encourage oral stimulation. Children with advanced CKD who receive appropriate oral stimulation and attempts with feeding, even if unsuccessful in infancy, are more likely to be able to quickly advance to an oral diet posttransplant or in later childhood [120]. Gentle, positive touches around the mouth and face, caregiver kisses, and nonnutritive sucking (e.g., pacifier) can all promote positive oral-nasal stimuli. Working through specific problems, such as adjusting nipple size or flow, external pacing, dipping a pacifier in baby foods, and other techniques, is an easy intervention to encourage. It is important to introduce solids and advance textures at age-appropriate times, to prevent further delays, unless there is a medical contraindication to do so [119].

Renal-specific or renal-associated gastrointestinal problems are another barrier for adequate oral intake and solid food intake. Gastroesophageal reflux disease is present in over 70% of children with CKD [121], and emesis, delayed gastric emptying, and abnormal stooling patterns are additional common problems [122, 123]. Uremia, taste changes, and decreased appetite are renal-specific challenges [71]. Up to a third of the feeding may also be lost through emesis [124]. Techniques to reduce losses such as changing the timing, rate or amounts of feeds, use of medications, and optimizing dialysis to reduce uremia are options to pursue. Fundoplication or gastro-jejunal feeding may be used in extreme cases [121–123].

Breastmilk is ideal for infants and young children with CKD because of its bioavailability, whey content, easy digestibility, and low mineral and electrolyte content. Whey proteins may aid with reflux and gastric emptying symptomology [125, 126]. Breastmilk and other products high in whey content are naturally low in aluminum. Aluminum toxicity, especially in the long term, is a concern for persons with CKD [126]. While feeding at the breast, or pumped breastmilk, is ideal and should be supported by the clinician, receipt of breastmilk may not be realistic for all infants with CKD. Maternal stressors, which may reduce milk supply, such as the emotions related to having a child with a chronic illness, are reasons that breastmilk may not be available, or at least not available in adequate amounts. Additionally, the infant may not be able to feed at the breast due to poor suck, naso-oral medical devices, or related effects from prematurity. A motivated mother should consult a lactation specialist early and often to overcome these barriers to breastfeeding; however, supplementing or fortifying breastmilk may be necessary if there is inadequate volume or if the child is unlikely to take enough volume to meet caloric needs.

If formula is used, the product should meet the nutritional needs of the individual child. Sometimes more than one product may need to be used to provide for specific needs, or medications such as sodium chloride, sodium bicarbonate, or phosphate supplements may be used to fill nutritional gaps in sodium or phosphorus intake that may be limited in the formula. Usually, a low potassium formula and often a low phosphorus formula are necessary. Sodium supplementation is often necessary for children with renal tubular disorders, although sodium limitation is more commonly necessary for the child who does not have a sodium-losing condition and who is hypertensive. As noted previously, the infant renal formula Similac PM 60/40® is often used as a base formula with modular or other products added to it. Pediatric renal formulas designed to modulate other products, including Renastart® or Nephea Kid®, are becoming increasingly popular. Not sole-source nutrition, these can be added to other renal products or regular formulas. These products are also higher in sodium than Similac PM 60/40® and their addition can help supplement sodium when necessary, as well as reduce acid load and potassium [127].

On occasion, "adult" renal products, such as Suplena (Abbott Nutrition, Columbus OH), have been diluted and provided to infants to control potassium levels [128]. However, some components of the micronutrient profile may be undesirable for the pediatric population. Adding fat and carbohydrate modulars to formula or breastmilk to increase calorie content with a minimal increase in renal solute and mineral load may be more desirable. The use of protein modulars may also help achieve protein needs, especially in the case of the infant on peritoneal dialysis. Although formulas not designed to meet renal needs (e.g., soy formulas) may be considered depending on the patients' biochemical profile and stage of CKD, the long-term effects of the increased aluminum, vitamin A, and other mineral load inherent in these formulas generally make their selection less desirable as an option. Soy and elemental formulas are high in phosphorus, potassium, and aluminum. Consequently, soy formulas should be avoided and elemental formulas should only be used when absolutely medically necessary. Cow's milk is not recommended for any child younger than age 1 and typically is not appropriate for the toddler with CKD due to the high renal solute load and high potassium and phosphorus content [1].

Children (Ages 4–12)

Children with CKD may suffer from poor appetite for multiple reasons including uremia, dietary restrictions, and developmental feeding-related delays that persist from infancy. Processed foods, fast food, and other foods with high phosphorus and sodium content are commonly preferred by children, but they are usually restricted because of the child's CKD status. In turn, children may learn to self-induce vomiting through vigorous crying, coughing, or retching to avoid eating food selected and offered by caregivers. The patient with a poor appetite may respond favorably to frequently scheduled small meals and snacks.

Regular, structured times for meals and snacks are important to encourage developmentally appropriate eating behaviors and to prevent further suppression of appetite by "grazing." Parents may be tempted to only give favorite foods or allow eating on demand to indulge the child with a chronic illness. This can limit nutrient dense intake, exacerbate electrolyte problems, and discourage advancement in the acceptance of a varied diet. The primary caregiver needs guidelines for setting limits around food and eating behavior, and they require support from the healthcare team, especially dietitians, to consistently enforce them. The family or team should educate other caregivers working with the child such as school personnel, grandparents, and childcare staff to provide consistency in care [129].

Some children may remain on supplemental tube feeding for an extended period of time. In these cases, it is important to encourage hunger by providing tube or other supplemental formula feedings after meals and snacks or overnight to promote transition to a normal oral feeding regimen [1]. As children become older, they ideally should be granted some autonomy in making appropriate food choices, but also need to be counseled about their diets so that they can recognize and refuse restricted foods offered by others. It is important to recognize that children with CKD may feel like they stand out to other children if their food choices are different or modified, and they may feel a desire to eat other preferred foods consumed at social events [129]. Finding ways to adjust the home diet to allow for some social eating opportunities may be especially helpful for the child dealing with food restrictions. Communication with school or daycare providers by the dietitian, nurse, or physician may sometimes be necessary to emphasize the importance of the dietary restrictions without making the child feel uneasy.

Pica and the use of herbal supplements and alternative medications may be additional topics that need to be addressed. Children, especially those on hemodialysis, appear to be at high risk for pica, with 46% of children on dialysis at one center reporting pica [130]. Although the majority of these children were found to exhibit "ice" pica (compulsive consumption of ice), 12.6% ingested items such as chalk or soap, indicative of "hard" pica. Pica is a concern not only for the common comorbidity of iron deficiency anemia, but also because of the potential for the ingestion of harmful, toxic substances.

Adolescents (Ages 13 and Older)

Teenagers and emerging adults are a special challenge for the clinician for multiple reasons, including blossoming independence, developmental barriers, changing nutritional needs, and life transitions [131, 132]. The adolescent will often resent being spoken to as a child and needs to learn to make decisions and take ownership of his/her healthcare needs. However, some children and adolescents with CKD will have poor executive functioning skills, which may lead to poor decision-making [131], and others may have development delays related to their underlying disorder. Thus, finding the balance between promoting the teen's independence and autonomy with the need for thorough education is an important treatment goal. Repeated education (without being patronizing), multisensory approaches, hands-on teaching, and face-to-face interaction are techniques that may help improve adolescent adherence to treatment recommendations [133].

Some adolescents may be faced with the need to increase caloric intake, especially males and athletes, while some adolescents may struggle with excess weight gain and obesity, especially if they have finished development or have received steroids as part of their medical treatment. The larger adolescent may have higher protein and other nutrient needs as well [131]. A PEW picture, even in the obese patient, may be present in those with minimal appetite and limited physical activity [44].

A recent study indicated that many children and teens that had elevated serum phosphorus levels felt they were making appropriate choices in terms of phosphorus intake [134]. Nonetheless, 88% of adolescents on dialysis had elevated serum phosphorus levels [134]. Clearly, there can be a disconnect between understanding and adherence. The struggle may be related to the hidden sources of phosphorus in the diet [111]. The aforementioned approach to teach patients to self-dose binders based on phosphorus meal content may empower adolescents to have further health independence in a successful manner [115]. Other techniques may include negotiation – an adolescent may be willing to make more renal-friendly diet choices at home, so they can eat more freely with peers. It is also important to acknowledge that children with CKD often have different priorities than healthcare providers whose main focus is the prevention of morbidity and mortality. The child or adolescent with CKD may care more about quality of life and lifestyle issues [135]. Thus, identifying motivators that are important to the patients and his or her family, and making connections with dietary and other health changes, may be the most fruitful.

Enteral Nutrition

Oral Supplementation

The KDOQI guidelines recommend supplemental nutritional support when growth is poor or calorie or protein intake is less than needs. Oral supplementation should be considered as the preferred form of nutrition support [1]. Use of high calorie supplements in existing foods, such as powders or added fats, is an option, as well as homemade high calorie or commercial beverages. Modifications to liquid feedings often require minimizing volume to maintain fluid balance, optimizing tolerance, and keeping the total hours of feeding manageable for the family.

Infants and toddlers may need calorie fortification of breastmilk or infant formula regardless of whether they are fed orally or by tube. Typically, the caloric concentration of these items is 0.67 kcal/mL or 20 kcal/oz. Concentration of the formulas, within the parameters of balancing the concentration of undesirable nutrients and promoting tolerance, is an option. The addition of macronutrient modulars to the breastmilk or formula is an additional option. Step-wise increases of 2–4 kcal/oz, every few days, may improve tolerance [127, 136]. Some children may, however, not tolerate very concentrated formulas and tolerance of each stepwise increase must be assessed carefully before consideration is given to concentrating the solution further. Intolerance may present as increased wretching or emesis, abdominal pain, or stool changes.

Increasing the energy density by concentrating the base formula is often not possible because of the accompanying increase in sodium, potassium, phosphorus, and other vitamins and minerals. Therefore, fat and/or carbohydrate modules are often used. Whereas protein modulars are typically added and adjusted based on protein needs, they may contribute somewhat to the caloric concentration as well. The choice of which macronutrient to add is based upon the serum glucose and lipid profiles, presence or absence of malabsorption or respiratory disease (carbohydrate metabolism increases CO_2 production), and cost. In addition, lipid modulars may impair gastric emptying, while excessive carbohydrate modulars may increase stools. Lipid modulars often do not mix well with formula, especially if some or all of the formula is given via tube [127]. Inexpensive, heart-healthy oils may be given orally to flavor foods or as an addition to the formula, but typically they do not work well for tube feeding due to separation. Excessive use of oils provided by the oral route may also make the formula unpalatable. However, an emulsified oil such as Microlipid® (Novartis Medical Nutrition, Freemont, Michigan) can be used in a tube feeding to prevent oil from separating out during continuous feedings. Solcarb® (Medica Nutrition) is a common carbohydrate modular. Duocal® (Nutricia, Rockville, MD) is a combined fat and carbohydrate modular. Keeping a balance between carbohydrate and fat is important to remain within acceptable macronutrient distribution ranges [127].

When weaning from tube feeding to an oral diet, use of energy-dense foods, such as homemade low phosphorus and potassium shakes, high-calorie beverages, energy-dense bars, high-calorie grain products, and the aforementioned healthy oils, may be useful in meeting caloric needs. The clinician must be careful to taper these foods as transition takes place to avoid creating an affinity for high calorie foods in the long term, as overweight and obesity are increasing in the CKD and transplant populations [14].

Nonrenal pediatric products often have a micronutrient profile that may be undesirable for children with CKD, including higher amounts of phosphorus, calcium, potassium, and vitamin A. As oral supplements, these products are contraindicated in children with hyperphosphatemia and/or hyperkalemia. Modulation of such formulas with a pediatric renal product (indicated for ages 1–10) such as Renastart® or Nephea Kid®, to lower potassium, phosphate, and other select micronutrient levels is an option. Despite being an infant formula, Similac PM 60/40® is often used in children over the age of one, possibly in combination with a pediatric renal product as well. Adult renal products have been used in pediatrics as well. Nepro® (Abbott Nutrition, Columbus, Ohio) or NovaSource Renal® (Nestle Nutrition, Florham Park, NJ) are used by adults receiving dialysis; they are typically too high in protein for a young child, but may be used as a nutritional supplement for the adolescent on dialysis. Suplena® (Abbott Nutrition, Columbus, Ohio) or Renalcal® (Nestle Nutrition, Florham Park, NJ) are also sometimes used for younger ages as an enteral product. Suplena® may be better tolerated if diluted. Renalcal, which has minimal micronutrient content, is typically used as a supplement to other formulas or an oral diet. Magnesium levels may need to be closely monitored in children as the "adult" products typically are much higher in magnesium content than the pediatric products [127]. Enteral nutrition product options are summarized in Table 20.8.

Table 20.8 Enteral nutrition feeding options for pediatric renal patients in North America

Enteral feeding option	Comments:	Age range for use	Predialysis use?	Dialysis use?
Breastmilk	Biologically ideal for infant feeding and may be used for toddlers if available	If available, through at least 1 year of age; may continue if available and desired by family	Yes	Yes
Similac PM 60/40® (Abbott)	Only infant formula designed for CKD patients in North America. May need modulars to meet kcal and protein needs	Infancy and often used through age 3	Yes	Yes. May need protein modulars if patient is receiving PD
Renastart® (Vitaflo)	Pediatric renal formula (oral and enteral) low in potassium, chloride, vitamin A, protein, calcium, and phosphorus. Used to modulate/titrate other formulas. Not to be used as sole-source nutrition except for short term acute needs due to very low potassium and chloride content	Indicated for ages 1 and older, but used as infant formula in Europe	Yes	Yes
Nephea Kid® (Meta-X)	Only available in Canada. Pediatric renal formula (oral and enteral) low in potassium, chloride, vitamin A, protein, calcium, and phosphorus. Used to modulate/titrate other formulas. Not to be used as sole-source nutrition except for short-term acute needs due to very low potassium and chloride content	Indicated for ages 1 and older, but used as infant formula in Europe.	Yes	Yes
Nepro® (Abbott)	High protein "adult" product	Typically ages 10 and older.	No	Yes
Suplena® (Abbott)	Low protein "adult" product. Can be diluted for tolerance in younger ages	Typically ages 10 and older but has been used (often diluted) in younger ages including infants	Yes	Typically only in young children
Novasource Renal® (Nestle)	High protein "adult" product	Typically ages 10 and older	No	Yes
Renalcal® (Nestle)	Liquid modular supplement to other formulas due to minimal vitamin/mineral content. Not a stand-alone formula	Adult product, but has been used in younger ages to modulate formula	Yes	Yes

Abbreviation: *PD* peritoneal dialysis

Tube Feeding

Young children on dialysis typically only achieve 80% or less of their caloric needs when left to feed spontaneously [137]. The KDOQI guidelines recommend that tube feeding should be considered when oral feeding of the child with CKD is inadequate [1]. In addition to providing a means to enhance caloric intake, tubes may also provide access for additional fluid and sodium supplementation, and they are often used posttransplant for fluid needs and liquid medication administration [124]. Gastrostomy tubes (GTs) are preferred as nasogastric (NG) tubes may irritate the nose and throat and

Table 20.9 Suggested rates for initiating and advancing tube feedings

Age	Initial Hourly Infusion	Daily Increases	Goal[a]
Continuous feedings			
0–1 year	10–20 mL/h or 1–2 mL/kg/h	5–10 mL/8h or 1 mL/kg/h	21–54 mL/h or 6 mL/kg/h
1–6 years	20–30 mL/h or 2–3 mL/kg/h	10-15 mL/8h or 1 mL/kg/h	71–92 mL/h or 4–5 mL/kg/h
6–14 years	30–40 mL/h or 1 mL/kg/h	15–20 mL/8h or 0.5 mL/kg/h	108–130 mL/h or 3–4 mL/kg/h
>14 years	50 mL/h or 0.5–1 mL/kg/h	25 mL/8h or 0.4–0.5 mL/kg/h	125 mL/h
Bolus feedings			
0–1 year	60–80 mL q 4h or 10–15 mL/kg/feed	20–40 mL q 4h	80–240 mL q 4h or 20–30 mL/kg/feed
1–6 years	80–120 mL q 4h or 5–10 mL/kg/feed	40–60 mL q 4h	280–375 mL q 4h or 15–20 mL/kg/feed
6–14 years	120–160 mL q 4h or 3–5 mL/kg/feed	60–80 mL q 4h	430–520 mL q 4h or 10–20 mL/kg/feed
>14 years	200 mL q 4h or 3 mL/kg/feed	100 mL q 4h	500 mL q 4h or 10 mL/kg/feed

Note: Calculating rates based on age and per kilogram body weight is useful for small-for-age patients
Reprinted with permission from National Kidney Foundation [1]
[a]Goal is expected maximum that child will tolerate; individual children may tolerate higher rates or volumes. Proceed cautiously for jejunal feedings. Goals for individual children should be based on energy requirements and energy density of feeding and therefore may be lower than expected maximum tolerance

create oral-nasal trauma, in addition to the undesirable cosmetic issues. For children with significant gastrointestinal issues, gastro-jejunal (GJ) tubes may be helpful [138]. Formula choice to be used with tube feeding is determined by biochemistries, family and patient social needs, cost, and possible comorbidities such as gastrointestinal factors [117, 124, 139].

Both intermittent bolus feeds and continuous tube feeding can be used in children with CKD, depending on individual needs. Bolus feeding may allow for more physiological intake, patterned after the usual daytime meal and snack patterns. Overnight continuous feeding allows for time during the day when the child can develop hunger for oral and solid food feeding. A combination of these techniques is often used, to achieve adequate intake especially in infants. Some children with severe food intolerance or gastrointestinal issues may need continuous tube feeding over the course of the entire day and night [1, 118].

Tube feedings are initiated and advanced according to pediatric guidelines and tolerance (Table 20.9). Reported complications of tube feeding include emesis, exit-site infection, leakage, and displacement [140, 141]. For the patient on peritoneal dialysis, placement of GT or GJ-tubes should ideally occur prior to the initiation of PD to decrease the risk of peritonitis [140–142]. Even when children receive the vast majority of their feeding by tube, oral stimulation remains important, and use of appropriate oral stimulation has been reported by several centers to help facilitate transition from tube to oral feeding after transplantation [118, 143–145].

Parenteral Nutrition

Use of parenteral nutrition (PN) in children with CKD is uncommon, and pediatric studies are limited. Typically, PN would only be expected if a comorbidity was present impairing the GI tract. With the exception of IDPN, which is discussed later, use of PN is more common in the setting of acute kidney injury (AKI). Children who receive PN in association with HD or PD or with uncomplicated predialysis CKD require a PN prescription that is consistent with recommendations appropriate for patients with CKD, unless a comorbidity such as trauma, burns, or multiorgan involvement has resulted in increased kcal and protein needs. It is recommended to adjust caloric intake to 85% of estimated needs for all children on PN given that there is no thermal effect from feeding. The provision of adequate protein has been shown to reduce mortality risks and complications in children recovering from AKI [146]. Children on continuous renal replacement therapy (CRRT) as part of AKI management need at least 2.5 g/kg/day of protein and EER calorie needs, unless a secondary issue is present to modify this standard recommendation [147, 148].

When PN is prescribed, standard trace vitamin and mineral supplements may need to be given every other day to prevent excesses of those that are not cleared well when kidney function is impaired. The provision of water-soluble vitamins daily is optimal as a means of addressing the substantial dialysis-related losses. Children receiving CRRT may need additional supplemental nutrients such as zinc and selenium. Fluid restrictions will depend on the type of treatment and urine output. Those receiving more intense dialysis and/or who have greater urine output will need less fluid restriction [147–149]. Frequent laboratory monitoring and adjustment of PN in accordance with the patient's clinical and laboratory status are critical [147, 148, 150].

Intradialytic Parenteral Nutrition (IDPN)

IDPN may be used as a treatment for malnutrition/PEW for the patient receiving chronic hemodialysis. The KDOQI nutrition guidelines recommend the use of IDPN if oral supplementation and subsequent tube feeding do not meet the nutritional needs and goals of children with CKD [1]. In a similar manner, Juarez [151] has recommended IDPN when a child on HD has experienced more than a 10% weight loss in a 3 month or less period or the child is <90% IBW, in association with an inability to meet nutritional needs with enteral nutrition. The increase in protein that can be provided by IDPN may spare lean tissue and promote gains in body weight and/or BMI. Typically, side effects from IDPN are minor and may include hypophosphatemia, transient hyperglycemia, lipid intolerance, and mildly elevated liver function tests [152–154].

IDPN is typically given as a concentrated amino acid and dextrose solution, with lipids administered separately and based on the patients' tolerance and individual requirements. The primary goal of the therapy is an increase in protein intake with a modest increase in kcal intake [155]. A recent study of 15 pediatric dialysis patients using intralipid therapy alone to provide additional calories and spare caloric use from protein intake showed promising results and may be an alternative to IDPN. However, more evidence is needed before routine use of intralipids alone can be recommended [156].

Transplant

Transplant is the desired treatment option for children with ESKD to improve their quality of life and ideally, their longevity. Nutritional care may contribute to the duration of the functioning transplanted kidney and the overall health of the patient. At the same time, it must be recognized that medications necessary for the maintenance of the functioning allograft may be associated with side effects, such as nausea, diarrhea, mouth sores, and taste changes, which can have a negative impact on nutritional management [157]. These side effects may be of greatest concern when medication doses are highest, such as immediately posttransplant or when treating a rejection episode. Food safety is also of the utmost importance in this immune-compromised population, but it is all too often neglected as part of the posttransplant education [1, 158, 159]. The clinician must work with the patient and family to optimize good nutrition through these challenges.

Side effects of transplant medications that may impact nutritional management and outcomes include hypomagnesemia, hyperkalemia, hyperglycemia, hypertension, and gastrointestinal side effects such as diarrhea or nausea [160]. Weight gain and overweight posttransplant in association with corticosteroid usage is a major concern and often occurs rapidly. It is suspected that increased appetite, reduced diet restrictions, and improved affect are additional factors in play [161]. Newer immunuosuppressive regimens that are based on a steroid withdrawal or minimal steroid usage may help prevent excessive weight gain and other steroid-related side effects.

In addition to the issue of weight gain, when glucocorticosteroids are used, along with immunosuppressive agents such as tacrolimus, there can be impaired glucose tolerance, glycosuria, and a relative resistance to insulin, leading to diabetes in approximately 5–20% of children [162]. Reducing simple carbohydrates, weight control, and physical exercise are prescribed to assist in the management of steroid-induced diabetes. Excess concentrated sweets may also induce hyperglycemia, especially when medication doses are highest [1].

Almost 80% of children are hypertensive 1 month after transplantation due to the effects of many of the immunosuppressive medications, mandating dietary sodium restriction [163]. The risk of hypertension decreases over time, but many posttransplant patients will continue to have hypertension or need medication to control hypertension. The KDOQI guidelines recommend limiting sodium intake to the DRI for age in hypertensive children [1].

Adequacy of calcium and vitamin D intake is important, as bone mass continues to deteriorate in the first year posttransplant. Poor phosphate control prior to transplant may be to blame, and phosphorus wasting and elevated PTH values remain a year or more posttransplant [164–166]. According to the KDOQI guidelines, 100–200% of the DRI for calcium is appropriate, and supplementation of vitamin D is necessary if deficient.

Protein needs may be 125–150% of the DRI for healing immediately posttransplant, but both energy and protein needs are similar to healthy children in the long term [1, 167]. Macronutrient distribution should fall in the range of the AMDR, and heart healthy guidelines, such as limitation of saturated and trans fat, are encouraged [1]. Hyperlipidemia is a common side effect of the transplant-related medications used, and the provision of 3–4 g of omega-3 fatty acids has been shown to be effective in lowering lipids in adolescents [168].

With a well-rounded healthful diet, multivitamin therapy is not necessary for the transplant recipient because nutrient-rich diets are encouraged. However, if intake remains poor or the quality of the diet is less than desired, a general, age-appropriate multivitamin may be warranted.

It is important to correct any abnormal electrolyte levels. Magnesium and phosphorus wasting and potassium retention commonly occur in the early posttransplant period and need to be addressed [1, 163]. A liberal dietary intake of phosphorus-rich foods and fluids is often encouraged in the early transplantation period to help manage hypophosphatemia. A high fluid intake is required posttransplantation to maintain good perfusion of the transplanted kidney and to prevent toxicity from immunosuppressive agents due to dehydration [1, 167]. Young children with adult-sized transplanted kidneys may need a very high amount of fluid per body surface area to perfuse the large kidney. One protocol recommends 2500 mL of fluid × body surface area (2500 mL/m2 BSA) for 6–12 months posttransplant [169]. Young children who receive large kidneys may also require sodium supplementation to enhance renal perfusion. See Table 20.10 for a summary of nutrition needs for the pediatric kidney transplant.

Table 20.10 Nutrition for pediatric renal transplant

Energy	EER for age. Avoid excess weight gain
Protein	Initially 150% of the DRI for surgical healing, then DRI long term
Carbohydrates	AMDR, limit simple carbohydrates
Fat	AMDR, limit trans and saturated fat, especially in the presence of dyslipidemia
Sodium	Restrict to UL to prevent HTN except in young children with urinary losses. Young children may need supplementation to perfuse adult-sized kidneys
Potassium	Some may need restriction due to medication-related retention, particularly early posttransplant
Calcium	100–200% of DRI for age
Phosphorus	May need to supplement during initial posttransplant period
Magnesium	May need to supplement during initial posttransplant period
Vitamins	Supplement only if evidence of deficiency in diet. Some may need additional vitamin D
Other Minerals	Supplement only if evidence of deficiency in diet. Some may need additional iron
Fluid	1.5–4 L/day depending on urine output. Young children may need a high amount for their size to perfuse adult-sized kidneys

Data from National Kidney Foundation[1]

Abbreviations: *EER* estimated energy requirement, *DRI* dietary reference intake, *AMDR* acceptable macronutrient intake, *UL* upper limit, *HTN* hypertension

Transition

As technology and medical expertise for chronic illnesses such as CKD advances, children affected by it are no longer expected to expire before reaching adulthood. It is estimated that there are nearly 7000 adolescents on dialysis and 11,000 with kidney transplants in the age range of 15–24 years, which is considered the emerging adult phase [170]. This group provides multiple challenges as they prepare to move or "transfer" from pediatric-focused care to adult-focused care. In a recent survey of adult-focused dietitians, 22.1% reported seeing at least one pediatric patient on a monthly basis and 58% worked with pediatric patients at some point in their career [171]. This indicates that even adult-focused clinicians may have some familiarity with pediatric renal nutrition care and thus may help facilitate the transfer process. However, for this reason, the adult-focused clinician should ensure they have some comfort with pediatric care.

The process of "transition" is defined by Bell et al. [172] as "a deliberate, planned, and focused process, in which adolescents and emerging adults with chronic illness assume progressively increasing responsibility for the management of their health." The AAP recommends that planning for transition starts at age 14 and that this plan should be reviewed at least annually, with follow-up and review after the actual transfer to adult care has taken place [173]. Gradually shifting responsibility for nutritional and other medical care to the patient and focusing education and intervention toward the patient (versus the parent) should be done during this time [170].

When considering the emerging adult, it is important to remember that the typical primary cause of renal failure in this patient population is very different than in most adult patients. Comorbidities are typically related to urinary or bladder issues, the effects of autoimmune disorders, or cognitive delays, as opposed to manifestations of diabetes, hypertension, or other common adult causes of renal failure. Even as adults, challenges from these "pediatric" issues will need to be considered. Nutrition education must be conducted with this in mind.

Issues such as short stature, impaired self-esteem, and delays in sexual and developmental maturation may result in "juvenilization" – or treatment of these young adults as younger than they are. This can lead to healthcare providers and family members not expecting mature decision-making and health care responsibility by the adolescent or young adult, all of which can result in prolonged dependence and nonadherence. It is estimated that at least a third of adolescents with a transplant are nonadherent and adolescents and young adults account for the highest rates of acute and chronic rejection and graft loss [172, 174]. Executive functioning, the cognitive process which affects reasoning and decision-making, continues to develop well into the 20s. Therefore, cognition is an issue that must be accounted for in patient education pertaining to medication and nutritional management [170].

It is also important for the healthcare team to address concerns related to sexuality and reproduction in the context of the chronic medical condition. If reproduction is deemed a possibility, the dietitian should prepare nutritional counseling geared to such eventualities [172]. Risky behaviors affecting nutrition and medical care, such as alcohol or drug intake, must be addressed as well [175]. Self-identification is peaking at this time. Social issues such as employment, income, and obtaining self-insurance must be addressed, and they are paramount to adherence to nutritional and health regimens, as affordability of nutritious food, medication, and healthcare may be affected. Young adults are also more likely to question medical care recommendations. They may benefit from interactions with healthcare providers who are frank, who allow for questions, who are respectful of confidentiality, and who make the patient feel autonomous. It may take time to build trust and understanding [172, 175]. Pediatric dialysis and transplant centers also typically have a higher staff-to-patient ratio, and emerging adults may need greater individual attention, at least at first, after transfer to an adult-focused center [174]. A close working relationship between the transferring pediatric center and the accepting adult center is ideal, with communication between comparable clinicians. An official "transition clinic" to review healthcare needs, including nutrition, is recommended in settings that permit its development. In free-standing children's hospitals, occasional interaction between the adult care providers and the emerging adults prior to transfer, followed by attendance of a representative from the pediatric facility at the first visit of the patient to the adult center is beneficial. [175].

Conclusion

Nutrition is a key component of good medical management in children with CKD. Growth, psychosocial issues, and emotional development add challenges that must be taken into consideration as part of optimal nutrition management [176]. Frequent evaluation and adjustment are necessary, and changes in biochemical values, residual kidney function, dialysis prescription, and medications are important pieces to evaluate as part of the routine nutritional assessment.

Major publications on optimal care of pediatric dialysis patients recommend that pediatric renal dietitians with specialized training in the care and management of children are important members of the interdisciplinary team [3, 176]. Collaboration with physicians, nurses, social workers, and other staff, such as child life specialists or psychologists, can contribute to excellent, holistic care [1, 176, 177]. Input from the patient and family is without question of utmost importance as well. Insights derived from the patient and his/her family can not only positively impact nutrition, but can ideally ease the burden of pediatric kidney disease and improve health outcomes.

Case Study

A 3-day-old infant in the neonatal intensive care unit (NICU) has increasing BUN (48 mg/dL) and creatinine (2.2 mg/dL). He was born at 34 weeks gestation and was treated immediately for respiratory issues related to fluid collection and it is determined he has renal dysplasia. His other labs include K+ 6.3 mEq/L, Ca++ 8.9 mg/dL, and PO4 of 5.6 mg/dL. He has high urine output, and at PD catheter is placed for dialysis as well as a gastrostomy.

Case Questions and Answers

1. What infant feeding would you encourage immediately? What might you change postdialysis treatment? What parameters would you be mindful of during his course in the NICU?

    Answer: Breastmilk is ideal for both the infant with and without kidney disease and if the child is able to nurse at the breast or receive pumped breastmilk, that would be the best choice. If the mother and infant are unable or unwilling, an infant renal formula is typically necessary. Similac PM 60/40® is the only formula approved for children under the age of one available in North America. Alterations to either the breastmilk or formula may be necessary depending on course. Children with difficulty receiving enough calories may need modulars added to the breastmilk or formula to increase the calories. Alterations to the product to lower potassium content may be necessary if dialysis does not decrease serum potassium. When fluid limits, electrolytes or feeding tolerance is of concern, nutritional needs may not be met completely, often until dialysis is initiated. More options are available postdialysis in terms of increasing protein content of the formula. Additionally, biochemical values such as BUN, creatinine, and potassium may improve, limiting the need to treat these issues nutritionally. Biochemical trends, especially serum potassium, are very important to monitor. Also important to consider is the need for increased phosphorus and calcium in children who are born preterm. Higher calorie and protein requirements may be needed for the preterm infant and additional protein may be necessary when dialysis is initiated. With the high fluid output, the clinician must be mindful of all sources of fluid, including IV or boluses, and if these supports are tapered, adequate fluid must be considered as part of the nutrition prescription.

    Follow-Up: After acute dialysis in the NICU, renal function improved; however, the PD catheter was kept as the child is expected to eventually need to start maintenance dialysis. By 13 months of age, his GFR has dropped to approximately 28 mL/min/1.73 m². His PTH is 322 pg/mL, Ca++ 9.2 mg/dL, K+ 5.9 mEq/L, and his PO_4 is 6.1 mg/dL. He takes small amounts of solid foods and struggles with increasing texture but is interested in others' eating. He receives nocturnal feeds of 30 mL/hour for 8 hours and is offered feeds 5 times daily with the remainder of the goal not consumed given via GT. He drinks water after formula feeds are given. His pediatrician placed him on a standard pediatric enteral feeding product (e.g., Pediasure®) at 1 year of age. Both his weight and linear growth are slowing, and his weight/length has decreased from the 25th to 50th percentile to just above the 10th percentile.

2. What nutritional modifications would you suggest?

    Answer: The child should receive a low potassium, low phosphorus formula. The general pediatric formula could be blended with a pediatric renal product. The products available in the United States (Renastart®) and Canada (Nephea Kid®) are not stand-alone products, being too low in potassium and chloride, but are ideal for reducing the phosphorus and potassium content of a regular formula. Some children remain on Similac PM 60/40, possibly with the addition of a pediatric renal product to further lower the potassium content. However, since this child has already been switched to a general pediatric formula, it is likely easiest to only make one change, by adding the pediatric renal product. Additionally, the caloric content of these products is adjustable, which may allow for greater kcal intake to offset the poor growth. Although education on high versus low potassium and phosphorus foods may be necessary if biochemical values remain high, the use of modulating pediatric renal formulas allows for more freedom with a wider variety of oral foods. Increasing feedings to allow for more calories and use of fortifiers (such as oils, caloric modular, etc.) in the food may accomplish this. Also, evaluating emesis and other gastrointestinal habits may identify losses from emesis or other problems that could be treated medically. Oral stimulation and promotion of a variety of solid foods should continue to be promoted.

Follow-Up: At age 2 years, part-time day care will be starting at the same time as starting peritoneal dialysis. Rapid renal decline after a period of stable kidney function made pre-emptive transplant not possible.

3. What nutritional interventions will you consider?

Answer: The child may be eating more solid foods by this time, and appropriate and adequate intake will need to be considered. If he continues to need enteral product supplementation, evaluation of growth and biochemical values will help adjust the prescription as needed. A higher protein formula or protein modular will likely need to be added to offset protein losses from PD. Continued monitoring of electrolytes, especially potassium, is important to consider needs for adjustment. Dialysis transport will likely influence serum potassium. Other values such as BUN, serum albumin, and serum sodium also provide information about fluid and protein needs.

Follow-Up: After 9 months on PD, he receives a living-related donor kidney transplant. His urine output increases greatly with the adult-sized kidney he receives. He becomes hypertensive, hyperglycemic, hyperkalemic, hypophosphatemic, and hypomagnesemic on immunosuppressant therapy.

4. How will you adjust his nutritional regimen? What else needs monitoring long-term?

Answer: If he remains on enteral supplementation, once creatinine has improved and urine output is adequate, he can be advanced to a regular pediatric enteral product. A short-term period of the previous diet may be necessary if kidney function does not improve rapidly posttransplant. As soon as kidney function is in an appropriate range, if he is not yet on a full solid oral diet, his feeding should be converted back to a standard pediatric product, and any dietary phosphorus restriction should be discontinued.

If he is on an oral diet, or mostly oral diet, the family should be educated on limiting simple sugars, continuing to limit high potassium and sodium foods. Encouraging high magnesium and phosphorus foods can be beneficial, but supplementation through medication may be necessary.

If he is still receiving tube feedings, these should be gradually reduced to stimulate hunger until he is able to be weaned fully. A full oral diet is expected within 6 months posttransplant assuming the family offered oral stimulation prior to transplant.

Laboratory values should inform nutrition counseling and, as medication levels decrease, nutrition-related side effects should improve. Growth, including avoidance of excessive weight gain, should be monitored. An overall healthy diet with adequate fruits, vegetables, whole grains, dairy or dairy substitute for adequate calcium, and healthy fats should be encouraged to prevent long-term chronic diseases, of which risk is increased in children with kidney transplants. Adequate fluid intake is important for perfusion of the transplanted kidney.

References

1. National Kidney Foundation. KDOQI clinical practice guideline for nutrition in children with CKD: 2008 update. Am J Kidney Dis. 2009;53(suppl 2):S1–S124.
2. Kent PS, McCarthy MP, Burrowes JD, Pavlinac J, Goeddeke-Merickel CM, Wiesen K, et al. Academy of Nutrition and Dietetics and National Kidney Foundation: revised 2014 standards of practice and standards of professional performance for registered dietitian nutritionists (competent, proficient, and expert) in nephrology nutrition. J Ren Nutr. 2014;24(5):275–85.
3. Chand DH, Swartz S, Tuchman S, Valentini RP, Somers MJG. Dialysis in children and adolescents: the pediatric nephrology perspective. Am J Kidney Dis. 2017;69(2):288–6.
4. United States Renal Data System. 2018 USRDS annual data report: epidemiology of kidney disease in the United States. National Institutes of Health, National Institute of Diabetes and Digestive and Kidney Diseases, Bethesda, MD, 2017. Accessed at: https://www.usrds.org/2018/view/v1_06.aspx on 10 Feb 2019.
5. Becherucci F, Roperto RM, Materassi M, Romagnani P. Chronic kidney disease in children. Clin Kidney J. 2016;9:583–91.

6. North American Pediatric Renal Transplant Cooperative Study (NAPRTCS) annual report. 2011. Accessed at https://naprtcs.org/.
7. Chavers BM, Molony JT, Solid CA, Rheault MN, Collins AJ. One-year mortality rates in US children with end-stage renal disease. Am J Nephrol. 2015;41(2):121–8.
8. Thumfart J, Muller D, Wagner S, Jayanti A, Borzych-Duzalka D, Schaefer F, et al. Barriers for implementation of intensified hemodialysis: survey results from the International Pediatric Dialysis Network. Pediatr Nephrol. 2018;33(4):705–12.
9. Silverstein DM. Frequent hemodialysis: history of the modality and assessment of outcomes. Pediatr Nephrol. 2017;33:1293–300.
10. Warady BA, Fischbach M, Geary D, Goldstein SL. Frequent hemodialysis in children. Pediatrics. 2007;3:297–303.
11. Chavers BM, Rheult MN, Matas AJ, Jackson SC, Cook ME, Nevins TE, et al. Improved outcomes of kidney transplantation in infants (age <2 years). Transplantation. 2018;102(2):284–90.
12. Seikaly MG, Salhab N, Gipson D, Yiu V, Stablein D. Stature in children with chronic kidney disease: analysis of NAPRTCS database. Pediatr Nephrol. 2006;21:793–9.
13. United States Renal Data System. 2017 USRDS annual data report: epidemiology of kidney disease in the United States. National Institutes of Health, National Institute of Diabetes and Digestive and Kidney Diseases, Bethesda, MD, 2017. Accessed at: https://www.usrds.org/2017/view/v2_07.aspx on 11 Feb 2019.
14. Rodig N, McDermott K, Schneider M, Hotchkiss H, Yadin O, Seikaly M, et al. Growth in children with chronic kidney disease: a report from the chronic kidney disease in children study. Pediatr Nephrol. 2014;29:1987–95.
15. Wong CS, Gipson DS, Gillen DL, Emerson S, Koepsell T, Sherrard DJ, et al. Anthropometric measures and risk of death in children with end-stage renal disease. Am J Kidney Dis. 2000;36:811–9.
16. Rees L, Azocar M, Borzych D, Watson AR, Büscher A, Edefonti A, et al. Growth in very young children undergoing chronic peritoneal dialysis. J Am Soc Nephrol. 2011;22:2303–12.
17. Tom A, McCauley L, Bell L, Rodd C, Espinosa P, Yu G, et al. Growth during maintenance hemodialysis: impact of enhanced nutrition and clearance. J Pediatr. 1999;134:464–71.
18. Parekh RS, Flynn JT, Smoyer WE, Milne JL, Kershaw DB, Bunchman TE, et al. Improved growth in young children with severe chronic renal insufficiency who use specified nutritional therapy. J Am Soc Nephrol. 2001;12:2418–26.
19. Tonshoff B, Kiepe D, Ciarmatori S. Growth hormone/insulin-like growth factor system in children with chronic renal failure. Pediatr Nephrol. 2005;20:279–89.
20. Franke D, Zivienjak M, Ehrich JHH. Growth hormone treatment of renal growth failure during infancy and early childhood. Pediatr Nephrol. 2009;24:1093–6.
21. International Society of Nephrology. KDIGO clinical practice guideline for the diagnosis, evaluation, prevention, and treatment of chronic kidney disease – mineral and bone disorder (CKD-MBD). Kidney Int. 2009;76(S113):S1–130.
22. Fischbach M, Terzic J, Menouer S, Dheu C, Soskin S, Helmstetter A, et al. Intensified and daily hemodialysis in children might improve statural growth. Pediatr Nephrol. 2006;21:1746–52.
23. Warady BA, Fischbach M, Geary D, Goldstein SL. Frequent hemodialysis in children. Adv Chronic Kidney Dis. 2007;14(3):297–303.
24. Fischbach M, Fothergill H, Seuge L, Zaloszyc A. Dialysis strategies to improve growth in children with chronic kidney disease. J Ren Nutr. 2011;21(1):43–6.
25. Fouque D, Kalantar-Zadeh K, Kopple J, Cano N, Chauveau P, Cuppari L, et al. A proposed nomenclature and diagnostic criteria for protein-energy wasting in acute and chronic kidney disease. Kidney Int. 2008;73:391–9.
26. Mak RH, Cheung WW, Zhan JY, Shen Q, Foster BJ. Cachexia and protein-energy wasting in children with chronic kidney disease. Pediatr Nephrol. 2012;27:173–81.
27. Edefonti A, Mastrangelo A, Paglialonga F. Assessment and monitoring of nutrition status in pediatric peritoneal dialysis patients. Perit Dial Int. 2009;29(S2):S176–9.
28. Nourbakhsh N, Rhee CM, Kalantar-Zadeh K. Protein-energy wasting and uremic failure to thrive in children with chronic kidney disease: they are not small adults. Pediatr Nephrol. 2014;29:2249–52.
29. Abraham AG, Mak RH, Mitsnefes M, White C, Moxey-Mims M, Warady B, et al. Protein energy wasting in children with chronic kidney disease. Pediatr Nephrol. 2014;29(7):1231–8.
30. Becker PJ, Nieman Carney L, Corkins MR, Monczka J, Smith E, Smith SE, et al. Consensus statement of the Academy of Nutrition and Dietetics/American Society for Parenteral and Enteral Nutrition: indicators recommended for the identification and documentation of pediatric malnutrition (undernutrition). J Acad Nutr Diet. 2014;114(12):1988–2000.
31. Yildiz OI, Gurdol F, Kocak H, Oner P, Cetinalp-Demircan P, Caliskan Y, et al. Appetite-regulating hormones in chronic kidney disease patients. J Ren Nutr. 2011;21(4):316–21.
32. Naufel MFS, Bordon M, de Aquino TM, Ribeiro EB, de Abreu Carvalhaes JT. Plasma levels of acylated and total ghrelin in pediatric patients with chronic kidney disease. Pediatr Nephrol. 2010;25:2477–82.

33. Ayestaran FW, Schneider MF, Kaskel FJ, Srivaths PR, Seo-Mayer PW, Moxey-Mims M, et al. Perceived appetite and clinical outcomes in children with chronic kidney disease. Pediatr Nephrol. 2016;31:1121–7.

34. Srivaths PR, Wong C, Goldstein SL. Nutrition aspects in children receiving maintenance hemodialysis: impact on outcome. Pediatr Nephrol. 2009;24:951–7.

35. Hobbs DJ, Bunchman TE, Weismantel DP, Cole MR, Ferguson KB, Gast TR, et al. Megestrol acetate improves weight gain in pediatric patients with chronic kidney disease. J Ren Nutr. 2010;20(6):408–13.

36. Fischbach M, Dheu C, Seuge L, Orfanos N. Hemodialysis and nutritional status in children: malnutrition and cachexia. J Ren Nutr. 2009;19(1):91–4.

37. Yilmaz D, Sonmez F, Karakas S, Yavascan O, Aksu N, Omurlu IK, Yenisey C. Evaluation of nutritional status in children during predialysis, or treated by peritoneal dialysis or hemodialysis. J Trop Pediatr. 2016;62:178–84.

38. Schaefer F, Benner L, Borzych-Duzalka D, Zaritsky J, Xu H, Rees L, et al. Global variation of nutritional status in children undergoing chronic peritoneal dialysis: a longitudinal study of the international pediatric peritoneal dialysis network. Sci Rep. 2019;9:4886.

39. Bonthuis M, van Stralen KJ, Verrina E, et al. Underweight, overweight and obesity in paediatric dialysis and renal transplant patients. Nephrol Dial Transplant. 2013;28(suppl 4):iv195–204.

40. Skinner AC, Mayer ML, Flower K, Weinberger M. Health status and health care expenditures in a nationally representative sample: how do overweight and healthy-weight children compare? Pediatrics. 2008;121(2):269–77.

41. Wilson AC, Schneider MF, Cox C, Greenbaum LA, Saland J, White CT, et al. Prevalence and correlates of multiple cardiovascular risk factors in children with chronic kidney disease. Clin J Am Soc Nephrol. 2011;6:2759–65.

42. Foster BJ, Kalkwarf HJ, Shults J, Zemel BS, Wetzsteon RJ, Thayu M, Foerster DL, Leonard MB. Association of chronic kidney disease with muscle deficits in children. J Am Soc Nephrol. 2011;22:377–86.

43. Rashid R, Neill E, Smith W, King D, Beattie TJ, Murphy A, Ramage IJ, Maxwell H, Ahmed SF. Body composition and nutritional intake in children with chronic kidney disease. Pediatr Nephrol. 2006;21:1730–8.

44. Secker D, Jeejeebhoy KN. Subjective global nutritional assessment for children. Am J Clin Nutr. 2007;85:1083–9.

45. Rees L, Shaw V. Nutrition in children with CRF and on dialysis. Pediatr Nephrol. 2007;22:1689–702.

46. Baumgartner RN, Roche AF, Himes JH. Incremental growth tables: supplementary to previously published charts. Am J Clin Nutr. 1986;43:711–22.

47. Michael M, Brewer ED, Goldstein SL. Blood volume monitoring to achieve target weight in pediatric hemodialysis patients. Pediatr Nephrol. 2004;19:432–7.

48. Foster BJ, Leonard MB. Measuring nutritional status in children with chronic kidney disease. Am J Clin Nutr. 2004;80:801–14.

49. Cole TJ, Flegal KM, Nicholls D, Jackson AA. Body mass index cut offs to define thinness in children and adolescents: international survey. BMJ. 2007;335:194–202.

50. Sgambat K, Roem J, Mitsnefes M, Portale AA, Furth S, Warady BA, Moudgil A. Waist-to-height ratio, body mass index, and cardiovascular risk profile in children with chronic kidney disease. Pediatr Nephrol. 2018;33(9):1577–83.

51. Sgambat K, Clauss S, Moudgil A. Comparison of BMI, waist circumference, and waist-to-height ratio for identification of subclinical cardiovascular risk in pediatric kidney transplant recipients. Pediatr Transplant. 2018;1:1–8. https://doi.org/10.1111/petr.13300.

52. Juarez-Congelosi M, Orellana P, Goldstein R. nPCR and sAlb as nutrition status markers in pediatric hemodialysis patients. Hemodial Int. 2006;10(1):129.

53. Cano F, Azocar M, Cavada G, Delucchi A, Marin V, Rodriguez E. Kt/V and nPNA in pediatric peritoneal dialysis: a clinical or a mathematical association? Pediatr Nephrol. 2006;21:114–8.

54. Schaefer F, Klaus G, Mehls O. Peritoneal transport properties and dialysis dose affect growth and nutritional status in children on chronic peritoneal dialysis. J Am Soc Nephrol. 1999;10(8):1786–92.

55. Cano F, Marin V, Azocar M, Delucchi MA, Rodriguez EE, Diaz ED, et al. Adequacy and nutrition in pediatric peritoneal dialysis. Adv Perit Dial. 2003;19:273–8.

56. Mendley SR, Majkowski NL. Urea and nitrogen excretion in pediatric pertitoneal dialysis pateints. Kidney Int. 2000;58:2564–70.

57. Kong K, Zhang L, Huang L, Tao Y. Validity and practicability of smartphone-based photographic food records for estimating energy and nutrient intake. Asia Pac J Clin Nutr. 2017;26(3):396–401.

58. Secker D, Cornelius V, Teh JC. Validation of subjective global (nutritional) assessment (SGNA) in children with CKD. J Ren Nutr. 2011;21(2):207.

59. Brooks ER, Fatallah-Shaykh SA, Langman CB, Wolf KM, Price HE. Bioelectrical impedance predicts total body water, blood pressure, and heart rate during hemodialysis in children and adolescents. J Ren Nutr. 2008;18(3):304–11.

60. Eng CSY, Bhowruth D, Mayes M, Stronach L, Blaauw M, Barber A, et al. Assessing the hydration status of children with chronic kidney disease and on dialysis: a comparison of techniques. Nephrol Dial Transplant. 2018;33(5):847–55.

61. Verduzco JGDA, López EFH, Vázquez CP, de la Torre Serrano A, Velarde ER, Garibay EMV. Factors associated with anthropometric indicators of nutritional status in children with chronic kidney disease undergoing peritoneal dialysis, hemodialysis, and after kidney transplant. J Ren Nutr. 2018;28(5):352–8.

62. Ponton-Vazquez C, Vasquez-Garibay M, Hurtado-Lopez EF, de la Torre Serrano A, Garcia GP, Romero-Velarde E. Dietary intake, nutritional status, and body composition in children with end-stage kidney disease on hemodialysis or peritoneal dialysis. J Ren Nutr. 2017;27(3):207–15.

63. Apostolou A, Printza N, Karagiozoglou-Lampoudi T, Dotis J, Papachristou F. Nutrition assessment of children with advanced stages of chronic kidney disease – a single center study. Hippokratia. 2014;18(3):212–6.

64. Canpolat N, Caliskan S, Sever L, Tasdemir M, Ekmekci OB, Pehlivan G, et al. Malnutrition and its association with inflammation and vascular disease in children on maintenance dialysis. Pediatr Nephrol. 2013;28(11):2149–56.

65. Wong-Vega M, Srivaths PR. Air displacement plethysmography versus bioelectrical impedance to determine body composition in pediatric dialysis patients. J Ren Nutr. 2017;27(6):439–44.

66. Bakr AMAEB, Hasaneen BM, Bassiouni DARH. Assessment of nutritional status in children with CKD using hand grip strength tool. J Ren Nutr. 2018;28(4):265–9.

67. Anderson CE, Gilbert RD, Elia M. Basal metabolic rate in children with chronic kidney disease and healthy control children. Pediatr Nephrol. 2015;30:1995–2001.

68. de Aquino TM, Avesani CM, Brasileiro RS, de Abreu Carvalhaes JT. Resting energy expenditure of children and adolescents undergoing hemodialysis. J Ren Nutr. 2008;18(3):312–9.

69. Chen W, Ducharme-Smith K, Davis L, Hui WF, Warady BA, Furth SL, et al. Dietary sources of energy and nutrient intake among children and adolescents with chronic kidney disease. Pediatr Nephrol. 2017;32:1233–41.

70. Hui WF, Betoko A, Savant JD, Abraham AG, Greenbaum LA, Warady B, et al. Assessment of dietary intake of children with chronic kidney disease. Pediatr Nephrol. 2017;32:485–94.

71. Ku E, Kopple JD, McCulloch CE, Warady BA, Furth SL, Mak RH, et al. Associations between weight loss, kidney function decline and risk of ESRD in the chronic kidney disease in children (CKiD) cohort study. Am J Kidney Dis. 2018;71(5):648–56.

72. Edefonti A, Picca M, Damiani B, Loi S, Ghio L, Giani M, et al. Dietary prescription based on estimated nitrogen balance during peritoneal dialysis. Pediatr Nephrol. 1999;13:253–8.

73. Salusky IB, Fine RN, Nelson P, Blumenkrantz MJ, Kopple JD. Nutritional status of children undergoing continuous ambulatory peritoneal dialysis. Am J Clin Nutr. 1983;38:599–611.

74. Edefonti A, Paglialonga F, Picca M. A prospective multicenter study of nutritional status in children maintained on peritoneal dialysis. Nephrol Dial Transplant. 2006;21:1946–51.

75. Expert panel on integrated guidelines for cardiovascular health and risk reduction in children and adolescents: summary report. Pediatrics. 2009;128(5):S213–58.

76. Khurana M, Silverstein DM. Etiology and management of dyslipidemia in children with chronic kidney disease. Pediatr Nephrol. 2015;30:2073–84.

77. Querfeld U. Disturbance of lipid metabolism in children with chronic renal failure. Pediatr Nephrol. 1993;7:749–57.

78. Querfeld U, Salusky IB, Nelson P, Foley J, Fine RN. Hyperlipidemia in pediatric patients undergoing peritoneal dialysis. Pediatr Nephrol. 1988;2:447–52.

79. Kavey RW, Allada V, Daniels SR, Hayman LL, McCrindle BW, Newburger JW, et al. Cardiovascular risk reduction in high-risk pediatric patients: a scientific statement from the American Heart Association expert panel on population and prevention science; the councils on cardiovascular disease in the young, epidemiology and prevention, nutrition, physical activity and metabolism, high blood pressure research, cardiovascular nursing, and the kidney in heart outcomes research: endorsed by the American Academy of Pediatrics. Circulation. 2006;114:2710–38.

80. Kidney disease: improving global outcomes (KDIGO) lipid work group. KDIGO clinical practice guideline for lipid management in chronic kidney disease. Kidney Int. 2013;3(3):259–305.

81. Don T, Friedlander S, Wong W. Dietary intakes and biochemical status of B vitamins in a group of children receiving dialysis. J Ren Nutr. 2010;20(1):23–8.

82. Kriley M, Warady BA. Vitamin status of pediatric patients receiving long-term peritoneal dialysis. Am J Clin Nutr. 1991;53:1476–9.

83. Warady BA, Kriley M, Alon U. Vitamin status of infants receiving long-term peritoneal dialysis. Pediatr Nephrol. 1994;8:354–6.

84. Joyce T, Court Brown F, Wallace D, Reid CJD, Sinha MD. Trace element and vitamin concentrations in paediatric dialysis patients. Pediatr Nephrol. 2018;33:159–65.

85. Kjellstand C, Eaton J, Pru C. Vitamin C intoxication and hyperoxalemia in chronic hemodialysis patients. Nephron. 1985;39:112–6.

86. Fassinger N, Imam A, Klurfeld DM. Serum retinol, retionol-binding protein and transthyretin in children receiving dialysis. J Ren Nutr. 2010;20(1):17–22.

87. Manichkavasagar B, McArdle AJ, Yadav P, Shaw V, Dixon M, Blomhoff R, et al. Hypervitaminosis A is prevalent in children with CKD and contributes to hypercalcemia. Pediatr Nephrol. 2015;30:317–25.

88. Nemeth I, Turi S, Haszon I, Bereczki C. Vitamin E alleviates the oxidative stress of erythropoietin in uremic children on hemodialysis. Pediatr Nephrol. 2000;14:13–7.

89. Wagner CL, Greer FR. Prevention of rickets and vitamin D deficiency in infants, children and adolescents. Pediatrics. 2008;122:1142–52.

90. American Academy of Pediatrics. American Academy of Pediatrics Section on Breastfeeding. Breastfeeding and the use of human milk. Policy statement. Pediatrics. 2005;115(2):496–506.

91. Canadian Paediatric Society, Dietitians of Canada, Health Canada. Nutrition for healthy term infants. Ottawa: Minister of Public Works and Government Services; 1998.

92. Shroff R, Wan M, Nagler EV, Bakkaloglu S, Fischer DC, Bishop N, et al. Clinical practice recommendations for native vitamin D therapy in children with chronic kidney disease stages 2–5 and on dialysis. Nephrol Dial Transplant. 2017;32:1098–113.

93. Seeherunvong W, Abitbol CL, Chandar J, Zilleruelo G, Freunduch M. Vitamin D insufficiency and deficiency in children with early chronic kidney disease. J Pediatr. 2009;154(6):906–11.

94. Querfeld U, Mak RH. Vitamin D deficiency and toxicity in chronic kidney disease: in search of the therapeutic window. Pediatr Nephrol. 2010;25:2413–30.

95. Hari P, Gupta N, Hari S, Gulati A, Mahajan P, Bagga A. Vitamin D insufficiency and effect of cholecalciferol in children with chronic kidney disease. Pediatr Nephrol. 2010;25:2483–8.

96. Rodriguez-Soriano J, Arant BS. Fluid and electrolyte imbalances in children with chronic renal failure. Am J Kidney Dis. 1986;7:268–74.

97. Stallings VA, Harrison M, Oria M, Committee to Review the Dietary Reference Intakes for Sodium and Potassium, Food and Nutrition Board, Health and Medicine Division, National Academy of Sciences, Engineering, and Medicine. Dietary reference intakes for sodium and potassium. Washington, DC: National Academies Press; 2019.

98. Mattes RD, Donnelly D. Relative contributions of dietary sodium sources. J Am Coll Nutr. 1991;10(4):383–93.

99. Beto J, Bansal VK. Hyperkalemia: evaluating dietary and nondietary etiology. J Ren Nutr. 1992;2(1):28–9.

100. Bunchman TE, Wood EG, Schenck MH, Weaver KA, Klein BL, Lynch RE. Pretreatment of formula with sodium polystyrene sulfonate to reduce dietary potassium intake. Pediatr Nephrol. 1991;5:29–32.

101. Rivard AL, Raup SM, Beilman GJ. Sodium polystyrene sulfonate used to reduce the potassium content of a high-protein enteral formula: a quantitative analysis. JPEN. 2004;28(2):76–8.

102. Taylor JM, Oladitan L, Carlson S, Hamilton-Reeves JM. Renal formulas pretreated with medications alters the nutrient profile. Pediatr Nephrol. 2015;30:1815–23.

103. Le Palma K, Rampolla-Pavlick E, Copelovitch L. Pretreatment of enteral nutrition with sodium polystyrene sulfonate: effective, but beware of high prevalence of electrolyte derangements in clinical practice. Clin Kidney J. 2018;11(2):166–71.

104. Chua AN, Warady BA. Care of the pediatric patient on chronic dialysis. Adv Chronic Kidney Dis. 2017;24(6):388–97.

105. National Kidney Foundation. K/DOQI clinical practice guidelines for bone metabolism and disease in children with chronic kidney disease. Am J Kidney Dis. 2005;46(4, Suppl 1):S1–121.

106. Haffner D, Schaefer F. Searching the optimal PTH target range in children undergoing peritoneal dialysis: new insights from international cohort studies. Pediatr Nephrol. 2013;28(4):537–45.

107. Kidney disease: improving global outcomes (KDIGO) CKD-MBD Update Work Group. KDIGO 2017 clinical practice guideline update for the diagnosis, evaluation, prevention, and treatment of chronic kidney disease-mineral bone disorder (CKD-MBD). Kidney Int. 2017;7(suppl 1):1–59.

108. Shinaberger CS, Kopple JD, Van Wyck D, Mehrotra R, Kovesdy CP, Kalantar-Zadeh K. Is controlling phosphorus by decreasing dietary protein intake beneficial or harmful in persons with chronic kidney disease? Am J Clin Nutr. 2008;88:1511–8.

109. Sedlacek M, Dimaano F, Uribarri J. Relationship between phosphorus and creatinine clearance in peritoneal dialysis: clinical implications. Am J Kidney Dis. 2000;36(5):1020–4.

110. Uribarri J, Calvo MS. Hidden sources of phosphorus in the typical American diet: does it matter in nephrology? Semin Dial. 2003;16(3):186–8.

111. Sullivan CM, Leon JB, Sehgal AR. Phosphorus-containing food additives and the accuracy of nutrient databases: implications for renal patients. J Ren Nutr. 2007;17(5):350–4.

112. Moe SM, Zidehsarai MP, Chambers MA, Jackman LA, Radcliffe JS, Trevino LL, et al. Vegetarian compared with meat dietary protein source and phosphorus homeostasis in chronic kidney disease. Clin J Am Soc Nephrol. 2011;6:257–64.

113. Abercrombie EL, Greenbaum LA, Baxter DH, Hopkins B. Effect of intensified diet education on serum phosphorus and knowledge of pediatric peritoneal dialysis patients. J Ren Nutr. 2010;20(3):193–8.

114. Raaijmakers R, Willems J, Houkes B, Heuval CS, Monnens LA. Pretreatment of various dairy products with sevelamer: effective P reduction but also a rise in pH. Perit Dial Int. 2008;29:S15A.

115. Ahlenstiel T, Pape L, Ehrich JHH, Kuhlmann MK. Self-adjustment of phosphate binder dose to meal phosphorus content improves management of hyperphosphataemia in children with chronic kidney disease. Nephrol Dial Transplant. 2010;25:3241–9.

116. Coleman JE, Norman LJ, Watson AR. Provision of dietetic care in children on chronic peritoneal dialysis. J Ren Nutr. 1999;9(3):145–8.

117. Coleman J, Watson A, Rance C, Moore E. Gastrostomy buttons for nutritional support on chronic dialysis. Nephrol Dial Transplant. 1998;13:2041–6.

118. Warady BA, Kriley M, Belden B, Hellerstein S, Alon U. Nutritional and behavioural aspects of nasogastric tube feeding in infants receiving chronic peritoneal dialysis. Adv Perit Dial. 1990;6:265–8.

119. Samaan S, Secker D. Oral feeding challenges in infants with chronic kidney disease. Infant Child Adolesc Nutr. 2014;6(3):164–71.

120. Pugh P, Watson A. Transition from gastrostomy to oral feeding following renal transplantation. Adv Perit Dial. 2006;22:153–7.

121. Ruley EJ, Bock GH, Kerzner B, Abbott AW, Majd M, Chatoor I. Feeding disorders and gastroesophageal reflux in infants with chronic renal failure. Pediatr Nephrol. 1989;3:424–9.

122. Ravelli AM, Ledermann S, Bissett W, Trompeter R, Barratt T, Milla P. Foregut motor function in chronic renal failure. Arch Dis Child. 1992;67:1343–7.

123. Ravelli AM. Gastrointestinal function in chronic renal failure. Pediatr Nephrol. 1995;9:756–62.

124. Rees L, Brandt M. Tube feeding in children with chronic kidney disease: technical and practical issues. Pediatr Nephrol. 2010;25:699–704.

125. Fried M, Khoshoo V, Secker D, Gilday D, Ash J, Pencharz P. Decrease in gastric emptying time and episodes of regurgitation in children with spastic quadriplegia fed a whey-based formula. J Pediatr. 1992;120(4 Pt 1):569–72.

126. Hawkins NM, Coffey S, Lawson MS, Delves HT. Potential aluminum toxicity in infants fed special infant formulas. J Pediatr Gastroenterol Nutr. 1994;19:377–81.

127. Nelms CL. Optimizing enteral nutrition for growth in pediatric chronic kidney disease (CKD). Front Pediatr. 2018;6:214.

128. Hobbs DJ, Gast TR, Ferguson KB, Bunchman TE, Barletta GM. Nutritional management of hyperkalemic infants with chronic kidney disease, using adult renal formulas. J Ren Nutr. 2010;20(2):121–6.

129. Lum A, Wakefield CE, Donnan B, Burns MA, Fardell JE, Marshall GM. Understanding the school experiences of children and adolescents with serious chronic illness: a systematic meta-review. Child Care Health Dev. 2017;43(5):645–62.

130. Katsoufis CP, Kertis M, McCullough J, Pereira T, Seeherunvong W, Chandar J, et al. Pica: an important and unrecognized problem in pediatric dialysis patients. J Ren Nutr. 2012;22(6):567–71.

131. Chen K, Didsbury M, van Zwieten A, Howell M, Kim S, Tong A, et al. Neurocognitive and educational outcomes in children and adolescents with CKD. Clin J Am Soc Nephrol. 2018;13:387–97.

132. de Ferris MEDG, Del Villar-Vilchis M, Guerrero R, Barajas-Valencia VM, Vander-Schaaf EB, de Pomposo A, et al. Self management and health care transition among adolescents and young adults with chronic kidney disease: medical and psychosocial considerations. Chronic Kidney Dis. 2017;24(6):405–9.

133. Rondon S, Sassi FC, de Andrade CRF. Computer game-based and traditional learning method: a comparison regarding students' knowledge retention. BMC Med Educ. 2013;13:1–8.

134. Taylor JM, Oladitan L, Degnan A, Henderson S, Honying D, Warady BA. Psychosocial factors that create barriers to managing serum phosphorus levels in pediatric dialysis patients: a retrospective analysis. J Ren Nutr. 2016;26(4):270–5.

135. Tong A, Manns B, Wang AYM, Hemmelgarn B, Wheeler DC, Gill J, et al. Implementing core outcomes in kidney disease: report of the Standardized Outcomes in Nephrology (SONG) implementation workshop. Kidney Int. 2018;94(6):1058–68.

136. Yiu VW, Harmon WE, Spinozzi N, Jonas M, Kim MS. High-calorie nutrition for infants with chronic renal disease. J Ren Nutr. 1996;6(4):203–6.

137. Paglialonga F, Edefonti A. Nutrition assessment and management in children on peritoneal dialysis. Pediatr Nephrol. 2009;24:721–34.

138. Monczka J. Enteral nutrition support: determining the best way to feed. In: Corkins MR, editor. The American Society for Parenteral and Enteral Nutrition pediatric nutrition support core curriculum. 2nd ed. Silver Spring: The American Society for Parenteral and Enteral Nutrition; 2015. p. 256–82.

139. Ledermann SE, Shaw V, Trompeter RS. Long-term enteral nutrition in infants and young children with chronic renal failure. Pediatr Nephrol. 1999;13(9):870–5.

140. Ramage IJ, Harvey E, Geary DF, Hebert D, Balfe JA, Balfe JW. Complications of gastrostomy feeding in children receiving peritoneal dialysis. Pediatr Nephrol. 1999;13(3):249–52.

141. Ledermann SE, Spitz L, Moloney J. Gastrostomy feeding in infants and children on peritoneal dialysis. Pediatr Nephrol. 2002;17:246–50.
142. Warady BA. Gastrostomy feedings in patients receiving peritoneal dialysis. Perit Dial Int. 1999;19(3):204–6.
143. Dello Strologo L, Principato F, Sinibaldi D, Appiani AC, Terzi F, Dartois AM, et al. Feeding dysfunction in infants with severe chronic renal failure after long-term nasogastric tube feeding. Pediatr Nephrol. 1997;11(1):84–6.
144. Coleman JE, Watson AR. Growth post transplantation in children previously treated with chronic dialysis and gastrostomy feeding. Adv Perit Dial. 1998;14:269–73.
145. Kari JA, Gonzalez C, Ledermann SE, Shaw V, Rees L. Outcome and growth of infants with severe chronic renal failure. Kidney Int. 2000;57(4):1681–7.
146. Kyle UG, Akcan-Arikan A, Silva JC, Goldsworthy M, Shekerdemian LS, Coss-Bu JA. Protein feeding in pediatric acute kidney injury is not associated with a delay in renal recovery. J Ren Nutr. 2017;27:8–15.
147. Zappitelli M, Goldstein SL, Symons JM, Somers MJ, Baum MA, Brophy PD, et al. Protein and calorie prescription for children and young adults receiving continuous renal replacement therapy; a report from the Prospective Pediatric Continuous Renal Replacement Therapy Registry Group. Pediatr Crit Care Med. 2008;36:3239–45.
148. Maxvold NJ, Smoyer WE, Custer JR, Bunchman TE. Amino acid loss and nitrogen balance in critically ill children with acute renal failure; a prospective comparison between classic hemofiltration and hemofiltration with dialysis. Crit Care Med. 2000;28(4):1161–5.
149. Spinozzi NS, Nelson P. Nutrition support in the newborn intensive care unit. J Ren Nutr. 1996;6(4):188–97.
150. Nakamura AT, Btaiche IF, Pasko DA, Jain JC, Mueller BA. In vitro clearance of trace elements via continuous renal replacement therapy. J Ren Nutr. 2004;14(4):214–9.
151. Juarez MD. Intradialytic parenteral nutrition in pediatrics. Front Pediatr. 2018;6:267.
152. Krause I, Shamir R, Davidovits M, Frishman S, Cleper R, Gamzo Z, et al. Intradialytic parenteral nutrition in malnourished children treated with hemodialysis. J Ren Nutr. 2002;12(1):55–9.
153. Goldstein SL, Baronette S, Vital Gambrell T, Currier H, Brewer ED. nPCR assessment and IDPN treatment of malnutrition in pediatric hemodialysis patients. Pediatr Nephrol. 2002;17:531–4.
154. Orellana P, Juarez-Congelosi M, Goldstein S. Intradialytic parenteral nutrition and biochemical marker assessment for malnutrition in adolescent maintenance hemodialysis patients. J Ren Nutr. 2005;15(3):312–7.
155. Council on Renal Nutrition of New England. Intradialytic parenteral nutrition. In: Renal nutrition handbook for renal dietitians. Massachusetts National Kidney Foundation; 1993. p. 86–98.
156. Haskin O, Sutherland SM, Wong CJ. The effect of intradialytic intralipid therapy in pediatric hemodialysis patients. J Ren Nutr. 2017;27:132–7.
157. McPartland KJ, Pomposelli JJ. Update on immunosuppressive drugs used in solid-organ transplantation and their nutrition implications. Nutr Clin Pract. 2007;22:467–73.
158. Obasyashi PAC. Food safety for the solid organ transplant patient: preventing foodborne illness while on chronic immunosuppressive drugs. Nutr Clin Pract. 2012;27(6):758–66.
159. Food safety for transplant recipients. https://www.fda.gov/food/people-risk-foodborne-illness/food-safety-transplant-recipients. Accessed 10 Jan 2019.
160. Coelho T, Tredger M, Dhawan A. Current status of immunosuppressive agents for solid organ transplantation in children. Pediatr Transplant. 2012;16:106–22.
161. Hanevold CD, Ping-Leung H, Talley L, Mitsnefes MM. Obesity and renal transplant outcome: a report of the North American Pediatric Renal Transplant Cooperative Study. Pediatrics. 2005;115(2):352–6.
162. Greenspan L, Gitelman S, Leung M, Glidden D, Mathias R. Increased incidence in post-transplant diabetes mellitus in children: a case-control analysis. Pediatr Nephrol. 2002;17:1–5.
163. Kasiske BL, Vazquez MA, Harmon WE, Brown RS, Danovitch GM, Gaston RS, et al. Recommendations for the outpatient surveillance of renal transplant recipients. J Am Soc Nephrol. 2000;11(Suppl 15):S1–86.
164. Guzzo I, Di Zazzo G, Laurenzi C, Ravà L, Giannone G, Picca S, et al. Parathyroid hormone levels in long-term renal transplant children and adolescents. Pediatr Nephrol. 2011;25:2051–7.
165. Ebbert K, Chow J, Krempien J, Matsuda-Abedini M, Dionne J. Vitamin D insufficiency and deficiency in pediatric renal transplant recipients. Pediatr Transplant. 2015;19:492–8.
166. Wessling-Perry K, Pereira RC, Tsai E, Ettenger R, Jüppner H, Salusky IB. FGF23 and mineral metabolism in the early post-renal transplantation period. Pediatr Nephrol. 2013;28:2207–15.
167. Asfaw M, Mingle J, Hendricks J, Pharis M, Nucci AM. Nutrition management after pediatric solid organ transplantation. Nutr Clin Pract. 2014;29(2):192–200.
168. Filler G, Weiglein G, Gharib MT, Casier S. Omega three fatty acids may reduce hyperlipidemia in pediatric renal transplant recipients. Pediatr Transplant. 2012;16:835–9.
169. Salvatierra O Jr, Singh T, Shifrin R, Conley S, Alexander S, Tanney D, et al. Successful transplantation of adult-sized kidneys into infants requires maintenance of high aortic blood flow. Transplantation. 1998;66:819–23.
170. Ferris ME, Bell LE. Transitioning the adolescent dialysis patient to adult care. In: Warady BA, Schaefer FS, Fine RN, Alexander SR, editors. Pediatric dialysis. 1st ed. Dordrecht: Springer; 2012.

171. Nelms CL, Johnson E, Peseski S. Determination of renal nutrition training and education need for pediatric-focused and adult-focused clinicians: the North American Pediatric Renal Nutrition Education Survey (NAPRNES). J Ren Nutr. 2018;S1051-2276(18):30130–4. https://doi.org/10.1053/j.jrn.2018.05.009. [Epub ahead of print].
172. Bell LE, Ferris ME, Fenton N, Hooper SR. Health care transition for adolescents with CKD - the journey from pediatric to adult care. ACKD. 2011;18(5):384–90.
173. American Academy of Pediatrics, American Academy of Family Physicians, American College of Physicians-American Society of Internal Medicine. A consensus statement on health care transitions for young adults with special health care needs. Pediatrics. 2002;110(6):1304–6.
174. Bell LE, Bartosh SM, Davis CL, Dobbels F, Al-Uzri A, Lotstein D, et al. Adolescent transition to adult care in solid organ transplantation: a consensus conference report. Am J Transplant. 2008;8(11):2230–42.
175. Bell LE, Sawyer SM. Transition of care to adult services for pediatric solid-organ transplant recipients. Pediatr Clin North Am. 2010;57(2):593–610.
176. Warady BA, Neu AM, Schaefer F. Optimal care of the pediatric end-stage renal disease patient on dialysis: 2014 update. Am J Kidney Dis. 2014;64(1):128–42.
177. Harvey E, Secker D, Braj B, Picone G, Balfe JW. The team approach to the management of children on chronic peritoneal dialysis. Adv Renal Replacement Ther. 1996;3(1):1–14.
178. Institute of Medicine. Dietary references intakes for energy, carbohydrates, fiber, fat, protein and amino acids (macronutrients). Washington, DC: National Academy of Sciences; 2002.

Chapter 21
The Aging Adult and Chronic Kidney Disease

D. Jordi Goldstein-Fuchs

Keywords Kidney senescence · Gernontology · Geriatric nephrology · Older adult · Nutrition

> **Key Points**
> - The population of the elderly with chronic kidney disease will continue to grow over the next 15–20 years. It is essential that medical providers and the community are available to support and meet their unique needs.
> - The aging process imparts particular stresses to the kidney that impact progression of disease and outcomes of the elderly on renal replacement therapy.
> - The elderly individual living with chronic kidney disease is particularly vulnerable to food and medication insecurity, social isolation, and depression.
> - Conversations to include quality of life with elderly individuals who have progressive chronic kidney disease and need to consider renal replacement therapy or alternatives such as hospice need to be implemented by the renal care team.

Introduction

The demographics of population growth in the United States is shifting. From 2002 to 2016, the population grew from 287 million to 323 million and life expectancy increased from 76.8 to 78.8 years [1]. Within this growth, there has been a drop in both fertility rate and mortality rate, resulting in significant growth of the elderly population. As reported by the US Census Bureau [2], by the year 2030, all baby boomers will be older than age 65. The size of the older population will grow such that by 2035, there will be 78 million people 65 years and older compared to 76.7 million under the age of 18. The report goes on to say that for the first time in US history, the number of older people will outnumber children [2].

The aging of the US population has important ramifications for the disease burden of chronic kidney disease (CKD) in the United States. In 2011, the US Renal Data System (USRDS) reported that adults older than 65 years of age are the most rapidly growing subset of the end-stage renal

The editors acknowledge the contribution of Denis Fouque and Julie Barboza to this chapter in *Nutrition in Kidney Disease, Second Edition*, Nutrition and Health, DOI https://doi.org/10.1007/978-1-62703-685-6_1, © Springer Science+Business Media New York 2014.

D. J. Goldstein-Fuchs (✉)
Department of Pediatric Nephrology, Lucile Packard Hospital Stanford, Palo Alto, CA, USA
e-mail: dgoldsteinfuchs@stanfordchildrens.org

disease (ESRD) patient population [3]. Individuals 60 years of age and older have the highest prevalence of CKD [4]. The 2018 USRDS report found that age had the highest correlation with low estimated glomerular filtration rate (eGFR) with an odds ratio of 70 in the 2013–2016 cohort [5]. The average eGFR for people 60 years of age and older was approximately 20 ml/min/1.73 m^2 [5]. In addition, the number of elderly treated for ESRD has doubled over the past 25 yrs [5]. As the number of older individuals presenting with CKD including end stage kidney failure is increasing in our medical environment, we need to be prepared to address their unique needs to optimize life quality during the older years through end of life. How CKD and aging impacts morbidity and mortality risk, or metabolism and nutrition needs is not totally clear. In addition, the complications of aging imposed by increased frailty and debility, loss of physical function, cognitive changes, psychosocial factors, all impacting nutritional status and quality of life, further challenge the complex needs of the older adult with chronic and end-stage kidney disease. This chapter will address these issues beginning with a discussion regarding alterations in kidney structure and assessment of renal functional in the aging kidney.

Kidney Senescence: Loss of Glomeruli and Functioning Nephrons

The aging of the normal kidney, described as a loss of nephrons and decline in GFR or kidney senescence [6], involves histological and physiological alterations. Renal mass decreases between the ages of 30 and 80 years, the largest decline occurring after age 50 [7]. There is an association of aging with an increase in globally sclerotic glomeruli. Fat and fibrotic scarring is found in the renal cortex. The scarring is hypothesized to negatively impact mechanisms promoting maximal urine concentrating. By age 75, approximately 30% of glomeruli are destroyed and display diffuse glomerular sclerosis [6, 7]. Other glomeruli exhibit impaired filtering ability. Interstitial fibrosis, moderate tubular atrophy, increased mesangial matrix, and ischemic injury are all seen in the glomerulus. The aging kidney experiences a loss of nephrons and hypofiltration [6]. It appears that the number of functioning nephrons present at birth and the rate of loss of nephrons with advanced aging impact the number of functioning glomeruli that remain available. When nephron loss occurs, a compensatory mechanism is not usually observed in the aging kidney, unlike in disease states [6].

Renal Functional Changes Associated with Aging

The average decline in renal function starting around age 30 has been reported to be 0.75–1.0 ml/min/1.73 m^2/year, or by about 8 ml/min/1.73 per decade of life [6–8] with an acceleration in the rate of decline in individuals over 80 yrs of age. These studies underlined the traditional consensus that a decline in kidney function is an inevitable part of the aging process. Results from the Baltimore Longitudinal Studies evaluated renal function decline in 254 normal men, followed over a period of 5–14 years [9] and noted the average clearance declined with age, as evidenced by a lower measured creatinine clearance with no change in serum values. This observation was more consistent in older individuals with hypertension. However, approximately one-third of the subjects had a stable creatinine clearance that did not decline with age [7, 8]. These studies revealed that while kidney function does decline with age, the decline is heterogeneous and is influenced by the presence or absence of vascular disease such as arteriosclerosis and hypertension [7, 8]. An increase in filtration fraction has been described with aging that is reported to be due to a fall in renal plasma flow that is relative to GFR [7]. This is observed in kidneys in 60- to

70-year-olds, despite the fact that the decline in eGFR is reported to start in the approximate third decade of life.

Estimates of Kidney Function

Chronic kidney disease, defined as an eGFR<60 ml/min per 1.73 m^2, is more prevalent in the elderly [7]. The prevalence of CKD in the older adult >65 years of age has been reported to be as high as 44%, and 46.8% in those older than 70 years of age [1, 7, 8, 10].

Equations to estimate the glomerular filtration rate for the general population have not been optimized for use in the older adult. This is in part due to the reliance on measuring creatinine dynamics and not being able to adjust for body composition. Creatinine generation, which is impacted by muscle mass, declines with age, and these equations tend to underestimate eGFR in the older adult. One of the earliest equations developed, The Cockcroft and Gault equation [11], overestimates eGFR in obese and edematous patients [12]. The equation for estimating GFR from the Modification of Diet in Renal Disease (MDRD) Study has been found to be less accurate in patients with normal kidney function, the elderly, kidney transplant recipients, and type 1 diabetes (DM) [1, 12, 13]. The MDRD equation tends to underestimate eGFR in the elderly. The Chronic Kidney Disease Epidemiology Collaborative (CKD-EPI) equations were developed with the intent to improve eGFR accuracy in adults >70 years of age [10, 12–14]. It is reported to be equivalent to the MDRD equation for patients with an eGFR <60 and more accurate than the MDRD equation at higher GFRs [1, 10, 12–16]. There are also equations that include cystatin-C and cystatin-C with creatinine (CKD-EPIcys; CKD-EPIcr-cys) [11–16]. Cystatin C is not dependent on musculature and is less influenced by age, gender, and race. However, the level of cystatin C can be affected by the presence of inflammation, thyroid disease, and steroids. While the CKD-EPIcys equation might be more accurate, the original studies had few participants older than 70 years of age. New equations specific for the elderly have recently been reported in the Berlin Initiative Study [16]. These studies were completed from data obtained in 610 individuals, mean age 78.5 years. The equations that include cystatin C and creatinine, or cystatin C alone, were found to be more accurate. However, validation in a more heterogeneous population is pending. For current clinical evaluation of kidney function in the elderly, the KDIGO (Kidney Disease: Improving Global Outcomes, 2012) CKD Workgroup [18] recommends utilization of the CKD-EPI equations in the elderly. See Table 21.1 for a summary of the equations most widely used for calculation of estimated glomerular filtration rates.

Identification of a reduced eGFR in the elderly is not uncommon and has been described as being "over-represented" in the elderly, in part due to the methodological limitation of kidney function

Table 21.1 Equations most widely used for calculation of estimated glomerular filtration rates

Equation	Evaluations
MDRD study	Less accurate at eGFR >60 ml/min/1.73 m^2 and older age
Cockcroft-Gault	Decreased accuracy at lower levels of CKD
CKD-EPI Scr	Overestimates CKD in older individuals
CKD-EPI cystatin C	Better for older individuals and those with reduced muscle mass
CKD-EPI Cr-cystatin C	Performs better than all above in estimating GFR. Better in elderly

Modified from Refs. [8, 14, 18]

Abbreviations: *MDRD Study* Modification of Diet in Renal Disease, *CKD-EPI Scr* Chronic Kidney Disease Epidemiology Collaboration serum creatinine, *CKD-EPI cystatin C* Chronic Kidney Disease Epidemiology Collaboration cystatin C, *CKD-EPI Cr-cystatin* Chronic Kidney Disease Epidemiology Collaboration creatinine cystatin C assessment described above [15–19]. Other factors cited as contributing to this observation include the dominance of type 2 diabetes and atherosclerosis, both of which affect the kidney as well as vascular, tubular, and glomerular changes. The risk for CKD was reported in the USRDS 2015 report to be 8 times higher in individuals over 60 years of age [3]. The National Health and Nutrition Examination Survey (NHANES) data from 1999 to 2004 reported using the CKD-EPI equation that the prevalence of CKD in participants 70 years of age and older was 46.8% compared to 6.71% in those between 40 and 59 years of age [19]. However, there are debates as to whether all levels of eGFR without proteinuria or other markers of kidney damage truly reflect disease or are within a benign range of kidney senescence [7, 20, 21]. This continues to be a challenge. Some report the risk of death in older adults with CKD is greater than that of ESRD and the eGFR threshold marking a greater ESRD risk versus mortality is lower than earlier reports [22]. In patients 45–65 years of age, rates of ESRD surpassed mortality only if eGFR was <30 ml/min/1.73 m^2 and for patients 65–75 years of age only when eGFR was <15 ml/min per 1.73 m^2 [13]. The question remains, in the absence of vascular and other diseases, as to what level of decreased eGFR accurately reflects normal kidney decline versus one that puts an older individual at risk of ESRD. The majority of older adults with reduced eGFR have a mortality event before reaching ESRD [8, 13, 21, 22]. In addition to comorbid conditions such as cardiovascular disease (CVD), psychosocial components including lifestyle might impact risk for CKD progression in an older person. Examples include polypharmacy, dehydration, cognitive decline, physical inactivity, debility, frailty and malnutrition, and overall all-cause mortality risk associated with aging.

Aging and CKD Risk

The etiology of CKD in the elderly population is not clear; however, vascular disease is thought to be a primary causal factor [19]. Risk factors for CVD in the elderly with CKD that might present themselves earlier in life include diabetes, hypertension, and obesity [1, 8, 13, 19]. These vascular risks are associated with kidney biopsy findings that can include respectively glomerulosclerosis, nephroarteriolar sclerosis, and focal segmental glomerulosclerosis (FSGS) [6, 7, 22]. However, as observations only, they do not rule out the possibility that older patients without these diagnoses may have subclinical vascular changes that are associated with the normal process of aging resulting in reduced GFR and glomerulosclerosis. The presence of albuminuria with or without a reduced eGFR is associated with a risk of adverse outcome in the elderly including ESRD and all-cause mortality [8, 19, 22]. The higher risk of acute cerebrovascular disease, hypertension, medication nephrotoxicity, and acute kidney injury, all place a higher risk of the elderly CKD patient toward progressing to ESRD [19]. Modifiable traditional and non-traditional risk factors and non-modifiable risk factors for CKD in the elderly have been described [14]. A discussion pertaining to those that involve nutrition intervention now follows.

Risk Reduction of CKD and ESRD in the Older Adult

Treat and Control Hypertension

Blood pressure goals for the older adult with CKD consider recommendations from The Eighth Report of the Joint National Committee on Prevention, Detection, Evaluation, and Treatment of High Blood Pressure [23], the 2013 KDIGO guidelines [24], and the American College of Cardiology/ American Heart Association (ACC/AHA) Guidelines published in 2018 [25]. Blood pressure targets are ≤140/90 mmHg if albuminuria is <30 mg per day and a blood pressure ≤130/80 mmHg if albuminuria is >30 mg/day. While selecting blood pressure–lowering medications such as angiotensin-converting enzyme (ACE) inhibitors and angiotensin receptor blockers (ARBs), the risk of potential adverse events such as hyperkalemia and worsening kidney function need to be considered. Close monitoring of the older patient's laboratory values is warranted. Nutrition recommendations include a low sodium diet and a diet pattern of eating that promotes intake of fresh fruits and vegetables, whole grains, avoidance of red meats, and nonfat dairy products. Physical activity as assessed individually is also encouraged as part of lifestyle modifications. All recommendations are individualized in accordance to nutrition assessment and laboratory findings [23–26].

Treat Hyperlipidemia

Treatment for dyslipidemia in the elderly with CKD is based on the guidelines of KDOQI [27], KDIGO [28], and the ACC/AHA guidelines [29]. A main change to the guidelines is a shift from a focus on low-density lipoprotein cholesterol (LDL-C) targets to the use of a statin to treat dyslipidemia. KDIGO recommends that all adults ≥50 years of age with CKD, but not those on dialysis, be treated with statin therapy. In addition, for adults in the same age group with an eGFR <60 ml/min/m^2, combination of a statin with ezetimibe is also recommended [27–29]. Nutrition therapy includes the use of omega-9 and omega-3 fatty acids containing oils as part of lifestyle modifications [30].

Diabetes Management

Chronic kidney disease resulting from microvascular injury to the kidneys from diabetes or diabetic nephropathy is reported to be responsible for approximately 40–50% of the CKD patient population [1, 8]. There is a growing incidence of diabetes in the United States and particularly within the elderly [1, 7, 8, 13]. The Centers for Disease Control and Prevention (CDC) reported an increased incidence of diabetes in individuals aged 65–79 years of age from 6.9 per 1000 in 1980 to 15.4 per 1000 in 2011 [14]. Diabetic nephropathy typically develops over a >5-year period, offering a window of time during adult years to reduce risk through optimizing blood glucose management and lifestyle modifications. Specific suggestions for diet modification of the individual with CKD and diabetes are available and encourage a diet pattern of eating that promotes fresh fruits and vegetables, whole grains, nonfat dairy products, and lean meats. Avoidance of higher ranges of protein intake defined as 20% of total calories or >1.3 gm protein/kg/day is suggested [30]. Individualization of guidelines to meet the unique needs of the elderly adult is recommended. Of note, tight blood glucose control is not recommended for the older adult with target HgbA1c goals increased to 7% to reduce the risk of nocturnal hypoglycemia [30].

Frailty

Older adults with CKD tend to have multiple comorbidities, which coupled with the effect of aging, can leave the individual more frail than their peers [31–33]. Changes in the musculoskeletal system with aging as well as chronic disease can have a negative impact on physiological function and can lead to frailty that is a precursor for disability [31–33]. Frailty is characterized by self-reported weakness, fatigue, balance or gait disorders, undernutrition, and an impaired ability to recover from insult, leading to impaired homeostatic reserve, malnutrition, decreased mobility, or functional loss related to diseases such as cerebrovascular accident (CVA), Parkinson's disease, or arthritis [33]. Shlipak found that elderly persons with CKD were three times more likely to be frail than their counterparts with normal kidney function [33]. The incidence of frailty within the CKD population is higher than that of the generalized population [31–33]. An analysis of data from the Third NHANES [31] was used to estimate the prevalence of frailty among persons with CKD; the overall prevalence of frailty was 2.8%. However, among persons with moderate to severe CKD (i.e., eGFR < 45 mL/min/1.73 m^2), the incidence of frailty was 20.9%. The odds of frailty were significantly increased among all stages of CKD, and were only marginally attenuated with additional adjustment for sarcopenia, anemia, acidosis, inflammation, vitamin D deficiency, hypertension, and CVD [31]. Frailty and CKD were independently associated with mortality [31, 32]. A recent meta-analysis on frailty and CKD in the elderly in 36,076 individuals aged 50–83 years reported that prevalence of frailty ranged from 7% in CKD stages 1–4 of elderly living in the community to 73% in a cohort of patients on hemodialysis [32]. The incidence of frailty increased with reduced GFR. Frailty was associated with adverse outcomes including increased risk of mortality and hospitalization [32]. The etiology of frailty is unclear [31]. However, nutrition, protein intake, and bone health and maintaining physical functioning as part of a healthy lifestyle are important considerations when caring for the elderly patient with CKD [31, 34].

Increased Falls Risk

Falls risk can be related to polypharmacy, impaired mobility, DM with impaired sensory neuropathy, autonomic neuropathy and/or visual impairment, orthostatic hypotension, renal osteodystrophy, and/or the risk of osteoporosis [35–37]. In addition, depression can impact judgment and safety awareness, which can increase falls risk. Falls risk in elderly dialysis patients is high with a 4.4 relative risk of hip fracture and the resultant mortality at 1 year being 2.5 times greater; the fall rates in this group are close to the rates in nursing homes [37, 38]. Falls can also lead to further decreases in mobility, which can directly impact ADLs and instrumental activities of daily living such as shopping and meal preparation. Maintenance of physical exercise and functioning is crucial for the elderly CKD patient.

Vascular Dementia

Vascular dementia increases in CVD with CKD, DM, and increased age [7, 8, 13, 39, 40]. The individual with vascular dementia will have areas of intact function contrasted with others of profound impairment and task-specific disabilities based on the location of the vascular event in the brain [41]. The Kidney Disease Quality of Life Cognitive Function (KDQOL-CF) subscale can be used to screen for cognitive function and help determine who needs further work-up [41]. Dementia is associated with malnutrition and an increased risk of mortality [7, 8, 13, 19].

Review of Normal Physiological Changes Associated with Aging

The aging process affects all body systems lending complications to maintaining an active and acceptable quality of life. These are reviewed in detail in the geriatric literature [42–48]. Summarized here are the elements of the aging process that are particularly challenging to maintain adequate nutritional status, including hydration, electrolyte balance, and a feeling of vitality to support daily functioning

Table 21.2 Nutrients potentially interfacing with traditional and nontraditional modifiable risk factors for chronic kidney, cardiovascular, and other chronic diseases

Traditional risk factors, modifiable	Nontraditional risk factors, modifiable	Interfacing nutrients; lifestyle factors
High-protein diet	Anemia, hyperuricemia,hyperphosphatemia	Dietary protein, type and quantity; including dairy products
Cardiovascular disease; hyperlipidemia	Nephrotoxic herbs	Fat: amount and type
Diabetes		Refined sugars, physical activity, BMI
Obesity		Total calories and diet composition; activity level
Proteinuria		BMI; diabetes control
Metabolic acidosis		Emerging data; diet; low intake of fresh fruits and vegetables, high animal protein intake
Smoking		Smoking cessation
Nutrition and herbal supplements and products		Avoid supplement products with unknown risk:benefit ratio

in the older adult with CKD. Nutrition intervention is important in the elderly as diet therapy interfaces with traditional and nontraditional modifiable risk factors for CKD, CVD, and other chronic diseases (Table 21.2) [26, 30, 34].

Nutritional Deficits in the Elderly

The US Dietary Guidelines (2015–2020) reported inadequate intake of several nutrients among older adult Americans including vitamin D, calcium, potassium, and dietary fiber. Moreover, the elderly are at risk for marginal intakes of omega-3 fatty acids; folate; vitamins B_6, B_{12}, C, D, E, and K; magnesium; and zinc [26]. Higher intakes of dietary protein in older adults aged 70–79 have been associated with a 40% reduced loss of lean muscle compared to those with lower intakes. Adequate dietary protein intake may be protective from risk of sarcopenia. The current recommendation for dietary protein is the same for all adults; it is possible that a higher range of intake is needed by the older adult. Contributing factors for a possible higher dietary protein need in the older adult may include a loss in the efficiency of overall metabolism for protein, fat, and carbohydrates among a milieu of inadequate dietary cofactors such as B vitamins. Physical activity is also an important consideration toward the risk of sarcopenia. It is possible that maintaining optimal nutrition throughout the adult aging process and physical activity contributes to a decreased risk of frailty and sarcopenia in the older years, when corrected for comorbid conditions and smoking. This relationship is further complicated in CKD where reports of a potential for accelerated aging of body symptoms is observed in younger adults (<ages 40) who are on renal replacement therapy [21, 49]. The malnutrition inflammation syndrome (MIS) and known protein energy wasting (PEW) that is observed in CKD patients, particularly those on renal replacement therapy, also impacts outcomes such as frailty, sarcopenia, cognitive health, and quality of life [26, 49, 50].

Medical Nutrition Therapy for the Older Adults with Chronic Kidney Disease

A complete nutritional assessment involves a review of documented medical problems to determine nutritional needs, risks, and barriers to obtaining a consistent adequate dietary intake. While older adults may already have established chronic disease such as hypertensive arteriosclerosis or diabetic nephropathy, nutrition therapy is important to reduce risk of exacerbation of disease and to contribute to overall physical well-being. Awareness of the behavioral health status of the older adult, whether living alone or as part of a household, is important for the healthcare team to maintain. Anxiety, depression, and dementia are all contributing factors to overall decline of health and well-being. Suicide rates are disproportionately high in the older population [51] and in individuals with CKD [52]. A team member that includes a psychologist and social worker who are specially trained in providing interventions for depression and anxiety is important.

Polypharmacy is another important consideration that impacts nutritional status and consistency of adequate intake. In addition to nutrient–drug interactions that can result in nutrient deficiencies, the interaction of drug classes themselves as well as individual agents can lead to fluid and electrolyte imbalances, dysgeusia, anorexia, xerostomia, hyposmia, diarrhea, and constipation. Completion of medication validation to be sure older adults are only taking the prescribed medications they need is a critical part of medical and nutrition management. This includes checking for excessive or inadequate use of nutrition supplements or inappropriate use of herbal formulations and other over-the-counter items. (See Chap. 9 on drug–nutrient interactions and Chap. 32 on complementary and alternative medicine.)

Renal Replacement Therapy

While CKD is more common in the older adult, the overall risk of mortality exceeds the risk for the development of ESRD. It has been reported that it is not until the eGFR drops to lower levels, approximately 15 ml/min/1.73 m^2 in 64- to 84-year-old adults [8], that the risk of developing ESRD is higher than mortality. After age 85, overall mortality risk again exceeds risk of progressing to end-stage disease, requiring renal replacement therapy. When renal replacement therapy is being considered, important factors impact the decision to initiate. Reduced life span cardiovascular morbidity, overall morbidity, adverse events such as hypotension, exacerbation of anemia, and fatigue are medical considerations. Obstacles regarding transportation, family/community support, integrity of vascular access are other concerns. Involvement of the elderly with Advanced Directives and Living Will details with discussions involving family members mediated by an experienced nephrology social worker are important. There are no data available demonstrating that renal replacement therapy in the elderly improves or worsens quality of life. While it has been reported that elderly who received renal replacement therapy versus maximum conservative management had a survival benefit, (37.8 months vs. 13.9 months), those on renal replacement therapy spent more time in the hospital, 173 days versus 16 days [7]. Those receiving conservative management were four times more likely to die at home or in a hospice [7].

Conclusion

The older adult is projected to outnumber the population of children in the United States. Specifically, there will be 78 million people 65 years and older compared to 76.7 million people who will be younger than this age threshold; this is an unprecedented statistic [2]. The new profile of the US population has significance for the burden of CKD and ESRD in the United States. Efforts to improve the diagnosis and treatment of a reduced eGFR in the elderly population are ongoing challenges. Kidney senescence involves functional and physiological modification to kidney tissue, which impacts accurate diagnosis and subsequent treatment approach. Development of equations to assess kidney function accurately within the confines of reduced musculature and other variables characterizing the older adult are reported to be in progress [1, 8, 12]. Medical nutrition therapy is an important component of care for the older adult with CKD as there is the potential to decrease chronic disease risk factors associated with CKD progression through diet modification [30, 53]. Specific nutrients that have been identified to be inadequately represented in the diet of the older adult can be incorporated into daily meal plans. In addition, maintaining optimal physical functionality and avoidance of frailty and sarcopenia are important for risk reduction of overall mortality. Nutrition integrity and consistency including diets enriched as appropriate with protein, vitamin D, and calcium have a role in maintaining physical health. Socioeconomics and community support systems influence medical outcomes. Behavioral health of the older adult is imperative to monitor and address as poor quality of life, depression, anxiety, and loneliness can all have a negative impact on dietary intake, nutritional status, and overall mortality risk. All of these factors need to be intertwined with metabolic and physiological challenges that confront the older adult and need to be considered when approaching end-of-life care, including decision to decline or initiate renal replacement therapy.

Case Study

C.M.D. is an 80-year-old Hispanic female, widower, with CKD late stage 4, early stage 5 (eGFR 12–16%), a history of hypertension (HTN), congestive heart failure stage 3, atrial fibrillation, mitral valve stenosis – not an operable candidate, and failure to thrive. Her oxygenation is stable on room air. C.M.D. does have a reported residual kidney and produces a urine output of approximately 650 cc per day. She lives with her daughter's family, which includes her son-in-law and three young grandchildren. There is a reported concern of food insecurity by the social worker. C.M.D. denies nausea, vomiting, diarrhea, abdominal pain, or any symptoms of acute illness. Her prescribed medications are as follows: 40 mg furosemide twice daily, sevelamer carbonate 800 mg three times daily with meals, metoprolol 25 mg qd, spirolactone 25 mg per day, apixaban 2.5 mg twice daily, nephrovite one tablet daily, and cholecalciferol 2000 units daily. C.M.D. has verbalized that she is unsure if she wants to start renal replacement therapy and does not understand what dialysis will do for her.

Objective– height: 64 inches; weight: 128 lb; reported weight change is 10 lb of unintentional weight gain over the past 2 weeks. She reports that her appetite is improving. Her sitting blood pressure is 128/60 mmHg. Labs: BUN 65 mg/dL, Cr 3.6 mg/dL, Na^+ 136 mEq/L, K^+4.8 mEq/L, CO_2 22 mEq/L, RBC 3.80, Hgb 11.1 g/dL, Hct 34.4%, total cholesterol 201 mg/dL, TRG 180 mg/dL, HDL 40 mg/dL, LDL 130 mg/dL, Ca^{2+}9.0 mg/dL, phosphate 6.0 mg/dL, albumin 2.5 gm/dL, serum parathyroid hormone 475 pg/mL, and vitamin D level (25OH) 24 ng/mL.

Case Questions and Answers

1. What are some of the immediate factors that need to be considered in completing C.M.D.'s nutrition assessment?
   Answer:

   - Recent weight gain; need to evaluate volume status; is this loss of residual renal function, worsening CHF, exacerbated by high sodium intake, non adherence to medications; does C.M.D. have insurance adequate to purchase medications and are they being purchased and taken?
   - Hypoalbuminemia: is dilution a factor if patient is hypervolemic?
   - Is diuresis being accomplished?
   - What is C.M.D.'s magnesium level? Why is magnesium important?

- When did C.M.D. last have evaluation by cardiology?
- Obtaining a 24-hour urine collection for creatinine clearance would be helpful in evaluating C.M.D.'s overall kidney function. Her weight is up on diuretics and if her residual kidney function has declined and she cannot obtain a negative fluid balance, renal replacement therapy is a consideration while undergoing above assessments.
- What is C.M.D.'s overall adequacy of nutrient intake?
- Definition of C.M.D.'s sodium intake and total fluid intake needs to be quantified.

2. Which eGFR equation would be ideal to use for estimate C.M.D.'s kidney function and why?
   Answer: CKD-EPI cystatin C or CKD-EPI Cr-cystatin C: more accurate choice for elderly and individuals with reduced mass.
3. What are some areas of concern related to this patient's psychosocial situation?
   Answer:

- Financial support: Does patient have financial support to purchase medications? Food?
- Education regarding renal replacement therapy is needed with patient and family for C.M.D. to decide whether to pursue dialysis. This evaluation is recommended to include the cardiologist to ascertain cardiovascular mortality risk and prognosis while C.M.D. is considering decisions regarding end-of-life care and quality of life. If C.M.D. decides to pursue renal replacement therapy, home peritoneal dialysis in addition to home and in-center hemodialysis are best to be included. C.M.D. may benefit from peritoneal dialysis due to her cardiovascular status. Code status and Advanced Directives are recommended to be identified and documented.

4. What nutrition assessment and therapies are indicated based on this presenting information?
   Answer:

- Evaluation of food intake for estimation of quality and quantity of nutrients.
- Determine if a fluid restriction is indicated by evaluating total fluid intake.
- How is her dental health? Can C.M.D. chew food properly?
- Evaluate visceral muscle stores with anthropometrics.
- Evaluate for frailty.
- Evaluate for sarcopenia – grip strength could prove helpful.
- Is protein intake adequate? What about calories?
- Is phosphorus elevated due to diet intake, lack of binders, needing more binders, high phosphorus food intake?
- Is vitamin D low due to not taking the supplement or not having the supplement to take or does C.M.D. need more vitamin D?

References

1. Bowe B, Xie Y, Li T, Mokdad AH, Xian H, Yan Y, et al. Changes in the US burden of chronic kidney disease from 2002 to 2016. An analysis of the global burden of disease study. JAMA Netw Open. 2018;1(17):e184412. https://doi.org/10.1001/jamanetworkopen.2018.4412.
2. The United States Census. Census.gov. 2018. Release #CB18-41, Tuesday, March 13, 2018. Accessed 1/6/2019.
3. U.S. Renal Data System. USRDS 2015 annual data report. National Institutes of Health, National Institute of Diabetes and Digestive and Kidney Diseases; 2016. www.USRDS.org/adr.htm. Accessed Jan 15 2019.
4. U.S. Renal Data System. USRDS 2018 annual data report: volume 1: CKD in the United States. In: Chapter 4: Cardiovascular disease in patients with CKD. Bethesda: National Institutes of Health, National Institute of Diabetes and Digestive and Kidney Diseases; 2016.www.USRDS.org/adr.htm. Accessed 2 Feb 2019.
5. U.S. Renal Data System. USRDS 2018 annual data report: volume 1: CKD in the United States. In: Chapter 3: Morbidity and mortality in patients with CKD. Bethesda: National Institutes of Health, National Institute of Diabetes and Digestive and Kidney Diseases; 2016. www.USRDS.org/adr.htm. Accessed 2 Feb 2019.

6. Glassock R, Denic A, Rule A. The conundrums of chronic kidney disease and aging. J Nephrol. 2017;30(4):477–83.
7. Nitta K, Okada K, Yanai M, Takahashi S. Aging and chronic kidney disease. Kidney Blood Press Res. 2013;38:109–20.
8. Maw T, Fried L. Chronic kidney disease in the elderly. Clin Geriatr Med. 2013;29:611–24.
9. Lindeman RD, Tobin J, Shock NW. Longitudinal studies on the rate of decline in renal function with age. J Am Geriatr Soc. 1985;33:278–5.
10. Vanita J. Chronic kidney disease in the elderly. ASN Kidney News; 2011.
11. Cockcroft DW, Gault M. Prediction of creatinine clearance from serum creatinine. Nephron. 1976;16:31–41.
12. Wieneke M, Grootendorst D, Verduijn M, Elliot E, Dekker F, Krediet T. Performance of the Cockcroft-Gault, MDRD, and new CKD-EPI formulas in relation to GFR, age, and body size. Clin J Am Soc Nephrol. 2010;5(6):1003–9.
13. Stevens L, Viswanathan G, Weiner D. CKD and ESRD in the elderly: current prevalence, future projections, and clinical significance. Adv Chronic Kidney Dis. 2010;17(4):293–301.
14. Mallappallil M, Friedman E, Delano B, McFarlane S, Salifu M. Chronic kidney disease in the elderly: evaluation and management. Clin Pract (Lond). 2014;11(5):525–35.
15. Garasto S, Fusco S, Corica F, Rosignuolo M, Marino A, Montesanto A, et al. Estimating glomerular filtration rate in older people. Biomed Res Int. 2014. Article ID 916542. https://doi.org/10.1155/2014/916542.
16. Fan L, Levey AS, Gudnason V, Eiriksdottir G, Andresdottir MB, Gudmundsdottir H, et al. Comparing GFR estimating equations using cystatin C and creatinine in elderly individuals. J Am Soc Nephrol. 2015;26(8):1982–9. https://doi.org/10.1681/ASN.2014060607.
17. Schaeffner E. Determining the glomerular filtration rate-an overview. J Ren Nutr. 2017;27(6):375–80.
18. KDIGO 2012 clinical practice guideline for the evaluation and management of chronic kidney disease. Kidney Int. 2013;1(3):1–150.
19. Stevens LA, Li S, Wang C, Huang C, Becker BN, Bomback AS, et al. Prevalence of CKD and comorbid illness in elderly patients in the United States: results from the Kidney Early Evaluation Program (KEEP). Am J Kidney Dis. 2010;55(3 suppl 2):s23–33. https://doi.org/10.1053/j.ajkd.2009.09.035.
20. Raman M, Green D, Middleton R, Kalra P. Comparing the impact of older age on outcome in chronic kidney disease of different etiologies: a prospective cohort study. J Nephrol. 2018;31:931–9.
21. Kooman P, van der Sand F, Leunissen K. Kidney disease and aging: a reciprocal relation. Exp Gerontol. 2017;87:156–9.
22. O'Hare AM, Bertenthal D, Covinsky KE, Landefeld CS, Sen S, Mehta K, et al. Mortality risk stratification in chronic kidney disease: one size for all ages? J Am Soc Nephrol. 2006;17(3):846–53.
23. James PA, Oparil S, Carter BL, Cushman WC, Dennison-Himmelfarb C, Handler J, et al. 2014 evidence-based guideline for the management of high blood pressure in adults report from the panel members appointed to the Eighth Joint National Committee (JNC 8). JAMA. 2014;311(5):507–20. https://doi.org/10.1001/jama.2013.284427.
24. K/DOQI clinical practice guidelines. National Kidney Foundation, 2000–2004. https://www.kidney.org/professionals/guidelines. Accessed 2 May 2020.
25. Whelton P, Carey R, Aronow WS, Casey DE Jr, Collins KJ, Dennison Himmelfarb C, et al. A report of the American College of Cardiology/American Heart Association task force on clinical practice guidelines. J Am Coll Cardiol. 2018;71:19.
26. Eggersdorfer M, Akobundu U, Bailey R, Shlisky J, Beaudreault AR, Bergeron G, et al. Hidden hunger: solutions for America's aging populations. Nutrients. 2018;10:1210. https://doi.org/10.3390/nu10091210; 1–15.
27. Sarnak MJ, Bloom R, Muntner P, Rahman M, Saland JM, Wilson PW, et al. KDOQI US commentary on the 2013 KDIGO clinical practice guideline for lipid management in CKD. Am J Kidney Dis. 2015;65(3):354–66.
28. Kidney disease: improving global outcomes (KDIGO) lipid work group. KDIGO clinical practice guideline for lipid management in chronic kidney disease. Kidney Int. 2013;Suppl. 3:259–305.
29. Grundy SM, Stone NJ, Bailey AL, et al. AHA/ACC/AACVPR/AAPA/ABC/ACPM/ADA/AGS/APhA/ASPC/NLA/PCNA guideline on the management of blood cholesterol. J Am Coll Cardiol Nov. 2018;2018:25709. https://doi.org/10.1016/j.jacc.2018.11.003.
30. Tuttle KR, Bakris GL, Bilous RW, Chiang JL, de Boer IH, Goldstein-Fuchs J, et al. Diabetic kidney disease: a report from an ADA consensus conference. Am J Kidney Dis. 2014;64(4):510–33.
31. Wilhelm-Leen E, Hall Y, Manjula T, Chertow G. Frailty and chronic kidney disease: the third national health and nutrition evaluation survey. Am J Med. 2009;122(7):664–71.
32. Chowdhury R, Peel NM, Krosch M, Hubbard RE. Frailty and chronic kidney disease: a systematic review. Arch Gerontol Geriatr. 2017;68:135–42.
33. Shlipak MG, Stehman-Breen C, Fried LF, Song X, Siscovick D, Fried LP, et al. The presence of frailty in elderly persons with chronic renal insufficiency. Am J Kidney Dis. 2004;43:861–7.
34. Magalhaes F, Goulart R, Prearo L. The impact of a nutrition intervention program targeting elderly people with chronic kidney disease. Cien Saude Colet. 2018;23(8):2555–64.
35. Singh P, Germain J, Cohen L, Unruh M. The elderly on diaysis: geriatric considerations. Nephrol Dial Transplant. 2014;29:990–6. https://doi.org/10.1093/ndt/gft246.

36. Roberts RG, Kenny RA, Brierley EJ. Are elderly haemodialysis patients at risk of falls and postural hypotension? Int Urol Nephrol. 2003;35:415–21.
37. Sims RJ, Cassidy MJ, Masud T. The increasing number of older patients with renal disease. BMJ. 2003;327:463–4.
38. Desmet C, Beguin C, Swine C, Jadoul M. Falls in hemodialysis patients: prospective study of incidence, risk factors and complications. Am J Kidney Dis. 2005;45:148–53.
39. Pereira AA, Weiner DE, Scott T, Sarnack MJ. Cognitive function in dialysis patients. Am J Kidney Dis. 2005;45:448–62.
40. Kurella M, Chertow GM, Luan J, Yaffe K. Cognitive impairment in chronic kidney disease. J Am Geriatr Soc. 2004;52:1863–9.
41. Kurella M, Luan J, Yaffe K, Chertow GM. Validation of kidney disease quality of life (KDQOL) cognitive function subscale. Kidney Int. 2004;66:2361–7.
42. Institute of Medicine. Cognitive aging: progress in understanding and opportunities for action. Washington, DC: The National Academies Press; 2015. https://doi.org/10.17226/21693.
43. Burke MM, Laramie J. Sensory impairment. In: A primary care of the older adult: a multidisciplinary approach. St. Louis: Mosby; 2000. p. 439–52.
44. Burke MM, Laramie J. Aging skin. In: A primary care of the older adult: a multidisciplinary approach. St. Louis: Mosby; 2000. p. 142–60.
45. Burke MM, Laramie J. Respiratory. In: A primary care of the older adult: a multidisciplinary approach. St. Louis: Mosby; 2000. p. 161–201.
46. Burke MM, Laramie J. The aging cardiovascular system. In: A primary care of the older adult: a multidisciplinary approach. St. Louis: Mosby; 2000. p. 202–53.
47. Burke MM, Laramie J. Gastrointestinal conditions. In: A primary care of the older adult: a multidisciplinary approach. St. Louis: Mosby; 2000. p. 254–68.
48. Burke MM, Laramie J. Musculoskeletal: common injuries. In: A primary care of the older adult: a multidisciplinary approach. St. Louis: Mosby; 2000. p. 302–53.
49. De Nicola L, Minutolo R, Chidin P, Borrelli S, Zoccali C, Postorino M, et al. Italian Society of Nephrology Study group Target Blood Pressure Levels (TABLE) in CKD. The effect of increasing age on the prognosis of non-dialysis patients with chronic kidney disease receiving stable nephrology care. Kidney Int. 2012;82:482–8.
50. Carrero J, Stenvinkel P, Cuppari L, Ikizler TA, Kalantar-Zadeh K, Kaysen G, et al. Etiology of the protein-energy wasting syndrome on chronic kidney disease: a concensus statement from the International Society of Renal Nutrition & Metabolism (ISRNM). J Ren Nutr. 2013;23(2):77–90.
51. Conejero I, Olie E, Courtet P, Calati R. Suicide in older adults: current perspectives. Clin Interv Aging. 2018;13:691–9.
52. Jhee J, Lee E, Cha MU, Lee M, Kim H, Park S, et al. Prevalence of depression and suicidal ideation increases proportionally with renal function decline, beginning from early stages of chronic kidney disease. Medicine (Baltimore). 2017;96(44):e8476.
53. Turgut F, Yesil Y, Balogun RA, Abdel-Rahman E. Hypertension in the elderly: unique challenges and management. Clin Geriatr Med. 2013;29:593–609.

Part VI
Nutritional Management of Other Disorders that Impact Kidney Function

The amount and the composition of diet have a profound impact on numerous homeostatic processes and affect the development and progression of several disease states, many of which are critically important in determining outcomes in patients with chronic kidney disease (CKD). Furthermore, proper nutrition is indispensable in the maintenance of the health and well-being of patients with CKD and end-stage renal disease (ESRD). Deficiencies in both the amount and quality of consumed nutrients can facilitate the development of protein-energy wasting (PEW), which is one of the most powerful determinants of poor outcomes in these populations. Nutritional interventions can thus be used to affect these processes and disease states and ultimately to improve outcomes in patients with CKD. Chronic inflammation is extremely common in patients with CKD and ESRD and has an impact on both the progression of CKD and on the development of comorbidities such as cardiovascular disease. Avesani et al. describe the etiology and pathophysiology of chronic inflammation in CKD, its role in the development of PEW, and the various dietary interventions that can be used to mitigate both its development and its adverse consequences. CKD-associated mineral and bone disorders (CKD-MBD) are extremely common in patients with CKD and ESRD and are associated with important adverse outcomes. McCann provides a summary of the conditions characteristic of CKD-MBD, their role in the development of CKD-associated adverse outcomes, and the various therapies (nutritional and pharmacological) used to treat them. Nephrotic syndrome characteristically develops in patients with glomerular diseases, and its salient features are high-grade proteinuria, edema, hyperlipidemia, and hypercoagulability. Ananthakrishnan et al. provide a general description of this disease state and discuss the pharmacologic and dietary interventions used to treat them. Nephrolithiasis affects about 9% of the general population and is a result of both genetic and environmental factors, with nutritional risk factors featuring prominently among the latter. Han et al. describe the causes and consequences of kidney stones, summarize diagnostic modalities used in the evaluation of patients with nephrolithiasis, and review therapeutic approaches used for kidney stones, including nutritional interventions. Finally, acute kidney injury (AKI) represents the sudden loss of kidney function that is commonly observed among hospitalized patients. AKI results in numerous complications that culminate on poor clinical outcomes in affected individuals, and it represents a unique nutritional challenge due to the highly catabolic states that these patients often suffer from, which is compounded by the presence of dialytic therapies. Grguric provides a description of the metabolic complications typically seen with AKI, the various interventions used in these patients including various types of renal replacement therapy, and the nutritional requirements and interventions typically observed in patients with AKI.

Chapter 22
Protein-Energy Wasting/Malnutrition and the Inflammatory Response

Carla Maria Avesani, Bengt Lindholm, and Peter Stenvinkel

Keywords Protein-energy wasting · Sarcopenia · Obesity · Malnutrition · Inflammation · Protein catabolism · Gut microbiome · Fibers · Probiotic · Prebiotic · Symbiotic · Antioxidants · Potassium · Healthy dietary pattern · Intradialytic oral supplementation · Intradialytic parenteral nutrition · Bioactive compounds · Energy intake · Protein intake

Key Points
- Patients with chronic kidney disease (CKD) often have systemic low-grade inflammation.
- Low-grade inflammation present in CKD patients can lead to nutritional disturbances such as protein-energy wasting (PEW) and sarcopenia. In addition, inflammation in end-stage renal disease (ESRD) patients is associated with cardiovascular events and higher mortality rates.
- Several non-CKD-related, CKD-related, and dialysis-related risk factors activate the immune response in the uremic *milieu*. These factors represent potential targets for treatments to diminish inflammation in CKD patients.
- The uremic-gut dysbiosis is recently recognized as a factor that activates the immune response and causes inflammation in CKD patients.
- A less restrictive diet with fruits, vegetables, nuts, beans and whole grains as sources of fiber, antioxidants, vitamins, and bioactive compounds should be encouraged in CKD, as it may have beneficial effects on the uremic gut dysbiosis and, therefore, could potentially diminish the inflammatory response. Serum potassium should be closely monitored to avoid hyperkalemia and, if present, the diet should only contain fruits and vegetables with low potassium content.
- Supplementation with prebiotics, probiotics, and symbiotics may potentially diminish uremic inflammation. However, interventional, randomized, and controlled studies with long follow-up time are needed to demonstrate such beneficial effects.

The editors acknowledge Kamyar Kalantar-Zadeh's contribution to this chapter in *Nutrition in Kidney Disease, Second Edition*, Nutrition and Health, DOI https://doi.org/10.1007/978-1-62703-685-6_1, © Springer Science+Business Media New York 2014.

C. M. Avesani
Nutrition Institute, Rio de Janeiro State University, Rio de Janeiro, Brazil

Department of Renal Medicine, Karolinska Institutet, and Baxter Novum, Stockholm, Sweden

B. Lindholm
Department of Renal Medicine, Karolinska Institutet, and Baxter Novum, Stockholm, Sweden

P. Stenvinkel (✉)
Department of Renal Medicine, Karolinska Institutet, Stockholm, Sweden
e-mail: peter.stenvinkel@ki.se

- Whether foods rich in bioactive compounds may ameliorate muscle catabolism in CKD remains to be studied in interventional randomized controlled studies.
- Energy and protein supplementation to reverse PEW should be implemented in patients with PEW or sarcopenia.
- Intradialytic oral supplementation and intradialytic parenteral nutrition to HD patients with PEW may ameliorate nutritional status.
- The combination of non-pharmacological (such as nutritional and lifestyle factors) and pharmacological strategies should be considered to diminish the systemic low-grade inflammation in CKD.

Introduction

The importance of enhanced inflammatory response as a leading cause of diminished reserves of protein stores in chronic kidney disease (CKD) has been extensively described as part of the uremic phenotype in the last 20 years [1, 2]. The persistent low-grade inflammation observed in end-stage renal disease (ESRD) patients plays a crucial role in protein-energy wasting (PEW) by promoting increased energy expenditure and protein catabolism while decreasing protein synthesis. This cycle can result in a negative nitrogen balance with loss of muscle mass and consequent wasting [2, 3]. In addition, inflammation, which has a pivotal role in the atherogenic process, worsens cardiovascular mortality and can further aggravate the detrimental outcomes, especially if wasting is present [4]. The cardiovascular mortality of ESRD patients is further increased in those with inflammation (C-reactive protein [CRP] ≥ 10 mg/L) and malnutrition (assessed by subjective global assessment (SGA)), as compared to those with only inflammation or malnutrition, or in the absence of both conditions [2]. Since inflammation is believed to be a leading cause of PEW and cardiovascular disease (CVD) in ESRD, and inflammation therefore represents a potential target for therapeutic – pharmacological as well as nonpharmacological – interventions, this chapter aims to review the interrelation between inflammation and nutritional disorders, especially PEW, and to discuss potential strategies of treatment targeting inflammation, PEW, and sarcopenia.

Interrelation Between Nutritional Disturbances and Inflammation in CKD

Defining and understanding well the different nutritional disorders that patients with CKD are exposed to is important for screening and planning of interventional studies, and for choosing which nutritional markers to target and to use as measurement of effectiveness after an intervention. In this regard, in 2007, the Expert Panel of the *International Society of Renal Nutrition and Metabolism* (ISRNM) released a publication addressing the definition of terminologies related to malnutrition, inflammation, and wasting in CKD that brought some light to this area [5]. *Malnutrition* was defined as a condition in which the total energy and nutrient intake, specially of protein, is insufficient to fulfill the energy and nutrient needs. As a result, there is an unintentional loss of body weight and body fat and, if maintained for a long period, loss of protein stores as well. If inflammation is present, a condition with increased production of pro-inflammatory cytokines, such as tumor necrosis factor (TNF), interleukin 6 (IL-6), and others, this will promote protein catabolism and also diminish appetite. This condition, defined as *wasting,* is characterized by higher blood concentration of inflammatory markers and by a loss of protein stores (i.e., diminished muscle mass). As CKD patients are exposed to many different factors that may induce an increased inflammatory response, and to other noninflammatory conditions that can lead to increased protein catabolism and diminished protein anabolism, the ISRNM expert committee proposed the use of the terminology *protein-energy wasting*

(PEW) to describe the nutritional disturbances observed in CKD [5]. In fact, in dialysis patients, those who were malnourished as assessed by SGA had higher concentrations of inflammatory markers (CRP, IL-6, and TNF) than the well-malnourished patients [6].

Another common feature of the uremic phenotype is sarcopenia. For decades, *sarcopenia* was defined as the loss of muscle mass that occurred primarily with aging [7], but since the publication of consensus reports on sarcopenia by different societies [8–12], especially by the *European Working Group on Sarcopenia in Older People* (EWGSOP) [8], a new definition was proposed. The EWGSOP from 2010 defines sarcopenia as a condition of diminished muscle mass and muscle strength (or muscle function) that could be primarily related to aging, but also secondary to other conditions, such as organ failure diseases or diseases that lead to increased inflammatory response (e.g., cancer, CKD, chronic obstructive pulmonary, congestive heart failure, HIV, and others), especially in those exposed also to long bed rest, chronic sedentary lifestyle, inadequate dietary intake, and nutrients malabsorption [8]. This definition was useful to bring awareness to screen and treat sarcopenia. In addition, the occurrence of sarcopenia was shown to be associated with higher levels of inflammatory markers and worse outcomes in CKD, such as higher mortality rates, more hospitalization events, and worse quality of life [13–15]. More recently, the revised EWGSOP consensus kept the same definition, but emphasized low muscle strength and not low muscle mass as the key characteristic for sarcopenia [16].

Lastly, but also important, obesity comes as another nutritional disturbance present in CKD that can be related to both systemic and local adipose tissue inflammation [17–19]. Obesity is defined as abnormal or excessive fat accumulation that is associated with increased mortality risk in the general population [20]. In obese individuals, the excessive adipocytes release TNF and IL-6 by macrophages infiltrating the adipose tissue [21]. As a result, there is a close association between obesity and increased concentration of proinflammatory interleukins as demonstrated by studies in CKD patients [17, 19, 22, 23]. Of note, obesity commonly coexists with PEW and sarcopenia, a condition called "sarcopenic obesity" [24].

As shown in Table 22.1, the prevalence of nutritional disturbances in CKD patients is elevated and, therefore, nutritional problems should as a rule be monitored and addressed when treating nondialysis, hemodialysis (HD), peritoneal dialysis (PD), and renal transplant patients. Taking all together, it becomes clear that CKD patients are exposed to a chronic state of low-grade inflammation and that this condition is closely related to the nutritional disturbances observed in CKD. Figure 22.1 summarizes the interrelation between the main nutritional disturbances with inflammation in CKD.

Table 22.1 Prevalence of protein-energy wasting, sarcopenia, and obesity in CKD

Nutritional disturbance	Prevalence (%)				References
	CKD stages 3–5 Non-dialysis	Hemodialysis	Peritoneal dialysis	Renal transplant	
PEW (SGA or MIS)	11–54%	28–54%		28–52%	Carrero et al. [84]
Sarcopenia (low muscle mass and low muscle strength)	8–16%	8–37%	11–15.5%	11.8%	Pereira et al. [15], Giglio et al. [14], Zhou et al. [85], Kittiskulnam et al. [86], Kim et al. [87], Isoyama et al. [13], Abro et al. [88], Yanishi et al. [89]
Obesity (excessive body fat percentage)	40–71%	27–65%			Sharma et al. [24], Agarwal et al. [90] Rodrigues et al. [91], Gracia-Iguacel et al. [92]

Abbreviations: *PEW* protein-energy wasting, *SGA* subjective global assessment, *MIS* malnutrition inflammation index

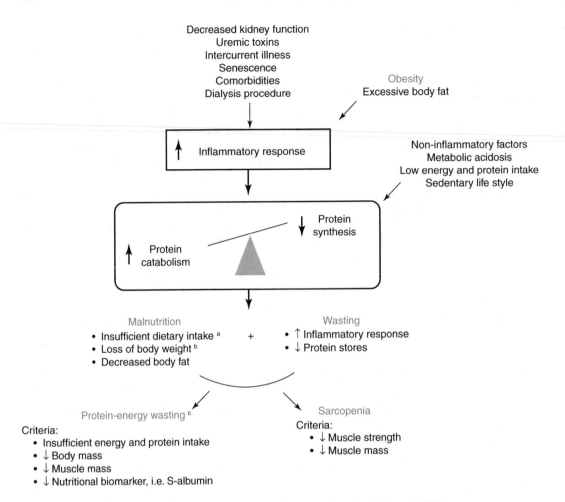

Fig. 22.1 Interrelation between the main nutritional disturbances with inflammation in CKD. Criteria for protein-energy wasting [5]. Criteria for sarcopenia [16]

Causes of Inflammation in CKD

The increased inflammatory response in ESRD is an established feature of CKD and a nontraditional risk factor for CVD [25]. On the one hand, the acute inflammatory process starts as a protective mechanism to defend the host against infectious pathogens, and it has a number of important functions, such as to allow tissue-repair response, to adapt to stress, and to restore the homeostatic state [26]. However, when a chronic deregulated inflammatory response occurs, there is high cost for the host, by compromising physiologic processes and impairing body functions needed to maintain nitrogen balance, which will lead to catabolism and sarcopenia [2]. A chronic state of low-grade inflammation is associated with a cluster of burden of lifestyle diseases that accumulate with age ("inflammaging"), including ischemic heart disease, congestive heart failure, periodontitis, osteoporosis, dementia, cancer, depression, and others [25, 27].

In the clinical situation, the systemic low-grade inflammation is assessed most commonly by CRP, which is produced and released from the hepatocytes, and rapidly increases after an inflammatory stimulus, resulting in an elevation of circulating IL-6, which induces the production of CRP in the

Table 22.2 Etiologic factors of inflammation in CKD

Non-CKD related
Intercurrent events and illnesses
Periodontitis and poor oral health
Senescence
Obesity (mainly central obesity)
Altered gut microbe bacterial composition
CKD related
Reduction in renal function
Dialysis procedure related
Vascular access by catheters
Nonbiocompatible membranes
Frequency and duration of the dialysis
Capacity to filter medium and large molecules
Non sterile dialysate solution and impure dialysate
Increased volume overload

liver during the acute phase of inflammation [28]. Since high-sensitivity (hs) CRP is a strong predictor of CVD events and mortality, hsCRP has become the standard method to assess inflammation in the clinic [29, 30]. The mean CRP levels in dialysis patients normally varies from 4–5 mg/L and was shown to be higher in HD than in PD patients [28, 31, 32]. In patients with CKD stages 3–5 (not on dialysis), more than 50% had CRP levels >2.1 mg/L [33].

The etiologic factors of this enhanced inflammatory condition in CKD are multiple and it may not be meaningful to address single factors, as many risk factors occur concomitantly and act together [25, 28]. In a didactic approach, inflammatory etiologic factors can be classified as those that are *CKD-unrelated*, *CKD-related*, and *dialysis-related*, i.e., due to the dialysis procedure *per se* (Table 22.2). Accumulating evidence suggests that cellular senescence – and the subsequent senescence-associated secretary phenotype (SASP) causing chronic inflammation – appears to play a fundamental role in both initiation and progression of uremic inflammation [34]. Intercurrent events and illnesses such as periodontitis and poor oral health and obesity (mainly central obesity) are examples of nonrelated CKD causes. More recently, the gastrointestinal tract has been shown to play an important role in the increase of inflammatory mediators in CKD [35–37]. The gut microbiome of CKD patients is markedly altered; this is in part a consequence of an increased influx of circulating urea and other uremic toxins to the colon lumen, promoting the growth of bacteria that express ureases. In addition, the dietary restrictions aiming to control for plasma potassium and phosphorous lead to a diet with an overall low intake of fruits, vegetables, grains, and whole cereals, and thus a low fiber intake [38]. Of note, this dietary profile was linked to a proinflammatory diet pattern, with increased CRP concentration in HD patients [39]. This change in dietary pattern can further worsen the bacterial composition of the gut microbiome, affecting enterocyte health [35–37].

Another potentially modifiable factor is progression of CKD, since the reduction in kidney function results in accumulation of circulating cytokines, advanced glycation end-products, and pro-oxidants, which are well-known CKD-related components of the inflammatory uremic *milieu* [25, 28]. Finally, low-grade inflammation is caused by the dialysis procedure in HD because of the vascular access by catheters, which is a common portal for infections, and the use of nonbiocompatible membranes, use of membranes with low capacity to filter larger molecules, contact of the blood with nonsterile dialysate solutions, and impure dialysate; these factors are influenced by the frequency and duration of the dialysis session [25, 28]. In addition, increased volume overload that commonly occurs in patients undergoing dialysis treatment can lead to endotoxin translocation from the gut, immune-activation and increased cytokine production [40]. Among the above-mentioned causes of inflammation in CKD, the altered gut microbiota deserves attention, as it is closely related to dietary intake and nutritional status.

Gut Microbiota in CKD: The Crosstalk Between Nutrition and Inflammation

The large intestine is colonized by trillions of microbes that carry many genes from what is called the microbiome. The microbiome in turn has unique metabolic properties, including the fermentation of nutrients and synthesis of vitamins. It also exerts a fundamental influence on local and systemic processes, such as immunity [35].

In the colon, the bacteria that participate in the digestion of food by catabolic pathways are categorized as saccharolytic (i.e., predominantly fermenting carbohydrates) or proteolytic (i.e., predominantly fermenting proteins). Nutritional intake is a key component regulating the intestinal microbiome and the intestinal microbial composition and metabolism. For instance, a healthy and balanced diet, with adequate intake of fibers provides substrate to the colon to ferment fibers to short-chain fatty acid (SCFA) by saccharolytic bacteria. The SCFA, in turn, have an important role in energy homeostasis, regulation of the epigenome, gut epithelial integrity, and is also known to exert a protective action and a positive immune-modulating activity [41]. The current Western diet, on the other hand, is characterized by a decrease in the intake of foods with a high fiber content (fruits, vegetables, grains, and whole cereals), and an increased intake of protein and fat. This unhealthy dietary pattern is not well received by the colon and leads to detrimental protein and choline fermentation instead of a beneficial fermentation coming from the carbohydrates provided by fibers. In addition, a diet poor in fibers augments the colonic transit time, which also has a negative impact on the colonic microbiome composition. Under this condition, the deprivation of carbohydrates in the colon (coming from a diet with low fiber intake), induces the growth of proteolytic species (proteolytic bacteria) and results in increased generation and uptake of end-products of bacterial protein fermentation (such as ammonia, amines, thiols, phenols, and indols) and to a "disturbed gut" with an altered microbial composition and metabolism, known as *gut dysbiosis* [37, 41, 42].

The uremic phenotype is characterized by an altered gut microbiome, i.e., dysbiosis, because of the slow colonic transit, high luminal pH, and poor dietary intake with diminished intake of fibers, vitamins, and antioxidants. A main culprit is the use of dietary restrictions aiming at preventing hyperkalemia and hyperphosphatemia [37, 41, 42]. Moreover, the uremic *milieu* can lead to gut dysbiosis by increasing the influx of circulating urea and other toxins to the gut lumen, favoring the growth of bacteria that express urease. Combined with poor fiber intake, this results in increased production of uremic toxins from the gut microbiota, among them, the p-cresyl sulfate, indoxyl sulfate, and trimethylamine-N-oxide (TMAO), which are protein-bound toxins that are difficult to remove by conventional dialysis [36, 37, 41, 42]. In addition, ESRD patients show a decreased production of bacteria that can ferment (saccharolytic bacteria) fibers to SCFA, which also contributes to gut dysbiosis. Finally, the gut dysbiosis in uremia may lead to disruption of the colonic epithelial tight junctions, inducing an increase in intestinal permeability, leading to bacterial translocation from the gut to the bloodstream and increased exposure to endotoxins, a condition called the "leaky gut" [43]. Of note, endotoxins are potent immune system activators, which induce inflammatory cascades and systemic, low-grade inflammation. Similarly, the increased production of uremic toxins coming from the gut microbiota can also induce proinflammatory responses and leukocytosis. CKD progression constitutes another factor that can amplify and perpetuate alterations in the gut microbiome and intestinal barriers, forming a vicious circle [36, 37]. Figure 22.2 summarizes the crosstalk between the uremia-gut dysbiosis, inflammation, and nutrition.

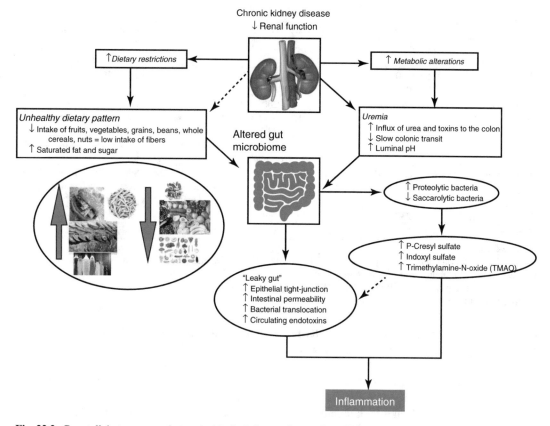

Fig. 22.2 Crosstalk between uremia-gut dysbiosis, inflammation, and nutrition

Proinflammatory Dietary Pattern: Another Factor Exacerbating Uremic Inflammation

The current dietary guidelines for nutrition focus on treating the main nutritional disturbances present in CKD, such as, reversing PEW, delaying the progression of CKD and avoiding or managing the occurrence of hyperkalemia and hyperphosphatemia [44–46]. In order to address the management of the nutritional problems in this complex setting, the proposed guidelines rely on recommendations focusing on the intake of energy, macronutrients, minerals, and vitamins to achieve the optimal or at least the minimal amount required of these nutrients, by the diet or by oral supplementation, and, if necessary, by employing enteral or intradialytic parenteral nutrition [44–46]. The current energy, protein, and mineral recommendations by CKD treatment modality is summarized in Table 22.3. Although patients must receive adequate information so that they ingest sufficient amounts of energy and nutrients to cover the minimal needs to maintain adequate nutritional status, recent observational studies have shown that the combination of these dietary recommendations into a healthy dietary pattern is equally important [47]. This can impose a dilemma for dietitians when planning the diet of CKD patients; for example, providing the minimum intake of energy, protein, and fibers may be in conflict with the need to reduce the intake of potassium and phosphorus if hyperkalemia and hyperphosphatemia is present. In other words, if not carefully designed, building the dietary plan based solely on energy, nutrients, and minerals as recommended by guidelines may lead to an unhealthy dietary pattern with low intake of fibers, but high intake of saturated fat and energy, and with low, moderate, or high intake of protein depending on the CKD stage [48]. In

Table 22.3 Nutritional recommendations to CKD patients

	CKD Stages 3 to 5 not on dialysis	Hemodialysis	Peritoneal dialysis
Energy (kcal/kg[a]/day)	25–35[b]	25–35[b]	25–35[b] Individualized
Protein (g/kg[a]/day)	0.55–0.60[b] 0.8–1.0[c]	1.0–1.2[b] >1.1[d]	1.0–1.2[b]
Potassium (mg/day)	To be adjusted to mantain adequate serum potassium levels[b]	2000–3000 (if serum K >6 mmol/L)[d] or to be adjusted to mantain adequate serum potassium levels[b]	2000–3000 (if serum K >6 mmol/L)[d] or to be adjusted to maintain adequate serum potassium levels[b]
Phosphorus (mg/day)	To be adjusted to mantain adequate serum phosphate levels[b]	800–1000[d] or to be adjusted to maintain adequate serum phosphate levels[b]	800–1000[d] or to be adjusted to mantain adequate serum phosphate levels[b]
Sodium (mg/day)	2000–2300	2000–2300	Individualized
Liquids	Individualized	500 ml + diuresis[d]	Individualized

[a]Body weight
[b]National Kidney Foundation Kidney Disease Outcomes Quality Initiative and the Academy of Nutrition and Dietetics Clinical Practice Guidelines for Nutrition in Chronic Kidney Disease [45]
[c]Kidney Disease Improving Quality Outcomes (KDIGO) [46]
[d]European Best Practice Guideline on Nutrition [44]

addition, these recommendations typically result in monotonous diets with limited food variety [49], inadequate content of vitamins, and an inflammatory dietary pattern.

The dietary inflammatory index (DII) is a relatively new tool for studying the effect of a diet, including the combined intake of macronutrients, micronutrients, flavonoids, and some food groups, on six inflammatory markers (IL-1β, IL-4, IL-6, IL-10, TNF, and CRP). The DII generates a score where a higher score indicates an inflammatory dietary pattern [50]. By using the DII, Kizil et al. [39] showed that in HD patients the DII was associated with higher CRP levels and PEW. In a subsequent study including nondialyzed CKD patients (CKD 3–5), a higher DII was associated with lower intake of the food groups (grains, vegetables, and fruits). Moreover, the risk of having more advanced CKD was higher among patients in the higher DII tertile in crude and adjusted models [51]. Of note, in another study including HD patients, it was shown that only half of the studied patients ate one to two servings/day of vegetables and 53% ate two servings/day of fruit, indicating a limited intake of fibers. Moreover, the most consumed vegetables (potato, carrot, onion) and fruits (apple, lemon, mandarin) were those with low amounts of antioxidants [52]. Recent research has outlined the importance of the uremic gut dysbiosis as a factor leading to inflammation [35–37], and a dietary intake characterized by a decreased intake of fruits, vegetables, whole grains, beans, and nuts can further worsen the uremic gut dysbiosis [41, 42]. Therefore, it seems reasonable to consider a paradigm shift in the recommended dietary plans for CKD patients. Perhaps it is time to replace the restricted, unbalanced, and potentially unhealthy diets currently recommended for uremic patients with diets with a more healthy dietary pattern. However, studies are needed to evaluate if such a change is safe and effective.

Food as Medicine: Using Food as a Therapeutic Approach to Control Inflammation

As inflammation appears to play a pivotal role in the uremic phenotype, characterized by the presence of PEW, CVD, sarcopenia, and obesity, which are associated with deleterious outcomes, including higher risk for premature CVD and increased all-cause mortality [25, 28], anti-inflammatory therapies should be developed to avoid and treat this condition. As previously described, there are many preexisting conditions leading to low-grade systemic inflammation in CKD (see Table 22.2), and ideally each of these factors should be targeted with appropriate treatments. Complementing these approaches, nutritional interventions have been showing favorable results on biomarkers of inflammation in nondialysis CKD patients and in ESRD patients in clinical trials [42, 53, 54]. Although these trials had small sample sizes, with relatively short follow-up, the results are promising as they suggest that nutritional interventions may have beneficial effects on uremic inflammation.

Low-Protein Diet to Nondialyzed CKD Patients

High-protein diets in patients with CKD stages 3–5 have been shown to increase glomerular hyperfiltration and proteinuria, accelerate the progression of CKD, and reduce the time until start of dialysis becomes necessary [55]. In addition, high-protein diets to nondialysis CKD patients increase the amino acid load that enhances advanced glycation end-product formation and are associated with higher production of gut-derived uremic toxins such as p-cresyl sulfate, hippuric acid, and phenylacetylglutamine, which are retained and therefore increase in the circulation as glomerular filtration decreases [56]. Therefore, one can expect that a low-protein diet can partially reverse the increased production of gut-uremic toxins, by diminishing the influx of urea into the gut and diminishing the proteolytic fermentation that generates gut-uremic toxins [37]. This was observed in a study by Marzocco et al. [57], showing that a very low protein diet supplemented with keto-analogues diminished the production of indoxyl sulfate levels. Moreover, Rossi et al. [58] showed that in nondialyzed CKD patients, diets exhibiting a high fiber intake in relation to protein intake was associated with lower circulating concentrations of p-cresyl sulfate and indoxyl sulfate. Since indoxyl sulfate can decrease the transcription of nuclear factor-erythroid 2 related factor 2 (Nrf2), a factor involved in the anti-inflammatory response, a low-protein diet that would increase Nrf2 has been proposed as an anti-inflammatory approach in nondialyzed CKD patients [59]. Recently, it was shown that after 6 months on a low-protein diet, there was a significant increase in Nrf2 mRNA expression, albeit no change in inflammatory markers was reported [60]. As low-protein diets are accompanied by a decrease in energy intake, it is important that patients receive an adequate intake of energy as this is of importance to avoid PEW.

Higher Intake of Fruits, Vegetables, Whole Grains, Beans, Nuts, Prebiotics, and Probiotics

A diet with a high intake of fruits, vegetables, and whole grains has a high content of fibers. A high intake of fibers, in turn, is associated with lower inflammatory markers as demonstrated by studies both in the general population and in CKD patients [61, 62]. Although the anti-inflammatory mechanism(s) behind this finding remains to be elucidated, the fermentation of soluble fiber and resistant starch by the saccharolytic bacteria in the colon to SCFA, the diminished production of gut-derived uremic toxins, and the higher intake of antioxidants with bioactive compounds that increase the transcription of Nrf2 are probably important contributing factors involved in the role of a healthy dietary pattern in diminishing inflammation [63]. A list of foods with increased amounts of bioactive compounds are shown in Table 22.4 with the corresponding amount of potassium, phosphorous, and fibers that could be incorporated to the daily diet of CKD patients.

In addition, fibers are sources of prebiotics, defined as a nondigestible food by the host that has a beneficial effect by stimulating the growth or activity of health-promoting bacteria. The prebiotics include inulin, fructo-oligosaccharides, galacto-oligosaccharides, soya-oligosaccha-

Table 22.4 Foods rich in bioactive compounds with the respective potassium content

	Bioactive compound	Potassium (mg)	Phosphorous (mg)	Total fibers (g)
Green and red grapes Serving (50 g, 10 grapes) 100 g	Resveratrol, anthocyanins	94 191	10 20	0.4 0.9
Cranberry juice Serving (240 ml) 100 g	Resveratrol, anthocyanins	29 12	NA NA	0 0
Blackberry Serving (144 g, 1 cup) 100 g	Anthocyanins	233[a] 162	32 22	7.6 5.3
Strawberry Serving (140 g, 1 cup) 100 g	Anthocyanins	210[a] 150	31 22	4.1 2.9
Cherries Serving (140 g, 1 cup) 100 g	Anthocyanins	169 121	NA NA	2.0 1.4
Avocado Serving (1/2 unit, 68 g) 100 g	Polyphenols	345[a] 507	37 54	4.6 6.8
Acai puree 100 g	Anthocyanins	60	16	3.0
Pomegranate Serving (140 g, 1/2 unit) 100 g	Polyphenols	333[a] 236	51 36	5.5 4.0
Tomato Serving (62 g, 1 unit) 100 g	Lycopene	147 237	15 24	0.7 1.2
Broccoli (cooked) Serving (85 g, ½ cup) 100 g	Sulforaphane	292[a] 343	70 82	2.4 2.8
Cabbage (raw) Serving (70 g, 1 cup) 100 g	Sulforaphane	170 243	21 30	1.5 2.1
Kale (raw) Serving (20 g, 1 cup) 100 g	Sulforaphane	73 348	12 55	0.9 4.1
Brussels sprouts (cooked) Serving (80 g, ½ cup) 100 g	Sulforaphane	247[a] 317	44 56	2.0 2.6
Garlic Serving (9 g, 3 clove) 100 g	Allicin	36 401	14 153	0.2 2.1
Brazilian nuts Serving (2 units, 10 g) 100 g	Selenium	65.1 651	85.3 853	0.79 7.9

Source of nutrients: United States Department of Agriculture, Agricultural Research Service, USDA Food Composition Databases, except for Acai puree, in which the source of nutrients was the Brazilian Food Composition Tables
[a]In patients with hyperkalemia, the administration of these foods should be carefully controlled due to their high content of potassium per serving (>200 mg/serving)

rides, xylo-oligosaccharides, and pyrodextrins. Studies with prebiotic supplementation for 4–6 weeks have been shown to decrease inflammatory markers in nondialyzed and dialyzed CKD patients [53, 54]; however, it should be noted that other studies failed to reproduce such findings [64, 65].

Probiotics, defined as "live microorganisms," confer health benefits on the host as they may promote a better composition of the gut microbiota when administrated in adequate amounts. The benefits are mediated by improvement in gut barrier integrity and function, in the activity of the gut immune system resulting in lower inflammatory response, and in the control of photobionts (i.e., the photosynthetic component of a lichen) overgrowth [36, 37]. In a systematic review including seven interventional trials, a significant reduction in CRP, but not in TNF, was observed after 2 months of probiotic supplementation in ESRD patients compared to the control group [66]. Another promising approach is the combination of pro- and prebiotics (symbiotics) that might result in a synergistic effect on gastrointestinal function. Rossi et al. [67] showed improvements in the production of gut-uremic toxins, but not in diminishing inflammatory markers, when supplementing with symbiotics for 6 weeks in CKD nondialysis patients. Whereas Viramontes-Hörner et al. [68] found that supplementation with a symbiotic gel for 2 months diminished the severity of gastrointestinal symptoms in HD patients, no significant changes on inflammatory markers were observed. Therefore, more studies are needed to confirm whether symbiotic supplementation can diminish the low-grade inflammation in CKD. In summary, the interventional studies testing the effects of prebiotics, probiotics, and/or symbiotics supplementation (>1 week) on inflammatory markers in adults with CKD show promising results. But, since a recent meta-analysis showed lack of conclusive results, it can currently not be recommended in CKD until randomized and controlled studies show positive results following interventions with pre-, pro-, or symbiotic, and which type, dose, and time of intervention that are required to gain positive results as regards to inflammation [69].

Polyunsaturated Fatty Acid Supplementation

There are three main types of fatty acids of special relevance for humans: saturated fatty acids, monounsaturated fatty acids (MUFAs), and polyunsaturated fatty acids (PUFAs). PUFAs are subclassified into n-3 (omega 3, i.e., eicosapentaenoic acid – EPA, docosahexaenoic acid – DHA), n-6 (omega 6, i.e., linoleic acid – LA, and α-linolenic acid – ALA), and n-9 (omega 9) [70]. Food sources of EPA and DHA are oily fish, other sea food, seaweed and krill oil, while food sources of LA and ALA are sunflower seeds, corn, soya, sesame, canola, safflower, and their oils [71]. Almost 20 years ago, studies showed that the contents of n-6 PUFA and EPA in the diet of HD patients are low and, therefore, not in line with a healthy dietary pattern in regards to fat [72, 73]. In fact, there are studies showing a low intake of fish (a source of EPA) and a high intake of food sources rich in saturated fatty acids by individuals with CKD, both nondialysis and dialysis patients [48, 74]. This – in addition to the low intake of fiber typical of CKD patients – indicates a dietary pattern not compatible with a heart-friendly diet. Particularly regarding the low intake of food sources of n-3 PUFA and n-6 PUFA, it has been shown in vivo and in vitro and in clinical studies that PUFAs exert anti-inflammatory properties and the balance between n-3 PUFA and n-6 PUFA in the diet is important to exert an anti-inflammatory effect [71]. The anti-inflammatory effects of *n*-3 PUFAs include attenuation of endothelial adhesiveness, activation of leukocytes and resident macrophages, leukocyte–endothelial interaction, leukocyte transmigration, and the release of substances that lead to tissue injury [71]. In CKD patients there are interventional studies showing that supplementation of n-3 PUFA has the potential to reduce inflammation (hsCRP, IL-6 and TNF) [71]. Although clinical trials do not support or recommend supplementation of n3-PUFA to CKD patients in clinical practice due lack of evidence (which may be due to inappropriate design, small sample size, and short follow-up time), these findings reinforce the idea of substituting food sources of saturated fatty acids (from red meats, cheeses, butter, and palm oil) to unsaturated fatty acids (PUFA and MUFA) to provide a healthy dietary pattern that potentially could exert protective effects in diminishing inflammation and CVD in CKD patients.

Energy and Protein Supplementation to Reverse PEW

An early, individualized and balanced nutritional counseling considering (1) the patient's food habits, (2) cultural and social economic condition, (3) the nutritional status, (4) the ability of chewing and swallowing food and liquids, and (5) the presence of comorbidities (which increase protein catabolism and energy expenditure as well as modify nutrient digestion and absorption) should be considered when planning the diet for CKD patients. For patients with PEW and sarcopenia, appetite and food preferences should be explored to enhance total energy and protein intake. According to specific guidelines for CKD and ESRD patients, the energy intake recommendation for metabolically stable adult CKD patients should be between 25 and 35 kcal/kg body weight/day depending on age, gender, level of physical activity, weight status goals, concurrent illness, or presence of inflammation. For protein, the recommended intake for metabolically stable adult CKD patients ranges from 0.55 to 0.60 g/kg body weight/day in CKD 3–5 not on dialysis without diabetes, 0.6–0.8 g/kg body weight/day for CKD 3–5 not on dialysis who have diabetes, and from 1.0 to 1.2 g/kg body weight/day for HD and PD patients [44–46]. Since low energy and protein intake are among the causes leading to PEW and sarcopenia, and may occur concomitantly with low-grade inflammation due to diminished appetite triggered by low-grade inflammation [28], the dietitian should explore options from the patients' food preferences to enhance the total intake. However, if this is not achieved after 2 weeks, and if nutritional status continues to deteriorate, an oral supplement should be considered [75].

Formulas designed for dialysis patients that combine a high amount of energy and protein with controlled amounts of potassium and phosphorus entail options for use in dialysis clinics. In a study including HD patients with serum albumin <35 g/L, intradialytic oral supplementation with formulas designed for dialysis patients resulted in an increase in serum albumin and in the normalized protein equivalent of nitrogen appearance (nPNA), a proxy of dietary protein intake, with no change in intradialytic body weight gain. In addition, a reduced number of missed dialysis treatments as compared to the control group not receiving the supplementation was reported [76]. Similarly, Weiner et al. [77] observed that intradialytic oral supplementation for 3 months was associated with a 29% reduction in the hazard ratio for all-cause mortality – a result not mediated by changes in serum albumin levels. In another study in HD patients, supplementation with soy or whey protein during the dialysis session was compared with no supplementation for 6 months. After the intervention, a significant decrease in IL-6 levels and an increase in gait speed and shuttle walk test was observed in the groups receiving whey protein and soy protein in comparison with the control group [78]. Despite these positive effects, the use of oral supplements for periods longer than 3 months is limited due to low adherence because of monotonous taste of the formulas. For this reason, some studies investigated the use of intradialytic enriched protein meals during the dialysis treatment. In a metabolic study, it was shown that when patients were fed with a meal enriched in energy and protein during the dialysis procedure, an improvement in nitrogen balance was observed, whereas a negative balance was observed when patients were fasting [79]. More recently, in a prospective study, Caetano et al. [80] showed positive results in HD patients after 6 months of intradialytic meals with enriched protein. Compared to the control group, patients in the intervention group showed an increase in spontaneous protein intake, body fat percentage, and no changes in serum potassium, phosphorous, and CRP levels. Finally, intradialytic parenteral nutrition (IDPN) can be used if the above approaches fail to reverse or arrest PEW. In addition, IDPN should be recommended when the spontaneous energy intake is below 20 kcal/kg/day and protein intake below 0.8–0.9 g/kg/day [75]. IDPN consists of a mixture of amino acids, glucose, and lipid in emulsions administrated in the extracorporeal circulation during the dialysis session. For safety, the IDPN supplementation should not exceed 1 liter of fluids, 1000 kcal, and 50 g of amino acids per dialysis session in a person weighing approximately 75 kg [75]. Ideally, IDPN should be gradually discontinued when the patients increase their oral intakes (with or without oral supplementation). The criteria to discontinue IDPN include an increase in serum albumin (>38 g/L for

3 months), an improvement in SGA or malnutrition inflammation (MIS) score, and an increase in energy and protein intake to >30 kcal/kg/day and >1 g/kg/day, respectively [75]. If the gastrointestinal tract is not functioning, total parenteral nutrition (TPN) should be considered. The benefits of using IDPN over oral intradialytic supplementation are inconclusive. In a prospective, randomized, and controlled trial including 186 patients on HD with PEW, Cano et al. [81] showed that when comparing controls with the group receiving oral intradialytic supplementation, IDPN was not associated with improvement in 2-year mortality rate, but showed significant improvement in serum pre-albumin and albumin concentrations, in addition to reduced rates of hospitalization and improved well-being. In a metabolic study investigating protein and energy homeostasis during HD, the use of IDPN was able to reverse the negative energy and nitrogen balance caused by the dialysis procedure, demonstrating a positive effect on metabolic parameters and nitrogen balance [82]. Intradialytic oral nutrition seems to offer similar benefits to IDPN in reversing and arresting PEW [83].

Taken together, nutritional interventions should be monitored using various markers before, during, and after energy and protein supplementation to assess effectiveness. The criteria for diagnosing PEW (see Fig. 22.1), complemented if possible by use of SGA or MIS, can be easily adopted in clinical practice [75]. Also, of importance, the energy and protein supplementation should be done in combination with a healthy dietary pattern as previously discussed. Close monitoring of potassium and phosphorus intake, and particularly for HD patients, control of intradialytic weight gain should also be implemented.

Conclusion

The low-grade inflammation present in CKD has multifactorial causes and leads to increased protein catabolism and diminished muscle mass. This condition, combined with the sedentary lifestyle in many dialysis patients, contributes to diminished muscle strength and physical performance. Diminished muscle strength and muscle mass reflects a process of sarcopenia and, therefore, PEW and sarcopenia may occur concomitantly. Moreover, obesity can also coexist with PEW and sarcopenia and, therefore, overweight and obese individuals should also be screened for PEW.

Target treatments to diminish low-grade inflammation should include nutritional and nonnutritional approaches. The implementation of a healthier dietary pattern with the inclusion of food sources of fiber, antioxidants, and bioactive compounds seems to be a potential approach to slow down low-grade inflammation in CKD, mediated by ameliorating uremic-gut dysbiosis. Although we still lack interventional, controlled, and randomized studies investigating the role of less-restrictive diets to reverse PEW and inflammation, it is reasonable to plan for diets enriched in energy and protein and that also offer replacement of ultra-processed food with food that is minimally processed and includes fruits, vegetables, and home-cooked meals. Finally, a careful assessment and monitoring of nutritional status should be performed before, during, and after nutritional counseling to evaluate the effectiveness of the intervention.

References

1. Stenvinkel P, Heimbürger O, Lindholm B, Kaysen GA, Bergström J. Are there two types of malnutrition in chronic renal failure? Evidence for relationships between malnutrition, inflammation and atherosclerosis (MIA syndrome). Nephrol Dial Transplant. 2000;15(7):953–60.
2. Avesani CM, Carrero JJ, Axelsson J, Qureshi AR, Lindholm B, Stenvinkel P. Inflammation and wasting in chronic kidney disease: partners in crime. Kidney Int. 2006;70:S8–S13.

3. Utaka S, Avesani CM, Draibe SA, Kamimura MA, Andreoni S, Cuppari L. Inflammation is associated with increased energy expenditure in patients with chronic kidney disease. Am J Clin Nutr. 2005;82(4):801–5.

4. Sun J, Axelsson J, Machowska A, Heimbürger O, Bárány P, Lindholm B, et al. Biomarkers of cardiovascular disease and mortality risk in patients with advanced CKD. Clin J Am Soc Nephrol. 2016;11(7):1163–72.

5. Fouque D, Kalantar-Zadeh K, Kopple J, Cano N, Chauveau P, Cuppari L, et al. A proposed nomenclature and diagnostic criteria for protein-energy wasting in acute and chronic kidney disease. Kidney Int. 2008;73(4):391–8.

6. Dai L, Mukai H, Lindholm B, Heimbürger O, Barany P, Stenvinkel P, et al. Clinical global assessment of nutritional status as predictor of mortality in chronic kidney disease patients. PLoS One. 2017;12(12):e0186659.

7. Rosenberg IH. Sarcopenia: origins and clinical relevance. J Nutr. 1997;127(5 Suppl):990S–1S.

8. Cruz-Jentoft AJ, Baeyens JP, Bauer JM, Boirie Y, Cederholm T, Landi F, et al. Sarcopenia: European consensus on definition and diagnosis: report of the European Working Group on sarcopenia in older people. Age Ageing. 2010;39(4):412–23.

9. Fielding RA, Vellas B, Evans WJ, Bhasin S, Morley JE, Newman AB, et al. Sarcopenia: an undiagnosed condition in older adults. Current consensus definition: prevalence, etiology, and consequences. International working group on sarcopenia. J Am Med Dir Assoc. 2011;12(4):249–56.

10. Morley JE, Abbatecola AM, Argiles JM, Baracos V, Bauer J, Bhasin S, et al. Sarcopenia with limited mobility: an international consensus. J Am Med Dir Assoc. 2011;12(6):403–9.

11. Muscaritoli M, Anker SD, Argilés J, Aversa Z, Bauer JM, Biolo G, et al. Consensus definition of sarcopenia, cachexia and pre-cachexia: joint document elaborated by Special Interest Groups (SIG) "cachexia-anorexia in chronic wasting diseases" and "nutrition in geriatrics". Clin Nutr. 2010;29(2):154–9.

12. Studenski SA, Peters KW, Alley DE, Cawthon PM, McLean RR, Harris TB, et al. The FNIH sarcopenia project: rationale, study description, conference recommendations, and final estimates. J Gerontol A Biol Sci Med Sci. 2014;69(5):547–58.

13. Isoyama N, Qureshi AR, Avesani CM, Lindholm B, Bàràny P, Heimbürger O, et al. Comparative associations of muscle mass and muscle strength with mortality in dialysis patients. Clin J Am Soc Nephrol. 2014;9(10):1720–8.

14. Giglio J, Kamimura MA, Lamarca F, Rodrigues J, Santin F, Avesani CM. Association of sarcopenia with nutritional parameters, quality of life, hospitalization, and mortality rates of elderly patients on hemodialysis. J Ren Nutr. 2018;28(3):197–207.

15. Pereira RA, Cordeiro AC, Avesani CM, Carrero JJ, Lindholm B, Amparo FC, et al. Sarcopenia in chronic kidney disease on conservative therapy: prevalence and association with mortality. Nephrol Dial Transplant. 2015;10(30):1718–25.

16. Cruz-Jentoft AJ, Bahat G, Bauer J, Boirie Y, Bruyère O, Cederholm T, et al. Sarcopenia: revised European consensus on definition and diagnosis. Age Ageing. 2019;48(1):16–31.

17. Lin CC, Kardia SL, Li CI, Liu CS, Lai MM, Lin WY, et al. The relationship of high sensitivity C-reactive protein to percent body fat mass, body mass index, waist-to-hip ratio, and waist circumference in a Taiwanese population. BMC Public Health. 2010;10:579.

18. Cordeiro AC, Qureshi AR, Stenvinkel P, Heimbürger O, Axelsson J, Bárány P, et al. Abdominal fat deposition is associated with increased inflammation, protein-energy wasting and worse outcome in patients undergoing haemodialysis. Nephrol Dial Transplant. 2010;25(2):562–8.

19. Axelsson J, Rashid Qureshi A, Suliman ME, Honda H, Pecoits-Filho R, Heimbürger O, et al. Truncal fat mass as a contributor to inflammation in end-stage renal disease. Am J Clin Nutr. 2004;80(5):1222–9.

20. World Health Organization Expert Committee on Physical Status. The use and interpretation of anthropometry. Physical Status: The use and interpretation of Anthropometry. Report of a WHO Expert Committee. World Health Organ Tech Rep Ser; 2012. Geneva: WHO; 1995.

21. Wellen KE, Hotamisligil GS. Obesity-induced inflammatory changes in adipose tissue. J Clin Invest. 2003;112(12):1785–8.

22. Sanches FM, Avesani CM, Kamimura MA, Lemos MM, Axelsson J, Vasselai P, et al. Waist circumference and visceral fat in CKD: a cross-sectional study. Am J Kidney Dis. 2008;52(1):66–73.

23. Carvalho LK, Barreto Silva MI, da Silva Vale B, Bregman R, Martucci RB, Carrero JJ, et al. Annual variation in body fat is associated with systemic inflammation in chronic kidney disease patients stages 3 and 4: a longitudinal study. Nephrol Dial Transplant. 2012;27(4):1423–8.

24. Sharma D, Hawkins M, Abramowitz MK. Association of sarcopenia with eGFR and misclassification of obesity in adults with CKD in the United States. Clin J Am Soc Nephrol. 2014;9(12):2079–88.

25. Jankowska M, Cobo G, Lindholm B, Stenvinkel P. Inflammation and protein-energy wasting in the uremic milieu. Contrib Nephrol. 2017;191:58–71.

26. Medzhitov R. Origin and physiological roles of inflammation. Nature. 2008;454(7203):428–35.

27. Stenvinkel P, Block GA, Chertow GM, Shiels PG. Understanding the role of the cytoprotective transcription factor NRF2 – lessons from evolution, the animal kingdom and rare progeroid syndromes. Nephrol Dial Transplant. 2019. https://doi.org/10.1093/ndt/gfz120.

28. Carrero JJ, Stenvinkel P. Inflammation in end-stage renal disease--what have we learned in 10 years? Semin Dial. 2010;23(5):498–509.
29. Mendall MA, Strachan DP, Butland BK, Ballam L, Morris J, Sweetnam PM, et al. C-reactive protein: relation to total mortality, cardiovascular mortality and cardiovascular risk factors in men. Eur Heart J. 2000;21(19):1584–90.
30. Tice JA, Browner W, Tracy RP, Cummings SR. The relation of C-reactive protein levels to total and cardiovascular mortality in older U.S. women. Am J Med. 2003;114(3):199–205.
31. Yong K, Dogra G, Boudville N, Lim W. Increased inflammatory response in association with the initiation of hemo-dialysis compared with peritoneal dialysis in a prospective study of end-stage kidney disease patients. Perit Dial Int. 2018;38(1):18–23.
32. Snaedal S, Qureshi AR, Lund SH, Germanis G, Hylander B, Heimbürger O, et al. Dialysis modality and nutritional status are associated with variability of inflammatory markers. Nephrol Dial Transplant. 2016;31(8):1320–7.
33. Avesani CM, Draibe SA, Kamimura MA, Colugnati FA, Cuppari L. Resting energy expenditure of chronic kidney disease patients: influence of renal function and subclinical inflammation. Am J Kidney Dis. 2004;44(6):1008–16.
34. Hobson S, Arefin S, Kublickiene K, Shiels PG, Stenvinkel P. Senescent cells in early vascuylar ageing and bone disease of chronic kidney disease – a novel target for treatment. Toxins (Basel). 2019;11(2):pii E82.
35. Ramezani A, Raj DS. The gut microbiome, kidney disease, and targeted interventions. J Am Soc Nephrol. 2014;25(4):657–70.
36. Lau WL, Kalantar-Zadeh K, Vaziri ND. The gut as a source of inflammation in chronic kidney disease. Nephron. 2015;130(2):92–8.
37. de Andrade LS, Ramos CI, Cuppari L. The cross-talk between the kidney and the gut: implications for chronic kidney disease. Forum Nutr. 2017;42:27.
38. St-Jules DE, Goldfarb DS, Sevick MA. Nutrient non-equivalence: does restricting high-potassium plant foods help to prevent hyperkalemia in hemodialysis patients? J Ren Nutr. 2016;26(5):282–7.
39. Kizil M, Tengilimoglu-Metin MM, Gumus D, Sevim S, Turkoglu İ, Mandiroglu F. Dietary inflammatory index is associated with serum C-reactive protein and protein energy wasting in hemodialysis patients: a cross-sectional study. Nutr Res Pract. 2016;10(4):404–10.
40. Dekker MJE, van der Sande FM, van den Berghe F, Leunissen KML, Kooman JP. Fluid overload and inflammation axis. Blood Purif. 2018;45(1–3):159–65.
41. Montemurno E, Cosola C, Dalfino G, Daidone G, De Angelis M, Gobbetti M, et al. What would you like to eat, Mr CKD microbiota? A mediterranean diet, please! Kidney Blood Press Res. 2014;39(2–3):114–23.
42. Mafra D, Borges N, Alvarenga L, Esgalhado M, Cardozo L, Lindholm B, et al. Dietary components that may influ-ence the disturbed gut microbiota in chronic kidney disease. Nutrients. 2019;11(3):496.
43. Vaziri ND, Yuan J, Rahimi A, Ni Z, Said H, Subramanian VS. Disintegration of colonic epithelial tight junction in uremia: a likely cause of CKD-associated inflammation. Nephrol Dial Transplant. 2012;27(7):2686–93.
44. Fouque D, Vennegoor M, ter Wee P, Wanner C, Basci A, Canaud B, et al. EBPG guideline on nutrition. Nephrol Dial Transplant. 2007;22(Suppl 2):ii45–87.
45. Ikizler TA, Burrowes J, Byham-Gray L, Campbell K, Carrero JJ, Chan W, et al. KDOQI Nutrition in CKD Guideline Work Group. KDOQI clinical practice guideline for nutrition in CKD: 2020 update. Am J Kidney Dis. 2020; in press.
46. Kidney disease: improving global outcomes (KDIGO) 2012 clinical practice guideline for the evaluation and man-agement of chronic kidney disease (CKD). Kidney Int Suppl. 2013;3(1):1–163.
47. Campbell KL, Carrero JJ. Diet for the management of patients with chronic kidney disease; it is not the quantity, but the quality that matters. J Ren Nutr. 2016;26(5):279–81.
48. Luis D, Zlatkis K, Comenge B, García Z, Navarro JF, Lorenzo V, et al. Dietary quality and adherence to dietary recommendations in patients undergoing hemodialysis. J Ren Nutr. 2016;26(3):190–5.
49. Fernandes AS, Ramos CI, Nerbass FB, Cuppari L. Diet quality of chronic kidney disease patients and the impact of nutritional counseling. J Ren Nutr. 2018;28(6):403–10.
50. Shivappa N, Steck SE, Hurley TG, Hussey JR, Hébert JR. Designing and developing a literature-derived, population-based dietary inflammatory index. Public Health Nutr. 2014;17(8):1689–96.
51. Rouhani MH, Najafabadi MM, Surkan PJ, Esmaillzadeh A, Feizi A, Azadbakht L. Dietary inflammatory index and its association with renal function and progression of chronic kidney disease. Clin Nutr ESPEN. 2019;29:237–41.
52. Maraj M, Kuśnierz-Cabala B, Dumnicka P, Gala-Błądzińska A, Gawlik K, Pawlica-Gosiewska D, et al. Malnutrition, inflammation, atherosclerosis syndrome (MIA) and diet recommendations among end-stage renal disease patients treated with maintenance hemodialysis. Nutrients. 2018;10(1):69.
53. Tayebi Khosroshahi H, Vaziri ND, Abedi B, Asl BH, Ghojazadeh M, Jing W, et al. Effect of high amylose resistant starch (HAM-RS2) supplementation on biomarkers of inflammation and oxidative stress in hemodialysis patients: a randomized clinical trial. Hemodial Int. 2018;22(4):492–500.
54. Xie LM, Ge YY, Huang X, Zhang YQ, Li JX. Effects of fermentable dietary fiber supplementation on oxidative and inflammatory status in hemodialysis patients. Int J Clin Exp Med. 2015;8(1):1363–9.

55. Hahn D, Hodson EM, Fouque D. Low protein diets for non-diabetic adults with chronic kidney disease. Cochrane Database Syst Rev. 2018;10:CD001892.

56. Pignanelli M, Bogiatzi C, Gloor G, Allen-Vercoe E, Reid G, Urquhart BL, et al. Moderate renal impairment and toxic metabolites produced by the intestinal microbiome: dietary implications. J Ren Nutr. 2019;29(1):55–64.

57. Marzocco S, Dal Piaz F, Di Micco L, Torraca S, Sirico ML, Tartaglia D, et al. Very low protein diet reduces indoxyl sulfate levels in chronic kidney disease. Blood Purif. 2013;35(1–3):196–201.

58. Rossi M, Johnson DW, Xu H, Carrero JJ, Pascoe E, French C, et al. Dietary protein-fiber ratio associates with circulating levels of indoxyl sulfate and p-cresyl sulfate in chronic kidney disease patients. Nutr Metab Cardiovasc Dis. 2015;25(9):860–5.

59. Anjos JS, Cardozo LFMF, Esgalhado M, Lindholm B, Stenvinkel P, Fouque D, et al. Could low-protein diet modulate Nrf2 pathway in chronic kidney disease? J Ren Nutr. 2018;28(4):229–34.

60. Anjos JSD, Cardozo LFMF, Black AP, Santos da Silva G, Vargas Reis DCM, Salarolli R, et al. Effects of low protein diet on nuclear factor erythroid 2-related factor 2 gene expression in nondialysis chronic kidney disease patients. J Ren Nutr. 2019;pii: S1051–2276(19):30005–6.

61. Krishnamurthy VM, Wei G, Baird BC, Murtaugh M, Chonchol MB, Raphael KL, et al. High dietary fiber intake is associated with decreased inflammation and all-cause mortality in patients with chronic kidney disease. Kidney Int. 2012;81(3):300–6.

62. McLoughlin RF, Berthon BS, Jensen ME, Baines KJ, Wood LG. Short-chain fatty acids, prebiotics, synbiotics, and systemic inflammation: a systematic review and meta-analysis. Am J Clin Nutr. 2017;106(3):930–45.

63. Wu M, Cai X, Lin J, Zhang X, Scott EM, Li X. Association between fibre intake and indoxyl sulphate/P-cresyl sulphate in patients with chronic kidney disease: meta-analysis and systematic review of experimental studies. Clin Nutr. 2018;pii: S0261–5614(18):32453–1.

64. Ramos CI, Armani RG, Canziani MEF, Dalboni MA, Dolenga CJR, Nakao LS, et al. Effect of prebiotic (fructooligosaccharide) on uremic toxins of chronic kidney disease patients: a randomized controlled trial. Nephrol Dial Transplant. 2019;34:1876–84.

65. Salmean YA, Segal MS, Palii SP, Dahl WJ. Fiber supplementation lowers plasma p-cresol in chronic kidney disease patients. J Ren Nutr. 2015;25(3):316–20.

66. Thongprayoon C, Kaewput W, Hatch ST, Bathini T, Sharma K, Wijarnpreecha K, et al. Effects of probiotics on inflammation and uremic toxins among patients on dialysis: a systematic review and meta-analysis. Dig Dis Sci. 2019;64(2):469–79.

67. Rossi M, Johnson DW, Morrison M, Pascoe EM, Coombes JS, Forbes JM, et al. Synbiotics easing renal failure by improving gut microbiology (SYNERGY): a randomized trial. Clin J Am Soc Nephrol. 2016;11(2):223–31.

68. Viramontes-Hörner D, Márquez-Sandoval F, Martín-del-Campo F, Vizmanos-Lamotte B, Sandoval-Rodríguez A, Armendáriz-Borunda J, et al. Effect of a symbiotic gel (Lactobacillus acidophilus + Bifidobacterium lactis + inulin) on presence and severity of gastrointestinal symptoms in hemodialysis patients. J Ren Nutr. 2015;25(3):284–91.

69. McFarlane C, Ramos CI, Johnson DW, Campbell KL. Prebiotic, probiotic, and synbiotic supplementation in chronic kidney disease: a systematic review and meta-analysis. J Ren Nutr. 2019;29(3):209–20.

70. The nomenclature of lipids (recommendations 1976). IUPAC-IUB Commission on Biochemical Nomenclature. J Lipid Res. 1978;19(1):114–28.

71. Huang X, Lindholm B, Stenvinkel P, Carrero JJ. Dietary fat modification in patients with chronic kidney disease: n-3 fatty acids and beyond. J Nephrol. 2013;26(6):960–74.

72. Peck LW, Monsen ER, Ahmad S. Effect of three sources of long-chain fatty acids on the plasma fatty acid profile, plasma prostaglandin E2 concentrations, and pruritus symptoms in hemodialysis patients. Am J Clin Nutr. 1996;64(2):210–4.

73. Friedman AN, Moe SM, Perkins SM, Li Y, Watkins BA. Fish consumption and omega-3 fatty acid status and determinants in long-term hemodialysis. Am J Kidney Dis. 2006;47(6):1064–71.

74. Santin F, Canella DS, Avesani CM. Food consumption in chronic kidney disease: association with sociodemographic and geographical variables and comparison with healthy individuals. J Ren Nutr. 2019;29(4):333–42.

75. Sabatino A, Regolisti G, Karupaiah T, Sahathevan S, Sadu Singh BK, Khor BH, et al. Protein-energy wasting and nutritional supplementation in patients with end-stage renal disease on hemodialysis. Clin Nutr. 2017;36(3):663–71.

76. Benner D, Brunelli SM, Brosch B, Wheeler J, Nissenson AR. Effects of oral nutritional supplements on mortality, missed dialysis treatments, and nutritional markers in hemodialysis patients. J Ren Nutr. 2018;28(3):191–6.

77. Weiner DE, Tighiouart H, Ladik V, Meyer KB, Zager PG, Johnson DS. Oral intradialytic nutritional supplement use and mortality in hemodialysis patients. Am J Kidney Dis. 2014;63(2):276–85.

78. Tomayko EJ, Kistler BM, Fitschen PJ, Wilund KR. Intradialytic protein supplementation reduces inflammation and improves physical function in maintenance hemodialysis patients. J Ren Nutr. 2015;25(3):276–83.

79. Veeneman JM, Kingma HA, Boer TS, Stellaard F, De Jong PE, Reijngoud DJ, et al. Protein intake during hemodialysis maintains a positive whole body protein balance in chronic hemodialysis patients. Am J Physiol Endocrinol Metab. 2003;284(5):E954–65.

80. Caetano C, Valente A, Silva FJ, Antunes J, Garagarza C. Effect of an intradialytic protein-rich meal intake in nutritional and body composition parameters on hemodialysis patients. Clin Nutr ESPEN. 2017;20:29–33.
81. Cano NJ, Fouque D, Roth H, Aparicio M, Azar R, Canaud B, et al. Intradialytic parenteral nutrition does not improve survival in malnourished hemodialysis patients: a 2-year multicenter, prospective, randomized study. J Am Soc Nephrol. 2007;18(9):2583–91.
82. Pupim LB, Majchrzak KM, Flakoll PJ, Ikizler TA. Intradialytic oral nutrition improves protein homeostasis in chronic hemodialysis patients with deranged nutritional status. J Am Soc Nephrol. 2006;17(11):3149–57.
83. Dukkipati R, Kalantar-Zadeh K, Kopple JD. Is there a role for intradialytic parenteral nutrition? A review of the evidence. Am J Kidney Dis. 2010;55(2):352–64.
84. Carrero JJ, Thomas F, Nagy K, Arogundade F, Avesani CM, Chan M, et al. Global prevalence of protein-energy wasting in kidney disease: a meta-analysis of contemporary observational studies from the international society of renal nutrition and metabolism. J Ren Nutr. 2018;28(6):380–92.
85. Zhou Y, Hellberg M, Svensson P, Höglund P, Clyne N. Sarcopenia and relationships between muscle mass, measured glomerular filtration rate and physical function in patients with chronic kidney disease stages 3–5. Nephrol Dial Transplant. 2018;33(2):342–8.
86. Kittiskulnam P, Carrero JJ, Chertow GM, Kaysen GA, Delgado C, Johansen KL. Sarcopenia among patients receiving hemodialysis: weighing the evidence. J Cachexia Sarcopenia Muscle. 2017;8(1):57–68.
87. Kim JK, Choi SR, Choi MJ, Kim SG, Lee YK, Noh JW, et al. Prevalence of and factors associated with sarcopenia in elderly patients with end-stage renal disease. Clin Nutr. 2014;33(1):64–8.
88. Abro A, Delicata LA, Vongsanim S, Davenport A. Differences in the prevalence of sarcopenia in peritoneal dialysis patients using hand grip strength and appendicular lean mass: depends upon guideline definitions. Eur J Clin Nutr. 2018;72(7):993–9.
89. Yanishi M, Kimura Y, Tsukaguchi H, Koito Y, Taniguchi H, Mishima T, et al. Factors associated with the development of sarcopenia in kidney transplant recipients. Transplant Proc. 2017;49(2):288–92.
90. Agarwal R, Bills JE, Light RP. Diagnosing obesity by body mass index in chronic kidney disease: an explanation for the "obesity paradox?". Hypertension. 2010;56(5):893–900.
91. Rodrigues J, Santin F, Brito FSB, Carrero JJ, Lindholm B, Cuppari L, et al. Sensitivity and specificity of body mass index as a marker of obesity in elderly patients on hemodialysis. J Ren Nutr. 2016;26(2):65–71.
92. Gracia-Iguacel C, Qureshi AR, Avesani CM, Heimbürger O, Huang X, Lindholm B, et al. Subclinical versus overt obesity in dialysis patients: more than meets the eye. Nephrol Dial Transplant. 2013;28(Suppl 4):iv175–81.

Chapter 23
Bone and Mineral Disorders

Linda McCann

Keywords Uremic or renal osteodystrophy (RO) · Chronic kidney disease-mineral and bone disorder (CKD-MBD) · Vitamin D · 1,25-Dihydroxyvitamin D · Secondary hyperparathyroidism · Parathyroid hormone (PTH) · Phosphate · Calcium · Vitamin D analogs · Calcimimetics · FGF23 · Klotho · Vitamin D receptor (VDR) · Calcium-sensing receptor (CaSR) · Calcidiol · Nutritional vitamin D · KDOQI · KDIGO · Evidence-based practice guidelines

---

Key Points
- To identify mechanisms of CKD-mineral and bone disorder (CKD-MBD)
- To describe consequences of bone and mineral abnormalities in CKD
- To identify the clinical, biochemical, bone, and physiologic indicators for the presence and progression of CKD-MBD
- To discuss current therapies and treatment recommendations for bone and mineral abnormalities in CKD

Introduction

Abnormal bone and altered mineral metabolism are common complications of chronic kidney disease (CKD) and have been the subject of concern and controversy throughout the world [1–5]. Mounting evidence suggests that disorders of bone and mineral metabolism are associated with an increased risk for cardiovascular calcification, morbidity, and mortality [6, 7]. As kidney function declines, mineral homeostasis deteriorates, leading to changes in the levels of various hormones, such as parathyroid hormone (PTH), 25-hydroxyvitamin D, 1,25-dihydroxyvitamin D, other vitamin D metabolites, fibroblastic growth factor-23 (FGF23), FGF co-receptor Klotho, and growth hormone. Eventually, serum and tissue concentrations of calcium and phosphate become abnormal. The discovery of FGF23 and its co-receptor, Klotho, has changed the understanding of abnormal phosphate and vitamin D metabolism in CKD.

Increased secretion of $1,25(OH)_2D$ and high dietary phosphate intake are the main stimuli of FGF23 secretion [8]. FGF23 levels increase early (CKD stages 2 or 3) and steadily increase as CKD progresses. This hormone stimulates an appropriate physiologic adaptation to maintain normal phosphate balance. It helps to augment urinary phosphate excretion (although hindered by low Klotho levels), increase PTH levels, and lower $1,25(OH)_2D$ production. Over time this adaptation fails, caus-

---

L. McCann (✉)
Nephrology Nutrition Consultant/Speaker, Eagle, ID, USA

© Springer Nature Switzerland AG 2020
J. D. Burrowes et al. (eds.), *Nutrition in Kidney Disease*, Nutrition and Health,
https://doi.org/10.1007/978-3-030-44858-5_23

ing a progressive decline in $1,25(OH)_2D$ levels with additional long-term consequences such as secondary hyperparathyroidism (SHPT). High FGF23 levels have been independently linked to adverse outcomes in CKD, such as cardiovascular disease and mortality. Additionally, treatment with activated vitamin D compounds stimulates FGF23. This finding has reinforced the need to consider the risks and benefits of using activated vitamin D and to determine the optimal doses [8].

With the decreased conversion of 25-hydroxyvitamin D to the active form, intestinal calcium absorption drops and PTH secretion increases. The diseased kidney does not respond appropriately to PTH or FGF23. There is also evidence of downregulation of vitamin D receptors (VDRs) and resistance to the actions of PTH at the tissue level. While all the interrelated mechanisms and consequences are not fully understood, the import of these abnormalities has generated considerable interest and controversy [2, 9, 10].

Evidence-based practice guidelines for the management of CKD-mineral bone disease (MBD) were published by the National Kidney Foundation (NKF) Kidney Disease Outcomes Quality Initiative (KDOQI) in 2003 [1]. In 2005, an international group, Kidney Disease Improving Global Outcomes (KDIGO), sponsored a controversies conference entitled "Definition, Evaluation and Classification of Renal Osteodystrophy" [9]. The resulting position statement, published in 2006, provided a broader definition of bone and mineral abnormalities which was labeled as CKD-MBD [9]. CKD-MBD was defined as a systemic disorder of mineral and bone metabolism due to CKD manifested by one or a combination of (1) abnormal calcium, phosphate, PTH, or vitamin D metabolism; (2) abnormalities of bone turnover, mineralization, volume, linear growth, or strength; and (3) vascular or other soft tissue calcification. It was suggested that the term renal osteodystrophy (RO) be applied only to alterations in CKD bone morphology that are quantifiable by histomorphometry of bone biopsy. There was also agreement within the consensus group that an international guideline was warranted to help clinicians understand and treat this disorder [9]. KDIGO evidence-based practice guidelines for CKD-MBD were developed and published in 2009 [2]. These guidelines were reviewed and embraced by experts around the world [2–5], noting the areas where financial limitations or lack of available therapies might alter the complete adoption of the guidelines. Review of evidence during a second consensus conference in 2013 determined an update of the guideline was warranted [11]. The updated version was published in 2017 [12], addressing primarily the guideline statements and recommendations that had new or stronger evidence to support them. The guidelines continue to recommend monitoring mineral metabolism parameters, but suggest a more individualized approach considering the risks (such as hypercalcemia) and the lack of evidence for better outcomes (meeting specific biochemical targets) with various treatment options [2, 12]. KDOQI (guideline group that determines the appropriateness of international CKD guidelines in the USA) reviewed the KDIGO guidelines and essentially agreed that the majority of the international guidelines were applicable to the US CKD population [13], but noted that a large number of the recommendations continue to be opinion based due to the lack of high-quality evidence.

In the years since dialysis became routinely available, the profile of bone and mineral abnormalities has changed, molded by the dialysis process and various therapies. The focus on hyperparathyroid bone disease and osteomalacia has expanded to include concern for low-turnover bone abnormalities, mixed bone disease, and soft tissue mineralization [1, 2, 9]. Abnormalities of bone and mineral metabolism, in those individuals on dialysis therapy, are typically asymptomatic until late in the course of the disease, and even then, symptoms may be nonspecific and unobtrusive [10, 14]. Common symptoms such as pruritus, bone pain, fractures, deformities, and muscle weakness [2, 9, 10] have been overshadowed by metastatic and extraskeletal calcifications, which have the potential to affect many areas of the body. Extraskeletal calcification can be localized in arteries, eyes, visceral organs, skin, and around joints [1, 2]. Manifestations of abnormal bone and mineral metabolism can be found in Table 23.1 [2, 7, 10, 12, 14, 15]. It is important to understand the widespread incidence and impact of bone and mineral abnormalities in CKD and to use caution in applying therapies, always weighing the risks and benefits.

Table 23.1 Manifestations of abnormal bone and mineral metabolism

Manifestation	Characteristics/Description
Altered vitamin D metabolism	Elevated FGF23 Decreased Klotho Deficiency of calcitriol Defective intestinal absorption of calcium Hypocalcemia Stimulation of PTH
Abnormal handling of calcium, phosphate, magnesium by the kidneys	Elevated FGF23 Hyperphosphatemia Hypocalcemia
Secondary hyperparathyroidism (SHPT)	Decreased skeletal response to PTH Altered degradation of PTH Abnormal regulation of calcium-dependent secretion Increased parathyroid chief cell proliferation Increased bone turnover Bone disease (osteitis fibrosa)
Metastatic and extraskeletal calcifications	Calcification of coronary arteries and cardiac valves Potential skin ulceration and soft tissue necrosis Increased risk for cardiovascular events/mortality
Fractures	Incidence is increased in CKD and associated with poorer outcomes (need for assisted living, mortality)
Bone pain	Not as common with the decrease is aluminum-associated bone disease, expressed as a general ache
Pruritus	Previously associated with high PTH, high calcium-phosphorus product, metastatic calcification; research patient-reported associations are inconsistent; postulated to link to immune response
Dialysis-related amyloidosis	Disabling arthropathy after years-long dialysis therapy
Calcific uremic arteriolopathy (calciphylaxis)	Characterized by microvascular occlusion in subcutaneous adipose tissue and dermis, which result in lesions or ulcers; rare but life-threatening
Proximal myopathy and muscle weakness	Usually limited to proximal muscles and thought to be caused by SHPT, phosphorus depletion, aluminum toxicity or low vitamin levels

Data from Refs. [1, 2, 7, 10, 48, 49, 52]

Abbreviations: *FGF23* fibroblastic growth factor, *PTH* parathyroid hormone, *CKD* chronic kidney disease, *SHPT* secondary hyperparathyroidism

Pathogenesis of Bone and Mineral Abnormalities in CKD

Progressive loss of kidney function causes disturbances in mineral metabolism and bone integrity. The cascade of events that leads to bone and mineral abnormalities begins early in CKD. The kidneys help maintain the balance of calcium and phosphate in the body by regulating the net excretion of these minerals in the urine. Balance is also maintained by changes in calcium and phosphate absorption in the gastrointestinal (GI) tract and through the exchange of ions between bone and the extracellular fluid. Bone-level calcium and phosphate stores help support metabolic and homeostatic requirements. PTH, calcitriol, and phosphatonins like FGF23, along with its co-regulator, Klotho, coordinate the responses of the kidneys, intestines, and bones [1, 2, 10, 15–17].

Mineral and endocrine derangements begin earlier in CKD than bone-level changes [9]. In response to increasing phosphate load and decreasing calcitriol levels, FGF23 and PTH increase the per-nephron phosphate excretion via sodium-dependent phosphate cotransporters NPT2a and NPT2c [16, 17], although low Klotho levels in CKD hinder the phosphaturic effect of FGF23. FGF23 and PTH levels increase as CKD progresses (stage G2 CKD) with compensatory adaptations striving to maintain normophosphatemia [16, 17]. In healthy volunteers, dietary phosphate loading stimulates FGF23 synthesis, while restricting dietary phosphate has the opposite effect [18]. Increased FGF23 is an early biochemical marker of mineral derangement, although commercial assays for FGF23 or its biologic activator, Klotho, are not yet available for routine clinical use [19]. In the prospective Chronic Renal Insufficiency Cohort (CRIC) [20], elevated FGF23 was independently associated with mortality risk at all stages of CKD and with risk of progression to requiring kidney replacement therapy in those individuals with baseline glomerular filtration rate (GFR) $\geq$30 mL/min. The role of FGF23 in the development of SHPT is due to both direct and indirect effects. FGF23 has a counter-regulatory effect on calcitriol; thus, in CKD it has the potential to reduce vitamin D activity. It can also stimulate local expression of 1α-hydroxylase in the parathyroid (PT) glands, which may indirectly downregulate PTH synthesis through increased local production of calcitriol [21]. There is also a downregulation of the FGF23 signaling pathway in the PT glands with a decreased expression of fibroblast growth factor receptor 1 and Klotho. Klotho, a single-pass transmembrane protein, has wide biologic effects and is expressed mainly in the kidneys and the PT glands but has also been detected in other tissues. It is central to FGF23 biologic activity and seems to be required for the FGF23-mediated receptor activation that stimulates phosphorylation pathways. Klotho also has a role in regulation of phosphate and calcium metabolism leading to increased calcium reabsorption [21] and directly regulates PTH synthesis [22]. Many general metabolism roles have also been attributed to Klotho, and it is believed that others will be identified in the future [21].

Once the GFR drops below 60 (stage G3 CKD), PTH levels begin to rise in the blood [2, 10], setting in motion the development of SHPT [9]. This rise in PTH appears to be in response to several factors, including increasing FGF23 levels, vitamin D deficiency, increasing phosphate retention, and a skeletal resistance to PTH, all of which lead to hypocalcemia and further stimulation of PTH. With progressive loss of kidney function, there seems to be a decrease in the number of vitamin D receptors (VDRs) and calcium-sensing receptors (CaSRs) in the PT glands, making them resistant to the actions of vitamin D and calcium. It has been suggested that dietary phosphate modification may modulate PTH [10, 14, 18] and FGF23 [8, 9, 18] levels even when serum phosphate levels are within the normal range. However, a recent Cochrane review indicates that there is only low-quality evidence that dietary intervention positively affects CKD-MBD biomarkers [22]. Hyperphosphatemia occurs later in the progression of CKD, usually when GFR drops to about 20–30 mL/m^3, and significantly influences the function and growth of parathyroid glands [1, 10, 14].

By the time dialysis is required, most CKD patients have some degree of SHPT which is characterized by hypersecretion of PTH and eventually hyperplasia of the parathyroid glands. The historic trade-off hypothesis [1, 2, 8, 14] suggests that as GFR declines, production of calcitriol is inadequate to meet physiologic needs, serum calcium levels decline, phosphate excretion declines, and serum phosphate levels increase. Reduced calcitriol levels hinder the absorption of calcium from the intestines. These factors lead to hypocalcemia, a primary stimulus for increased production and secretion of PTH. Increased PTH levels stimulate phosphate excretion and calcitriol production to correct the hypocalcemia. However, research on FGF23 challenges this trade-off hypothesis and indicates that elevated FGF23 is one of the first abnormalities, and that it decreases 1,25-vitamin D production and starts the cascade of events that lead to SHPT [8].

In the later stages of CKD, increased PTH production and secretion can no longer counterbalance the abnormal serum levels of calcium, phosphate, and FGF23 [1, 8, 10, 14]. Increased PTH production and secretion along with decreased PTH degradation lead to SHPT [4, 9, 10].

Phosphate is a key element for many physiologic pathways, such as skeletal development, bone mineralization, membrane composition, nucleotide structure, maintenance of plasma pH, and cellular signaling [21, 22]. The kidneys are central to its regulation, mainly through two hormonal regulators, FGF23 and PTH. Both hormones have hypophosphatemic effects through decreased phosphate tubular reabsorption. The third regulator of phosphate metabolism is 1,25-vitamin D, which increases intestinal calcium and phosphate absorption and inhibits PTH synthesis [21, 23]. Hyperphosphatemia helps regulate the production of calcitriol by reducing the activity of the enzyme that activates 25(OH) vitamin D [24]. Hyperphosphatemia also influences PTH gene expression and indirectly increases PTH production [25]. In those without CKD, higher PTH levels, along with increased FGF23 levels

[21], increase phosphate excretion to restore serum phosphate levels to normal. In the late stages of CKD, this compensatory mechanism is inadequate to maintain the serum phosphate levels [21, 25]. Additionally, with significant SHPT, phosphate is released directly from the bone into the blood contributing to hyperphosphatemia [26]. Chronically elevated phosphate levels are associated with parathyroid gland size and parathyroid gland hyperplasia with continued high PTH levels that may eventually require surgical intervention [10, 20, 21].

In CKD, production of calcitriol by the kidney is reduced in response to high FGF23 [8]. Low levels of calcitriol contribute to SHPT both directly and indirectly [27, 28]. Calcitriol exerts a direct negative feedback control on the parathyroid gland, inhibiting preproPTH production and gene transcription [10, 14]. Indirectly, low calcitriol levels hinder the absorption of calcium from the intestine and mobilization of calcium from the bone. These actions suggest that calcium, rather than vitamin D, predominantly regulates PTH [29].

Hypocalcemia results from increased calcium-phosphate complexes and from a decrease in absorption of dietary calcium from the intestine [28–30]. In addition, the ability of the bone to release calcium into the blood is hindered. The calcium-sensing receptor (CaSR) provides a regulatory mechanism involving release of PTH to maintain calcium homeostasis [24]. Even slight physiologic, within normal range, changes in serum calcium seem to modulate the development of SHPT.

Skeletal resistance to the calcemic action of PTH is also a factor in the development of SHPT. As CKD progresses, increasingly higher levels of PTH are needed to induce PTH effects and to maintain normal bone remodeling activity [31]. Skeletal resistance is thought to be multifactorial, perhaps from altered regulation of PTH receptors in the bone that makes them less sensitive to PTH as well as from phosphate retention and calcitriol deficiency [14, 32–34].

As hypocalcemia, hyperphosphatemia, increased FGF23, and calcitriol deficiency continue, the parathyroid glands continually increase production of PTH, leading to parathyroid cell hypertrophy. With chronic stimulation, the parathyroid cells proliferate, and diffuse hyperplasia develops. This proliferation of parathyroid cells makes it difficult to modulate PTH levels. Nodular hyperplasia is characterized by cells with fewer CaSRs and VDRs and is significantly resistant to vitamin D therapy [26, 27]. The effects of calcimimetics on gland hyperplasia are still being investigated; however, calcimimetics may have the potential to reduce the need for parathyroidectomy [22].

Bone Manifestations

The traditional types of RO have been defined based on turnover, mineralization, and volume (TMV). Two general characteristics define the state of the bone – high-turnover and low-turnover. High-turnover bone states, including osteitis fibrosa and mixed bone disorders, are characterized by abnormal and increased bone remodeling. Low-turnover bone states, including osteomalacia and adynamic bone disorder, are characterized by decreased bone mineralization and formation, including osteomalacia and adynamic bone disorder (ABD) [1, 9, 10]. The spectrum of possible bone changes, from low-to high-turnover, from low- to high-volume, and with or without mineralization abnormalities, can be found in Table 23.2 [2, 9, 28]. The incidence and profile of bone abnormalities is varied and has changed in response to available therapies, dialysis techniques, and patient populations.

Osteitis fibrosa is caused by SHPT and historically has been the most common form of bone abnormality in CKD [9, 29]. It is characterized by marrow fibrosis and increased bone turnover due to both bone resorption and bone formation. Bone resorption is caused by an increase in the number and activity of osteoclasts, and changes in bone formation are due to increased osteoblasts and osteoid deposition [10, 14]. While mixed bone disease has features of both high- and low-turnover abnormalities, it is generally classified as a high-turnover disease. Mixed bone disease has been associated with aluminum accumulation, hypocalcemia, and variable levels of serum phosphate [9, 10, 28].

Table 23.2 Types and characteristics of renal osteodystrophy

Type	Bone turnover	Mineralization	Volume
Mild SHPT	Slightly high	Normal	Normal
Osteitis fibrosa	High	Normal	High
Osteomalacia	Low	Abnormal	Normal
Adynamic bone disorder	Low	Normal/Acellularity	Low
Mixed	High	Abnormal	Normal

These are general characteristics that may vary over time and with the duration of the abnormality. Bone strength can be impaired in any of the above [2, 9, 10]

Abbreviation: *SHPT* secondary hyperparathyroidism

Osteomalacia, characterized by low bone turnover, due to aluminum overload was common in the 1970s and early 1980s secondary to aluminum levels in the dialysate and the use of aluminum hydroxide phosphate binders. With the change in dialysate standards and limitations of aluminum ingestion, aluminum-related osteomalacia is uncommon, but toxicity can still occur [9, 10, 29]. KDIGO guidelines suggest avoiding long-term exposure to aluminum sources (binders and dialysate) and indicate toxicity can be diagnosed with a bone biopsy [2].

There is also a potential for developing osteomalacia related to vitamin D deficiency, metabolic acidosis, hypophosphatemia, and deficiencies in the trace elements, fluoride and strontium [10]. Osteomalacia is characterized by a decreased bone formation rate, widened osteoid seams, and decreased formation and resorption surfaces [9, 10].

ABD is characterized by a lack of new bone formation, low cellular activity, low numbers of osteoblasts, and normal or reduced osteoclasts. Increased bone matrix is the primary defect. Mineralization is usually decreased, without excess osteoid deposition or abnormal thickness. The reduction in osteoblasts and limited bone formation may be a result of a relative deficiency in PTH. Other systemic PTH inhibitory factors may also play a role in ABD [9, 29, 35, 37]. Several subgroups of CKD stage 5D may be more likely to develop ABD. These include those who are treated with peritoneal dialysis, the elderly, and those with diabetes mellitus [36, 38].

Plasma levels of PTH are generally higher than normal in CKD, even when associated with ABD. In uremia, a relative reduction in PTH can induce a low-turnover bone state even at laboratory normal PTH levels [37, 38]. There are also racial differences in response to PTH. Blacks tend to have reduced skeletal sensitivity to PTH and less likelihood of developing overt osteitis fibrosa despite higher plasma levels of PTH [39].

Most of the studies of bone histomorphometry have not been designed to fully evaluate the relationship between fractures and types of renal osteodystrophy. Evidence is mixed regarding the relationship between low-turnover bone state and increased fractures, but some research suggests that fractures are more common in osteomalacia and adynamic bone state. It is well established that fractures in those with CKD are associated with poorer outcomes and a higher mortality rate [2].

In addition to bone abnormalities, extraskeletal calcification is a significant finding in CKD-MBD [2, 9]. Arterial calcification is found early in CKD and progresses over time. Early research suggests that coronary calcification is more likely to occur in individuals who have higher serum phosphate, higher calcium times phosphate product (CaP) levels, and a higher daily calcium load [40, 41]. Guérin et al. found that the severity of calcification is correlated with age, dialysis vintage, fibrinogen levels, and the prescribed dose of calcium-based phosphate binders [42]. Vascular calcification is associated with increased stiffness of the large capacity arteries such as the carotid artery and the aorta [41–43]. Other research shows that the presence and severity of arterial calcifications predict cardiovascular and all-cause mortality [43]. The full pathology of extraskeletal calcification in CKD is not fully understood, but FGF23 is also considered to be contributory to this process [44, 45].

Calcific uremic arteriolopathy (CUA), previously termed calciphylaxis, is a rare but severe form of medial calcification of the small, cutaneous arteries. It is associated with painful skin lesions, subcutaneous nodules, tissue ischemia, and necrosis of the skin or subcutaneous tissue of the extremities. Disturbances in mineral metabolism, SHPT, and vascular calcification appear to play a role in the genesis of CUA [46–49]. Proposed risk factors for calciphylaxis include female gender, Caucasian ethnicity, obesity, diabetes, liver disease, local trauma, hypotension, hypoalbuminemia, elevated mineral levels, protein C and protein S deficiencies, malnutrition, iron deposition, and hyperparathyroidism. There are discrepancies in reported risk factors because of the relatively small numbers of patients in many of the studies [49]. While the incidence of CUA is low and limited research has failed to fully explain the mechanisms, it can be a life-threatening complication of bone and mineral abnormalities in CKD [10].

Another abnormality in CKD is atypical accumulation of β_2-microglobulin (β_2MA), a polypeptide that is involved in a lymphocyte-mediated immune response. Accumulation is progressive due to decreased catabolism and excretion by the kidneys. Symptoms seldom occur until the patient has been on dialysis therapy for a long time, i.e., 5–15 years. The most common first symptom is carpal tunnel syndrome. Kidney transplantation is currently the only therapy that stops the progression of β_2MA. Current treatment focuses the use of biocompatible dialyzer membranes to enhance clearance of β_2MA during dialysis and on easing joint pain and inflammation [50–52].

Osteoporosis is a skeletal disorder commonly found in older individuals. Since a large percentage of those receiving dialysis are over the age of 65, osteoporosis may occur as an adjunct problem to CKD-MBD. Diagnosis of osteoporosis in CKD is more complicated since CKD-MBD may have similar manifestations [53, 54]. KDIGO suggests that patients in stages 1 to 3 with osteoporosis or high risk of fracture be treated in accordance with World Health Organization (WHO) recommendations for the general public [12]. The 2017 guidelines expand osteoporosis treatment options to include Stage G5D, stating that with biochemical abnormalities of CKD-MBD, low bone mineral density (BMD), and/or fragility fractures, treatment choices should be made with consideration of the magnitude and reversibility of the biochemical abnormalities and the progression of CKD, with consideration of a bone biopsy [12]. The rationale warns that when osteoporosis treatment choices are considered, their specific side effects must be considered especially since the underlying bone phenotype may be unclear [12].

Bone Biopsy

Bone biopsy is the most accurate diagnostic tool for determining bone lesions in CKD. All other assessment parameters should be compared to bone biopsy as the gold standard for assessing bone metabolism [1, 2, 12]. Historically, bone biopsy has been viewed as significantly invasive and potentially painful. Additionally, appropriate sample processing techniques, expert interpretation, and standardized reporting terminology have been lacking. Biopsy with tetracycline labeling allows the classification of bone pathology based on static and dynamic parameters that diagnose RO [12]. Routine bone biopsy is not recommended for CKD stage 5D patients unless the identification of bone histology has potential to alter treatment decisions [2, 12]. However, the KDIGO continues to encourage biopsy with the expectation that it might help establish the reliability of coexisting biochemical parameters.

Radiography, Pulse Pressure, and Electron Beam Computed Tomography

While X-rays provide limited information on CKD stage 5D-specific bone abnormalities, they do help in the assessment and identification of extraskeletal calcification and osteoporosis. Lateral abdominal X-rays are a simple low-cost way to detect vascular calcification [2, 10]. Pulse pressure (PP) (the difference between systolic and diastolic blood pressure) has been shown to predict arterial stiffness, and cardiac calcification contributes to arterial stiffness in CKD and dialysis patients. Increased pulse pressure in dialysis patients is also associated with increased mortality risk. PP may help identify CKD patients with subclinical coronary artery calcification (CAC) who need further evaluation. High PP indicates vessel wall alterations that may lead to adverse outcomes [42, 43].

Another method of identifying soft tissue calcification is electron beam computed tomography (EBCT); however, EBCT is not routinely available. EBCT studies have shown that dialysis patients have CAC scores that are several folds higher than individuals without CKD [2, 42, 43].

Bone Mineral Density

BMD is most commonly measured by dual energy X-ray absorptiometry (DEXA). This procedure measures the mineral content and the density of the bone but does not predict bone turnover, bone histology, or identify the type of lesion in CKD stage 5D [54]. However, KDIGO suggests that with evidence of CKD-MBD or risk factors for osteoporosis, BMD testing should be conducted to assess fracture risk, if the results will affect treatment decisions [12].

Biochemical Markers of Bone and Mineral Metabolism in CKD

With some limitations, a number of biochemical parameters can assist in the diagnosis and management of CKD-MBD. Much of the current research is focused on correlating specific biochemical parameters to bone biopsy, thus enhancing their clinical value. Concomitant, serial monitoring of biomarkers is useful. These include total and corrected serum calcium, serum phosphate, alkaline phosphatase, and plasma PTH [2, 10, 12].

Ionized calcium is the fraction of blood calcium that is critical to physiologic processes. It is more difficult to accurately measure than total calcium but is the most indicative of the physiologic effects of calcium in the circulation. Routine monitoring of total calcium over ionized is recommended because it is usually more reproducible, less affected by timing of processing, less costly, and adequate in the presence of normal plasma proteins [2, 10, 55].

Total calcium may underrepresent ionized calcium in protein-compromised patients. Since a significant portion of serum calcium is bound to protein, predominately albumin, it has been suggested that correcting total calcium for low albumin may more accurately estimate ionized calcium. There are multiple formulas that have been proposed, but their accuracy is questionable in ESRD. Most major renal laboratories correct total calcium for low measured albumin, and while recent data does not show any superiority of using corrected calcium over total calcium alone, the KDIGO work group did not recommend abandoning this practice [2]. Adjusting total calcium downward when albumin levels are greater than 4.0 g/dL is not appropriate [10].

High serum calcium is associated with bone abnormalities as well as morbidity and mortality in CKD patients on dialysis [1, 6, 10]. KDIGO recommends avoiding hypercalcemia, as opposed to the earlier recommendation to maintain calcium within the normal range. This change was precipitated by research indicating that calcium loading to correct hypocalcemia may not be appropriate or warranted in many situations [12, 13]. The guidelines suggest treating hyperphosphatemia with phosphate binders but suggest restricting the use of calcium-based binders [12]. Although none of the studies indicate an explicit maximum calcium load, the KDIGO work group wanted to acknowledge the potential for a safe upper limit that may differ from that in the general population [12]. After an exhaustive review of the literature, the Institute of Medicine (IOM) recognized that excessive calcium intake can lead to hypercalcemia, hypercalciuria, vascular and soft tissue calcification, nephrolithiasis, prostate cancer, interactions with iron and zinc, progression of CKD, and constipation. It is noted that excessive calcium intake is rarely from foods alone but is more likely to be from medications, supplements, and calcium-fortified foods. The report notes that those with CKD may be more sensitive or susceptible to the effects of excess calcium or vitamin D intakes [56]. Thus, it is reasonable for those with CKD to limit excessive calcium load by restricting the dose of calcium-based phosphate binders [12]. The upper tolerable limit specifies the level above which the risk for harm begins to increase or the highest average daily intake that is not likely to pose a risk of adverse health effects in the general population. The IOM tolerable upper limits for elemental calcium for adults is 2000–2500 mg/d depending on age range [56]. In view of the common use of active vitamin D (i.e., to increase calcium absorption), increased incidence of cardiovascular calcification, and the minimal calcium excretion in CKD, it may be more prudent to observe the Dietary Reference Intake (DRI) recommendations for calcium, which for adult women and those older than 70 years of age is 1200 mg/d and for adult men age 70 or younger is 1000 mg/d [56].

Phosphate, one of the most common chemical elements in the body, is involved in a wide variety of metabolic and enzymatic processes. It circulates and is measured as phosphate ions in the serum but is usually reported as elemental phosphate concentrations [15]. Concentration of phosphate in the serum varies significantly depending on the time of day and recent dietary phosphate intake. This may help explain the significantly high and variable levels seen in individual CKD patients. Fasting phosphate measures are ideal but unlikely in chronic dialysis patients. Falsely high levels may be due to breakdown of blood cells if specimens are processed incorrectly [12]. Chronic hyperphosphatemia is associated with bone and mineral abnormalities, worsening SHPT, as well as morbidity and mortality [2, 60]. Hyperphosphatemia is also aggravated by severe SHPT, where bone phosphate is released directly into the blood and is unavailable to phosphate binders [14]. KDIGO suggests that decisions about phosphate lowering treatment should be based on progressively or persistently elevated serum phosphate [12]. This modified recommendation is the result of new pathophysiologic insights into phosphate regulation and the roles of FGF23 and soluble Klotho in early CKD without elevated serum phosphate levels. In a randomized controlled trial (RCT) by Block [57], predialysis patients' G3b-G4 were exposed to three different phosphate binders (sevelamer, lanthanum, or calcium acetate) compared to matching placebos. The study explored the effects of the treatments on serum phosphate levels, urinary phosphate excretion, serum FGF23 levels, vascular calcification, bone density, etc. While there was a small decrease in serum phosphate over the 9-month follow-up, there was no significant change in FGF23 levels compared to placebo. Progression of coronary and aortic calcification was observed in the active binder treatment groups but not in the placebo groups [57]. This study is supported by another study (that did not meet the criteria for inclusion in the KDIGO evidence review) where the use of calcium-based binders increased the risk of hypercalcemia [58]. One small group of CKD G3b-G4 patients had 1.5 grams of calcium carbonate added to a metabolic diet containing 1 gram of calcium and 1.5 grams of phosphate. The addition of the 1.5 grams of calcium carbonate had no effect on the baseline neutral phosphate balance, but caused a significant positive calcium balance, at least in the short-term [58]. These studies suggested phosphate-lowering therapies may not be indicated in normophosphatemia and provided doubt that phosphate binders are interchangeable. Binders may have potential risk even if they are calcium-free (nonphosphate effects such as adverse GI symptoms, nutrient binding, changes in the gut microbiome) [59]. The use of phosphate binders in normophosphatemic CKD patients has been studied with variable results [60]. Thus, the 2017 guideline suggests that phosphate-lowering therapies are indicated in persistent or progressive hyperphosphatemia, which reinforces that benefit versus risk must be considered [12].

The calcium times phosphate product has predictive power for abnormal mineral metabolism, morbidity, and mortality [2, 6, 7]. However, KDIGO recommends evaluating the individual values of serum calcium and phosphate together rather than using the mathematical construct of calcium times phosphate [2].

PTH is an important biomarker for the evaluation of CKD-MBD even though standardization of assays to measure serum levels is lacking. Additionally, serum levels change quickly in response to changes in ionized calcium, and it is possible to see wide variations in the values from measurement to measurement. KDIGO recommends using trends rather than single values to guide therapy [2, 12]. PTH plays a critical role in the regulation of mineral and bone homeostasis, and its secretion is regulated by serum-ionized calcium. Levels of phosphate and vitamin D also affect synthesis and secretion of PTH. There are some studies that relate intact PTH levels to various states of bone turnover. Qi et al. found significant predictive power for high-turnover bone state at iPTH level >450 pg/mL, and low-turnover bone state when iPTH levels are within or below the normal range [61]. However, when the iPTH is between 65 and 450 pg/mL, a definitive analysis of turnover requires a bone biopsy [1, 15, 61]. There are inconsistencies in published data correlating PTH levels to bone turnover. Qi et al. found that PTH failed to predict bone turnover in 30% of hemodialysis (HD) patients and 51% of peritoneal dialysis (PD) patients [61]. Biologically active PTH (1–84) polypeptide is synthesized and secreted by the parathyroid cells. However, along with 1–84 PTH, PTH fragments are also released [14, 29, 60]. As previously discussed, many factors modulate PTH gene expression, PTH production, PTH secretion, and parathyroid cell proliferation [62]. Calcium is the primary determinant of minute-to-minute PTH secretion, whereas calcium, FGF23, phosphate, and vitamin D levels regulate PTH production and cell proliferation. Degradation of PTH is modulated by parathyroid cells and serum calcium concentration. PTH fragments have varying half-lives; they also have diverse biologic activity on PTH receptors. Elimination of PTH fragments is primarily through glomerular filtration and tubular degradation; therefore, they accumulate in CKD. These variable circumstances have generated questions regarding the predictive value and interpretation of plasma PTH [14, 61].

It is known that second-generation iPTH assays capture both 1–84 and other fragments. The metabolic significance of PTH fragments is not fully understood. The action of the largest known PTH fragment (7–84) may oppose the action of the 1–84 molecule and contribute to the PTH resistance seen in CKD stage 5D. The third-generation or bio-intact or whole PTH assays are reported to overcome the capture of fragments and are generally about 40–50% lower than iPTH. The iPTH assay continues to be the most widely used [2, 62–64]. Further research is needed to fully elucidate the opposing action of PTH fragments and to correlate second-generation and third-generation assay results to bone histology [2, 62–65].

The normal range of iPTH, ~10–65 pg/mL (1.1–7.0 pmol/L), reflects normal bone turnover in those without CKD. In CKD, with progressive skeletal resistance to PTH, normal bone turnover more closely correlates with higher plasma iPTH levels. Thus, a normal PTH is not normal in CKD patients on dialysis [61]. While the optimal PTH level is not known, on the basis of observational studies, the KDIGO work group considered that levels less than two or greater than nine times the upper normal limit for the PTH assay in use represent extreme ranges of risk for those on dialysis [2, 12], but states that significant changes even within that range should trigger evaluation and intervention to avoid those extremes [2]. The optimal PTH levels for those individuals not on dialysis (Stages G3b-G5) is unknown.The updated guideline suggests treatment only when PTH levels are progressively or persistently elevated and does not recommend routine use of active vitamin D or analogs in this population. This change acknowledges that some changes in PTH for G3-G5 CKD may be appropriate adaptive responses [12]. In spite of a reported trend toward rising PTH values in dialysis populations, there was not enough high-quality evidence to change the 2009 recommendation [12].

Alkaline phosphatase (AP) can also add information about the state of bone turnover [2, 12]. AP is an isoenzyme that is produced primarily in the liver and by osteoblasts in the bone. Other sites of AP production are the intestines, placenta, and kidneys, although these sources contribute negligible amounts under normal conditions. With normal liver function, AP is a useful indicator of bone cell activity. Most research indicates that in CKD, elevated serum AP levels are due to bone AP and correlate with other markers of high-turnover bone disease [66]. The KDIGO guidelines suggest using total AP as an adjunct test to PTH in providing information about the state of bone turnover, particularly when PTH levels are high [2]. Parallel consideration of AP with PTH has the potential to increase the predictive power of PTH; however, the specificity and sensitivity for identifying RO with AP alone

Table 23.3 Comparison of KDIGO guideline biochemical targets: 2009 and 2017

Parameter	Stage	KDIGO 2009	KDIGO 2017	Rationale
Calcium	G3a-5	Suggest maintaining serum calcium in the normal range	Suggest avoiding hypercalcemia; maintain children in age-appropriate range	Mild, asymptomatic hypocalcemia in the context of calcimimetics can be tolerated to avoid inappropriate calcium loading in adults
	G5D	Suggest maintaining serum calcium in the normal range	Same as above	Same as above; suggest restricting dose of calcium-based binders
Phosphorus	G3a-5	Suggest maintaining serum levels within the normal range	Suggest lowering elevated levels toward the normal range	Absence of data showing efforts to maintain WNL are beneficial; some safety concerns with use of phosphorus lowering meds
	G5D	Suggest lowering elevated levels toward normal range	Unchanged	Treatment should aim at overt hyperphosphatemia
iPTH	G3a-5	Optimal iPTH is not known; suggest those with iPTH levels above the normal limit be evaluated for modifiable factors	In adults not on dialysis, optimal iPTH is not known; suggest iPTH levels that are *progressively rising* or *persistently above normal limit*, first be evaluated and correct modifiable factors	Modest increases in PTH may represent an adaptive response to declining kidney function; revised to include progressive and persistent; do not modify treatment based on a single measurement
	G5D	Between 2–9× upper normal limit	Unchanged	Although recognized that global PTH levels are rising, there was insufficient evidence to change this recommendation

Adapted with permission from Ref. [12]

Abbreviations: *KDIGO* Kidney Disease Improving Global Outcome, *iPTH* intact parathyroid hormone, *PTH* parathyroid hormone, *WNL* within normal limits

or together with PTH have not been fully demonstrated [2]. Bone-specific AP (BSAP) is the fraction of AP that is generated by the osteoblasts. BSAP correlates well with iPTH and other indices of SHPT where markedly high or low values may predict underlying bone turnover [12].

In the past, aluminum exposure was a complicating factor in CKD-mineral and bone disorder. Primary causes of aluminum toxicity in CKD have been eliminated; thus, serum aluminum is measured less frequently than in the past. Measures of serum aluminum reflect recent aluminum exposure and the potential for accumulation. They may identify hidden sources of aluminum to which a patient is exposed. In CKD patients on dialysis, serum aluminum levels of >60 µg/L have notable specificity, sensitivity, and predictive value for the diagnosis of aluminum-related bone disease [1, 2].

FGF23 and Klotho levels are important markers in current research, but assays for routine clinical use are not yet available. Table 23.3 compares biochemical targets between the 2009 and 2017 KDIGO guidelines.

Treatment of CKD-MBD

Evidence-based practice guidelines serve to promote standardized, best practice management of bone and mineral abnormalities to improve patient outcomes [12, 67]. They are meant to help clinicians in decision-making, but not to dictate practice or set absolute standards. KDIGO found a paucity of high-quality evidence to support generally accepted practice patterns for the treatment of CKD-MBD. The KDIGO clinical practice guidelines for bone and mineral disorder allow flexibility for clinicians to apply those guidelines and recommendations in view of an individual patient's status and needs [2,

12]. They also recognize and address the difference in practice patterns and availability of therapies around the world. In some cases, recommendations recognize that while not ideal, a specific treatment may be better than no treatment at all [12].

Treatment approaches are intended to normalize phosphate and calcium and to optimize PTH levels for normal bone turnover while minimizing complications such as extraskeletal calcification. The evidence that achieving very specific target ranges of these biochemical markers will absolutely alter hard outcomes is lacking [2, 12]. However, treating high levels of calcium and phosphorus to move them toward the normal ranges seems reasonable to prevent or reduce progression of CKD-MBD [2, 10–12]. Table 23.4 summarizes interventions that are commonly used to treat CKD-MBD.

Table 23.4 Summary of common recommendations for treating CKD-MBD

Nutrition/dietary intake	
Educate the patient on methods to:	Reduce high dietary phosphate intake, but maintain good nutritional status. Limit or avoid sources of inorganic phosphate (high bioavailable) like food additives; utilize plant-based proteins (lower phosphate bioavailability) within other dietary modifications. Avoid hidden sources of phosphate and calcium from medications, supplements, water.
Pharmacologic	Base on serial measurements and trends of CKD-BMD biological parameters .
25(OH)D	Test and correct 25 hydroxy vitamin D (Calcidiol) insufficiencies/deficiencies in accordance with recommendations for the general public. Nutritional vitamin D has the potential to delay rising PTH in CKD G3b-G4.
Phosphate binding agents	Use to avoid hyperphosphatemia but restrict calcium-based binders/calcium load. Choice of agent: tolerable to the individual; comes in an acceptable form; avoids high pill burden; avoids excessive GI symptoms; considers the CKD-MBD biochemical profile. Monitor response and adherence to the prescription before changing doses or compounds. Proactive binder use in CKD stages G3b-G4 normophosphatemic individuals may not be without risk. Phosphate control with diet and/or binders will be hindered by high PTH from release of bone phosphate.
Calcitriol/analogs	Prescribe and titrate calcitriol or its analogs to help control PTH[a]/progression of SHPT; alter or discontinue doses if hypercalcemia or hyperphosphatemia occur. Reserve treatment in stages G3b-G4 to those with a PTH that is persistently and progressively rising above the upper normal limit for the assay.
Calcimimetics	Prescribe and titrate calcimimetics to control PTH[a]/progression of SHPT but alter or discontinue the dose if symptomatic hypocalcemia occurs. IV calcimimetics are indicated for in-center hemodialysis patients and have the advantage of in-clinic administration that minimizes patient nonadherence.
Combination (Active D and calcimimetics)	Consider using active vitamin D and calcimimetics together, coordinating their actions for optimal clinical response without exacerbation of negative side effects.[b]
Dialytic therapy	Optimize dialytic therapy for phosphorus removal and symptom control; may require longer duration and/or more frequent dialysis. Maintain dialysate calcium between 2 and 3 mEq/L (1.25–1.5 mmol/L).
Surgical	Parathyroidectomy may be warranted in those who are unable to control PTH/SHPT with pharmacological therapies or if surgery is deemed most appropriate.
Lateral abdominal radiographic/ECHO	May be helpful to detect/track the presence of vascular/valvular calcification, which indicates higher cardiovascular risk.
Bone mineral density	May help predict fracture risk in those with CKD-MBD or osteoporosis.
Bone biopsy	Should be considered if results will affect treatment decisions.

Abbreviations: *CKD-MBD* chronic kidney disease mineral bone disorder, *PTH* parathyroid hormone, *SHPT* secondary hyperparathyroidism, *ECHO* echocardiogram
[a]Recognize the limitations of PTH measurements and their differences in specific populations. Attempt to achieve PTH levels that have the potential to promote normal bone turnover, avoiding the extremes of less than two or greater than nine times the upper limit of the assay being used. Actively treat trends that move toward the upper or lower thresholds but avoid relying on single values
[b]Consider the effects of various therapies and their risk-to-benefit profiles. Treatment of one abnormal parameter can negatively affect others

Dietary Modification

Adequate and appropriate nutrition is a cornerstone of treatment in CKD. In relation to CKD-MBD, the primary dietary focus has been on excesses of phosphate intake and excessive calcium load.

Modifying dietary phosphate can be a challenge when combined with meeting protein needs for those on dialysis [1, 2, 68]. Primary food sources of organic dietary phosphate are phosphate protein-rich foods such as dairy products, meat, poultry, eggs, fish, legumes, and nuts. Food additives supply significant amounts of inorganic phosphate. Typically, about 30–60% of organic phosphate is hydrolyzed in the gastrointestinal tract and then absorbed into the circulation as inorganic phosphate [68, 69]. Absorption rates are affected by the digestibility of dietary nutrients and bioavailability of dietary phosphate as well as the degree of activation of vitamin D receptors (VDR) in the GI tract. The presence of compounds that bind phosphate or interfere with GI absorption, such as phosphate binders, also affects absorption rates [68–71].

Most of the dietary phosphate in the typical western diet comes from animal proteins which have a higher bioavailability than plant-based proteins. The phosphate in animal proteins is easily hydrolyzed and readily absorbed [69–72]. The phosphate-to-protein ratio is also quite variable [2] but needs to consider bioavailability as well as content [72]. Additionally, meat and dairy products often contain phosphate additives which add to the total phosphate content [69].

While most fruits and vegetables have small amounts of organic phosphate, others such as plant seeds, nuts, and legumes are quite high in phosphate. Plant-based organic phosphates, especially in beans, peas, nuts, and cereals, are generally in the form of phytic acid or phytate [70–72]. Phytate is the primary storage form of both phosphate and inositol in plant seeds. The bioavailability of plant-based organic phosphate is limited, usually less than 50%, because humans do not make phytase, the enzyme needed to degrade phytate. This complex renders plant-based, high-phosphate foods less phosphatemic than animal-based protein sources [70, 71]. Despite reported high-phosphate content of many plant protein sources in food composition databases, patients (mean GFR 32 mL/min) who consumed a metabolic lab-prepared vegetarian diet (grain and soy based) for 1 week had significantly lower serum phosphate and FGF23 levels than those consuming equivalent protein and calories in a meat- and dairy-based diet [73]. Thus, plant sources of protein may have lower phosphate bioavailability than their in vitro-measured phosphate content. More research is required to fully understand the variability of phosphate bioavailability and patient-specific absorption [68, 70, 72].

While phosphate from plant-based proteins is generally less available, there are exceptions such as leavened breads that contain yeast-based phytase. Probiotics may also enhance phytase-associated phosphate release and availability. Processing techniques, such as soaking, germination, malting, and fermentation, reduce phytate content by increasing activity of naturally present phytase. Phytic acid also has potential to reduce the digestibility and utilization of protein and various minerals [70–72]. One must also consider that plant-based proteins generally have a lower biological value than animal proteins; thus, care must be taken to ensure adequate protein intake in CKD patients if shifting toward a diet of mainly plant derivative foods [72]. It is important to note that use of plant-based proteins may be limited by the increased load of other nutrients like potassium.

Phosphate, in its inorganic form, is the main component of food additives and preservatives that are used to extend shelf life, improve color, retain moisture, and enhance flavors of processed foods [72]. Because the inorganic phosphate in additives is not protein bound, the salts break apart and become readily absorbed in the GI tract. These additives are commonly used in processed foods, frozen meals, enhanced meats, colas, snack bars, cereals, spreadable cheese, instant products, and many bakery products. Unfortunately, there is very little information to estimate the amount of phosphate that is contributed by additives, nor is there a method to fully distinguish between organic and additive-based inorganic phosphate that is contained in traditional foods. Inorganic phosphate is estimated to be over 90% absorbed, while about 40–60% of animal-based phosphate and even less plant-based phosphate is absorbed [76].

It is difficult to accurately assess dietary phosphate intake due to the outdated values in food composition tables and other databases [74–76]. The IOM guidance for phosphate intake, which has not been revised since 1997 and does not address the specific needs of CKD patients, provides an estimated average requirement of 580 mg/day and a recommended daily allowance of 700 mg/day for all adults [77]. The upper tolerable limit, 4000 mg/day, should not be approached even by those without CKD given recent information that associates high phosphate intake and cardiovascular disease in the general public. Since intakes exceeding metabolic requirements directly increase serum phosphate, it is important to advise CKD patients on dietary choices that avoid excess phosphate loads [77].

Improving awareness of foods high in phosphate and understanding differences in phosphate absorption between animal, plant, and additive sources is essential for the dietitian [69, 72]. Dietitians are key to patient education about the dangers of bone and mineral abnormalities in CKD. While there is little evidence for long-term success of educational interventions to improve serum phosphate, several studies have shown at least short-term success [2, 12]. The extent to which dietitian-to-patient staffing ratios support intense CKD-MBD management and intense counseling is important, but not easily quantified. While dietitians have an active role in treating hyperphosphatemia with phosphate binders, dietary counseling becomes more important when the phosphate intake is high. Education should focus on the significant contribution of food additives, bioavailability of phosphate from different foods, and the complementary actions of phosphate binders and reduction of high intake. The amounts of phosphate in foods is underrepresented in nutrition labels and databases [68, 69, 72]. Significant underestimations of phosphate content by as much as 350 mg/day have been reported in Europe, Japan, and the USA [72, 74–76]. Analysis of chicken products in the USA showed actual phosphate contents exceeding those estimated from a nutrient database [69]. The use of additives that increase phosphate by two-fold or more, together with a lack of information on the nutritional label, has motivated nephrology dietitians and other groups to discourage manufacturers' indiscriminate use of phosphate additives and to call for greater transparency regarding the phosphate content of foods [69, 72].

A common dialysis treatment regimen, 4 hours three times per week, is unlikely to maintain a net zero balance between phosphate intake and clearance for most individuals. Approximately 800–1000 mg of phosphate (2400–3000 mg/week) is removed by high-flux dialysis each treatment [81]. Even if the dietary intake is limited to 800 to 1000 mg/day, there is still a significant positive phosphate balance which generally requires the use of phosphate binders and/or additional dialysis therapy to control serum levels in both PD and HD [81].

Calcium balance is complex in CKD and normal serum levels do not necessarily mean that this mineral is in balance [58, 78, 79]. There is concern with excess calcium even in the general public [77]. While calcium content of the traditional "renal" diet is low due to limits on dairy products, calcium-fortified foods may add to the daily calcium load. Large amounts of calcium-based binders are the most common source of excess calcium load in CKD, often exceeding the upper tolerable limit of elemental calcium [77, 78]. While the KDIGO work group members could not make an explicit recommendation for a maximum dose of calcium-based binders or total elemental calcium, they wanted to acknowledge the potential existence of a safe upper limit by suggesting that the dose of calcium-based binders be restricted [12]. They also noted that calcium loading to correct low serum calcium levels may not be effective, nor appropriate, especially in the presence of calcimimetics [12].

Pharmacologic Treatments

Phosphate Binders

There are many choices and different forms of phosphate binders which work in combination with limiting high dietary phosphorus sources and appropriate dialysis prescriptions [12, 80, 81]. The most appropriate phosphate binders are patient-specific and readily available. They must be well tolerated, without creating other problems or adding an excessive pill burden [1, 2]. Appropriate prescription of phosphate binders requires an assessment of dietary phosphate intake, modification of that phosphate intake as appropriate, and titration of the dose to avoid hyperphosphatemia and move serum phosphate toward the normal range [12]. Prior to each modification of the binder prescription, it is critical to assess patient adherence to that binder prescription. The binder dose should be titrated to the phosphate content of the meal(s) and include binders for additional sources of phosphate such as snacks. It is also well-recognized that uncontrolled hyperparathyroidism will hinder the control of serum phosphorus due to phosphorus release from the bone to the blood. Routinely increasing binder doses without considering the source of hyperphosphatemia could create an unnecessary patient burden and the potential for negative side effects from the binders. For those with CKD stages G3b-G4, it is suggested that phosphate binders be used with caution and primarily to treat persistent or progressive hyperphosphatemia, since some research calls into question the safety profile of binder use in normophosphatemic individuals [12, 57]. Commonly available phosphate-binding compounds can be found in Table 23.5.

Table 23.5 Common phosphate binders

Binder source	Rx	Available forms	Mineral content	Potential advantages	Potential disadvantages
Aluminum hydroxide	No	Liquid, tablet, capsule	Aluminum, varies 100 to >200 mg	Very effective binding power, inexpensive	Potential for aluminum toxicity, not recommended for long-term use
Calcium acetate	Yes	Tablet, liquid	169 mg elemental calcium per 667 mg pill	Effective; potentially better binding than carbonate, less calcium absorption	Increased cost over carbonate, potential for excess calcium load, hypercalcemia/vascular calcification, GI symptoms, constipation
Calcium carbonate	No	Tablet, liquid, chewable, capsule, gum	40% elemental Ca 200 mg calcium/500 mg CaCO$_3$	Effective, inexpensive, readily available	Potential for excess calcium load, hypercalcemia/vascular calcification; GI symptoms, constipation
Ferric citrate	Yes	Tablet	No calcium, 1 gm = 210 mg ferric acid	Effective, improves iron parameters	Cost, GI side effects, not to be used in iron overload, discolored feces
Lanthanum carbonate	Yes	Wafer, can be chewed/crushed	250–500 mg elemental lanthanum	Effective binding power, lower pill burden	Cost, potential for lanthanum accumulation with unknown long-term effects, GI symptoms
Magnesium and calcium carbonate	No	Tablet 300 400Rx	~101 mg elemental Ca, 86 mg mag	Effective	Monitor for hypermagnesemia, GI side effects, calcium load, 400 Rx not for nondialysis,
(MagneBind™)	Yes		~80 mg elemental Ca, 112 mg mag		
Sevelamer Carbonate	Yes	Tablet, powder	None	Effective, avoids decrease in bicarbonate levels, no calcium or metals	Cost, GI symptoms, pill burden
Sevelamer HCL	Yes	Caplet	None, ion exchange resin	Effective, no calcium or metal	Cost, GI symptoms, pill burden, potential for decreased bicarbonate levels, contraindicated in bowel obstruction
Sucroferric Oxyhydroxide	Yes	Tablet, chewable, crushable	500 mg iron	Very effective, potential for reduced pill burden, noncalcium	Cost, GI symptoms, contraindicated in iron overload

Outside USA: Bixalomer (Kilkin™) 250 mg capsule of an amine functional polymer, similar profile to Sevelamer (Japan)
Calcium acetate and magnesium carbonate (OsvaRen™) Tablet 425/235; ~ 106 mg calcium, 65 mg magnesium
Abbreviations: *CaCO$_3$* calcium carbonate, *GI* gastrointestinal

Calcium-based binders are also addressed in the recommendation to avoid hypercalcemia. The KDIGO recommendation to avoid hypercalcemia is based primarily on a consensus of expert opinion and retrospective studies that suggested potential for higher mortality with elevated serum calcium and phosphate [2, 12]. Avoiding hypercalcemia requires several interventions, including regulating the calcium in the dialysate as well as monitoring and modifying the calcium load from the diet and medications such as calcium-based binders or antacids [12]. It is important that patients be made aware of calcium sources (diet, medications, supplements, calcium fortified foods, dialysate) to help avoid hypercalcemia. This change from "maintain serum levels in the normal range" was in part stimulated by the observation that those on calcimimetics may tolerate lower blood calcium levels without symptoms of hypocalcemia. There is also recognition that the potential for extraskeletal calcification increases with excess calcium loads that might be given to normalize serum calcium [12].

Generally, the use of 2.5 mEq/L dialysate calcium concentration minimizes the movement of calcium from blood to dialysate or dialysate to blood [12, 82]. With 3.5 mEq/L calcium dialysate concentrations, most patients have a positive flux of calcium. Conversely, lower concentrations of dialysate calcium promote negative calcium flux. As with phosphate, the movement of calcium depends on serum levels, dialysate levels, and the duration of exposure to dialysate. Serum calcium is affected by calcium load, the presence of active vitamin D, and circulating PTH. Severe SHPT promotes release of calcium from the bone, adding another source for hypercalcemia. Serum calcium may also be elevated when PTH levels are low and blood calcium is not being incorporated into the bone [9, 10].

Vitamin D and Analogs

Active vitamin D or analogs are commonly used to control PTH levels in CKD-MBD [2, 83, 84]. Active forms of vitamin D_2 including calcitriol, paricalcitol, and doxercalciferol are most commonly used in the USA. Active forms of vitamin D_3 include maxacalcitol, 1-alpha-calcidiol, and 22-oxacalcitriol. PTH-lowering therapies, including active vitamin D, analogs, and calcimimetics along with some of their biologic effects can be found in Table 23.6. All these therapies are available in oral or IV forms. Each of the active vitamin D products has specific structure and actions. In SHPT, active vitamin D/analog doses are typically based on the elevation of plasma PTH. They also have the potential for increasing calcium and phosphate absorption in the GI tract and cause increased levels of both these minerals in the serum. Studies vary as to which of the active vitamin D medications is most calcemic. Calcitriol (1,25-dihydroxycholecalciferol or 1,25(OH)2D3) is a synthetic active vitamin D[83].

Paricalcitol [19-nor-1,25(OH)$_2$] is a sterol derived from vitamin D_2 and is available in oral or IV formulation. It is missing a carbon-19 methylene group that is present in all natural vitamin D metabolites. Paricalcitol has been reported to have a lower calcemic effect through VDR selectivity at the tissue level of bone and intestine, while having greater activity in the parathyroid tissue. Clinical trials have demonstrated the effectiveness of paricalcitol at controlling PTH [83, 84]. An observational study suggests that the use of paricalcitol provides a survival advantage over calcitriol; however, this has not been confirmed by studies using more rigorous research standards such as an RCT [85].

Doxercalciferol (1α-hydroxyvitamin D_2) is a prohormone that requires hepatic conversion to its active form, 1,25(OH)$_2$D$_2$. Doxercalciferol has also been shown to be clinically effective in controlling PTH in CKD patients [86, 87].

Dihydrotachysterol$_2$ (DHT$_2$) is one of the first vitamin D derivatives used to treat CKD-MBD. It is available for oral administration in tablet and liquid form outside the USA [83]. There are several other vitamin D products that are used outside the USA, which will not be discussed here but can be reviewed in the literature [83].

Table 23.6 PTH-lowering therapies

Vitamin D/Analogs (Oral) (Calcitriol, paricalcitol, doxercalciferol) USA[a]	Vitamin D/Analogs (IV) (Calcitriol, paricalcitol, doxercalciferol)	Calcimimetics (Oral) (Cinacalcet)	Calcimimetics (IV) (Etelcalcetide)
Indication for G3b-G5D	Indication for in-center HD	Indication for CKD on dialysis	Indication for in-center HD
Acts on the VDR to reduce PTH synthesis and secretion, stimulates calcium and phosphate absorption	Acts on the VDR, same as oral	Acts on the surface transmembrane of the CaSR to reduce PTH synthesis and secretion, is associated with reductions in serum levels of calcium and phosphate	Acts on the extracellular domain of the CaSR to reduce PTH synthesis and secretion, is associated with reductions in serum levels of calcium and phosphate
NA	Little or no loss to dialysate, but some PI recommend administer at end of dialysis	NA	Dialyzable, requires specific timing of administration to the dialysis circuit after rinse back
Onset of action/peak serum concentrations 3–8 hours Doxercalciferol 11–22 hours	Doxercalciferol 11–22 hours	Nadir PTH 2–6 hours post dose, steady state within 7 days	PTH decrease within 30 minutes, steady state 7–8 weeks
Elimination half-life[b] depends on the agent/dose Calcitriol 5–8 hours Paracalcitol Doxercalciferol 11–12 hours	Calcitriol Doxercalciferol 32–37 hours, up to 90 hours Paracalcitol 14–20 hours	Elimination half-life 30–40 hours	Elimination half-life 3–5 days
Little or no effect on nodular or hyperplasic PT glands	Little or no effect on nodular or hyperplasic PT glands	Potential to suppress PTH even when glands are nodular, may inhibit gland hyperplasia	Potential to suppress PTH even when glands are nodular, may inhibit gland hyperplasia

Abbreviations: *USA* United States, *IV* intravenous, *HD* hemodialysis, *CKD* chronic kidney disease, *VDR* vitamin D receptor, *CaSR* calcium sensing receptor, *PTH* parathyroid hormone, *NA* not applicable, *PT* parathyroid, *PI* package insert

[a]Maxacalcitol, alfacacidol outside USA

[b]The biological or elimination half-life is the time it takes for bioactivity of the drug to reduce by 50% of its initial value
https://wikem.org/wiki/Dialyzable_drugs

Nutritional Vitamin D

Commonly available forms of nutritional vitamin D are ergocalciferol (D_2) and cholecalciferol (D_3). Kandula et al. performed a systematic review and meta-analysis of both observational and randomized controlled trials in respect to nutritional vitamin D supplementation in CKD [88]. The prevalence of vitamin D deficiency is well documented in the general public and increases with extremes of age, postmenopausal state, Black race, women, and the presence of CKD. It is estimated that as many as 80% of those with CKD around the world are vitamin D deficient. Although the kidneys are the primary site for hydroxylation of vitamin D to its active form, many other extrarenal conversion sites have been identified, including the parathyroid gland. There is renewed interest in the use of calciferols to affect bone and mineral metabolism in CKD. The interest has been intensified by studies demonstrating nonskeletal benefits of vitamin D. An association between mortality and vitamin D deficiency has been shown in those with CKD, both before and after dialysis dependence. The observational and randomized controlled studies indicate that vitamin D supplementation improves biochemical end points (increased 25(OH)D and 1,25(OH)$_2$D levels) and delays the rise in PTH levels in CKD (G3–G4) without increasing the frequency of hypercalcemia or hyperphosphatemia. Like other interventions, future research will need to determine whether supplementation can improve biochemical end points and translate into better cardiovascular and skeletal outcomes in CKD [88, 89].

Nutritional vitamin D is not commonly found in plants and animal food sources except for oily fish and those foods that are vitamin D fortified. Nutritional vitamin D is obtained through ultraviolet B radiation acting on the 7-dehyrdrocholesterol in the skin to form previtamin D$_3$, which is quickly converted to D$_3$. The aggressive use of sunscreen and reported effects of pollution have been associated with the very common deficiencies seen in the general population. Additionally, many of those with CKD on dialysis have fewer opportunities for sun exposure. Vitamin D$_2$ is similarly produced by solar irradiation of marine plankton or yeasts and molds. Because of the endocrine functions and the ability of mammals to synthesize nutritional vitamin D, it is not truly a vitamin but a prehormone [89].

Nutritional vitamin D, whether ingested or derived from the skin, is hydroxylated to 25-hydroxyvitamin D$_2$ or D$_3$ in the liver. 25-hydroxy vitamin D ((25(OH)D)) concentration in the blood is a reliable measure of nutritional deficiency because it is stable in the circulation and has a half-life of about 2 weeks. The major site of activation is the kidneys, but there are other sites for vitamin D activation, all of which are influenced by serum levels of PTH, FGF23, calcium, and phosphate. The IOM was charged with conducting a review of existing literature to determine the optimal intake of vitamin D and calcium for the general public. There were pitfalls with each of the potential outcome measures (variability of PTH level and assays, fractures, calcium absorption) as well as a mixture of study designs without the ability to factor in the effect of sun exposure and seasonal variations [72]. The IOM found a paucity of data demonstrating any causal benefit of vitamin D for most health outcomes, but suggested that most children and adults would have adequate vitamin D levels (20 ng/mL) with 600 IU/day for those between 1 and 70 years of age (800 IU/day for those over 70). Many have taken issue with this recommendation and suggest that it is too low. Vitamin D intoxication is rare in adults who are supplemented with 1000–2000 IU vitamin D daily. Hypercalcemia, the primary manifestation of toxicity, is generally not seen until vitamin D levels exceed 115–200 ng/mL (375–500 nmol/L). Without more definitive research, the IOM recommendations may be reasonable, but as clinicians we must consider individual patient characteristics that might dictate a different approach [77, 88, 89]. It is recommended that 25(OH) D levels be tested and supplementation be considered to raise low levels; however, the exact dose, form, and optimal blood levels are unknown for CKD [12].

Calcimimetics

Calcimimetics are a class of compounds that act on the CaSRs in the parathyroid cells, differing from the active vitamin D or analogs. They lower the threshold for receptor activation by extracellular calcium ions and suppress PTH secretion. Unlike vitamin D products, calcimimetics reduce plasma PTH with either no change or a decrease in serum calcium and phosphate levels. Cinacalcet HCl (Sensipar™) has been shown to be effective in lowering PTH, even in patients who have been unresponsive to vitamin D due to gland hyperplasia. The action of cinacalcet is rapid with peak reduction of PTH levels in 2–6 hours after administration. The drug is taken orally and is generally well tolerated [90–93]. The current IV calcimimetic (etelcalcetide/Parsabiv™) is indicated for those being treated with in-center hemodialysis and is administered at the end of treatment to avoid loss to dialysate. Staff administration has the potential to minimize issues with non-adherence to the oral form [93]. Phase III trials also show that IV calcimimetics extend the duration of action with steady state being reached in 7–8 weeks versus 7 days for the oral calcimimetic [93]. Both of these calcimimetics directly target the CaSR, but the IV form binds directly to the extracellular domain of the calcium-sensing receptor, a different site than the oral calcimimetic. Thus, they are not the same and cannot be used together [94]. There must be at least a 7-day interval after stopping oral calcimimetics before starting IV to avoid compounding the hypocalcemic effects. The longer half-life of the IV formulation allows it to be dosed three times per week rather than the daily dosing of oral calcimimetics [Parsabiv™ Package Insert].

With the potential decrease in serum calcium, it is important for patients to have normal serum calcium levels before starting any calcimimetic therapy. Patient response to calcimimetics is varied, and biochemical markers must be measured routinely: calcium and phosphate within 1 week and PTH within 1–4 weeks after initiation or dose adjustment. The initial dose of cinacalcet is 30 mg/day with titration every 4 weeks up to a maximum dose of 180 mg/day. The initial dose of etelcalcetide is 5 mg, 3 times per week with a maximum dose of 15 mg three times per week. Cinacalcet and etelcalcetide can be used in conjunction with phosphate binders and vitamin D products to maximize treatment of CKD-MBD. Both oral and IV calcimimetics combined with low-dose vitamin D were more effective in lowering PTH than vitamin D analogs alone [94–97].

Alternative Dialysis Therapies

More frequent hemodialysis sessions and longer session lengths may offer improved phosphate control and potentially improvements in bone and mineral status. An analysis of the Frequent Hemodialysis Network (FHN) Daily and Nocturnal Trials examined the effects of treatment assignment on predialysis serum phosphate and on prescribed dose of phosphate binder [98]. While frequent hemodialysis did not have major effects on calcium or PTH, these trials showed that frequent hemodialysis helps control serum phosphate, and extended session lengths may allow more liberal diets and freedom from phosphate binders. Of the therapies offered, more frequent, long nocturnal dialysis had the most profound effect and eventually required more than 40% of patients to have phosphate added to the dialysate to maintain normal serum phosphate levels [98].

Phosphate removal on dialysis depends on the serum phosphate concentration at the beginning of treatment, the ultrafiltration rate, the dialyzer capabilities, as well as the frequency and duration of dialysis. Most phosphate clearance takes place early in the treatment and is followed by a slow equilibrium from the intracellular compartment. While phosphate removal continues throughout the treatment, it is removed more slowly as serum concentrations decline [81]. Patients who are unable to control serum phosphate with a conventional dialysis schedule may benefit from one or more extra days of dialysis [81]. While phosphate clearance is better with more frequent dialysis, phosphate binder doses may not change since many of these patients eat more heartily [98].

Patient Education

Patient education is a vital part of the long-term management of CKD-MBD. Adherence to treatment regimens depends partially on the patient's understanding of the treatment advice and potential consequences of non-adherence. While the ultimate choice of following the advice of the healthcare team resides with the patient, the clinical team must provide information at the level the patient can understand, utilizing a common message and varied teaching techniques including patient engagement techniques.

Parathyroidectomy (PTX)

PTX, subtotal or total, is an option for those patients who do not respond to medical or pharmacologic management of SHPT [1, 2] and those for whom surgery is deemed best. Postsurgical management of the patient is critical [99, 100]. With the sudden reduction in plasma PTH after surgery, flux of calcium and phosphate into the bone can be remarkable. This condition is referred to as "hungry bone syndrome," which results in significant hypocalcemia that requires close monitoring and often IV calcium and vitamin D administration [99, 100].

Treatment Options for Adynamic Bone

Patients with adynamic bone have an increased risk for fracture [2, 6], hypercalcemia, and extraskeletal calcifications. In dialysis patients with biopsy-documented adynamic bone or iPTH levels below 100 pg/mL, bone turnover can be stimulated by allowing the iPTH to rise. This may be accomplished by decreasing the total calcium load and serum calcium, and/or by reducing or discontinuing agents that suppress PTH synthesis and secretion [35–37]. The off-label use of teriparatide (PTH1-34) has been reported to improve static and dynamic bone parameters of bone formation in case reports and pilot studies, but needs further research with larger populations to confirm its value for routine practice [101].

Conclusion

Whether treating biopsy-documented RO or CKD-MBD, identified by abnormal biomarkers, bone and mineral abnormalities, or extraskeletal calcifications, the issues are extremely complex. There have been significant advances in the understanding of bone and mineral abnormalities in CKD patients, including the significant potential for increasing morbidity and mortality. Additionally, techniques for monitoring and treating these abnormalities continue to evolve. Improving patient outcomes requires early identification of abnormalities and appropriate utilization of all the therapeutic options– nutritional, pharmacologic, and dialytic – to minimize the progression and complications of CKD-MBD. Furthermore, successful management of bone and mineral abnormalities in CKD requires the full commitment and participation from the entire healthcare team, including the patient.

Case Study

The patient is a 55-year-old male who has been on dialysis for 3 years in a US outpatient center. He has had a slow decline in urine output, and a recent collection shows that the output is now insignificant. He has been adherent to his in-center hemodialysis prescription and medication regimens. His bone and mineral parameters have been well controlled as shown in Table 23.7, with the following medications: sevelamer carbonate 800 3 per meal and 2.5 µg oral doxercalciferol per day.

Table 23.7 History of biochemical parameters for the case patient

Date	Calcium mg/dL	Phosphorus mg/dL	Alkaline phosphatase U/L	iPTH pg/mL
7/1/2018	8.8 (2.2 mmol/L)	4.5 (1.45 mmol/L)	92 (1.53 µkat/L)	215 (22.7 pmol/L)
10/4/2018	9.0 (2.3 mmol/L)	4.6 (1.48 mmol/L)	89 (1.48)	206 (21.8)
1/7/2019	8.9 (2.2 mmol/L)	4.8 (1.54 mmol/L)	102 (1.7)	243 (25.7)
4/5/2019	8.4 (2.1 mmol/L)	5.5 (1.77 mmol/L)	120 (2.0)	310 (32.9)
Recent				
7/12/2019	8.5 (2.1 mmol/L)	6.5 (2.1 mmol/L)	130 (2.2)	520 (55.7)

Abbreviation: *iPTH* intact parathyroid hormone

Case Question and Answer

1. Considering KDIGO recommendations (assuming no financial limits) and based on his most recent biochemical parameters, what action(s) would you take (USA)?
   Answer
   Action 1: Evaluate phosphate intake, evaluate adherence and tolerance of current binder prescription, change and/or increase binders if appropriate.
   Action 2: Start cinacalcet at 30 mg/day.
   Action 3: Reduce oral doxercalciferol to 1 µgper day.
   Key
   1. Based on 2017 KDIGO guidelines, the most appropriate actions are 1 and 2. His serum phosphate is increasing, possibly from dietary intake and loss of urinary phosphate clearance. His phosphate intake should be evaluated, and he should be counseled to eliminate significant sources of phosphate while maintaining other recommended nutrient levels. Binder therapy can be assessed and modified for better phosphorus control.
   2. The iPTH has had a significant change even though it does not exceed either extreme limit (high or low). KDIGO strongly suggests using PTH trends and treating to AVOID the extremes. Some misinterpretation of the PTH recommendations led clinicians to wait until the patient exceeded the iPTH extremes before initiating or changing treatment. The increasing alkaline phosphatase in alignment with increasing PTH in this case suggests increased bone turnover. Thus, additional suppression of iPTH is warranted to avoid the upper extreme level. Additionally, the 2017 guidelines list calcimimetics along with calcitriol and vitamin D analogs as a first-line therapy. It is recognized that calcitriol and vitamin D analogs may increase absorption of phosphate and raise serum levels. Calcimimetics suppress PTH while also lowering serum phosphate and calcium. Since his blood calcium level is above the lab lower limit, it is acceptable to start calcimimetics and monitor serum calcium and phosphate levels (at 1 week and with any dose change). Manufacturers' information warns against starting calcimimetics if the blood calcium is below the lower limit of normal and stopping the drug if blood calcium levels drop below 7.5 mg/dL. The package inset (PI) also provides measures to increase the serum calcium with a significant drop or any hypocalcemic symptoms. The KDIGO guidelines suggest that mild and asymptomatic hypocalcemia in the context of calcimimetic treatment can be tolerated to avoid inappropriate calcium loading in adults. Reducing or holding the calcimimetic will typically allow serum calcium levels to move back to an acceptable range [12].
   3. Some might recommend decreasing the doxercalciferol dose to limit phosphate absorption; however, there is a known drop in blood calcium levels with calcimimetics, thus it would be acceptable to wait for the weekly calcium level after the initiation calcimimetics before decreasing the dose of the vitamin D analog.

4. If the patient is nonadherent, not responding, or develops side effects that limit his ability to take a sufficient oral dose, he should switch to an IV calcimimetic (etelcalcetide) since he is being treated in-center on hemodialysis where it can be administered by the hemodialysis staff during or after rinse-back.

5. It is important to note that countries or regions outside the USA have differing formularies, drug availability, and financial resources that limit or prevent the use of calcimimetics and certain phosphate binders. Calcimimetics are also not indicated for children. In those cases, it would be important to (1) evaluate and modify dietary intake to eliminate high phosphate foods and additives; (2) increase phosphate-lowering medications to control serum phosphate while attempting to increase active vitamin D or analogs to suppress PTH. A significant contribution to high serum phosphate is the release of phosphate from the bone, stimulated by the high PTH. It may be difficult or impossible to control serum phosphate if the high PTH is not addressed.

References

1. National Kidney Foundation. KDOQI clinical practice guidelines for bone metabolism and disease in chronic kidney disease. Am J Kidney Dis. 2003;42(Suppl 3):S1–202.
2. Kidney disease: improving global outcomes (KDIGO) CKD–MBD work group. KDIGO clinical practice guideline for the diagnosis, evaluation, prevention, and treatment of chronic kidney disease–mineral and bone disorder (CKD–MBD). Kidney Int. 2009;76(Suppl 113):S1–130.
3. Uhlig K, Berns JS, Kestenbaum B, Kumar R, Leonard MB, Martin KJ, et al. KDOQI US commentary on the 2009 KDIGO clinical practice guideline for the diagnosis, evaluation, and treatment of CKD-MBD. Am J Kidney Dis. 2010;55(5):773–99.
4. Manns BJ, Hodsman A, Zimmerman DL, Mendelssohn DC, Soroka SD, Chan C, et al. Canadian Society of Nephrology commentary on the 2009 KDIGO clinical practice guideline for the diagnosis, evaluation, and treatment of CKD-mineral and bone disorder (CKD-MBD). Am J Kidney Dis. 2010;55(5):800–12.
5. Goldsmith DJA, Covic A, Fouque D, Locatelli F, Olgaard K, Rodriquez M, et al. Editorial review: endorsement of the kidney disease improving global outcomes (KDIGO) chronic kidney disease–mineral and Bone disorder (CKD-MBD) guidelines: a European Renal Best Practice (ERBP) commentary statement. Nephrol Dial Transplant. 2010;10:1093.
6. Block GA, Klassen PS, Lazarus JM, Ofsthun N, Lowrie E, Chertow GM. Mineral metabolism, mortality, and morbidity in maintenance hemodialysis. J Am Soc Nephrol. 2004;15:2208–18.
7. Young EW, Akia T, Albert J, McCarthy J, Kerr PG, Mendelssohn DC, et al. Magnitude and impact of abnormal mineral metabolism in hemodialysis patients on Dialysis Outcomes and Practice Patterns Study (DOPPS). Am J Kidney Dis. 2004;44:S34–8.
8. Gutierrez OM. Fibroblast growth factor 23 and disordered vitamin D metabolism in chronic kidney disease: updating the "trade-off" hypothesis. Clin J Am Soc Nephrol. 2010;5(9):1710–6.
9. Moe S, Drueke T, Cunningham J, Goodman W, Martin K, Olgaard K, et al. Definition, evaluation, and classification of renal osteodystrophy: a position statement from Kidney disease: Improving Global Outcomes (KDIGO). Kidney Int. 2006;69:1945–53.
10. Olgaard K, editor. Clinical guide to bone and mineral metabolism in CKD. New York: National Kidney Foundation; 2006.
11. Ketteler M, Elder GJ, Evenepoel P, Ix JH, Jamal SA, Lafage-Proust MH, et al. Revisiting KDIGO clinical practice guideline on chronic kidney disease-mineral and bone disorder: a commentary from a Kidney Disease: Improving Global Outcomes controversies conference. Kidney Int. 2015;87(3):502–28. https://doi.org/10.1038/ki.2014.425.
12. Kidney disease: improving global outcomes (KDIGO) CKD-MBD update work group. KDIGO 2017 clinical practice guideline update for the diagnosis, evaluation, prevention, and treatment of chronic kidney disease-mineral bone disorder (CKD-MBD) Kidney Int Suppl. 2017;7:1–59.
13. Isakova T, Nickolas TL, Denburg M, Yarlagadda S, Weiner DE, Gutiérrez OM, et al. KDOQI US commentary on the 2017 KDIGO clinical practice guideline update for the diagnosis, evaluation, prevention, and treatment of chronic kidney disease–mineral and bone disorder (CKD-MBD). Am J Kidney Dis. 2017;70(6):737–51.
14. Llach F, Yudd M. Pathogenic, clinical, and therapeutic aspects of secondary hyperparathyroidism. Am J Kidney Dis. 1998;32(Suppl 2):S3–12.

15. Malluche H, Faugere D. Hyperphosphatemia: pharmacologic intervention yesterday, today, and tomorrow. Clin Nephrol. 2000;54(4):309–17.

16. Kurosu H, Ogawa Y, Miyoshi M, Yamamoto M, Nandi A, Rosenblatt KP, et al. Regulation of fibroblast growth factor-23 signaling by Klotho. J Biol Chem. 2006;281:6120–3.

17. Jüppner H. Phosphate and FGF23. Kidney Int. 2011;79(Suppl 121):S24–7.

18. Burnett SM, Gunawardene SC, Bringhurst FR, Jüppner H, Lee H, Finkelstein JS. Regulation of C-terminal and intact FGF23 by dietary phosphate in men and women. J Bone Miner Res. 2006;21(8):1187–96.

19. Isakova T, Gutierrez OM, Wolf M. A blueprint for randomized trials targeting phosphate metabolism in chronic kidney disease. Kidney Int. 2009;76(7):705–16.

20. Isakova T, Xie H, Yang W, Xie D, Anderson AH, Scialla J, et al. Chronic renal insufficiency cohort (CRIC) study group. Fibroblast growth factor 23 and risks of mortality and end-stage renal disease in patients with chronic kidney disease. JAMA. 2011;305(23):2432–9.

21. Bacchetta J, Fouque D. FGF23 and Klotho. 2011. https://www.researchgate.net/publication/267845497_FGF23_and_Klotho.

22. Bergwitz C, Jüppner H. Regulation of phosphate homeostasis by PTH, vitamin D, and FGF23. Annu Rev Med. 2010;61:91–104.

23. Razzaque MS. Klotho and Na$^+$, K$^+$-ATPase activity: solving the calcium metabolism dilemma. Nephrol Dial Transplant. 2008;23:459–61.

24. Silver J, Levi R. Cellular and molecular mechanisms of secondary hyperparathyroidism. Clin Nephrol. 2005;63(2):119–26.

25. Slatopolsky E, Finch J, Denda M, Ritter C, Zhong M, Dusso A, et al. Phosphate restriction prevents parathyroid gland growth. High phosphate directly stimulates PTH secretion in vitro. J Clin Invest. 1996;97(11):2534–40.

26. Drueke T, Martin D, Rodriguez M. Can calcimimetics inhibit parathyroid hyperplasia? Evidence from preclinical studies. Nephrol Dial Transplant. 2007;22(7):1828–39. https://doi.org/10.1093/ndt/gfm177.

27. Ballinger AE, Palmer SC, Nistor I, Craig JC, Strippoli GFM. Calcimimetics for secondary hyperparathyroidism in chronic kidney disease patients. Cochrane Database Syst Rev. 2014;(12). Art. No.: CD006254. https://doi.org/10.1002/14651858.CD006254.pub2.

28. Malluche HH, Mawad H, Monier-Faugere M-C. Effects of treatment of renal osteodystrophy on bone histology. Clin J Am Soc Nephrol. 2008;3(Suppl 3):S157–63.

29. Sutton AL, Cameron EC. Renal osteodystrophy: pathophysiology. Semin Nephrol. 1992;12(2):91–100.

30. Slatopolsky E, Brown A, Dusso A. Calcium, phosphate, and vitamin D disorders in uremia. Contrib Nephrol. 2005;149:261–71.

31. Coburn JW, Koeppel MH, Brickman AS, Massry SG. Study of intestinal absorption of calcium in patients with renal failure. Kidney Int. 1973;3:264–72.

32. Rodriguez M, Martin-Malo A, Martinez ME, Torres A, Felsenfeld AJ, Llach F. Calcemic response to parathyroid hormone in renal failure: role of and its effect on calcitriol. Kidney Int. 1991;40:1055–62.

33. Massry SG, Stein R, Garty J, Arieff AI, Coburn JW, Norman AW, et al. Skeletal resistance to the calcemic action of parathyroid hormone in uremia: role of 1,25 (OH)$_2$ D$_3$. Kidney Int. 1976;9:467–74.

34. Hoyland JA, Picton ML. Cellular mechanisms of renal osteodystrophy. Kidney Int Suppl. 1999;73:S8–13.

35. Couttenye MM, D'Haese PC, Verschoren WJ, Behets GJ, Schrooten I, De Broe ME. Low bone turnover in patients with renal failure. Kidney Int Suppl. 1999;73:S70–6.

36. Salusky IB, Goodman WG. Adynamic renal osteodystrophy: is there a problem? J Am Soc Nephrol. 2001;12:1978–85.

37. Coen G. Adynamic bone disease: an update and overview. J Nephrol. 2005;18(2):117–22.

38. Sanchez C, Auziliadora BM, Selgas R, Mate A, Millán I, Eugenia Martínez M, et al. Parathormone secretion in peritoneal dialysis patients with adynamic bone disease. Am J Kidney Dis. 2000;36(5):953–61.

39. Gupta A, Kallenback LR, Zasuwa G, Devine GW. Race is a major determinant of secondary hyperparathyroidism in uremic patients. J Am Soc Nephrol. 2000;11(2):330–4.

40. Galassi A, Spiegel DM, Bellasi A, Block GA, Raggi P. Accelerated vascular calcification and relative hypoparathyroidism in incident hemodialysis diabetic patients receiving calcium binders. Nephrol Dial Transplant. 2006;21(11):3215–22.

41. Goodman WG, Goldin J, Kuizon BD, Yoon C, Gales B, Sider D, et al. Coronary artery calcification in young adults with end stage renal disease who are undergoing hemodialysis. N Engl J Med. 2000;342:1478–83.

42. Guérin AP, London GM, Marchais SJ, Metivier F. Arterial stiffening and vascular calcifications in end stage renal disease. Nephrol Dial Transplant. 2000;15:1014–21.

43. Blacher J, Guérin AP, Pannier B, Marchais SJ, London GM. Arterial calcification, arterial stiffness, and cardiovascular risk in end stage renal disease. Hypertension. 2001;38:938–42.

44. Desjardins L, Liabeuf S, Renard C, Lenglet A, Lemke HD, Choukroun G, et al. FGF23 is independently associated with vascular calcification but not bone mineral density in patients at various CKD stages. Osteoporos Int. 2012;23(7):2017–25.

45. Memon F, El-Abbadi M, Nakatani T, Taguchi T, Lanske B, Razzaque MS. Does FGF23-klotho activity influence vascular and soft tissue calcification through regulating phosphate homeostasis? Kidney Int. 2008;74(5): 566–70.

46. Mazhar AR, Johnson RJ, Gillen D, Stivelman JC, Ryan MJ, Davis CL, et al. Risk factors and mortality associated with calciphylaxis in end stage renal disease. Kidney Int. 2001;60:324–32.

47. Ahmed S, O'Neill KD, Hood AF. Calciphylaxis is associated with hyperphosphatemia and increased osteopontin expression by vascular smooth muscle cells. Am J Kidney Dis. 2001;37(6):1267–76.

48. Rogers NM, Teubner DJ, Coates PT. Calcemic uremic arteriolopathy: advances in pathogenesis and treatment. Semin Dial. 2007;20(2):150–7.

49. Fine A, Zacharias J. Calciphylaxis is usually non-ulcerating: risk factors, outcome, and therapy. Kidney Int. 2002;61:2210–7.

50. Kuchle C, Fricke H, Held E, Schiffl H. High-flux hemodialysis postpones clinical manifestation of dialysis related amyloidosis. Am J Nephrol. 1996;16(6):484–8.

51. Ayli M, Ayli D, Azak A, Yuksel C, Atilgan G, Dede F, Akalin T, Abayli E, Camlibel M. The effect of high-flux hemodialysis on dialysis-associated amyloidosis. Ren Fail. 2005;27(1):31–4.

52. Yamamoto S, Kazama JJ, Narita I, Naiki H, Gejyo F. Recent progress in understanding dialysis-related amyloidosis. Bone. 2009;45(Suppl 1):S39–42.

53. Moe SM, Drüeke TB. Controversies in bone and mineral metabolism in CKD. A bridge to improving healthcare outcomes and quality of life. Am J Kidney Dis. 2004;43(3):552–7.

54. Miller PD. Treatment of osteoporosis in chronic kidney disease and end-stage renal disease. Curr Osteoporos Rep. 2005;3(1):5–12.

55. Toffaletti JG. Calcium: is ionized calcium always right and total calcium always wrong? Clin Lab News. 2011;37(9):8–10.

56. Ross AC, Taylor CL, Yaktine AL, Del Valle HB, editors; Committee to Review Dietary Reference Intakes for Vitamin D and Calcium; Institute of Medicine; Dietary reference intakes for calcium and vitamin D. The National Academies Press, Washington, DC; 2011.

57. Block GA, Wheeler DC, Persky MS, Kestenbaum B, Ketteler M, Spiegel DM, et al. Effects of phosphate binders in moderate CKD. J Am Soc Nephrol. 2012;23:1407–15.

58. Hill KM, Martin BR, Wastney ME, McCabe GP, Moe SM, Weaver CM, et al. Oral calcium carbonate affects calcium but not phosphorus balance in stage 3–4 chronic kidney disease. Kidney Int. 2013;83:959–66.

59. Biruete M, Hill Gallant KM, Lindemann SR, Wiese GN, Chen NX, Moe SM. Phosphate binders and nonphosphate effects in the gastrointestinal tract. J Ren Nutr. 2020;30:4–10.

60. Martin KJ, González EA. Prevention and control of phosphate retention/hyperphosphatemia in CKD-MBD: what is normal, when to start, and how to treat? Clin J Am Soc Nephrol. 2011;6(2):440–6.

61. Qi Q, Monier-Faugere MC, Geng Z, Malluche HH. Predictive value of serum parathyroid hormone levels for bone turnover in patients on chronic maintenance dialysis. Am J Kidney Dis. 1995;26(4):622–31.

62. Martin KJ, Hruska KA, Lewis J, Anderson C, Slatopolsky E. The renal handling of parathyroid hormone. Role of peritubular uptake and glomerular filtration. J Clin Invest. 1977;60:808–14.

63. Martin KJ, Akhtar I, Gonzalez EA. Parathyroid hormone: new assays, new receptors. Semin Nephrol. 2004;24:3–9.

64. Goodman WG, Salusky IS, Jüppner H. New lessons from old assays: parathyroid hormone (PTH), its receptors, and the potential biological relevance of PTH fragments. Nephrol Dial Transplant. 2002;17(10):1731–6.

65. Joly D, Drueke TB, Alberti C, Houillier P, Lawson-Body E, Martin KJ, et al. Variation in serum and plasma PTH levels in second-generation assays in hemodialysis patients: a cross-sectional study. Am J Kidney Dis. 2008;51(6):987–95.

66. Canavese C, Barolo S, Gurioli L, Cadario A, Portigliatti M, Isaia G, et al. Correlations between bone histopathology and serum biochemistry in uremic patients on chronic hemodialysis. Int J Artif Organs. 1998;21:443–50.

67. Moe SM, Drueke T. Improving global outcomes in mineral and bone disorders. Clin J Am Soc Nephrol. 2008;3(Suppl 3):S127–30.

68. Uribarri J. Phosphorus homeostasis in normal health and in chronic kidney disease patients with special emphasis on dietary phosphorus intake. Semin Dial. 2007;20(4):295–301.

69. Sullivan CM, Leon JB, Sehgal AR. Phosphorus-containing food additives and the accuracy of nutrient databases: implications for renal patients. J Ren Nutr. 2007;17(5):350–4.

70. Carnovale E, Lugaro E, Lombardi-Boccia G. Phytic acid in faba bean and pea: effect on protein availability. Cereal Chem. 1988;65(2):114–7.

71. Vikas Kumar V, Sinha AK, Hariner PS, Becker K. Dietary roles of phytate and phytase in human nutrition: a review. Food Chem. 2010;120(4):945–59.

72. Kalantar-Zadeh K, Gutekunst L, Mehrotra R, Kovesdy CP, Bross R, Shinaberger CS, et al. Understanding sources of dietary phosphorus in the treatment of patients with chronic kidney disease. Clin J Am Soc Nephrol. 2010;5(3):519–30.

73. Moe SM, Zidehsarai MP, Chambers MA, Jackman LA, Radcliffe JS, Trevino LL, et al. Vegetarian compared with meat dietary protein source and phosphorus homeostasis in chronic kidney disease. Clin J Am Soc Nephrol. 2011;6(2):257–64.

74. Oenning LL, Vogel J, Calvo MS. Accuracy of methods estimating calcium and phosphorus intake in daily diets. J Am Diet Assoc. 1988;88(9):1076–80.

75. Zhang ZW, Shimbo S, Miyake K, Watanabe T, Nakatsuka H, Matsuda-Inoguchi N, et al. Estimates of mineral intakes using food composition tables vs measures by inductively-coupled plasma mass spectrometry: part 1. Calcium, phosphorus and iron. Eur J Clin Nutr. 1999;53(3):226–32.

76. Moreno-Torres R, Ruiz-Lopez MD, Artacho R, Oliva P, Baena F, Baro L, et al. Dietary intake of calcium, magnesium and phosphorus in an elderly population using duplicate diet sampling vs food composition tables. J Nutr Health Aging. 2001;5(4):253–5.

77. US National Academy of Sciences, Institute of Medicine, Food and Nutrition Board. Dietary reference intakes for calcium, phosphorus, magnesium, vitamin D, and fluoride. 1997. https://www.nal.usda.gov/sites/default/files/fnic_uploads/calcium_full_doc.pdf. Accessed May 10, 2020.

78. Langman CB, Cannata-Andia JB. Calcium in chronic kidney disease: myths and realities. Clin J Am Soc Nephrol. 2010;5(Suppl 1):S1–2.

79. Moe SM. Confusion on the complexity of calcium balance. Semin Dial. 2010;23(5):492–7.

80. Goodman WG. Medical management of secondary hyperparathyroidism in chronic renal failure. Nephrol Dial Transplant. 2003;18(3):iii2–8.

81. Gutzwiller JP, Schneditz D, Huber AR, Schindler C, Gutzwiller F, Zehnder CE. Estimating phosphate removal in haemodialysis: an additional tool to quantify dialysis dose. Nephrol Dial Transplant. 2002;17:1037–44.

82. Malberti F, Ravani P. The choice of dialysate calcium concentration in the management of patients on haemodialysis and haemodiafiltration. Nephrol Dial Transplant. 2003;18(Suppl 7):vii37–40.

83. Brown AJ. Vitamin D analogues. Am J Kidney Dis. 1998;32(4 Suppl 2):S25–39.

84. Llach F, Keshav G, Goldblat MV, Lindberg JS, Sadler R, Delmez J, et al. Suppression of parathyroid hormone secretion in hemodialysis patients by a novel vitamin D analog: 19-Nor-1,25-dihydroxyvitamin D_2. Am J Kidney Dis. 1998;32(4 Suppl 2):S48–54.

85. Teng M, Wolf M, Lowrie E, Ofsthun N, Lazarus JM, Thadhani R. Survival of patients undergoing hemodialysis with paricalcitol or calcitriol therapy. N Engl J Med. 2003;349:446–56.

86. Frazzo JM, Elangovan L, Maung HM, Chesney RW, Acchiardo SR, Bower JD, et al. Intermittent doxercalciferol (1α hydroxyvitamin D2) therapy for secondary hyperparathyroidism. Am J Kidney Dis. 2000;36:550–61.

87. Morii H, Ishimura E, Inoue T, Tabata T, Morita A, Nishii Y, et al. History of vitamin D treatment of renal osteodystrophy. Am J Nephrol. 1997;17:382–6.

88. Kandula P, Dobre M, Schold JD, Schreiber MJ Jr, Mehrotra R, Navaneethan SD. Vitamin D supplementation in chronic kidney disease: a systematic review and meta-analysis of observational studies and randomized controlled trials. Clin J Am Soc Nephrol. 2011;6(1):50–62.

89. Monk RD, Bushinsky DA. Making sense of the latest advice on vitamin D therapy. J Am Soc Nephrol. 2011;22:994–8.

90. Block GA, Martin KJ, de Francisco ALM, Turner SA, Avram MM, Suranyi MG, et al. Cinacalcet for secondary hyperparathyroidism in patients receiving hemodialysis. N Engl J Med. 2004;350:1516–25.

91. Nemeth EF, Heaton WH, Miller M, Fox J, Balandrin MF, Van Wagenen BC, et al. Pharmacodynamics of type II calcimimetic compound cinacalcet HCL. J Pharmacol Exp Ther. 2004;308:627–35.

92. Goodman WG. Calcimimetics: a remedy for all problems of excess parathyroid hormone activity in chronic kidney disease? Curr Opin Nephrol Hypertens. 2005;14(4):355–60.

93. Block GA, Bushinsky DA, Cunningham J, Drueke TB, Ketteler M, Kewalramani R, et al. Effect of etelcalcetide vs. placebo on serum parathyroid hormone in patients receiving hemodialysis with secondary hyperparathyroidism: two randomized clinical trials. JAMA. 2017;317:146–55.

94. Block GA, Bushinsky DA, Cheng S, Cunningham J, Dehmel B, Drueke TB, et al. Effect of etelcalcetide vs cinacalcet on serum parathyroid hormone in patients receiving hemodialysis with secondary hyperparathyroidism: a randomized trial. JAMA. 2017;317:156–64.

95. Messa P, Macário F, Yaqoob M, Bouman K, Braun J, von Albertini B, et al. The OPTIMA study: assessing a new cinacalcet (Sensipar/Mimpara) treatment algorithm for secondary hyperparathyroidism. Clin J Am Soc Nephrol. 2008;3(1):36–45.

96. Fishbane S, Shapiro WB, Corry DB, Vicks SL, Roppolo M, Rappaport K, et al. Cinacalcet HCl and concurrent low-dose vitamin D improves treatment of secondary hyperparathyroidism in dialysis patients compared with vitamin D alone: the ACHIEVE study results. Clin J Am Soc Nephrol. 2008;3(6):1718–25. https://doi.org/10.2215/CJN.01040308.

97. Pereira L, Meng C, Marques J, Frazao JM. Old and new calcimimetics for treatment of secondary hyperparathyroidism; impact on biochemical and relevant clinical outcomes. Clin Kidney J. 2018;11(1):80–8.

98. Daugirdas JT, Chertow GM, Larive B, Pierratos A, Greene T, Ayus JC, et al. Frequent Hemodialysis Network (FHN) trial group. Effects of frequent hemodialysis on measures of CKD mineral and bone disorder. J Am Soc Nephrol. 2012;23(4):727–38.
99. Mittendorf EA, Merlino JI, McHenry CR. Post-parathyroidectomy hypocalcemia: incidence, risk factors, and management. Am Surg. 2004;70(2):114–9.
100. Richards ML, Wormuth J, Bingener J, Sirinek K. Parathyroidectomy in secondary hyperparathyroidism: is there an optimal operative management? Surgery. 2006;139(2):174–80.
101. Palcu P, Dion N, St-Marie LG. Teriparatide and bone turnover and formation in a hemodialysis patient with low-turnover bone disease: a case report. Am J Kidney Dis. 2015;65(6):933–6.

Chapter 24
Nephrotic Syndrome

Shubha Ananthakrishnan, Jane Y. Yeun, and George A. Kaysen

Keywords Nephrotic syndrome · Complications · Treatment · Protein restriction · Renin-angiotensin blockade · Dietary treatment

> **Key Points**
> - Identify nephrotic syndrome, its causes, and its complications.
> - Describe the pharmacologic management of nephrotic syndrome.
> - Discuss the nutritional management of nephrotic syndrome.

Introduction

Nephrotic syndrome is defined as proteinuria >3.5 g/day for an adult, hypoalbuminemia, edema, hyperlipidemia, and lipiduria. While there is a myriad of causes, the complications result from the severity of proteinuria and the accompanying changes in plasma protein composition that occur. Complications include atherosclerosis, vascular thrombosis, anasarca, infection, nutritional depletion, and progressive kidney injury. Reducing proteinuria is critical. When specific therapy targeting the underlying etiology fails, blocking the renin-angiotensin system will reduce proteinuria, enhanced by concomitant moderate protein restriction. Plant sources of protein may offer additional benefit in reducing proteinuria and hyperlipidemia. Vitamin D, iron, and zinc deficiency may occur due to urinary loss of carrier proteins and are treated with appropriate dietary supplementation.

The editors acknowledge Kumar Dinesh's contribution to this chapter in *Nutrition in Kidney Disease, Second Edition*, Nutrition and Health, DOI 10.1007/978-1-62703-685-6_1, © Springer Science+Business Media New York 2014

S. Ananthakrishnan (✉)
Division of Nephrology, Department of Medicine, UC Davis Medical Center, Sacramento, CA, USA
e-mail: sananthakrishnan@ucdavis.edu

J. Y. Yeun
Nephrology Section, Sacramento Veterans Administration Medical Center, Mather, CA, USA

Division of Nephrology, UC Davis Health, Sacramento, CA, USA

G. A. Kaysen
Department of Medicine, Division of Nephrology, Genome University of California, Davis, and Biomedical Sciences Facility, Davis, CA, USA

© Springer Nature Switzerland AG 2020
J. D. Burrowes et al. (eds.), *Nutrition in Kidney Disease*, Nutrition and Health,
https://doi.org/10.1007/978-3-030-44858-5_24

Definition of Nephrotic Syndrome

Nephrotic syndrome results from excessive urinary losses of albumin and other plasma proteins of similar mass and is characterized by edema, hyperlipidemia, and hypoalbuminemia (Table 24.1) [1, 2]. At least 3.5 grams of protein per 1.73 m^2 of body surface area must be present in a 24-hour urine collection to make the diagnosis, although most patients have, on average, 6–8 grams of proteinuria a day. Over 80% of the urinary protein is albumin, reflecting plasma protein composition. The remainder of the urinary protein is comprised of other plasma proteins such as immunoglobulins, binding proteins, complements, and coagulation factors [2].

Causes of Nephrotic Syndrome

A wide range of glomerular diseases can cause nephrotic syndrome and may be primary (idiopathic) in nature, genetically inherited, or secondary to a systemic disease or medication [1–3]. Primary or idiopathic glomerular diseases that result in nephrotic syndrome include minimal change disease (MCD), membranous nephropathy, and focal segmental glomerulosclerosis (FSGS) (Table 24.2) [1–3]. The incidence of FSGS has been rising likely because it is the common final pathway for a variety of insults to the glomeruli, while that of membranous nephropathy is waning [1, 2]. The diagnosis is made on the basis of the histologic appearance of the kidney tissue. Recent studies have also identified several gene mutations that result in glomerular injury and nephrotic syndrome, manifesting histologically as minimal change disease, FSGS, and membranous nephropathy [4, 5]. The majority of these genes encode podocyte and slit diaphragm proteins, which are critical to the integrity of the glomerular filtration barrier.

Systemic diseases or medications also can cause nephrotic syndrome (see Table 24.2). Of these causes, diabetic nephropathy is the most common. Certain connective tissue diseases, infections, chronic inflammatory states, malignancies, drugs, and plasma cell dyscrasias can also give rise to

Table 24.1 Manifestations of nephrotic syndrome

≥3.5 grams proteinuria/1.73 m^2/day
Hypoalbuminemia
Edema
Hyperlipidemia
Lipiduria
Hypercoagulability

Table 24.2 Causes of nephrotic syndrome

Primary or idiopathic	Secondary to systemic diseases	
Membranous nephropathy (30%–35%)	Diabetes mellitus	Infections
Focal segmental glomerulosclerosis (FSGS) (30%–35%)	Connective tissue disease	HIV
Minimal change disease (15%)	Systemic lupus erythematosus	Hepatitis B
IgA nephropathy (5%–10%)	Amyloidosis	Hepatitis C
Membranoproliferative glomerulonephritis (5%–10%)	Dysproteinemias	Syphilis
Other (2%–5%)	Multiple myeloma	Malaria
	Other light-chain-mediated disease	Drugs
	Other malignancy (not exhaustive)	NSAID
	Adenocarcinomas	Interferon
	Lymphoma	Pamidronate

nephrotic syndrome [1–3]. Diagnosis is made on the basis of a thorough history, careful physical examination, and selected tests guided by the history and examination. A kidney biopsy is sometimes required for further classification as in the case of lupus nephritis or to exclude other types of glomerular diseases, especially when hematuria is prominent [3]. Whatever the underlying cause, injury to the podocyte is what ultimately alters the permselective properties of the glomerular barrier and results in massive urinary protein loss [4–6].

Complications of Nephrotic Syndrome

Regardless of the etiology of nephrotic syndrome, the clinical sequelae are identical (Table 24.3). All of the adverse effects discussed below result directly or indirectly (through decreased levels of albumin or of other specific plasma proteins, and/or oncotic pressure) from urinary protein losses [1–3]. Therefore, management of nephrotic patients targets reduction of proteinuria to modify the complications of nephrotic syndrome.

Sodium Retention (Edema)

Edema is a common clinical manifestation in nephrotic syndrome and occurs because of accumulation of fluid in the interstitial space. Two mechanisms are thought to be responsible for the edema [7–9]: (1) avid renal sodium retention, resulting in "overfilling" of the vascular space and

Table 24.3 Systemic complications and clinical sequelae of nephrotic syndrome

Complication	Mechanism	Clinical Sequelae
Sodium retention	Atrial natriuretic peptide resistance ↓ Plasma oncotic pressure ↑ Urine plasmin → ENaC activation	Edema → Skin breakdown → Cellulitis Pleural effusion → Shortness of breath Ascites → Spontaneous bacterial peritonitis
Hypercoagulable state	Loss of anti-thrombin III ↓ Plasma proteins C and S ↑ Plasma fibrinogen Thrombosis ↑ Platelet aggregation	Deep venous thrombosis Pulmonary embolism Renal vein thrombosis
Infection	Loss of immunoglobulins Loss of complement	Spontaneous bacterial peritonitis Other infections with encapsulated organisms
Hyperlipidemia	Altered lipoprotein metabolism: ↑ Pro-atherogenic lipoproteins Oxidized high density lipoprotein ↑ Triglycerides	Accelerated atherosclerosis
Progressive renal injury	Iron-induced oxidative injury Lipid peroxidation Complement-mediated injury	Interstitial fibrosis Chronic kidney disease
Nutritional depletion	Loss of tissue proteins Loss of erythropoietin Loss of plasma binding proteins	Tissue proteins → Muscle wasting Anemia Transferrin → Iron deficiency anemia Thyroglobulin binding protein → Hypothyroidism Vitamin D binding protein → Hypocalcemia, rickets Zinc (bound to albumin) → Zinc deficiency

consequent edema because of increased hydrostatic pressure; (2) decrease in plasma oncotic pressure when serum albumin levels fall below 1.5–2.0 g/dL, resulting in translocation of fluid into the interstitial space because of reduced oncotic pressure [1–3, 8, 9]. Current evidence suggests that avid renal sodium retention is the most important mechanism. Plasma serine protease precursors such as plasminogen appear in nephrotic urine and undergo cleavage to activated plasmin. Plasmin, in turn, activates the epithelial sodium channels (ENaCs) in the cortical collecting tubule, enhancing sodium absorption and consequent edema [7, 8]. In addition, nephrotic kidneys are less responsive to atrial natriuretic peptide (ANP) due to reduced expression of tubular corin, an enzyme that converts pro-ANP to ANP [9]. Regardless of the mechanisms, the consequences are edema, pleural effusions, and ascites. Skin breakdown from tense edema and the presence of ascites predispose to infection.

Hypercoagulability (Thrombophilia)

Patients with nephrotic syndrome are prone to develop deep venous thrombosis, pulmonary embolism, renal vein thrombosis and, occasionally, sagittal sinus thrombosis and arterial thrombosis. The incidence of thromboembolic disease is estimated variably at 7% to 20% in patients with nephrotic syndrome, but may be as high as 50% in those with membranous nephropathy. The higher the urinary protein losses and the lower the serum albumin level, the higher is the risk of thromboembolism [10, 11]. The underlying mechanism for hypercoagulability in nephrotic syndrome is incompletely understood, but appears to derive from an imbalance in the levels of procoagulants and anticoagulants, reduced thrombolysis, and enhanced platelet numbers as well as function (see Table 24.3) [10–12]. Urinary loss of anticoagulant factors such as anti-thrombin III and proteins C and S, combined with increased liver synthesis of fibrinogen and other procoagulants, tip the balance in favor of thrombosis [10, 11]. An altered structure of the fibrin clot and urinary loss of plasminogen in nephrotic syndrome may reduce fibrinolysis, further contributing to the problem [10]. Recent data suggest that urinary loss of an inhibitory polypeptide may be responsible for the observed thrombocytosis and increased platelet adherence [12]. Finally, the glomerular endothelial cell may be contributing directly to the hypercoagulable state through increased release of thrombotic regulators, disturbed cytokine profiles, and disrupted interaction with other cells in the glomerulus [13].

Hyperlipidemia

Nephrotic syndrome is characterized by hypoalbuminemia and increased lipid levels. The mechanisms responsible for their increase are a combination of increased rate of synthesis of the associated apolipoproteins and decreased clearance [14]. Increased levels of low-density lipoproteins (LDL) result, at least in part, from increased synthesis, while increases in the levels of very low density lipoproteins (VLDL) as well as apo E are a consequence of reduced clearance. In contrast to the negative acute phase proteins, such as serum albumin and transferrin, and the positive acute phase proteins, such as fibrinogen and other associated clotting factors, the rates of synthesis of apo B associated with LDL does not appear to be statistically linked to that of serum albumin [14, 15], nor is it regulated at the level of transcription [15], suggesting a different triggering mechanism. Reduced clearance must also contribute to increased LDL levels because of the linkage to increased levels of proprotein convertase subtilisin/kexin type 9 (PCSK9) [16] providing a mixed mechanism for increased LDL levels.

PCSK9 is increased in animals with experimentally induced nephrotic syndrome and decreases in remission of proteinuria in nephrotic patients [16], consistent with a link between PCSK9 expression and proteinuria, although the linkage between the rate of transcription of albumin and PCSK9 has not been explored. At least part of the mechanism increasing PCSK9 expression is increased hepatic transcription in nephrotic syndrome [17]. As a result of the impaired uptake of LDL by the liver, enzymes that synthesize cholesterol are upregulated and enzymes that catabolize cholesterol by diverting it to bile synthesis are downregulated, further aggravating the hyperlipidemia. Increased LDL levels are not reduced significantly by the use of statins, and instead are more closely associated with serum albumin levels [18].

In contrast to LDL, triglyceride levels and reduced clearance of VLDL is not a consequence of hypoalbuminemia [14, 19], but instead appears to be a direct effect of proteinuria [14, 20]. The link between albuminuria and decreased clearance of triglyceride-rich lipoproteins is a consequence of delivery of free fatty acids bound to filtered albumin to podocytes, causing the release of angiopoietin-like 4, a strong inhibitor of lipoprotein lipase (LPL) [20, 21]. Although the observation that VLDL clearance is as defective in rats with hereditary analbuminemia as in rats with a normal albumin gene [19] suggests that albumin need not be the molecule delivering the free fatty acids to podocytes to trigger this cycle. Levels of pro-atherogenic lipoprotein Lp (a) [22] are also increased in nephrotic syndrome [23, 24]. Increased levels of Lp(a) are a consequence of increased synthesis and not decreased clearance [25–27]. While high-density lipoprotein (HDL) levels are either normal or slightly decreased, it is the small, dense, and less protective HDL particles that accumulate [23, 24]. Urinary loss of lecithin cholesterol acyl transferase (LCAT) in massive proteinuria interferes further with normal HDL maturation, resulting in reduced HDL-mediated scavenging of cholesterol [23, 24, 28].

Progressive Renal Injury

Proteinuria is not only a marker for kidney disease but it is also involved in the progression of the underlying kidney disease [29]. Studies also show that reduction in proteinuria is associated with slowing of kidney function decline [30, 31]. Prolonged and massive proteinuria leads to progressive renal injury with interstitial fibrosis and glomerular sclerosis. In heavy proteinuric states, the proximal tubule is overloaded with resorption of filtered albumin, along with protein-bound products, such as free fatty acids that can cause tubulointerstitial injury [32] and tubular cell apoptosis. Filtered plasma proteins themselves that get reabsorbed in the proximal tubular cells, as well as filtered complement components such as C3, upregulate inflammatory and profibrotic events in the kidney [33]. The sum of these events results in tubulointerstitial inflammation, fibrosis, and apoptosis.

Infection

There is an increased risk of infectious events among patients with nephrotic syndrome [34–36] and is a significant risk factor for acute kidney injury (AKI) [37]. There are a variety of predisposing factors increasing risk, including the use of immunosuppressive therapy to treat the underlying kidney disease [38, 39], as well as low serum immunoglobulin G (IgG) levels [40] resulting from the urinary loss of IgG [41], which unlike liver-derived proteins is not replaced by increased synthesis. Infection risk has been demonstrated in some cases to be reduced by immunoglobulin infusion [42]. Immunoglobulin levels are closely associated with those of albumin in patients with nephrotic syndrome [43], although the effect is partially dependent upon IgG class [44].

Nutritional Depletion

The primary cause of nephrotic syndrome is the urinary loss of a variety of serum proteins, many accompanied by bound metal ions, nutrients, and vitamins, as well as the obligate loss of protein. Since albumin makes up approximately half of the total serum protein, the majority of amino acids lost in the urine are contributed by the loss of this protein. The rate of synthesis of proteins lost in the urine –albumin, transferrin –are increased [45, 46]. Total protein synthesis is unchanged in nephrotic patients [47], so that amino acid losses must be accompanied by decreased amino acid stores elsewhere. Muscle protein synthesis is impaired in rats with nephrotic syndrome [48]. Dietary protein restriction results in a decline in urinary albumin losses [49, 50], and despite a decline in albumin synthetic rate [51, 52] and gene transcription [53], an increase in serum albumin concentration is observed in both experimental models of nephrotic syndrome in the rat [51] and in humans [52]. Urinary protein losses in nephrotic syndrome lead to muscle wasting presumably due to shunting of amino acid building blocks to the liver to enhance plasma protein synthesis, in the absence of a compensatory decrease in total body protein turnover [24, 25].

Loss of erythropoietin and binding proteins that transport iron, vitamin D, and thyroxine may result in anemia and iron deficiency [54, 55], hypocalcemia and rickets, and hypothyroidism, respectively [1, 3, 56]. Anemia management may require iron supplementation as well as administration of erythropoietin even in patients with otherwise normal renal function [57]. Nephrotic range proteinuria has been shown to result in negative zinc and copper balance in experimental animals [58]. Sustained and massive proteinuria may lead also to zinc deficiency because two-thirds of circulating zinc is bound to albumin [59] and copper depletion through the urinary loss of ceruloplasmin [60]. These trace element deficiencies can induce skin rashes [61] and may result in neutropenia and anemia [60]. Deficiency in vitamins B6 and B12 may be associated with increased levels of homocysteine and thrombosis [62].While vitamin D supplementation has been recommended to protect bone in children with nephrotic syndrome during steroid treatment [63], high doses of vitamins D, C, and A as well as a variety of plant supplements have been demonstrated to be harmful [64]. Long-term efficacy of doses even as low as 400 IU per day of vitamin D3 have been questioned [65]. The primary therapeutic efficacy of vitamin D replacement may be related to improvement in the adverse effect of steroids on bone density [66].

Patients with progressive loss of kidney function may develop metabolic acidosis, particularly when the glomerular filtration rate falls below 30 mL/min [67]. Potential adverse effects of metabolic acidosis include increased muscle catabolism, growth retardation in children, exacerbation of bone disease, impaired glucose tolerance, and reduced albumin synthesis which predisposes to hypoalbuminemia [67]. In addition, a low serum bicarbonate (<22 vs. 25–26 mEq/L) may confer an increased risk for progression of CKD [68], because compensatory mechanisms to augment ammonium production and urinary acidification through activation of aldosterone and kidney endothelin production may lead to increased urinary protein losses and interstitial fibrosis [69, 70]. Enhanced ammonium production is also thought to activate the alternative complement pathway, further aggravating inflammation and interstitial fibrosis [68–70].

Treatment of Nephrotic Syndrome

The main goal in treating nephrotic syndrome is to reduce or eliminate proteinuria to blunt or prevent the development of associated complications, to protect kidney function, and to reduce the risk for accelerated atherosclerosis. Dietary management and pharmacologic management (Table 24.4) each plays a major and complementary role in this endeavor.

Table 24.4 Treatment considerations for patients with nephrotic syndrome

Dietary		Pharmacologic/other
Calorie	35 kcal/kg/d	Remove underlying cause
Protein	0.8 g/kg/d	Start immunosuppressive drugs
	Soy protein -? more beneficial	Reduce proteinuria
Fat	< 30% of total calories	Angiotensin converting enzyme inhibitor
	Cholesterol <200 mg/d	Angiotensin receptor blocker
Minerals	Sodium <2 g/day	Nonsteroidal anti-inflammatory drugs[a]
	Iron, if clearly iron deficient	Spironolactone
	Zinc, if zinc deficient (220 mg/d)	Statin therapy for hyperlipidemia
Vitamins	Vitamin D, if deficient	Anticoagulation for hypercoagulability
		Antibiotics for infection
Fluid	Fluid restriction, if massive edema or hyponatremia	Diuretics for edema

[a]Although NSAIDs may reduce urinary protein loss, they increase the risk of loss of renal function and may increase sodium retention and blood pressure and should not be used in clinical practice to reduce urinary protein losses

Specific Treatment

If possible, treatment of nephrotic syndrome is directed at the underlying cause (see Table 24.2). In the cases of drug-induced nephrotic syndrome, the offending drug is stopped. Chemotherapy, radiation therapy, and/or surgical resection of the responsible cancer may lead to resolution of malignancy-related nephrotic syndrome. Antibiotics or antiviral drugs are used when the suspect cause of the underlying nephrotic syndrome is an infection. For idiopathic nephrotic syndrome, depending upon the presenting histology, suppressing the immune system with drugs such as steroids, cyclophosphamide, mycophenolate, rituximab, or other immunomodulating drugs may result in complete resolution of nephrotic syndrome. A full discussion of the immunosuppressive treatment of glomerular diseases is beyond the scope of this chapter.

Nonspecific Treatment

If nephrotic syndrome does not respond to removal of the offending agent or immunosuppressive therapy, then nonspecific measures are employed to reduce proteinuria.

Pharmacologic Management

Angiotensin-converting enzyme inhibitors (ACEI), angiotensin receptor blockers (ARB), cyclosporine, nonsteroidal anti-inflammatory drugs (NSAIDs), cyclooxygenase 2 (COX 2) inhibitors all help reduce glomerular capillary pressure, and, therefore, proteinuria (see Table 24.4). Combination of ACEI and ARB showed greater reduction in proteinuria than either agent alone and was previously considered safe and useful in the management of proteinuric states [71]. However, more recent studies showed increased incidence of hyperkalemia, hypotension, and acute renal failure, particularly in patients with diabetes and vascular disease on dual therapy [72, 73]. At the present time, combination of ACEI and ARB therapy is not recommended. The combination of an ACEI or an ARB with spironolactone or eplerenone, further reduces proteinuria [74, 75], but there is risk of worsening hyperkalemia. There is also uncertainty regarding long-term benefits, such as mortality and long-term renal function, with such combinations [76]. NSAIDs and COX 2 inhibitors reduce proteinuria [77, 78], but are rarely used in treating nephrotic syndrome because of the increased risk of acute renal failure and gastrointestinal bleeding, as well as their association with the risk of chronic kidney disease [79]. Of special note is that increased salt intake blunts the beneficial effect of ACE inhibition in proteinuric kidney disease. Therefore, salt restriction is also indicated in the management of these patients [80].

Statins help improve the hyperlipidemia seen in nephrotic syndrome (see Table 24.4). They are indicated if the dyslipidemia persists despite treatment of the underlying nephrotic syndrome. They may also have reno-protective effects because of their lipid-lowering and anti-inflammatory effects [81, 82].

Use of diuretics may be necessary when edema becomes symptomatic, but kidney function must be monitored carefully because of potential for precipitating acute renal failure. Patients with nephrotic syndrome often require higher doses of diuretics or combination of diuretics to achieve adequate diuresis [83]. If other complications of nephrotic syndrome develop (hypothyroidism, thromboembolic disease, infection), therapy targeted at the complication is started (see Table 24.4).

Nutritional Management

Nephrotic syndrome is characterized by the urinary loss of protein, predominantly albumin, as well as a variety of other proteins, several of which have the capacity to bind, and thus result in the urinary loss of micronutrients, in addition to the obligate amino acid loss driven by urinary protein losses. While the rate of albumin synthesis may increase in response to urinary losses accompanied by increased dietary protein intake, urinary albumin excretion increases as well [51, 84]. A high-protein diet in nephrotic syndrome will increase urinary protein excretion and lead to a decline in serum albumin concentration through its adverse effects on glomerular hemodynamics [49]. In contrast, protein restriction, especially when combined with ACEI and/or ARB therapy, will reduce proteinuria [85]. Nephrotic proteinuria has no net effect on whole body protein synthesis [47], so that the urinary losses result in negative overall protein balance. Although some studies suggest that severe protein restriction to 0.3 g/kg/day supplemented with amino acids is of additional benefit [86], most experts recommend moderate (0.7–0.8 g/kg/day) protein restriction because of concern about precipitating malnutrition [3, 29].

The type of dietary protein is also important. Recent studies suggest that chicken and fish sources of protein may be of more benefit than pork or beef [87]. Vegetarian sources of protein such as soy [88–90] and flaxseed [91] reduce proteinuria and hyperlipidemia more than animal proteins. Studies of nephrotic rats suggest that the benefit derived from soy protein is due to a direct effect on the kidneys possibly to reduce nitrotyrosine formation rather than through changes in hepatic lipid metabolism [90, 92]. Soy protein may also reduce inflammatory cytokines, further ameliorating progressive kidney injury [89]. The types of amino acids present in plant proteins may be responsible for their beneficial effects, rather than the change in dietary lipid content, because branched chain and gluconeogenic amino acids (such as arginine and glutamate) do not increase proteinuria in animal models while other amino acids do [93, 94]. Since diets that contain animal protein also are relatively high in acid, the greater acid load accompanying greater protein loads may be contributing to progressive kidney injury. Not all amino acids exert the proteinuric effect observed as a consequence of increasing dietary protein. Branch chain amino acids [93], arginine, proline, glutamate, and aspartate [94] have no effect in experimental models even when administered at 30% of total intake, while a combination of other amino acids results in an increase in urinary protein losses. Soy protein or vegetarian diets have been found to reduce urinary protein excretion in humans [95], but it is unclear whether the control diet and the vegetarian diet were isonitrogenous or whether the effect was simply that of dietary protein restriction. If the diets were isonitrogenous it may be possible to identify specific protein sources that are less injurious. In contrast, cow's milk protein has been found to be injurious in some subjects, although this may be associated with an allergic phenomenon [96].

If iron deficiency is clearly present, then cautious oral iron repletion is indicated, keeping in mind that filtered iron may exacerbate renal injury (see Table 24.4) [97]. Patients who are hypocalcemic because of vitamin D deficiency should receive oral vitamin D and calcium supplements (see Table 24.4). Other than correction of hypocalcemia, vitamin D repletion in patients with proteinuria may have beneficial effects on albuminuria [98]. Sodium and fluid restrictions will help reduce edema and hyponatremia, especially when used in conjunction with diuretics. Although lowering dietary lipids alone will not correct the observed hyperlipidemia, its effect on lipids is additive when used with statins [99]. Finally, bicarbonate supplementation to correct metabolic acidosis may delay progression of kidney failure and improve nutritional status among patients with CKD [100–102].

Conclusion

Although nephrotic syndrome may begin with severe proteinuria, it quickly becomes a multisystem disease. Despite the diverse causes of nephrotic syndrome, the common thread is massive urinary loss of proteins leading to an increased risk for cardiovascular disease, vascular thrombosis, anasarca, infection, nutritional depletion, and progressive kidney injury. Treatment is targeted at reducing proteinuria in order to prevent progressive kidney injury and to reduce associated complications. Pharmacologic and dietary management of nephrotic syndrome are complementary, with the mainstay of therapy being the use of ACEI or an ARB, alone or in combination with spironolactone, statin, and moderate protein restriction (preferably with plant or soy protein) to reduce proteinuria and hyperlipidemia, while waiting for immunosuppression to control the underlying cause.

References

1. Hull RP, Goldsmith DJ. Nephrotic syndrome in adults. BMJ. 2008;336(7654):1185–9.
2. CG SK, Marsden PA, Taal MW, ASL Y, editors. Brenner and Rector's the kidney. 10th ed. Philadelphia: Elsevier; 2016.
3. de Seigneux S, Martin PY. Management of patients with nephrotic syndrome. Swiss Med Weekly. 2009;139(29–30):416–22.
4. Sharif B, Barua M. Advances in molecular diagnosis and therapeutics in nephrotic syndrome and focal and segmental glomerulosclerosis. Curr Opin Nephrol Hypertens. 2018;27(3):194–200.
5. Couser WG. Primary membranous nephropathy. Clin J Am Soc Nephrol. 2017;12(6):983–97.
6. Mundel P, Reiser J. Proteinuria: an enzymatic disease of the podocyte? Kidney Int. 2010;77(7):571–80.
7. Teoh CW, Robinson LA, Noone D. Perspectives on edema in childhood nephrotic syndrome. Am J Physiol Renal Physiol. 2015;309(7):F575–82.
8. Siddall EC, Radhakrishnan J. The pathophysiology of edema formation in the nephrotic syndrome. Kidney Int. 2012;82(6):635–42.
9. Klein JD. Corin: an ANP protease that may regulate sodium reabsorption in nephrotic syndrome. Kidney Int. 2010;78(7):635–7.
10. Kerlin BA, Ayoob R, Smoyer WE. Epidemiology and pathophysiology of nephrotic syndrome-associated thromboembolic disease. Clin J Am SocNephrol. 2012;7(3):513–20.
11. Loscalzo J. Venous thrombosis in the nephrotic syndrome. N Engl J Med. 2013;368(10):956–8.
12. Eneman B, Freson K, van den Heuvel L, van Hoyweghen E, Collard L, Vande Walle J, et al. Pituitary adenylate cyclase-activating polypeptide deficiency associated with increased platelet count and aggregability in nephrotic syndrome. J Thromb Haemost. 2015;13(5):755–67.
13. Chen G, Liu H, Liu F. A glimpse of the glomerular milieu: from endothelial cell to thrombotic disease in nephrotic syndrome. Microvasc Res. 2013;89:1–6.
14. de Sain-van der Velden MG, Kaysen GA, Barrett HA, Stellaard F, Gadellaa MM, Voorbij HA, et al. Increased VLDL in nephrotic patients results from a decreased catabolism while increased LDL results from increased synthesis. Kidney Int. 1998;53(4):994–1001.

15. Sun X, Jones H Jr, Joles JA, van Tol A, Kaysen GA. Apolipoprotein gene expression in analbuminemic rats and in rats with Heymann nephritis. Am J Phys. 1992;262(5 Pt 2):F755–61.

16. Haas ME, Levenson AE, Sun X, Liao WH, Rutkowski JM, de Ferranti SD, et al. The role of proprotein convertase subtilisin/kexin type 9 in nephrotic syndrome-associated hypercholesterolemia. Circulation. 2016;134(1):61–72.

17. Liu S, Vaziri ND. Role of PCSK9 and IDOL in the pathogenesis of acquired LDL receptor deficiency and hyper-cholesterolemia in nephrotic syndrome. Nephrol Dial Transplant. 2014;29(3):538–43.

18. Hari P, Khandelwal P, Satpathy A, Hari S, Thergaonkar R, Lakshmy R, et al. Effect of atorvastatin on dyslipidemia and carotid intima-media thickness in children with refractory nephrotic syndrome: a randomized controlled trial. Pediatr Nephrol. 2018;33(12):2299–309.

19. Davies RW, Staprans I, Hutchison FN, Kaysen GA. Proteinuria, not altered albumin metabolism, affects hyperlip-idemia in the nephrotic rat. J Clin Invest. 1990;86(2):600–5.

20. Clement LC, Avila-Casado C, Mace C, Soria E, Bakker WW, Kersten S, et al. Podocyte-secreted angiopoietin-like-4 mediates proteinuria in glucocorticoid-sensitive nephrotic syndrome. Nat Med. 2011;17(1):117–22.

21. Mace C, Chugh SS. Nephrotic syndrome: components, connections, and angiopoietin-like 4-related therapeutics. J Am Soc Nephrol. 2014;25(11):2393–8.

22. Wanner C, Rader D, Bartens W, Krämer J, Brewer HB, Schollmeyer P, et al. Elevated plasma lipoprotein(a) in patients with the nephrotic syndrome. Ann Intern Med. 1993;119(4):263–9.

23. Vaziri ND. Molecular mechanisms of lipid disorders in nephrotic syndrome. Kidney Int. 2003;63(5):1964–76.

24. Kronenberg F. Dyslipidemia and nephrotic syndrome: recent advances. J Renal Nutr. 2005;15(2):195–203.

25. Stenvinkel P, Berglund L, Ericsson S, Alvestrand A, Angelin B, Eriksson M. Low-density lipoprotein metabolism and its association to plasma lipoprotein(a) in the nephrotic syndrome. Eur J Clin Investig. 1997;27(2):169–77.

26. De Sain-Van Der Velden MG, Reijngoud DJ, Kaysen GA, Gadellaa MM, Voorbij H, Stellaard F, et al. Evidence for increased synthesis of lipoprotein(a) in the nephrotic syndrome. J Am Soc Nephrol. 1998;9(8):1474–81.

27. Shearer GC, Kaysen GA. Proteinuria and plasma compositional changes contribute to defective lipoprotein catab-olism in the nephrotic syndrome by separate mechanisms. Am J Kidney Dis. 2001;37(1 Suppl 2):S119–22.

28. Vaziri ND, Liang K, Parks JS. Acquired lecithin-cholesterol acyltransferase deficiency in nephrotic syndrome. Am J Physiol Renal Physiol. 2001;280(5):F823–8.

29. Wilmer WA, Rovin BH, Hebert CJ, Rao SV, Kumor K, Hebert LA. Management of glomerular proteinuria: a com-mentary. J Am Soc Nephrol. 2003;14(12):3217–32.

30. Peterson JC, Adler S, Burkart JM, Greene T, Hebert LA, Hunsicker LG, et al. Blood pressure control, pro-teinuria, and the progression of renal disease. The modification of diet in renal disease study. Ann Intern Med. 1995;123(10):754–62.

31. Ruggenenti P, Perna A, Remuzzi G, Investigators GG. Retarding progression of chronic renal disease: the neglected issue of residual proteinuria. Kidney Int. 2003;63(6):2254–61.

32. Moorhead JF, Chan MK, El-Nahas M, Varghese Z. Lipid nephrotoxicity in chronic progressive glomerular and tubulo-interstitial disease. Lancet. 1982;2(8311):1309–11.

33. Abbate M, Zoja C, Remuzzi G. Progression of renal injury toward interstitial inflammation and glomerular scle-rosis is dependent on abnormal protein filtration. Nephrol Dial Transplant. 2014;30(5):706–12.

34. Li J, Zhang Q, Su B. Clinical characteristics and risk factors of severe infections in hospitalized adult patients with primary nephrotic syndrome. J Int Med Res. 2017;45(6):2139–45.

35. Trivin C, Tran A, Moulin B, Choukroun G, Gatault P, Courivaud C, et al. Infectious complications of a rituximab-based immunosuppressive regimen in patients with glomerular disease. Clin Kidney J. 2017;10(4):461–9.

36. Groves AP, Reich P, Sigdel B, Davis TK. Pneumococcal hemolytic uremic syndrome and steroid resistant nephrotic syndrome. Clin Kidney J. 2016;9(4):572–5.

37. Rheault MN, Zhang L, Selewski DT, Kallash M, Tran CL, Seamon M, et al. AKI in children hospitalized with nephrotic syndrome. Clin J Am Soc Nephrol. 2015;10(12):2110–8.

38. Alfakeekh K, Azar M, Sowailmi BA, Alsulaiman S, Makdob SA, Omair A, et al. Immunosuppressive burden and risk factors of infection in primary childhood nephrotic syndrome. J Infect Public Health. 2019;12(1):90–4.

39. Aljebab F, Choonara I, Conroy S. Long-course oral corticosteroid toxicity in children. Arch Dis Child. 2016;101(9):e2.

40. Afroz S, Roy DK, Khan AH. Low serum immunglobulin G (IgG) during nephrosis is a predictor of urinary tract infection (UTI) in children with nephrotic syndrome. Mymensingh Med J. 2013;22(2):336–41.

41. al-Bander HA, Martin VI, Kaysen GA. Plasma IgG pool is not defended from urinary loss in nephrotic syndrome. Am J Phys. 1992;262(3 Pt 2):F333–7.

42. Ogi M, Yokoyama H, Tomosugi N, Hisada Y, Ohta S, Takaeda M, et al. Risk factors for infection and immuno-globulin replacement therapy in adult nephrotic syndrome. Am J Kidney Dis. 1994;24(3):427–36.

43. Han JW, Lee KY, Hwang JY, Koh DK, Lee JS. Antibody status in children with steroid-sensitive nephrotic syn-drome. Yonsei Med J. 2010;51(2):239–43.

44. Warshaw BL, Check IJ. IgG subclasses in children with nephrotic syndrome. Am J Clin Pathol. 1989;92(1):68–72.

45. de Sain-van der Velden MG, Kaysen GA, de Meer K, Stellaard F, Voorbij HA, Reijngoud DJ, et al. Proportionate increase of fibrinogen and albumin synthesis in nephrotic patients: measurements with stable isotopes. Kidney Int. 1998;53(1):181–8.
46. Prinsen BH, de Sain-van der Velden MG, Kaysen GA, Straver HW, van Rijn HJ, Stellaard F, et al. Transferrin synthesis is increased in nephrotic patients insufficiently to replace urinary losses. J Am Soc Nephrol. 2001;12(5):1017–25.
47. de Sain-Van Der Velden MG, de Meer K, Kulik W, Melissant CF, Rabelink TJ, Berger R, et al. Nephrotic proteinuria has no net effect on total body protein synthesis: measurements with (13)C valine. Am J Kidney Dis. 2000;35(6):1149–54.
48. Kaysen GA, Carstensen A, Martin VI. Muscle protein synthesis is impaired in nephrotic rats. Miner Electrolyte Metab. 1992;18(2–5):228–32.
49. Kaysen GA. Albumin metabolism in the nephrotic syndrome: the effect of dietary protein intake. Am J Kidney Dis. 1988;12(6):461–80.
50. Giordano M, De Feo P, Lucidi P, DePascale E, Giordano G, Cirillo D, et al. Effects of dietary protein restriction on fibrinogen and albumin metabolism in nephrotic patients. Kidney Int. 2001;60(1):235–42.
51. Kaysen GA, Kirkpatrick WG, Couser WG. Albumin homeostasis in the nephrotic rat: nutritional considerations. Am J Phys. 1984;247(1 Pt 2):F192–202.
52. Kaysen GA, Gambertoglio J, Felts J, Hutchison FN. Albumin synthesis, albuminuria and hyperlipemia in nephrotic patients. Kidney Int. 1987;31(6):1368–76.
53. Sun X, Martin V, Weiss RH, Kaysen GA. Selective transcriptional augmentation of hepatic gene expression in the rat with Heymann nephritis. Am J Phys. 1993;264(3 Pt 2):F441–7.
54. Iorember F, Aviles D. Anemia in nephrotic syndrome: approach to evaluation and treatment. Pediatr Nephrol. 2017;32(8):1323–30.
55. Brown EA, Sampson B, Muller BR, Curtis JR. Urinary iron loss in the nephrotic syndrome--an unusual cause of iron deficiency with a note on urinary copper losses. Postgrad Med J. 1984;60(700):125–8.
56. Taal MWCG, Marsden PA, Skorecki K, Yu ASL, Brenner BM, editors. Brenner and Rector's the kidney. 9th ed. Philadelphia: Elsevier Saunders; 2011.
57. Ishimitsu T, Ono H, Sugiyama M, Asakawa H, Oka K, Numabe A, et al. Successful erythropoietin treatment for severe anemia in nephrotic syndrome without renal dysfunction. Nephron. 1996;74(3):607–10.
58. Pedraza-Chaverri J, Torres-Rodriguez GA, Cruz C, Mainero A, Tapia E, Ibarra-Rubio ME, et al. Copper and zinc metabolism in aminonucleoside-induced nephrotic syndrome. Nephron. 1994;66(1):87–92.
59. Bovio G, Piazza V, Ronchi A, Montagna G, Semeraro L, Galli F, et al. Trace element levels in adult patients with proteinuria. Minerva Gastroenterol Dietol. 2007;53(4):329–36.
60. Niel O, Thouret MC, Berard E. Anemia in congenital nephrotic syndrome: role of urinary copper and ceruloplasmin loss. Blood. 2011;117(22):6054–5.
61. Shah KN, Yan AC. Acquired zinc deficiency acrodermatitis associated with nephrotic syndrome. Pediatr Dermatol. 2008;25(1):56–9.
62. Podda GM, Lussana F, Moroni G, Faioni EM, Lombardi R, Fontana G, et al. Abnormalities of homocysteine and B vitamins in the nephrotic syndrome. Thromb Res. 2007;120(5):647–52.
63. Choudhary S, Agarwal I, Seshadri MS. Calcium and vitamin D for osteoprotection in children with new-onset nephrotic syndrome treated with steroids: a prospective, randomized, controlled, interventional study. Pediatr Nephrol. 2014;29(6):1025–32.
64. Brown AC. Kidney toxicity related to herbs and dietary supplements: online table of case reports. Part 3 of 5 series. Food Chem Toxicol. 2017;107(Pt A):502–19.
65. Banerjee S, Basu S, Sen A, Sengupta J. The effect of vitamin D and calcium supplementation in pediatric steroid-sensitive nephrotic syndrome. Pediatr Nephrol. 2017;32(11):2063–70.
66. Gulati S, Sharma RK, Gulati K, Singh U, Srivastava A. Longitudinal follow-up of bone mineral density in children with nephrotic syndrome and the role of calcium and vitamin D supplements. Nephrol Dial Transplant. 2005;20(8):1598–603.
67. Kraut JA, Madias NE. Consequences and therapy of the metabolic acidosis of chronic kidney disease. Pediatr Nephrol. 2011;26(1):19–28.
68. Shah SN, Abramowitz M, Hostetter TH, Melamed ML. Serum bicarbonate levels and the progression of kidney disease: a cohort study. Am J Kidney Dis. 2009;54(2):270–7.
69. de Brito-Ashurst I, Varagunam M, Raftery MJ, Yaqoob MM. Bicarbonate supplementation slows progression of CKD and improves nutritional status. J Am Soc Nephrol. 2009;20(9):2075–84.
70. Wesson DE, Simoni J, Broglio K, Sheather S. Acid retention accompanies reduced GFR in humans and increases plasma levels of endothelin and aldosterone. Am J Physiol Renal Physiol. 2011;300(4):F830–7.

71. MacKinnon M, Shurraw S, Akbari A, Knoll GA, Jaffey J, Clark HD. Combination therapy with an angiotensin receptor blocker and an ACE inhibitor in proteinuric renal disease: a systematic review of the efficacy and safety data. Am J Kidney Dis. 2006;48(1):8–20.

72. ONTARGET Investigators, Yusuf S, Teo KK, Pogue J, Dyal L, Copland I, et al. Telmisartan, ramipril, or both in patients at high risk for vascular events. N Engl J Med. 2008;358(15):1547–59.

73. Susantitaphong P, Sewaralthahab K, Balk EM, Eiam-ong S, Madias NE, Jaber BL. Efficacy and safety of combined vs. single renin-angiotensin-aldosterone system blockade in chronic kidney disease: a meta-analysis. Am J Hypertens. 2013;26(3):424–41.

74. Bianchi S, Bigazzi R, Campese VM. Long-term effects of spironolactone on proteinuria and kidney function in patients with chronic kidney disease. Kidney Int. 2006;70(12):2116–23.

75. Epstein M, Williams GH, Weinberger M, Lewin A, Krause S, Mukherjee R, et al. Selective aldosterone blockade with eplerenone reduces albuminuria in patients with type 2 diabetes. Clin J Am Soc Nephrol. 2006;1(5):940–51.

76. Navaneethan SD, Nigwekar SU, Sehgal AR, Strippoli GF. Aldosterone antagonists for preventing the progression of chronic kidney disease: a systematic review and meta-analysis. Clin J Am Soc Nephrol. 2009;4(3):542–51.

77. Vriesendorp R, Donker AJ, de Zeeuw D, de Jong PE, van der Hem GK. Antiproteinuric effect of naproxen and indomethacin. A double-blind crossover study. Am J Nephrol. 1985;5(4):236–42.

78. Vogt L, de Zeeuw D, Woittiez AJ, Navis G. Selective cyclooxygenase-2 (COX-2) inhibition reduces proteinuria in renal patients. Nephrol Dial Transplant. 2009;24(4):1182–9.

79. Nelson DA, Marks ES, Deuster PA, O'Connor FG, Kurina LM. Association of nonsteroidal anti-inflammatory drug prescriptions with kidney disease among active young and middle-aged adults. JAMA Netw Open. 2019;2(2):e187896.

80. Vegter S, Perna A, Postma MJ, Navis G, Remuzzi G, Ruggenenti P. Sodium intake, ACE inhibition, and progression to ESRD. J Am Soc Nephrol. 2012;23(1):165–73.

81. Fried LF. Effects of HMG-CoA reductase inhibitors (statins) on progression of kidney disease. Kidney Int. 2008;74(5):571–6.

82. Bianchi S, Bigazzi R, Caiazza A, Campese VM. A controlled, prospective study of the effects of atorvastatin on proteinuria and progression of kidney disease. Am J Kidney Dis. 2003;41(3):565–70.

83. Wilcox CS. New insights into diuretic use in patients with chronic renal disease. J Am Soc Nephrol. 2002;13(3):798–805.

84. Kaysen GA, Gambertoglio J, Jimenez I, Jones H, Hutchison FN. Effect of dietary protein intake on albumin homeostasis in nephrotic patients. Kidney Int. 1986;29(2):572–7.

85. Don BR, Kaysen GA, Hutchison FN, Schambelan M. The effect of angiotensin-converting enzyme inhibition and dietary protein restriction in the treatment of proteinuria. Am J Kidney Dis. 1991;17(1):10–7.

86. Walser M, Hill S, Tomalis EA. Treatment of nephrotic adults with a supplemented, very low-protein diet. Am J Kidney Dis. 1996;28(3):354–64.

87. Jenkins DJ, Kendall CW, Marchie A, Jenkins AL, Augustin LS, Ludwig DS, et al. Type 2 diabetes and the vegetarian diet. Am J Clin Nutr. 2003;78(3 Suppl):610S–6S.

88. Taku K, Umegaki K, Sato Y, Taki Y, Endoh K, Watanabe S. Soy isoflavones lower serum total and LDL cholesterol in humans: a meta-analysis of 11 randomized controlled trials. Am J Clin Nutr. 2007;85(4):1148–56.

89. Azadbakht L, Atabak S, Esmaillzadeh A. Soy protein intake, cardiorenal indices, and C-reactive protein in type 2 diabetes with nephropathy: a longitudinal randomized clinical trial. Diabetes Care. 2008;31(4):648–54.

90. Pedraza-Chaverri J, Barrera D, Hernandez-Pando R, Medina-Campos ON, Cruz C, Murguía F, et al. Soy protein diet ameliorates renal nitrotyrosine formation and chronic nephropathy induced by puromycin aminonucleoside. Life Sci. 2004;74(8):987–99.

91. Velasquez MT, Bhathena SJ, Ranich T, Schwartz AM, Kardon DE, Ali AA, et al. Dietary flaxseed meal reduces proteinuria and ameliorates nephropathy in an animal model of type II diabetes mellitus. Kidney Int. 2003;64(6):2100–7.

92. Tovar AR, Murguia F, Cruz C, Hernández-Pando R, Aguilar-Salinas CA, Pedraza-Chaverri J, et al. A soy protein diet alters hepatic lipid metabolism gene expression and reduces serum lipids and renal fibrogenic cytokines in rats with chronic nephrotic syndrome. J Nutr. 2002;132(9):2562–9.

93. Kaysen GA. al-Bander H, Martin VI, Jones H, Jr., Hutchison FN. Branched-chain amino acids augment neither albuminuria nor albumin synthesis in nephrotic rats. Am J Phys. 1991;260(2 Pt 2):R177–84.

94. Kaysen GA, Martin VI, Jones H Jr. Arginine augments neither albuminuria nor albumin synthesis caused by high-protein diets in nephrosis. Am J Phys. 1992;263(5 Pt 2):F907–14.

95. Gentile MG, Fellin G, Cofano F, Delle Fave A, Manna G, Ciceri R, et al. Treatment of proteinuric patients with a vegetarian soy diet and fish oil. Clin Nephrol. 1993;40(6):315–20.

96. Sieniawska M, Szymanik-Grzelak H, Kowalewska M, Wasik M, Koleska D. The role of cow's milk protein intolerance in steroid-resistant nephrotic syndrome. Acta Paediatr. 1992;81(12):1007–12.

97. Alfrey AC. Toxicity of tubule fluid iron in the nephrotic syndrome. Am J Phys. 1992;263(4 Pt 2):F637–41.

98. Agarwal R. Vitamin D, proteinuria, diabetic nephropathy, and progression of CKD. Clin J Am Soc Nephrol. 2009;4(9):1523–8.
99. Rayner BL, Byrne MJ, van Zyl Smit R. A prospective clinical trial comparing the treatment of idiopathic membranous nephropathy and nephrotic syndrome with simvastatin and diet, versus diet alone. Clin Nephrol. 1996;46(4):219–24.
100. Sahni V, Rosa RM, Batlle D. Potential benefits of alkali therapy to prevent GFR loss: time for a palatable 'solution' for the management of CKD. Kidney Int. 2010;78(11):1065–7.
101. Phisitkul S, Khanna A, Simoni J, Broglio K, Sheather S, Rajab MH, et al. Amelioration of metabolic acidosis in patients with low GFR reduced kidney endothelin production and kidney injury, and better preserved GFR. Kidney Int. 2010;77(7):617–23.
102. Goraya N, Simoni J, Jo CH, Wesson DE. Treatment of metabolic acidosis in patients with stage 3 chronic kidney disease with fruits and vegetables or oral bicarbonate reduces urine angiotensinogen and preserves glomerular filtration rate. Kidney Int. 2014;86(5):1031–8.

Chapter 25
Nephrolithiasis

Haewook Han

Keywords Nephrolithiasis · Kidney stone · Hypercalciuria · Hyperoxaluria · Dietary risk factors of kidney stone · Prevention of recurrence of stone disease · American Urology Association (AUA) guidelines

> **Key Points**
> - Kidney stones are prevalent in about 9% of the population and the incidence is on the rise with calcium stones being the most common type of stone.
> - Risk factors can be environmental, genetic, dietary, and medical.
> - Evaluation of kidney stones is done through imaging, stone analysis, and metabolic workup. The 24-hour urine test is the most important in identifying the risk factors for stone formation and guiding dietary and medical therapy.
> - Therapy for prevention of kidney stone formation can be medical with treating the underlying disease or dietary by modifying the risk factors.
> - Most of the time, dietary prevention is the primary intervention and focuses on modifying dietary habits.

Introduction

Nephrolithiasis (kidney stones, urolithiasis) is the formation of stone-like concretions in the urinary system caused by the precipitation of calcium, phosphate, urate, and other molecules. The incidence and prevalence of nephrolithiasis among adults in the USA have been increasing for 30 years. According to the National Health and Nutrition Examination Survey (NHANES 2007–2010), current

The editors acknowledge Julian L. Seifter's contribution to this chapter in *Nutrition in Kidney Disease*, *Second Edition*, Nutrition and Health, DOI: https://doi.org/10.1007/978-1-62703-685-6_1, © Springer Science+Business Media, New York, 2014.

H. Han (✉)
Atrius Health, Department of Nephrology, Boston, MA, USA

MS/DI Program Director, Tufts University Friedman School, Boston, MA, USA

Tufts Medical Center, Division of Nephrology, Boston, MA, USA
e-mail: haewook.han@tufts.edu

© Springer Nature Switzerland AG 2020
J. D. Burrowes et al. (eds.), *Nutrition in Kidney Disease*, Nutrition and Health,
https://doi.org/10.1007/978-3-030-44858-5_25

Table 25.1 Types of stones

Types	Frequency	Gender	Shape	Radiography
Ca stones (mixed)	80%	M > F	Envelope	Round, radiodense, sharply outlined
CaP (brushite)		F > M	Amorphous	Small, radiodense, sharply outlined
Uric acid	9%	M = F	Diamond shape	Round/staghorn, radiolucent, filling defect
Struvite	10%	F > M	Coffin lid	Staghorn, laminated radiodense
Cystine	1%	M > F	Hexagon	Staghorn, radiodense

Adapted from [12, 14]

prevalence is estimated at 8.8% among adults [1] as compared to a prevalence of 5.2% in 1994 [2]. More than $5.3 billion is spent directly and indirectly on treatment for nephrolithiasis annually in the USA [3]. Kidney stones are more prevalent in men than women with a lifetime risk of 12% in men and 6% in women [4]. As many as 20% of patients present with renal colic and require urological intervention [5].

Obesity and the metabolic syndrome are important risk factors for nephrolithiasis [6, 7]. In fact, increased incidence of nephrolithiasis is observed with the obesity epidemic in the USA [8, 9]. Also, climate and temperature-related changes may be contributing factors [10, 11].

About 80% of stones contain calcium, primarily calcium oxalate (CaOx), with a small percentage of calcium phosphate (CaP) as apatite [5, 12, 13]. CaP stones are more prevalent among younger female stone formers [14]. Uric acid (UA) stones account for only about 9% of stones and are more prevalent in individuals older than 50 years of age. The remaining 10% of stones are composed of a variety of substances including struvite, often associated with infection, and 1% are cysteine stones due to inborn errors of metabolism [15]. Although each stone type has unique pathophysiologic features, the final common pathway of stone formation is supersaturation (SS) of the relevant components. This chapter will discuss assessment, risk factor identification, and nutritional interventions for different types of stones (Table 25.1 and Fig. 25.1).

Pathophysiology

Supersaturation and Stone Formation

Stone formation is a multistep process. Crystal formation occurs when the solute concentration in the urine exceeds its solubility product; this is defined as supersaturation (SS). With low urine volume, SS of calcium, oxalate, and uric acid promotes stone formation. Solute concentration also increases due to increased absolute excretion in the urine. Increased excretion of solutes can occur in genetic diseases such as cystinuria and primary hyperoxalruia or in some disease states such as inflammatory bowel disease (IBD), which results in secondary hyperoxaluria [5, 16]. Hyperparathyroidism and sarcoidosis can increase the excretion of calcium in the urine [17, 18].

Nucleation and growth of crystals require the presence of crystal-forming substances at concentrations above their solubility [19, 20]. The saturation status of the urine depends on the combined excretion of water and lithogenic substances [21]. Different stone types precipitate depending on the pH of the urine. Normal urine pH is about 6. Uric acid and CaOx stones form in low urine pH whereas CaP stones tend to form in high urine pH. Most uric acid stone formers have a relatively low urine pH, while CaP stone formers generally have higher urine pH (often persistently >6.2).

There are a number of substances in the urine such as citrate, pyrophosphate, osteopontin, anduromodulin, and glycosaminoglycans that can decrease stone formation by inhibiting nucleation, aggregation, and growth of Ca stones in vitro [22, 23]. However, citrate is the only inhibitor in clinical use.

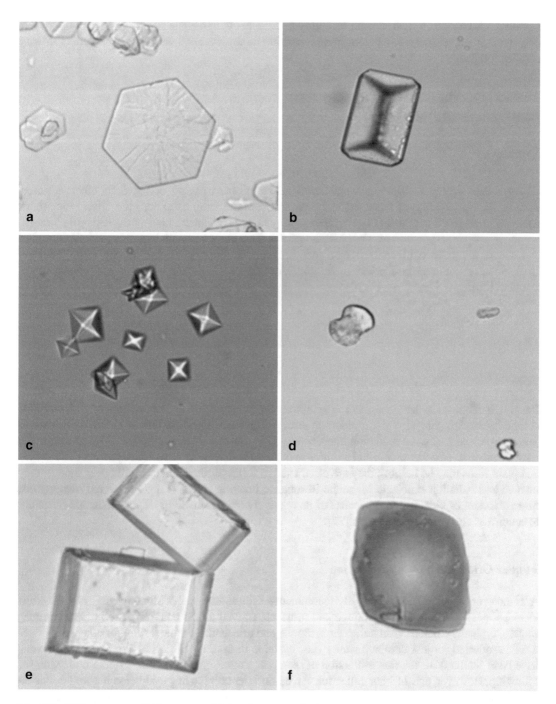

Fig. 25.1 Different types of kidney stones. Light microscopy of urine crystals: (**a**) hexagonal cystine crystals (200_); (**b**) coffin-lid-shaped struvite crystals (200_); (**c**) pyramid-shaped calcium oxalate dehydrate crystals (200_); (**d**) dumbbell-shaped calcium oxalate monohydrate crystal (400_); (**e**) rectangular uric acid crystals (400_); and (**f**) rhomboidal uric acid crystals (400_). (From Asplin JR. Evaluation of the kidney stone patient. Seminars in Nephrology 28(2); 99–110, 2008. Reprinted with permission from John R. Asplin and Elsevier Limited)

Citrate binds calcium, which reduces its ability to complex with oxalate and form stones. It may also play a role in preventing non-calcium stone formation through various mechanisms including urinary alkalization [24].

Symptoms and Diagnosis

Symptoms

Kidney stones may be asymptomatic and found incidentally on imaging tests done for other purposes. Patients develop symptoms when the stone passes from the renal calyx into the ureter, sometimes resulting in obstruction of urine. The symptoms may include ipsilateral flank pain, hematuria, nausea, vomiting, and urinary tract infection [25].The pain is often severe enough to warrant emergency ward care where the patient is usually treated with intravenous fluids, pain control, and alpha blockers. Urologic intervention is required when the stone does not pass spontaneously with conservative management [26].

Diagnosis

Imaging

Imaging is required in the assessment of symptomatic stone disease and to evaluate for stone-related complications. Imaging also gives important information regarding stone burden and it can be used to follow the success of stone reduction interventions [26]. Computed tomography (CT) is generally the most sensitive imaging technique but it is more expensive and involves radiation exposure. Ultrasounds and plain films may be helpful; they are often used to follow stone burden serially over time as they involve less radiation exposure. Magnetic Resonance Imaging (MRI) is not a preferred imaging test for assessment of kidney stones because of its relatively lower sensitivity, higher cost, and difficulty to acquire as compared to a CT scan [27].

24-hour Urine Test and Interpretation

A 24-hour urine collection is generally recommended for assessment of stone forming risk. The test includes measurement of urine volume and urine pH as well as the daily excretion of various substances, typically calcium, oxalate, sodium, citrate, and uric acid. Specific testing for other substances can be requested for less common stones (i.e., cysteine in cystinuria).Two 24-hour urine collections have been standard for the first evaluation of recurrent stone formers and one 24-hour collection for follow-up. However, one 24-hour collection can be sufficient for the first evaluation if a well-collected sample is done [28].

Adequacy of Urine Sample

Adequacy of the 24-hour collection can be done by checking 24-hour urine creatinine excretion. Male creatinine excretion is 20–25 mg/kg/day while females excrete 15–20 mg/kg/day [29]. Elevated levels suggest either an over-collection (more than 24 hours) or elevated creatinine production (as in a muscular patient). If the value obtained is below normal, malnourishment and/or low muscle mass should be suspected. It is advisable to obtain the 24-hour urine collection when kidney function is stable to ensure a steady daily solute excretion.

Interpretation of 24-hour Urine Collection

The 24-hour collection should report, at a minimum, urine volume, calcium, phosphorus, oxalate, citrate, pH, and uric acid. An estimate of SS for each compound or electrolyte is helpful. Also, measurements of urinary sodium, sulfate, potassium, magnesium, and urea can be used to evaluate dietary risk factors. Dietary factors such as sulfates from animal protein (e.g., the acid ash diet) and sodium can alter urinary calcium excretion. Urea nitrogen may be used to estimate protein catabolic rate (PCR), which is usually indicative of dietary protein intake. The urinary nitrogen appearance can be used to calculate estimated dietary protein intake [30] and it will be discussed later in the chapter.

In an individual patient, normal ranges reported by the laboratory may not be optimum for stone prevention; this usually requires clinician interpretation [31]. Follow-up urine testing can help determine if dietary and medical therapies are effective.

The 24-hour urine collection should be done several weeks after any urological procedure (i.e., 6–8 weeks after lithotripsy) to minimize interference by infection, blood, or acute kidney injury, which may be present after a urologic procedure. Infection, for example, can change the pH and citrate levels. Also, the patient may not be feeling well and may not be consuming typical nutrients and fluids. It is important that patients continue with their usual diet and activities during the collection period [26].

The clinician uses the results of the 24-hour urine to evaluate dietary nutrients and fluid intake as targets for intervention. For example, normal urinary calcium levels are <250 mg/day for men and <200 mg/day for women. High urinary calcium can be caused by idiopathic hypercalciuria (IH), hyperparathyroidism, or high sodium or protein diet. On the other hand, low urinary calcium may be caused by malabsorption or underlying bone disease. Normal urinary oxalate excretion is 20–40 mg/day and high levels may be due to increased absorption as in high oxalate diet and IBD or increased endogenous production of oxalate as in primary hyperoxaluria and high vitamin C consumption. Normal urinary citrate excretion is >450 mg/day for men and >550 mg/day for women. A high animal protein diet or renal tubular acidosis (RTA) can increase acid production, decrease urinary pH and lower urinary citrate levels [30]. Table 25.2 provides a summary of the normal values of the 24-hour urine collection and interpretation and causes of abnormal values [32].

Table 25.2 Summary of the normal values of the 24-hour urine collection, interpretation of and causes of abnormal values

Test (24-hour urine)	What to assess with the tests?	Reference value	Possible causes of abnormal values
Urine volume	Daily urine flow	>2500 mL/day	↓ With low fluid intake
Creatinine (Cr/kg)	Adequate urine collection	18–24 mg/kg for males 15–20 mg/kg for females	↑ With more than 24-hour collection ↓ With under-collection
Calcium	Risk of calcium stones	<250 mg/day for males <200 mg/day for females	↑ Idiopathic hypercalciuria, high-Na diet (high urine Na), high-protein diet, primary hyperparathyroidism. ↓ With bone disease
Phosphorus	Primary hyperparathyroidism, malnutrition or malabsorption	0.6–1.2 g/day	↓ With bowel disease, malnutrition, ↑ With large amount of food intake

(continued)

Table 25.2 (continued)

Test (24-hour urine)	What to assess with the tests?	Reference value	Possible causes of abnormal values
pH	Risk for different types of certain stones	5.8–6.2	↓ RTA, urea splitting infection, acidosis, high animal protein intake (high purine content), <5.5 increase uric acid stone risk ↑ >6.5 increase calcium phosphate risk, vegetarian diet, high citrus consumption
Oxalate	Calcium oxalate stone risk	20–40 mg/day	↑ With high oxalate diet, high vitamin C consumption, if >80, intestinal (inflammatory bowel disease), malabsorptive states or oxalosis
Citrate	Risk of calcium oxalate, uric acid stones	>450 mg/day males >550 mg/day females	↓ RTA, hypokalemia, high animal protein diet, acidosis, diarrhea
Uric acid	Uric acid stone	<0.8 g/day males <0.75 g/day females	↑ With high animal protein diet (high purine), alcoholic beverages, overproduction, diabetes, and use of SGLT2 inhibitors
Magnesium	Magnesium binds oxalate Assess Ca stone risks	30–120 mg/day	↓ With some laxatives, malnutrition, malabsorption, increase risk for calcium stones as more oxalate is available
Sodium	Estimate of sodium intake	50–150 mEq/day (1150–3450 mg)	↑ With high Na diet ↓ With bowel disease
Potassium	Evaluate risk of hypocitraturia and to follow medication compliance, if started on diuretics	20–100 mEq/day	Less than 20, bowel disease, diuretics, laxatives
Urea nitrogen	Evaluate total protein metabolism	6–14 g/kg/day	↑ With high protein diet
Sulfate	Assessment of protein intake especially animal protein	20–80 mEq/day	↑ With high protein especially animal protein diet
Ammonium	Evaluation of infection, and medical condition	15–60 mM/day	↑ pH >7 urea splitting infection, ↓ pH <5.5 CKD, uric acid stones, gout
Protein catabolic rate (PCR)	Total protein intake to assess adequate amount	0.8–1.4 g/kg/day	↑ With high protein diet
Supersaturation	Determines the risk of crystal formation in the urine	Reference values vary with different labs SSCaOx, SSCaP, SSUA	↑ of each supersaturation: increase CaOx, CaP, and uric acid stone risks

Adapted from [32]

Abbreviations: *RTA* renal tubular acidosis, *SSCaOx* supersaturation of calcium oxalate, *SSCaP* supersaturation of calcium phosphate, *SSUA* supersaturation of uric acid

Risk Factors

Genetic Risk Factors

There are various genetic disorders that can cause kidney stones. Monogenic causes include cystinuria, distal RTA, variants of Bartter's syndrome, familial hypomagnesemia with hypercalciuria and nephrocalcinosis, Dent's disease, hypophosphatemic rickets with hypercalciuria, autosomal dominant hypoparathyroidism, and Lowe syndrome [33].

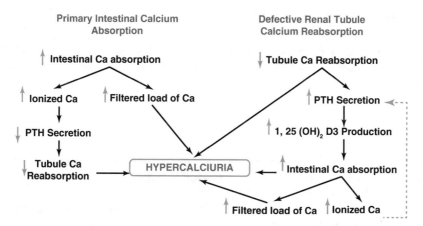

Fig. 25.2 Model of idiopathic hypercalciuria

Idiopathic hypercalciuria (IH) is a common disorder found in about 50% of calcium stone formers (Fig. 25.2) [34].There is an increased incidence of hypercalcuria in first-degree relatives of patients with this condition but it appears to be complex and likely polygenic [5]. IH involves abnormal metabolism of calcium absorption by the gastrointestinal (GI) tract, kidney, and bone. In addition to having decreased ability of renal calcium reabsorption, patients with IH often have elevated 1, 25-dihydroxy vitamin D levels, which increases intestinal absorption of calcium [35].

Primary hyperoxaluria is a rare genetic defect resulting in overproduction of oxalate in the liver. Hyperoxaluria causes high urinary SS of CaOx, which promotes stone formation, or can even cause acute and chronic renal failure by progressive nephrocalcinosis, tubular damage, and interstitial fibrosis [36]. Progression to end-stage kidney disease (ESKD) is common in this disorder.

Cystinuria is another rare genetic disorder resulting in nephrolithiasis. Cystine is the homo-dimer of the amino acid cysteine. Due to one of two possible renal transporter defects, reabsorption of filtered cystine is decreased and urinary cystine level is elevated [37]. These high excretion rates lead to cystine SS and cystine stones. Patients with cystinuria have a higher incidence of CKD than the general population and progression to ESKD is possible [38, 39].

Environmental Risk Factors

Hot climates have been associated with an increased risk of kidney stone formation. For example, in the USA, the Southeast region has a significantly higher prevalence (up to 50% in some analyses) than the Northwest [2, 10, 40]. This data are further supported by the Second Cancer Prevention Survey (CPS II), which shows that the highest prevalence of kidney stones in the USA is in six Southeastern states: Tennessee, Alabama, Mississippi, Georgia, North Carolina, and South Carolina, also known as the "Kidney Stone Belt" [40]. It has been hypothesized that inadequate fluid intake in these hot climates may lead to an increase of urinary electrolyte concentrations and lower urine pH, which promotes stone formation [41, 42]. However, other risk factors that may co-segregate with warm regions need to be considered.

Dietary Risk Factors

Dietary factors are thought to play an important role in the formation of kidney stones and composition of the urine. These factors include dietary intake of calcium, sodium, oxalate, protein (especially animal protein), fructose, fluids (including water and other beverages), nutritional supplements and vitamins. Measurement and modification of such factors is limited by largely retrospective study data that are often confounded by recall bias, since stone formers frequently change their diet prior to enrollment in studies [4]. In addition, studies are limited by their inability to measure concentrations of the different molecular components in food that may have multiple and contradictory effects on stone formation.

Fluid Intake

High fluid intake leads to an increase in urine volume and a decrease in urinary SS of any lithogenic solute. Fluid intake is probably the most important modifiable risk factor among stone formers because of its relative safety, low cost, and ability to decrease the risk of any stone type. The benefit of increased fluid intake on decreasing the risk of stone formation has been shown in multiple observational and randomized controlled trials [43–45]. It is important to note that any fluid, regardless of specific content, will augment urine output and urine free water excretion.

There are lingering misconceptions about the proper choice of fluid for stone formers. For example, coffee may increase urine calcium and some guidelines suggest avoiding coffee; however observational studies have found that tea, coffee, beer, wine, soda, and orange juice are not associated with any increased risk of nephrolithiasis [44, 46, 47]. Recently, Ferraro et al. concluded that there is actually a decreased risk of kidney stone formation with coffee consumption [47]. Although the mechanisms remain unclear, decreased stone risk may be related to the protective properties of other unmeasured components or a diuretic effect of coffee [48, 49].

Calcium

Historically, there has been concern that higher dietary calcium may increase calcium stone risk. However, most data points in the opposite direction. For example, a study with a large cohort of greater than 50,000 male health professionals showed that men with a higher intake of dietary calcium were found to actually have a lower risk of kidney stones when adjusted for other risk factors [50]. Higher dietary calcium was also found to decrease stone risk in women as well in a more recent analysis of men [45, 51, 52]. It is possible that dietary calcium is protective because low calcium intake leads to increased oxalate absorption and urinary excretion [53]. Consistent with the data above, higher dietary calcium intake (800–1200 mg/day), specifically from dairy products, has been associated with decreased stone formation [50]. However, excess calcium supplementation beyond standard recommendations for bone health is not recommended for stone patients (especially calcium stone formers) because it may increase urinary calcium excretion especially if taken without meals [51]. A randomized trial conducted by Borghi et al. that compared two diets (normal calcium: 30 mmol vs. low calcium: 10 mmol) in patients with IH and calcium oxalate stones, showed a 50% reduction in the rate of recurrence among the normal calcium intake group [54]. Given the current state of research, a calcium-restricted diet is not recommended for calcium-based stone formers. Patients should consume a "normal" calcium diet in line with standard dietary recommendations (1000–1200 mg/day) to ensure bone health.

Oxalate

The role of dietary oxalate in modifying the risk of CaOx stone formation is not clear for several reasons. First, the amount of urinary oxalate derived from dietary intake is relatively small (ranging from 10% to 50%) [55]. Second, some portion of urinary oxalate comes from GI absorption and there is also a significant contribution from endogenous metabolism. Third, dietary oxalate has variable bioavailability and may not be absorbed easily from some foods. One consistent finding is that oxalate absorption is higher in those with GI diseases such as IBD, and in those with gastric bypass surgery [56–58]. A low oxalate diet is often recommended for CaOx stone formers with high urinary oxalate levels, but practical dietary modification is hampered by a lack of reliable information on the oxalate content of foods. Another clinical concern is that high oxalate foods are also an important part of heart-healthy diets, such as the Dietary Approaches to Stop Hypertension (DASH) Diet, which is designed to decrease cardiovascular risk. A more accurate measurement of oxalate is necessary to support the dietary oxalate restriction in CaOx stone formers [59–61].

Sodium

A high sodium intake and urinary sodium excretion is associated with higher urinary calcium excretion. The high calcium excretion in IH is especially sensitive to dietary intake of sodium [60, 61]. Observational and experimental studies have demonstrated that calcium excretion rises more steeply in IH than in normal subjects for a given increase in sodium excretion [62]. Dietary sodium restriction decreases urinary calcium excretion, which lowers the risk of CaOx stone formation [54]. A low-sodium diet is a reasonable strategy to prevent hypercalciuria and may have independent benefits for patients with hypertension or congestive heart failure.

Protein and Uric Acid Stones

Protein restriction (especially animal protein which is high in purine) reduces hypercalciuria by increasing urinary citrate and pH, and may be of benefit for uric acid stone formers [54]. Dietary protein intake and excretion may be estimated from a 24-hour urine by calculating the urea nitrogen appearance (UNA) and the protein catabolic rate (PCR). In a healthy steady state, intake of protein is equivalent to protein catabolism; therefore, PCR determines the nitrogen balance from a 24-hour urine urea concentration using the following formula:

$$PCR = \left[6.25 \left(\{24 \text{ h urea N}\} + \{0.031 \times \text{weight}\} \right) \right] / \text{weight}$$

Patients who have severe medical conditions such as cancer, kidney disease, or acute or chronic infection are often malnourished and remain in a catabolic state and protein/nitrogen excretion will exceed intake.

A high protein intake generates an acid load, which is excreted largely as urinary ammonium (NH_4). Generally, the higher the protein intake, the higher the urinary ammonium. Urinary ammonium levels may be lower in patients who take alkali therapy or who have certain kinds of RTA. High ammonium and sulfate are indicators of a high-protein diet, especially animal protein [63]. Also, a high-protein diet (≥ 1.5 g/kg/day) can reduce urine pH; therefore, a moderate- to low-protein diet (0.8–1.2 g/kg/day) [30] is recommended for recurrent nephrolithiasis patients with hypocitraturia. Patients with low citrate levels who take alkali therapy may lower urinary ammonium and increase pH, decreasing the risk of uric acid and CaOx stones.

High-protein, low-carbohydrate diets designed for weight loss are popular but not recommended for the patients with history of kidney stones. Such diets may increase hypercalciuria, lower urine pH, and increase uric acid levels.

Vegetable proteins are thought to be less lithogenic than animal proteins; however, Massey et al. studied stone risk in beef vs. plant protein-based diets and concluded that lower protein intake, regardless of source, had the same effect in reducing CaOx stone risk [64]. Also, another recent epidemiologic study showed that animal protein intake was not independently associated with the incidence of nephrolithiasis among a large cohort of postmenopausal women [65]. The amount of protein may be more important than the source.

Low urinary pH is a significant risk factor for uric acid stones since the solubility of uric acid is decreased in acid urine. The prevalence of uric acid stones is about 5–10% of total kidney stone disease. Measurements of urinary calcium, uric acid, and post-prandial urine pH are used to assess the uric acid stone risk. The average adult consumes about 2 mg of purine/kg/day, which produces 200–300 mg of uric acid, and endogenous production is about 300 mg/day, totaling 500–600 mg/day. In one study, normal uric acid excretion was 5.6 mg/kg/day [66], with total excretion of uric acid less than 800 mg/day. Dietary consumption of purine varies daily by individuals but elevated levels of urine uric acid are thought to contribute to uric acid stone formation [67]. Ingestion of alcohol can increase urinary uric acid excretion. Kessler et al. conducted a cross-sectional study by using bicarbonate-rich mineral water and various types of juices on uric acid stone formation. They found that black currant juice decreased uric acid stone risk by increasing the urine pH [68, 69]. If patients have gout, allopurinol is usually prescribed along with a low-purine diet to reduce blood uric acid and may be tried to decrease uricosuria [66, 70]. Interestingly, evidence that allopurinol prevents calcium stones is stronger than for uric acid stones [71].

Potassium

Potassium is abundant in most fruits and vegetables, and potassium intake appears to decrease calcium excretion and increase urinary citrate [72]. Studies have shown that dietary potassium supplementation decreases stone risk in men and older women [45, 50, 51]. Monitoring 24-h urinary excretion of potassium is important to evaluate compliance with diet and medications. Taylor et al. analyzed the 24-h urine of individuals who followed the DASH diet and found that a higher DASH score (consuming more fruits and vegetables) was associated with a decreased risk of stone formation. Since foods with a higher DASH score are high in potassium, magnesium, and phosphorus, these foods may increase urine pH, resulting in decreased SS of CaOx and uric acid in urine as well as increased urine volume and citrate [73, 74]. If patients have chronic kidney disease (CKD) or take medications that impair the action of aldosterone such as angiotensin converting enzyme inhibitors (ACEI) or angiotensin receptor blockers (ARBs), serum potassium levels should be monitored closely.

Magnesium

Magnesium reduces oxalate absorption by forming a complex with oxalate in the GI tract. This makes magnesium an attractive tool to reduce urinary oxalate. Although randomized trials examining the effect of magnesium supplementation on stone recurrence showed beneficial effects, the results have been confounded by concurrent treatment with thiazide diuretics and/or citrate supplementation [4]. Other prospective studies showed reduction of stone risk in men but not in women with magnesium supplementation [45, 51, 52].

Phytates

Phytates are a storage form of phosphorus abundant in plants. They may also have an important role in stone prevention. Cold cereal, dark bread, and beans are high in phytates. It is believed they form insoluble complexes with calcium in the GI tract and prevent calcium reabsorption that results in a decrease in urinary calcium excretion [45]. However, this proposed mechanism may result in increased oxalate reabsorption from the GI tract, since calcium is bound to phytates and not available to bind oxalate. A different hypothesis is that phytates inhibit CaOx crystal formation in the urine [75]. Indirect evidence of the role of phytates in stone formation include a finding that urinary phytate levels were significantly lower in calcium stone formers compared with healthy controls, and levels were normalized with phytate supplementation [76]. In addition, secondary analysis of the Nurses' Health Study (NHS) II showed a 36% lower risk of nephrolithiasis in women with the highest quintile of phytate intake [45].

Vitamin and Herbal Supplements

Ascorbic acid (vitamin C) is metabolized to oxalate in the body. Researchers have shown that 1000 mg of twice-daily vitamin C supplementation in normal subjects and in prior calcium oxalate stone formers increased urinary oxalate excretion by 20% and 33%, respectively, without a change in urinary pH [77]. Other observational studies showed that supplemental and dietary vitamin C intake elevated the risk for calcium oxalate nephrolithiasis among men, but not in women, after controlling for potassium intake [52, 78].

Vitamin B6 is a co-factor in oxalate metabolism. Low vitamin B6 levels can lead to increased oxalate excretion in the urine [46, 79, 80]. However, there is no evidence that supplementation of vitamin B6 can lower CaOx stone formation. Higher natural intake of vitamin B6 may reduce the risk of stone formation in women, but not in men [79, 80].

Vitamin D increases both calcium and phosphorus absorption in the GI tract. Many patients currently take vitamin D supplements based on blood vitamin D levels or for general presumed health benefits. Although a small study of vitamin D repletion in healthy women did not increase urine calcium excretion [81, 82], recent data showed that vitamin D alone or calcium with vitamin D supplements with high serum 25-hydroxyvitamin D levels may have increased urinary calcium excretion among stone formers [83]. Therefore, use of vitamin D supplementation among stone formers should be individualized and requires close monitoring of blood and urine calcium levels.

Herbal supplements are often used in conjunction with other complementary and alternative medicine (CAM) supporting therapies such as meditation, cleansing, food systems, yoga and acupuncture. These herbal formulae have multiple spectrums of intended action, including analgesic, anti-inflammatory, antimicrobial, anti-spasmodic, anti-calcifying, diuretic, or litholytic, but there is little scientific evidence to support these claims. Use of herbal supplements for stone prevention should be used with caution [84–86].

Table 25.3 summarizes the genetic, environmental, and dietary risk factors of kidney stones.

Table 25.3 Risk factors of kidney stone

Genetic and other disease related		Environmental and diet related	
Genetic	Idiopathic hypercalciuria Hyperoxalosis Cystinuria Dent's disease	Climate	Heat Water loss, sweating
Kidney disease related	Medullary sponge kidney PKD (10% develop stones) Horseshoe Metabolic causes: hypercalcemia, hyperparathyroidism, DM and obesity	Dietary	High sodium Oxalate Protein (animal) Acid/ alkaline ash diet Fluid
Systemic disease	GI, inflammatory bowel diseases (Ox and UA stones)		Potassium and citrate Fluid
Hyperparathyroidism	CaP stone		Vitamins (C, D)
Renal tubular acidosis (RTA)	Hypercalcemic states, Ca phosphate		Ca supplement Low Ca diet
Sarcoidosis	Hypercalciuria, CaOx stone		High-protein weight loss diet

Abbreviations: *PKD* polycystic kidney disease, *DM* diabetes mellitus, *GI* gastrointestinal, *Ox* oxalate, *UA* uric acid, *CaP* calcium phosphate, *CaOx* calcium oxalate

Types of Stones and Treatment

Urologic Management of Stones: Surgical Removal of Stones

Most kidney stones will spontaneously pass, but between 10% and 20% of stone patients will need (urologic) surgical intervention [87, 88]. For some stones, such as struvite and staghorn stones, the primary intervention is surgical.

Common reasons for stone surgery include intractable pain, kidney failure, infection associated with a kidney or ureteral stone, failure of a ureteral stone to pass, or management of a large kidney stone. Surgical management of stones includes extracorporeal shockwave lithotripsy (ESWL), ureteroscopy (URS), or percutaneous nephrolithotomy (PCNL). Today, open surgical procedures are rarely performed [87, 89].

Medical and Dietary Interventions of Various Types of Kidney Stones

Calcium stones (calcium oxalate, calcium phosphate) account for 80% of all stones, followed by uric acid stones (5–10%), with cystine, struvite, and ammonium acid stones constituting most of the remainder [16]. Often, patients are referred to the nephrology and nutrition departments after stone removal procedures. The primary purpose of medical and dietary interventions is to prevent stone recurrence. All stone formers should be evaluated for medical conditions that might predispose to recurring stones. A 24-hour urine collection is important to assess stone forming and nutritional risk factors. The American Urology Association (AUA) provides guidelines for standard treatment and prevention of kidney stones [90].

General Nutrition Assessment

The dietitian should assess nutritional risk factors by dietary intake assessments and provide therapeutic recommendations based on identified risk factors. Specifically, the dietitian should evaluate dietary intake of calcium, oxalate, sodium, protein (both animal and plant), dietary supplements, and fluid intake since these can either promote or inhibit stone formation. However, the assessment of dietary oxalate intake is very difficult because the database for oxalate content of foods is inconsistent, and dietary analysis programs do not support this data. Therefore, dietitians should use their own judgment in estimating the patient's oxalate consumption along with other dietary intake analysis.

The most commonly used dietary assessment methods are the 24-hour recall, food record, diet history, and food frequency questionnaire. The 24-hour urine collection provides important data to assess the patients' diet 1–2 days before the urine collection and it is useful to monitor changes over time. Dietary records provide information on intake of foods, beverages, and dietary supplements over specific periods. The best diet assessment for kidney stones is the food record before and during a 24-hour urine collection. Data should be recorded 1–2 days before the collection and throughout the duration of the collection. The food record should be analyzed to evaluate intake of protein, sodium, potassium, calcium, phosphorus, magnesium, uric acid, oxalate, and fluid. Based on the food intake and 24-hour urine test, the clinician provides practical advice that can be reassessed at a future date.

Calcium Stones: Calcium Oxalate and Calcium Phosphate Stones

Calcium Oxalate Stones

Calcium-containing stones are the most common type of stones representing about 70% to 80% of identified stones and may be comprised of calcium oxalate or calcium phosphate. Recurrence is common and about 10% of patients with calcium-type stones will have episodes of symptomatic stones [91] more than three times throughout their lives.

Medical Management

Hypercalciuria is associated with calcium stone formation but the relationship with calcium intake is complex. Paradoxically, reducing calcium intake may increase the risk of calcium oxalate stone formation [53]. Dietary management of hypercalciuria starts by reducing sodium intake. If dietary intervention does not lower urinary calcium excretion, medical management may be considered by using thiazide diuretics, which tend to lower urine calcium. Of note, thiazides may elevate serum calcium and lower serum potassium, so these laboratory studies should be monitored [92]. Also, if patients have normal blood pressure, thiazide diuretics can cause hypotension, so blood pressure should be monitored.

Potassium citrate can be prescribed for CaOx stone formers with low urine citrate and low urinary pH. Patients should be monitored for gastrointestinal complaints [93]. If the patient is taking ACEI or ARBs for blood pressure control, blood potassium levels should be monitored for hyperkalemia. If potassium citrate is not tolerated or if patients have elevated serum potassium levels, sodium bicarbonate may be used to increase urinary citrate levels and reduce SS of CaOx, but it is not as effective as potassium citrate and represents a sodium load [94]. In patients with high urinary pH and hypercalciuria, potassium citrate may further increase the pH and increase the risk of CaP stones. Usually, the addition of lemon juice is recommended to help increase urinary citrate, and studies using commercial fruit juices such as orange, cranberry, or apple have shown significant increases in urinary citrate levels [95]. However, due to their high caloric content, these beverages should be consumed with caution in patients with metabolic syndrome and they may increase serum potassium levels.

Certain gut bacteria can increase oxalate breakdown and thus decrease oxalate gut absorption and subsequently reduce oxalate excretion in the urine. The gut microbiome may play a role in influencing alkali absorption and increase citrate concentration in the urine, which may reduce stone formation [96].

One organism, *Oxalobacter formigenes*, uses oxalate as a carbon source and promotes oxalate release in the gut by stimulating its transport through the gut epithelium, potentially reducing gut oxalate absorption. One study revealed that colonizing the gut with this bacteria reduced the risk of recurrent stones in stone-forming patients [97, 98]. Therefore, *Oxalobacter formigenes* therapy may be considered for patients with primary hyperoxaluria to reduce urinary oxalate [99]. However, there was no difference in urinary oxalate excretion in a randomized placebo controlled trial in patients with primary hyperoxaluria [100]. Therefore, the clinical application of probiotics in calcium stone disease is still uncertain.

Nutritional Management

Fluid

Increasing urine volume is key to stone prevention generally and daily fluid intake is the most important determinant of urinary volume. The AUA guidelines recommend adequate fluid intake to produce at least 2.5 liters of urine daily [90]. Almost all beverages, including alcoholic beverages, coffee (both caffeinated and decaffeinated), tea, wine, and orange juice, are associated with lower risk of stones [44, 46, 101]; however, some specific fluids such as sugar-sweetened drinks, soda, and grapefruit juice are associated with increased stone risk [44, 48]. Most patients require three liters or more of fluid intake per day to reach this urine volume to the goal, but this varies with patients and other factors including insensible water loss from sweat or the GI tract as in diarrhea.

Dietary and Supplemental Calcium Intake

Low calcium diets may increase the risk of calcium oxalate stone formation by increasing oxalate absorption and subsequent excretion [90]. A study comparing dietary calcium intake of <800 mg/day showed a higher incidence of kidney stones than individuals who consumed "adequate" dietary calcium, defined as 1000–1200 mg/day for most adults [65]. If dietary intake is low, supplemental calcium is reasonable to prevent bone loss, especially among postmenopausal women. However, supplemental calcium has been correlated with a higher risk of kidney stone formation in older women. In the Women's Health Initiative clinical trial, calcium supplementation exceeding the recommended upper limit of 1200 mg daily for adults increased the risk of kidney stones [102, 103]. If calcium supplements are used it may be better to take them with meals in order to bind to the oxalate in the food. The AUA recommends that total daily calcium intake from both diet and supplements should not exceed the adequate range of about 1000–1200 mg daily for adults. SS levels on 24-hour urine collections may help determine whether calcium supplements are beneficial or problematic for this patient group [90]. The clinician ultimately must weigh the risks and benefits of calcium supplementation by considering bone health and stone risk together.

Dietary Sodium

Dietary sodium may increase stone risk by increasing urinary calcium. Often sodium and animal protein are found in the same foods. In a study of calcium oxalate stone formers, a low-salt diet alone decreased urinary calcium and oxalate excretion but it was not designed to look for a reduction in the incidence of kidney stones [104]. One other study showed that a low-sodium and low non-dairy animal protein diet with an adequate calcium intake reduced urinary calcium excretion in hypercalciuric stone formers [54]. The AUA recommends dietary sodium allowance for stone formers should be no more than 100 mEq or 2300 mg daily for most adults [90].

The DASH diet may be appropriate for most stone formers [105]. It is supported by observational studies that demonstrated reduced risk of kidney stones in groups consuming the DASH diet [73]. The DASH diet consists of low sodium, low nondairy animal protein, which is higher in fruits, vegetables, nuts, legumes, whole grains, and dairy products, compared to a typical Western diet. The DASH diet provides about 4–6 oz of animal protein per day, which is adequate for most people. The DASH diet also has benefits in reducing risk of CKD, type 2 diabetes, cardiovascular disease, and stroke, which may coexist in stone formers [106].

Dietary Oxalate

If patients have adequate calcium intake but urinary oxalate levels are elevated, dietary oxalate restriction is appropriate for calcium oxalate stone formers. There are databases of oxalate content of foods, but the values are inconsistent. The Harvard School of Public Health maintains an extensive online oxalate database to provide guidance in managing a low oxalate diet restriction [90].

Tables 25.4 and 25.5 show examples of high oxalate foods and content.

Table 25.4 Oxalate content of foods

Food item (100 g)	Range of oxalate values (mg)	Food item (100 g)	Range of oxalate values (mg)	Food item (100 g)	Range of oxalate values (mg)
Flours and grains		**Herbs and spices**		**Vegetables**	
Barley flour	56	Black pepper	419	Amaranth leaves, raw	1090
Buckwheat flour	269	Caraway seeds	890–900	Asparagus, raw	130
Bulgur, cooked	47	Cardamom, green	4000-4014	Bamboo shoots, raw	23
Cornmeal	54	Coriander seeds	995–1005	Beet leaves, raw	121–916
Couscous	10–65	Cumin	1500-1505	Beet root, boiled	76–675
Grits, corn	57	Curry powder	1065-1070	Bitter melon, raw	71
Millet, cooked	36	Ginger	1480-1488	Broccoli, raw	190
Oats	16	Nutmeg	200–201	Brussel sprouts, raw	360
Rice, basmati	17	Turmeric powder	1910–1914	Cabbage, Chinese, raw	6
Rice, brown, cooked	12			Cabbage, green, raw	100
Rice flour, brown	37	**Legumes**		Carrot, raw	500
Rice bran	238	Anasazi beans, boiled	80	Cassava root, raw	1260
Rye flour, dark	51	Azuki beans, boiled	25	Cauliflower, raw	150
Semolina flour	48	Black beans, boiled	72	Celery	190
Wheat flour, white unbleached	40	Cowpeas, boiled	4	Chicory, raw	210
Wheat flour, whole	67	Fava beans, boiled	22	Chives, raw	1480
Wheat bran	457	Garbanzo beans, boiled	9	Collard greens, raw	450
Wheat germ	44–269	Great Northern beans, boiled	75	Coriander, raw	10
Fruit		Kidney beans, boiled	16	Corn, raw	10
Apple	9–11	Lentils, boiled	8–118	Cucumber, raw	20
Apricot	48–50	Lima beans, boiled	8	Eggplant, raw	190
Avocado	18	Mung beans, boiled	5	Endive, raw	110
Blackberries	19	Navy beans, boiled	57	Garlic, raw	360
Blueberries	15	Peas, green, raw	50	Kale, raw	20
		Peas, split, green, boiled	6	Kale, Chinese, raw	23
Cherries, canned	8	Peas, split, yellow, boiled	5	Leek, raw	89
Currants	19	Pink beans, boiled	75	Lettuce, raw	330
Date	100	Pinto beans, boiled	27	Okra, raw	50

(continued)

Table 25.4 (continued)

Food item (100 g)	Range of oxalate values (mg)	Food item (100 g)	Range of oxalate values (mg)	Food item (100 g)	Range of oxalate values (mg)
Feijoa	60	Red beans, boiled	35	Olives	44
Figs, dried	57	Soybeans, boiled	56	Onion, raw	50
Figs, fresh	18	White beans, small, boiled	78	Parsley, raw	150–1700
Goji berries	138			Parsnip, raw	40
Gooseberries, green	88	**Nuts**		Pepper, raw	40
Grapes, Concord	25	Almonds, roasted	431–490	Potato, raw	50
Grapefruit	10	Cashews, roasted	262–2310	Purslane, raw	850–1310
Guava	17–18	Hazelnuts, raw	167–222	Radish, raw	480
Kiwifruit	23	Macadamia nuts, raw	42	Rutabaga, raw	30
Lemon peel	83	Peanuts, raw	96–705	Snap beans, raw	360
Lime peel	110	Peanut butter	81–705	Spinach, raw	400–970
Mango	10–12	Pecans, raw	64	Squash, raw	20
Orange	21	Pine nuts, raw	198	Sweet potato, raw	240
Papaya	5	Pine nuts, roasted	140	Swiss chard, raw	800–812
Pineapple, canned	26	Pistachio nuts, roasted	49–57	Tomato, raw	50
Pineapple, dried	38	Pumpkin seeds, roasted	14	Tomato, sauce	14
Prunes, dried	34	Sunflower seeds, roasted	9	Turnip, raw	210
Raspberries, black	55	Walnuts, raw	74	Turnip greens, raw	50
Raspberries, red	15			Watercress, raw	310
Rhubarb, raw	260–1235	**Soy-based products**		Yams, cooked	59
Star fruit	80–730	Miso	15	Yard long beans, raw	38
Strawberries	15–25	Soy beverage (240 ml)	5–336		
		Soy flour	107–183	**Other foods**	
		Soy protein	15–496	Chocolate, milk (240 ml)	7
		Soy sauce	11	Chocolate, milk, candy	42–123
		Soy yogurt	47	Chocolate syrup	97
		Soynuts, roasted	1400	Cocoa powder	170–623
		Soynut butter	38–63	Tea (100 ml), black, brewed	48–92
		Tempeh	28		
		Textured vegetable protein	58–584	Tea (100 ml), green, brewed	6–26
		Tofu	2–280	Tea (100 ml) herbal, brewed	0–8

Table 25.5 Oxalate content of foods by common portion size

Food group	Food	Portion size	Oxalate content (mg)	Food group	Food	Portion size	Oxalate content (mg)
Beverages	Hot chocolate	1 cup	65	Potatoes	French fries	4 oz or ½ cup	51
	Tea, brewed	1 cup	14		Baked potato with skin	1 medium	97
	Tomato juice	1 cup	14		Mashed potato	1 cup	29
	Prune juice	1 cup	18		Potato chip	1 oz	21
	Lemonade (frozen concentrate)	8 floz	15		Sweet potato	1 cup	28
Nuts and seeds	Almonds	1 oz or 22 kernels	122	Meat and substitute	Tofu	3.5 oz	13
	Candies with nuts	2 oz	38		Veggie burger	1 patty	24
	Cashews	1 oz or 18 kernels	49		Soy burger	3.5 oz	12
	Peanuts	1 oz	27	Bread, grains, starch	English muffin, whole wheat	1 muffin	12
	Pistachios	1 oz	14		All-purpose flour	1 cup	17
	Mixed nuts with peanuts	1 oz	39		Brown rice, cooked	1 cup	24
	Trail mix	1 oz	15		Buckwheat groats	1 cup, cooked	133
	Walnuts	1 oz or 7 nuts	31		Bulgur, cooked	1 cup	86
	Pecans	1 oz or 15 halves	10		Corn grits	1 cup	97
Vegetables	Bamboo shoots	1 cup	35		Cornmeal	1 cup	64
	Beets	½ cup	76		Couscous	1 cup	15
	Fava beans	½ cup	20		Millet, cooked	1 cup	62
	Navy beans	½ cup	76		Miso	1 cup	40
	Okra	½ cup	57		Soy flour	1 cup	94
	Parsnip	½ cup	15		Whole flour, whole grain	1 cup	29
	Red kidney beans	½ cup	15	Fruits	Dates	1 date	24
	Rhubarb	½ cup	541		Grape fruit	½ fruit	12
	Spinach cooked	½ cup	755		Kiwi	1	16
	Spinach, raw	1 cup	656		Orange	1 fruit	29
	Tomato sauce	½ cup	17		Raspberries	1 cup	48
	Turnip	½ cup mashed	30		Canned pineapple	½ cup	24
	Yams	½ cup	40	Miscellaneous	Peanut butter	1 Tbsp	13
Cakes and cookies	Brownies	1 oz or ½	31		Coco powder	4 tsp	67
	Chocolate syrup	1 Tbsp	38		Miso soup	1 cup	111
	Chocolate chip cookies	1 cookie	11		Lentil soup	1 cup	39

Data source: https://regepi.bwh.harvard.edu/health/Oxalate/files

Complicating the problem are large variations in the oxalate content of foods themselves [107, 108]. For example, the oxalate content of foods vary with the ripeness of the fruit or vegetable when picked and the soil characteristics [107, 108]. Due to the difficulties in restricting dietary oxalate, hyperoxaluria treatment is often focused on adequate calcium intake to modulate oxalate absorption rather than decreased oxalate in the diet [109, 110]. Generally speaking, an adequate amount of calcium, along with lower nondairy animal protein and sodium, and higher amounts of fruits and vegetables and plant-based proteins reduce the risk of calcium oxalate stone formation and recurrence [73]. Although the DASH diet is probably high in oxalate, it contains high fiber and phytates that help to lower oxalate absorption in the GI tract. Patients with IBD and gastric bypass surgery such as Roux-en-Y have enteric hyperoxaluria and absorb excessive amounts of oxalate because of fat malabsorption [58, 111]. For these patients, a more restrictive oxalate diet may provide benefit to decrease hyperoxaluria. An adequate amount of calcium intake and lower fat intake may also help prevent increased oxalate absorption among malabsorption conditions. In addition, calcium supplements taken with meals promote oxalate binding of free oxalate and, therefore, decrease oxalate absorption in the GI tract. Some dietary supplements can elevate urinary oxalate excretion. High doses of ascorbic acid from supplements is metabolized to oxalate [112], and turmeric and cranberry supplements have been associated with higher oxalate levels in the urine [113, 114]. The AUA advises avoiding vitamin C supplements due to calcium oxalate stone risk.

Acid-Forming Foods or Animal Protein

Diets rich in animal protein are associated with increased net acid excretion and a low urinary pH. Low urinary pH is associated with hypocitraturia and, among calcium stone formers, 20–60% of patients have hypocitraturia [115]. Citrate in the urine is a very important inhibitory factor for calcium stone formation [116]. Medical conditions that alter urine pH, and some medications such as acetazolamide and valproic acid, can cause hypocitraturia. Foods with a high potential renal acid load (PRAL) such as meats, fish, poultry, cheese, eggs, and white grains promote acidosis and a low urinary pH. In contrast, fruits and vegetables provide alkali, which can help lower stone formation risk [117]. Some dairy products and lipid-rich foods are considered neutral PRAL [118, 119].

Patients with hypocitraturia and consumption of high PRAL foods can benefit from increasing consumption of fruits and vegetables and decreasing animal protein sources [120]; however, calories need to be adjusted to prevent weight gain. To improve hypocitraturia, both dietary intake of citrate and prescription of potassium or sodium citrate are recommended [121]. In practice, lemon or lime juice is recommended for patients with hypocitraturia with similar pharmacologic effects [101]. Three tablespoons of concentrated lemon juice from two medium-sized fresh lemons added in 1 L water consumed daily can provide a comparable amount of citrate to what is present in 30 milliequivalents (mEq) of potassium citrate divided in three doses with lower cost and possibly less GI side effects [122].

Acidic urine with low pH is a risk factor of uric acid stones and is favorable for CaOx stone formation with hypercalciuria. Usually, 30% of total urinary uric acid is from dietary sources in the Western diet that is primarily from animal protein with a high purine content [123].

Table 25.6 shows acid and alkaline ash foods.

Table 25.6 Acid-ash and alkaline-ash foods

Acid-ash foods		Alkaline ash foods	
Meat	Beef, fish, shellfish, egg, fowl, pork, chicken, veal	Dairy, nuts and protein-rich foods	Butter milk, goat cheese, almonds, chestnuts, pine nuts, Brazil nuts, pecans, tofu, most beans
Dairy and nuts	Most dairy products including milk, cheese especially processed cheese Sweetened yogurt Cottage cheese Nuts: peanuts, pistachio, walnuts		
Fat	Bacon, lard	Fat	Coconuts, sunflower oil, pumpkin seed oil, grape seed oil, canola oil
Starch	All types of bread, especially white, whole wheat products Crackers, cereal, macaroni, spaghetti, noodles (all white flour products), white rice, corn and lentils	Starch	Most beans Taro roots Brown rice Buckwheat
Vegetables	None	Vegetables	All vegetables, including fresh corn
Fruits	Fruit juice with sugar Prunes, cranberry Dried fruits	Fruits	All fresh fruits except cranberry and prunes
Other	Soft drinks, liquor, malt, sugar (white and brown), wine, artificial sweeteners, cocoa, pastries, coffee, fructose, table salt	Other	Garlic Spices: ginger, herbal tea

Adapted from Krause's Food, nutrition & diet therapy, 12th ed. Philadelphia: Saunders; 2008: 952

Calcium Phosphate Stones

Calcium phosphate stones are the second most common type of stones after calcium oxalate stones, but their incidence may be increasing. They are associated with an alkaline urine [124]. If urine is more alkaline (pH > 6.2) with hypercalciuria, SS of CaP is elevated. Also, CaP stones have been seen with primary hyperparathyroidism and RTA without metabolic acidosis. Treatment is aimed at decreasing the SS of CaP by lowering hypercalciuria and increasing fluid intake. When a patient is treated for hypocitraturia, urine pH can be elevated and, therefore, a CaP stone can be formed in this environment [5].

In summary, the primary intervention of recurrent calcium stones is nutritional therapy (low sodium, low protein, and increasing fluid intake); however, thiazide diuretics may be considered with consistent hypercalciuria, especially in IH. Citrate supplementation may be used when hypocitraturia is present or the urine pH is low. Pharmacological treatment should be used with nutritional management to prevent calcium stones.

Uric Acid Stones

In the USA, the incidence of uric acid stones has risen in the past few decades, and the management strategies should include alkalization with a decrease of urine uric acid and an increase of urine volume.

Medical Management

Urine alkalization is the primary treatment for uric acid stones. Uric acid is soluble in alkaline pH>6.5; thus, higher pH is better to prevent uric acid stones [125].

Urinary alkalization is typically achieved with potassium citrate. However, potassium citrate may be costly, and may elevate serum potassium levels especially in patients with impaired kidney function, patients on ACEI or ARBs, and transplant patients on calcineurin inhibitors [126]. In addition, the GI side effects from potassium citrate make patients reluctant to take this preventive medicine.

In a 24-hour urine study, potassium citrate dosing is dependent on urine pH and SS of uric acid. A daily average dose of 60 mEq potassium citrate, divided twice or thrice a day, is a reasonable starting point [127, 128]. Once initiated, a dose adjustment is based on the urinary pH, keeping in mind that a very high urine pH in some individuals may predispose to CaP stone development [127, 129].

Sodium citrate is an alternative medication used to increase urine pH especially in patients who have volume depletion and low sodium in the urine due to GI disease. A study compared the use of sodium citrate and potassium citrate for patients with urolithiasis and both raised urinary pH [127, 130]. However, urinary calcium levels were higher with sodium citrate in contrast to potassium citrate, most likely due to the calciuric effect of increased urinary sodium excretion [127]. Therefore, sodium citrate could be used mainly for volume-depleted patients to help improve citrate and pH.

Sodium bicarbonate is another potential treatment to alkalize the urine [131]. A high dose of sodium bicarbonate should be avoided because it can increase urinary calcium and may contribute to volume overload in susceptible patients. Allopurinol is the most commonly used xanthine oxidase inhibitor to treat gout and prevent uric acid stones. Xanthine oxidase inhibitors such as allopurinol or febuxostat reduce xanthine and hypoxanthine conversion to uric acid, and xanthine oxidase decreases uric acid excretion in the urine [132, 133].

Nutritional Management

The typical American diet has a high purine content from animal protein, which produces approximately 300–400 mg of uric acid per day [127]. Two-thirds of the uric acid produced is excreted in the urine [67]. The urine uric acid concentration is often high (>600 mg/dL) among uric acid stone formers [125]. Exogenous sources of uric acid is from dietary purine (a precursor of uric acid), which is abundant in the typical Western diet and produced by the metabolism of animal protein such as meats, fish, shellfish, and poultry. A diet high in animal protein is also associated with a more acidic urine as discussed previously. Therefore, a diet high in animal protein produces more uric acid and an acidic urine, both risk factors for uric acid stones. A moderate amount of total protein with less animal protein (less than 1.2 g/kg/day) is advisable for uric acid stone formers [134]. Reduction of uric acid excretion and increase of urine pH are major goals in uric acid stone formers [125, 127].

Beer has a high purine content [135], and elevated levels of serum uric acid have been observed with beer consumption but not with small amounts of wine [135, 136]. Whether this contributed to uric acid stones is not known and there is no direct association between alcohol consumption and nephrolithiasis.

Citric acid from the diet can reduce uric acid stone risk by increasing urine pH. A vegetarian diet is low in purine, high in other fiber (phytate), and higher in citrate and produces alkaline ash. Citrus fruits such as lemons, oranges, and limes are rich in citrate. A study conducted by Odvina et al. compared orange juice and lemonade consumption over a week to monitor impact on kidney stone risk factors. Orange juice compared to lemonade resulted in the greatest increase in urinary pH and citrate [137]. A concern about recommending orange juice is its high caloric content for people with diabetes and obesity. Another study was conducted to monitor the effect of long-term consumption of lemonade compared with potassium citrate. The changes of urinary pH was higher in the potassium citrate consumption group but the urinary citrate levels were similar in both groups (700 mg/day for lemonade vs. 800 mg/day for potassium citrate group) [101].

The effect of beverage choice on uric acid stone risk is not clear. Choi et al. showed that coffee and tea intake were associated with lower levels of serum uric acid but the study did not measure urine uric acid [138].

Mineral water contains various levels of bicarbonate [127]. Heilberg et al. evaluated the effects of mineral water on urine pH among calcium oxalate stone formers and found that urine pH and citrate levels were higher with significantly lower SS of uric acids among individuals who consumed mineral water for 3 days than the group that consumed regular water [127, 139, 140].

Consumption of fructose, especially high concentrated fructose corn syrup, has increased in the past decade. When metabolized, fructose is transformed into purine, the precursor of uric acid. Observational studies showed that hyperuricemia and gout were positively associated with increased fructose consumption [141]. Also, in a large prospective study, Taylor et al. concluded that fructose was an independent risk factor for kidney stones but nonfructose carbohydrates did not show the associations [142]. Fructose infusion in animal studies increased insulin resistance and it was postulated that fructose can be a primary contributor of lower urine pH and possible kidney stone risk factor [127, 142, 143].

A vegetarian diet and the DASH diet, which are rich in citrate, can generate an alkaline urine which has beneficial effects for the prevention of uric acid stones [127]. A study conducted by Heilberg et al. showed higher urine citrate and pH levels following the DASH diet, but the study did not measure the stone risk [73, 139]. In addition, the DASH diet has other health benefits such as weight loss, which possibly improves metabolic syndrome and insulin sensitivity, and increased urine pH.

Cystine Stones

Cystine stones are rare and represent about 1% of all stones in adults and 5% and 10% in children [39, 144]. They are formed when the amino acid cystine is highly concentrated in the urine and occur exclusively in patients with the genetic condition of cystinuria, which has a prevalence of about 1/7000 [145]. Cystinuria is caused by a genetic disorder related to defective transport of cystine in the kidney, leading to excretion of a large amount of cystine and other cationic amino acids (ornithine, arginine, and lysine or COAL) in the urine. Nephrolithiasis is the dominant clinical feature; however, about 6% of patients with cystinuria do not present with stone disease [145].

The normal excretion of cystine is less than 30 mg/day. However, in patients with cystinuria, cystine excretion often exceeds 400 mg/day [146]. Cystine stones are seen from infancy to the fifth decade of life but the median age of presentation is 12 years [146, 147]. Eighty percent of symptomatic cystine stone formers had a first stone episode in the second decade [147]. In addition to having stones at an earlier age, cystinuria patients tend to have more bilateral, more frequent, and more staghorn calculi than other stone formers [38, 148, 149].

Cystinuria is diagnosed with high urine cystine levels and all patients with cystinuria should complete a 24-hour urine test to assess other metabolic stone risk factors. Urine pH and urine volume are the most important factors to determine cystine stones.

Cystine is soluble in high urine pH, especially at pH of 7 or higher. At a pH of 7, cystine is soluble at a concentration of 250 mg/L. This doubles to 500 mg/L at pH 7.5 and goes up further at pH of 8 [150–152].

Medical Management

Patients often have recurrent and multiple stones and many patients require urological procedures [150]. Despite the fact that medical therapy reduces the number of recurrent stones and removal procedures up to 78% and 52%, respectively, medical therapy compliance is poor for cystinuria patients [38, 150]. Urine alkalization, high urine volume, and cystine-binding medications are the mainstay of medical management.

Potassium citrate is the mainstay of treatment to alkalinize the urine. Sodium bicarbonate can be used but it can increase sodium load. Acetazolamide can also be used as a last choice, but it is poorly tolerated and may have adverse effects on bone health due to metabolic acidosis [152].

High fluid intake (>3–4 L/day) can lower concentration of cystine. Tolvaptan, an anti-diuretic hormone receptor antagonist, has been proposed as an option in patients with low urine volume; however, it is very expensive and has risk of liver disease [153].

When patients fail to achieve urine alkalization and fluid intake, CBTDs are recommended. These drugs form a complex with cystine monomer that is 50 times more soluble than cystine and thus prevent crystallization [154, 155]. D-penicillamine and 2-meracptopropionylglycine (tiopronin) are used in clinical practice but tiopronin has less side effects and is better tolerated among cystine stone formers [156]. Several studies were conducted to compare CBTD use with conservative managements, and the former group showed reduced recurrence of stones by 32% to 65% and a reduction of stone size as well as better dissolution [152, 157].

Nutritional Management

The goal of nutritional management is to increase fluid intake and to decrease cystine concentration to less than 300 mg/L, but this may be hard to achieve in clinical practice and requires vigilance with scheduled fluid intake [158]. A low animal protein diet is also recommended to help urine alkalization and to lower cystine production from methionine, a precursor of cystine, which is abundant in animal protein [159]. However, methionine is an essential amino acid especially for children and adolescents who require normal protein intake for overall growth. Also, a low-sodium diet can lower cystine concentration in urine but the mechanism is unknown [160]. Lastly, fruit and vegetable intake are recommended as well as the DASH diet to increase urine pH [120].

Struvite/Staghorn Calculi

Struvite stones are composed of magnesium ammonium phosphate that is usually formed secondary to genitourinary infection and urinary stasis. Other risk factors include urinary tract obstruction, indwelling catheters, neurogenic bladder, and immobility [161, 162]. Struvite stones are more common in women probably because of their increased risk of urinary tract infection. They often form staghorn calculi, which are large stones that branch into the urinary space. While documented urinary tract infection is common in patients with staghorn calculi, which is present in 59% to 68% of all patients and 74% in women with bilateral staghorn calculi [163, 164], recent data suggest that staghorn calculi are not necessarily related to infection and are not necessarily composed of struvite. A study looking at staghorn calculi showed that only about half are struvite while the rest consist of calcium phosphate, calcium oxalate, uric acid, or cystine [164].

The standard treatment of struvite and staghorn calculi is surgical, but metabolic evaluation may be warranted in some patients because such stones can be associated with metabolic abnormalities. The use of antibiotics and documented clearance of infection are also important for the prevention of struvite stones [162], but the data are scarce regarding the choice and duration of antibiotics [165].

Nutritional Management

There is no specific dietary modification that can help lower the recurrence of struvite stones. However, since staghorn stones are made from various stone types, 24-hour urine analysis and general nutritional guidelines such as increasing fluid intake to >3 L/day, a low-sodium diet, and moderate protein consumption would be appropriate.

Table 25.7 presents a summary of current nutritional guidelines from AUA and Table 25.8 shows a general diet guideline for stone prevention.

Table 25.9 presents a summary of medical and nutritional recommendations for different types of stones.

Table 25.7 Nutrient recommendation for kidney stones

Nutrients	Recommendation
Calcium	1000–1200 mg/day
Oxalate	40–50 mg/day
Sodium	<2300 mg/day
Protein	0.8–1.4 g/kg/day
Fluid	>3 L/day to produce urine volume >2.5 L
Vitamin D	Low dose if vitamin D insufficiency or deficiency (1000 IU/day)
Vitamin C	Dietary reference intake (DRI)

Adapted from [90]

Table 25.8 General diet guidelines for stone prevention

Drink plenty of fluid: at least 3 L/day or more
  Any type of fluids such as water, coffee, and lemonade except grapefruit juice and soda have shown beneficial effect.
  Produce less concentrated urine with good volume (*at least 2.5 L/day*).

Avoid foods with high oxalate
  Spinach, lot of berries, chocolate, wheat bran, nuts, beets, and rhubarb should be eliminated from the diet if possible.
  Discuss with nutritionist for more questions.

Consume adequate amount of dietary calcium
  Three servings of dairy consumption per day will help lower the risk of calcium stones.
  Consume with meals.

Avoid extra calcium supplements
  Calcium supplement should be individualized by physician.

Avoid high-protein diet
  With high protein intake, kidney will excrete more calcium; therefore it will form more stones in the kidney.
  Cut down animal protein to lower renal acid load.

Avoid high salt diet
  High sodium diet can increase calcium in the urine so increase the stone risk.
  Blood pressure control is also important for stone formation and high salt diet can lead to high blood pressure.

Avoid high dose of vitamin C supplement
  Recommend to take 60 mg/day (US dietary reference intake).
  Excess amount (1000 mg/day) may produce more oxalate in the body.

Developed by H. Han, at Harvard Vanguard Medical Associates (Atrius Health), Department of Nephrology

Table 25.9 Nutritional and medical recommendation for different types of stones

Type	Medical	Nutrition
CaOx	Treatment of hypercalciuria Low urine pH: K-citrate Prebiotics/ probiotics	Fluid: >3 L: all types except soda/sugar-containing fluid Ca: Ca-rich foods 1000–120 mg Avoid low Ca intake or high-Ca supplement Low Na: 2300 mg (100 mEq) Oxalate: Avoid very high oxalate foods. If consuming a small amount, consume with Ca-rich foods at the same time Moderate amount of animal protein (acid-forming foods)
CaP	Monitor primary hyperparathyroidism and RTA	High fluid intake Individualize with urinary Ca and medical condition
Uric acid	Urine alkalization K-citrate Na-citrate Sodium bicarbonate Xanthine oxidase inhibitor	Fluid >3 L include mineral water, citrate rich sources Moderate protein especially animal protein DASH diet Cut down high fructose consumption Vegetarian diet
Cystine	Urine alkalization (pH higher is better) High urine volume Cystine-binding thiol drugs (CBTDs)	Fluid >3–4 L Low to moderate animal protein esp low methionine Low sodium: 2300 mg DASH/high fruit and vegetable intake
Struvite	Use of antibiotic to avoid infection	Fluid >3 L Low sodium: 2300 mg

Abbreviations: *CaOx* calcium oxalate stone, *CaP* calcium phosphate stone, *RTA* renal tubular acidosis

Special Considerations

Diabetes Mellitus

According to the NHS I and II and the Health Professionals Follow-up Study [HPFS]), there is a higher prevalence of kidney stone formation among diabetics than nondiabetics [6]. This may be due to defective renal acid excretion in diabetics, leading to uric acid stone formation. A study demonstrated that patients with glucose intolerance and type 2 diabetes have more pure uric acid stones than CaOx stones [166, 167]. Other studies have shown that patients with diabetes have more uric acid stones than those without diabetes (28.5%–33% vs. 6.2%–13%, respectively) [166–169]. Diabetes may also contribute to calcium stone risk. In normal subjects, postprandial insulinemia is associated with increased calcium and phosphorus excretion. Postprandial hyperinsulinemia may play an important physiologic role in the regulation of renal tubular calcium reabsorption [35].

Hypertension

According to a study by Soucie et al., there was a higher prevalence of kidney stones in hypertensive versus normotensive subjects [42]. A large prospective cohort study of 51,529 men also showed an association between nephrolithiasis and hypertension. In this study, most (79.5%) of the stone patients reported that nephrolithiasis occurred either prior to or concomitant with the diagnosis of hypertension [170]. Some have hypothesized that nephrolithiasis may increase the risk of hypertension [171]. Conversely, interference of calcium metabolism is frequent among patients with essential hypertension [172–174], and it can lead to hypercalciuria. In addition, there was an independent association of hypocitraturia and hypertension in the large observational study via evaluation of 24-hour urine collections [175]. Apler et al. postulated that uric acid stone risk is higher in both adults and pediatric hypertension patients with elevated blood uric acid levels [176]. At this point there remains an association without enough data to establish cause and effect.

Cardiovascular Disease

The association between cardiovascular disease and nephrolithiasis is not very well known. It was first reported in a longitudinal study with a 20-year follow-up where a significant association was found between kidney stones and subclinical carotid atherosclerosis [177]. A population-based study that used ultrasounds to determine carotid thickness and stenosis found an association between increased carotid thickness and symptomatic kidney stone formation. Also, Hamano et al. reported that calcium oxalate stone cases were higher among those with a history of coronary artery disease patients than normal subjects [178]. Rule's more recent study revealed an increased risk (31%) of myocardial infarction in stone formers, after adjustment for other comorbidities associated with myocardial infarction [179]. Whether this represents a causal connection or an association based on shared risk factors remains unknown.

Chronic Kidney Disease

Although nephrolithiasis is not commonly recognized as a cause of CKD in the absence of obstructive uropathy, there are studies that show an association between the development of CKD and nephrolithiasis [180]. After adjusting the common causes of CKD and ESKD such as diabetes, hypertension, and cardiovascular disease, there was an independent risk of CKD among stone formers [181, 182]. According to data collected from NHANES III, stone formers who are overweight or obese (BMI $\geq$ 27 kg/m^2) have a higher prevalence of lower glomerular filtration rate (GFR) than normal BMI subjects. Overweight stone formers have more stage 3 CKD (GFR: 30–59 mL/min/1.73m^2) with relative risk ratio of 1.87 than overweight non-stone formers [183]. As with hypertension and cardiovascular disease, it is not clear if this represents shared risk factors or if the lithogenic process causes subtle renal damage [170].

Gastrointestinal Disease–Related Medical Conditions, Gastric Bypass Surgery, and Kidney Stones

Gastrointestinal Disease

GI disease can cause low urine volume, which leads to concentrated urine and increases all types of stone risks [58]. This may be due to an inadequate intake of fluid (due to nausea and vomiting) or to loss of fluid from diarrhea. A high fluid intake is the most important recommendation of stone prevention in this population [16, 56, 184].

GI disease can also lead to increased oxalate absorption and secondary hyperoxaluria. Unlike primary hyperoxaluria, which is a genetic defect of liver oxalate metabolism, secondary hyperoxaluria is caused by a high dietary oxalate, fat malabsorption, alterations in the gut microbiome, and/or genetic variations in oxalate transporters in the gut.

Under normal conditions, calcium binds to dietary oxalate in the distal intestine forming a complex that is excreted in the stool. Other nutrients such as magnesium, fatty acids, phytate, and bile salts also bind oxalate alter absorption [184]. In patients with GI disease, calcium binds malabsorbed fat instead of oxalate, which increases free oxalate absorption. Also, inflammation increases the permeability of the intestinal mucosa allowing excess oxalate absorption. These combined processes are referred to as enteric hyperoxaluria [185]. GI disease may also result in disruption of normal enteric bacteria. *Oxalobacter formigens* is normal fecal flora and it metabolizes oxalate to carbon dioxide and formate, decreasing available oxalate for absorption [186].

Bariatric Surgery

Obesity is a risk factor of nephrolithiasis; some might think that weight loss related to bariatric surgery would decrease stone risk. However, risk of stone formation among bariatric surgery patients increases significantly due to malabsorption of all nutrients, macronutrients, and essential vitamins and minerals, which may occur with substantial weight loss [57]. Fat malabsorption may be present and contribute to calcium binding in a manner similar to patients with GI disease [187]. Supporting this hypothesis, a low fat diet showed lower urinary oxalate levels than a normal fat intake [188]. Vitamin B deficiencies due to malabsorption, which are co-factors of oxalate metabolism, may increase urinary oxalate levels. Although the microbiome alteration after bariatric surgery is not well characterized, a decrease in oxalate-degrading bacteria such as *Oxalobacter formigens* in patients after gastric bypass was observed [189]. Hypocitraturia is also seen with gastric bypass surgery with acidosis. A combination of various factors after bariatric surgery can lead to increased free oxalate absorption and causes enteric hyperoxaluria [190, 191].

Conclusion

Risk factors of kidney stone formation include various genetic, medical, environmental, and dietary causes. Most nephrolithiasis patients have recurrent kidney stones throughout their lifetime. Kidney stone prevention strategies should be individualized based on stone type when known and assessment of stone risk factors. A 24-hour urine collection is particularly useful and provides information on specific data about urine composition. Dietary interventions based on the clinical assessment and 24-hour urine studies are first line to prevent recurrence. Pharmaceutical interventions are also appropriate in certain circumstances. In general, prevention of kidney stones includes fluid intake adequate to produce more than 2.5 L urine output per day, calcium intake to achieve the standard daily allowance of 1000–1200 mg/day, a moderate amount of protein especially animal protein, moderate oxalate intake, and low-sodium diet. In addition, appropriate medical treatment with thiazides, citrate salts, and other medications may be helpful to prevent further stone formation. All interventions should be individualized based on multiple and serial 24-hour urine collections.

Practical Rules of Thumb

- Do not discuss risks in general BEFORE the DATA (i.e., 24-hour urinalysis)
  - People make stones for different reasons.
  - There are different types of stone risks and some individuals like to follow a diet to prevent all types of stones, which can lead to inaccurate stone risk analysis.
  - There may be bias when the patients collect the urine. A collection should be done without changing the diet and fluid intakes.
  - Patients often have unnecessary restrictions of their diet, which have effects on the cause of stone risks.

- Do not treat without DATA
  - Prescribing thiazides without a low-sodium (Na) diet or with low urine Ca:

    24-h urine analysis should be performed before prescribing thiazides. If the patient has a high urinary Na with elevated Ca levels, a low-Na diet should be instructed first in an effort to lower urinary calcium.

    If a thiazide is prescribed without a low-Na diet, the patient can have polyuria until the body reaches a steady state with hypokalemia, which can lower citrate levels in the urine, which then lowers pH and eventually increases SS CaOx.

  - Prescribing citrate without knowing Ca and pH.

    Citrate will increase urine pH; therefore, urinary Ca and pH should be evaluated first. If the patient has a high urinary Ca with normal pH and citrate is prescribed, urine pH may rise too much, which will increase risk of CaP stones.

- Use of allopurinol for gout and stone risk

    - Allopurinol is commonly used for treatment of gout. If a patient is taking allopurinol, a low purine diet should be prescribed, and urine pH should be monitored to prevent uric acid stones.
    - Allopurinol is generally second-line therapy for uric acid stones after failure of urinary alkalization.

- Using sodium citrate instead of potassium citrate

    - If the patient has GI disorders such as IBD, the patient may have GI loss of Na, low volume status, and high oxalate absorption, which leads to increased risk of CaOx stones. When the patient has a low urine output, low urinary Na, and high urinary oxalate with low urine pH, sodium citrate is a better choice than potassium citrate to increase pH and Na status, which will improve volume status.

- Low urinary Ca

    - If the patient has a low urinary Ca level, it may decrease the risk of Ca stones, but the patient should be evaluated for negative Ca balance or bone disease.

- Hyperparathyroidism increases calcium and phosphorus excretion

    - If hyperparathyroidism is observed in the absence of vitamin D deficiency (and especially with hypercalcemia or hypercalciuria) consider primary hyperparathyroidism.

Acknowledgement

Dr. Han is grateful for the contributions and support of Drs. Mutter and Nasser to this chapter.

Case Studies

Case 1

The following 24-h urine values were observed in a 45-year-old man.

	Volume	Ca	Oxalate	Citrate	Uric acid	pH	Creatinine	Na	Phos	NH$_4$
Results	2.506	364 mg	77 mg	1278 mg	1.806 g	5.1	3040 mg	426 mEq	1.5 g	108 mM
Ref value	>2.5 L	<250	<40	200–1000	<0.8	5.8–6.2		<150	<1.2	<60

Case Questions and Answers

1. What type of stone risk does this patient have?

    (a) Calcium oxalate
    (b) Uric acid
    (c) Struvite
    (d) Cysteine

    Answer: The answer is A and B – CaOx and uric acid stone. Calcium and oxalate levels are high. Also, uric acid level is very high with low pH.

2. What would be the preferred treatment strategy for the patient in case 1?

   (a) Allopurinol
   (b) Na citrate
   (c) K citrate and increase urine volume to 3 L
   (d) Na and protein-restricted and low oxalate diet
   (e) Thiazide diuretics

   Answer: The answer is D – sodium and protein-restricted and low oxalate diet.

   - The patient has a large excretion rate of sodium, which will increase urinary calcium excretion.
   - He also has high urinary oxalate, which increases CaOx stone risk with low urine pH.
   - High protein intake is suggested by the elevated ammonium, uric acid, and phosphate in the urine, as well as by the high creatinine excretion.
   - One would need to confirm that this is not an over-collection.

Case 2

A 45-year-old woman is referred for recurrent oxalate stone formation. The following is her 24-h urine result.

	Vol	SSCaOx	Ca	Ox	Cit	SSCa	UpH	SSUA	UA
Results	1.52	10.04	40	143	23	0.09	5.5	0.53	0.202
Ref value	>2.5	6–10	<200	20–40	>550	0.5–2	5.8–6.2	0–1	<0.75

Case Questions and Answers

1. What is the likely cause of her disorder?

   (a) Renal tubular acidosis resulting in hypocitraturia
   (b) Dietary excess of nuts, chocolate, and berries
   (c) Hyperparathyroidism
   (d) Crohn's disease
   (e) Oxalosis

   Answer: The answer is D – Crohn's disease causing low urinary calcium excretion.

   - There is low citrate, high oxalate, and low volume in this intestinal malabsorptive condition.
   - RTA does not explain increased urine oxalate.
   - Nuts, etc., do not explain the degree of hyperoxaluria.
   - Oxalosis does not explain low urine citrate and low urine calcium.

2. The preferred treatment for the patient in case 2 would include all except the following:

   (a) Na citrate
   (b) Ca supplementation with meals
   (c) Cholestyramine
   (d) K citrate
   (e) Dietary oxalate restriction

Answer: The answer is D. K citrate is not ideal.

- In this case of volume depletion associated with intestinal disorders, alkali therapy with sodium salts is preferable as it may increase the extracellular volume and urine output.
- Restrict dietary oxalate.
- Use cholestyramine to bind intestinal oxalate.
- Calcium with meals binds intestinal oxalate.

References

1. Scales CD Jr, Smith AC, Hanley JM, Saigal CS, Urologic Diseases in America Project. Prevalence of kidney stones in the United States. Eur Urol. 2012;62(1):160–5.
2. Stamatelou KK, Francis ME, Jones CA, Nyberg LM, Curhan GC. Time trends in reported prevalence of kidney stones in the United States: 1976-1994. Kidney Int. 2003;63(5):1817–23.
3. Saigal CS, Joyce G, Timilsina AR, Urologic Diseases in America Project. Direct and indirect costs of nephrolithiasis in an employed population: opportunity for disease management? Kidney Int. 2005;68(4):1808–14.
4. Curhan GC. Epidemiology of stone disease. Urol Clin N Am. 2007;34(3):287–+.
5. Worcester EM, Coe FL. Nephrolithiasis. Prim Care. 2008;35(2):369–91, vii.
6. Taylor EN, Stampfer MJ, Curhan GC. Diabetes mellitus and the risk of nephrolithiasis. Kidney Int. 2005;68(3):1230–5.
7. Taylor EN, Stampfer MJ, Curhan GC. Obesity, weight gain, and the risk of kidney stones. JAMA. 2005;293(4):455–62.
8. Carbone A, Al Salhi Y, Tasca A, et al. Obesity and kidney stone disease: a systematic review. Minerva Urol Nefrol. 2018;70(4):393–400.
9. Kelly C, Geraghty RM, Somani BK. Nephrolithiasis in the obese patient. Curr Urol Rep. 2019;20(7):36.
10. Brikowski TH, Lotan Y, Pearle MS. Climate-related increase in the prevalence of urolithiasis in the United States. Proc Natl Acad Sci U S A. 2008;105(28):9841–6.
11. Pearle MS, Calhoun EA, Curhan GC, Urologic Diseases of America Project. Urologic diseases in America project: urolithiasis. J Urol. 2005;173(3):848–57.
12. Coe FL, Evan A, Worcester E. Kidney stone disease. J Clin Invest. 2005;115(10):2598–608.
13. Costa-Bauza A, Ramis M, Montesinos V, et al. Type of renal calculi: variation with age and sex. World J Urol. 2007;25(4):415–21.
14. Lieske JC, Rule AD, Krambeck AE, et al. Stone composition as a function of age and sex. Clin J Am Soc Nephrol. 2014;9(12):2141–6.
15. Daudon M, Frochot V, Bazin D, Jungers P. Drug-induced kidney stones and crystalline nephropathy: pathophysiology. Prev Treat Drugs. 2018;78(2):163–201.
16. Moe OW. Kidney stones: pathophysiology and medical management. Lancet. 2006;367(9507):333–44.
17. Kato Y, Taniguchi N, Okuyama M, Kakizaki H. Three cases of urolithiasis associated with sarcoidosis: a review of Japanese cases. Int J Urol. 2007;14(10):954–6.
18. Sharma OP. Hypercalcemia in granulomatous disorders: a clinical review. Curr Opin Pulm Med. 2000;6(5):442–7.
19. Qiu SR, Wierzbicki A, Orme CA, et al. Molecular modulation of calcium oxalate crystallization by osteopontin and citrate. Proc Natl Acad Sci U S A. 2004;101(7):1811–5.
20. Qiu SR, Orme CA. Dynamics of biomineral formation at the near-molecular level. Chem Rev. 2008;108(11):4784–822.
21. Coe FL, Parks JH, Nakagawa Y. Inhibitors and promoters of calcium oxalate crystallization their relationship to the pathogenesis and treatment of nephrolithiasis. 1992:757–800.
22. Aggarwal KP, Narula S, Kakkar M, Tandon C. Nephrolithiasis: molecular mechanism of renal stone formation and the critical role played by modulators. Biomed Res Int. 2013;2013:292953.
23. De Yoreo JJ, Qiu SR, Hoyer JR. Molecular modulation of calcium oxalate crystallization. Am J Physiol Renal Physiol. 2006;291(6):F1123–31.
24. Rimer JD, An Z, Zhu Z, et al. Crystal growth inhibitors for the prevention of L-cystine kidney stones through molecular design. Science. 2010;330(6002):337–41.
25. Ingimarsson JP, Krambeck AE, Pais VM Jr. Diagnosis and management of nephrolithiasis. Surg Clin North Am. 2016;96(3):517–32.
26. Lynch M NS. Evaluation of Patients with Nephrolithiasis. In: Han H MW, Nasser S, ed. Nutritional and Medical Management of Kidney Stones. Switzerland: Humana Press/Springer; 2019:63–81.

27. Brisbane W, Bailey MR, Sorensen MD. An overview of kidney stone imaging techniques. Nat Rev Urol. 2016;13(11):654–62.

28. Castle SM, Cooperberg MR, Sadetsky N, Eisner BH, Stoller ML. Adequacy of a single 24-hour urine collection for metabolic evaluation of recurrent nephrolithiasis. J Urol. 2010;184(2):579–83.

29. Reilly RF, Perazella MA. Nephrology in 30 days. 2nd ed. New York: McGraw-Hill; 2014.

30. Asplin JR. Evaluation of the kidney stone patient. Semin Nephrol. 2008;28(2):99–110.

31. Curhan GC, Taylor EN. 24-h uric acid excretion and the risk of kidney stones. Kidney Int. 2008;73(4):489–96.

32. Asplin JR. Hyperoxaluric calcium nephrolithiasis. Endocrinol Metab Clin N Am. 2002;31(4):927–+.

33. Vezzoli G, Terranegra A, Arcidiacono T, Soldati L. Genetics and calcium nephrolithiasis. Kidney Int. 2011;80(6):587–93.

34. Coe FL, Parks JH, Moore ES. Familial idiopathic hypercalciuria. N Engl J Med. 1979;300(7):337–40.

35. Worcester EM, Gillen DL, Evan AP, et al. Evidence that postprandial reduction of renal calcium reabsorption mediates hypercalciuria of patients with calcium nephrolithiasis. Am J Physiol Renal Physiol. 2007;292(1):F66–75.

36. Worcester EM, Evan AP, Coe FL, et al. A test of the hypothesis that oxalate secretion produces proximal tubule crystallization in primary hyperoxaluria type I. Am J Physiol Renal Physiol. 2013;305(11):F1574–84.

37. Worcester E. Pathophysiology of Kidney Stone Formation. In: Han H MW, Nasser S, ed. Nutritional and Medical Management of Kidney Stones. Switzerland: Humana Press, Springer; 2019:21–42.

38. Worcester EM, Coe FL, Evan AP, Parks JH. Reduced renal function and benefits of treatment in cystinuria vs other forms of nephrolithiasis. BJU Int. 2006;97(6):1285–90.

39. Prot-Bertoye C, Lebbah S, Daudon M, et al. CKD and its risk factors among patients with cystinuria. Clin J Am Soc Nephrol. 2015;10(5):842–51.

40. Soucie JM, Thun MJ, Coates RJ, McClellan W, Austin H. Demographic and geographic variability of kidney stones in the United States. Kidney Int. 1994;46(3):893–9.

41. Robertson WG, Peacock M, Heyburn PJ, Hanes FA. Epidemiological risk factors in calcium stone disease. Scand J Urol Nephrol Suppl. 1980;53:15–30.

42. Soucie JM, Coates RJ, McClellan W, Austin H, Thun M. Relation between geographic variability in kidney stones prevalence and risk factors for stones. Am J Epidemiol. 1996;143(5):487–95.

43. Borghi L, Meschi T, Amato F, Briganti A, Novarini A, Giannini A. Urinary volume, water and recurrences in idiopathic calcium nephrolithiasis: a 5-year randomized prospective study. J Urol. 1996;155(3):839–43.

44. Curhan GC, Willett WC, Speizer FE, Stampfer MJ. Beverage use and risk for kidney stones in women. Ann Intern Med. 1998;128(7):534–+.

45. Curhan GC, Willett WC, Knight EL, Stampfer MJ. Dietary factors and the risk of incident kidney stones in younger women – nurses' health study II. Arch Intern Med. 2004;164(8):885–91.

46. Curhan GC, Willett WC, Rimm EB, Spiegelman D, Stampfer MJ. Prospective study of beverage use and the risk of kidney stones. Am J Epidemiol. 1996;143(3):240–7.

47. Ferraro PM, Taylor EN, Gambaro G, Curhan GC. Caffeine intake and the risk of kidney stones. Am J Clin Nutr. 2014;100(6):1596–603.

48. Ferraro PM, Taylor EN, Gambaro G, Curhan GC. Soda and other beverages and the risk of kidney stones. Clin J Am Soc Nephrol. 2013;8(8):1389–95.

49. Paleerath P, Visith T. Caffeine in kidney stone disease: risk or benefit? Adv Nutr. 2018;9(4):419–24.

50. Curhan GC, Willett WC, Rimm EB, Stampfer MJ. A prospective-study of dietary calcium and other nutrients and the risk of symptomatic kidney-stones. N Engl J Med. 1993;328(12):833–8.

51. Curhan GC, Willett WC, Speizer FE, Spiegelman D, Stampfer MJ. Comparison of dietary calcium with supplemental calcium and other nutrients as factors affecting the risk for kidney stones in women. Ann Intern Med. 1997;126(7):497–+.

52. Taylor EN, Stampfer MJ, Curhan GC. Dietary factors and the risk of incident kidney stones in men: new insights after 14 years of follow-up. J Am Soc Nephrol. 2004;15(12):3225–32.

53. Bataille P, Charransol G, Gregoire I, et al. Effect of calcium restriction on renal excretion of oxalate and the probability of stones in the various pathophysiological groups with calcium stones. J Urol. 1983;130(2):218–23.

54. Borghi L, Schianchi T, Meschi T, et al. Comparison of two diets for the prevention of recurrent stones in idiopathic hypercalciuria. N Engl J Med. 2002;346(2):77–84.

55. Holmes RP, Assimos DG. The impact of dietary oxalate on kidney stone formation. Urol Res. 2004;32(5):311–6.

56. Fink HA, Akornor JW, Garimella PS, et al. Diet, fluid, or supplements for secondary prevention of nephrolithiasis: a systematic review and meta-analysis of randomized trials. Eur Urol. 2009;56(1):72–80.

57. Wong YV, Cook P, Somani BK. The association of metabolic syndrome and urolithiasis. Int J Endocrinol. 2015;2015:570674.

58. Worcester EM. Stones from bowel disease. Endocrinol Metab Clin N Am. 2002;31(4):979–+.

59. Siener R, Honow R, Voss S, Seidler A, Hesse A. Oxalate content of cereals and cereal products. J Agric Food Chem. 2006;54(8):3008–11.

60. Lemann J, Piering WF, Lennon EJ. Possible role of carbohydrate-induced calciuria in calcium oxalate kidney-stone formation. N Engl J Med. 1969;280(5):232–&.

61. Muldowney FP, Freaney R, Moloney MF. Importance of dietary-sodium in the hypercalciuria syndrome. Kidney Int. 1982;22(3):292–6.

62. Coe F, Worcester EM. Idiopathic hypercalciuria. In: Coe F, Worcester EM, Lingeman JE, Evan AP, editors. Kidney stones: medical and surgical management. 2nd ed. New Delhi: Jaypee Brother Medical Publishers; 2018. p. 276–302.

63. Cameron MA, Maalouf NM, Adams-Huet B, Moe OW, Sakhaee K. Urine composition in type 2 diabetes: predisposition to uric acid nephrolithiasis. J Am Soc Nephrol. 2006;17(5):1422–8.

64. Massey LK, Kynast-Gales SA. Diets with either beef or plant proteins reduce risk of calcium oxalate precipitation in patients with a history of calcium kidney stones. J Am Diet Assoc. 2001;101(3):326–31.

65. Sorensen MD, Kahn AJ, Reiner AP, et al. Impact of nutritional factors on incident kidney stone formation: a report from the WHI OS. J Urol. 2012;187(5):1645–9.

66. Moran ME. Uric acid stone disease. Front Biosci Landmark. 2003;8:S1339–55.

67. Maiuolo J, Oppedisano F, Gratteri S, Muscoli C, Mollace V. Regulation of uric acid metabolism and excretion. Int J Cardiol. 2016;213:8–14.

68. Kessler T, Hesse A. Cross-over study of the influence of bicarbonate-rich mineral water on urinary composition in comparison with sodium potassium citrate in healthy male subjects. Br J Nutr. 2000;84(6):865–71.

69. Kessler T, Jansen B, Hesse A. Effect of blackcurrant-, cranberry- and plum juice consumption on risk factors associated with kidney stone formation. Eur J Clin Nutr. 2002;56(10):1020–3.

70. Kenny J-ES, Goldfarb DS. Update on the pathophysiology and management of uric acid renal stones. Curr Rheumatol Rep. 2010;12(2):125–9.

71. Fink HA, Wilt TJ, Eidman KE, Garimella PS, MacDonald R, Rutks IR. Medical management to prevent recurrent nephrolithiasis in adults: a systematic review for an American College of Physicians Clinical Guideline (vol 158, pg 535, 2013). Ann Intern Med. 2013;159(3):230.

72. Lemann J, Pleuss JA, Gray RW, Hoffmann RG. Potassium administration increases and potassium deprivation reduces urinary calcium excretion in healthy-adults. Kidney Int. 1991;39(5):973–83.

73. Taylor EN, Fung TT, Curhan GC. DASH-style diet associates with reduced risk for kidney stones. J Am Soc Nephrol. 2009;20(10):2253–9.

74. Taylor EN, Stampfer MJ, Mount DB, Curhan GC. DASH-style diet and 24-hour urine composition. Clin J Am Soc Nephrol. 2010;5(12):2315–22.

75. Grases F, Garcia-Gonzalez R, Torres JJ, Llobera A. Effects of phytic acid on renal stone formation in rats. Scand J Urol Nephrol. 1998;32(4):261–5.

76. Grases F, March JG, Prieto RM, et al. Urinary phytate in calcium oxalate stone formers and healthy people – dietary effects on phytate excretion. Scand J Urol Nephrol. 2000;34(3):162–4.

77. Traxer O, Huet B, Poindexter J, Pak CYC, Pearle MS. Effect of ascorbic acid consumption on urinary stone risk factors. J Urol. 2003;170(2):397–401.

78. Ferraro PM, Curhan GC, Gambaro G, Taylor EN. Total, dietary, and supplemental vitamin C intake and risk of incident kidney stones. Am J Kidney Dis. 2016;67(3):400–7.

79. Curhan GC, Willett WC, Speizer FE, Stampfer MJ. Intake of vitamins B6 and C and the risk of kidney stones in women. J Am Soc Nephrol. 1999;10(4):840–5.

80. Curhan GC, Willett WC, Rimm EB, Stampfer MJ. A prospective study of the intake of vitamins C and B6, and the risk of kidney stones in men. J Urol. 1996;155(6):1847–51.

81. Penniston KL, Nakada SY, Hansen KE. Vitamin D repletion does not alter urinary calcium excretion in postmenopausal women. J Urol. 2008;179(4):504–5.

82. Gupta M, Korets R, Leaf DE, et al. Vitamin D repletion does not increase calcium excretion among patients with kidney stones. J Endourol. 2011;25:A245–6.

83. Letavernier E, Daudon M. Vitamin D, hypercalciuria and kidney stones. Nutrients. 2018;10(3):366.

84. Kasote DM, Jagtap SD, Thapa D, Khyade MS, Russell WR. Herbal remedies for urinary stones used in India and China: a review. J Ethnopharmacol. 2017;203:55–68.

85. Kieley S, Dwivedi R, Monga M. Ayurvedic medicine and renal calculi. J Endourol. 2008;22(8):1613–6.

86. Miyaoka R, Monga M. Use of traditional chinese medicine in the management of urinary stone disease. Int Braz J Urol. 2009;35(4):396–405.

87. Assimos D, Krambeck A, Miller NL, et al. Surgical management of stones: American Urological Association/Endourological Society guideline, part I. J Urol. 2016;196(4):1153–60.

88. Smith-Bindman R, Aubin C, Bailitz J, et al. Ultrasonography versus computed tomography for suspected nephrolithiasis. N Engl J Med. 2014;371(12):1100–10.

89. Alivizatos G, Skolarikos A. Is there still a role for open surgery in the management of renal stones? Curr Opin Urol. 2006;16(2):106–11.

90. Pearle MS, Goldfarb DS, Assimos DG, et al. Medical management of kidney stones: AUA guideline. J Urol. 2014;192(2):316–24.
91. Strohmaier WL. Course of calcium stone disease without treatment. What can we expect? Eur Urol. 2000;37(3):339–44.
92. Bergsland KJ, Worcester EM, Coe FL. Role of proximal tubule in the hypocalciuric response to thiazide of patients with idiopathic hypercalciuria. Am J Physiol Renal Physiol. 2013;305(4):F592–9.
93. Phillips R, Hanchanale VS, Myatt A, Somani B, Nabi G, Biyani CS. Citrate salts for preventing and treating calcium containing kidney stones in adults. Cochrane Database Syst Rev. 2015;10.
94. Pinheiro VB, Baxmann AC, Tiselius H-G, Heilberg IP. The effect of sodium bicarbonate upon urinary citrate excretion in calcium stone formers. Urology. 2013;82(1):33–7.
95. Pachaly MA, Baena CP, Buiar AC, de Fraga FS, Carvalho M. Effects of non-pharmacological interventions on urinary citrate levels: a systematic review and meta-analysis. Nephrol Dial Transplant. 2016;31(8):1203–11.
96. Lieske JC. Probiotics for prevention of urinary stones. Ann Transl Med. 2017;5(2):29.
97. Kaufman DW, Kelly JP, Curhan GC, et al. Oxalobacter formigenes may reduce the risk of calcium oxalate kidney stones. J Urol. 2009;181(2):676.
98. Adnan W NS. Calcium Stone: Pathophysiology, Prevention and Medical Management. In: Han H MW, Nasser S, ed. Nutritional and Medical Management of Kidney Stones. Switzerland: Humana Press/Springer; 2019:93–106.
99. Hoppe B, Beck B, Gatter N, et al. Oxalobacter formigenes: a potential tool for the treatment of primary hyperoxaluria type 1. Kidney Int. 2006;70(7):1305–11.
100. Milliner D, Hoppe B, Groothoff J. A randomised Phase II/III study to evaluate the efficacy and safety of orally administered Oxalobacter formigenes to treat primary hyperoxaluria. Urolithiasis. 2018;46(4):313–23.
101. Kang DE, Sur RL, Haleblian GE, Fitzsimons NJ, Borawski KM, Preminger GM. Long-term lemonade based dietary manipulation in patients with hypocitraturic nephrolithiasis. J Urol. 2007;177(4):1358–62.
102. Jackson RD, LaCroix AZ, Gass M, et al. Calcium plus vitamin D supplementation and the risk of fractures. N Engl J Med. 2006;354(7):669–83.
103. Wallace RB, Wactawski-Wende J, O'Sullivan MJ, et al. Urinary tract stone occurrence in the Women's Health Initiative (WHI) randomized clinical trial of calcium and vitamin D supplements. Am J Clin Nutr. 2011;94(1):270–7.
104. Nouvenne A, Meschi T, Prati B, et al. Effects of a low-salt diet on idiopathic hypercalciuria in calcium-oxalate stone formers: a 3-mo randomized controlled trial. Am J Clin Nutr. 2010;91(3):565–70.
105. Noori N, Honarkar E, Goldfarb DS, et al. Urinary lithogenic risk profile in recurrent stone formers with hyperoxaluria: a randomized controlled trial comparing DASH (dietary approaches to stop hypertension)-style and low-oxalate diets. Am J Kidney Dis. 2014;63(3):456–63.
106. Rebholz CM, Crews DC, Grams ME, et al. DASH (dietary approaches to stop hypertension) diet and risk of subsequent kidney disease. Am J Kidney Dis. 2016;68(6):853–61.
107. Attalla K, De S, Monga M. Oxalate content of food: a tangled web. Urology. 2014;84(3):555–9.
108. Massey LK. Food oxalate: factors affecting measurement, biological variation, and bioavailability. J Am Diet Assoc. 2007;107(7):1191–4.
109. Taylor EN, Curhant GC. Oxalate intake and the risk for nephrolithiasis. J Am Soc Nephrol. 2007;18(7):2198–204.
110. Taylor EN, Curhan GC. Determinants of 24-hour urinary oxalate excretion. Clin J Am Soc Nephrol. 2008;3(5):1453–60.
111. Hylander E, Jarnum S, Nielsen K. Calcium treatment of enteric hyperoxaluria after jejunoileal bypass for morbid-obesity. Scand J Gastroenterol. 1980;15(3):349–52.
112. Baxmann AC, Mendonca CDG, Heilberg IP. Effect of vitamin C supplements on urinary oxalate and pH in calcium stone-forming patients. Kidney Int. 2003;63(3):1066–71.
113. Tang M, Larson-Meyer DE, Liebman M. Effect of cinnamon and turmeric on urinary oxalate excretion, plasma lipids, and plasma glucose in healthy subjects. Am J Clin Nutr. 2008;87(5):1262–7.
114. Terris MK, Issa MM, Tacker JR. Dietary supplementation with cranberry concentrate tablets may increase the risk of nephrolithiasis. Urology. 2001;57(1):26–9.
115. Zuckerman JM, Assimos DG. Hypocitraturia: pathophysiology and medical management. Rev Urol. 2009;11(3):134–44.
116. Ryall RL. Urinary inhibitors of calcium oxalate crystallization and their potential role in stone formation. World J Urol. 1997;15(3):155–64.
117. Adeva MM, Souto G. Diet-induced metabolic acidosis. Clin Nutr. 2011;30(4):416–21.
118. Remer T, Manz F. Potential renal acid load of foods and its influence on urine pH. J Am Diet Assoc. 1995;95(7):791–7.
119. Trinchieri A, Lizzano R, Marchesotti F, Zanetti G. Effect of potential renal acid load of foods on urinary citrate excretion in calcium renal stone formers. Urol Res. 2006;34(1):1–7.

120. Meschi T, Maggiore U, Fiaccadori E, et al. The effect of fruits and vegetables on urinary stone risk factors. Kidney Int. 2004;66(6):2402–10.

121. Sakhaee K, Alpern R, Poindexter J, Pak CYC. Citraturic response to oral citric-acid load. J Urol. 1992;147(4):975–6.

122. Aras B, Kalfazade N, Tugcu V, et al. Can lemon juice be an alternative to potassium citrate in the treatment of urinary calcium stones in patients with hypocitraturia? A prospective randomized study. Urol Res. 2008;36(6):313–7.

123. Bobulescu A, Moe OW. Renal transport of uric acid: evolving concepts and uncertainties. Adv Chronic Kidney Dis. 2012;19(6):358–71.

124. Bushinsky DA, Asplin JR. Thiazides reduce brushite, but not calcium oxalate, supersaturation, and stone formation in genetic hypercalciuric stone-forming rats. J Am Soc Nephrol. 2005;16(2):417–24.

125. Coe FL, Kassirer JP, Shields M, et al. Uric-acid and calcium-oxalate nephrolithiasis. Kidney Int. 1983;24(3): 392–403.

126. Wang L, Cui Y, Zhang J, Zhang Q. Safety of potassium-bearing citrate in patients with renal transplantation: a case report. Medicine. 2017;96(42):e6933.

127. Mitra S CR. Medical Management of Uric Acid Stone. In: Han H MW, Nasser S, ed. Nutritional and Medical Management of Kidney Stones. Switzerland: Humana Press, Springer; 2019:117–22.

128. Pak CYC, Sakhaee K, Fuller C. SUccessful management of uric-acid nephrolithiasis with potassium citrate. Kidney Int. 1986;30(3):422–8.

129. Cameron M, Maalouf NM, Poindexter J, Adams-Huet B, Sakhaee K, Moe OW. The diurnal variation in urine acidification differs between normal individuals and uric acid stone formers. Kidney Int. 2012;81(11):1123–30.

130. Riese RJ, Sakhaee K. Uric-acid nephrolithiasis – pathogenesis and treatment. J Urol. 1992;148(3):765–71.

131. McKenzie DC. Changes in urinary ph following bicarbonate loading. Can J Sport Sci Revue Canadienne Des Sciences Du Sport. 1988;13(4):254–6.

132. Anderson EE, Rundles RW, Silberman HR, Metz EN. Allopurinol control of hyperuricosuria – a new concept in prevention of uric acid stones. J Urol. 1967;97(2):344–+.

133. Becker MA, Schumacher HR, Wortmann RL, et al. Febuxostat compared with allopurinol in patients with hyperuricemia and gout. N Engl J Med. 2005;353(23):2450–61.

134. Han H, Segal AM, Seifter JL, Dwyer JT. Nutritional management of kidney stones (nephrolithiasis). Clin Nutr Res. 2015;4(3):137–52.

135. Yu K-H, See L-C, Huang Y-C, Yang C-H, Sun J-H. Dietary factors associated with hyperuricemia in adults. Semin Arthritis Rheum. 2008;37(4):243–50.

136. Choi HK, Liu SM, Curhan G. Intake of purine-rich foods, protein, and dairy products and relationship to serum levels of uric acid – the Third National Health and Nutrition Examination Survey. Arthritis Rheum. 2005;52(1): 283–9.

137. Odvina CV. Comparative value of orange juice versus lemonade in reducing stone-forming risk. Clin J Am Soc Nephrol. 2006;1(6):1269–74.

138. Choi HK, Curhan G. Coffee, tea, and caffeine consumption and serum uric acid level: the Third National Health and Nutrition Examination Survey. Arthritis Rheum. 2007;57(5):816–21.

139. Heilberg IP. Treatment of patients with uric acid stones. Urolithiasis. 2016;44(1):57–63.

140. Karaguelle O, Smorag U, Candir F, et al. Clinical study on the effect of mineral waters containing bicarbonate on the risk of urinary stone formation in patients with multiple episodes of CaOx-urolithiasis. World J Urol. 2007;25(3):315–23.

141. Rho YH, Zhu Y, Choi HK. The epidemiology of uric acid and fructose. Semin Nephrol. 2011;31(5):410–9.

142. Taylor EN, Curhan GC. Fructose consumption and the risk of kidney stones. Kidney Int. 2008;73(2):207–12.

143. Daly M. Sugars, insulin sensitivity, and the postprandial state. Am J Clin Nutr. 2003;78(4):865S–72S.

144. Knoll T, Zollner A, Wendt-Nordahl G, Michel M, Alken P. Cystinuria in childhood and adolescence: recommendations for diagnosis, treatment, and follow-up. Pediatr Nephrol. 2005;20(1):19–24.

145. Eggermann T, Zerres K, Nunes V, et al. Clinical utility gene card for: cystinuria. Eur J Hum Genet. 2012;20(2).

146. Fattah H, Hambaroush Y, Goldfarb DS. Cystine nephrolithiasis. Transl Androl Urol. 2014;3(3):228–33.

147. Lambert EH, Asplin JR, Herrell SD, Miller NL. Analysis of 24-hour urine parameters as it relates to age of onset of cystine stone formation. J Endourol. 2010;24(7):1179–82.

148. Cranidis AI, Karayannis AA, Delakas DS, Livadas CE, Anezinis PE. Cystine stones: the efficacy of percutaneous and shock wave lithotripsy. Urol Intern. 1996;56(3):180–3.

149. Rhodes HL, Yarram-Smith L, Rice SJ, et al. Clinical and genetic analysis of patients with cystinuria in the United Kingdom. Clin J Am Soc Nephrol. 2015;10(7):1235–45.

150. Barbey F, Joly D, Rieu P, Mejean A, Daudon M, Jungers P. Medical treatment of cystinuria: critical reappraisal of long-term results. J Urol. 2000;163(5):1419–23.

151. Mattoo A, Goldfarb DS. Cystinuria. Semin Nephrol. 2008;28(2):181–91.
152. Agrawal N Z-NK. Cystine Stones. In: Han H MW, Nasser S, ed. Nutritional and Medical Management of Kidney Stones. Switzerland: Humana Press; 2019:141–7.
153. Torres VE, Chapman AB, Devuyst O, et al. Tolvaptan in patients with autosomal dominant polycystic kidney disease. N Engl Med. 2012;367(25):2407–18.
154. Pereira DJ, Schoolwerth AC, Pais VM. Cystinuria: current concepts and future directions. Clin Nephrol. 2015;83(3):138–46.
155. Andreassen KH, Pedersen KV, Osther SS, Jung HU, Lildal SK, Osther PJ. How should patients with cystine stone disease be evaluated and treated in the twenty-first century? Urolithiasis. 2016;44(1):65–76.
156. Pak CY, Fuller C, Sakhaee K, Zerwekh JE, Adams BV. Management of cystine nephrolithiasis with alpha-mercaptopropionylglycine. J Urol. 1986;136(5):1003–8.
157. Moe OW, Pearle MS, Sakhaee K. Pharmacotherapy of urolithiasis: evidence from clinical trials. Kidney Int. 2011;79(4):385–92.
158. Rogers A, Kalakish S, Desai RA, Assimos DG. Management of cystinuria. Urol Clin N Am. 2007;34(3):347–+.
159. Rodman JS, Blackburn P, Williams JJ, Brown A, Pospischil MA, Peterson CM. The effect of dietary-protein on cystine excretion in patients with cystinuria. Clin Nephrol. 1984;22(6):273–8.
160. Jaeger P, Portmann L, Saunders A, Rosenberg LE, Thier SO. Anticystinuric effects of glutamine and of dietary-sodium restriction. N Engl J Med. 1986;315(18):1120–3.
161. Gnessin E, Mandeville JA, Handa SE, Lingeman JE. Changing composition of renal calculi in patients with mus-culoskeletal anomalies. J Endourol. 2011;25(9):1519–23.
162. Healy KA, Ogan K. Pathophysiology and management of infectious staghorn calculi. Urol Clin N Am. 2007;34(3):363–+.
163. Resnick MI, Boyce WH. Bilateral staghorn calculi – patient-evaluation and management. J Urol. 1980;123(3):338–41.
164. Viprakasit DP, Sawyer MD, Herrell SD, Miller NL. Changing composition of staghorn calculi. J Urol. 2011;186(6):2285–90.
165. Chamberlin JD, Clayman RV. Medical treatment of a staghorn calculus: the ultimate noninvasive therapy. J Endourol Case Rep. 2015;1(1):21–3.
166. Sakhaee K. Nephrolithiasis as a systemic disorder. Curr Opin Nephrol Hypertens. 2008;17(3):304–9.
167. Sakhaee K. Epidemiology and clinical pathophysiology of uric acid kidney stones. J Nephrol. 2014;27(3):241–5.
168. Daudon M, Lacour B, Jungers P. High prevalence of uric acid calculi in diabetic stone formers. Nephrol Dial Transpl. 2005;20(2):468–9.
169. Pak CYC, Sakhaee K, Moe O, et al. Biochemical profile of stone-forming patients with diabetes mellitus. Urology. 2003;61(3):523–7.
170. William J. Epidemiology of Kidney Stones in the United States. In: Han H MW, Nasser S, ed. Nutritional and Medical Management of Kidney Stones. Switzerland: Humana Press, Springer; 2019:3–17.
171. Madore F, Stampfer MJ, Willett WC, Speizer FE, Curhan GC. Nephrolithiasis and risk of hypertension in women. Am J Kidney Dis. 1998;32(5):802–7.
172. Cutler JA, Brittain E. Calcium and blood-pressure – an epidemiologic perspective. Am J Hypertens. 1990;3(8):S137–46.
173. McCarron DA, Morris CD, Henry HJ, Stanton JL. Blood-pressure and nutrient intake in the United-States. Science. 1984;224(4656):1392–8.
174. Strazzullo P, Mancini M. Hypertension, calcium-metabolism, and nephrolithiasis. Am J Med Sci. 1994;307:S102–6.
175. Taylor EN, Mount DB, Forman JP, Curhan GC. Association of prevalent hypertension with 24-hour urinary excretion of calcium, citrate, and other factors. Am J Kidney Dis. 2006;47(5):780–9.
176. Alper AB, Chen W, Yau L, Srinivasan SR, Berenson GS, Hamm LL. Childhood uric acid predicts adult blood pressure – the Bogalusa Heart Study. Hypertension. 2005;45(1):34–8.
177. Reiner AP, Kahn A, Eisner BH, et al. Kidney stones and subclinical atherosclerosis in young adults: the CARDIA Study. J Urol. 2011;185(3):920–5.
178. Hamano S, Nakatsu H, Suzuki N, Tomioka S, Tanaka M, Murakami S. Kidney stone disease and risk factors for coronary heart disease. Int J Urol. 2005;12(10):859–63.
179. Rule AD, Roger VL, Melton LJ III, et al. Kidney stones associate with increased risk for myocardial infarction. J Am Soc Nephrol. 2010;21(10):1641–4.
180. Rule AD, Krambeck AE, Lieske JC. Chronic kidney disease in kidney stone formers. Clin J Am Soc Nephrol. 2011;6(8):2069–75.

181. El-Zoghby ZM, Lieske JC, Foley RN, et al. Urolithiasis and the risk of ESRD. Clin J Am Soc Nephrol. 2012;7(9):1409–15.
182. Rule AD, Bergstralh EJ, Melton LJ III, Li X, Weaver AL, Lieske JC. Kidney stones and the risk for chronic kidney disease. Clin J Am Soc Nephrol. 2009;4(4):804–11.
183. Gillen DL, Worcester EM, Coe FL. Decreased renal function among adults with a history of nephrolithiasis: a study of NHANES III. Kidney Int. 2005;67(2):685–90.
184. Robijn S, Hoppe B, Vervaet BA, D'Haese PC, Verhulst A. Hyperoxaluria: a gut-kidney axis? Kidney Int. 2011;80(11):1146–58.
185. Tappenden KA. Pathophysiology of short bowel syndrome considerations of resected and residual anatomy. JPEN J Parenter Enteral Nutr. 2014;38:14S–22S.
186. Mittal RD, Kumar R, Bid HK, Mittal B. Effect of antibiotics on Oxalobacter formigenes colonization of human gastrointestinal tract. J Endourol. 2005;19(1):102–6.
187. Nasr SH, D'Agati VD, Said SM, et al. Oxalate nephropathy complicating Roux-en-Y gastric bypass: an under-recognized cause of irreversible renal failure. Clin J Am Soc Nephrol. 2008;3(6):1676–83.
188. Lieske JC, Kumar R, Collozo-Clovell ML. Nephrolithiasis after bariatric surgery for obesity. Semin Nephrol. 2008;28(2):163–73.
189. Canales BK, Gonzalez RD. Kidney stone risk following Roux-en-Y gastric bypass surgery. Transl Androl Urol. 2014;3(3):242–9.
190. Abegg K, Gehring N, Wagner CA, et al. Roux-en-Y gastric bypass surgery reduces bone mineral density and induces metabolic acidosis in rats. Am J Physiol Regul Integr Comp Physiol. 2013;305(9):R999–R1009.
191. Froeder L, Arasaki CH, Malheiros CA, Baxmann AC, Heilberg IP. Response to dietary oxalate after bariatric surgery. Clin J Am Soc Nephrol. 2012;7(12):2033–40.

Chapter 26
Acute Kidney Injury

Laryssa Grguric

Keywords Acute kidney injury · Acute renal failure · Nutrient requirements · Parenteral nutrition · Enteral nutrition · Metabolism

> **Key Points**
> - Identify metabolic changes that occur with acute kidney injury (AKI).
> - List the impact of renal replacement therapy options for the patient with AKI.
> - Evaluate nutritional requirements for the patient with AKI.
> - Define modalities used for the provision of specialized nutrition support for the patient with AKI.
> - Identify considerations in the provision of nutrition support for the patient with AKI.

Function of the Kidneys

The primary function of the kidneys is to excrete end products of metabolism, to regulate electrolytes and mineral concentrations, and to maintain fluid and electrolyte balance [1]. Other functions include urine production, dilution, and concentration; maintenance of blood pressure; concentration of extracellular and intracellular fluids; gluconeogenesis; maintenance of calcium phosphorus balance; and activation of vitamin and hormone synthesis [1].

The kidney has approximately one million nephrons, each of which is composed of several functional segments, including the glomeruli, the proximal tubules, the distal tubules, the loop of Henle, and the collecting duct, which drains into the renal pelvis. The nephron clears plasma of the end products of metabolism (urea, creatinine, uric acid, inorganic and organic acids). Electrolytes (sodium, potassium, chloride, bicarbonate), minerals (calcium, phosphorus, magnesium), and micronutrients (zinc, selenium) are filtered through the glomeruli and are reabsorbed or excreted based on needs. Small nutrients such as glucose, small proteins, amino acids, and vitamins are filtered through the glomerulus and reabsorbed via active transport in the proximal tubule of the kidney [1].

The editors acknowledge Marcia A. Kalista-Richards' contribution to this chapter in *Nutrition in Kidney Disease*, *Second Edition*, Nutrition and Health, DOI: https://doi.org/10.1007/978-1-62703-685-6_1, © Springer Science+Business Media, New York, 2014.

L. Grguric (✉)
Formerly Nassau University Medical Center, Currently Working in Home Infusion for Coram/CVS Specialty Infusion Services, Miramar, FL, USA
e-mail: Laryssa.grguric@coramhc.com

© Springer Nature Switzerland AG 2020
J. D. Burrowes et al. (eds.), *Nutrition in Kidney Disease*, Nutrition and Health,
https://doi.org/10.1007/978-3-030-44858-5_26

Acute Kidney Injury

Acute kidney injury (AKI) is characterized by an abrupt reduction of kidney function over hours to days, which results in failure to maintain electrolyte, acid–base, and fluid homeostasis. AKI can occur in up to 20% of all hospitalized patients [2]. Several complications can occur in AKI, including hyperkalemia, hyperphosphatemia, glucose intolerance, fluid overload, and azotemia [3]. It may present with normal or abnormal urine outputs with abnormal levels being classified according to the following urine volumes: anuria (<100 mL/day), oliguria (100–400 mL/day), and nonoliguria (>400 mL/day) [4, 5]. AKI can also occur as a result of multiple organ dysfunction syndrome (MODS) or it may be restricted to the kidney alone. Depending on the etiology, permanent damage can occur or, if the underlying problem is corrected, the nephrons can recover. AKI can occur along with preexisting chronic kidney disease (CKD). Mortality is highly associated with the diagnosis [4, 6–9].

Categories of AKI include prerenal, renal (intrarenal and intrinsic), and postrenal. Decreased renal perfusion related to volume depletion or redistribution, burns, pancreatitis, peritonitis, hypoalbuminemia, and decreased cardiac output or embolus are related to the onset of prerenal AKI [4]. Early diagnosis and improving glomerular filtration and blood flow are beneficial in reversing prerenal AKI, unless the patient had underlying preexisting kidney disease or experience a considerable decline of baseline kidney function [10]. People taking certain medications such as nonsteroidal antiinflammatory drugs (NSAIDs), angiotensin-converting enzyme (ACE) inhibitors, or angiotensin 2 receptor blockers (ARB); the elderly; those with renal insufficiency and liver disease are high-risk groups [6]. Nutritional requirements and the need for specialized nutrition support would be based on concurrent diagnosis and patient status [11].

Urinary tract obstruction is a frequent cause of postrenal AKI. The most common reason for obstruction is bladder outlet obstruction, typically due to prostate pathology, such as benign prostatic hypertrophy (BPH). Other causes may include stricture, malignancy or inflammatory processes, vascular diseases, papillary necrosis, or intratubular crystals [4]. The goal is to reverse what has caused the postrenal AKI and manage any complications that may result from postobstructive diuresis. Nutrition intervention would be directed towards any other comorbid factors associated with the development of postrenal AKI [12].

Intrarenal AKI (also referred to as intrinsic AKI) is associated with renal parenchyma damage. Prerenal AKI can trigger the problem, but a major cause of intrarenal AKI is acute tubular necrosis (ATN) and damage to the renal tubules as a result of ischemia or nephrotoxins [4]. Predisposing factors to ATN are renal ischemia from prolonged prerenal azotemia, nephrotoxins such as radiocontrast and chemotherapy agents, interstitial nephritis, infections, and pigmenturia [4]. Trauma, major surgery, hypotension, and sepsis are also associated with ATN [4, 10].

International experts representing intensive care and nephrology societies collaborated to establish the Acute Dialysis Quality Initiative (ADQI). ADQI developed a definition and staging system known as the RIFLE system, which classifies AKI into three severity categories based on increased serum creatinine and urine output: R = risk, I = injury, and F = failure, and two clinical categories, L = loss and E = end-stage renal disease [12, 13]. The Acute Kidney Injury Network (AKIN) later made modifications to the RIFLE categories and established a three-level staging system based on serum creatinine and urine output [13, 14]. More recently, international guidelines by the Kidney Disease: Improving Global Outcomes (KDIGO) unified the ADQI and AKIN guidelines with the goal to establish a global definition and guidelines [13, 14] (Tables 26.1 and 26.2).

AKI commonly occurs with a combination of disease states associated with critically ill patients, including sepsis and hypotension; it can also be caused by exposure to nephrotoxic drugs [3]. Treatment for AKI includes elimination of the causative factor, treatment of the disease process, volume repletion in hypovolemic patients, use of renal replacement therapy (RRT), and maintenance of nutritional status [11].

Table 26.1 AKI definition [13]

Increase in SCr by ≥0.3 mg/dL (≥26.5 μmol/L) within 48 hours
Increase in SCr to ≥1.5 times baseline, which is known or presumed to have occurred within the prior 7 days (or)
Urine volume of <0.5 mL/kg/hour for 6 hours

Source: http://www.kdigo.org

Table 26.2 Staging of AKI [13]

Stage	Serum creatinine	Urine output
1	1.5–1.9 times baseline	<0.5 mL/kg/hour for 6–12 hours
	or	
	≥0.3 mg/dL (≥26.5 μmol/L) increase	
2	2.0–2.9 times baseline	<0.5 mL/kg/hour for ≥12 hour
3	≥3.0 times baseline	<0.3 mL/kg/hour for ≥24 hours
	or	or
	Increase in serum creatinine to ≥4.0 mg/dL (≥353.65 μmol/L)	Anuria for ≥12 hours
	or	
	Initiation of renal replacement therapy	
	or	
	In patients <18 years, decrease in eGFR to <35 mL/min per 1.73 m^2	

Source: http://www.kdigo.org

In the past, nutrition intervention in its various forms was often delayed so not to worsen the kidney failure in nondialyzed patients with hopes to delay the start of dialysis or avoid it all together [9]. Given the catabolic nature of AKI and comorbidities, it is now recognized that nutrition supplementation should not be withheld. Up to 75% of patients in AKI are considered to have varying degrees of wasting or malnourishment [3, 15].Patients who exhibit loss of fat and/or muscle mass are at an increased risk of death and, therefore, early nutritional interventions to stave off excessive losses has become imperative in the treatment of AKI [3, 15]. The development and utilization of RRT over the years has permitted the judicious use of nutrition support while limiting or removing previous concerns [9]. It has been shown that nutrition support may promote renal function; however, the success of the therapy is dependent on the ability to resolve the underlying cause of AKI [3].

Renal Replacement Therapy

RRT options in AKI include continuous or intermittent therapy. Continuous renal replacement therapy (CRRT) refers to outside the body purification therapy and is applied, as its name implies, continuously, if tolerated by the patient. CRRT includes continuous venovenous hemodialysis (CVVHD), continuous venovenous hemofiltration (CVVHF), continuous venovenous hemodiafiltration (CVVHDF), and slow continuous ultrafiltration (SCUF) [10].

Intermittent therapy or hemodialysis treatments, also an outside the body purification therapy, is administered three times per week or more as needed. Each type of RRT requires special consideration in the nutrition prescription; for example, CRRT may require less restrictions versus intermittent hemodialysis, due to increased losses during therapy.

Nutrition Management of the AKI Patient

Nutrition Assessment

It is agreed that the diagnosis of AKI creates numerous metabolic derangements that can lead to deterioration of an individual's nutritional status; therefore, a referral should be made to the dietitian for evaluation [14]. Frequent nutrition assessments should be performed to help guide the appropriate nutrition plan and to monitor its effectiveness and appropriateness. No one tool or parameter can be used in the evaluation of the patients' nutritional status. Available parameters require analysis of trends and an evaluation of how the underlying disease state will potentially skew results of such values. This is particularly important for the individual with AKI [11].

Due to the nature of renal disease, fluid accumulation may occur due to oliguria or anuria, which should be taken into consideration when evaluating weight status. When treatment in the form of RRT is applied, significant reductions in the patient's weight may occur; however, this loss correlates with fluid removal and not loss of muscle or fat mass. When estimating nutrient needs, particularly when using a weight-based formula, the current weight is likely inaccurate and should be avoided; usual or dry weight should be used if available. If the patient is obtunded and a weight history is unavailable, ideal body weight (IBW) can be calculated using the patient's height.

A nutrition-focused physical exam is imperative to the nutrition assessment and it is particularly useful in the patient with AKI. Fluid status may mask some signs of muscle and fat wasting. For example, a patient may present with lower extremity edema yet have muscle or fat wasting, as evidenced by temporal indentation or prominence of the rib cage. Techniques for physical examination include inspection, palpation, percussion, and auscultation. Skin alterations including lesions, wounds, and pressure ulcers must be factored into the assessment for accurate determination of nutritional requirements, as wound healing requires additional nutrient provision of both macro- and micronutrients. Refer to Chap. 6 for the nutrition-focused physical exam.

Bioimpedance analysis is widely used to assess total body water, intracellular water, and lean body mass but due to fluid shifts seen in AKI, results should be interpreted with caution. Midarm muscle circumference may be used as a surrogate for total body protein and lean body mass but it also has limitations. Subjective Global Assessment (SGA), which is a validated tool for malnutrition screening, may be helpful for those with renal dysfunction; however, it may also have limitations in the critically ill patient population [2]. Caution should be taken while interpreting SGA results in AKI. In the ICU, screening tools such as the Nutrition Risk in Critically Ill (NUTRIC) and Nutrition Risk Screening 2002 (NRS 2002) are useful [3], but may be cumbersome to calculate. The NUTRIC includes Acute Physiology and Chronic Health Evaluation (APACHE) II score, Sequential Organ Failure Assessment (SOFA) score, and serum interleukin 6 (IL-6) [16], which may not be readily available.

Laboratory parameters are of value in the nutrition assessment but they are not without limitations. Serum albumin is a prognostic indicator of overall disease-related outcome; however, profound hypoalbuminemia occurs in a critically ill patient and, once albumin is adjusted for inflammatory markers, it loses its predictive value [3]. Serum albumin, thyroxine-binding prealbumin (PA), retinol-binding protein (RBP), and transferrin are negative acute phase reactants that will decrease as a result of the stress and inflammatory response related to injury and illness [11]. C-reactive protein (CRP) and serum ferritin levels are positive acute phase reactants that inversely increase during stress and inflammation. These important parameters are related to inflammatory metabolism, which contributes to anorexia, lean body mass loss, risk for complications including infection, increased length of stay, and mortality [13]. Cytokines, including interleukin 1 (IL-1), IL-6, and tumor necrosis factor α (TNF-α), may also be measured; however, interpretation of these results in the AKI patient have not been standardized [11]. It is possible that inflammation itself may be a predictor for poor outcomes in this patient population.

Table 26.3 Urea nitrogen appearance and protein catabolic rate equations [17, 18]

Urea nitrogen appearance, g/day = UUN + [(BUN2 − BUN1) × 0.6 × BW1] + [BW2 − BW1 × BUN2]
Where net protein breakdown = UNA × 6.25
BUN1 = initial concentration of BUN, postdialysis (g/L)
BUN2 = final concentration of BUN, predialysis (g/L)
BW1 = postdialysis weight (kg)
BW2 = predialysis weight (kg)
PCR, g/day = UNA × 6.25

UUN urine urea nitrogen; *BUN* blood urea nitrogen; *BW* body weight; *UNA* urea nitrogen appearance; *PCR* protein catabolic rate

A nitrogen balance evaluation can be used to help determine the degree of catabolism and establish protein goals for the critically ill patient. A creatinine clearance of >50 mL/min/1.78 m² is needed for accurate determination [17], therefore limiting the use of this parameter to the patient with oliguria and anuria. Nitrogen balance can be determined by calculating the urea nitrogen appearance (UNA) or the protein catabolic rate (PCR) in patients with AKI receiving RRT [7, 17–19]. However, it also has limitations due to protein fluctuations and catabolism that can result in errors with interpretation [17] (Table 26.3).

Blood urea nitrogen values reflect the rate of urea synthesis by the liver and excretion by the kidney. Creatinine is proportional to the body's muscle mass [20].

Electrolyte balance is affected by AKI and requires careful evaluation. Metabolic acidosis and other abnormalities can result in hyperkalemia, and hyponatremia may occur with overhydration. Changes in glomerular function, medications, exogenous sources of electrolytes, quality of urine production, nutrition support, and RRT will each alter serum values [11].

Oral Intake and Supplements

In patients with AKI who can consume an oral diet, there are several factors that may affect their ability to obtain adequate nutrition such as taste changes, gastrointestinal (GI) disorders, or conditions related to their comorbid disease. If intake is compromised by poor appetite, overly restrictive diets should be avoided to help ensure adequate intake of nutrients. There are several oral supplements available commercially for patients with AKI. Each product will need to be evaluated for its appropriateness in the individual patient. If appetite remains poor, appetite stimulants may be prescribed. If all other interventions fail, or if there is a physical reason as to why the patient cannot consume an oral diet (e.g., dysphagia or need to protect the airway with mechanical ventilation), alternative means of nutrition support should be considered.

Specialized Nutrition Support

If the patient is unable to consume an adequate diet by mouth and is unable to meet nutrient demands with oral supplements, nutrition support using enteral or parenteral nutrition is warranted. Adequate nutrition support will help to mitigate the metabolic and immunologic disturbances and improve outcomes. Malnutrition has been identified as a predictor of hospital mortality for AKI patients independent of complications and comorbidities [21]. Enteral nutrition support is the preferred route of feeding for these patients provided GI function is adequate. This method has been associated with fewer metabolic complications and increased immunological benefits in comparison with parenteral nutrition (PN) [14, 22–24]. However, recent studies debate whether infection rates increase with PN

[25]. The literature suggests that supplemental PN may be beneficial to meet nutrient demands [26]. An individual's clinical condition, the presence and severity of malnutrition, the degree of food inadequacy, and time period (days to weeks) that oral intake is less than optimal will influence when enteral tube feeding should be initiated. Guidelines from the Society of Critical Care Medicine (SCCM) and the American Society of Parenteral and Enteral Nutrition (ASPEN) suggest that enteral nutrition is considered safe and practical. The guidelines recommend that in critically ill patients, enteral nutrition should be started within the first 24–48 hours after admission once the patient is hemodynamically stable [22]. Patients who require high-dose vasopressors and volume resuscitation may be able to tolerate trophic feeding of 10–20 mL per hour; however, absolute contraindications to enteral feeding include bowel perforation, obstructions, and proximal high-output fistulas [27].

The route of enteral support can either be gastric or into the small bowel based on the patients' GI anatomy, current disease state, and motility function. Gastric feedings rely on adequate GI function without problems of delayed gastric emptying, obstruction, or fistula [28]. For individuals with gastroparesis, gastric reflux conditions, gastric outlet obstruction, pancreatitis, those at risk of aspiration, or small bowel feedings should be considered. Critically ill patients who are being fed into the small bowel and who require simultaneous gastric decompression can utilize a dual-lumen gastrojejunal tube [28].

Tolerance to tube feedings is assessed by the presence of abdominal distention, rigidity, or firmness; absence of stools; or vomiting [28]. The use of gastric residual volumes to determine feeding intolerance has recently been debated [29]. The ability to reinitiate enteral feeding should be reevaluated regularly. Prokinetic drugs can be used to help promote feeding tolerances; however, renal doses should be provided if indicated [30].

Tube-Feeding Formulas

Formulas used for tube-feeding range from those that require complete digestion to predigested formulas that are developed for individuals with digestive disorders such as malabsorption or short gut syndrome. There are various enteral nutrition products available that will provide anywhere from 1.0 to 2.0 kcal/mL. Products have also been developed to meet specialty needs of individuals with disease-specific disorders, such as liver or kidney disease. However, there has been no clear benefit demonstrated for the routine use of disease-specific tube feeding products and, therefore, a standard polymeric formula may be the most appropriate enteral product for patients with AKI [27]. Some facilities may use volume-based protocols to help ensure adequate delivery of the enteral prescription. These protocols are beneficial as they highlight the importance and benefits of early enteral nutrition. The prescribed volume is determined by the weight of the patient and initiated within the first 24–48 hours of admission when possible. The protocol will also determine the enteral formula that is initiated. The patient's specific enteral need is then reevaluated by the unit dietitian for its appropriateness based on formula type and volume provided. Run rates are not static in the volume-based enteral prescription, which allows the bedside nurse to adjust the rate based on the volume already infused and the number of hours remaining in the day. This allows the healthcare team to provide appropriate interventions that require withholding enteral nutrition without sacrificing adequate nutrition support [31].

Enteral products developed specifically for renal patients on dialysis require digestion and they are lower in sodium, potassium, and phosphorus with a concentrated source of calories and protein. An individualized approach to the tube feeding prescription is imperative as there is not a "one size fits all" approach. There should be careful daily laboratory monitoring when using renal-specific formulas to ensure adequate provision of electrolytes. Hypokalemia may occur due to low potassium content in the formula when a restriction is not required. Adjustments should be made to the enteral nutrition prescription to address such concerns. Hyperphosphatemia can often be resolved with the addition of phosphorus binders to the patient's medication regimen. The powder form of sevelamer carbonate can be successfully provided to the patient via feeding tube for their desired effect. However, adequate flush protocols should be implemented to maintain tube patency. The use of phosphorus binders with meals or enteral feeding will reduce hyperphosphatemia, which will help facilitate the use of protein [3]. Furthermore, the concentrated renal-specific formula may also not be appropriate for the patient with AKI as the etiology of AKI may be severe volume depletion, which can be reversed with additional fluid to improve volume status [32]. Vitamin and mineral contents of renal-specific formulas are designed to match the needs of the dialysis patient with added amounts of folic acid and pyridoxine, and limited amounts of vitamins C and A. However, vitamin and mineral deficiencies may be common in patients with AKI due to anorexia prior to the current state. Moreover, the process of dialysis, if initiated, may cause further deficiencies [33]. Renal function should be considered when making recommendations for vitamin and mineral supplementation [27]. The Dietary Reference Intakes (DRIs) for most nutrients are met using 1 L of formula. It may be necessary to calculate the micronutrients provided by the volume of enteral nutrition delivered prior to adding additional supplements to the nutrition prescription. Enteral formulas contain vitamin K; this should be considered for patients receiving warfarin. The dose of warfarin may need to be adjusted and coagulation protocols monitored with tube feedings, any oral intake, or transition to oral intake [34].

Renal products should be used cautiously or replaced with non-renal-specific products when an individual has been undernourished and is at risk for refeeding syndrome. Individuals with a history of poor dietary intakes, chronic alcoholics, and malnourished patients, particularly those with marasmus or obese patients with significant weight loss, are at risk for refeeding syndrome [35]. This syndrome can be defined as severe electrolyte and fluid shifts associated with metabolic abnormalities in malnourished patients undergoing aggressive refeeding, whether enterally or parenterally [35]. Hypokalemia, hypophosphatemia, hypomagnesemia, abnormal glucose metabolism, and fluid balance abnormalities may occur. Prevention of refeeding syndrome includes the slow administration of nutrients at a caloric level below maintenance needs, with careful attention to phosphorus, potassium, and magnesium, as it should be anticipated that these values will drop [35–38]. Low serum potassium, magnesium, or phosphorus is generally not expected in patients with kidney disease; therefore, it is of particular importance to be aware of the problems related to refeeding syndrome. Early and aggressive supplementation of electrolytes may be required. The lower potassium, phosphorus, and magnesium content of renal formulas may exacerbate a serious decline in serum electrolytes once nutrition support is initiated. It is advantageous if the clinician is familiar with the individual's previous dietary intake before the start of nutrition support in order to select the most appropriate product, and to manage the patient wisely by initiating nutrition support "low and slow" with adequate supplementation of thiamine [38]. However, knowing the patient's nutritional status prior to admission may not always be possible. If characteristics of refeeding syndrome are present (e.g., low serum magnesium, potassium, and phosphorus), then a standard formula should be used rather than a renal product that is low in electrolytes. The need for a renal-specific formula can be reassessed by monitoring lab values and considering other aspects of the patient's case. Other non-renal concentrated formulas that provide 1.5–2 kcal/mL may also be used depending on the individual's status, RRT, fluid, and laboratory results. Many volume-based feeding protocols will also include regular monitoring of electrolytes for 72 hours after the start of enteral nutrition. Modular protein sources are available and can be used to tailor individual needs; they can also be used during trophic feeding to help meet protein goals until the patient becomes more stable to tolerate goal volumes or rates.

Closed enteral systems contain sterile tube feeding; they are ready-to-hang for up to 24 to 72 hours and they have been associated with less contamination when compared to open enteral systems. These products also require less nursing intervention time [39].

Tube-Feeding Management

While feeding enterally via a nasogastric or gastrostomy tube, management of GI complications, including diarrhea, malabsorption, nausea, and vomiting, along with mechanical complications such as tube occlusions, are similar in any individual who requires enteral support. The AKI patient requires close monitoring of fluid status, electrolyte management, and GI status. The amount of free-water flushes with feedings may need to be reduced. The administration of medications introduces a source of free water that should be taken into consideration.

Tube occlusions are a potential problem particularly when the tube is used for the administration of medications. Clog prevention strategies should be implemented more often in patients receiving tube feedings. Ideally, feeding tubes should be flushed routinely with about 20–30 mL of water every 4 hours during continuous feeding. The feeding tube should also be flushed at the beginning of any tube feeding withholding period, as well as after, prior to resumption of feeding. This includes stoppage for medication administration [37, 40]. Flushes contribute extra water and can be a challenge for the renal patient. Maintaining continuous feedings, particularly for small-bore feeding tubes, may help to ensure continued feeding tube patency. In addition to water, carbonated beverages such as cola and cranberry juice have been used to flush feeding tubes; however, these products are not recommended as they can exacerbate existing clogs [37] and can negatively change serum potassium and phosphorus levels. Liquid irrigants, enzyme solutions, and mechanical devices have been used to unclog a tube [37]. Gentle flushing with warm water is often the preferred method to unclog tubes.

Fluid restriction is determined by (1) whether the patient is anuric, oliguric, or has some residual renal function; (2) the ability of the type of RRT to remove unwanted fluid; and (3) other comorbid factors ranging from heart failure to the presence of an ileostomy. Strict fluid restrictions would require the use of 1.5–2 kcal/mL formula; serum potassium and phosphorus values would dictate which enteral product would best meet the needs of the patient. GI losses can decrease serum potassium levels and increase free-water requirements, which need to be factored into the selection of an enteral product.

Gastroparesis is common in individuals with diabetes and is associated with dialytic procedures, elevated BUN values, and hyperglycemia, thereby necessitating close monitoring of the tolerance to enteral tube feedings [37]. Metabolic intolerance to tube feeding may be related to underlying stress of critical illness and can be controlled with insulin protocols. Placement of the tube in the small bowel may be indicated if the patient demonstrates gastric feeding intolerances. Promotility agents such as metoclopramide or erythromycin can be used to promote gastric emptying and, in turn, promote tolerance to the enteral feeding [37]. The patient's position during dialysis should be considered to determine whether tube feeding can be given. For example, if a patient needs to be in a supine position because of hypotensive episodes during dialysis, the feeding may need to be held in order to prevent the risk of aspiration. A semi-recumbent position (>30° elevation) is recommended to prevent aspiration for individuals requiring tube feeding [37]. However, postpyloric feeding tube placement may decrease the risk of aspiration [41].

AKI may require medications with noted side effects such as constipation, diarrhea (defined as multiple stools >5/24-hour period), nausea, or vomiting. Tube feedings have been associated with similar side effects; therefore, it is important to identify the etiology of the symptoms and to treat the problem based on the actual cause rather than an assumption. Prokinetic agents, medications containing sorbitol, and *Clostridium difficile* colitis are also common causes of diarrhea [40]. Feedings may be held inappropriately because of symptoms that may be incorrectly attributed to the enteral feeding. Holding feedings should be deferred until other causes are ruled out successfully to minimize calorie and protein deficits.

Metabolic complications can occur in individuals on tube feedings. The healthcare team must assess each laboratory value independently with a baseline metabolic panel that is obtained at the initiation of enteral feeding. Follow-up parameters should be obtained based on the individual's needs and clinical condition.

Guidelines for Administration

Initiation of enteral feeding rates may be static or they may change based on the protocol. Generally, goal feeding tube rates are well tolerated without the need for ramp up [42, 43]. It should be noted that rate does not equal the same protein and calorie provision, as the same volume from each enteral product will have different compositions. If the goal is to minimize the patient's fluid intake, then a more calorically dense product may be required. For example, 1000 mL of a 2 kcal/mL product will provide 2000 calories, whereas a 1.2 kcal/mL product will provide only 1200 calories. Therefore, decreasing the rate from 40 mL/h to 20 mL/h will severely compromise delivery of adequate nutrients.

Parenteral Nutrition Support

Use of Parenteral Nutrition

Parenteral nutrition (PN) is the administration of nutrients using an intravenous (IV) method intended for individuals who do not have a functional GI tract or in situations where administration of nutrients using the GI tract is not tolerated or could not be safely used. There is some evidence to support the addition of PN to the already existing nutrition regimen if the original intervention is unable to meet the nutrition prescription [26]. Parenteral nutrition can be administered either centrally or peripherally. Generally, due to fluid limitations, central access may be required to administer PN in the AKI patient. However, it could be possible to provide adequate nutrients via the peripheral route if required in the short-term.

PN solutions may be provided as a "2-in-1" solution where the carbohydrate, protein, vitamins, electrolytes, minerals, additives, and sterile water are combined in one solution. Intravenous fat emulsions (IVFEs) also known as intravenous lipid emulsions (ILE) can be administered separately from the "2-in-1" solution. When ILE is added to the PN solution, it forms a total nutrient admixture (TNA) or a "3-in-1" solution [11].

Nutrient Substrates

Protein

Protein is provided in the PN formula to provide a source of nitrogen. Crystalline amino acid (AA) is a source of protein with commercial solutions available in concentrations of 3.5–20%. The concentration used will be based on an individual's protein requirements, fluid allowance, and availability in the formulary. Generally, 10% and 15% base amino acid solutions are utilized. Occasionally, 20% base solutions, if required due to fluid restrictions, may be available for use. The AKI patient with increased protein requirements and limited fluid allowance generally would use the most concentrated solution available. Standard AA solutions include a balance of essential amino acids (EAA) and nonessential amino acids (NEAA) and they are appropriate for the AKI patient. There is insufficient evidence to support the use of only EAA solutions in the treatment of AKI [23]. EAA use alone does not offer benefits and, in fact, has been noted to be potentially harmful to patients due to hyperammonemia and metabolic encephalopathy [40]. NEAA including ornithine, citrulline, and arginine are needed to enable detoxification of ammonia via the urea cycle [23].

Carbohydrate

Carbohydrates provide a source of calories that are supplied as an anhydrous dextrose monohydrate in sterile water. It is available in concentrations ranging from 5% to 70% and provides 3.4 kcal/g of dextrose [11]. Dextrose supports the energy needs of the individual but requires careful consideration to achieve glycemic control. Overfeeding can be avoided by minimizing the carbohydrate load. Although exact carbohydrate requirements have not been clearly identified, a minimum of 50 g/day is required to avoid ketone production [44]. Suggested carbohydrate intake for critically ill patients is ≤4 mg/kg/min/day [45]. Fluid limits and the targeted plasma glucose of 150–180 mg/dL (8.3–10.0 mmol/L) [13] may affect dosing of dextrose grams and total volume used. Intensive glycemic control may result in hypoglycemia in patients with AKI. Therefore, tight glycemic control should be avoided because of the increased risk of hypoglycemic events [13].

Fat

Lipids provide a source of essential fatty acids and a concentrated source of calories. Traditionally, long-chain fatty acid emulsions were from either soybean oil or a combination of safflower and soybean oils. Recently, there has been an increased availability of lipid types in the United States, which include a blend of fats (soybean, medium chain triglyceride (MCT), olive oil, and fish oil) or solely fish oil. ILE are available as either 10%, 20%, or 30% solutions; the 30% solution is reserved for TNA. ILE contains egg phospholipids as an emulsifier with glycerol to adjust the osmolarity; therefore, they may be contraindicated in individuals who have an egg allergy or potential soy allergy. A test dose in a controlled setting may be necessary to determine tolerance of the lipid infusion in order to help meet nutrient demands. ILE contributes to the phosphorus and vitamin K intake.

Soy-based lipids are generally dosed at 1 g/kg/day. Newer lipids such as Smoflipid® (SMOF®) [46] and Omegaven® [47] have recently become commercially available in the United States. SMOF requires higher dosing, up to 2 g/kg/day, to meet essential fatty acid requirements. Omegaven is only indicated in those pediatric patients with parenteral-nutrition-associated cholestasis (PNAC) as treatment [47]. These newer lipids boast a higher omega-3 content versus their primarily omega-6 soy predecessors [46–48]. Triglycerides should be monitored to assess lipid clearance; desired values are less than 400 mg/dL in adult patients [40]. Overfeeding or rapid infusion of ILE can cause hypertriglyceridemia, leading to altered immune and pulmonary response, and increased risk of pancreatitis [49].

Other lipid sources, such as propofol, contribute fat calories as propofol utilizes a 10% soy-based ILE as the medication vehicle and should be calculated into the individual's overall caloric and lipid intake. Propofol provides 1.1 kcal/mL and 0.1 g fat/mL [11].

Parenteral Additives

Fluid and Electrolytes

Impaired kidney function impacts the kidney's ability to maintain normal fluid and electrolyte balance. Daily fluid intake allowance usually corresponds to fluid output. If urine output is less than 1 L/day, fluid intake of 1–1.5 L/day is recommended [50]. In patients who are oliguric (i.e., urine output declines to ≤400 mL/day) or anuric (urine output <100 mL/day), tighter fluid management is needed [11].

Electrolyte requirements have been established for individuals with normal kidney function along with suggested values for individuals with kidney failure [51]. Body weight, nutritional status, residual kidney function, comorbid diseases, and medications can influence both fluid and electrolyte status. Serum potassium, magnesium, and phosphorus levels will likely increase with poor kidney function due to impaired excretion. Management of electrolytes requires careful monitoring of laboratory values to minimize the potential risk of complications and to meet the patient's needs [11].

Sodium and potassium may be available as chloride, acetate, or phosphate; calcium gluconate and magnesium sulfate are preferred [52]. Parenteral AA solutions may include small amounts of electrolytes and acetate, which need to be calculated into the total solution. Acetate, a bicarbonate precursor, is used for PN rather than bicarbonate itself because of potential pH changes and the risk of insoluble precipitation with calcium and magnesium [52]. Acetate can be metabolized to bicarbonate by the liver. Individuals with acidosis may be treated with the addition of acetate; however, the amount will be dependent on sodium and potassium additives. Bicarbonate may also be used to treat acidosis but would require access using a separate line. The amount of calcium and phosphorus requires careful monitoring as excess amounts added to the PN solution can result in insoluble precipitation, causing crystal deposition that may lead to death [52]. Solubility curves are available to graph calcium and phosphorus based on type of AA used [53].

Vitamins and Trace Minerals

The American Medical Association (AMA) Nutrition Advisory Committee has made recommendations for the inclusion of multivitamins (MVI) and trace elements (TE) in PN [40]. In commercially available PN formulations, adult preparations contain 12 or 13 of the known vitamins. Vitamin K has been added to create MVI 13, which contains 150 µg vitamin K. ILE also contains vitamin K from soybean or safflower oils. Daily vitamin K requirements for adults receiving PN is 150 µg [34]; however, use of coagulation therapy needs to be considered with vitamin K use.

Parenteral MVI contains 1 mg vitamin A, whereas oral vitamins used for dialysis patients do not contain vitamin A. Total vitamin A intake, whether oral or parenteral, should be monitored, particularly in individuals who require long-term PN support as toxicity may develop. Adult MVI preparations contain 200 mg vitamin C [52], whereas an oral renal vitamin contains 60–100 mg [54].

Daily TE supplementation for adult PN formulations have also been established [40]; however, exact requirements for AKI patients have not been made. TE may be withheld, given several times per week or administered in a half dose. Select TE may be ordered based on route of excretion, risk for toxicity, or the patient's needs. A combination of clinical judgment, assessment of symptoms, and evaluation of laboratory data are needed when deciding to administer TE and their dosage. Ongoing research and reporting of outcomes and observations which help strengthen evidence-based guidelines are needed in this area [11].

Initiation and Monitoring of Parenteral Nutrition Support

Parenteral nutrition orders should consider the patient's fluid, electrolyte, and acid–base balance status; glycemic control; access availability; and risk for refeeding syndrome when starting and monitoring PN. The total volume can be delivered safely; however, hypervolemic patients with fluid limits are likely to be restricted to 1–1.5 L/day. Achievement of RRT goals, urinary output, and overall hydration status will determine fluid allowances when starting PN to help identify a safe total volume allowance. The initial adult carbohydrate dose is usually 150–200 g/day; for those with diabetes mellitus or hyperglycemia the recommendation is 100–150 g/day [40]. However, those patients who are stable may be able to initiate PN at a moderate dose of 4.3 g/kg/day. Provision of at least 2.88 g/kg/day provides maximal suppression of gluconeogenesis. In adults, the maximum dose of dextrose administration is 7.2 g/kg/day [55]. Lower dextrose may be required for those who are at risk of refeeding syndrome. When determining grams of dextrose, other sources of dextrose from CRRT, intravenous piggy back medications, and other medication drips that are reconstituted in 5% dextrose should be taken into consideration [56]. PN can be increased to meet nutritional requirements to achieve goals in 72–96 hours [45] as long as metabolic tolerance to the solution is demonstrated.

Correction of electrolyte disturbances is recommended prior to starting PN. Refeeding syndrome can be avoided by limiting the amount of carbohydrate in feedings, which can cause laboratory abnormalities [40]. However, RRT may correct some of these abnormalities and should be monitored as the nutrition support formula is developed. For example, if an individual is at risk for refeeding syndrome (which can lower serum potassium), the same individual may have hyperkalemia because of kidney failure; therefore, the dialysate solution can be adjusted to a low potassium bath. Caution should be taken that the potassium does not fall to an undesirable level with the initiation of PN. Thus, it is important to assess the whole picture [11].

Protein can be administered at full dose without dose reduction. ILE may be started at full dose provided serum triglyceride levels are within normal range [52].

Acid–base abnormalities may be the result of the individual's underlying condition, although nutrition support can also influence the values. Manipulation of the acetate and chloride content of the PN may aid in the correction of such abnormalities [57].

Discontinuing Parenteral Nutrition

Abrupt discontinuation of PN should be avoided, if possible, to prevent hypoglycemia. However, in stable patients, there is no evidence of significant differences in mean glucose, epinephrine, norepinephrine, insulin, glucagon, growth hormone, cortisol, symptom scores, and vital signs following abrupt discontinuation [58].Therefore, it is likely that stable patients can tolerate interruptions in PN and abrupt discontinuation of the solution. To prevent hypoglycemia, some institutions may implement strategies such as making 10% dextrose solutions readily available and monitoring glucose levels via fingersticks. In addition, prior to tapering PN, other modalities of nutrition support such as oral feedings or enteral nutrition should be in place to help ensure nutrition provision remains adequate.

Monitoring Clinical and Laboratory Parameters

General guidelines for monitoring clinical and laboratory parameters in patients receiving PN include obtaining a baseline comprehensive metabolic panel, daily weights, intakes and output, daily laboratory values until stable then weekly thereafter, and serum glucose three times per day until stable. Serum triglyceride levels should be checked prior to the infusion of lipids. Liver enzymes, bilirubin, and a complete blood count (CBC) should be checked when PN is initiated, then two to three times per week until stable, then weekly thereafter [51]. Frequency of monitoring will be based on acuity and results. Less frequent monitoring can be used as stabilization occurs [11].

Nutritional Requirements in AKI

It has been well established that AKI presents with protein-calorie malnutrition and an inflammatory and pro-oxidative state with all of its known complications [13, 24, 59–61]. Nutrition support should be aimed towards attenuating and counteracting the negative nitrogen balance and loss of lean body mass that occurs in most patients with critical illness. The goals of nutrition support for the AKI patient are similar if not the same as for other ICU patients with normal renal function. Obviously, renal impairment adds challenges while attempting to provide nutritional adequacy, prevent malnutrition, support immune function, accelerate recovery, and prevent mortality.

In patients with AKI who are critically ill, catabolism is multifactorial and may include sepsis, trauma, and surgical interventions [62, 63]. The underlying comorbid conditions and degree of critical illness will impact the overall level of catabolism of the patient. Negative nitrogen balance also results from uremic toxins, endocrine factors, metabolic acidosis, inadequate protein intake, and RRT loses [62, 63].

Impaired lipolysis causes plasma lipid changes with noted decreased production of lipoprotein lipase, especially with acidosis and hepatic triglyceride lipase reduction [62–64]. This is of particular importance when PN containing ILE or lipid-based medication use is required. The triglyceride content of lipoproteins including very-low-density and low-density lipoprotein levels is increased with AKI, and total cholesterol and high-density lipoproteins are decreased [62].

Insulin resistance occurs with AKI, leading to an imbalance of glycemic parameters. Hyperglycemia complications include risk of infection, poor wound healing, and mortality [65]. Glycemic control is recommended and fluctuations to hypoglycemia should be avoided [13].

Energy Requirements

It has been determined that inflammation caused by AKI can increase caloric needs up to 30% [13]. Energy needs may be further increased due to concurrent medical conditions or surgical interventions [3, 23]. Indirect calorimetry should be performed if it is available and if there are no barriers to performing a study. Indirect calorimetry is a noninvasive means for measuring oxygen consumed compared with carbon dioxide expired to calculate resting metabolic rate [23]. Barriers to performing indirect calorimetry include the presence of air leaks, chest tubes, supplemental oxygen, or continuous renal replacement therapy [27], which may be therapies applied to the patient with AKI. If indirect calorimetry is not available, or if it is not appropriate due to the aforementioned factors, applying alternative methods to determine energy needs for the critically ill patient may be appropriate. There are several predictive equations; however, ASPEN and SCCM recommend the use of a weight-based formula of 25–30 kcal/kg/day [27]. The 2012 KDIGO Guidelines recommend 30–35 kcal/kg/day [13]. When calorie levels of 40 kcal/kg/day were used in comparison to 30 kcal/kg/day combined with 1.5 g/protein/kg/day, the higher calorie infusion did not show differences in positive nitrogen balance, but did result in elevated glucose and triglyceride levels along with insulin needs [59].

Protein Requirements

Protein losses in AKI are increased due to compromised homeostasis and RRT [33]. Noncatabolic, nonoliguric, milder cases of AKI that require RRT, and are likely to regain renal function within a short period of time, can generally receive up to 0.8 g/kg/day of protein provided adequate calories are delivered (30 kcal/kg/day) [23, 62, 66]. KDIGO also supports administering 0.8 to 1.0 g/kg/day of protein in noncatabolic AKI patients who are not in need of dialysis [12]. Consideration must be given to concurrent events that may increase needs based on protein breakdown or losses. Protein restriction with the intent of preventing or delaying initiation of RRT should be avoided [13].

Losses of protein and amino acids via the extracorporeal circulation of RRT are approximately 0.2 g amino acid per liter of ultrafiltrate or up to 20 g amino acid per day [24, 64, 66]. An added 5–10 g of protein is needed per day above the 1.5 g/kg/day for AKI to replace losses when treatments are daily or when high flux filters and/or high-efficiency modalities including CRRT and sustained low-efficiency dialysis (SLED) are used [24, 64, 66].

KDIGO recommendations include1.0 to 1.5 g/kg/day protein in AKI patients on RRT, and up to a maximum of 1.7 g/kg/day in patients on CRRT and in hypercatabolic states [13]. ASPEN/SCCM recommends an increased protein load of 1.5–2 g/kg/day of protein up to a maximum of 2.5 g/kg/day in order to achieve positive nitrogen balance with CRRT treatments [22, 23, 67, 68]. Other studies have suggested that protein intake during CRRT should range between 1.8 and 2.5 g/kg/day [23]. Protein intake of 2.5 g/kg/day has been found to be associated with positive nitrogen balance [33]. The patient's catabolic rate, renal function, and dialysis losses should be evaluated to best determine protein needs in order to promote positive nitrogen balance [23].

Fat Requirements

Lipid requirements parallel those that avoid development of essential fatty acid deficiency (EFAD) in at-risk patients receiving PN and to avoid overfeeding. Lipids are recommended at 1 g/kg/day or 30–35% of total energy in the critically ill patient and should not exceed 2.5 g/kg/day in parenteral solutions [40]. Use of propofol or amphotericin B housed in a lipid emulsion needs to be factored into the lipid dose provided [11].

Vitamins and Trace Elements

There are numerous consequences of AKI, including an imbalance in both vitamins and TE. Various recommendations have been made for fat-soluble vitamins. Plasma levels of vitamins A and E were found to be low in experimental models of AKI [13, 59] and the kidney's inability to degrade RBP may lead to increased retinol levels [63]. Oral renal MVI do not contain vitamin A; however, adult multivitamin preparations contain 1 mg or 3300 IU of vitamin A as retinol. Current evidence does not support added supplementation of vitamins A or E, and retinol may require limitations [69]. Vitamin K levels may be normal or elevated [13] and vitamin D3 activation is impaired in AKI [24, 62, 66].

Water-soluble vitamins including vitamin C, thiamine, and folic acid levels may be lower due to extracorporeal excretion [63]. Vitamin C losses can be up to 100 mg per day during RRT [64]. Vitamin C supplementation in the critically ill patient may be associated with lower 28-day mortality and, therefore, increased vitamin C provided in the MVI may be favorable [69]. However, vitamin C should be limited to 100 mg with intermittent hemodialysis and should not exceed 200 mg with CRRT, as oxalate may accumulate in the heart, kidney, and blood vessels with excessive supplementation [60, 62, 70]. However, the high-dose vitamin C that is now provided in some sepsis protocols is short-term and has not been found to increase the risk of oxalate formation [71].Thiamine losses may be up to 1.5 times the daily amount provided in standard parenteral MVI [72]. The addition of 100 mg of thiamine into the PN solution may be appropriate. Recent interest has been circulating in regard to thiamine supplementation in critically ill patients. There has been an association between decreased mortality in septic patients with thiamine deficiency [71, 73, 74]. Thiamine deficiency may also predispose patients to increased oxalate excretion [71].

Numerous factors that impact the need for TE in the AKI patient should be evaluated. These include the route of excretion, use of solutions containing contaminant or TE sources, TE in PN solution, GI excretory or protein-bound losses, conditions that require elimination due to potential of toxicity, illness-related deficiencies, and the use of RRT. Both TE and vitamins can be altered with the AKI inflammatory activity. Another concern is that although it is known that AKI patients are at risk for depletion, exact requirements have not been established [64].

PN commonly contains zinc, copper, chromium, manganese, and selenium. In cases of cholestasis, copper and manganese are reduced or removed due to the excretion route and toxicity potential. Fluids used in CRRT may be contaminated with TE. The CRRT fluid does not have an appreciable amount of selenium or copper, but losses occur in the effluent [73, 75]. If the copper has been removed due to cholestasis and the patient requires continued RRT, deficiency may be of concern [64]. Zinc is found in effluent fluid in CVVHDF. Patients may also be in positive zinc balance after receiving zinc from several sources such as replacement fluids, anticoagulants and PN [64]. Patients who have concurrent GI problems such as diarrhea or colocutaneous fistula may require increased zinc supplementation based on such losses. Selenium levels have been noted to be low in patients with AKI [69]. Losses of selenium may occur during CRRT or result from increases in output [75, 76].

Fluid, Electrolytes, and Mineral Needs

The amount of fluid that can be excreted by the injured kidney and the selection of RRT dictate the daily fluid intake. Intermittent dialysis generally necessitates fluid limits, whereas the use of continuous therapy allows for a full nutrition support prescription to be given [11].

AKI causes electrolyte imbalances that can be related to the underlying disease, hypermetabolic conditions, medications, nutritional refeeding issues, kidney failure, RRT, and the use of specialized nutritional support. Standard daily electrolyte requirements have been published for adult EN and PN formulations [40].

Hyperkalemia is common in AKI with acidosis and reduced kidney clearance; however, gastrointestinal disease can cause potassium losses. In the absence of RRT, potassium may need to be restricted. AKI can cause hypocalcemia related to hyperphosphatemia, hypoalbuminemia, losses with CRRT, and citrate anticoagulation [77]. The renal replacement prescription can be used to manage potassium and calcium levels. Hyperphosphatemia seen in AKI can be treated using phosphorus binders and restricting intake. Hypermagnesemia occurs with AKI due to impaired excretion requiring limits of intake; however, the use of CRRT typically causes loss of phosphorus and magnesium requiring supplementation [17]. Recommendations for electrolyte and micronutrient requirements are based on serum concentrations [23].

Conclusion

Nutrition support in the patient with AKI has been demonstrated to help prevent deterioration of nutritional status during the catabolic events of multiple organ dysfunction syndrome. There are alterations in the metabolism of protein, carbohydrate, and fat, and changes in fluid and electrolyte balance caused by AKI. A thorough nutritional assessment needs to be performed with the development of a nutrition care plan based on individual needs and limitations of AKI. Specialized nutrition support requires skillful monitoring with ongoing evaluation of the patient's status to avoid complications.

Acknowledgments A special thank you is reserved for Lisa Musillo for her support and critical review of this chapter.

Case Study

Background A 58-year-old male patient has been admitted to your hospital's medical intensive care unit with urosepsis. His medical history consists of transient ischemic attack and coronary artery disease. The patient has experienced acute hypoxemia and respiratory failure leading to cardiac arrest. He is currently experiencing metabolic acidosis, ischemic hepatitis, and acute kidney injury. He is anuric and there is concern for anoxic brain injury. The patient remains on mechanical ventilation, but he has been stable on vasopressors. A central venous catheter and a nasogastric tube are in place for administration of medications. The team is asking for a recommendation to start nutrition. The modality of RRT the team is utilizing for this case is CVVHD. Of note, the patient's family at the bedside report that prior to this event the patient was in his normal state of health and had no prior issues with dietary intake. The daughter guesses the patient is about 160 lb but she is not sure. She also denies any weight loss prior to admission. Skin is intact of pressure ulcers.

Physical assessment Recumbent height measure: 5′6″. Patient does not present with any obvious signs of bony prominences. There is upper and lower bilateral edema but the patient's abdomen is flat and soft.

Labs WBC 18.45 thousand/μL, K 5.2 mmol/L (↑), HCO3 15 mmol/L (↓), Alb 1.9 (↓) g/dL, Glu 244 mg/dL (↑), Ca 7.3 (↓) mg/dL, Ionized Ca normalized 4.08 mg/dL (↓), BUN 52 mg/dL (↑), Crt 6.3 mg/dL (↑), P 6.6 mg/dL (↑). Last four fingerstick glucose checks: 278, 186, 255, and 243 mg/dL.

Medications Vasopressin (stable at 12 ml/h to maintain mean arterial pressure >60 mmHg), vancomycin, meropenem, levetiracetam, esomeprazole, hydrocortisone, atorvastatin.

Urine output via Foley catheter 0–5 ml/h.

Case Questions and Answers

1. The dietitian performs an assessment and finds the patient is not at risk of refeeding syndrome based on history provided by the patient's family. Do you agree with this assessment? Why?
   Answer: Yes – this seems like an accurate assessment as the patient's physical exam does not indicate any fat or muscle loss. It is true that edema may mask some signs of muscle or fat loss. However, the patient's daughter was able to give information that seems to indicate the patient was not at nutritional risk prior to admission.

2. What is the appropriate recommendation for protein and energy prescription for this patient? Justify your answer.
   Answer: Up to 30 calories per kilogram/day and 2 grams of protein per kilogram/day are appropriate recommendations. This patient has AKI and is on CVVHD. He is also septic and on a ventilator in the ICU. Increased calories and protein per kilogram are appropriate for this type of case due to increased energy expenditure caused by critical illness. In addition, there is increased proteolysis

in AKI. A higher dose of protein may help achieve nitrogen balance. The ASPEN/SCCM Critical Care Guidelines suggest that weight-based estimates should be used for estimation of energy needs in lieu of indirect calorimetry. There is evidence of edema and, therefore, the weight estimated by the daughter is likely to be more reflective of the patient's dry or true weight and thus it should be used to calculate nutrient requirements.

3. Is enteral or parenteral nutrition the appropriate modality of nutrition support for this patient? Justify your response.

   Answer: Enteral feeding. While the patient is in the ICU, there is no contraindication to initiation of enteral feeding as the enteral tract has not been compromised. The patient is hemodynamically stable, but still requires vasopressor support. Therefore, it may be most appropriate to start the enteral feeding at a trophic rate and supplement additional protein via a modular protein supplement to meet the estimated protein requirement. The case should be regularly reevaluated to determine if an increase to goal enteral nutrition rate is feasible. Once the requirement for vasopressors decreases, the patient may be able to tolerate goal rate. The patient may have enteral intolerance issues that can be resolved with prokinetic medications, however, if intolerance persists, initiation of parenteral nutrition can be considered.

4. Taking into consideration the patient's laboratory values, determine what would be the best type of parenteral/enteral formula for this patient and why?

   Answer: The patient is currently hyperkalemic and has hyperphosphatemia as evidenced by his labs. In addition, the patient is anuric. For this particular case, it may be beneficial to utilize a renal-specific formula that provides less potassium and phosphorus than the standard formula. Regular monitoring of laboratory values is required to ensure continued appropriateness of the renal-specific formula. If potassium and and/or phosphorus trends down towards normal or below normal limits, it may be appropriate to change the formula type. If the patient becomes hypokalemic but continues to experience hyperphosphatemia, a standard formula with the introduction of phosphorus binders in powder form (sevelamer carbonate) may be appropriate.

References

1. Biggs JP, Kriz W, Schnermann JB. Overview of kidney function and structure. In: Greenberg A, editor. Primer on kidney disease. 4th ed. Philadelphia: Elsevier Saunders; 2005. p. 2–19.
2. Cruz DN, Ronco C. Acute kidney injury in the intensive care unit: current trends in incidence and outcome. Crit Care. 2007;11(4):149. PMCID:PMC2206527.
3. Sarav M, Kovesdy CP. Renal disease. In: The ASPEN adult nutrition support core curriculum. 3rd ed. Silver Spring: American Society for Parenteral and Enteral Nutrition; 2017.
4. Holley JL. Clinical approach to the diagnosis of acute renal failure. In: Greenberg A, editor. Primer on kidney disease. 4th ed. Philadelphia: Elsevier Saunders; 2005. p. 287–92.
5. Peacock PR, Sinert R. Renal failure, acute. Emedicine from WebMD.
6. Campbell D. How acute renal failure puts the brakes on kidney function. Nursing. 2003;33:59–64.
7. Goldstein-Fuchs DJ, McQuiston B. Renal failure. In: Matarese LE, Gottschlich MM, editors. Contemporary nutrition support practice: a clinical guide. 2nd ed. Philadelphia: Saunders; 2003. p. 460–83.
8. Chertow GM, Soroko SH, Paganin EP, Cho KC, Himmelfarb J, Ikizler TA, et al. Mortality after acute renal failure: models for prognostic stratification and risk adjustment. Kidney Int. 2006;70:1120–6.
9. Star RA. Treatment of acute renal failure. Kidney Int. 1998;54(6):1817–31.
10. Mindell JA, Chertow GM. A practical approach to acute renal failure. Med Clin North Am. 1997;81(3):731–48.
11. Kalista-Richards MA. Acute kidney injury. In: Byham-Gray LD, Burrowes JD, Chertow GM, editors. Nutrition in kidney disease. Humana Press; 2014. p. 233–45.
12. Bellamo R, Ronco C, Kellum JA, Mehta RL, Palevsky P, ADQI Workgroup. Acute renal failure—definition, outcome measures, animal models, fluid therapy and information technology needs: the Second International Consensus Conference of the Acute Dialysis Quality Initiative (ADQI) group. Crit Care. 2004;8(4):R204–12.

13. Kidney Disease: Improving Global Outcomes (KDIGO) Acute Kidney Injury Work Group. KDIGO Clinical Practice Guideline for Acute Kidney Injury. Kidney Int, Suppl. 2012;2:1–138.

14. Lewington A, Kanagasundaram S. Renal Association Clinical Practice Guidelines on acute kidney injury. Nephron Clin Pract. 2011;118(Suppl 1):c349–90.

15. Fouque D, Kalantar-Zadeh K, Kopple J, Cano N, Chauveau P, Cuppari L, et al. A proposed nomenclature and diagnostic criteria for protein–energy wasting in acute and chronic kidney disease. Kidney Int. 2008;73(4):391–8.

16. Jeong DH, Hong S-B, Lim C-M, Koh Y, Seo J, Kim Y, et al. Comparison of accuracy of NUTRIC and modified NUTRIC scores in predicting 28-day mortality in patients with sepsis: a Single Center Retrospective Study. Nutrients. 2018;17:10(7).

17. Gervasio JM, Garmon WP, Holowaty M. Nutrition support in acute kidney injury. Nutr Clin Pract. 2011;26:374–80.

18. Blumenkrantz MJ, Kopple JD, Gutman RA, Chan YK, Barbour GL, Roberts C, et al. Methods for assessing nutritional status of patients with renal failure. Am J Clin Nutr. 1980;3:1567–85.

19. Druml W. Nutrition support in acute renal failure. In: Mitch WE, Klahr S, editors. Handbook of nutrition and the kidney. 4th ed. Philadelphia: Lippincott, Williams & Wilkins; 2002. p. 191–213.

20. Traub S. The kidneys. In: Traub SL, editor. Basic skills in interpreting laboratory data. 2nd ed. Bethesda: American Society of Health-System Pharmacist; 1996. p. 131–57.

21. Fiaccadori E, Lombardi M, Leonardi S, Rotelli CF, Tortella G, Borghetti A. Prevalence and clinical outcome associated with pre-existing malnutrition in acute renal failure: a prospective cohort study. J Am Soc Nephrol. 1999;10:581–93.

22. McClave SA, Martindale RG, Vanek VW, McCarthy M, Roberts P, Taylor B, Ochoa JB, Napolitano L, Cresci G, A.S.P.E.N. Board of Directors; American College of Critical Care Medicine; Society of Critical Care Medicine. Guidelines for the provision and assessment of nutrition support therapy in the adult critically ill patient: Society of Critical Care Medicine (SCCM) and American Society for Parenteral and Enteral Nutrition (A.S.P.E.N.). JPEN J Parenter Enteral Nutr. 2009;33(3):277–313.

23. Brown RO, Compher C, American Society for Parenteral and Enteral Nutrition (A.S.P.E.N.) Board of Directors. A.S.P.E.N. clinical guidelines: nutrition support in adult acute and chronic renal failure. JPEN J Parenter Enteral Nutr. 2010;34(4):366–77.

24. Cano N, Fiaccadori E, Tesinski P, Toigo G, Druml W, DGEM, Kuhlmann M, Mann H, Horl WH. ESPEN guidelines on enteral nutrition: adult renal failure. Clin Nutr. 2006;25:295–310.

25. Harvey SE, Parrott F, Harrison DA, Bear DE, Segaran E, Beale R, et al. Trial of the route of early nutritional support in critically ill adults. N Engl J Med. 2014;371(18):1673–84.

26. Wischmeyer PE, Hasselmann M, Kummerlen C, Kozar R, Kutsogiannis DJ, Karvellas CJ, et al. A randomized trial of supplemental parenteral nutrition in underweight and overweight critically ill patients: the TOP-UP pilot trial. Crit Care. 2017;21(1):142.

27. McClave SA, Taylor BE, Martindale RG, Warren MM, Johnson DR, Braunschweig C, et al. Guidelines for the provision and assessment of nutrition support therapy in the adult critically ill patient. JPEN J Parenter Enteral Nutr. 2016;40(2):159–211.

28. A.S.P.E.N. enteral access devices: selection, insertion, maintenance, and complications. In: Boullata J, Nieman Carney L, Guenter P, editors. Enteral nutrition handbook. Silver Spring: The American Society for Parenteral and Enteral Nutrition; 2010: 159–203.

29. Parrish CR, McClave SA. Checking gastric residual volumes: a practice in search of science? Pract Gastroenterol. 2008;67:33–47.

30. Lewis K, Alqahtani Z, Mcintyre L, Almenawer S, Alshamsi F, Rhodes A, et al. The efficacy and safety of prokinetic agents in critically ill patients receiving enteral nutrition: a systematic review and meta-analysis of randomized trials. Crit Care [Internet]. 2016;20. Available from: https://www.ncbi.nlm.nih.gov/pmc/articles/PMC4986344/.

31. McClave SA, Saad MA, Esterle M, Anderson M, Jotautas AE, Franklin GA, et al. Volume-based feeding in the critically ill patient. JPEN J Parenter Enteral Nutr. 2015;39(6):707–12.

32. Harty J. Prevention and management of acute kidney injury. Ulster Med J. 2014 Sep;83(3):149–57.

33. Patel JJ, McClain CJ, Sarav M, Hamilton-Reeves J, Hurt RT. Protein requirements for critically ill patients with renal and liver failure. Nutr Clin Pract. 2017;32(1S):101S–11S.

34. Singh H, Duerksen DR. Vitamin K and nutrition support. Nutr Clin Pract. 2003;18:359–65.

35. Crook MA, Hally V, Panteli JV. The importance of the refeeding syndrome. Nutrition. 2001;17:632–7.

36. Task Force for the Revision of Safe Practices for Parenteral Nutrition. Safe practices for parenteral nutrition. JPEN J Parenter Enteral Nutr. 2004;28:S39–70.

37. Lord L, Harrington M. Enteral nutrition implementation and management. In: Merritt R, editor. A.S.P.E.N. nutrition support practice manual. 2nd ed. Silver Spring: The American Society for Parenteral and Enteral Nutrition; 2006. p. 76–89.

38. Mehanna H, Nankivell PC, Moledina J, Travis J. Refeeding syndrome – awareness, prevention and management. Head Neck Oncol. 2009;1:4.

39. Vanek WV. Closed versus open enteral delivery systems: a quality improvement study. Nutr Clin Pract. 2000;15:234–43.

40. A.S.P.E.N. Board of Directors and the Clinical Guidelines Task Force. Guidelines for the use of parenteral and enteral nutrition in adult and pediatric patients. JPEN J Parenter Enteral Nutr. 2002;26(Suppl 1):1SA–138SA.

41. Jiyong J, Tiancha H, Huiqin W, Jingfen J. Effect of gastric versus post-pyloric feeding on the incidence of pneumonia in critically ill patients: observations from traditional and Bayesian random-effects meta-analysis. Clin Nutr. 2013;1:32(1).

42. Heyland DK, Cahill N, Day AG. Optimal amount of calories for critically ill patients: depends on how you slice the cake!*. Crit Care Med. 2011;39(12):2619–26.

43. Heyland DK, Cahill NE, Dhaliwal R, Wang M, Day AG, Alenzi A, Aris F, et al. Enhanced protein—energy provision via the enteral route in critically ill patients: a single center feasibility trial to the PEP uP protocol. Crit Care. 2010;14(2):R78.

44. Ling P, McCowen KC. Carbohydrates. In: Gottschlich MM, editor. The A.S.P.E.N. nutrition support core curriculum: a case-based approach-the adult patient. Silver Spring: The American Society for Parenteral and Enteral Nutrition; 2007. p. 33–47.

45. A.S.P.E.N. how to write parenteral nutrition orders. In: Canada T, Grill C, Guenter P, editors. A.S.P.E.N. parenteral nutrition handbook. Silver Spring: The American Society for Parenteral and Enteral Nutrition; 2009: 163–85.

46. SMOFLIPID (lipid injectable emulsion) [Internet]. Available from: https://www.accessdata.fda.gov/drugsatfda_docs/label/2016/207648lbl.pdf.

47. OMEGAVEN (fish oil triglyceries) injectable emulsion, for intravenous use [Internet]. Available from: https://www.accessdata.fda.gov/drugsatfda_docs/label/2018/0210589s000lbledt.pdf.

48. Driscoll DF. Lipid injectable emulsions. Nutr Clin Pract. 2006;21:381–6.

49. A.S.P.E.N. complications of parenteral nutrition. In: Canada T, Grill C, Guenter P, editors. A.S.P.E.N. parenteral nutrition handbook. Silver Spring: The American Society for Parenteral and Enteral Nutrition; 2009: 197–234.

50. Fuhrman MP. Parenteral nutrition in kidney disease. In: Byham-Gray L, Wiesen K, editors. Clinical guide to nutrition in kidney disease. 1st ed. Chicago: The American Dietetic Association; 2004. p. 159–74.

51. Skipper A. Parenteral nutrition. In: Matarese LE, Gottschlich MM, editors. Contemporary nutrition support practice: a clinical guide. 2nd ed. Philadelphia: Saunders; 2003. p. 227–41.

52. A.S.P.E.N. parenteral nutrition formulations. In: Canada T, Grill C, Guenter P, editors. A.S.P.E.N. parenteral nutrition handbook. Silver Spring: The American Society for Parenteral and Enteral Nutrition; 2009: 129–61.

53. Baxter Healthcare Corporation. Travasol calcium phosphate solubility curves. 1995.

54. National Kidney Foundation. Nutrient prescription. In: McCann L, editor. Pocket guide to nutrition assessment of the patient with chronic kidney disease. 4th ed. New York: National Kidney Foundation; 2009. p. 4-1–4-18.

55. Hertz DE, Karn CA, Liu YM, Liechty EA, Denne SC. Intravenous glucose suppresses glucose production but not proteolysis in extremely premature newborns. J Clin Invest. 1993;92(4):1752–8.

56. Borum PR, editor. Nutrition support dietetics core curriculum. 2nd ed. 1993.

57. Kingley J. Fluid and electrolyte management in parenteral nutrition. 2005;27(6):15.

58. Eisenberg PG, Gianino S, Clutter WE, Fleshman JW. Abrupt discontinuation of cycled parenteral nutrition is safe. Dis Colon Rectum. 1995;38(9):933–9.

59. Fiaccadori E, Maggiore U, Rotelli C, Giacosa R, Picett E, Parenti E, et al. Effects of different energy intakes on nitrogen balance in patients with acute renal failure: a pilot study. Nephrol Dial Transplant. 2005;20:1976–80.

60. Fiaccadori E, Parenti E, Maggiore U. Nutrition support in acute kidney injury. J Nephrol. 2008;21:645–56.

61. Heng AE, Cano NJM. Nutritional problems in adult patients with stage 5 chronic kidney disease on dialysis (both haemodialysis and peritoneal dialysis). NDT Plus. 2010;3:109–17.

62. Druml W. Nutrition management of acute renal failure. Am J Kidney Dis. 2001;37(1 Suppl 2):S89–94.

63. Kopple JD. Nutrition management. In: Massry SG, Glassock RJ, editors. Massry & Glassock's textbook of nephrology. 4th ed. Philadelphia: Lippincott Williams & Wilkins; 2000. p. 1449–73.

64. Fiaccadori E, Regolisti G, Cabassi A. Specific nutritional problems in acute kidney injury, treated with non-dialysis and dialytic modalities. NDT Plus. 2010;3:1–7.

65. van den Berghe G, Woutersn P, Weekers F, Verwaest C, Bruyninckx F, Schetz M, et al. Intensive insulin therapy in the critically ill patients. N Engl J Med. 2001;345:1359–67.

66. Cano N, Aparicio M, Brunori G, Carrero JJ, Cianciaruso B, Fiaccadori E, et al. ESPEN guidelines on parenteral nutrition. Parenteral nutrition in adult renal failure. Clin Nutr. 2009;28(4):401–14.

67. Wooley JA, Btaiche IF, Good KL. Metabolic and nutritional aspects of acute renal failure in critically ill patients requiring continuous renal replacement therapy. Nutr Clin Pract. 2005;20(2):176–91.

68. Frankenfield DC, Reynolds HN. Nutritional effect of continuous hemodiafiltration. Nutrition. 1995;11(4):388–93.

69. Metnitz GH, Fischer M, Bartens C, Steltzer H, Lang T, Druml W. Impact of acute renal failure on antioxidant status in multiple organ failure. Acta Anaesthesiol Scand. 2000;44:236–40.

70. Strejc JM. Considerations in the nutritional management of patients with acute renal failure. Hemodial Int. 2005;9:135–42.

71. Moskowitz A, Andersen LW, Huang DT, Berg KM, Grossestreuer AV, Marik PE, et al. Ascorbic acid, corticosteroids, and thiamine in sepsis: a review of the biologic rationale and the present state of clinical evaluation. Crit Care [Internet]. 2018 [cited 14 Mar 2019]; 22.

72. Fiaccadori E, Cremaschi E, Regolisti G. Nutritional assessment and delivery in renal replacement therapy patients. Semin Dial Wiley Online Library. 2011;24(2):169–75.

73. Berger MM, Shenkin A, Revelly JP, Roberts E, Cayeux MC, Baines M, et al. Copper, selenium, zinc and thiamine balances during continuous venovenous hemodiafiltration in critically ill patients. Am J Clin Nutr. 2004;80(2):410–6.

74. Heyland D, Stoppe C, Benstoem C, Lemieux M. Systematic reviews Critical Care Nutrition [Internet]. [cited 28 Feb 2019]. Available from: https://criticalcarenutrition.com/systematic-reviews.

75. Story DA, Ronco C, Bellomo R. Trace element and vitamin concentration and losses in critically ill patients treated with continuous venovenous hemofiltration. Crit Care Med. 1999;27:220–3.

76. Jin J, Mulesa L, Carrilero RM. Trace elements in parenteral nutrition: considerations for the prescribing clinician. Nutrients. 2017;28:9(5).

77. Fall P, Szerlip HM. Continuous renal replacement therapy: cause and treatment of electrolyte complications. Semin Dial. 2010;23(6):581–5.

Part VII
Additional Nutritional Considerations in Kidney Disease

This last section of the text represents additional nutrition-related topics that are of keen interest to the practicing health professional working with patients diagnosed with kidney disease and are organized into three overarching themes: (1) physiological and metabolic changes that occur in kidney disease; (2) the role of complementary and alternative therapies, such as physical activity and exercise as well as dietary supplements; and lastly (3) key resources that assist the practitioner in the education and counseling of patients diagnosed with kidney disease as part of a multicultural society.

In terms of physiological and metabolic changes that occur in kidney disease, Mafra and Borges begin this section describing the gut microbiome in both health and in disease. Dysbiosis, or microbial imbalance or maladaptation, readily occurs in kidney disease and is associated with an increased risk for cardiovascular disease. The authors present the latest research evidence related to pre-, pro-, and synbiotics, which are theorized to improve the gut microbiota in this vulnerable group. Protein-energy wasting, a syndrome exhibited in kidney disease that includes malnutrition, is widely prevalent across the globe. Guebre-Egziabher suggests that some of the factors related to a suboptimal oral intake are secondary to impaired appetite regulation. Besides alterations in neuroendocrine or central nervous system pathways, the existence of uremia, chronic inflammation, as well as behavioral and environmental factors are other key components that shape eating habits and patterns. Lastly, Biruete and Uribarri explore the latest science regarding the role of advanced glycation end products (AGEs) which are pro-oxidative and pro-inflammatory metabolites that have been linked to kidney disease progression. AGEs may be either of endogenous or exogenous sources. The authors give a thorough explanation of the metabolic implications for AGEs as well as offer practical guidance on how to lower the AGEs content in the diet among persons at considerable risk for kidney disease.

Complementary and alternative therapies comprise biologically based (e.g., dietary supplements) and manipulative or body-based practices (e.g., physical activity and exercise). Persons diagnosed with kidney disease are known to have declining functional status secondary to the loss of muscle mass resulting in sarcopenia. Such deleterious effects of inactivity can be reversed with exercise. Meade and Wilund provide an overview of the importance for routine physical activity and structured exercise in patients diagnosed with kidney disease and how health professionals can help to make these lifestyle changes achievable. In regard to biologically based practices, Radler describes some of the dietary supplements that may either provide protective benefits to kidney function or may be potentially harmful or associated with known drug interactions. The author also discusses health policy and regulations related to dietary supplements and encourages health professionals to engage their patients so they feel comfortable disclosing the use of any substances. Steiber et al. complete a comprehensive review of micronutrients often of concern in kidney disease. The authors identify how micronutrient imbalances may occur either during the disease course or its management, and evaluate the current level of evidence on appropriate interventions aimed at improving nutrient status across the spectrum of disease.

Patient-centered care requires that health professionals educate and counsel individuals about their disease so that they can make informed decisions about their treatment. Isoldi describes several theoretical models and counseling approaches that will assist the health professional in communicating effectively with their clients. The author also provides illustrative examples on how to apply these techniques into practice. Regardless whether in the United States or across the globe, health professionals must be cognizant of practices that may impact food selection, dietary intake, and adherence. Burrowes discusses the social determinants of health (e.g., economics, environment, culture) and how these factors can affect the ability of the individual to adhere to therapeutic lifestyle changes, specifically as it relates to diet. In addition, the author establishes some practical ways to improve dietary adherence in patients diagnosed with kidney disease. In the chapter on **Dietary Patterns**, Kelly further emphasizes the importance of adopting a heart healthy approach to food selection and eating. The author reviews the level of evidence supporting plant-based diets and the mindful considerations when implementing them in practice. To further assist the health professional, Prest provides a thorough list of invaluable resources that are available to the practitioner related to diet and nutrition in kidney disease. Lastly, Byham-Gray encourages that health professionals integrate a patient-centered approach when evaluating the effectiveness of diet and nutrition interventions in this population. The author provides examples on how health professionals can measure the impact that they make on patient outcomes and offers an overview of the steps in the research process within the practice-based setting.

Chapter 27
The Gut Microbiome

Denise Mafra and Natália Alvarenga Borges

Keywords Gut microbiota · Microbiome · Chronic kidney disease · Dysbiosis · Probiotic · Prebiotic Synbiotic · Uremic toxins · Diet · Nutrients

---

Key Points
- The gut microbiota interact with the host in a continuous relationship indispensable to the host homeostasis.
- There is a bidirectional cause-effect relationship between chronic kidney disease (CKD) and the gut microbiota.
- The modulation of the gut microbiota composition and function has been targeted to improve the metabolic repercussions of CKD.
- Pre-, pro-, and synbiotics have been proposed as potential therapeutic strategies in CKD patients.

Introduction

Microbiome refers to the genes encoded in the microbiota genome that are about three million, in contrast to the human cells genes that are around 23,000 [1]. The microbiome is recognized as our "second genome," a connotation that refers to the complex biochemical and metabolic role of the gut bacteria in the human body [2].

The gut is the most colonized place (1.5 kg of bacteria) in the human body with trillions of microbes (majority composed by anaerobes), which contains two big phyla: *Bacteroidetes* and *Firmicutes*, but *Proteobacteria*, *Verrucomicrobia*, *Actinobacteria*, *Fusobacteria*, and *Cyanobacteria* can also be present [1, 2].

The composition of the human gut microbiota is influenced by multiple factors, including type of delivery, duration of breastfeeding, hygiene and use of antibiotics. Infants, exclusively breastfed, have a microbiota dominated by bifidobacteria, and, due to physiological changes and dietary habits, the gut microbiota change.

Diet is the first modulator of microbiota profile in the gastrointestinal tract. Some nutrients from foods reach the colon and are metabolized by these bacteria. For example, carbohydrate fermentation in the colon form hydrogen, methane, and short-chain fatty acids (SCFA), such as

---

D. Mafra (✉)
Department of Clinical Nutrition, Federal University Fluminense, Niterói, Rio de Janeiro, Brazil

N. A. Borges
Institute of Nutrition, Rio de Janeiro State University (UERJ), Rio de Janeiro, RJ, Brazil

© Springer Nature Switzerland AG 2020
J. D. Burrowes et al. (eds.), *Nutrition in Kidney Disease*, Nutrition and Health,
https://doi.org/10.1007/978-3-030-44858-5_27

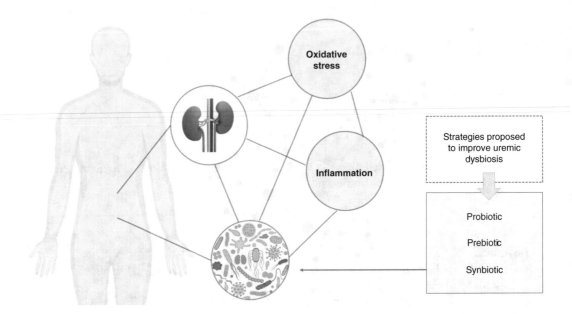

Fig. 27.1 The network among the gut microbiota, kidney, inflammation, and oxidative stress in chronic kidney disease (CKD) and some therapeutic strategies proposed to modulate gut microbiota with possible effects in all interrelated factors

butyrate, propionate, and acetate. Many of these end products are generally accepted to be beneficial to the host. On the other hand, end products from proteins' fermentation, including metabolites such as ammonia, amines, thiols, phenols, and indoles, are potentially toxic [3]. Additionally, the enzymatic activity of gut bacteria contribute to the breakdown of the oligomeric and polymeric polyphenols into low-molecular-weight phenolic metabolites, increasing their bioavailability [4]. Thus, nutrients impact diversity, density, and functionality of the gut microbiota, while microbiota-derived metabolites connect the gut microbiota with distant organs, impacting health and disease.

Under normal conditions, the gut microbiota and the host are in a continuous relationship indispensable to the host homeostasis. Metabolites from microbiota such as SCFA and vitamins enter the bloodstream and promote benefits to the host. In contrast, when there are abnormalities in the gut barrier or even in the microbiota composition, some toxins from the gut can reach the blood-like lipopolysaccharide (LPS) and uremic toxins, leading to oxidative stress and inflammation [5, 6].

Dysbiosis is found to be closely related to chronic kidney disease (CKD) complications and some strategies have been proposed to decrease this gut microbiota imbalance like the use of probiotic, prebiotic, or synbiotic supplementation (Fig. 27.1). However, there is still no consensus by the clinical guidelines on which type of supplementation is better for CKD patients. In this chapter, we will describe practical applications of nutritional strategies to modulate the gut microbiota in CKD patients.

Gut Microbiota in CKD

In CKD patients, the uremic milieu seems to impair the structure and function of the gut microbiota and epithelial barrier, promoting inflammation and oxidative stress and disturbing the metabolism. There is a bidirectional cause-effect relationship between CKD and the gut microbiota. With the loss of kidney function, there is an accumulation of a range of molecules in the blood, among them urea, which has been identified as a substance harmful to the intestinal barrier, compromising its integrity. In addition, the accumulation of urea in the gut lumen disturbs the gut environment, leading to changes in the composition and functionality of the gut microbiota. On the other hand, these disorders in the gut microbiota, promoted by CKD, lead to increased production of substances resulting from gut microbial metabolism, as uremic toxins such as indoxyl sulfate (IS), p-cresyl sulfate (p-CS), indole-3-acetic acid (IAA), and trimethylamine-N-oxide (TMAO), which accumulate in the blood, aggravating the state of inflammation in these patients by activating the immune system. Thus, the gut microbiota may be seen as the cross-road between CKD and the phenotype of inflammation and oxidative stress, typical of these patients [7, 8].

Nutrients influence the composition of the gut microbiota in CKD patients, and in addition, intestinal bacteria also promote the conversion of dietary components leading to the formation of a wide variety of metabolites, which may have beneficial or adverse effects on human health.

High-protein diets lead to a high amount of protein in the colon, resulting in increased fermentation of products that include nitrogenous metabolites detrimental to the integrity of the intestinal microbiota [9].

The amino acid tryptophan can be metabolized to indole by tryptophanase in the large intestine by intestinal bacteria, such as *Escherichia coli*. Indole is absorbed into the blood, undergoing oxidation and sulfation in the liver and then is metabolized to indoxyl sulfate. The accumulation of indoxyl sulfate is associated with high concentrations of interlukin-6 (IL-6), stimulates progressive tubulointerstitial fibrosis, glomerular sclerosis, and progression of CKD by increasing expression of transforming growth factor (TGF)-β1 that works by inhibiting the production of metalloproteinase (TIMP) 1 and pro-α 1 (I) collagen, leading to loss of nephrons and completing a vicious cycle of renal injury [10].

The uremic toxin indole-3-acetic acid (IAA) is also produced from tryptophan being metabolized to indole directly in the intestine or tissue via tryptamine. IAA is commonly excreted in the urine and accumulates in the blood of patients with CKD. It is an aryl hydrocarbon receptor (AhR) transcription agonist, which regulates cell response by means of xenobiotics, such as tetrachlorodibenzo-p-dioxin. Activation of AhR by exogenous ligands promotes vascular inflammation, oxidative stress, and atherosclerosis, and plays an important role in the development of cardiovascular disease (CVD) [11].

On the other hand, the amino acids tyrosine and phenylalanine from dietary protein undergo conversion to 4-hydroxyphenylacetic acid by putrefactive bacteria of the intestinal microbiota, which is then decarboxylated to p-cresol by an enzyme that has been shown to be present in *Clostridium difficile*. In addition, the gut microbiota can convert dietary choline and L-carnitine into trimethylamine (TMA), which in the liver is metabolized into trimethylamine *N*-oxide (TMAO), associated with atherosclerosis risk in CKD patients [12].

Research has shown a relationship between dysbiosis and increased cardiovascular risk and mortality in CKD patients, and some strategies are proposed to reduce this risk such as pre-, pro-, or synbiotic supplementation.

Probiotics

According to the WHO, probiotics are live microorganisms with beneficial effects on the health of the host [13]. In recent years, there was a rapid increase in the use of probiotics that affected the intestinal ecology, physiology, and metabolism [6]. Probiotic functions vary according to the specific strain, but in CKD patients their effects remain controversial [14, 15].

The strains most commonly used are *B. bifidum, B. bifidus, B. lactis, B. longum, B. breve (Yakult)*, and *B. infantis* [6]. Administration of some probiotics may ameliorate the metabolic changes, but positive results have to be further confirmed in CKD patients in well-designed clinical trials. Probiotics have contributed to a reduction in uremic toxins, inflammatory markers, and urea [15, 16], but some other reports have shown opposite results or no benefits at all [14, 17–19].

When we think about the use of probiotics as a therapeutic alternative to restore the gut microbiota of CKD patients, uremia should be considered because it alters the intestinal biochemical environment and does not promote a hospitable environment, which compromises the efficacy of this therapy [7, 14]. Supplementation of a single probiotic strain or a combination of different strains is another issue to consider because bacteria may behave differently when combined with others [20]. In addition, according to Tsai et al. [6], special care should be taken in the use of probiotics in patients with severe immunodeficiency, malnutrition, and cancer.

Since the effect of probiotics is controversial in CKD patients, their prescription as the only intervention is not recommended. The combination of probiotics with other strategies to benefit the gut ecosystem, such as a healthy diet rich in prebiotics and bioactive compounds, for example, could be more effective [14, 15, 21]. Then, more randomized controlled clinical trials are needed to clarify the role of probiotics as a good therapeutic strategy for CKD patients.

Prebiotics

Prebiotics are nondigestible food ingredients that are fermented by the gut microbiota in the colon and show beneficial effects on the host. Dietary fibers are among the most known prebiotics, including:

Resistant starch (RS), defined as the starch fraction that is resistant to the pancreatic α-amylase hydrolysis and reaches the large bowel, is available as substrate for bacterial fermentation [22]. There are four different types of resistant starch: RS 1, physically inaccessible whole or partly, abundant in milled grains, seeds, and legumes; RS 2, present in raw potato, green banana, some legumes, and high-amylose starches; RS 3, also called retrograded starch (cooked and cooled) from potato, bread, and cornflakes; and RS 4, etherized, esterified, or cross-bonded starches present in processed foods.

Nonstarch polysaccharides, a large variety of polysaccharide molecules excluding RS: celluloses (vegetables), hemicelluloses (cereal grains), pectins (fruits, vegetables, legumes, sugar beet, potato), gums (leguminous seed plants, seaweed extracts, microbial gums), and mucilage (plant extracts) [23].

Inulin is a water-soluble storage polysaccharide belonging to a group of nondigestible carbohydrates called fructans. It is naturally found in chicory (the richest source), garlic, asparagus, onion, banana and wheat [24].

Oligosaccharides are composed of up to twenty monosaccharides. The most popular are fructooligosaccharides (FOS), fructose units polymerized present in wheat, rye, honey, onion, garlic, and banana; galactooligosaccharides (GOS), complex oligosaccharide compound in greater quantity by galactose units occurring naturally in mammalian milk; and xylooligosaccharides (XOS), composed of chains of xylose moieties. These are found in plant sources like Bengal gram husk, wheat bran and straw, spent wood, barley hulls, brewery spent grains, almond shells, bamboo, and corn cob [25].

Fibers are the main source of energy for the gut microbiota and promote growth of *Bifidobacteria* and *Lactobacilli* species that synthetize SCFA as acetate, propionate, and butyrate, which confer a health benefit, including immunomodulatory effects.

Little is known about the clinical effects of prebiotics in CKD patients and only few select prebiotics have been studied. Some positive results on uremic toxins and inflammatory or oxidative stress markers have been reported. Meijers et al. [26] observed that supplementation for hemodialysis (HD) patients of 10–20 g/d of oligofructose-enriched inulin for 4 weeks caused reduction of 20% on p-CS plasma levels. In another study conducted by Sirich et al. [27], it was observed that 15 g/d of resistant starch for 6 weeks promoted reduction in IS plasma levels. In the study by Esgalhado et al. [28], 16 g/d of RS supplementation for 4 weeks reduced IS plasma levels and also IL-6 and TBARS (an oxidative stress marker) in hemodialysis (HD) patients.

Although few studies have evaluated the effects of prebiotics directly on the gut microbiota, the results observed possibly reflect gut microbiota modulation and restoration of the intestinal barrier promoted by prebiotics. Therefore, CKD patients may benefit from intake of prebiotic-rich foods.

Synbiotics

Synbiotics refer to food ingredients composed of probiotics and prebiotics, and their effects depend on the combination of both. The most common are *Bifidobacterium* or *Lactobacillus* with fructooligosaccharides (FOS), which have the potential to stimulate growth of these strains [6]. Thus, theoretically, the use of synbiotics may have better health effects compared with isolated use of pre- or probiotics. Synbiotics seem promising in CKD; however, studies on synbiotics in CKD are few and have analyzed inulin, FOS, and GOS, generally with small amounts compared to studies with isolated prebiotic supplementation, associated with different strains across the *Lactobacillus*, *Bifidobacteria*, and *Streptococcus* genera. They have observed different parameters or outcomes, but generally with positive results. However, there is limited evidence to support the recommendation of synbiotic use in CKD patients [29, 30].

Diet Composition

Some nutrients from the diet, when not absorbed or when escaping the absorption process, are able to be processed by the gut microbiota. There is a body of evidence that dysbiosis can be caused by food ingredients and it is associated with several complications. For example, around 12–18 g of residual dietary proteins reach the colon every day and they are metabolized by the gut microbiota; they produce toxic substances like ammonia, amines, phenols, thiols, and indols [9], mainly when this protein comes from red meat [31]. Studies on vegetarian or low-protein diets in which red meat intake is reduced have been shown to be effective in decreasing uremic toxins in CKD patients [32, 33].

As food is the first modulator of the gut microbiota, more attention should be paid to that. There are no studies on the effects of the amount of salt and sugar in the diet on the gut microbiota in CKD patients, but recent studies suggest that both may alter the gut microbiota composition [34, 35]. The same with polyphenol-rich foods like grapes, red wine, pomegranate, garlic, green tea, chocolate, turmeric, blueberry, and cranberry that may modify the composition of the gut microbiota, but no study has been published in CKD patients. Artificial sweeteners (saccharin, sucralose, aspartame, and acesulfame K) may increase *Firmicutes*, which are involved in the inhibition of anaerobic fermentation of glucose [36]. Also, food-emulsifying agents and food additives may alter the gut microbiota diversity.

Conclusion

Gut microbiota studies in CKD are highly relevant; however, more studies about the effects of prebiotics/probiotics/synbiotics or other diet components on amelioration of CKD complications are necessary. Synbiotics or even prebiotics may be a good alternative strategy to restore the gut microbiota profile in CKD patients, but there is no set recommendation for dietary intake of these compounds in this population.

References

1. Qin J, Li R, Raes J, Arumugam M, Burgdorf KS, Manichanh C, et al. A human gut microbial gene catalogue established by metagenomic sequencing. Nature. 2010;464(7285):59–65.
2. Grice EA, Segre JA. The human microbiome: our second genome. Annu Rev Genomics Hum Genet. 2012;13:151–70.
3. Evenepoel P, Meijers BK, Bammens BR, Verbeke K. Uremic toxins originating from colonic microbial metabolism. Kidney Int Suppl. 2009;114:S12–9.
4. Cardona F, Andrés-Lacueva C, Tulipani S, Tinahones FJ, Queipo-Ortuño MI. Benefits of polyphenols on gut microbiota and implications in human health. J Nutr Biochem. 2013;24(8):1415–22.
5. Pisano A, D'Arrigo G, Coppolino G, Bolignano D. Biotic supplements for renal patients: a systematic review and meta-analysis. Nutrients. 2018;10(9). pii: E1224.
6. Tsai YL, Lin TL, Chang CJ, Wu TR, Lai WF, Lu CC, et al. Probiotics, prebiotics and amelioration of diseases. J Biomed Sci. 2019;26(1):3.
7. Vaziri ND, Zhao YY, Pahl MV. Altered intestinal microbial flora and impaired epithelial barrier structure and function in CKD: the nature, mechanisms, consequences and potential treatment. Nephrol Dial Transplant. 2015;31(5):737–46.
8. Khodor SA, Shatat IF. Gut microbiome and kidney disease: a bidirectional relationship. Pediatr Nephrol. 2016;32(6):921–31.
9. Mafra D, Barros AF, Fouque D. Dietary protein metabolism by gut microbiota and its consequences for chronic kidney disease patients. Future Microbiol. 2013;8(10):1317–23.
10. Niwa T. Role of indoxyl sulfate in the progression of chronic kidney disease and cardiovascular disease: experimental and clinical effects of oral sorbent AST-120. Ther Apher Dial. 2011;15(2):120–4.
11. Brito JS, Borges NA, Esgalhado M, Magliano DC, Soulage CO, Mafra D. Aryl hydrocarbon receptor activation in chronic kidney disease: role of uremic toxins. Nephron. 2017;137(1):1–7.
12. Borges NA, Stenvinkel P, Bergman P, Qureshi AR, Lindholm B, Moraes C, et al. Effects of probiotic supplementation on trimethylamine-N-oxide plasma levels in hemodialysis patients: a pilot study. Probiotics Antimicrob Proteins. 2019;11:648–54.
13. Hill C, Guarner F, Reid G, Gibson GR, Merenstein DJ, Pot B, et al. The International Scientific Association for Probiotics and Prebiotics consensus statement on the scope and appropriate use of the term probiotic. Nat Rev Gastroenterol Hepatol. 2014;11(8):506–14.
14. Borges NA, Carmo FL, Stockler-Pinto MB, de Brito JS, Dolenga CJ, Ferreira DC, et al. Probiotic supplementation in chronic kidney disease: a double-blind, randomized, placebo-controlled trial. J Ren Nutr. 2018;28(1):28–36.
15. Sánchez B, Delgado S, Blanco-Miguez A, Lourenço A, Gueimonde M, Margolles A. Probiotics, gut microbiota, and their influence on host health and disease. Mol Nutr Food Res. 2017;61(1):1–15
16. Wang IK, Wu YY, Yang YF. The effect of probiotics on serum levels of cytokine and endotoxin in peritoneal dialysis patients: a randomized, double-blind, placebo controlled trial. Benef Microbes. 2015;6(4):423–30.
17. Eidi F, Gholi FP, Ostadrahimi A, Dalili N, Samadian F, Barzegari A. Effect of Lactobacillus Rhamnosus on serum uremic toxins (phenol and P-Cresol) in hemodialysis patients: A double blind randomized clinical trial. Clin Nut ESPEN. 2018;28:158–64.
18. Shariaty Z, Mahmoodi GR, Farajollahi M, Amerian M, Behnam PN. The effects of probiotic supplement on hemoglobin in chronic renal failure patients under hemodialysis: a randomized clinical trial. J Res Med Sci. 2017;22:74.
19. Barros AF, Borges NA, Nakao LS, Dolenga CJ, Carmo FL, Ferreira DC, et al. Effects of probiotic supplementation on inflammatory biomarkers and uremic toxins in non-dialysis chronic kidney patients: a double-blind, randomized, placebo-controlled trial. J Funct Foods. 2018;46:378–83.
20. Gareau MG, Sherman P, Walker WA. Probiotics and the gut microbiota in intestinal health and disease. Nat Rev Gastroenterol Hepatol. 2010;7(9):503–14.
21. Lozupone CA, Stombaugh JI, Gordon JI, Jansson JK, Knight R. Diversity, stability and resilience of the human gut microbiota. Nature. 2012;489(7415):220–30.
22. Moraes C, Borges NA, Mafra D. Resistant starch for modulation of gut microbiota: promising adjuvant therapy for chronic kidney disease patients? Eur J Nutr. 2016;55(5):1813–21.
23. Dhingra D, Michael M, Rajput H, Patil RT. Dietary fiber in foods: a review. J Food Sci Technol. 2011;49(3):255–66.
24. Shoaib M, Shehzad A, Omar M, Rakha A, Raza H, Sharif HR, et al. Inulin: properties, health benefits and food applications. Carbohydr Polym. 2016;147:444–54.
25. Belorkar AS, Gupta AK. Oligosaccharides: a boon from nature's desk. AMB Express. 2016;6(1):82.
26. Meijers BK, De Preter V, Verbeke K, Vanrenterghem Y, Evenepoel P. p-Cresyl sulfate serum concentrations in haemodialysis patients are reduced by the prebiotic oligofructose-enriched inulin. Nephrol Dial Transplant. 2010 Jan;25(1):219–24.
27. Sirich TL, Plummer NS, Gardner CD, Hostetter TH, Meyer TW. Effect of increasing dietary fiber on plasma levels of colon-derived solutes in hemodialysis patients. Clin J Am Soc Nephrol. 2014;9(9):1603–10.

28. Esgalhado M, Kemp JA, Azevedo R, Paiva BR, Stockler-Pinto MB, Dolenga CJ, et al. Could resistant starch supplementation improve inflammatory and oxidative stress biomarkers and uremic toxins levels in hemodialysis patients? A pilot randomized controlled trial. Food Funct. 2018;9(12):6508–16.

29. Rossi M, Johnson DW, Morrison M, Pascoe EM, Coombes JS, Forbes JM, et al. Synbiotics Easing Renal Failure by Improving Gut Microbiology (SYNERGY): a randomized trial. Clin J Am Soc Nephrol. 2016;11(2):223–31.

30. Dehghani H, Heidari F, Mozaffari-Khosravi H, Nouri-Majelan N, Dehghani A. Synbiotic supplementations for azotemia in patients with chronic kidney disease: a randomized controlled trial. Iran J Kidney Dis. 2016;10(6):351–7.

31. Mafra D, Borges NA, Cardozo LFMF, Anjos JS, Black AP, Moraes C, et al. Red meat intake in chronic kidney disease patients: two sides of the coin. Nutrition. 2018;46:26–32.

32. Black AP, Anjos JS, Cardozo L, Carmo FL, Dolenga CJ, Nakao LS, et al. Does low-protein diet influence the uremic toxin serum levels from the gut microbiota in nondialysis chronic kidney disease patients? J Ren Nutr. 2018;28(3):208–14.

33. Kandouz S, Mohamed AS, Zheng Y, Sandeman S, Davenport A. Reduced protein bound uraemic toxins in vegetarian kidney failure patients treated by haemodiafiltration. Hemodial Int. 2016;20(4):610–7.

34. Hu J, Luo H, Wang J, Tang W, Lu J, Wu S, et al. Enteric dysbiosis-linked gut barrier disruption triggers early renal injury induced by chronic high salt feeding in mice. Exp Mol Med. 2017;49(8):e370–0.

35. Rinninella E, Mele M, Merendino N, Cintoni M, Anselmi G, Caporossi A, et al. The role of diet, micronutrients and the gut microbiota in age- related macular degeneration: new perspectives from the gut–retina Axis. Nutrients. 2018;10(11):1677.

36. Wang Q-P, Browman D, Herbert H, Gregory Neely G, Virolle M-J. Non-nutritive sweeteners possess a bacteriostatic effect and alter gut microbiota in mice. PLoS One. 2018;13(7):e0199080.

Chapter 28
Appetite Regulation

Fitsum Guebre-Egziabher

Keywords Appetite · Hypothalamus · GI motility · Orexigenic pathway · Anorexigenic pathway Chronic kidney disease · Food intake · Food preference · Neurohormonal circuits

Key Points
- The brain, especially the hypothalamus, plays a key role in the control of food intake.
- The gut-brain axis ensures the coupling between nutrient intake, feeding behaviors, and activity of the reward system.
- Peripheral hormones modulate feeding behaviors via direct or indirect central signaling pathways.
- Gastrointestinal hormones and signaling metabolites are secreted in response to mechanical and chemical properties of ingested food, and most of them with the exception of ghrelin restrain further food intake.
- Chronic kidney disease (CKD) often exhibits symptoms of anorexia.
- CKD-associated alteration of appetite is complex and multifactorial.
- Impaired neuroendocrine or central factors that regulate appetite, accumulation of uremic toxins, inflammation, and neurological dysfunction may all play a critical role in CKD-associated anorexia.
- Behavioral and environmental factors may also be key players shaping eating behavior in CKD.

Introduction

Malnutrition and overnutrition are both related to inadequate energy intake, and they are the major public health issues worldwide. Health is influenced by diet composition as well as total energy consumption. All diets contain a mixture of the three macronutrients (protein, carbohydrate, and fat), with varying proportions from one diet or another. Food intake is regulated by complex neurohormonal circuits that can be impaired in metabolic diseases. Peripheral hormones participate in the regulation of energy homeostasis via direct or indirect central signaling pathways. Food preferences are formed by multiple factors, including social, environmental, and genetic determinants. Individual food preferences are prominent determinants of food intakes and subsequently may have implications for the

F. Guebre-Egziabher (✉)
Department of Nephrology, Dialysis and Hypertension, Hospices Civils de Lyon, Hôpital Edouard Herriot, Laboratoire CarMeN, INSERM u1060, Université Lyon-1, Lyon, France

Faculté de Médecine Lyon-Est, Université Lyon-1, Lyon, France
e-mail: fitsum.guebre-egziabher@chu-lyon.fr

© Springer Nature Switzerland AG 2020
J. D. Burrowes et al. (eds.), *Nutrition in Kidney Disease*, Nutrition and Health,
https://doi.org/10.1007/978-3-030-44858-5_28

development of long-term chronic diseases such as obesity, diabetes, and chronic kidney diseases (CKD) that are increasingly prevalent.

The development of CKD may further impair appetite regulation that impacts the neuroendocrine or central factors that regulate appetite. These alterations might explain the increased prevalence of protein-energy wasting (PEW) during CKD.

Role of the Central Nervous System

The central nervous system (CNS) plays an important role in energy metabolism, through the regulation of appetite and the circuits that control hunger, food seeking, and the hedonic aspect of feeding (Fig. 28.1). Neural centers in the hypothalamus regulate food intake and body weight in response to hormones and other neural stimuli.

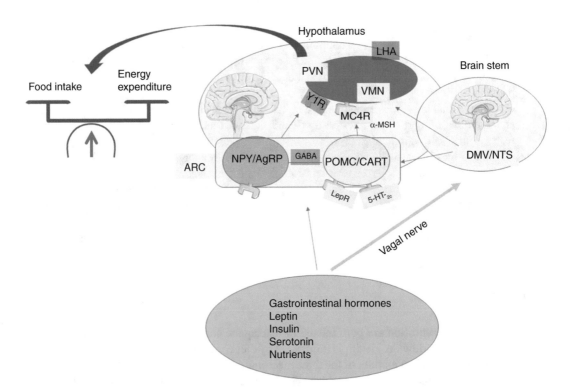

Fig. 28.1 Schematic representation of central regulation of appetite. Hypothalamic arcuate nucleus (ARC) receives direct stimulation from the peripheral hormones and signaling molecules through its incomplete blood-brain barrier or indirectly from the brainstem (through the vagal nerve). In the ARC two populations of neurons coexist: orexigenic (containing neuropeptide Y (NPY) or agouti-related peptide (AgRP)) and anorexigenic (containing cocaine- and amphetamine-related transcript (CART) and proopiomelanocortin (POMC), the precursor of α-melanocyte-stimulating hormone). α-MSH signals through melanocortin receptor 4 (MC4-R) and NPY through neuropeptide YY$_1$ receptor (Y1R). NPY/AgRP neurons have axon terminals that release the inhibitory neurotransmitter GABA. Activation of ventromedial (VMN) or paraventricular nucleus (PVN) of the hypothalamus causes hypophagia, increased energy expenditure, and weight loss, while lateral hypothalamic area (LHA) is reported to induce hyperphagia, decreased energy expenditure, and weight gain. PVN paraventricular nucleus, VMN ventromedial nucleus, DMV dorsal motor nucleus of the vagus nerve, LHA lateral hypothalamic area, ARC arcuate nucleus, NPY neuropeptide Y, AgRP agouti-related protein, NTS nucleus of the solitary tract, POMC proopiomelanocortin, α-MSH α-melanocyte-stimulating hormone, MC4-R melanocortin receptor 4, LepR leptin receptor, 5-HT-$_{2C}$ hypothalamic serotonin receptor

Hypothalamic lesioning experiments in rodents allowed the identification of key brain areas associated with energy balance and food intake. Bilateral lesions of the ventromedial nucleus (VMN) or paraventricular nucleus (PVN) of the hypothalamus cause hyperphagia, decreased energy expenditure, and weight gain, while lesions of the lateral hypothalamic area (LHA) are reported to induce hypophagia, increased energy expenditure, and weight loss [1]. Two distinct populations of neurons with opposite function on feeding behavior are located in the arcuate nucleus of the hypothalamus (ARC): the orexigenic neuropeptide Y (NPY)/agouti-related peptide (AgRP) neurons and the anorexigenic proopiomelanocortin (POMC) neurons. Food restriction studies in rodents have shown an increased expression of mRNA encoding anabolic peptides, NPY, AgRP, melanin-concentrating hormone (MCH) and orexin, and decreased mRNA expression for catabolic peptides, such as corticotropin-releasing hormone (CRH) and POMC which is the precursor of melanocortin [2–4]. Furthermore, central injections of NPY, AgRP, MCH, and orexin increase food intake [3, 5–7], whereas CRH and α-melanocyte-stimulating hormone (α-MSH) which derives from POMC decrease food intake [8, 9]. One of the key players is melanocortin receptor 4 (MC4-R) found in neurons of the paraventricular region which upon activation suppress food intake. MC4-R is activated by α-MSH or when NPY and AgRP are inhibited. AgRP is an endogenous antagonist of melanocortin receptors in the brain and, consequently, increases food intake by blocking the anorectic action of α-MSH [6]. NPY/AgRP neurons have axon terminals that release the inhibitory neurotransmitter gamma-aminobutyric acid (GABA).

In the arcuate nucleus of the hypothalamus (ARC), there are two populations of neurons expressing POMC – one expressing leptin receptor (LepR) and the other expressing a subtype of serotonin receptors. Serotonin is a neurotransmitter that modulates neural activity through receptors that are expressed in all brain regions. Brain serotonergic activity has been reported to be implicated in appetite and reward regulation by modulating the anorexigenic POMC pathway through hypothalamic 5-HT-$_{2C}$ receptors [10]. Treatment with 5-HT-$_{2C}$ agonist in humans has been reported to suppress appetite and decrease energy intake and body weight [11–13].

Another important mediator of feeding is the central reward system, which promotes adaptive actions such as consuming palatable nutrients by associating them with pleasure. Neural circuits involving the hypothalamus, brainstem, and mesolimbic system play a role in the regulation of eating behavior. Furthermore, there is evidence in favor of preferences for different nutrients that may impact both total energy intake and food choices [14–19], but the underlying mechanisms are not well defined.

Central melanocortin signaling has been reported to be involved in food preference in rodent models [14, 15]. In humans, there is evidence suggesting that food preferences are partly under genetic control [16]. Fat mass and obesity-associated (FTO) gene variants have been shown to associate with elevated dietary protein intake in adults [20, 21] and energy dense food in children [22]. MC4-R deficiency in humans was reported to be associated with an increased preference for high fat and reduced preference for sucrose rich food, mirroring the effects that were reported in MC4-R KO rodent models [17, 18]. Lastly, variants at the chromosome 19 locus were reported to be correlated with increased carbohydrate but decreased protein and fat intake. The candidate gene encodes a circulating liver-derived fibroblast growth factor (FGF)-21 and is involved in lipid and glucose metabolism [19, 20].

Role of the Gastrointestinal System

A primary function of the gut is to achieve food efficiency through nutrient digestion and absorption that can be optimized via gastrointestinal (GI) motility and secretion. GI hormones and signaling metabolites are secreted in response to mechanical and chemical properties of ingested food, and most of them restrain further food intake.

Foods are sensed in the oral cavity by receptors present on the surface of taste bud cells, which transduce signals generated during feeding to the brain by fibers of the cranial nerves VII, IX, and X. These gustatory messages enter the nucleus of the solitary tract (NTS).

As the core of appetite regulation lies in the gut-brain axis, efficient coupling between nutrient intake and activity of the reward system is needed to prevent eating disorders. Satiation signals arise from multiple sites in the GI system, including the stomach, proximal small intestine, distal small intestine, colon, and pancreas. The hindbrain is the principal central site receiving short-acting satiation signals, which are transmitted both by neural circuits (vagal afferents) and by gut peptides acting directly on the area postrema (AP).

Gastric Signaling

Gastric satiation signals arise primarily from mechanical distention and are relayed to the brain through vagal and spinal sensory nerves via neurotransmitters and neuromodulators, including glutamate, acetylcholine, nitric oxide, calcitonin gene-related peptide, substance P, galanin, and cocaine- and amphetamine-related transcript [23, 24].

Ghrelin

Ghrelin is a 28 amino acid (aa) peptide that is predominantly secreted by the stomach; it is the only known circulating orexigenic factor that stimulates appetite and promotes adiposity [25]. Ghrelin requires a posttranslational modification: octanoylation by ghrelin O-acyltransferase (GOAT), for full activity and signaling through the growth hormone secretagogue receptor (GHSR) [26, 27]. Blood levels of ghrelin increase and peak preprandially followed by a rapid postprandial reduction. At the periphery, ghrelin increases GI motility and inhibits insulin secretion. In the brain, ghrelin activates neurons that are involved in appetite regulation: arcuate nucleus (ARC), VMN, and PVN of the hypothalamus. Ghrelin has also been shown to be involved in reward processes in rodents [28]. Humans with exogenous administration of ghrelin report hunger and an increase in food intake [29]. However, the loss of function of ghrelin or its signaling in rodent models did not result in a striking phenotype alteration [27]. Recent experimental studies reported that ghrelin signaling in early life influences neural development and is important in shaping later-life susceptibilities to metabolic disorders [30].

Intestinal Signaling

Intestinal satiety signaling arises primarily from the chemical effect of food. The mediators are gut peptides secreted by neuroendocrine cells or metabolites derived from the digestion of food. These mediators signal through the activation of nearby fibers or function as hormones by entering into the bloodstream.

Upper Intestinal Signaling

Cholecystokinin (CCK)

CCK is produced by I cells in the duodenum and jejunum and other organs such as the brain and enteric nervous system. CCK preproprotein is processed by endoproteolytic cleavage into at least six peptides of 8–83 aa. Intestinal CCK is secreted in response to luminal nutrients, especially lipids and proteins, and interacts with two receptors expressed in the gut (CCK receptor 1) and brain (CCK2R). The bioactive forms share a common carboxyl terminal octapeptide. CCK might relay satiation signals to the brain both directly (through a receptor located in the hindbrain region) and indirectly (inhibition of gastric emptying, activation of vagal afferents). CCK administration decreases food intake acutely in humans by shortening meals [31, 32], but these effects dissipate after 24 hours of continuous infusion with the development of a rapid tolerance of the behavioral effect of CCK [33]. Trials with CCK1R agonist administration as anti-obesity therapeutics have been unsuccessful to date.

At the central level, the short-term effect of the peripherally secreted CCK is attributed to stimulation of vagal sensory neurons influencing the brainstem. CCK is also synthesized within the brain by a subset of cells located in the NTS. These CCK secreting cells are responsive to nutritional state and relay the signal to the hypothalamus. Experimental studies have shown that activation of NTS cells containing CCK reduces appetite and body weight in mice [34] through a circuit involving the PVH and MC4-R pathway.

Lower Intestinal Signaling

Glucagon-Like Peptide-1 (GLP-1)

GLP-1 is a peptide expressed in the gut, pancreas, and brain and derives from the cleavage of proglucagon by a prohormone convertase which also generates other peptides: glucagon, oxyntomodulin, GLP-2, and glicentin. In the intestine, GLP-1 is produced by L cells present in the ileum and colon, and its secretion is stimulated through the direct and indirect effect of ingested nutrients, especially fat and carbohydrate. GLP-1 signals via receptors: GLP1R expressed by the gut, pancreatic islet, brainstem, hypothalamus, and vagal afferent nerves and kidney. Bioactive GLP-1 exists as two equipotent circulating molecular forms, GLP-1(7–37) and GLP-1(7–36) amide. GLP-1(7–36) amide represents the majority of circulating active GLP-1 in human plasma. In the circulation, GLP-1 is rapidly inactivated by dipeptidyl peptidase 4 (DPP4), an essential enzyme regulating the degradation of both glucose-dependent insulinotropic polypeptide (GIP) and GLP-1. GLP-1 is also rapidly cleared from the circulation via the kidney [24]. Plasma levels of GLP-1 rise rapidly within minutes of food intake and exert antidiabetic effects through the stimulation of glucose-dependent insulin release, inhibition of glucagon secretion, and stimulation of pancreatic cell growth. GLP-1 administration decreases gastric emptying and food intake in animals and humans through vagal or direct central pathways [35]. Clinical studies have confirmed that long-acting GLP-1 agonists have a powerful antidiabetic effect and cause weight loss [36]. In rodents, GLP-1 induces the development of a conditioned taste aversion that is mediated by neuronal GLP1R [37]. Aversive and anorectic actions of GLP-1 are mediated by different regions in the CNS [35].

Oxyntomodulin

Like GLP-1, oxyntomodulin derives from proglucagon, and its secretion is stimulated by nutrient intake. In rodents and humans, exogenous administration decreases food intake while increasing energy expenditure, and chronic injections reduce body weight gain [38]. These effects are partially mediated through GLP1R and activation of neurons in the hypothalamic region [24].

Peptide PYY

Peptide PYY3–36 is a 36 aa peptide. It is a member of the neuropeptide Y and is secreted by L cells in the distal intestine which coexpress GLP-1. The secretion is stimulated mainly during feeding predominantly by fat. Secreted PYY delays gastric emptying and reduces food intake. The central anorectic effect is mediated through Y2 receptors in the hypothalamic arcuate nucleus and the inhibition of neurons that express both NPY and AgRP [24]. Peripheral administration of PYY in humans has been shown to decrease appetite and calorie intake in both lean and obese subjects [39].

Pancreas Signaling

Pancreatic Polypeptide

Pancreatic peptide (PP) is produced in specialized islet cells, and its secretion is stimulated postprandially in proportion to caloric load that is under vagal control. PP has a role in GI motility, biliary and exocrine pancreatic function, and gastric acid secretion. Its role in appetite regulation is unclear, but exogenous peripheral administration of this peptide reduces appetite and food intake in humans independently of gastric emptying [24, 39].

Amylin

Amylin is a peptide that is co-secreted with insulin after ingestion of meal. Its effect on appetite regulation is mediated via the decrease of food intake primarily on the AP and gastric emptying [24]. Recent studies reported that the activation of hindbrain neural circuitry by amylin modulates hypothalamic signaling and responsiveness to the anorectic effect of leptin, an adipose-derived anorexigenic hormone [40].

Insulin

Insulin is secreted by the pancreas postprandially and stimulates glucose uptake and utilization in target organs among other functions. At the central level, insulin binds to its receptors on the surface of POMC neurons to promote the release of α-MSH, which signals to decrease food intake through the inhibition of AgRP/NPY neurons in the hypothalamus [41].

Role of Ingested Food-Derived Metabolites

The digestion of macronutrients generates compounds in the digestive lumen that may mediate appetite regulation. Specific nutrients may activate GI function or serve as precursors for neurotransmitters that regulate GI motility and appetite.

Metabolites Derived from Protein Metabolism

L-tryptophan is an aromatic amino acid that derives from protein digestion. There is evidence for the role of L-tryptophan in the inhibition of food intake as it is a potent stimulator of GI function and serves as a precursor of serotonin, which is a key regulator of appetite. The majority of serotonin is released from intestinal enterochromaffin cells. Upon feeding, the activation of taste bud cells on the tongue causes serotonin release onto sensory afferent nerves and transmits taste to the CNS. In the GI tract, serotonin stimulates secretion and motility [10]. The combined intraduodenal administration of L-tryptophan and lauric acid (a fatty acid metabolite) reduces appetite in healthy subjects by stimulating CCK release and suppression of ghrelin release [42, 43].

Metabolites Derived from Fatty Acid Metabolism

Other potential mediators derive from fatty acid metabolism. The fat-specific satiety factor oleoyle-thanolamide (OEA), which derives from oleic acid, contributes to appetite regulation by modifying brain reward circuits with the activation of the vagus nerve. OEA promotes satiety through dopamine release from the dorsal striatum [44]. In the GI tract, OEA stimulates the secretion of GLP-1 [45].

CB_1 cannabinoid receptor and its endogenous ligands, the endocannabinoids (EC), are involved in controlling energy balance. Activation of the CB_1 receptor subtype, which is particularly abundant in the brain and spinal cord, increases food intake, and it enhances reward aspects of eating through neural pathways. Precursor molecules for EC ligands of the cannabinoid receptor are derived from the polyunsaturated fatty acid (PUFA), arachidonic acid (20:4n-6) [45].

Metabolites Derived from Carbohydrate Metabolism

High carbohydrate and ketogenic diets have been reported to induce the liver-derived FGF-21 secretion, which in turn plays an important role in eating behavior (e.g., reducing sweet preference). The liver has been hypothesized to regulate nutrient-specific appetite since it receives information about nutrient supply in the portal vein. In recent years, the observation that FGF-21 knockout mice had increased sugar intake has raised the possibility that this predominantly liver-derived hormone could regulate nutrient-specific appetite by acting on the reward system [46, 47]. The modulation of sugar intake by FGF-21 has been confirmed in mice and humans through a negative feedback loop between the liver and the brain [48]. This effect involves FGF-21 co-receptor β-Klotho in the CNS and correlates with reductions in dopamine concentrations in the nucleus accumbens [47, 48].

Role of Adipose Tissue

White adipose tissue secretes a large variety of compounds named adipokines among which leptin, a 167 aa peptide, exhibits pleiotropic metabolic effects.

Leptin

Leptin is an anorexigenic hormone that is secreted in proportion of fat mass with additional effects on the regulation of energy homeostasis and metabolism, inflammation, and the cardiovascular system. Leptin belongs to the interleukin-6 family of proinflammatory cytokines that is regulated by acute changes in calorie intake. Leptin binds to its receptors (LepR) located throughout the central nervous system, as well as in several peripheral tissues to exert its effects. In patients with congenital leptin deficiency, which is characterized by hyperphagia and severe, early-onset obesity, treatment with leptin results in decreased food intake and weight loss [49]. The central effect of leptin is mediated through GABAergic presynaptic neurons found in the hypothalamic ARC. Leptin reaches the brain by a saturable transport through the blood-brain barrier. It suppresses food intake by activating neurons that express POMC and cocaine- and amphetamine-regulated transcript (CART), thereby enhancing their antiorexigenic action [50] and the inhibition of AgRP/NPY.

Leptin may also act synergistically with GI hormones in the NTS where LepR-expressing neurons have also been found and include subpopulations that express POMC, proglucagon/GLP-1, and CCK [51] to promote satiety. Leptin administration to rodents has been found to enhance the anorexic and weight loss responses to intraperitoneally administered CCK, GLP-1, and amylin [40, 52, 53].

Leptin also influences the hedonic aspects of feeding via interactions with the mesolimbic dopaminergic system, which is known to regulate reward [54]. These data suggest that leptin decreases both the incentive to feed and pleasure from eating.

Nesfatin-1

Nesfatin-1 is an adipokine that is also expressed in other tissues (pancreas, CNS, pituitary, stomach). Nesfatin-1 was reported to have a role in satiety through leptin-independent mechanisms in rodents when administered centrally [55]. However, there is still a lack of data confirming its role in appetite regulation in humans.

Role of Inflammation

Various inflammatory cytokines (interleukins 1, 6, and 8, tumor necrosis α, and interferon α) inhibit appetite in healthy conditions and various diseases (cancer, sepsis, cardiac cachexia, chronic pulmonary disease) by acting on meal size, duration, and frequency through the central pathway [56].

Behavioral and Environmental Factors

One aspect of appetite regulation that needs to be addressed is the socially driven food intake. In humans, food intake depends on the social environment and social interaction. It has been reported that men and women consume less food in the presence of a stranger of the opposite sex, and there is a positive correlation between group size and meal duration [57]. Cultural habits, accessibility of food, and financial constraints are among the critical factors that shape feeding behaviors.

Appetite Regulation in Chronic Kidney Disease

The development of chronic kidney disease (CKD) is associated with a significant reduction in food intake and an increased risk of nutritional deficiencies. There are different mechanisms that can induce decreased food intake and anorexia during CKD including the alteration of taste, nausea, stomach

Table 28.1 Peripheral appetite-regulating hormones and their modifications during chronic kidney disease

Site of production	Hormones	Effects	Levels in CKD
Stomach	Ghrelin	Increased GI motility ↑ Food intake and hunger	Increased ↑ Food intake in CKD patients, with short-term administration
Testin: duodenum, jejunum	CCK	↓ Gastric emptying Activates vagal afferents ↑ Satiety and fullness ↓ Good intake	Increased Associated with ↑ fullness and ↓ hunger perception in PD patients
Intestine: ileum, colon	GLP-1 Oxyntomodulin Peptide YY	↓ Gastric emptying ↓ Food intake ↑ Satiety and fullness ↓ Food intake ↑ NRJ expenditure ↓ Gastric emptying ↓ Food intake	Increased
Pancreas	Insulin Amylin Pancreatic peptide	↓ Food intake ↓ Food intake and gastric emptying ↓ Appetite and food intake	Increased
Adipose tissue	Leptin Nesfatin-1	↓ Food intake ↑ NRJ expenditure ↑ Satiety ↓ Pleasure from eating ↑ Satiety	Increased ↓ Food intake through central effect on MC4-R signaling in rodent models of CKD

Abbreviations: *CCK* cholecystokinin, *GLP-1* glucagon-like peptide-1, *CKD* chronic kidney disease, *PD* peritoneal dialysis, *NRJ* energy, *MC4-R* melanocortin receptor 4

irritation and pain, altered GI motility, chronic inflammation, accumulation of unidentified anorexigenic molecules, altered levels of circulating molecules known to mediate appetite, as well as psychological and economic factors (Table 28.1).

Taste and Olfactory Function Alterations and Modifications of Eating Preferences

Potential causes of anorexia in CKD patients include a decreased ability to distinguish flavors (i.e., abnormal taste) and altered palatability. Palatability may influence food choice as it influences the pleasure from eating a specific food. Studies have reported taste abnormalities affecting food palatability and intake in dialysis patients [58, 59]. Aguilera et al. reported differences in food preference when comparing peritoneal dialysis patients to healthy subjects with a trend toward carbohydrate preference, refusal of red meat, and attraction to citric and strong flavors [60]. This was reported by others in hemodialysis (HD) and peritoneal dialysis (PD) subjects [61] with red meat being the most unpopular food in both groups. In this latter study, the most common factor affecting dietary intake was a loss of interest in food and/or cooking. Furthermore, Wright et al. reported that a HD session reduces hunger and desire to eat. After a dialysis session, there is a reduction of food intake related to increased fullness [62].

Olfaction plays an important role in the identification of food and appetite regulation. CKD is associated with altered olfactory function that may thus partly explain food aversion [63]. Potential mechanisms include altered regeneration of olfactory cells related to uremic toxins or neurological dysfunction since these alterations are reported to correlate with the degree of renal impairment and improved after kidney transplantation [63–65]. Odor identification was reported to be altered in the majority of CKD (70%) and end-stage renal disease (ESRD) (HD and PD) (90%) patients using a validated test (i.e., the University of Pennsylvania Smell Identification Test [UPSIT]) compared to controls [66]. Altered olfactory function was associated with malnutrition as assessed by the subjective global assessment (SGA) score [66, 67]. In a proof of concept trial, 6 weeks' intranasal theophylline administration (which has been proven to improve olfactory function in other diseases) in ESRD patients with at least mild odor identification deficit improved their olfactory functions [66].

Altered Central Regulation of Appetite

Results from rodent models of CKD indicate that CKD causes a defect in the ability of AgRP to block MC4-R in the hypothalamus. Cheung et al. reported that AgRP injected centrally into the lateral ventricle of CKD mice resulted in growth improvement with increased food intake and decreased resting metabolic rate. Furthermore, MC4-R knockout mice were resistant to the cachectic effect of uremia [68]. This was further supported by the observation that the peripheral administration of NBI-12i, a small molecule antagonizing MC4-R, was able to improve uremic cachexia in mice [69]. In PD patients, low serum levels of NPY have been reported to be associated with anorexia [70]. Whether this reflects a decreased central NPY signaling is unclear.

Altered Levels of Circulating Molecules Known to Mediate Appetite

The hypothesis that circulating molecules are implicated in the reduction of food intake during CKD has been raised. Studies showed that middle-sized molecule fractions isolated from uremic ultrafiltrate of end-stage renal disease (ESRD) patients and normal urine were associated with decreased food intake in rats [71]. These results suggested that the accumulation of middle-sized compounds which are normally excreted in the urine suppresses food intake.

Leptin

Experimental and clinical studies demonstrated that serum levels of leptin are significantly increased in CKD mainly due to a lack of renal clearance [72–74], but it does not seem to be the only mechanism explaining the development of hyperleptinemia in CKD. In vitro studies demonstrated that uremic plasma can induce overproduction of leptin from adipocyte primary culture and 3T3 cell lines [75, 76]. In ESRD patients, other mechanisms such as increased fat mass, hyperinsulinemia, and inflammation may also contribute to hyperleptinemia through an increased production of leptin [77–80]. Experimental uremic anorexia in mice CKD models can be improved by blocking leptin signaling pathway through the MC4-R [68, 69]. Human data on leptin and uremic cachexia are so far inconclusive. Clinical studies found conflicting results, some reporting that increased leptin concentration is associated with anorexia and muscle mass loss [81–83], and others did not find any correlation between leptin concentration and the nutritional status of uremic patients [84–86].

Ghrelin

Ghrelin is the only GI-released peptide that is known to stimulate food intake and is considered as one potential treatment in multiple disease states associated with anorexia, malnutrition, or cachexia. In CKD, the plasma level of ghrelin is elevated above normal and has been reported to correlate with fat mass, plasma insulin, and serum leptin levels [84]. Both acyl ghrelin and des-acyl ghrelin are increased in nondialysis-dependent CKD patients [87]. In hemodialysis, an increased level of des-acyl ghrelin and normal level of acyl ghrelin have been reported [88]. In contrary, others have reported a 70% decrease of des-acyl ghrelin by hemodialysis without effect on acyl ghrelin levels [87]. A small study in hemodialysis patients reported that higher levels of ghrelin were associated with poor appetite [86]. In rodent models of CKD, administration of ghrelin or ghrelin receptor agonists resulted in increased food intake and improved lean mass [89]. Short-term administration of ghrelin in malnourished hemodialysis or peritoneal dialysis patients was associated with increased appetite and energy intake [90, 91]. Whether this effect is sustained in the long term and improves PEW needs further investigations.

Others

Visfatin

Visfatin, also called nicotinamide phosphoribosyltransferase (NAMPT), is an insulin-sensitizing adipokine enzyme. The extracellular form, eNAMPT, has been demonstrated to modulate the pathways involved in the pathophysiology of obesity. Serum visfatin concentrations were reported to be negatively correlated with serum aa levels and increased in nondialysis ESRD patients with worsening appetite [92]. However, the causal role of visfatin in the dysregulated appetite in CKD patients needs to be fully established.

GLP-1

GLP-1 level is increased in CKD patients (hemodialysis) and is an independent predictor of mortality. Uremic serum stimulates GLP-1 in vitro, suggesting that increased GLP-1 in CKD is the sum of increased secretion and decreased renal clearance [93]. The link between increased endogenous GLP-1 and decreased appetite has never been reported in CKD patients. Altered GI motility with delayed gastric emptying is one of the symptoms reported in nondialysis CKD stages 4–5 patients [94] and improved by dialysis treatment [95]. A recent human study has shown that an increase in ghrelin and a decrease in GLP-1 might be a mechanism associated with improved gastric slow wave in hemodialysis patients when compared to nondialysis CKD subjects [95]. Exogenous administration of GLP-1 agonists in stages 3–4 diabetic CKD patients retains similar weight loss effect (approximately 2 kg at 12 months) compared to non-CKD diabetic patients [96].

CCK

The concentrations of circulating CCK molecules are increased in dialysis patients resulting from decreased clearance but also increased production [70]. Increased CCK has been reported to be associated with increased fullness and decreased hunger perception in PD patients [97].

FGF-21

FGF-21 has been reported to be disproportionately elevated in CKD patients (20 times higher in ESRD patients) [98, 99]. This increase is not explained solely by the reduction of renal clearance and correlates with poor metabolic profile, inflammation, higher morbidity, and mortality [98, 99]. Whether this increased FGF-21 level has a role in the appetite regulation of CKD patients is unclear.

Inflammation

Chronic inflammation is a common feature in CKD patients. A strong association of inflammatory markers (C-reactive protein, interleukin-6, and tumor necrosis factor-α) and decreased appetite has been shown in hemodialysis [100] and peritoneal dialysis patients [70].

Altered Amino Acid Profile

There is a modification in the aa pattern in CKD with reduced essential/nonessential aa ratio and lower branched chain aa (BCAA) levels [101]. One hypothesis is that low levels of BCAA and essential aa in plasma and cerebrospinal fluid would favor tryptophan transport across the blood-brain barrier causing an increase in serotonin and reduced appetite. However, in dialysis subjects, poor appetite was correlated with lower BCAA but not with higher free tryptophan levels [86]. Hiroshige et al. gave BCAA to malnourished elderly HD patients and observed an improvement in appetite and nutritional status [102].

Conclusion

Despite a tremendous progress in the understanding of appetite regulation and the complex neurohormonal circuit, mechanisms that govern appetite dysregulation in CKD are still unclear. Disorders in GI-derived hormones, retention of inflammatory or anorexigenic products, and changes in central nervous system circuits may all play a role. Other behavioral and environmental factors may also be key players shaping eating behavior in CKD and need to be specifically addressed.

References

1. Bernardis LL, Bellinger LL. The lateral hypothalamic area revisited: neuroanatomy, body weight regulation, neuroendocrinology and metabolism. Neurosci Biobehav Rev. 1993;17(2):141–93.
2. Brady LS, Smith MA, Gold PW, Herkenham M. Altered expression of hypothalamic neuropeptide mRNAs in food-restricted and food-deprived rats. Neuroendocrinology. 1990;52(5):441–7.

3. Qu D, Ludwig DS, Gammeltoft S, Piper M, Pelleymounter MA, Cullen MJ, et al. A role for melanin-concentrating hormone in the central regulation of feeding behaviour. Nature. 1996;380(6571):243–7.

4. Hahn TM, Breininger JF, Baskin DG, Schwartz MW. Coexpression of Agrp and NPY in fasting-activated hypothalamic neurons. Nat Neurosci. 1998;1(4):271–2.

5. Morley JE, Levine AS, Gosnell BA, Kneip J, Grace M. Effect of neuropeptide Y on ingestive behaviors in the rat. Am J Physiol. 1987;252(3 Pt 2):R599–609.

6. Rossi M, Kim MS, Morgan DG, Small CJ, Edwards CM, Sunter D, et al. A C-terminal fragment of Agouti-related protein increases feeding and antagonizes the effect of alpha-melanocyte stimulating hormone in vivo. Endocrinology. 1998;139(10):4428–31.

7. Sakurai T, Amemiya A, Ishii M, Matsuzaki I, Chemelli RM, Tanaka H, et al. Orexins and orexin receptors: a family of hypothalamic neuropeptides and G protein-coupled receptors that regulate feeding behavior. Cell. 1998;92(4):573–85.

8. Britton DR, Koob GF, Rivier J, Vale W. Intraventricular corticotropin-releasing factor enhances behavioral effects of novelty. Life Sci. 1982;31(4):363–7.

9. Tsujii S, Bray GA. Acetylation alters the feeding response to MSH and beta-endorphin. Brain Res Bull. 1989;23(3):165–9.

10. Berger M, Gray JA, Roth BL. The expanded biology of serotonin. Annu Rev Med. 2009;60:355–66.

11. Martin CK, Redman LM, Zhang J, Sanchez M, Anderson CM, Smith SR, et al. Lorcaserin, a 5-HT(2C) receptor agonist, reduces body weight by decreasing energy intake without influencing energy expenditure. J Clin Endocrinol Metab. 2011;96(3):837–45.

12. Tuccinardi D, Farr OM, Upadhyay J, Oussaada SM, Mathew H, Paschou SA, et al. Lorcaserin treatment decreases body weight and reduces cardiometabolic risk factors in obese adults: a six-month, randomized, placebo-controlled, double-blind clinical trial. Diabetes Obes Metab. 2019;21(6):1487–92.

13. Bohula EA, Scirica BM, Fanola C, Inzucchi SE, Keech A, McGuire DK, et al. Design and rationale for the Cardiovascular and Metabolic Effects of Lorcaserin in Overweight and Obese Patients-Thrombolysis in Myocardial Infarction 61 (CAMELLIA-TIMI 61) trial. Am Heart J. 2018;202:39–48.

14. Mul JD, van Boxtel R, Bergen DJM, Brans MAD, Brakkee JH, Toonen PW, et al. Melanocortin receptor 4 deficiency affects body weight regulation, grooming behavior, and substrate preference in the rat. Obesity. 2012;20(3):612–21.

15. Panaro BL, Cone RD. Melanocortin-4 receptor mutations paradoxically reduce preference for palatable foods. Proc Natl Acad Sci U S A. 2013;110(17):7050–5.

16. Pallister T, Sharafi M, Lachance G, Pirastu N, Mohney RP, MacGregor A, et al. Food preference patterns in a UK twin cohort. Twin Res Hum Genet. 2015;18(6):793–805.

17. van der Klaauw AA, Keogh JM, Henning E, Stephenson C, Kelway S, Trowse VM, et al. Divergent effects of central melanocortin signalling on fat and sucrose preference in humans. Nat Commun. 2016;7:13055.

18. van der Klaauw A, Keogh J, Henning E, Stephenson C, Trowse VM, Fletcher P, et al. Role of melanocortin signalling in the preference for dietary macronutrients in human beings. Lancet. 2015;385 Suppl 1:S12.

19. Tanaka T, Ngwa JS, van Rooij FJA, Zillikens MC, Wojczynski MK, Frazier-Wood AC, et al. Genome-wide meta-analysis of observational studies shows common genetic variants associated with macronutrient intake. Am J Clin Nutr. 2013;97(6):1395–402.

20. Chu AY, Workalemahu T, Paynter NP, Rose LM, Giulianini F, Tanaka T, et al. Novel locus including FGF21 is associated with dietary macronutrient intake. Hum Mol Genet. 2013;22(9):1895–902.

21. Qi Q, Kilpeläinen TO, Downer MK, Tanaka T, Smith CE, Sluijs I, et al. FTO genetic variants, dietary intake and body mass index: insights from 177,330 individuals. Hum Mol Genet. 2014;23(25):6961–72.

22. Cecil JE, Tavendale R, Watt P, Hetherington MM, Palmer CNA. An obesity-associated FTO gene variant and increased energy intake in children. N Engl J Med. 2008;359(24):2558–66.

23. Ritter RC. Gastrointestinal mechanisms of satiation for food. Physiol Behav. 2004;81(2):249–73.

24. Cummings DE, Overduin J. Gastrointestinal regulation of food intake. J Clin Invest. 2007;117(1):13–23.

25. Kojima M, Hosoda H, Date Y, Nakazato M, Matsuo H, Kangawa K. Ghrelin is a growth-hormone-releasing acylated peptide from stomach. Nature. 1999;402(6762):656–60.

26. Gutierrez JA, Solenberg PJ, Perkins DR, Willency JA, Knierman MD, Jin Z, et al. Ghrelin octanoylation mediated by an orphan lipid transferase. Proc Natl Acad Sci U S A. 2008;105(17):6320–5.

27. Sun Y, Wang P, Zheng H, Smith RG. Ghrelin stimulation of growth hormone release and appetite is mediated through the growth hormone secretagogue receptor. Proc Natl Acad Sci U S A. 2004;101(13):4679–84.

28. Abizaid A, Liu Z-W, Andrews ZB, Shanabrough M, Borok E, Elsworth JD, et al. Ghrelin modulates the activity and synaptic input organization of midbrain dopamine neurons while promoting appetite. J Clin Invest. 2006;116(12):3229–39.

29. Wren AM, Seal LJ, Cohen MA, Brynes AE, Frost GS, Murphy KG, et al. Ghrelin enhances appetite and increases food intake in humans. J Clin Endocrinol Metab. 2001;86(12):5992.

30. Steculorum SM, Collden G, Coupe B, Croizier S, Lockie S, Andrews ZB, et al. Neonatal ghrelin programs development of hypothalamic feeding circuits. J Clin Invest. 2015;125(2):846–58.

31. Kissileff HR, Pi-Sunyer FX, Thornton J, Smith GP. C-terminal octapeptide of cholecystokinin decreases food intake in man. Am J Clin Nutr. 1981;34(2):154–60.

32. Kissileff HR, Carretta JC, Geliebter A, Pi-Sunyer FX. Cholecystokinin and stomach distension combine to reduce food intake in humans. Am J Physiol Regul Integr Comp Physiol. 2003;285(5):R992–8.

33. Crawley JN, Beinfeld MC. Rapid development of tolerance to the behavioural actions of cholecystokinin. Nature. 1983;302(5910):703–6.

34. D'Agostino G, Lyons DJ, Cristiano C, Burke LK, Madara JC, Campbell JN, et al. Appetite controlled by a cholecystokinin nucleus of the solitary tract to hypothalamus neurocircuit. Elife. 2016;14:5.

35. Drucker DJ. The biology of incretin hormones. Cell Metab. 2006;3(3):153–65.

36. Marso SP, Daniels GH, Brown-Frandsen K, Kristensen P, Mann JFE, Nauck MA, et al. Liraglutide and cardiovascular outcomes in type 2 diabetes. N Engl J Med. 2016;375(4):311–22.

37. Sisley S, Gutierrez-Aguilar R, Scott M, D'Alessio DA, Sandoval DA, Seeley RJ. Neuronal GLP1R mediates liraglutide's anorectic but not glucose-lowering effect. J Clin Invest. 2014;124(6):2456–63.

38. Bagger JI, Holst JJ, Hartmann B, Andersen B, Knop FK, Vilsbøll T. Effect of Oxyntomodulin, glucagon, GLP-1, and combined glucagon +GLP-1 infusion on food intake, appetite, and resting energy expenditure. J Clin Endocrinol Metab. 2015;100(12):4541–52.

39. Batterham RL, Cohen MA, Ellis SM, Le Roux CW, Withers DJ, Frost GS, et al. Inhibition of food intake in obese subjects by peptide YY3-36. N Engl J Med. 2003;349(10):941–8.

40. Mietlicki-Baase EG, Olivos DR, Jeffrey BA, Hayes MR. Cooperative interaction between leptin and amylin signaling in the ventral tegmental area for the control of food intake. Am J Physiol Endocrinol Metab. 2015;308(12):E1116–22.

41. Baldini G, Phelan KD. The melanocortin pathway and control of appetite-progress and therapeutic implications. J Endocrinol. 2019;241(1):R1–33.

42. Steinert RE, Luscombe-Marsh ND, Little TJ, Standfield S, Otto B, Horowitz M, et al. Effects of intraduodenal infusion of L-tryptophan on ad libitum eating, antropyloroduodenal motility, glycemia, insulinemia, and gut peptide secretion in healthy men. J Clin Endocrinol Metab. 2014;99(9):3275–84.

43. McVeay C, Fitzgerald PCE, Ullrich SS, Steinert RE, Horowitz M, Feinle-Bisset C. Effects of intraduodenal administration of lauric acid and L-tryptophan, alone and combined, on gut hormones, pyloric pressures, and energy intake in healthy men. Am J Clin Nutr. 2019;109(5):1335–43.

44. Hankir MK, Seyfried F, Hintschich CA, Diep T-A, Kleberg K, Kranz M, et al. Gastric bypass surgery recruits a gut PPAR-α-striatal D1R pathway to reduce fat appetite in obese rats. Cell Metab. 2017;25(2):335–44.

45. DiPatrizio NV, Piomelli D. Intestinal lipid–derived signals that sense dietary fat. J Clin Invest. 2015;125(3):891–8.

46. Talukdar S, Owen BM, Song P, Hernandez G, Zhang Y, Zhou Y, et al. FGF21 regulates sweet and alcohol preference. Cell Metab. 2016;23(2):344–9.

47. von Holstein-Rathlou S, BonDurant LD, Peltekian L, Naber MC, Yin TC, Claflin KE, et al. FGF21 mediates endocrine control of simple sugar intake and sweet taste preference by the liver. Cell Metab. 2016;23(2):335–43.

48. Søberg S, Sandholt CH, Jespersen NZ, Toft U, Madsen AL, von Holstein-Rathlou S, et al. FGF21 Is a sugar-induced hormone associated with sweet intake and preference in humans. Cell Metab. 2017;25(5):1045–1053.e6.

49. Farooqi IS, Matarese G, Lord GM, Keogh JM, Lawrence E, Agwu C, et al. Beneficial effects of leptin on obesity, T cell hyporesponsiveness, and neuroendocrine/metabolic dysfunction of human congenital leptin deficiency. J Clin Invest. 2002;110(8):1093–103.

50. Vong L, Ye C, Yang Z, Choi B, Chua S, Lowell BB. Leptin action on GABAergic neurons prevents obesity and reduces inhibitory tone to POMC neurons. Neuron. 2011;71(1):142–54.

51. Garfield AS, Patterson C, Skora S, Gribble FM, Reimann F, Evans ML, et al. Neurochemical characterization of body weight-regulating leptin receptor neurons in the nucleus of the solitary tract. Endocrinology. 2012;153(10):4600–7.

52. Kanoski SE, Ong ZY, Fortin SM, Schlessinger ES, Grill HJ. Liraglutide, leptin and their combined effects on feeding: additive intake reduction through common intracellular signalling mechanisms. Diabetes Obes Metab. 2015;17(3):285–93.

53. Matson CA, Reid DF, Ritter RC. Daily CCK injection enhances reduction of body weight by chronic intracerebroventricular leptin infusion. Am J Physiol Regul Integr Comp Physiol. 2002;282(5):R1368–73.

54. Dardeno TA, Chou SH, Moon H-S, Chamberland JP, Fiorenza CG, Mantzoros CS. Leptin in human physiology and therapeutics. Front Neuroendocrinol. 2010;31(3):377–93.

55. Stengel A, Taché Y. Minireview: nesfatin-1—an emerging new player in the brain-gut, endocrine, and metabolic axis. Endocrinology. 2011;152(11):4033–8.

56. Plata-Salamán CR. Cytokines and feeding. Int J Obes Relat Metab Disord. 2001;25(Suppl 5):S48–52.

57. Olszewski PK, Levine AS. Basic research on appetite regulation: social context of a meal is missing. Pharmacol Biochem Behav. 2016;148:106–7.

58. Hylander B, Barkeling B, Rössner S. Changes in patients' eating behavior: in the uremic state, on continuous ambulatory peritoneal dialysis treatment, and after transplantation. Am J Kidney Dis. 1997;29(5):691–8.

59. McMahon EJ, Campbell KL, Bauer JD. Taste perception in kidney disease and relationship to dietary sodium intake. Appetite. 2014;83:236–41.

60. Aguilera A, Codoceo R, Bajo MA, Iglesias P, Diéz JJ, Barril G, et al. Eating behavior disorders in uremia: a question of balance in appetite regulation. Semin Dial. 2004;17(1):44–52.

61. Dobell E, Chan M, Williams P, Allman M. Food preferences and food habits of patients with chronic renal failure undergoing dialysis. J Am Diet Assoc. 1993;93(10):1129–35.

62. Wright MJ, Woodrow G, O'Brien S, King NA, Dye L, Blundell JE, et al. A novel technique to demonstrate disturbed appetite profiles in haemodialysis patients. Nephrol Dial Transplant. 2001;16(7):1424–9.

63. Landis BN, Marangon N, Saudan P, Hugentobler M, Giger R, Martin P-Y, et al. Olfactory function improves following hemodialysis. Kidney Int. 2011;80(8):886–93.

64. Griep MI, Van der Niepen P, Sennesael JJ, Mets TF, Massart DL, Verbeelen DL. Odour perception in chronic renal disease. Nephrol Dial Transplant. 1997;12(10):2093–8.

65. Bomback AS, Raff AC. Olfactory function in dialysis patients: a potential key to understanding the uremic state. Kidney Int. 2011;80(8):803–5.

66. Nigwekar SU, Weiser JM, Kalim S, Xu D, Wibecan JL, Dougherty SM, et al. Characterization and correction of olfactory deficits in kidney disease. J Am Soc Nephrol. 2017;28(11):3395–403.

67. Raff AC, Lieu S, Melamed ML, Quan Z, Ponda M, Meyer TW, et al. Relationship of impaired olfactory function in ESRD to malnutrition and retained uremic molecules. Am J Kidney Dis. 2008;52(1):102–10.

68. Cheung W, Yu PX, Little BM, Cone RD, Marks DL, Mak RH. Role of leptin and melanocortin signaling in uremia-associated cachexia. J Clin Invest. 2005;115(6):1659–65.

69. Cheung WW, Kuo H-J, Markison S, Chen C, Foster AC, Marks DL, et al. Peripheral administration of the melanocortin-4 receptor antagonist NBI-12i ameliorates uremia-associated cachexia in mice. J Am Soc Nephrol. 2007;18(9):2517–24.

70. Aguilera A, Codoceo R, Selgas R, Garcia P, Picornell M, Diaz C, et al. Anorexigen (TNF-alpha, cholecystokinin) and orexigen (neuropeptide Y) plasma levels in peritoneal dialysis (PD) patients: their relationship with nutritional parameters. Nephrol Dial Transplant. 1998;13(6):1476–83.

71. Anderstam B, Mamoun AH, Södersten P, Bergström J. Middle-sized molecule fractions isolated from uremic ultrafiltrate and normal urine inhibit ingestive behavior in the rat. J Am Soc Nephrol. 1996;7(11):2453–60.

72. Cumin F, Baum HP, Levens N. Leptin is cleared from the circulation primarily by the kidney. Int J Obes Relat Metab Disord. 1996;20(12):1120–6.

73. Sharma K, Considine RV, Michael B, Dunn SR, Weisberg LS, Kurnik BR, et al. Plasma leptin is partly cleared by the kidney and is elevated in hemodialysis patients. Kidney Int. 1997;51(6):1980–5.

74. Meyer C, Robson D, Rackovsky N, Nadkarni V, Gerich J. Role of the kidney in human leptin metabolism. Am J Physiol. 1997;273(5):E903–7.

75. Aminzadeh MA, Pahl MV, Barton CH, Doctor NS, Vaziri ND. Human uraemic plasma stimulates release of leptin and uptake of tumour necrosis factor-alpha in visceral adipocytes. Nephrol Dial Transplant. 2009;24(12):3626–31.

76. Kalbacher E, Koppe L, Zarrouki B, Pillon NJ, Fouque D, Soulage CO. Human uremic plasma and not urea induces exuberant secretion of leptin in 3T3-L1 adipocytes. J Ren Nutr. 2011;21(1):72–5.

77. Stenvinkel P, Heimbürger O, Lönnqvist F. Serum leptin concentrations correlate to plasma insulin concentrations independent of body fat content in chronic renal failure. Nephrol Dial Transplant. 1997;12(7):1321–5.

78. Heimbürger O, Lönnqvist F, Danielsson A, Nordenström J, Stenvinkel P. Serum immunoreactive leptin concentration and its relation to the body fat content in chronic renal failure. J Am Soc Nephrol. 1997;8(9):1423–30.

79. Pecoits-Filho R, Nordfors L, Heimbürger O, Lindholm B, Anderstam B, Marchlewska A, et al. Soluble leptin receptors and serum leptin in end-stage renal disease: relationship with inflammation and body composition. Eur J Clin Invest. 2002;32(11):811–7.

80. Mak RH, Cheung W, Cone RD, Marks DL. Leptin and inflammation-associated cachexia in chronic kidney disease. Kidney Int. 2006;69(5):794–7.

81. Daschner M, Tönshoff B, Blum WF, Englaro P, Wingen AM, Schaefer F, et al. Inappropriate elevation of serum leptin levels in children with chronic renal failure. European Study Group for Nutritional Treatment of Chronic Renal Failure in Childhood. J Am Soc Nephrol. 1998;9(6):1074–9.

82. Odamaki M, Furuya R, Yoneyama T, Nishikino M, Hibi I, Miyaji K, et al. Association of the serum leptin concentration with weight loss in chronic hemodialysis patients. Am J Kidney Dis. 1999;33(2):361–8.

83. Castaneda-Sceppa C, Sarnak MJ, Wang X, Greene T, Madero M, Kusek JW, et al. Role of adipose tissue in determining muscle mass in patients with chronic kidney disease. J Ren Nutr. 2007;17(5):314–22.

84. Rodriguez Ayala E, Pecoits-Filho R, Heimbürger O, Lindholm B, Nordfors L, Stenvinkel P. Associations between plasma ghrelin levels and body composition in end-stage renal disease: a longitudinal study. Nephrol Dial Transplant. 2004;19(2):421–6.

85. Chudek J, Adamczak M, Kania M, Hołowiecka A, Rozmus W, Kokot F, et al. Does plasma leptin concentration predict the nutritional status of hemodialyzed patients with chronic renal failure? Med Sci Monit. 2003;9(8):CR377–82.

86. Bossola M, Scribano D, Colacicco L, Tavazzi B, Giungi S, Zuppi C, et al. Anorexia and plasma levels of free tryptophan, branched chain amino acids, and ghrelin in hemodialysis patients. J Ren Nutr. 2009;19(3):248–55.
87. Gupta RK, Kuppusamy T, Patrie JT, Gaylinn B, Liu J, Thorner MO, et al. Association of plasma des-acyl ghrelin levels with CKD. Clin J Am Soc Nephrol. 2013;8(7):1098–105.
88. Mafra D, Guebre-Egziabher F, Cleaud C, Arkouche W, Mialon A, Drai J, et al. Obestatin and ghrelin interplay in hemodialysis patients. Nutrition. 2010;26(11–12):1100–4.
89. Deboer MD, Zhu X, Levasseur PR, Inui A, Hu Z, Han G, et al. Ghrelin treatment of chronic kidney disease: improvements in lean body mass and cytokine profile. Endocrinology. 2008;149(2):827–35.
90. Ashby DR, Ford HE, Wynne KJ, Wren AM, Murphy KG, Busbridge M, et al. Sustained appetite improvement in malnourished dialysis patients by daily ghrelin treatment. Kidney Int. 2009;76(2):199–206.
91. Wynne K, Giannitsopoulou K, Small CJ, Patterson M, Frost G, Ghatei MA, et al. Subcutaneous ghrelin enhances acute food intake in malnourished patients who receive maintenance peritoneal dialysis: a randomized, placebo-controlled trial. J Am Soc Nephrol. 2005;16(7):2111–8.
92. Carrero JJ, Witasp A, Stenvinkel P, Qureshi AR, Heimbürger O, Bárány P, et al. Visfatin is increased in chronic kidney disease patients with poor appetite and correlates negatively with fasting serum amino acids and triglyceride levels. Nephrol Dial Transplant. 2010;25(3):901–6.
93. Lebherz C, Schlieper G, Möllmann J, Kahles F, Schwarz M, Brünsing J, et al. GLP-1 levels predict mortality in patients with critical illness as well as end-stage renal disease. Am J Med. 2017;130(7):833–841.e3.
94. Hirako M, Kamiya T, Misu N, Kobayashi Y, Adachi H, Shikano M, et al. Impaired gastric motility and its relationship to gastrointestinal symptoms in patients with chronic renal failure. J Gastroenterol. 2005;40(12):1116–22.
95. Wu G-J, Cai X-D, Xing J, Zhong G-H, Chen JDZ. Circulating motilin, ghrelin, and GLP-1 and their correlations with gastric slow waves in patients with chronic kidney disease. Am J Physiol Regul Integr Comp Physiol. 2017;313(2):R149–57.
96. Tuttle KR, Lakshmanan MC, Rayner B, Busch RS, Zimmermann AG, Woodward DB, et al. Dulaglutide versus insulin glargine in patients with type 2 diabetes and moderate-to-severe chronic kidney disease (AWARD-7): a multicentre, open-label, randomised trial. Lancet Diabetes Endocrinol. 2018;6(8):605–17.
97. Wright M, Woodrow G, O'Brien S, Armstrong E, King N, Dye L, et al. Cholecystokinin and leptin: their influence upon the eating behaviour and nutrient intake of dialysis patients. Nephrol Dial Transplant. 2004;19(1):133–40.
98. Stein S, Bachmann A, Lössner U, Kratzsch J, Blüher M, Stumvoll M, et al. Serum levels of the adipokine FGF21 depend on renal function. Diabetes Care. 2009;32(1):126–8.
99. de PGA S, de Paula RB, Sanders-Pinheiro H, Moe OW, Hu M-C. Fibroblast growth factor 21 in chronic kidney disease. J Nephrol. 2019;32(3):365–77.
100. Kalantar-Zadeh K, Abbott KC, Salahudeen AK, Kilpatrick RD, Horwich TB. Survival advantages of obesity in dialysis patients. Am J Clin Nutr. 2005;81(3):543–54.
101. Carr SJ, Layward E, Bevington A, Hattersley J, Walls J. Plasma amino acid profile in the elderly with increasing uraemia. Nephron. 1994;66(2):228–30.
102. Hiroshige K, Sonta T, Suda T, Kanegae K, Ohtani A. Oral supplementation of branched-chain amino acid improves nutritional status in elderly patients on chronic haemodialysis. Nephrol Dial Transplant. 2001;16(9):1856–62.

Chapter 29
Advanced Glycation End Products

Annabel Biruete and Jaime Uribarri

Keywords Advanced glycation end products · Chronic kidney disease · Diabetes mellitus · Oxidative stress · Inflammation · Carboxymethyllysine · Pentosidine · Methylglyoxal · Diet · Nutritional intervention

Key Points
- Advanced glycation end products (AGEs) can be produced endogenously or obtained exogenously from the diet.
- AGEs have been associated with kidney damage and, thus, progression of chronic kidney disease.
- Cooking methods where high heat and low moisture are used increase the formation of AGEs.
- Interventions with a low dietary AGE have been shown to reduce circulating AGEs and markers of oxidative stress and inflammation.
- Diets low in AGEs should be recommended for patients at high risk of CKD.

Introduction

Advanced glycation end products (AGEs) play a major role in diabetic vascular complications, such as chronic kidney disease (CKD), by activating pro-oxidant and pro-inflammatory responses [1, 2]. Although traditionally AGEs have been associated with uncontrolled hyperglycemia of diabetes mellitus, there is increasing evidence that exogenous AGEs from diet have an important contribution to these processes [3, 4]. The reduction of dietary AGE intake has been demonstrated to prevent or diminish pro-oxidant and pro-inflammatory responses in several clinical trials [5–10]. These trials have also demonstrated that dietary AGE restriction is simple, feasible, and safe to apply clinically, even in CKD patients. In this chapter, we will summarize the current data on the use of this intervention in clinical practice with particular emphasis on CKD patients.

A. Biruete
Division of Nephrology, Department of Medicine, Indiana University School of Medicine, Indianapolis, IN, USA

J. Uribarri (✉)
Department of Medicine, Icahn School of Medicine at Mount Sinai, New York, NY, USA
e-mail: Jaime.uribarri@mssm.edu

© Springer Nature Switzerland AG 2020
J. D. Burrowes et al. (eds.), *Nutrition in Kidney Disease*, Nutrition and Health,
https://doi.org/10.1007/978-3-030-44858-5_29

What Are Advanced Glycation End Products (AGEs) and How Do They Cause Disease?

AGEs are a very large and heterogeneous group of compounds originating from the spontaneous reaction of reducing sugars with free amino groups in amino acids in the so-called Maillard or browning reaction. Although a lot of attention has been devoted to this reaction, we currently know that AGEs can be formed through many other reactions, such as oxidation of sugars, lipids, and amino acids that creates reactive aldehydes that in turn form AGEs. Carboxymethyllysine (CML), carboxyethyllysine (CEL), methylglyoxal-derivatives (MG), and pentosidine are some commonly measured and well-described AGEs in biological studies.

AGEs form continuously in the body through a variety of spontaneous reactions, which are markedly increased in conditions of hyperglycemia or elevated oxidative stress, such as in CKD; these are the endogenous AGEs. Of note, however, AGEs can also form outside of the body in any system as long as the required reagents are available. For example, we know they form spontaneously in food, especially when processed and cooked with heat; these are the exogenous AGEs [11, 12]. In a fraction of ingested food, AGEs will get absorbed and incorporated into the body AGE pool, where they are indistinguishable from their endogenous counterparts, both in structure and function [13].

AGEs, endogenous or exogenous, lead to tissue injury by at least two mechanisms: (1) by causing protein cross-linking, inducing direct modifications of protein structure and, therefore, function and (2) by activating pro-inflammatory and pro-oxidative cellular signaling pathways through receptor- and non-receptor-mediated mechanisms. For example, direct cross-linking of collagen may be responsible for arterial wall stiffness, and glycation of specific amino acids in a protein molecule could affect the binding of this protein to receptors.

AGE binding to the receptor of AGEs (RAGE) or Toll-like receptors (TLRs) 2 and 4 initiates intracellular signaling that leads to the activation of several pro-inflammatory and pro-oxidative stress responses [14]. In contrast, AGE binding and activation of the AGE receptor 1 (AGER1) initiate AGE breakdown and diminish the RAGE-mediated activation of nuclear factor-kappa B (NF-κB) [15].

Increased oxidative stress and inflammation are the underlying mechanisms of many chronic diseases, including diabetes, cardiovascular disease, and CKD. The kidneys are the major players in maintaining AGE homeostasis. AGE peptides undergo filtration followed by partial tubular reabsorption and possibly also secretion after tubular uptake from the peritubular blood flow [16]. AGEs undergo variable degrees of catabolism within the renal tubules. Not surprisingly, an elevation of AGEs is characteristic of any reduction in kidney function [17] and may play a role in facilitating the progression of any underlying kidney condition. Circulating AGE levels are markedly increased in CKD of any etiology, before and after the initiation of dialysis [1, 18]. This increase of AGEs in CKD may play a role in the high prevalence of endothelial dysfunction and subsequent cardiovascular disease in this population [19].

Conventional hemodialysis (HD) of three times a week for 4 hours each is not very effective at removing AGEs [18], while short daily dialysis, hemodiafiltration, and hemofiltration have been shown to be more effective [20, 21]. At least in one study, hemodiafiltration significantly lowered serum AGE levels as compared to high-flux HD by the end of the treatment period [22]. Circulating AGE levels are also increased in peritoneal dialysis (PD) patients, but lower than in HD patients, and the amount seems to vary depending on the type of PD solution [18, 23, 24]. Importantly, circulating AGE levels fall significantly following a successful kidney transplantation [25].

Evidence Linking AGEs and Kidney Disease

In Vitro Studies

AGEs, through their cross-link of proteins in the kidney extracellular matrix, lead to many abnormalities: altered matrix protein structure and function, aberrant cell-matrix interactions that change cellular adhesion, altered cell growth, and loss of the epithelial phenotype [26, 27].

In vitro incubation of AGEs with every cell type within the kidneys has been shown to initiate potential mechanisms of cell injury [28]. For example, binding of AGEs to mesangial cells increases production of matrix proteins while decreasing expression of major metalloproteinases that normally would degrade matrix proteins [29]. Incubation of human glomerular endothelial cells with AGEs increases expression of vascular endothelial growth factor that attracts inflammatory cells [30]. RAGE activation changes the endothelium surface from an anticoagulant to a procoagulant state by reducing thrombomodulin activity and increasing tissue factor expression [31]. AGEs also affect podocytes inducing podocyte apoptosis and reducing expression of nephrin [32], providing a direct link between AGEs and kidney damage.

Animal Studies

There is strong experimental animal data supporting a role for AGEs causing kidney damage *in vivo*. A classic study showed that intraperitoneal administration of AGEs for 4 weeks into mice induced a marked increase in glomerular extracellular matrix $\alpha1(IV)$ collagen, laminin $\beta1$, and transforming growth factor β (TGFβ) [33]. Moreover, these changes diminished with the coadministration of aminoguanidine, a known AGE inhibitor [33]. In another study, long-term administration of intravenous AGE-albumin to normal rats induced albuminuria and morphologic changes of diabetic nephropathy, including glomerular hypertrophy, mesangial matrix expansion, and basement membrane thickening [34]. Overexpression of RAGE in diabetic mice increased the signs of kidney disease, while blockade of RAGE by a soluble truncated form of RAGE prevented structural and functional characteristics of nephropathy in db/db mice [35, 36]. Anti-AGE strategies, such as the administration of aminoguanidine, benfotiamine, pyridoxamine, OPB-9195, and AGE breakers, have all been shown to ameliorate diabetic nephropathy in rats without influencing glycemic control [37, 38].

A direct connection between dietary AGEs and the development of kidney disease was demonstrated when diabetic nephropathy, highly prevalent in non-obese diabetic mice with type 1 diabetes and db/db mice with type 2 diabetes, fed with regular chow (rich in AGEs through pellet formation and sterilization), was almost completely abrogated in the same groups of mice randomized to a low-AGE diet (which was a purified diet that does not need to be sterilized) [39].

Human Data

Effects of Acute Oral AGE Loads

Recently, an interesting study performed in healthy volunteers tested the acute effect of a protein load (1 g/kg) either high or low on AGEs on noninvasive parameters of kidney function [40]. The study suggests that it is the AGE content, not the total protein load, that is responsible for the observed renal hemodynamic modifications (increased renal perfusion and renal oxygen consumption). Extrapolating results one may assume that decreasing dietary AGE content may ameliorate glomerular hyperfiltration and perhaps progressive CKD, but long-term studies are lacking.

In the past, acute oral AGE loads have been shown to have endothelial effects on both healthy subjects and diabetic patients. In one study, a single oral dose of a high-AGE beverage was administered to both healthy subjects and patients with diabetes [41]. Within 2 hours, serum AGE levels increased in association with transient impairment of flow-mediated vasodilatation, a noninvasive test of endothelial function. Pretreatment of the subjects with benfotiamine, an inhibitor of glycation, prevented the endothelial effects [42]. In another study, a single high-AGE solid meal given to patients with diabetes was also followed by marked impairment of flow-mediated vasodilatation, as compared with an isocaloric low-AGE meal [43]. All of these results support a mechanistic link between dietary AGEs and cardio-vascular disease, since endothelial dysfunction is the earliest abnormality in atherosclerosis.

Observational Studies

There are several studies showing an association between levels of circulating AGEs and progression of CKD [44–47]. In a study in American Indians with type 2 diabetes, circulating AGEs (including CML and CEL) were inversely associated with glomerular filtration rate [44]. In a prospective cohort of individuals with CKD, MG was an independent risk factor for death, cardiovascular events, and/or end-stage kidney disease (ESKD) (which were the primary endpoints) [46]. Similarly, Semba et al. [45] showed that in a cohort of community-dwelling women from the Women's Health and Aging Study, circulating CML and the soluble RAGE were independently associated with lower glomerular filtration rate. Finally, circulating levels of soluble RAGE were positively associated with CKD and ESKD [47].

Clinical Trials with Dietary AGE Restriction

CKD Patients Without Diabetes

Two clinical trials have tested the effects of an AGE-restricted diet in patients with CKD in the absence of diabetes. In one of the studies, a group of stage 3 CKD patients was randomly assigned to either a regular diet or an isocaloric diet containing 50% lower AGEs for a period of 4 weeks [7]. Patients on the low-AGE diet exhibited a significant decrease of extracellular and intracellular markers of inflammation and oxidative stress, including AGEs, tumor necrosis factor (TNFα), vascular cell adhesion molecule 1 (VCAM-1), and RAGE compared to the regular diet group [7]. In a second trial, a group of patients with ESKD without diabetes on maintenance PD was randomized to follow either a regular or a low-AGE diet for 4 weeks [6]. The low-AGE diet group showed a significant decrease in the levels of circulating AGEs and high-sensitivity C-reactive protein (hsCRP) [6].

In the above studies, patients with CKD without diabetes were instructed to lower the dietary intake of AGEs, while maintaining the same baseline caloric and nutrient content. This was achieved by receiving detailed instructions on how to prepare their food at home by a study dietitian who was in frequent telephone contact with them.

Patients with Diabetes without CKD

A few trials on the effect of dietary AGE restriction have been performed in patients with diabetes without overt kidney disease. The first study was published in 2002 [5]. This was a crossover study between low and regular AGE diets for a period of 6 weeks. Meals were prepared in the clinical research unit metabolic kitchen and patients picked them up twice a week during the duration of the study. Levels of circulating AGEs (both CML and MG) as well as markers of endothelial function and inflammation such as VCAM-1, hsCRP and TNFα markedly decreased in patients during the low-AGE diet intervention. Circulating AGE levels decreased by as much as 40% during the study despite similar degree of diabetic control. Of importance, before this study was published, high serum AGE levels in patients with diabetes were thought to result exclusively from hyperglycemia-induced endogenous overproduction. Therefore, the observed fall of serum AGE levels while maintaining overall unchanged glycemic control, probably attributed to the restricted AGE diet, was a novel finding.

In a more recent study, a group of patients with type 2 diabetes were randomized to follow either a regular or a low-AGE diet for 4 months [8]. Circulating markers of AGEs, inflammation, and oxidative stress also decreased following the low-AGE diet, but more importantly the AGE-restricted diet decreased the homeostatic model assessment index (HOMA), a marker of insulin resistance [8]. This reduction of HOMA, which implies improvement of insulin sensitivity, brings up an important hypothesis: AGEs seem to have an important role in modifying insulin resistance itself and, therefore, diabetes. If this effect of the low-AGE diet is further confirmed, it opens a big opportunity for a safe, inexpensive, and effective dietary modulation to prevent or improve diabetes and, therefore, future development of CKD.

A low-AGE diet has also been shown to increase AGER1 and sirtuin 1 (SIRT1), two protective markers that tend to be suppressed in conditions of high oxidative stress, such as diabetes and CKD [48]. The restoration of their levels by the low-AGE diet suggests the previous suppression is due to an environmental factor, most likely the high AGE-induced oxidative stress.

A third published clinical trial performed in Mexico also demonstrated that a low-AGE diet decreased markers of inflammation and oxidative stress in a group of patients with type 2 diabetes [10]. Recently, a randomized controlled trial by Lopez-Moreno et al. [49] tested the effects of a high saturated fat diet, high monounsaturated fat diet, and low-fat high-complex carbohydrate diet with or without omega-3 fatty acids in individuals with metabolic syndrome. The authors showed that those in the high monounsaturated fat diet reduced circulating AGEs and expression of genes associated with AGEs in peripheral blood mononuclear cells, such as the receptor for RAGE [49]. Although none of the patients with diabetes included in the studies above had CKD, these studies are very pertinent to this chapter since diabetes is a major risk factor for CKD in the USA.

An Oral AGE Binder in CKD Patients with Diabetes

Two studies from the same group of investigators have been reported on the systemic effects of the use of sevelamer carbonate, proposed as an oral AGE binder, in CKD patients with diabetes [50]. Sevelamer is a nonselective anion binder, which is traditionally used as a phosphate binder, but may also bind other molecules, such as AGEs. The first study was a crossover study of 20 patients with diabetes and CKD comparing sevelamer carbonate versus calcium carbonate for 8 weeks, and the second study was a larger randomized study comparing sevelamer carbonate with calcium carbonate as parallel groups in 117 patients with type 2 diabetes and stages 2–4 CKD [51]. In both studies, attention was given to maintain dietary intake unchanged during the intervention period. The results in both studies were similar: sevelamer therapy, in contrast to calcium carbonate, reproduced all the findings observed with the low dietary AGE intervention described above, despite the unchanged dietary intake during the study period [50]. More specifically, the use of sevelamer was associated with reduced circulating levels of AGEs, 8-isoprostane, and TNFα, all of which were high and increased AGER1 and SIRT1, both of which were low. *In vitro* tests documented that sevelamer binds AGEs quite effectively, and presumably this was the explanation for the findings [50]. Of interest, in the second study, although the urinary albumin/creatinine ratio did not change in the overall group on sevelamer, subgroup analyses showed that the ratio was significantly decreased in subjects less than 65 years of age and in non-Caucasians [51]. Another randomized study from Japan looked at the effects of sevelamer versus calcium carbonate for 1 year in a group of 183 HD patients. Patients on sevelamer experienced decreased serum pentosidine levels and coronary artery calcium scores compared to those on calcium carbonate [42].

Healthy Subjects and Patients with the Metabolic Syndrome

A few studies done on healthy subjects [3, 7] and in patients with the metabolic syndrome [10, 52–54] have confirmed that the initiation of a low-AGE diet decreases circulating markers of AGEs, inflammation, oxidative stress, and more importantly, HOMA-IR index [10, 52–54].

How Does a Low-AGE Diet Work?

The exact mechanisms how dietary AGEs contribute to cardiovascular disease and CKD have not been precisely determined, but they may not just result from direct gastrointestinal absorption raising serum AGE levels that in turn induce elevated systemic oxidative stress and inflammation. In fact, only about 10% of dietary AGEs are absorbed [16]. However, it is also important to know that the amount of AGEs in foods far exceeds the amount of circulating AGEs and, thus, that 10% is a significant amount [16]. An action of unabsorbed dietary AGEs in the colon remains possible, including AGEs binding to RAGE or Toll-like receptors in the colon cells inducing a local inflammatory response with subsequent release of inflammatory mediators into the circulation or AGEs altering the microbiome profile in the gut leading to release of toxins into circulation. Yacoub et al. [55] assessed the effects of a low-AGE versus high-AGE diet for a month in peritoneal dialysis patients. They found that the dietary intervention altered the composition of the gut microbiota. Specifically, those in the AGE-restricted group had a reduction in the relative abundance of *Prevotella copri* and *Bifidobacterium animalis* and an increase in the relative abundance of *Alistipes indistinctus*, *Clostridium citroniae*, *Clostridium hathewayi*, and *Ruminococcus gauvreauii*. Recently, Snelson and Coughlan [13] reviewed the potential effects of AGEs on the gastrointestinal microbiome and metabolites produced by the microbiota. Interestingly, in experimental studies in rats, the use of heat-treated diets has been shown to decrease the cecal concentration of short-chain fatty acids, derived from the bacterial fermentation of carbohydrates and traditionally considered beneficial [13]. However, the long-term effects of these changes in the fecal microbiota and functional capacity of the microbiome in the context of CKD remain to be fully explored.

How to Implement and Recommend a Low-AGE Diet

Although the formation of AGEs is a complex process, dietary AGE intake is relatively easy to decrease. Additionally, a large database with the AGE content of common foods has been published and can be used to estimate dietary AGE intake as well as to give advice on how to reduce this intake [11, 12]. There are four main characteristics that affect the formation of AGEs in food: temperature, moisture, pH, and substrates for AGE formation (i.e., protein content) [11]. In terms of cooking foods, the basic concept of the low-AGE diet is that the same amount of a nutrient can provide very different amounts of oxidant substances depending on the cooking method. Unfortunately, there is no specific threshold temperature above which AGEs start to generate. Therefore, one can only make the general recommendation that the lower the temperature, the less the amount of AGEs generated. Cooking methods that use dry heat, such as broiling, searing, and frying, have been shown to have the highest content of AGEs [11]. Contrarily, methods that utilize a moisture-based heating process, such as poaching, stewing, steaming, and boiling, are lower in AGEs [11]. Thus, these methods should be preferred.

An acidic pH has also been shown to limit the formation of AGEs, whereas alkaline pH favors the Schiff base formation, one of the first reactions for AGE formation. Thus, the use of acidic foods, such as citrus foods or vinegars, as condiments can be recommended (i.e., marinade made with vinegar for high-protein foods, such as meats, is an easy way to incorporate into cooking). These culinary techniques have long been featured in the Mediterranean, Asian, and other cuisines throughout the world to create palatable, easily prepared meals, with an added benefit of limiting AGE formation.

The content of dietary protein is also a determinant of AGE formation, as it is the substrate of the amine group. Dietary protein intake is a cornerstone of the medical nutrition therapy in kidney diseases. While a low-protein diet is recommended in moderate-to-late stages of CKD, once patients transition into dialysis, dietary protein intake is recommended to increase. Unfortunately, to date, there are no studies that have assessed the effect of different amounts of dietary protein in nondialysis and dialysis-dependent CKD on circulating AGEs and AGE-mediated effects.

The immediate critique to a dietary intervention that relies on changing culinary technique is that patients will not follow it. The argument is often made that stewed chicken would be less tasty than fried chicken and, therefore, people will abandon this diet very easily. Based on our studies, however, consumers can be educated as to how to use low-AGE-generating cooking methods such as poaching, steaming, stewing, and boiling. Additionally, the use of herbs, condiments (free of sodium and potassium), and spices should be encouraged, as some may have intrinsic antiglycation activity. In addition, as mentioned above, the use of marinades based on citrus fruits and vinegars may also reduce the amount of AGEs formed. These recommendations would make the low-AGE diet appealing and flavorful.

Currently, no official recommendations exist which point out the acceptable range or identify the upper limit on dietary AGE intake. We have previously proposed that half of the current mean AGE intake, or about 7500 kU per day, is a realistic goal [11]. Studies have shown that dietary AGE reduction of this magnitude is feasible and can significantly alter levels of circulating AGEs, while at the same time reducing levels of markers of oxidative stress and inflammation and enhancing insulin sensitivity in patients with diabetes [5–9].

We propose a multipronged strategy, which is a food-first approach:

1. Decrease the intake of foods rich in AGEs (based on existing databases), taking into consideration cooking methods, moisture, pH, and protein [11, 18].
2. Increase the intake of fresh food, naturally high in polyphenols and antioxidants to counter the already high oxidative stress and inflammatory states in CKD.
3. Incorporate the use of herbs, spices, and condiments (with no sodium or potassium added) to improve the taste of food and which may also have antiglycation effect (curcumin, cinnamon, parsley, thyme, and clove) [56].
4. Although not a dietary intervention, avoid the use of cigarette as it is high in AGEs [56]. Additionally, supplementation with benfotiamine (a derivative of vitamin B1– thiamine) [43] and pyridoxamine (a form of vitamin B6) [57] has been shown in experimental and clinical studies to reduce AGE formation. We must state clearly, however, that we have tested only the AGE-restricted diet and we are assuming that the simultaneous application of points 2 through 4 will have beneficial and synergistic effects.

Conclusion

Dietary AGEs, abundantly present in the food commonly consumed in a typical American diet, contribute significantly to the body pool of AGEs, which in turn is at least partly responsible for the elevated oxidative stress and inflammation observed in patients with diabetes and CKD. A final proof of a therapeutic role for the low-AGE diet will require large, prospective, and randomized clinical trials, which indeed may never take place. In the meantime, however, we believe that a careful analysis of the current data makes it reasonable and prudent to advise the limitation of dietary AGEs in CKD patients. This is particularly important since consumption of lower-AGE foods and preparation methods can easily be integrated into dietary patterns that are consistent with current recommendations designed to promote public health and prevent cardiovascular disease, cancer, diabetes, and obesity.

References

1. Gugliucci A, Menini T. The axis AGE-RAGE-soluble RAGE and oxidative stress in chronic kidney disease. Adv Exp Med Biol. 2014;824:191–208.
2. Chilelli NC, Burlina S, Lapolla A. AGEs, rather than hyperglycemia, are responsible for microvascular complications in diabetes: a "glycoxidation-centric" point of view. Nutr Metab Cardiovasc Dis. 2013;23(10):913–9.
3. Uribarri J, Cai W, Peppa M, Goodman S, Ferrucci L, Striker G, et al. Circulating glycotoxins and dietary advanced glycation endproducts: two links to inflammatory response, oxidative stress, and aging. J Gerontol A Biol Sci Med Sci. 2007;62(4):427–33.
4. Vlassara H, Uribarri J. Advanced glycation end products (AGE) and diabetes: cause, effect, or both? Curr Diab Rep. 2014;14(1):453.
5. Vlassara H, Cai W, Crandall J, Goldberg T, Oberstein R, Dardaine V, et al. Inflammatory mediators are induced by dietary glycotoxins, a major risk factor for diabetic angiopathy. Proc Natl Acad Sci U S A. 2002;99(24):15596–601.
6. Uribarri J, Peppa M, Cai W, Goldberg T, Lu M, He C, et al. Restriction of dietary glycotoxins reduces excessive advanced glycation end products in renal failure patients. J Am Soc Nephrol. 2003;14(3):728–31.
7. Vlassara H, Cai W, Goodman S, Pyzik R, Yong A, Chen X, et al. Protection against loss of innate defenses in adulthood by low advanced glycation end products (AGE) intake: role of the antiinflammatory AGE receptor-1. J Clin Endocrinol Metab. 2009;94(11):4483–91.
8. Uribarri J, Cai W, Ramdas M, Goodman S, Pyzik R, Chen X, et al. Restriction of advanced glycation end products improves insulin resistance in human type 2 diabetes: potential role of AGER1 and SIRT1. Diabetes Care. 2011;34(7):1610–6.
9. Birlouez-Aragon I, Saavedra G, Tessier FJ, Galinier A, Ait-Ameur L, Lacoste F, et al. A diet based on high-heat-treated foods promotes risk factors for diabetes mellitus and cardiovascular diseases. Am J Clin Nutr. 2010;91(5):1220–6.
10. Luevano-Contreras C, Garay-Sevilla ME, Wrobel K, Malacara JM, Wrobel K. Dietary advanced glycation end products restriction diminishes inflammation markers and oxidative stress in patients with type 2 diabetes mellitus. J Clin Biochem Nutr. 2013;52(1):22–6.
11. Goldberg T, Cai W, Peppa M, Dardaine V, Baliga BS, Uribarri J, et al. Advanced glycoxidation end products in commonly consumed foods. J Am Diet Assoc. 2004;104(8):1287–91.
12. Uribarri J, Woodruff S, Goodman S, Cai W, Chen X, Pyzik R, et al. Advanced glycation end products in foods and a practical guide to their reduction in the diet. J Am Diet Assoc. 2010;110(6):911–16.e12.
13. Snelson M, Coughlan MT. Dietary advanced glycation end products: digestion, metabolism and modulation of gut microbial ecology. Nutrients. 2019;11(2)
14. Monden M, Koyama H, Otsuka Y, Morioka T, Mori K, Shoji T, et al. Receptor for advanced glycation end products regulates adipocyte hypertrophy and insulin sensitivity in mice: involvement of Toll-like receptor 2. Diabetes. 2013;62(2):478–89.
15. Cai W, Ramdas M, Zhu L, Chen X, Striker GE, Vlassara H. Oral advanced glycation endproducts (AGEs) promote insulin resistance and diabetes by depleting the antioxidant defenses AGE receptor-1 and sirtuin 1. Proc Natl Acad Sci U S A. 2012;109(39):15888–93.
16. He C, Sabol J, Mitsuhashi T, Vlassara H. Dietary glycotoxins: inhibition of reactive products by aminoguanidine facilitates renal clearance and reduces tissue sequestration. Diabetes. 1999;48(6):1308–15.
17. Vlassara H, Uribarri J, Cai W, Striker G. Advanced glycation end product homeostasis: exogenous oxidants and innate defenses. Ann N Y Acad Sci. 2008;1126:46–52.
18. Peppa M, Uribarri J, Cai W, Lu M, Vlassara H. Glycoxidation and inflammation in renal failure patients. Am J Kidney Dis. 2004;43(4):690–5.
19. Linden E, Cai W, He JC, Xue C, Li Z, Winston J, et al. Endothelial dysfunction in patients with chronic kidney disease results from advanced glycation end products (AGE)-mediated inhibition of endothelial nitric oxide synthase through RAGE activation. Clin J Am Soc Nephrol. 2008;3(3):691–8.

20. Fagugli RM, Vanholder R, De Smet R, Selvi A, Antolini F, Lameire N, et al. Advanced glycation end products: specific fluorescence changes of pentosidine-like compounds during short daily hemodialysis. Int J Artif Organs. 2001;24(5):256–62.

21. Gerdemann A, Wagner Z, Solf A, Bahner U, Heidland A, Vienken J, et al. Plasma levels of advanced glycation end products during haemodialysis, haemodiafiltration and haemofiltration: potential importance of dialysate quality. Nephrol Dial Transplant. 2002;17(6):1045–9.

22. Lin CL, Huang CC, Yu CC, Yang HY, Chuang FR, Yang CW. Reduction of advanced glycation end product levels by on-line hemodiafiltration in long-term hemodialysis patients. Am J Kidney Dis. 2003;42(3):524–31.

23. Friedlander MA, Wu YC, Schulak JA, Monnier VM, Hricik DE. Influence of dialysis modality on plasma and tissue concentrations of pentosidine in patients with end-stage renal disease. Am J Kidney Dis. 1995;25(3):445–51.

24. Vongsanim S, Fan S, Davenport A. Comparison of skin autofluorescence, a marker of tissue advanced glycation end-products in peritoneal dialysis patients using standard and biocompatible glucose containing peritoneal dialysates. Nephrology (Carlton). 2019;24(8):835–40.

25. Slowik-Zylka D, Safranow K, Dziedziejko V, Ciechanowski K, Chlubek D. Association of plasma pentosidine concentrations with renal function in kidney graft recipients. Clin Transpl. 2010;24(6):839–47.

26. Uribarri J, Tuttle KR. Advanced glycation end products and nephrotoxicity of high-protein diets. Clin J Am Soc Nephrol. 2006;1(6):1293–9.

27. Daroux M, Prevost G, Maillard-Lefebvre H, Gaxatte C, D'Agati VD, Schmidt AM, et al. Advanced glycation end-products: implications for diabetic and non-diabetic nephropathies. Diabetes Metab. 2010;36(1):1–10.

28. Zhou G, Li C, Cai L. Advanced glycation end-products induce connective tissue growth factor-mediated renal fibrosis predominantly through transforming growth factor beta-independent pathway. Am J Pathol. 2004;165(6):2033–43.

29. McLennan SV, Kelly DJ, Schache M, Waltham M, Dy V, Langham RG, et al. Advanced glycation end products decrease mesangial cell MMP-7: a role in matrix accumulation in diabetic nephropathy? Kidney Int. 2007;72(4):481–8.

30. Pala L, Cresci B, Manuelli C, Maggi E, Yamaguchi YF, Cappugi P, et al. Vascular endothelial growth factor receptor-2 and low affinity VEGF binding sites on human glomerular endothelial cells: biological effects and advanced glycosilation end products modulation. Microvasc Res. 2005;70(3):179–88.

31. Cerami C, Founds H, Nicholl I, Mitsuhashi T, Giordano D, Vanpatten S, et al. Tobacco smoke is a source of toxic reactive glycation products. Proc Natl Acad Sci U S A. 1997;94(25):13915–20.

32. Chuang PY, Yu Q, Fang W, Uribarri J, He JC. Advanced glycation endproducts induce podocyte apoptosis by activation of the FOXO4 transcription factor. Kidney Int. 2007;72(8):965–76.

33. Yang CW, Vlassara H, Peten EP, He CJ, Striker GE, Striker LJ. Advanced glycation end products up-regulate gene expression found in diabetic glomerular disease. Proc Natl Acad Sci U S A. 1994;91(20):9436–40.

34. Horie K, Miyata T, Maeda K, Miyata S, Sugiyama S, Sakai H, et al. Immunohistochemical colocalization of glycoxidation products and lipid peroxidation products in diabetic renal glomerular lesions. Implication for glycoxidative stress in the pathogenesis of diabetic nephropathy. J Clin Invest. 1997;100(12):2995–3004.

35. Yamamoto Y, Kato I, Doi T, Yonekura H, Ohashi S, Takeuchi M, et al. Development and prevention of advanced diabetic nephropathy in RAGE-overexpressing mice. J Clin Invest. 2001;108(2):261–8.

36. Wendt TM, Tanji N, Guo J, Kislinger TR, Qu W, Lu Y, et al. RAGE drives the development of glomerulosclerosis and implicates podocyte activation in the pathogenesis of diabetic nephropathy. Am J Pathol. 2003;162(4):1123–37.

37. Soulis T, Cooper ME, Sastra S, Thallas V, Panagiotopoulos S, Bjerrum OJ, et al. Relative contributions of advanced glycation and nitric oxide synthase inhibition to aminoguanidine-mediated renoprotection in diabetic rats. Diabetologia. 1997;40(10):1141–51.

38. Peppa M, Brem H, Cai W, Zhang JG, Basgen J, Li Z, et al. Prevention and reversal of diabetic nephropathy in db/db mice treated with alagebrium (ALT-711). Am J Nephrol. 2006;26(5):430–6.

39. Zheng F, He C, Cai W, Hattori M, Steffes M, Vlassara H. Prevention of diabetic nephropathy in mice by a diet low in glycoxidation products. Diabetes Metab Res Rev. 2002;18(3):224–37.

40. Normand G, Lemoine S, Villien M, Le Bars D, Merida I, Irace Z, et al. AGE content of a protein load is responsible for renal performances: a pilot study. Diabetes Care. 2018;41(6):1292–4.

41. Uribarri J, Stirban A, Sander D, Cai W, Negrean M, Buenting CE, et al. Single oral challenge by advanced glycation end products acutely impairs endothelial function in diabetic and nondiabetic subjects. Diabetes Care. 2007;30(10):2579–82.

42. Kakuta T, Tanaka R, Hyodo T, Suzuki H, Kanai G, Nagaoka M, et al. Effect of sevelamer and calcium-based phosphate binders on coronary artery calcification and accumulation of circulating advanced glycation end products in hemodialysis patients. Am J Kidney Dis. 2011;57(3):422–31.

43. Stirban A, Negrean M, Stratmann B, Gawlowski T, Horstmann T, Gotting C, et al. Benfotiamine prevents macro- and microvascular endothelial dysfunction and oxidative stress following a meal rich in advanced glycation end products in individuals with type 2 diabetes. Diabetes Care. 2006;29(9):2064–71.

44. Saulnier PJ, Wheelock KM, Howell S, Weil EJ, Tanamas SK, Knowler WC, et al. Advanced glycation end products predict loss of renal function and correlate with lesions of diabetic kidney disease in American Indians with type 2 diabetes. Diabetes. 2016;65(12):3744–53.

45. Semba RD, Ferrucci L, Fink JC, Sun K, Beck J, Dalal M, et al. Advanced glycation end products and their circulating receptors and level of kidney function in older community-dwelling women. Am J Kidney Dis. 2009;53(1):51–8.

46. Tezuka Y, Nakaya I, Nakayama K, Nakayama M, Yahata M, Soma J. Methylglyoxal as a prognostic factor in patients with chronic kidney disease. Nephrology (Carlton). 2019;24(9):943–50.

47. Rebholz CM, Astor BC, Grams ME, Halushka MK, Lazo M, Hoogeveen RC, et al. Association of plasma levels of soluble receptor for advanced glycation end products and risk of kidney disease: the Atherosclerosis Risk in Communities study. Nephrol Dial Transplant. 2015;30(1):77–83.

48. Uribarri J, Cai W, Pyzik R, Goodman S, Chen X, Zhu L, et al. Suppression of native defense mechanisms, SIRT1 and PPARgamma, by dietary glycoxidants precedes disease in adult humans; relevance to lifestyle-engendered chronic diseases. Amino Acids. 2014;46(2):301–9.

49. Lopez-Moreno J, Quintana-Navarro GM, Camargo A, Jimenez-Lucena R, Delgado-Lista J, Marin C, et al. Dietary fat quantity and quality modifies advanced glycation end products metabolism in patients with metabolic syndrome. Mol Nutr Food Res. 2017;61(8)

50. Vlassara H, Uribarri J, Cai WJ, Goodman S, Pyzik R, Post J, et al. Effects of sevelamer on HbA1c, inflammation, and advanced glycation end products in diabetic kidney disease. Clin J Am Soc Nephrol. 2012;7(6):934–42.

51. Yubero-Serrano EM, Woodward M, Poretsky L, Vlassara H, Striker GE, Group AG-lS. Effects of sevelamer carbonate on advanced glycation end products and antioxidant/pro-oxidant status in patients with diabetic kidney disease. Clin J Am Soc Nephrol. 2015;10(5):759–66.

52. Vlassara H, Cai W, Tripp E, Pyzik R, Yee K, Goldberg L, et al. Oral AGE restriction ameliorates insulin resistance in obese individuals with the metabolic syndrome: a randomised controlled trial. Diabetologia. 2016;59(10):2181–92.

53. Luevano-Contreras C, Gomez-Ojeda A, Macias-Cervantes MH, Garay-Sevilla ME. Dietary advanced glycation end products and cardiometabolic risk. Curr Diab Rep. 2017;17(8):63.

54. Kim Y, Keogh JB, Clifton PM. Effects of two different dietary patterns on inflammatory markers, advanced glycation end products and lipids in subjects without type 2 diabetes: a randomised crossover study. Nutrients. 2017;9(4)

55. Yacoub R, Nugent M, Cai W, Nadkarni GN, Chaves LD, Abyad S, et al. Advanced glycation end products dietary restriction effects on bacterial gut microbiota in peritoneal dialysis patients; a randomized open label controlled trial. PLoS One. 2017;12(9):e0184789.

56. Nagai R, Shirakawa J, Ohno R, Moroishi N, Nagai M. Inhibition of AGEs formation by natural products. Amino Acids. 2014;46(2):261–6.

57. Williams ME, Bolton WK, Khalifah RG, Degenhardt TP, Schotzinger RJ, McGill JB. Effects of pyridoxamine in combined phase 2 studies of patients with type 1 and type 2 diabetes and overt nephropathy. Am J Nephrol. 2007;27(6):605–14.

Chapter 30
Physical Activity and Exercise in Chronic Kidney Disease

Anthony Meade and Kenneth R. Wilund

Keywords Exercise · Physical activity · Resistance · Balance · Cardiovascular · Exercise history Exercise prescription · Nutrition support · Physical function · Rehabilitation · Chronic kidney disease Hemodialysis · Peritoneal dialysis · Weight loss · Sarcopenia

---

Key Points
- People with chronic kidney disease (CKD) are more sedentary than the general population.
- Exercise capacity is restricted by the effects of CKD on cardiovascular (CV) and muscle function.
- People with CKD often have multiple comorbid conditions that also impact their physical function and activity levels.
- Sarcopenia and muscle wasting are common but potentially reversible with resistance training.
- The volume and intensity of most exercise interventions to date may have been insufficient to elicit the true benefits of exercise training for CKD patients.
- Improvements in physical function through exercise training are associated with improved quality of life in CKD and dialysis.
- Clinicians should include exercise history in clinical assessment and exercise interventions in treatment plans.

Introduction

The chronic kidney disease (CKD) population is older, with common comorbidities such as diabetes, hypertension, and cardiovascular disease (CVD). Frailty [1–5], low levels of physical function [2, 6–8], and low levels of physical activity [9–11] are related to morbidity and

---

The editors acknowledge the contribution of Kirsten L. Johansen and Patricia Painter to this chapter in *Nutrition in Kidney Disease, Second Edition*, Nutrition and Health, DOI https://doi.org/10.1007/978-1-62703-685-6_1, © Springer Science+Business Media New York 2014.

A. Meade
Royal Adelaide Hospital, Central Northern Adelaide Renal and Transplantation Service, Adelaide, Australia

K. R. Wilund (✉)
Department of Kinesiology and Community Health, University of Illinois, Urbana, IL, USA
e-mail: kwilund@illinois.edu

mortality and are well documented in people with CKD. Obesity is common; however, sarcopenic obesity is increasingly recognized [12–15]. Although physical activity is generally recognized as important, self-perception of actual activity levels is often overstated [16]. Physical activity and exercise should be the core components of the management of people with CKD.

Physical activity has been defined as bodily movement produced by the contraction of skeletal muscle that increases energy expenditure above a basal level and generally refers to the physical activity that *enhances health. Exercise* is a form of physical activity that is planned, structured, repetitive, and performed with the goal of *improving* health or fitness. All exercise is physical activity, but not all physical activity is exercise [17].

The goals of physical activity and exercise can be broadly broken down into rehabilitation from illness or injury, general health maintenance, disease prevention (including depression, weight loss), optimizing overall health (physical and cognitive function, comorbidity management), and improving performance. In this chapter we will consider the different types of physical activity including aerobic, muscle strengthening, bone strengthening, balance, and flexibility.

Aerobic physical activity (also called endurance or cardiovascular (CV) activity) involves the body's large muscles moving in a rhythmic manner for a sustained period of time and improves cardiorespiratory fitness. When considering aerobic activity, there are three basic components: frequency (how often), duration (how long), and intensity (how hard is the activity).

Muscle-strengthening activities are also called strength training, resistance training, or muscular strength and endurance exercises. The aim of muscle-strengthening activities is to increase skeletal muscle strength, power, endurance, or mass. Muscle-strengthening activity has three basic components: frequency (how often), intensity (how much resistance or weight can be lifted), and sets and repetitions (how many times a person repeats the muscle-strengthening activity during a session, comparable to duration for aerobic activity).

Balance is a component of physical fitness closely related to muscle-strengthening activity that involves maintaining the body's equilibrium while stationary or moving. Balance training includes static and dynamic exercises that are designed to improve an individual's ability to resist forces that cause falls while a person is stationary or moving.

Bone-strengthening activity involves weight-bearing activities that produce an impact or tension force on bones to promote bone strength. *Flexibility* is a health- and performance-related component of physical activity that is intended to improve the range of motion of joints.

The basic principles of exercise prescription are overload, progression, and specificity. Overload is the amount of new activity added to a person's usual activity level. Progression is the process of overloading as the body adapts by increasing the intensity, duration, frequency, or amount of activity. Specificity is the principle that the benefits of the activity relate to the body systems doing the work (e.g., leg exercises to improve leg strength).

Benefits of Exercise

The benefits of exercise in the general population are discussed at length in the *Physical Activity Guidelines for Americans* [17] and other similar guidelines from Australia [18], the United Kingdom, and Canada. In brief, these guidelines suggest (1) moving more and sitting less throughout the day. Some physical activity is better than none, though doing moderate to vigorous activity provides even greater health benefits. (2) For more substantial benefits, 150–300 minutes/week of moderate intensity activity, and/or 75–150 minutes/week of vigorous activity, are recommended. (3) Additional benefits can accrue if moderate intensity activity for >300 minutes/week is done. (4) Adults should also do muscle-strengthening activities of moderate or greater intensity that involve all major muscle groups for 2 or more days a week. (5) Balance and flexibility activities several days a week will also

Table 30.1   Health benefits associated with regular physical activity [17]

Lower risk of all-cause mortality
Lower risk of cardiovascular disease mortality
Lower risk of cardiovascular disease (including heart disease and stroke)
Lower risk of hypertension
Lower risk of type 2 diabetes
Lower risk of adverse blood lipid profile
Lower risk of cancers of the bladder, breast, colon, endometrium, esophagus, kidney, lung, and stomach
Improved cognition
Reduced risk of dementia (including Alzheimer's disease)
Improved quality of life (QOL)
Reduced anxiety
Reduced risk of depression
Improved sleep
Slowed or reduced weight gain
Weight loss, particularly when combined with reduced calorie intake
Prevention of weight regain following initial weight loss
Improved bone health
Improved physical function
Lower risk of falls (older adults)
Lower risk of fall-related injuries (older adults)

provide benefits for many. Examples of the benefits from engaging in regular physical activity are described in Table 30.1.

Guidelines and Special Considerations for Exercise in CKD

Although CKD is not specifically recognized in the *Physical Activity Guidelines for Americans*, the evidence and recommendations support the benefits of exercise for the management of hypertension and diabetes, both risk factors for the development and progression of CKD, to lower the risk of CV mortality and disease progression. Considering the majority of people living with CKD are older adults, there are specific guidelines that recognize that the goals of exercise shift from disease prevention to management of chronic disease, healthy aging, optimizing physical function, and preventing physical and cognitive decline with increasing age. These guidelines also recognize the importance of considering the relative intensity of exercise and physical activity that should be matched to the individual's ability.

The evidence for the benefits of physical activity in the population with CKD is increasingly recognized in nephrology guidelines. The 2005 National Kidney Foundation Kidney Disease Outcomes Quality Initiative (NKF-KDOQI) guidelines for cardiovascular disease in dialysis patients [19] emphasized the importance of exercise for adults receiving dialysis, especially if attempting to manage CV risk factors. In 2013, Exercise and Sports Science Australia (ESSA) published a position statement encouraging regular exercise training to be a component of the management of patients with CKD to reduce the risk of CV complications [20]. The Kidney Disease Improving Global Outcomes (KDIGO) 2012 Clinical Practice Guideline for the Evaluation and Management of Chronic Kidney Disease [21] recommend that people with CKD be encouraged to undertake physical activity compatible with CV health and tolerance (aiming for at least 30 minutes 5 times per week). The exercise guidelines for CKD patients are similar to those for the general population in terms of the recommended frequency, intensity, and types of physical activity in which to engage [22]. This includes combinations of endurance, resistance, flexibility, and balance exercises at least several days a week. However, none of these guidelines address implementation, the cornerstone of activity counselling.

Although the general population physical activity guidelines appear appropriate for people with CKD, there are reasons why these recommendations need to be considered carefully in the CKD population. In CKD there are conditions resulting in loss of lean body mass unrelated to reduced nutrient intake. These include nonspecific inflammatory processes, intercurrent catabolic illnesses, nutrient losses into dialysate, acidosis, and endocrine disorders such as resistance to insulin, growth hormone, and insulin-like growth factor-1 (IGF-1) [23]. Inflammation can impair protein anabolism independently of whether adequate nutrition is present [23]. Acidosis is common and an established cause of increased protein catabolism, muscle wasting, and inhibition of anabolic signaling pathways [24]. Impaired insulin/IGF-1 intracellular signaling activates the ubiquitin-proteasome system (UPS) to stimulate muscle protein catabolism [25]. In addition, people with CKD have impaired muscle protein synthesis and muscle mitochondrial metabolism [26], and there are metabolic and structural abnormalities in muscle fibers [24] and increased arterial stiffness [27] that may limit the anabolic effectiveness of exercise independent of age, hemoglobin levels, and endothelial function. Peripheral neuropathy is a common complication of diabetes that can impair basic physical functions such as walking.

Before 1990 many considered the predominant cause of exercise limitation in CKD to be related to the associated anemia; however, the adoption of erythropoietin-stimulating agents in clinical practice failed to fully improve patient symptoms of well-being and functional capacity [28]. The implications of mild anemia on exercise capacity are perhaps understated. Poorly managed renal anemia is related to lethargy, decreased motivation, and reduced CV exercise capacity [29]. The ceiling exercise intensity may also be influenced by medications such as beta-blockers that limit maximum heart rate.

Another significant problem in people with CKD that may impact ability to exercise is chronic volume overload (VO). VO is a concern in all CKD patients, but it is an especially vexing problem in hemodialysis. It is the primary cause of hypertension and congestive heart failure, but also leads to intradialytic hypotension (IDH) and increased CV mortality [30]. VO is also highly correlated with fatigue [31] and also limits ability to exercise during dialysis [32].

Assessing Outcomes from Exercise Interventions

Aside from physical performance measures such as progression of intensity/loads, repetitions, and frequency, it is also useful to consider various physical assessments as outcome measures in research and clinical practice. Research studies can use computed tomography (CT) scanning to measure muscle cross-sectional area (CSA), magnetic resonance imaging (MRI) to measure muscle volume, or dual-energy X-ray absorptiometry (DXA) to measure lean mass, but these are usually not an affordable option in most healthcare settings. In the clinic, simple anthropometric measures such as upper and lower limb girths and validated tools such as Subjective Global Assessment (SGA) or Patient-Generated SGA (PG-SGA) and physical function assessment tools can also provide valuable insight into physical function and outcomes of exercise interventions. Bioimpedance spectroscopy (BIS) has also been used to assess body composition in the clinic, but its utility in CKD patients is questionable due to the effect of fluid shifts on the algorithms used to derive body composition estimates [33]. Lastly, a variety of objective and self-reported measures of physical function and physical activity can be utilized for patient assessments [34–36]. Cardiorespiratory fitness, measured by assessing maximal oxygen consumption during a graded endurance exercise protocol (VO$_2$max), is considered the gold standard method of assessing physical fitness. However, many CKD patients may have physical limitations as well as autonomic dysfunction, both of which may preclude them from achieving objective criteria required for these tests. As such, there are a variety of field tests that can be reliably used to assess physical function. The most common functional tests with demonstrated utility in CKD patients include the following: the 6-minute walk test (6MWT), intermittent shuttle walk, normal and fast gait speed, the chair stand ("sit to stand") test, the timed up and go (TUG), stair climb test, and short physical performance battery (SPPB). The relative merits and limitations of these objective tests, as well as self-reported measures of physical function and activity, have been reviewed extensively [34–36].

Benefits of Exercise in CKD and End-Stage Kidney Disease (ESKD)

In recent years, numerous systematic reviews and meta-analyses have detailed the benefits of exercise interventions in individuals with CKD [35–49]. This included data from interventions in non-dialysis CKD, dialysis, and transplant patients, using endurance training (ET), resistance training (RT), as well as combinations of ET and RT. Taken together, it is clear that exercise seems to improve the overall health and quality of life (QOL) in people with CKD, regardless of the stage of disease or the type of exercise intervention. Most of the data has been collected during "intradialytic exercise" in hemodialysis patients, specifically intradialytic cycling. However, there also does not appear to be large differences in benefits between intradialytic or out-of-center ("interdialytic") exercise training. Based on this literature, many have argued that exercise should be included in the standard of care for all CKD patients [50–53], and several guidelines and position statements have been published recommending CKD patients engage in regular exercise [20, 54–56].

While many studies indicate that exercise is clearly beneficial to individuals with CKD, it is important to recognize that the evidence does not appear to be as consistent or robust as the evidence of benefits in other populations [42, 57, 58]. This may be due to a variety of factors, including the poor physical health of many CKD patients which limits the volume and intensity of exercise they can perform. There is also a lack of high-quality, adequately powered randomized controlled trials (RCTs) of exercise in CKD, and this may also explain some of the inconsistent results. Both the benefits of different types of exercise in CKD and the deficiencies in the literature will be reviewed below to provide a better understanding of the complexities of exercise prescription in this population.

Endurance Exercise in CKD and Its Benefits

Endurance Exercise, Aerobic Capacity, and Physical Function

The majority of data examining the efficacy of exercise in CKD patients has come from studies incorporating primarily endurance training. Several recent reviews and meta-analyses have demonstrated benefits of short-term, supervised endurance exercise training on aerobic capacity (VO_{2peak}), muscle strength, physical function, and self-reported QOL across the spectrum of CKD patients [37–39, 41–48], although most of the data has been collected from studies in hemodialysis patients, specifically from studies utilizing "intradialytic" cycling exercise. It is important, however, to recognize that there are some inconsistencies and areas of concern in the literature that deserve further scrutiny. For example, one of the most consistently reported benefits of exercise is the improvements in aerobic capacity following endurance exercise in hemodialysis patients. In a review of 18 studies, Johansen found that the mean improvement in VO_{2peak} following endurance exercise training in hemodialysis patients was around 17%, and this occurred across a wide range of exercise prescriptions [59]. Despite these improvements, VO_{2peak} for most patients in these studies remained below age-adjusted norms [60]. Moreover, a recent review by Young et al. did not find significant improvements in VO_{2peak} following intradialytic cycling, which is the most common form of exercise employed in clinical practice in hemodialysis patients [42].

Much of the data assessing benefits of exercise have come from relatively small pilot studies, many of which lacked control groups or had other deficiencies. However, a few larger RCTs of endurance exercise in CKD have recently been published that are informative [61, 62]. In perhaps the largest exercise intervention in ESKD patients conducted to date ($n = 296$), Manfredini et al. showed that a 6-month, low-intensity, home-based walking program significantly improved walking performance and muscle strength by ~12% compared to usual care [62]. Moreover, there was a dose-response effect, where those with greater adherence to the exercise protocol had the largest improvements in function. These findings are both encouraging and generally consistent with other studies in the literature. However, it is also important to note that the magnitude of improvements was modest. For example, the average improvement in the 6-minute walk test in the exercise group was just 39 m, while changes in distance from 53 to 71 m are believed to be clinically meaningful in cardiopulmonary populations [63]. There also was a large dropout (31%) of participants in the exercise group (compared to 15% in the control group), and nearly 50% of those completing the intervention had low adherence to the exercise protocol (defined as completing <60% of sessions). The study also excluded patients with both low mobility and high fitness, reducing the external validity of the study. In another recent RCT, Koh et al. [61] compared the effects of 6 months of intradialytic or home-based endurance exercise to a control group receiving usual care ($n = 70$). Surprisingly, changes in physical function did not differ between the exercise and control groups. While there was a relatively high adherence to the exercise programs (70–75%), there was also a 29% dropout in the exercise groups. Similar to other studies in this population, the null findings may be partially due to the fact that the volume of exercise was very low (work rate was ~35 kcal/session at the end of the study). Taken together these studies highlight both the promise and challenges associated with implementing exercise programs in CKD patients.

Endurance Exercise and Markers of Cardiovascular Function and Risk

Data regarding the efficacy of exercise training in CKD patients on markers of CVD risk are also mixed. While most studies generally confirm a beneficial effect of exercise on traditional CVD risk factors such as plasma lipids and blood pressure [38], the apparent paradoxical association between many traditional CVD risk factors and adverse CV events in CKD makes these findings difficult to interpret [64]. In contrast, markers of cardiac function, endothelial function, and arterial stiffness have been consistently associated with CVD mortality in CKD patients [65, 66]. In non-dialysis CKD patients, recent data suggests no effect of endurance exercise training on blood pressure [67], endothelial function, or arterial stiffness [68]. However, Kirkman et al. recently showed that 12 weeks of endurance exercise training significantly improved microvascular function in CKD patients [69]. The data on arterial function in hemodialysis patients is also mixed. Studies by Koudi and Deligiannis et al. have demonstrated that 6–10 months of endurance training improves markers of cardiac function in hemodialysis patients [70, 71]. In addition, three small pilot studies noted modest improvements in markers of arterial stiffness following 3–4 months of intradialytic exercise [72–74]. However, a larger RCT conducted by Koh et al. [61] did not find reductions in markers of arterial stiffness after 6 months of either intradialytic or home-based aerobic exercise. A possible reason for the inconsistent effects of exercise on arterial health may be due to the significant vascular remodeling and calcification in CKD patients that may limit the vessels' ability to respond to exercise [75, 76].

Endurance Exercise and QOL

In chronic conditions such as CKD, functional limitations, disability, and comorbidity increase, often resulting in compromised physical, emotional, and psychological well-being. The increasing incidence of adults with CKD and other chronic disorders has directed public policy toward ways to maintain the independence, societal worth, and physical and mental well-being of this group. In essence, we have moved from simply trying to add quantity to life toward adding quality to those years of life. There is increasing evidence to suggest that physical activity interventions may represent an effective behavioral strategy for not only attenuating functional decline and reducing risk of disease and disability [77–79], but also for enhancing psychological well-being and QOL across the lifespan [80, 81]. Similar benefits on psychological well-being and QOL have been noted with intradialytic cycling in many studies in CKD patients [82–84], although the data are not entirely consistent. For example, a recent review suggests intradialytic cycling may not improve patient-reported physical function or QOL [42]. Moreover, in the RCT from Koh et al. [61], self-reported physical function actually regressed following 6 months of intradialytic cycling compared to a control group. One reason for the lack of clarity is the lack of large-scale, interdisciplinary RCTs targeting QOL outcomes [50]. An ongoing RCT in the United Kingdom called PEDAL (PrEscription of intra-Dialytic exercise to improve quAlity of Life in patients with chronic kidney disease) may help clarify this issue. Such research is needed to conclusively demonstrate the clinical importance of endurance exercise, which may influence current standard clinical practice among nephrologists and, as such, improve the health and QOL of this vulnerable cohort.

Resistance Exercise in CKD and Its Benefits

Muscle-strengthening or resistance exercise is increasingly recognized as important for maintaining physical function, balance, and resilience, particularly in older adults [17, 18, 85], but has been less well studied in CKD patients. Resistance training makes muscles do more work than they are accustomed to during activities of daily living. Table 30.2 shows examples of muscle-strengthening exercises. These exercises can be completed in supervised (e.g., gym, outpatient clinic) [85, 86] or unsupervised (e.g., gym or home) environments and incorporated into daily activities.

It is well established that advanced CKD is associated with significant protein-energy wasting (PEW) [87, 88]. Resistance training is known to be a more potent anabolic stimuli than endurance exercise, so may be especially important in CKD patients [89]. Indeed, several studies in non-dialysis CKD patients have demonstrated the benefits of RT. For example, resistance exercise has been shown to increase weight, muscle mass, and strength in non-dialysis CKD follow-

Table 30.2 Examples of muscle-strengthening activities

Lifting free weights
Using specific gym equipment
Working with resistance bands
Using body weight for resistance (such as push-ups, pull-ups, and planks)
Pilates
Climbing stairs
Carrying heavy loads

ing low-protein diets to preserve renal function [90]. In addition, Watson et al. [91] showed that 8 weeks of supervised progressive resistance exercise increased muscle anatomical cross-sectional area, muscle volume, knee extensor strength, and exercise capacity in non-dialysis CKD patients (see Table 30.2).

In dialysis patients, there are fewer studies on the benefits of resistance training than there are on endurance exercise. This may be due in part to perceived difficulty of performing resistance exercises during dialysis. Nonetheless, light free weights, resistance bands, and body weight exercises have been incorporated into intradialytic muscle-strengthening programs [92, 93]. Specific gym equipment designed to fit around hemodialysis chairs has also been used effectively [94]. However, it is often more practical to undertake muscle-strengthening exercises prior to dialysis sessions or outside of the clinic [95]. Successful programs often utilize the waiting time prior to dialysis as an opportunity to encourage resistance training. While most traditional strength training programs incorporate four to eight exercises with two to three sets of 8–12 repetitions, targeted single exercise programs have also proven effective in skeletal muscle protein accretion [96]. In practice, people with an arteriovenous fistula (AVF) should avoid static/isometric exercises, but should not be discouraged from participating in muscle-strengthening activities. One-armed resistance exercise can be performed with the non-AVF arm during hemodialysis, and with the AVF arm in the clinic waiting room or at home.

Several recent systematic reviews in dialysis patients indicate that progressive resistance training increases muscle hypertrophy, strength, and objective measures of physical function in most studies [35, 40]. In addition, a recent study by Chen et al. showed that even low-intensity strength training can yield modest improvements in muscle strength, physical function, and body composition [97]. Similar to the data with endurance training, benefits from many resistance training studies are either modest or inconsistent. For example, several resistance training interventions with the largest sample sizes and longest intervention periods have failed to yield increases in muscle hypertrophy [95, 98, 99]. In addition, several studies that have shown improved muscle size or composition in response to RT have failed to improve objective measures of physical function [98, 100, 101]. The modest or inconsistent results suggest that adjunct therapies may be needed to potentiate the benefits of RT in dialysis patients.

Studies Combining Endurance and Resistance Training

CKD patients often suffer from several comorbid conditions, so multiple therapeutic strategies may be needed to improve their health and QOL [102, 103]. For example, aerobic capacity is limited by both peripheral (skeletal muscle) and central CV factors, and aerobic training alone may not adequately improve peripheral oxygen uptake [104]. As a result, it has been hypothesized that combining endurance and resistance training may provide greater health benefits in CKD patients than either intervention alone. Indeed, a recent meta-analysis by Scapini et al. [49] found that studies combining endurance and resistance training in dialysis patients yield greater improvements in both aerobic capacity and blood pressure control than either modality alone. Few studies have assessed the efficacy of combining endurance and resistance training in non-dialysis CKD patients. However, a recent study by Watson et al. [105] showed that 12 weeks of combined resistance and aerobic training protocol improved muscle mass and strength more than aerobic training alone in pre-dialysis CKD patients. Yet once again, the data are not entirely consistent, as Kopple et al. [106] failed to find improvements in body composition after 6 months of isolated endurance or resistance training or a combination of the two modalities.

Studies Combining Exercise and Nutritional Supplementation

In the elderly, muscle is resistant to normally robust anabolic stimuli such as amino acids and resistance exercise [107]. However, combining resistance exercise with amino acid ingestion produces a potentiated anabolic response in the elderly, producing a "youthful" muscle more capable of hypertrophy and increased strength [107]. Similarly, CKD patients have alterations in muscle protein synthesis that may limit the effects of either supplemental protein or resistance exercise [88, 108]. However, it is uncertain if combining exercise and nutritional supplementation would help overcome this anabolic resistance in CKD. Early studies in hemodialysis patients showed that a single bout of either endurance or resistance exercise potentiates the anabolic response to nutritional supplementation [96, 109]. At least four long-term studies have combined various forms of nutritional supplementation and exercise training in hemodialysis patients for up to 6 months, but none demonstrated additive benefits on strength, function, or body composition [86, 95, 110, 111]. This suggests that a greater exercise stimulus or higher protein intake may be needed to demonstrate the potentiated anabolic response that is seen in the elderly or healthy controls.

Other Exercise Strategies

Balance Training

Postural control and walking performance [112] decline in people with CKD, which increases the risk of falls [113] and fall-related morbidity and mortality [114]. Balance training is a variation of muscle-strengthening exercise that can improve the ability to resist forces within or outside of the body that cause falls. Fall prevention programs that include balance training and other exercises to improve activities of daily living can also significantly reduce the risk of injury, such as bone fractures, if a fall does occur [17]. Balance training examples include standing on one leg, standing from a sitting position, and using unstable surfaces such as a wobble board. Although there is very little data in people with CKD, Frih et al. [115] recently demonstrated that incorporating balance training into a combined endurance/resistance training protocol could improve static and dynamic balance. The training included two weekly sessions lasting 30 minutes each and four types of exercises, including stance, transition, gait, and functional strength exercises. The protocol was modeled after balance training studies in other chronic diseases [116–118] and guidelines for fall prevention in older adults [119, 120]. Further research is needed to determine if balance training also reduces falls and fall-related injuries in CKD patients. Regardless, the evidence in support of balance activities in fall prevention in the general population is strong and should be encouraged as part of an overall physical activity program in CKD patients as well.

HIIT and SIT

Recent systematic reviews and meta-analyses have concluded that interval training (high-intensity interval training [HIIT] and sprint interval training [SIT]), or alternating periods of relatively intense exercise and recovery, can be a time-efficient strategy to enhance cardiorespiratory fitness (CRF), as determined by whole-body maximal oxygen uptake (VO_2max) [121–123]. Given that "lack of time" is a common barrier to regular physical activity in people with CKD and particularly dialysis, the identification of time-efficient exercise strategies that could confer health benefits favorably is worthy of investigation. Interesting, recent studies (in diabetes not including people with CKD) by Allison et al. [124] and Jenkins et al. [125], using 3× 60-second stair climbing "snacks", may prove beneficial for people with CKD due to the benefits for cardiorespiratory fitness and shorter time requirement.

Exercise for Weight Loss for Transplant

Although there is debate in the literature [126–132] as to the pros and cons of weight loss for renal transplant eligibility, there are no specific guidelines for exercise for weight loss in people with CKD. It would however be reasonable to defer to general population guidelines [17] for obesity which recommend >150 up to 300 minutes of exercise per week. Recent guidelines recognize that the recommendations for health-focused physical activity are inadequate to drive weight loss and that additional exercise will be required. A combination of aerobic and muscle-strengthening exercises is encouraged in order to preserve lean body mass while reducing adiposity. In addition, an individually planned exercise program designed in conjunction with the patient and an appropriately recognized exercise professional is advised [20].

Promoters and Inhibitors of Involvement in Exercise

Despite strong evidence to support physical activity and exercise, and recognition from patients of the benefits [133], there remain barriers to greater levels of activity and uptake of exercise programs in people with CKD [26, 91, 134–137]. Barriers include lack of medical [134, 138], nursing [136, 139], and allied health [140, 141] appreciation of the benefits of exercise, conservative nephrologist views about exercise and low levels of exercise discussion during clinic visits [134, 138, 142], and inadequately equipped staff who don't feel comfortable talking about or leading the conversation about exercise or have perceived bias due to their own exercise participation and experience [139, 141]. Barriers to exercise also include lack of encouragement to exercise, transportation and healthcare system issues [139, 140, 143], cost of equipment [26, 141], the use of exercise equipment that precludes participation by patients who recline during dialysis, and nursing concerns about equipment-related injury [136, 141].

Positive attitudes to exercise reflected autonomous motivations including exercising for health, enjoyment, and social interaction. Family support and goal-setting were seen as motivators for exercise, and the accessibility of local facilities influenced activity levels [143].

Debate continues around the ideal location for exercise programs. Outpatient [85, 91, 144, 145], in-center dialysis [86, 92, 94, 146–149] versus self-managed exercise/home-based therapies [61, 62, 150] have all been considered, although the majority of research has been completed in hemodialysis centers where the patient group is easily accessible. Patient preferences favor home-based programs [133]. While outcomes are comparable [61], recruitment to home-based programs has proven challenging [91]. The answer should be "where the patient feels most comfortable and has the greatest confidence in sustaining the program."

Several authors have reviewed the elements of sustainable exercise programs for people with CKD [137, 140]. Common elements include qualified exercise professional involvement, intradialytic physical activity, commitment from dialysis and medical staff, adequate equipment and space, interesting and stimulating programs, cost-effective and affordable, recognition that age is no barrier and exercise is not for everyone, and that exercise requires individual prescription. In addition, strategies are required to ensure that the healthcare system is actively promoting and routinely supporting exercise for all patients with CKD [133, 143], recognizing that the healthcare system is not always the best place for exercise programs.

Deficiencies in the Literature

It is widely acknowledged that there is a dearth of high-quality, adequately powered RCTs [42, 57, 58] in the exercise literature in CKD. This partially explains some of the modest or inconsistent benefits of exercise that have been seen. The most commonly cited concerns include short intervention durations, small and biased samples, a lack of adequate control groups, low exercise intensity, low compliance with the intervention, and high patient dropout rates. The majority of studies have also been conducted using in-center low-intensity endurance exercise in hemodialysis patients, with very few studies in non-dialysis CKD, peritoneal dialysis, and transplant recipients. The question of whether exercise can prevent a decline in health has rarely been addressed. To accomplish this, longer interventions including non-exercising control groups are needed. While this would allow researchers to capture health decline in a non-exercising control group, it is considered an unethical approach since it is generally acknowledged that all patients should be exercising. Many of the exercise studies in CKD also have focused on the healthier cohorts, therefore excluding the most deconditioned individuals that could potentially benefit the most from increased physical activity.

The reasons for all of these deficiencies in the literature are clearly multifactorial and complex. Poor overall health, lack of motivation for exercise training, as well as low recruitment and retention rates are common barriers to better research studies. Examining details from the EXCITE trial can help illustrate many of these points [62]. In many regards, this was one of the most impressive exercise interventions conducted to date in people with CKD. It was a relatively long-term intervention (6 months, low-intensity walking) with a large sample size ($n = 296$ patients) and included a non-exercising control group. By comparison, many exercise studies in the CKD literature include 10–20 patients in a 3- to 4-month intervention with or without a control group. However, details of the study protocol and adherence to the exercise intervention in the EXCITE trial also highlight many of the difficulties in conducting exercise trials in this population. For example, just 30% of patients at the participating clinics met the study inclusion criteria, and 36% of those refused to participate. This is despite the fact that the volume and intensity of exercise in the protocol were modest: requiring a maximum of 60 minutes per week of low-intensity walking, which represents about 40% of the recommended volume of aerobic exercise (150 minutes per week) in most published guidelines. Moreover, 31% of those randomized to the exercise group dropped out prematurely, and nearly 50% of those completing the intervention had low adherence to the exercise protocol (defined as completing <60% of sessions). In summary, for one reason or another, just 14% of the patients in the participating clinics were able to adhere to a 6-month walking program, that is 60% below the recommended volume of aerobic exercise in most physical activity guidelines. Unfortunately, the low volume and intensity of the exercise prescriptions, poor adherence, and high dropout rates are the norm, rather than the exception, in the CKD exercise literature [61, 62, 106]. These data speak to the difficulty of conducting robust exercise interventions in this critically ill patient population.

With these deficiencies in mind, it is clear that novel approaches to increasing physical activity and exercise training in people with CKD need to be considered. In particular, exercise prescriptions should be individualized so as to address patient-specific goals and barriers [151]. Research is also needed to evaluate the efficacy of interventions focused on minimizing sedentary behavior, ultimately progressing to targeted exercise training when appropriate. There are models for this approach in the CKD [152] and diabetes [153] literature, although more research in this area is clearly needed.

Table 30.3 Practice tips for supporting and encouraging physical activity in people with CKD

Discuss exercise and physical activity by including exercise history as part of routine clinical assessment
Screen for frailty risk factors and signs of physical deconditioning
Measure physical function using validated assessments such as 6MWT, STS, handgrip strength
Ask about intensity, duration, and frequency of exercise and physical activities
Discuss exercise training principles such as overload, variation, progression, and specificity
Be realistic about the differences between physical activity and exercise and the benefits to health, physical function, and well-being
Use techniques such as motivational interviewing to identify barriers and facilitators to encourage physical activity
Involve qualified exercise professionals for individualized exercise prescription [20] and include as part of medical and nutrition prescriptions
Work with patients to set exercise and physical activity goals and review these during follow-up consultations

Abbreviations: 6MWT = 6-minute walk test, STS = sit to stand

Conclusion and Future Directions

People with CKD often have multiple comorbid conditions that impact their physical function and activity levels. There is a wealth of data demonstrating benefits of exercise training in this population, although the benefits in many studies have been modest or inconsistent. More inclusive study protocols are needed that include all people with CKD regardless of functional status to assess the real benefits of exercise training.

It is possible that larger, longer RCTs with greater volumes and intensity of exercise may be needed to provide more robust and consistent benefits. Historically, one-size-fits-all approaches using mandated exercise prescriptions (e.g., progressive endurance or resistance training protocols) have been the standard in the CKD literature. In contrast, interventions designed to allow more flexibility to self-select types of activities in which they choose to engage should be encouraged. A liberalized activity prescription also may result in greater participation and more sustained and robust lifestyle changes in people with CKD. Studies testing the efficacy of comprehensive interventions that include physical activity, nutrition, and other behavioral modifications are needed.

Finally, all health professionals need to be able to assess and promote exercise and physical activity as a part of comprehensive clinical management of people with CKD; however, increased awareness and skills are needed. Table 30.3 outlines practice tips for supporting and encouraging physical activity in people with CKD.

Case Study

The following case study highlights some of the complexities related to exercise prescription in hemodialysis patients: A 44-year-old African-American male with ESKD has been on maintenance hemodialysis for 2 years. He is morbidly obese (BMI = 38.5 kg/m^2) and has been told he needs to lose ~ 50 pounds (20 kg) to become eligible for a transplant. He is hypertensive (pre-dialysis BP = 170/100), and his interdialytic weight gain for the past month has averaged 5.0 kg. He has occasional intradialytic hypotension and/or cramping during treatment, which is normally resolved by saline treatments or prematurely stopping ultrafiltration. The patient also complains of post-dialysis fatigue and poor sleep patterns. He acknowledges that he does not exercise. He also describes his diet as poor, including "a lot of fast food and frozen meals," and rarely cooks. He is divorced and lives with his 22-year-old son who is also overweight and does little exercise. The patient expresses that he is very motivated to lose the weight needed to become eligible for a transplant and has asked for help in developing an exercise program to assist with this.

Medications Darbepoetin, Amlodipine, Clonidine, Losartan, and sevelamer carbonate.

Laboratory Values Albumin, 3.8 mg/dL; hematocrit, 36.0%; hemoglobin, 10.8 g/dL; serum P, 4.8 mg/dL; serum K, 5.5 mmol.

Physical Evaluation

Physical activity history: The patient currently does not engage in any physical activity. He played football and basketball in high school, but has not been involved in any structured exercise program since then. He previously had a construction job and was fairly active at work, but he lost his job after starting dialysis and is now completely sedentary, except for occasional trips (once a month) to a grocery store that is just a few blocks from his home. He lives in a neighborhood in which he does not feel safe walking at night, but is comfortable walking during the day. He would like to join a gym but does not feel he can afford it.

Physical function testing:

Four-meter gait speed: 1.0 m/s < 1.1 m/s indicates impaired mobility [34]; 1.21 m/s is the average age/gender comfortable gait speed [154]; 0.98 m/s is average in 40- to 50-year-old hemodialysis patients [34]. Thus, his gait speed is 83% of expected.

Chair stands (time for five repetitions): 9.5 s > 13.7 s indicates impaired function [155]; 7.6 s is age-expected time [156]. Thus, his performance is 80% of expected.

Six-minute walk distance: 445 m < 460 m indicates impaired mobility [34]; 570 m is the average age-gender reported distance [157]. Thus, his distance is 78% of expected.

Patient-stated activity goals:

Short-term: Start lifting weights and/or walking to the store 3 days a week, preferably on non-dialysis days when he has the most energy.

Long-term: Lose 50 pounds to become eligible for a transplant.

Case Questions and Answers

1. Prior to developing a physical activity plan for this patient, what considerations would you have?
   Answer: Prior to developing a physical activity plan for this patient, it is important to assess his physical activity history, complete a functional assessment, and also identify activity-related goals and barriers.

2. Is exercise alone likely to help this patient achieve his weight loss goal?
   Answer: The situation outlined above is rather common. As stated above, there is debate in the literature as to the pros and cons of weight loss for renal transplant eligibility, and there are no clear guidelines for doing so [126–132]. Regardless, his goal of losing 50 pounds to become transplant eligible is unlikely to be resolved through exercise alone. According to the current physical activity recommendations, losing weight through exercise alone requires 60–90 minutes of daily exercise [158], which is an unrealistic expectation in any reasonable time frame. As such, some reduction in caloric intake is needed to facilitate the required weight loss.

   Complicating matters, the patient has excessive fluid intakes contributing to volume overload, and this is contributing to his intradialytic symptoms, including premature cessation of ultrafiltration, post-dialysis fatigue, and disturbed sleep patterns. Results from the physical function testing indicate he may have mildly impaired function, but is not frail, so should have few if any restraints on his physical activity.

3. What would be a realistic exercise prescription for this patient?
   Answer: An appropriate prescription for this patient should include a plan to slowly increase his physical activity levels, followed by structured exercise as he progresses. An excellent example of

a strategy to increase the patient's physical activity levels is outlined in the study by Tawney et al. [152]. A realistic initial goal could be to develop strategies for the patient to build toward accumulating at least 30 minutes of self-selected physical activity per day. Activity goals should be set that consider the patient's preference and lifestyle, barriers to physical activity should be identified, and supports for addressing these barriers, such as inclusion of family or other care providers, should be considered. An intriguing possibility would be to inquire if his son would be willing to exercise with him on occasion, especially since he also has a weight problem. For the first several weeks, modest goals such as walking around the neighborhood on his non-dialysis days should be considered, starting from modest goals of 10–15 minutes several days a week. As the patient has a goal of improving his strength, simple at-home exercises such as push-ups and body weight squats can be incorporated into his daily routine, perhaps while he watches television.

4. What dietary interventions would you suggest to support the exercise prescription?

   Answer: A dietitian should also be consulted to help safely manage his weight loss, which should include a focus on how to reduce his sodium intake to reduce interdialytic weight gain and chronic volume overload. This could include walking to the grocery store and tips on how to shop for low-sodium and lower-calorie food products, to help facilitate weight loss. Short-term weight loss goals should be considered, such as losing 1–2 pounds per week. This will be facilitated by changes in his diet that could result from purchasing more food at the grocery store and eating out less. A balanced approach to higher diet quality and less processed foods should be encouraged with an individualized lower-calorie plan including whole grains, legumes, dairy, fruits, and vegetables. Cooking is another form of physical activity that increases energy expenditure a modest amount and contributes to an overall activity plan.

5. How would you adjust the exercise prescription as the patient starts to make progress?

   Answer: As the patient sees progress, activity and nutrition goals can be adjusted as necessary. Aerobic activity should increase to at least 150 minutes per week. If the patient has reduced his dietary intake, specifically from calorically dense processed food, he should slowly start to lose weight, but in a reasonable manner that should help preserve lean mass. Incorporating some resistance training into his physical activity plan can also help maintain muscle. Moreover, reduced sodium intake from eating less processed food should reduce interdialytic weight gains (IDWGs) and subsequently ultrafiltration rates during dialysis. This should reduce post-dialysis fatigue and give him more energy to exercise, possibly even after dialysis.

This case study is meant to highlight the many complexities of prescribing exercise in dialysis patients. It is clear that a comprehensive approach to physical activity is required to significantly improve the health and QOL of many hemodialysis patients. Individualized approaches to an exercise prescription are needed, especially when weight loss is an objective.

References

1. Evans WJ. Protein nutrition, exercise and aging. J Am Coll Nutr. 2004;23(sup6):601S–9S.
2. Greco A, Paroni G, Seripa D, Addante F, Dagostino MP, Aucella F. Frailty, disability and physical exercise in the aging process and in chronic kidney disease. Kidney Blood Press Res. 2014;39(2–3):164–8.
3. Johansen KL, Dalrymple LS, Delgado C, Chertow GM, Segal MR, Chiang J, et al. Factors associated with frailty and its trajectory among patients on hemodialysis. Clin J Am Soc Nephrol. 2017;12(7):1100–8.
4. Laur CV, McNicholl T, Valaitis R, Keller HH. Malnutrition or frailty? Overlap and evidence gaps in the diagnosis and treatment of frailty and malnutrition. Appl Physiol Nutr Metab. 2017;42(5):449–58.
5. Sy J, Johansen KL. The impact of frailty on outcomes in dialysis. Curr Opin Nephrol Hypertens. 2017;26(6):537–42.
6. Kaysen GA, Larive B, Painter P, Craig A, Lindsay RM, Rocco MV, et al. Baseline physical performance, health, and functioning of participants in the Frequent Hemodialysis Network (FHN) trial. Am J Kidney Dis. 2011;57(1):101–12.

7. Marcus RL, LaStayo PC, Ikizler TA, Wei G, Giri A, Chen X, et al. Low physical function in maintenance hemodialysis patients is independent of muscle mass and comorbidity. J Ren Nutr. 2015;25(4):371–5.

8. Torino C, Manfredini F, Bolignano D, Aucella F, Baggetta R, Barilla A, et al. Physical performance and clinical outcomes in dialysis patients: a secondary analysis of the EXCITE trial. Kidney Blood Press Res. 2014;39(2–3):205–11.

9. Avesani CM, Trolonge S, Deléaval P, Baria F, Mafra D, Faxén-Irving G, et al. Physical activity and energy expenditure in haemodialysis patients: an international survey. Nephrol Dial Transplant. 2012;27(6):2430–4.

10. Baria F, Kamimura MA, Avesani CM, Lindholm B, Stenvinkel P, Draibe SA, et al. Activity-related energy expenditure of patients undergoing hemodialysis. J Ren Nutr. 2011;21(3):226–34.

11. Matsuzawa R, Matsunaga A, Wang G, Kutsuna T, Ishii A, Abe Y, et al. Habitual physical activity measured by accelerometer and survival in maintenance hemodialysis patients. Clin J Am Soc Nephrol. 2012;7:2010.

12. Carrero JJ. Misclassification of obesity in CKD: appearances are deceptive. Clin J Am Soc Nephrol. 2014;9(12):2025–7.

13. Kalantar-Zadeh K, Block G, Humphreys MH, Kopple JD. Reverse epidemiology of cardiovascular risk factors in maintenance dialysis patients. Kidney Int. 2003;63(3):793–808.

14. Kovesdy CP, Furth SL, Zoccali C. Obesity and kidney disease: hidden consequences of the epidemic. J Ren Care. 2017;43(1):3–10.

15. Sharma D, Hawkins M, Abramowitz MK. Association of sarcopenia with eGFR and misclassification of obesity in adults with CKD in the United States. Clin J Am Soc Nephrol. 2014;9(12):2079–88.

16. Panaye M, Kolko-Labadens A, Lasseur C, Paillasseur J-L, Guillodo MP, Levannier M, et al. Phenotypes influencing low physical activity in maintenance dialysis. J Ren Nutr. 2015;25(1):31–9.

17. U.S. Department of Health and Human Services. Physical Activity Guidelines for Americans, 2nd ed. Washington, DC: U.S. Department of Health and Human Services; 2018.

18. Brown WJ, Bauman AE, Bull FC, Burton NW. Development of evidence-based physical activity recommendations for adults (18–64 years). Report prepared for the Australian Government Department of Health, August 2012.

19. National Kidney Foundation. K/DOQI clinical practice guidelines for cardiovascular disease in dialysis patients. Am J Kidney Dis. 2005;45:16–153.

20. Smart NA, Williams AD, Levinger I, Selig S, Howden E, Coombes JS, et al. Exercise & Sports Science Australia (ESSA) position statement on exercise and chronic kidney disease. J Sci Med Sport. 2013;16(5):406–11.

21. KDIGO. Clinical practice guideline for the evaluation and management of chronic kidney disease. Kidney Int. 2012;3(1):1–150.

22. Piercy KL, Troiano RP, Ballard RM, Carlson SA, Fulton JE, Galuska DA, et al. The physical activity guidelines for Americans. JAMA. 2018;320(19):2020–8.

23. Fouque D, Kalantar-Zadeh K, Kopple J, Cano N, Chauveau P, Cuppari L, et al. A proposed nomenclature and diagnostic criteria for protein-energy wasting in acute and chronic kidney disease. Kidney Int. 2008;73(4): 391–8.

24. Clapp EL, Bevington A. Exercise-induced biochemical modifications in muscle in chronic kidney disease: occult acidosis as a potential factor limiting the anabolic effect of exercise. J Ren Nutr. 2011;21(1):57–60.

25. Workeneh BT, Mitch WE. Review of muscle wasting associated with chronic kidney disease. Am J Clin Nutr. 2010;91(4):1128S–32S.

26. Roshanravan B, Gamboa J, Wilund K. Exercise and CKD: skeletal muscle dysfunction and practical application of exercise to prevent and treat physical impairments in CKD. Am J Kidney Dis. 2017;69(6):837–52.

27. Van Craenenbroeck AH, Van Craenenbroeck EM, Van Ackeren K, Hoymans VY, Verpooten GA, Vrints CJ, et al. Impaired vascular function contributes to exercise intolerance in chronic kidney disease. Nephrol Dial Transplant. 2016;31(12):2064–72.

28. McMahon LP, McKenna MJ, Sangkabutra T, Mason K, Sostaric S, Skinner SL, et al. Physical performance and associated electrolyte changes after haemoglobin normalization: a comparative study in haemodialysis patients. Nephrol Dial Transplant. 1999;14(5):1182–7.

29. McMahon LP. Exercise limitation in chronic kidney disease: deep seas and new shores. Nephrol Dial Transplant. 2016;31(12):1975–6.

30. Zoccali C, Mallamaci F. Mapping progress in reducing cardiovascular risk with kidney disease: managing volume overload. Clin J Am Soc Nephrol. 2018;13(9):1432–4.

31. Tangvoraphonkchai K, Davenport A. Extracellular water excess and increased self-reported fatigue in chronic hemodialysis patients. Ther Apher Dial. 2018;22(2):152–9.

32. Moore GE, Painter PL, Brinker KR, Stray-Gundersen J, Mitchell JH. Cardiovascular response to submaximal stationary cycling during hemodialysis. Am J Kidney Dis. 1998;31(4):631–7.

33. Zhou Y, Hoglund P, Clyne N. Comparison of DEXA and bioimpedance for body composition measurements in nondialysis patients with CKD. J Ren Nutr. 2019;29(1):33–8.

34. Painter P, Marcus R. Assessing physical function and physical activity in patients with CKD. Clin J Am Soc Nephrol. 2013;8(5):861–72.

35. Clarkson MJ, Bennett PN, Fraser SF, Warmington SA. Exercise interventions for improving objective physical function in end-stage kidney disease patients on dialysis: a systematic review and meta-analysis. Am J Physiol Renal Physiol. 2019;316(5):F856–72.

36. Smart N, Steele M. Exercise training in haemodialysis patients: a systematic review and meta-analysis. Nephrology (Carlton). 2011;16(7):626–32.

37. Barcellos FC, Santos IS, Umpierre D, Bohlke M, Hallal PC. Effects of exercise in the whole spectrum of chronic kidney disease: a systematic review. Clin Kidney J. 2015;8(6):753–65.

38. Cheema BS, Singh MA. Exercise training in patients receiving maintenance hemodialysis: a systematic review of clinical trials. Am J Nephrol. 2005;25(4):352–64.

39. Heiwe S, Jacobson SH. Exercise training in adults with CKD: a systematic review and meta-analysis. Am J Kidney Dis. 2014;64(3):383–93.

40. Chan D, Cheema BS. Progressive resistance training in end-stage renal disease: systematic review. Am J Nephrol. 2016;44(1):32–45.

41. Wang Y, Jardine MJ. Benefits of exercise training in patients receiving haemodialysis: a systematic review and meta-analysis. Br J Sports Med. 2011;45(14):1165–6.

42. Young HML, March DS, Graham-Brown MPM, Jones AW, Curtis F, Grantham CS, et al. Effects of intradialytic cycling exercise on exercise capacity, quality of life, physical function and cardiovascular measures in adult haemodialysis patients: a systematic review and meta-analysis. Nephrol Dial Transplant. 2018;33(8):1436–45.

43. Sheng K, Zhang P, Chen L, Cheng J, Wu C, Chen J. Intradialytic exercise in hemodialysis patients: a systematic review and meta-analysis. Am J Nephrol. 2014;40(5):478–90.

44. Pu J, Jiang Z, Wu W, Li L, Zhang L, Li Y, et al. Efficacy and safety of intradialytic exercise in haemodialysis patients: a systematic review and meta-analysis. BMJ Open. 2019;9(1):e020633.

45. Gomes Neto M, de Lacerda FFR, Lopes AA, Martinez BP, Saquetto MB. Intradialytic exercise training modalities on physical functioning and health-related quality of life in patients undergoing maintenance hemodialysis: systematic review and meta-analysis. Clin Rehabil. 2018;32(9):1189–202.

46. Chung YC, Yeh ML, Liu YM. Effects of intradialytic exercise on the physical function, depression and quality of life for haemodialysis patients: a systematic review and meta-analysis of randomised controlled trials. J Clin Nurs. 2017;26(13–14):1801–13.

47. Heiwe S, Jacobson SH. Exercise training for adults with chronic kidney disease. Cochrane Database Syst Rev. 2011;10:CD003236.

48. Calella P, Hernandez-Sanchez S, Garofalo C, Ruiz JR, Carrero JJ, Bellizzi V. Exercise training in kidney transplant recipients: a systematic review. J Nephrol. 2019;32(4):567–79.

49. Scapini KB, Bohlke M, Moraes OA, Rodrigues CG, Inacio JF, Sbruzzi G, et al. Combined training is the most effective training modality to improve aerobic capacity and blood pressure control in people requiring haemodialysis for end-stage renal disease: systematic review and network meta-analysis. J Physiother. 2019;65(1):4–15.

50. Cheema BS, Smith BC, Singh MA. A rationale for intradialytic exercise training as standard clinical practice in ESRD. Am J Kidney Dis. 2005;45(5):912–6.

51. Painter P. Implementing exercise: what do we know? Where do we go? Adv Chronic Kidney Dis. 2009;16(6):536–44.

52. Deschamps T. Let's programme exercise during haemodialysis (intradialytic exercise) into the care plan for patients, regardless of age. Br J Sports Med. 2016;50(22):1357–8.

53. Johansen K, Painter P. Exercise for patients with CKD: what more is needed? Adv Chronic Kidney Dis. 2009;16(6):407–9.

54. Inker LA, Astor BC, Fox CH, Isakova T, Lash JP, Peralta CA, et al. KDOQI US commentary on the 2012 KDIGO clinical practice guideline for the evaluation and management of CKD. Am J Kidney Dis. 2014;63(5):713–35.

55. Koufaki P, Greenwood S, Painter P, Mercer T. The BASES expert statement on exercise therapy for people with chronic kidney disease. J Sports Sci. 2015;33(18):1902–7.

56. NKF. K/DOQI clinical practice guidelines for cardiovascular disease in dialysis patients. Am J Kidney Dis. 2005;45(4 Suppl 3):S1–153.

57. March DS, Graham-Brown MP, Young HM, Greenwood SA, Burton JO. 'There is nothing more deceptive than an obvious fact': more evidence for the prescription of exercise during haemodialysis (intradialytic exercise) is still required. Br J Sports Med. 2017;51(18):1379.

58. Johansen KL. Resistance exercise in the hemodialysis population – who should do the heavy lifting? Am J Nephrol. 2016;44(1):29–31.

59. Johansen KL. Exercise in the end-stage renal disease population. J Am Soc Nephrol. 2007;18(6):1845–54.

60. Johansen KL. Exercise and dialysis. Hemodial Int. 2008;12(3):290–300.

61. Koh KP, Fassett RG, Sharman JE, Coombes JS, Williams AD. Effect of intradialytic versus home-based aerobic exercise training on physical function and vascular parameters in hemodialysis patients: a randomized pilot study. Am J Kidney Dis. 2010;55(1):88–99.

62. Manfredini F, Mallamaci F, D'Arrigo G, Baggetta R, Bolignano D, Torino C, et al. Exercise in patients on dialysis: a multicenter, randomized clinical trial. J Am Soc Nephrol. 2017;28(4):1259–68.

63. ATS Committee on Proficiency Standards for Clinical Pulmonary Function Laboratories. ATS statement: guidelines for the six-minute walk test. Am J Respir Crit Care Med. 2002;166(1):111–7.

64. Park J, Ahmadi SF, Streja E, Molnar MZ, Flegal KM, Gillen D, et al. Obesity paradox in end-stage kidney disease patients. Prog Cardiovasc Dis. 2014;56(4):415–25.

65. Blacher J, Guerin AP, Pannier B, Marchais SJ, Safar ME, London GM. Impact of aortic stiffness on survival in end-stage renal disease. Circulation. 1999;99(18):2434–9.

66. Sato M, Ogawa T, Otsuka K, Ando Y, Nitta K. Stiffness parameter beta as a predictor of the 4-year all-cause mortality of chronic hemodialysis patients. Clin Exp Nephrol. 2013;17(2):268–74.

67. Vanden Wyngaert K, Van Craenenbroeck AH, Van Biesen W, Dhondt A, Tanghe A, Van Ginckel A, et al. The effects of aerobic exercise on eGFR, blood pressure and VO2peak in patients with chronic kidney disease stages 3-4: a systematic review and meta-analysis. PLoS One. 2018;13(9):e0203662.

68. Van Craenenbroeck AH, Van Craenenbroeck EM, Van Ackeren K, Vrints CJ, Conraads VM, Verpooten GA, et al. Effect of moderate aerobic exercise training on endothelial function and arterial stiffness in CKD stages 3-4: a randomized controlled trial. Am J Kidney Dis. 2015;66(2):285–96.

69. Kirkman DL, Ramick MG, Muth BJ, Stock JM, Pohlig RT, Townsend RT, et al. The effects of aerobic exercise on vascular function in non-dialysis chronic kidney disease: a randomized controlled trial. Am J Physiol Renal Physiol. 2019;316(5):F898–905.

70. Deligiannis A, Kouidi E, Tassoulas E, Gigis P, Tourkantonis A, Coats A. Cardiac effects of exercise rehabilitation in hemodialysis patients. Int J Cardiol. 1999;70(3):253–66.

71. Kouidi EJ, Grekas DM, Deligiannis AP. Effects of exercise training on noninvasive cardiac measures in patients undergoing long-term hemodialysis: a randomized controlled trial. Am J Kidney Dis. 2009;54(3):511–21.

72. Mustata S, Chan C, Lai V, Miller JA. Impact of an exercise program on arterial stiffness and insulin resistance in hemodialysis patients. J Am Soc Nephrol. 2004;15(10):2713–8.

73. Toussaint ND, Polkinghorne KR, Kerr PG. Impact of intradialytic exercise on arterial compliance and B-type natriuretic peptide levels in hemodialysis patients. Hemodial Int. 2008;12(2):254–63.

74. Cooke AB, Ta V, Iqbal S, Gomez YH, Mavrakanas T, Barre P, et al. The impact of intradialytic pedaling exercise on arterial stiffness: a pilot randomized controlled trial in a hemodialysis population. Am J Hypertens. 2018;31(4):458–66.

75. Briet M, Bozec E, Laurent S, Fassot C, London GM, Jacquot C, et al. Arterial stiffness and enlargement in mild-to-moderate chronic kidney disease. Kidney Int. 2006;69(2):350–7.

76. Garnier AS, Briet M. Arterial stiffness and chronic kidney disease. Pulse (Basel). 2016;3(3–4):229–41.

77. Keysor JJ. Does late-life physical activity or exercise prevent or minimize disablement? A critical review of the scientific evidence. Am J Prev Med. 2003;25(3 Suppl 2):129–36.

78. Singh MA. Exercise to prevent and treat functional disability. Clin Geriatr Med. 2002;18(3):431–62, vi–vii.

79. Miller ME, Rejeski WJ, Reboussin BA, Ten Have TR, Ettinger WH. Physical activity, functional limitations, and disability in older adults. J Am Geriatr Soc. 2000;48(10):1264–72.

80. McAuley E, Konopack JF, Motl RW, Morris KS, Doerksen SE, Rosengren KR. Physical activity and quality of life in older adults: influence of health status and self-efficacy. Ann Behav Med. 2006;31(1):99–103.

81. Rejeski WJ, Focht BC, Messier SP, Morgan T, Pahor M, Penninx B. Obese, older adults with knee osteoarthritis: weight loss, exercise, and quality of life. Health Psychol. 2002;21(5):419–26.

82. Kutner NG, Zhang R, McClellan WM. Patient-reported quality of life early in dialysis treatment: effects associated with usual exercise activity. Nephrol Nurs J. 2000;27(4):357–67; discussion 68, 424.

83. Painter P, Carlson L, Carey S, Paul SM, Myll J. Physical functioning and health-related quality-of-life changes with exercise training in hemodialysis patients. Am J Kidney Dis. 2000;35(3):482–92.

84. Suh MR, Jung HH, Kim SB, Park JS, Yang WS. Effects of regular exercise on anxiety, depression, and quality of life in maintenance hemodialysis patients. Ren Fail. 2002;24(3):337–45.

85. Greenwood SA, Lindup H, Taylor K, Koufaki P, Rush R, Macdougall IC, et al. Evaluation of a pragmatic exercise rehabilitation programme in chronic kidney disease. Nephrol Dial Transplant. 2012;27(suppl 3):iii126–i34.

86. Molsted S, Harrison AP, Eidemak I, Andersen JL. The effects of high-load strength training with protein- or nonprotein-containing nutritional supplementation in patients undergoing dialysis. J Ren Nutr. 2013;23(2):132–40.

87. Carrero JJ, Stenvinkel P, Cuppari L, Ikizler TA, Kalantar-Zadeh K, Kaysen G, et al. Etiology of the protein-energy wasting syndrome in chronic kidney disease: a consensus statement from the International Society of Renal Nutrition and Metabolism (ISRNM). J Ren Nutr. 2013;23(2):77–90.

88. Ikizler TA, Pupim LB, Brouillette JR, Levenhagen DK, Farmer K, Hakim RM, et al. Hemodialysis stimu-lates muscle and whole body protein loss and alters substrate oxidation. Am J Physiol Endocrinol Metab. 2002;282(1):E107–16.

89. Ikizler TA. Exercise as an anabolic intervention in patients with end-stage renal disease. J Ren Nutr. 2011; 21(1):52–6.

90. Castaneda C, Gordon PL, Uhlin KL, Levey AS, Kehayias JJ, Dwyer JT, et al. Resistance training to counteract the catabolism of a low-protein diet in patients with chronic renal insufficiency. A randomized, controlled trial. Ann Intern Med. 2001;135(11):965–76.

91. Watson EL, Greening NJ, Viana JL, Aulakh J, Bodicoat DH, Barratt J, et al. Progressive resistance exercise train-ing in CKD: a feasibility study. Am J Kidney Dis. 2015;66(2):249–57.

92. Olvera-Soto MG, Valdez-Ortiz R, López Alvarenga JC, Espinosa-Cuevas ML. Effect of resistance exercises on the indicators of muscle reserves and handgrip strength in adult patients on hemodialysis. J Ren Nutr. 2016;26(1):53–60.

93. Bullani R, El-Housseini Y, Giordano F, Larcinese A, Ciutto L, Bertrand PC, et al. Effect of intradialytic resis-tance band exercise on physical function in patients on maintenance hemodialysis: a pilot study. J Ren Nutr. 2011;21(1):61–5.

94. Bennett PN, Breugelmans L, Agius M, Simpson-gore K, Barnard B. A Haemodialysis exercise programme using novel exercise equipment: a pilot study. J Ren Care. 2007;33(4):153–8.

95. Dong J, Sundell MB, Pupim LB, Wu P, Shintani A, Ikizler TA. The effect of resistance exercise to augment long-term benefits of intradialytic oral nutritional supplementation in chronic hemodialysis patients. J Ren Nutr. 2011;21(2):149–59.

96. Majchrzak KM, Pupim LB, Flakoll PJ, Ikizler TA. Resistance exercise augments the acute anabolic effects of intradialytic oral nutritional supplementation. Nephrol Dial Transplant. 2008;23(4):1362–9.

97. Chen JL, Godfrey S, Ng TT, Moorthi R, Liangos O, Ruthazer R, et al. Effect of intra-dialytic, low-intensity strength training on functional capacity in adult haemodialysis patients: a randomized pilot trial. Nephrol Dial Transplant. 2010;25(6):1936–43.

98. Cheema B, Abas H, Smith B, O'Sullivan A, Chan M, Patwardhan A, et al. Progressive exercise for anabolism in kidney disease (PEAK): a randomized, controlled trial of resistance training during hemodialysis. J Am Soc Nephrol. 2007;18(5):1594–601.

99. Kopple JD, Cohen AH, Wang H, Qing D, Tang Z, Fournier M, et al. Effect of exercise on mRNA levels for growth factors in skeletal muscle of hemodialysis patients. J Ren Nutr. 2006;16(4):312–24.

100. Johansen KL, Painter PL, Sakkas GK, Gordon P, Doyle J, Shubert T. Effects of resistance exercise training and nandrolone decanoate on body composition and muscle function among patients who receive hemodialysis: a randomized, controlled trial. J Am Soc Nephrol. 2006;17(8):2307–14.

101. Kirkman DL, Mullins P, Junglee NA, Kumwenda M, Jibani MM, MacDonald JH. Anabolic exercise in haemodi-alysis patients: a randomised controlled pilot study. J Cachexia Sarcopenia Muscle. 2014;5(3):199–207.

102. Qunibi WY. Reducing the burden of cardiovascular calcification in patients with chronic kidney disease. J Am Soc Nephrol. 2005;16(Suppl 2):S95–102.

103. Cheema BS. Review article: tackling the survival issue in end-stage renal disease: time to get physical on haemo-dialysis. Nephrology (Carlton). 2008;13(7):560–9.

104. Painter P. Determinants of exercise capacity in CKD patients treated with hemodialysis. Adv Chronic Kidney Dis. 2009;16(6):437–48.

105. Watson EL, Gould DW, Wilkinson TJ, Xenophontos S, Clarke AL, Vogt BP, et al. Twelve-week combined resis-tance and aerobic training confers greater benefits than aerobic training alone in nondialysis CKD. Am J Physiol Renal Physiol. 2018;314(6):F1188–F96.

106. Kopple JD, Wang H, Casaburi R, Fournier M, Lewis MI, Taylor W, et al. Exercise in maintenance hemo-dialysis patients induces transcriptional changes in genes favoring anabolic muscle. J Am Soc Nephrol. 2007;18(11):2975–86.

107. Breen L, Phillips SM. Skeletal muscle protein metabolism in the elderly interventions to counteract the 'anabolic resistance' of ageing. Nutr Metab (Lond). 2011;8:68.

108. van Vliet S, Skinner SK, Beals JW, Pagni BA, Fang HY, Ulanov AV, et al. Dysregulated handling of dietary protein and muscle protein synthesis after mixed-meal ingestion in maintenance hemodialysis patients. Kidney Int Rep. 2018;3(6):1403–15.

109. Pupim LB, Flakoll PJ, Levenhagen DK, Ikizler TA. Exercise augments the acute anabolic effects of intra-dialytic parenteral nutrition in chronic hemodialysis patients. Am J Physiol Endocrinol Metab. 2004;286(4): E589–97.

110. Hristea D, Deschamps T, Paris A, Lefrancois G, Collet V, Savoiu C, et al. Combining intra-dialytic exercise and nutritional supplementation in malnourished older haemodialysis patients: towards better quality of life and auton-omy. Nephrology (Carlton). 2016;21(9):785–90.

111. Martin-Alemany G, Valdez-Ortiz R, Olvera-Soto G, Gomez-Guerrero I, Aguire-Esquivel G, Cantu-Quintanilla G, et al. The effects of resistance exercise and oral nutritional supplementation during hemodialysis on indicators of nutritional status and quality of life. Nephrol Dial Transplant. 2016;31(10):1712–20.
112. Kim JC, Kalantar-Zadeh K, Kopple JD. Frailty and protein-energy wasting in elderly patients with end stage kidney disease. J Am Soc Nephrol. 2013;24(3):337–51.
113. Cook WL, Tomlinson G, Donaldson M, Markowitz SN, Naglie G, Sobolev B, et al. Falls and fall-related injuries in older dialysis patients. Clin J Am Soc Nephrol. 2006;1(6):1197–204.
114. Li M, Tomlinson G, Naglie G, Cook WL, Jassal SV. Geriatric comorbidities, such as falls, confer an independent mortality risk to elderly dialysis patients. Nephrol Dial Transplant. 2008;23(4):1396–400.
115. Frih B, Mkacher W, Jaafar H, Frih A, Ben Salah Z, El May M, et al. Specific balance training included in an endurance-resistance exercise program improves postural balance in elderly patients undergoing haemodialysis. Disabil Rehabil. 2018;40(7):784–90.
116. Mkacher W, Mekki M, Tabka Z, Trabelsi Y. Effect of 6 months of balance training during pulmonary rehabilitation in patients with COPD. J Cardiopulm Rehabil Prev. 2015;35(3):207–13.
117. Beauchamp MK, Janaudis-Ferreira T, Parreira V, Romano JM, Woon L, Goldstein RS, et al. A randomized controlled trial of balance training during pulmonary rehabilitation for individuals with COPD. Chest. 2013;144(6):1803–10.
118. Capato TT, Tornai J, Avila P, Barbosa ER, Piemonte ME. Randomized controlled trial protocol: balance training with rhythmical cues to improve and maintain balance control in Parkinson's disease. BMC Neurol. 2015;15:162.
119. Panel on Prevention of Falls in Older Persons AGS, British Geriatrics S. Summary of the Updated American Geriatrics Society/British Geriatrics Society clinical practice guideline for prevention of falls in older persons. J Am Geriatr Soc. 2011;59(1):148–57.
120. Guideline for the prevention of falls in older persons. American Geriatrics Society, British Geriatrics Society, and American Academy of Orthopaedic Surgeons Panel on Falls Prevention. J Am Geriatr Soc. 2001;49(5):664–72.
121. Gibala MJ, Hawley JA. Sprinting toward fitness. Cell Metab. 2017;25(5):988–90.
122. Batacan RB, Duncan MJ, Dalbo VJ, Tucker PS, Fenning AS. Effects of high-intensity interval training on cardiometabolic health: a systematic review and meta-analysis of intervention studies. Br J Sports Med. 2017;51(6):494–503.
123. Gillen JB, Martin BJ, MacInnis MJ, Skelly LE, Tarnopolsky MA, Gibala MJ. Twelve weeks of Sprint interval training improves indices of cardiometabolic health similar to traditional endurance training despite a five-fold lower exercise volume and time commitment. PLoS One. 2016;11(4):e0154075.
124. Allison MK, Baglole JH, Martin BJ, Macinnis MJ, Gurd BJ, Gibala MJ. Brief intense stair climbing improves cardiorespiratory fitness. Med Sci Sports Exerc. 2017;49(2):298–307.
125. Jenkins EM, Nairn LN, Skelly LE, Little JP, Gibala MJ. Do stair climbing exercise "snacks" improve cardiorespiratory fitness? Appl Physiol Nutr Metab. 2019;44(6):681–4.
126. Lambert K, Beer J, Dumont R, Hewitt K, Manley K, Meade A, et al. Weight management strategies for those with chronic kidney disease: a consensus report from the Asia Pacific Society of Nephrology and Australia and New Zealand Society of Nephrology 2016 Renal Dietitians meeting. Nephrology (Carlton). 2018;23(10):912–20.
127. Lee RA, Deshmukh N, Deyo J, Andreoni K, Kozlowski T. Can obese kidney transplant candidates effectively use wait list time to improve BMI? – Experience of southeastern center. Am J Transplant. 2012;3:241–2.
128. Lentine KL. Pro: pretransplant weight loss: yes. Nephrol Dial Transplant. 2015;30(11):1798–803.
129. Marks WH, Florence LS, Chapman PH, Precht AF, Perkinson DT. Morbid obesity is not a contraindication to kidney transplantation. Am J Surg. 2004;187(5):635–8.
130. Sever MS, Zoccali C. Moderator's view: pretransplant weight loss in dialysis patients: cum grano salis. Nephrol Dial Transplant. 2015;30(11):1810–3.
131. Streja E, Molnar MZ, Kovesdy CP, Bunnapradist S, Jing J, Nissenson AR, et al. Associations of pretransplant weight and muscle mass with mortality in renal transplant recipients. Clin J Am Soc Nephrol. 2011;6(6):1463–73.
132. Teta D. Weight loss in obese patients with chronic kidney disease: who and how? J Ren Care. 2010;36(Suppl 1):163–71.
133. Moorman D, Suri R, Hiremath S, Jegatheswaran J, Kumar T, Bugeja A, et al. Benefits and barriers to and desired outcomes with exercise in patients with ESKD. Clin J Am Soc Nephrol. 2019;14(2):268–76.
134. Delgado C, Johansen KL. Barriers to exercise participation among dialysis patients. Nephrol Dial Transplant. 2012;27(3):1152–7.
135. Mallamaci F, Torino C, Tripepi G. Physical exercise in haemodialysis patients: time to start. Nephrol Dial Transplant. 2016;31(8):1196–8.
136. Kontos PC, Miller KL, Brooks D, Jassal SV, Spanjevic L, Devins GM, et al. Factors influencing exercise participation by older adults requiring chronic hemodialysis: a qualitative study. Int Urol Nephrol. 2007;39(4):1303–11.
137. Bennett PN, Breugelmans L, Barnard R, Agius M, Chan D, Fraser D, et al. Sustaining a hemodialysis exercise program: a review. Semin Dial. 2010;23(1):62–73.

138. Johansen KL, Sakkas GK, Doyle J, Shubert T, Dudley RA. Exercise counseling practices among nephrologists caring for patients on dialysis. Am J Kidney Dis. 2003;41(1):171–8.

139. Thompson S, Tonelli M, Klarenbach S, Molzahn A. A qualitative study to explore patient and staff perceptions of intradialytic exercise. Clin J Am Soc Nephrol. 2016;11(6):1024–33.

140. Capitanini A, Lange S, D'Alessandro C, Salotti E, Tavolaro A, Baronti ME, et al. Dialysis exercise team: the way to sustain exercise programs in hemodialysis patients. Kidney Blood Press Res. 2014;39(2–3):129–33.

141. Jhamb M, McNulty ML, Ingalsbe G, Childers JW, Schell J, Conroy MB, et al. Knowledge, barriers and facilitators of exercise in dialysis patients: a qualitative study of patients, staff and nephrologists. BMC Nephrol. 2016;17(1):192.

142. Aucella F, Valente GL, Catizone L. The role of physical activity in the CKD setting. Kidney Blood Press Res. 2014;39(2–3):97–106.

143. Clarke AL, Young HML, Hull KL, Hudson N, Burton JO, Smith AC. Motivations and barriers to exercise in chronic kidney disease: a qualitative study. Nephrol Dial Transplant. 2015;30(11):1885–92.

144. Willingham FC, Speelman I, Hamilton J, von Fragstein G, Shaw S, Taal MW. Feasibility and effectiveness of pre-emptive rehabilitation in persons approaching dialysis (PREHAB). J Ren Care. 2019;45(1):9–19.

145. Rossi AP, Burris DD, Lucas FL, Crocker GA, Wasserman JC. Effects of a renal rehabilitation exercise program in patients with CKD: a randomized, controlled trial. Clin J Am Soc Nephrol. 2014;9(12):2052–8.

146. Smart N, Steele M. Exercise training in haemodialysis patients: a systematic review and meta-analysis. Nephrology. 2011;16(7):626–32.

147. Hristea D, Deschamps T, Paris A, Lefrançois G, Collet V, Savoiu C, et al. Combining intra-dialytic exercise and nutritional supplementation in malnourished older haemodialysis patients: towards better quality of life and autonomy. Nephrology. 2016;21(9):785–90.

148. Groussard C, Rouchon-Isnard M, Coutard C, Romain F, Malardé L, Lemoine-Morel S, et al. Beneficial effects of an intradialytic cycling training program in patients with end-stage kidney disease. Appl Physiol Nutr Metab. 2015;40(6):550–6.

149. Bennett PN, Fraser S, Barnard R, Haines T, Ockerby C, Street M, et al. Effects of an intradialytic resistance training programme on physical function: a prospective stepped-wedge randomized controlled trial. Nephrol Dial Transplant. 2016;31(8):1302–9.

150. Kosmadakis GC, John SG, Clapp EL, Viana JL, Smith AC, Bishop NC, et al. Benefits of regular walking exercise in advanced pre-dialysis chronic kidney disease. Nephrol Dial Transplant. 2012;27(3):997–1004.

151. Valenzuela PL, de Alba A, Pedrero-Chamizo R, Morales JS, Cobo F, Botella A, et al. Intradialytic exercise: one size doesn't fit all. Front Physiol. 2018;9:844.

152. Tawney KW, Tawney PJ, Hladik G, Hogan SL, Falk RJ, Weaver C, et al. The life readiness program: a physical rehabilitation program for patients on hemodialysis. Am J Kidney Dis. 2000;36(3):581–91.

153. Balducci S, D'Errico V, Haxhi J, Sacchetti M, Orlando G, Cardelli P, et al. Effect of a behavioral intervention strategy on sustained change in physical activity and sedentary behavior in patients with type 2 diabetes: the IDES_2 randomized clinical trial. JAMA. 2019;321(9):880–90.

154. Bohannon RW, Wang YC. Four-meter gait speed: normative values and reliability determined for adults participating in the NIH toolbox study. Arch Phys Med Rehabil. 2019;100(3):509–13.

155. Guralnik JM, Ferrucci L, Simonsick EM, Salive ME, Wallace RB. Lower-extremity function in persons over the age of 70 years as a predictor of subsequent disability. N Engl J Med. 1995;332(9):556–61.

156. Bohannon RW, Bubela DJ, Magasi SR, Wang YC, Gershon RC. Sit-to-stand test: performance and determinants across the age-span. Isokinet Exerc Sci. 2010;18(4):235–40.

157. Casanova C, Celli BR, Barria P, Casas A, Cote C, de Torres JP, et al. The 6-min walk distance in healthy subjects: reference standards from seven countries. Eur Respir J. 2011;37(1):150–6.

158. Nelson ME, Rejeski WJ, Blair SN, Duncan PW, Judge JO, King AC, et al. Physical activity and public health in older adults: recommendation from the American College of Sports Medicine and the American Heart Association. Med Sci Sports Exerc. 2007;39(8):1435–45.

Chapter 31
Dietary Patterns

Jaimon T. Kelly

Keywords Dietary pattern · Diet exposure · Foods · DASH · Mediterranean · Vegetarian · Vegan
Plant · Plant-based · Dietary guidelines

> **Key Points**
> - Dietary patterns refer to the pattern of eating over time and can be healthy or unhealthy.
> - The key food components of healthy dietary patterns include being higher in fruits, vegetables, fish and omega-3 fatty acids, whole grains and fiber, and lower in sodium, red meat, and saturated fats.
> - Dietary patterns have strong evidence in cardiovascular disease prevention, which makes them promising in managing CKD complications and risk of disease progression.
> - Key dietary patterns considered healthy for preventing CKD include the DASH diet, the Mediterranean diet, and vegetarian diets.
> - Dietary patterns considered healthy for managing CKD include plant-based diets, Mediterranean diets, and diets consistent with the Dietary Guidelines for Americans.
> - Concerns of the safety profile of dietary patterns in the CKD patient can be attenuated by practical modifications and/or substitutions to the types of foods consumed.
> - Dietary pattern changes need to be closely monitored by the dietitian in the early stages of CKD, including transient changes in dietary intake and serum biochemistry.

Introduction

A number of dietary strategies are known to support the modification of chronic kidney disease (CKD), either in assisting in the control of risk factors associated with disease progression or supporting survival. Single-nutrient interventions have long been the center of the traditional renal diet; however, these isolated nutrient targets also follow substantial patient-reported burden. Furthermore, this "traditional" approach ignores the real world that people with CKD engage in and the way people truly eat. As people do not consume nutrients in isolation, whole food-based diet interventions reflect the synergistic effect of food and the combined nutrients within a pattern of eating. These combined interactions form the basis of the premise of dietary patterns and may contribute to better health outcomes; moreover, they are more likely to be comprehendible and applicable to people with CKD [1, 2].

J. T. Kelly (✉)
Griffith University, Menzies Health Institute Queensland, Gold Coast, QLD, Australia
e-mail: jaimon.kelly@griffith.edu.au

© Springer Nature Switzerland AG 2020
J. D. Burrowes et al. (eds.), *Nutrition in Kidney Disease*, Nutrition and Health,
https://doi.org/10.1007/978-3-030-44858-5_31

The US Department of Agriculture, the US Department of Health and Human Services, and the National Kidney Foundation all recommend plant-based diets for their cardioprotective benefits. These include the Dietary Approaches to Stop Hypertension (DASH) diet and the Mediterranean diet, which are high in fiber and low in saturated fat and processed meats; contain sources of potassium, phosphorus, magnesium, and calcium; and have low levels of sodium.

The potential role of a healthy dietary pattern is far more complex than delivering a combination of nutrients. Similarly, addressing overall health is more complex than addressing single risk factors. Therefore, the shift toward dietary patterns can be seen as the equivalent of the shift from evaluating single risk factors to evaluating total risk profiles in CKD.

While dietary pattern studies have gained appreciable traction in recent years across various chronic disease incidence and control, the evidence base for their effectiveness in CKD has not been fully elucidated in high-quality randomized controlled trials (RCTs). The majority of evidence on the possible associations to kidney outcomes predominantly comes from post hoc analyses from large cohort studies which are not designed to test these associations. Nonetheless, a meta-analysis combining the associations from all these cohort datasets demonstrates the role of healthy dietary patterns in reducing the risk of all-cause mortality in established CKD populations [3].

The opportunity to educate people with kidney disease to achieve a healthy dietary pattern presents itself with many benefits in comparison to isolated nutrient interventions. The translation of nutrient-based recommendations into practical day-to-day strategies is exceptionally challenging for patients without ongoing guidance and feedback from health professionals [4]. In contrast, behavioral counseling to achieve a desired pattern of eating can lead to better compliance due to offering flexibility, choices to suit individual preferences, and a manageable change to a multitude of nutrients within the whole diet concurrently [4].

In this chapter, we will overview the current evidence base for dietary patterns to CKD risk and risk of CKD progression, and will consider some of the key clinical practice strategies when working with patients adopting a healthy dietary pattern.

What Is a Dietary Pattern?

The Dietary Guidelines for Americans [5] define a dietary pattern as the quantities, proportions, variety or combination of different foods, drinks, and nutrients within an individual's diet and the frequency with which they are habitually consumed. As such, the study of dietary patterns considers the cumulative effect and synergy between the combinations of foods, drinks, and nutrients consumed day to day [6].

It is prudent to note, with this definition, that a dietary pattern can be considered "healthy" or "unhealthy." Examples of a "healthy" dietary pattern include diet approaches such as the DASH diet, the Mediterranean diet, vegetarian diet, and other patterns of eating consistent with the Dietary Guidelines for Americans [5]. Observational studies suggest these mentioned dietary patterns may be superior to single-nutrient interventions [7], particularly due to the cumulative effects of the multiple nutrients consumed through diets rich in fruits and vegetables, fish and omega-3 fatty acids, legumes, whole-grain cereals, and nuts and lower in sodium, red meat, saturated fats, and common phosphate additives [8]. The effects of dietary patterns on health outcomes have been linked to reduced inflammation from higher consumption of whole grains, reduced oxidative stress through increased consumption of fruits and vegetables [9], and decreased circulating concentrations of inflammatory markers through a higher consumption of unsaturated fats including nuts and seeds [10].

In contrast, examples of unhealthy dietary patterns include Western diets and high-fat and meat dietary patterns. These dietary patterns that are rich in refined carbohydrates, sodium, saturated fat, and protein from red meat, and low in fiber-rich foods, are generally associated with increased risk of CKD and a multitude of other chronic diseases. It is thought that diets high in refined starches, saturated fats, trans-fatty acids, and sodium, and lower in whole grains, fruits, vegetables, omega-3 fatty acids, and fiber, may heighten the inflammatory response [11]. Increased inflammatory markers, including C-reactive protein, are associated with glomerular damage and loss of kidney function as a result of renal cell injury and impaired vasodilation [12]. As elevations in inflammatory markers have been suggested as a biomarker for the incidence of CKD [13], a dietary approach which lowers inflammatory markers and dietary acid load may be important for reducing the incidence of CKD and potentially reducing the risk for disease progression.

Dietary Patterns and Incident CKD (Free from CKD Populations)

It is prudent to consider the distinction between primary and secondary prevention of CKD. Dietary pattern research commonly blends these approaches; however, the evidence base and likely mechanisms are appreciably different.

Healthy dietary patterns have an evidence base that supports the reduction in known risk factors for incident CKD. Existing observational studies have demonstrated significant associations between healthy dietary patterns and the primary prevention of health outcomes, including type 2 diabetes [14], cardiovascular disease (CVD) [15], hypertension, and metabolic syndrome [16], which are closely linked to incident CKD. Large meta-analyses of RCTs have demonstrated significant control of cardiovascular risk factors such as blood pressure control and unhealthy weight gain from following the DASH diet [17], glycemic and lipid profile control from following a vegetarian diet [18], and improved body mass, metabolic, and inflammatory risk parameters from following a Mediterranean diet [19].

There are a select number of studies evaluating the associations of long-term dietary pattern exposure to incident CKD. The overall evidence base predominately supports the prevention of CKD, albuminuria, and rapid decline in estimated glomerular filtration rate (eGFR) from the Mediterranean diet, the DASH diet, a lacto-vegetarian diet, and dietary patterns consistent with the Dietary Guidelines for Americans [20–23]. Collectively, these dietary patterns are higher in vegetables, fruits, legumes, nuts, whole grains, fish, and low-fat dairy, and lower in red and processed meats, sodium, and sugar-sweetened beverages. There have been no clinical trials conducted to date which test the effect of healthy dietary patterns and incident CKD. It is also unlikely that such a trial which is long enough in duration and adequately powered will ever be conducted, as chronic conditions develop over many years, and dietary trials are inherently resource intensive. As people with very early stages of kidney damage and those at high risk of CKD (such as those with hypertension and diabetes) would benefit from improving diet quality, dietary pattern approaches appear to be a safe and patient-centered approach that may prevent incident CKD.

CKD Incidence and the DASH Diet

The DASH diet emphasizes fruits, vegetables, low-fat dairy products, and whole-grain carbohydrates, and it limits large quantities of meats and discretionary choices. The DASH diet has a nutrient profile high in fiber, protein, magnesium, calcium, and potassium, yet it is low in total and saturated fats (Table 31.1). These characteristics have led to public health recommendations to advocate for the DASH diet in primary and secondary prevention of CVD, with the majority of the evidence base existing in blood pressure control [17]. Since up to 80% of people with CKD have comorbid hypertension,

Table 31.1 Characteristics of selected dietary patterns and comparison to CKD nutrition intake recommendations

Nutrients	US Dietary Guidelines[a]	DASH diet[b]	Mediterranean diet[c]	CKD diet stages 3–4[d]
Protein (%EEI)	10–35	18	19	10
Fat (%EEI)	20–35	27	35	<30
Saturated (%EEI)	<10	7	11	<7
Monounsaturated fat (%EEI)	11	10	15	>20
Polyunsaturated fat (%EEI)	NR	7	5	>10
Carbohydrates (%EEI)	45–65	58	44	50–60
Fiber (g/day)	28–34	30	37	20–30
Sodium (mg/day)	<2300	2890	3600	<2400
Potassium (mg/day)	4700	4590	6130	2000–4000
Phosphorous (mg/day)	700	1480	2230	800–1000
Calcium (mg/day)	1000	1220	1400	700
Food group serving suggestions with considerations for the CKD patient				
Vegetables	5/day	4–5/day	2/main meal	NR
		Suggest low potassium alternatives only if required		
Fruit	2/day	4–5/day	1–2/main meal	NR
		Suggest low potassium alternatives only if required		
Grains	3–6/day	6–8/day	1–2/main meal	NR
		At least 50% from whole-grain sources, aim for > 6 g fiber per 100 g		
Dairy	2/day	2–3/day	2/day	NR
		Monitor protein consumption; low-fat options: 250 mL milk, 40 g cheese, 200 g yogurt; nondairy substitutes are lower in phosphorous if required		
Meat/alternatives	2/day	<2/day	<2/week (red); 2/week (white)	NR
		Pre-dialysis: Limit animal protein servings to 2× 65 g (palm size) servings/day *Dialysis: 2× 125 g (hand size) servings/day*		
Nuts/seeds/legumes	NR	4–5/day	1–2/day	NR
		Monitor protein consumption; suggest unsalted; 30 g (small handful) is the equivalent of 1 meat serving		

Abbreviations: *DASH* Dietary Approaches to Stop Hypertension, *CKD* chronic kidney disease, *EEI* estimated energy intake, *g* gram, *mg* milligram, *NR* no recommendation
[a]As recommended by the Dietary Guidelines for Americans 2015–2020 [5]
[b]Serra-Majem et al. [91]
[c]American Heart Association Nutrition Committee [92]
[d]As recommended by K/DOQI guidelines [46]

the DASH diet has been hypothesized to be a dietary pattern which may reduce the risk of incident CKD if targeted toward people with hypertension.

Existing cohort studies demonstrate that the DASH dietary pattern is associated with preserved residual kidney function and reduced overall incidence of CKD in community-dwelling individuals [24–26]; however, the findings have been inconsistent. Seven studies from seven cohorts have been published to date [7, 20, 21, 26–29]; three of the studies demonstrated a significant association with reduced risk of incident CKD [20, 21, 26], and one of two studies showed significant reductions in albuminuria and eGFR decline [27, 30]. Preliminary data also suggest that adherence to the DASH diet may reduce the risk of incident end-stage kidney disease (ESKD) [31].

CKD Incidence and the Mediterranean Diet

The Mediterranean diet has no standardized approach. Rather, the widely used term "Mediterranean diet" reflects a variety of eating habits traditionally practiced by populations in countries surrounding the Mediterranean Sea, with considerable variability by location. The Mediterranean pattern of eating is in general rich in unsaturated fats, fruits, vegetables, legumes, and fiber and moderate in red wine consumption. The Mediterranean diet has long-standing associations with reduced CVD incidence and mortality in the non-CKD population [32–35].

Existing cohort studies demonstrate that the Mediterranean dietary pattern is associated with reduced risk of incident CKD and progression to ESKD in community-dwelling individuals. One of two studies has shown the Mediterranean diet to reduce the risk of incident CKD and rapid eGFR decline [23, 36]. Cross-sectional analysis from the large PREDIMED RCT demonstrated that 1-year adherence to the Mediterranean diet was associated with improved renal function [37].

CKD Incidence and Vegetarian/Plant-Based Diets

Plant-based diets, including lacto-ovo-vegetarian and vegan diets, are followed by approximately 5% of the population in Western countries. Vegetarianism encompasses the practice of following plant-based food consumption excluding foods from animal flesh. Lacto-ovo-vegetarian diets can include animal products, including eggs, milk, and honey, while vegan diets exclude all animal products. Vegetarian and plant-based diets are inherently higher in many nutrients, phytochemicals, and antioxidants, including complex carbohydrates, fiber, folic acid, and vitamin C. However, these dietary approaches can also be low in other nutrients, such as omega-3 fatty acids and vitamin B12 [38].

Several studies have shown that vegetarian diets are associated with lower prevalence of some of the most common reasons for CKD progression, including hypertension, diabetes, obesity, and metabolic syndrome [39]. One cohort study has been conducted to date establishing the association of a lacto-vegetarian diet and incident CKD [22]. A similar cohort study demonstrated that vegetable proteins are protective against incident CKD compared to red and processed meat proteins, which increase the risk of incident CKD [40].

CKD Incidence and Diets Consistent with the Dietary Guidelines for Americans

The Dietary Guidelines for Americans recommend a dietary pattern with serving suggestions that mirror the characteristics of the dietary patterns discussed previously. Specifically, the dietary patterns promote consumption of fruits, vegetables, whole grains, and low-fat dairy, and limit saturated fat, sodium, and sugar in foods/beverages. Given that the Dietary Guidelines for Americans were developed to meet the nutrition needs and health of the general population, the relationship between long-term adherence to a dietary pattern consistent with such guidelines and incident CKD is important to understand.

There have only been two cohort studies evaluating the associations of adherence to dietary guidelines and incident CKD. These studies analyzed the same cohort dataset, both demonstrating significant associations with reduced risk of incident CKD, albuminuria, and rapid eGFR decline [41, 42]. Although no RCT has been conducted to evaluate the effect of dietary guidelines on incident CKD, a small-scale RCT has established the effect of adherence to dietary guidelines on attenuating CVD [43].

Dietary Patterns in Established CKD Populations

Healthy dietary patterns have an evidence base that supports the reduction in known risk factors associated with CKD progression. To date, there have only been a select number of studies evaluating these associations with long-term exposure to dietary patterns. The overall evidence base supports the associations of healthy dietary patterns to reduce the risk of death from all causes across Mediterranean diets, plant-based diets, and diets consistent with the Dietary Guidelines for Americans [3].

CKD Outcomes and the DASH Diet

While the DASH diet has been proven to be effective in CVD protection in non-CKD populations, the safety profile and appropriateness of this dietary approach in the established CKD population remain controversial. These concerns are specifically related to the possible higher protein (approx. 14% total calories) and potassium (approx. 4500 mg/day) content in the DASH diet. However, many renal dietitians argue that the DASH dietary pattern can have important health benefits for the management of CKD and dialysis patients with some slight modifications possible to the typical DASH diet. In fact, best practice guidelines, such as the 2004 Kidney Disease Outcomes Quality Initiative (KDOQI) guidelines, deem the DASH pattern in early CKD a suitable method to increase fruit and vegetable intake and improve kidney outcomes [44, 45]. The 2007 KDOQI guidelines on nutrition in diabetes and CKD allude to a "DASH-type" diet which concludes that a protein intake of 15% total calories per day is "likely" safe, given an altered red meat-to-plant-based protein ratio as potentially "kidney sparing" [46].

Small single-arm studies of the DASH diet have recently been conducted in CKD patients, suggesting the DASH diet is safe [47]. Two studies, both of 5-week duration each, tested the safety of the DASH pattern (maintaining protein intake 1 g/kg/day and 1500 g sodium/day) in people with stage 3 CKD and hypertension. Both studies demonstrated that daily dietary sodium intake can be reduced by 1200 mg/day. Serum potassium, dietary potassium, and dietary protein intake did not significantly change throughout the study periods [47, 48].

In the absence of high-quality RCTs, recommendations concerning the DASH diet in established CKD populations are difficult. However, practical modifications still make achieving a "DASH-type" diet realistic in CKD, with practical suggestions for clinicians presented in Table 31.1.

CKD Outcomes and the Mediterranean Diet

The evidence for the Mediterranean diet suggests that it is likely a safe intervention for CKD populations. Although issues with recommending a Mediterranean diet to people with CKD can arise, many of the traditional food types and serving suggestions in the Mediterranean diet can conflict with the traditional dietary restrictions placed on the CKD patient. There are many favorable attributes to recommending a Mediterranean diet to the CKD patient, including a healthy protein and fat intake, low glycemic index foods, and moderate consumption of phenolic compounds in red wine, which collectively make this dietary pattern one of the most powerful combaters of inflammation and oxidative stress. Observational analyses have shown that the Mediterranean diet may delay the progression to ESKD in individuals with CKD [36]. One clinical trial demonstrated the effectiveness of the Mediterranean diet in reducing systemic inflammation and microalbuminuria [49]. Despite the benefits of certain foods emphasized in the Mediterranean diet that are not commonly included in current renal nutrition guidelines, this practical diet can be modified for use in the CKD patient (see Table 31.1).

CKD Outcomes and Plant-Based/Vegetarian Diets

There is limited evidence available on vegetarian diets in established CKD populations. One existing RCT demonstrated the efficacy of the vegetarian diet compared to an omnivorous diet through decreased serum phosphorus and fibroblast growth factor 23 in patients with stages 3–4 CKD [50]. The gut microbiota also likely benefits from a predominantly plant-based/vegetarian diet and, by association, reduced CVD risk. Populations consuming a predominantly plant-based diet have greater microbiome abundance and biodiversity compared with populations consuming a diet subject to processing and inadequate fiber, characteristic of Western omnivorous diets [51]. A diet high in animal protein promotes proteolytic (putrefaction) bacteria over saccharolytic (fermentation) bacteria, which in turn contributes to dysbiosis and a higher risk of CVD [52]. Protein metabolism in the gut leads to the breakdown of tyrosine, phenylalanine, and tryptophan, which are precursors for indole sulfate and p-crystal sulfate conversion; these are commonly associated with elevated CVD risk [52]. In contrast, a high-fiber vegetarian diet reduces the production of these cardiorenal toxic compounds, and the fermentation of fiber releases short-chain fatty acids that favor healthy microbial activity to control dysbiosis [53] (See Chap. 27 on the Gut Microbiome).

CKD Outcomes and Diets Consistent with Dietary Guidelines

The recommended food and nutrient intakes advised for people with CKD are mostly in line with the Dietary Guidelines for Americans, with relatively minor modifications for nondairy alternatives that are lower in calcium, and fruits/vegetables that are lower in potassium, if required [5] (see Table 31.1). Healthy dietary patterns promote higher plant-based food intake and less refined and processed foods that are higher in fruits and vegetables (with vitamins and antioxidants), fish and omega-3 fatty acids, legumes, whole-grain cereals, and nuts. At the same time, the dietary pattern promotes a lower consumption of sodium, red and processed meat, saturated fats, and common phosphate additives that are highly prevalent in the Australian food supply.

No one dietary guideline has been tested for its long-term exposure on CKD outcomes in existing observational studies. One cohort study evaluated the post hoc association of adherence to the Healthy Eating Index based on the Food Guide Pyramid and demonstrated a nonsignificant association to all-cause mortality [49]. One recent RCT conducted in people with stages 3–4 CKD demonstrated a diet consistent with the Australian Dietary Guidelines, which is similar to the Dietary Guidelines for Americans, to be safe and effective at reducing body weight and keeping patients motivated for dietary change [50].

Should the Renal Diet Be Liberalized in Line with a Healthy Dietary Pattern?

The dietary patterns tested in the CKD literature to date have similar characteristics which fundamentally are in line with the dietary advice given in the Dietary Guidelines for Americans to the general population [6]. Therefore, liberalizing the renal diet to allow for higher plant-based intake appears safe and likely associated with improved crude outcomes. However, it is still important for the clinician to consider that observational analyses in population samplings with low eGFR may not necessarily extrapolate to the commonly referred patient for dietary management. In fact, the current evidence base for healthy dietary patterns and CKD outcomes remains inconclusive at best, attributable to the reliance on data from small subgroups of large cohorts analyzing post hoc associations.

To understand the potential benefit of dietary patterns and to determine the mechanisms by which these dietary approaches may translate to improved outcomes in individual CKD patients, it may be beneficial to look at studies examining the key components (or characteristics) of healthy dietary patterns and how these influence clinical outcomes.

The Food Group Synergy of Healthy Dietary Patterns

Consumption of food from the core food groups as per the Dietary Guidelines for Americans [5] likely displays a cumulative benefit on outcomes through synergy when consumed as a healthy dietary pattern, superior to the effect of the individual food groups and nutrients.

Healthy Dietary Patterns Promote a Higher Intake of Fruits and Vegetables

Fruits and vegetables have many properties which make them appealing as an intervention in CKD. Fruits and vegetables release potassium salts, generating bicarbonate naturally, to decrease the renal acid load. In fact, a diet higher in fruits and vegetables has been shown to more effectively manage metabolic acidosis compared to standard bicarbonate prescriptions [54]. In contrast, sulfur-containing animal proteins naturally produce acid, which can exacerbate renal acidosis [31]. Fruits and vegetables also have a low bioavailability of dietary phosphorus and calcium, which means there is limited absorption [due to the presence of phytate in vegetable forms of phosphorous] following intake of these foods, despite their respective nutrient content [55], in comparison to higher animal protein diets [50].

Consuming more fruits and vegetables has been suggested to reduce the risk of all-cause mortality by 65% in stages 3–4 CKD and 20% in hemodialysis populations [56, 57]. A well-designed RCT also showed that adults with stage 4 CKD can safely increase their servings of fruits and vegetables without adverse hyperkalemia, while significantly reducing blood pressure and body weight [54]. The use of fruits and vegetables as a naturally occurring food option to manage conditions such as metabolic acidosis is appealing as it also promotes a higher intake of dietary fiber. Dietary fiber has a complex role in CKD, reducing inflammation and the risk of mortality in association studies [58, 59]. A recent meta-analysis demonstrated that consumption of dietary fiber of at least 25 g per day can also reduce serum urea and creatinine levels [60], and lead to greater diversity of the gut microbiome and attenuation of nephron-vascular uremic toxins.

Healthy Dietary Patterns Promote Complex Carbohydrates That Are Higher in Dietary Fiber

Traditional mechanisms underpinning the benefits of quality carbohydrates that are rich in dietary fiber, including improved glycemic control, cholesterol and lipid management, and weight control, are well established. In recent years, additional therapeutic benefits of complex carbohydrate consumption on renal outcomes are becoming better understood. A large meta-analysis encompassing 185 observational and 58 clinical trials provides compelling evidence for a daily consumption of 25 to 29 g fiber to reduce all-cause and cardiovascular-related mortality [59]. While specific studies relating to CKD are limited, there are indications that whole-grain carbohydrates may have a role in the development of CKD [61, 62] and influence outcomes (all-cause mortality) in established CKD [58, 63].

Healthy Dietary Patterns Promote Lower Intake of Red and Processed Meat and Have Higher Plant-Animal Protein Ratios

Meat intake is another food group commonly targeted in CKD dietary interventions. Restriction of this food group is based on the premise that a low-protein diet may attenuate the risk of CKD progression and complications (see Chap. 2). However, the evidence underpinning these benefits is conflicting at best, and low-protein diets are notoriously difficult for patients to follow [64]. Incorporating protein advice into food-based guidance has been suggested by patients to be more comprehendible. Furthermore, in recent years, it appears the type (or quality) of the food group (and by consequence, the quality of the protein) consumed may better associate with clinical outcomes in CKD. Lowering the red meat-to-plant-based protein ratio has been described as "kidney sparing" in CKD [46, 65]. The potential benefit of reducing red meat intake extends into the dialysis population, where balanced portions from red meat, fish, and plant-based sources may lower the risk of cardiovascular death compared to an unbalanced diet higher in red meat intake [66].

Existing cohorts have found varying degrees of risk to kidney function from diets high in red and processed meats. The Nurses' Health Study in the United States found that a typical Western-style diet may lead to a higher risk of decline in eGFR rate compared to a dietary pattern lower in red meat, but equal in overall protein [67].

In contrast, seminal data from the large Atherosclerosis Risk in Communities (ARIC) cohort study [40] showed that people consuming the highest quartile of vegetable protein had a reduced risk of incident CKD of 24% over a 23-year follow-up period. Across all levels of protein intake in this study, there was no significant association for delaying incident CKD. However, when the analysis targeted individual food groupings, there were significant increased risks of developing CKD for those who consumed more protein from red and processed meats, whereas the CKD risk was lower among those with a higher consumption of low-fat dairy proteins, nuts, and legumes [40]. Similarly, in the Singapore Chinese Health Study, high red meat intake was associated with increased risk of CKD progression [65]. Meat protein is usually accompanied by other nutrients that may be considered less healthy (saturated fat, salt, bioavailable phosphate), whereas plant protein may be accompanied by other salutary vitamins, minerals, fiber, and antioxidants, while also being inherently low in saturated fat, calories, and organic phosphate [68].

Healthy Dietary Patterns Promote Healthy Fats, Eggs, and Low-Fat Dairy

Eggs are an important source of protein, healthy fat, and key micronutrients. While no study has specifically examined the effect of eggs on CKD outcomes to date, some large cohort databases have reported no negative associations between dietary patterns rich in egg intake and CKD risk progression [3].

The total and type of dairy consumption have been a commonly debated topic, attributable to its high sources of protein, phosphorous, calcium, and overall saturated fat content. However, overall findings from longitudinal studies generally support the consumption of dairy that is in line with the Dietary Guidelines for Americans (i.e., approximately two and a half low-fat servings per day).

While renal nutrition guidelines have many isolated nutrient targets, dietary fat targets are not common features in these guidelines. This comes despite the fact that dietary fat intake is approximately 40% of total energy intake in CKD populations, with the majority of that being from saturated fat [69–72]. The issue with this is that a diet high in saturated fat has been shown to be associated with a higher incidence of albuminuria and risk factor for kidney disease progression [25].

Dietary omega-3 polyunsaturated fatty acids (PUFA) have gained interest in CKD for their anti-inflammatory properties and potentially beneficial effects on blood pressure, endothelial function, and proteinuria [73, 74] (see Chaps. 13 and 22). In the general population, omega-3 PUFA intake correlates with a lower incidence of CKD [75] and reduced risk of albuminuria in people with type 2 diabetes [76]. One meta-analysis demonstrated that any dose of omega-3 supplementation (compared to no supplementation) reduces the risk of proteinuria and CKD progression to ESKD [77]. However, many studies involve small sample sizes and short intervention periods and are observational in most cases, which renders this evidence inconclusive.

Healthy Dietary Patterns Are Inherently Lower in Sodium

As shown in Table 31.1, healthy dietary patterns are inherently low in sodium in comparison to the Western diet with an average of 8–12 g/day, mostly due to not promoting discretionary and processed food (which can be up to 80% of a patient's daily sodium intake) [78]. Good quality evidence from RCTs and large meta-analyses support the effectiveness of reduced sodium intake in improving a range of outcomes for people with CKD including blood pressure, volume control, and proteinuria (see Chap. 10). Aside from increases in blood pressure and cardiovascular morbidity and mortality, high dietary sodium intake is associated with increased proteinuria and accelerated decline in kidney function [79].

Healthy Dietary Patterns Are Abundant Sources of Polyphenols, Which May Reduce Cardiovascular Risks for CKD Progression

Polyphenols are only present in plant-based foods and have been associated with multiple health benefits, mostly due to their antioxidant and anti-inflammatory properties [80]. Healthy dietary patterns, such as the Mediterranean, DASH, and vegetarian diets, are inherently higher in antioxidants and have an abundant source of non-nutrient phytochemicals such as carotenoids and polyphenols, adding to their cardioprotective profile [81, 82]. Mounting evidence suggests a role for polyphenols in modulating cell signaling pathways and may play a role in controlling inflammation associated with cardiovascular complications and progression [80]. There is a collection of polyphenol supplementation studies that included grape juice powder, pomegranate juice, turmeric, and cocoa flavanols. These studies have shown promise in controlling oxidative stress and ameliorating inflammation in ESKD patients [83–85]. In CKD populations, polyphenols have been shown to significantly reduce oxidative stress and urinary albumin-creatinine ratios [86, 87]. It remains unclear, however, whether recommending higher amounts of antioxidant-containing vitamins and non-nutritive polyphenol food sources raises a safety concern to electrolyte profiles. Therefore, these interventions would require regular review by the clinician and monitoring changes in dietary intake and serum biochemistry.

Safety Profile of a Plant-Based Dietary Pattern in the Kidney Disease Population

Safety concerns regarding the various dietary patterns relate to the high fruit and vegetable intake and potential for excessive protein intake (greater than 1 g/kg/day). However, fruit and vegetable intake are typically low across the CKD spectrum, and unnecessary restriction may risk many vitamin and mineral insufficiencies [69]. While fruit and vegetable intake convey higher dietary potassium, it has been recently argued that this does not necessarily translate into hyperkalemia [88]. Careful planning and regular monitoring are essential in the absence of clinical trials; however, modifications proposed in this chapter suggest that these dietary patterns can be implemented in the CKD patient group. In addition, an increased fiber intake from a higher fruit and vegetable diet can prevent constipation in dialysis populations and facilitate fecal excretion of excess potassium, which can be up to 3.5 times greater than that of the general population [89]. This ability of intestinal potassium excretion to compensate for a reduction in renal potassium handling has called into question the priority for dietary restriction in hyperkalemic states [88].

While the dietary patterns discussed in this chapter can be higher in protein (as a percentage of total calories consumed), they contain higher plant-based protein ratios which may be kidney-sparing and cardiorenal protective [90]. The bioavailability of phosphorous and calcium from plant-based sources is typically poor, which strengthens the kidney-sparing potential these diets may possess [50]. Nonetheless, it is important for the renal dietitian to carefully plan the patient's diet, using the practical considerations presented in Table 31.1, and individualizing nutrition needs in line with best practice guidelines.

Conclusion

This chapter has discussed dietary patterns, which reflect a whole pattern of eating and have widely accepted evidence for reducing blood pressure and cardiovascular health. As dietary patterns are a whole food-based intervention and characteristically higher in fruits, vegetables, and whole grains, caution for potential electrolyte derangement has been advised in the CKD population. It is important to note that there have been no RCTs conducted to date to either support or refute these claims. While preliminary data shows there are no adverse effects from following a DASH or Mediterranean pattern in CKD, careful meal planning with experienced clinicians is vitally important. With this in mind, promoting a healthy dietary pattern should be achievable in the common CKD patient.

References

1. Schwingshackl L, Hoffmann G. Diet quality as assessed by the healthy eating index, the alternate healthy eating index, the dietary approaches to stop hypertension score, and health outcomes: a systematic review and meta-analysis of cohort studies. J Acad Nutr Diet. 2015;115(5):780–800.e5.
2. USDA. A series of systematic reviews on the relationship between dietary patterns and health outcomes. 2014.
3. Kelly JT, Palmer SC, Wai SN, Ruospo M, Carrero JJ, Campbell KL, et al. Healthy dietary patterns and risk of mortality and ESRD in CKD: a meta-analysis of cohort studies. Clin J Am Soc Nephrol. 2017;12(2):272–9.
4. Mozaffarian D. Dietary and policy priorities for cardiovascular disease, diabetes, and obesity a comprehensive review. Circulation. 2016;133(2):187–225.
5. U.S. Department of Health and Human Services and U.S. 2015 – 2020 Dietary Guidelines for Americans. 8th ed. Department of Agriculture; 2015.
6. Nutrition Evidence Library. Technical Expert Collaborative on Study of Dietary Patterns. U.S. Department of Agriculture; 2014.
7. Smyth A, Griffin M, Yusuf S, Mann JF, Reddan D, Canavan M, et al. Diet and major renal outcomes: a prospective cohort study. The NIH-AARP diet and health study. J Ren Nutr. 2016;26(5):288–98.
8. Kelly JT, Rossi M, Johnson DW, Campbell KL. Beyond sodium, phosphate and potassium: potential dietary interventions in kidney disease. Semin Dial. 2017;30(3):197–202.
9. Hermsdorff HHM, Barbosa KB, Volp ACP, Puchau B, Bressan J, Zulet MÁ, et al. Vitamin C and fibre consumption from fruits and vegetables improves oxidative stress markers in healthy young adults. Br J Nutr. 2012;107(8):1119–27.
10. Jiang R, Jacobs DR Jr, Mayer-Davis E, Szklo M, Herrington D, Jenny NS, et al. Nut and seed consumption and inflammatory markers in the multi-ethnic study of atherosclerosis. Am J Epidemiol. 2006;163(3):222–31.
11. Casas R, Estruch R. Dietary patterns, foods, nutrients and chronic inflammatory disorders. Immunome Res. 2016;12(2):1.
12. Tonelli M, Sacks F, Pfeffer M, Jhangri GS, Curhan G, Cholesterol and Recurrent Events (CARE) Trial Investigators. Biomarkers of inflammation and progression of chronic kidney disease. Kidney Int. 2005;68(1):237–45.
13. Fried L, Solomon C, Shlipak M, Seliger S, Stehman-Breen C, Bleyer AJ, et al. Inflammatory and prothrombotic markers and the progression of renal disease in elderly individuals. J Am Soc Nephrol. 2004;15(12):3184–91.
14. Huo R, Du T, Xu Y, Xu W, Chen X, Sun K, et al. Effects of Mediterranean-style diet on glycemic control, weight loss and cardiovascular risk factors among type 2 diabetes individuals: a meta-analysis. Eur J Clin Nutr. 2015;69(11):1200–8.
15. Panagiotakos DB, Pitsavos C, Arvaniti F, Stefanadis C. Adherence to the Mediterranean food pattern predicts the prevalence of hypertension, hypercholesterolemia, diabetes and obesity, among healthy adults; the accuracy of the MedDietScore. Prev Med. 2007;44(4):335–40.
16. Esposito K, Marfella R, Ciotola M, Di Palo C, Giugliano F, Giugliano G, et al. Effect of a Mediterranean-style diet on endothelial dysfunction and markers of vascular inflammation in the metabolic syndrome: a randomized trial. JAMA. 2004;292(12):1440–6.
17. Saneei P, Salehi-Abargouei A, Esmaillzadeh A, Azadbakht L. Influence of Dietary Approaches to Stop Hypertension (DASH) diet on blood pressure: a systematic review and meta-analysis on randomized controlled trials. Nutr Metab Cardiovasc Dis. 2014;24(12):1253–61.
18. Viguiliouk E, Kendall CW, Kahleová H, Rahelić D, Salas-Salvadó J, Choo VL, et al. Effect of vegetarian dietary patterns on cardiometabolic risk factors in diabetes: a systematic review and meta-analysis of randomized controlled trials. Clin Nutr. 2019;38(3):1133–45.
19. Dinu M, Pagliai G, Casini A, Sofi F. Mediterranean diet and multiple health outcomes: an umbrella review of meta-analyses of observational studies and randomised trials. Eur J Clin Nutr. 2018;72(1):30–43.
20. Yuzbashian E, Asghari G, Mirmiran P, Amouzegar-Bahambari P, Azizi F. Adherence to low-sodium dietary approaches to stop hypertension-style diet may decrease the risk of incident chronic kidney disease among high-risk patients: a secondary prevention in prospective cohort study. Nephrol Dial Transplant. 2018;33(7):1159–68.
21. Asghari G, Yuzbashian E, Mirmiran P, Azizi F. The association between Dietary Approaches to Stop Hypertension and incidence of chronic kidney disease in adults: The Tehran Lipid and Glucose Study. Nephrol Dial Transplant. 2017;32(suppl_2):ii224–30.
22. Asghari G, Momenan M, Yuzbashian E, Mirmiran P, Azizi F. Dietary pattern and incidence of chronic kidney disease among adults: a population-based study. Nutr Metab (Lond). 2018;15:88.
23. Asghari G, Farhadnejad H, Mirmiran P, Dizavi A, Yuzbashian E, Azizi F. Adherence to the Mediterranean diet is associated with reduced risk of incident chronic kidney diseases among Tehranian adults. Hypertens Res. 2017;40(1):96–102.
24. Crews DC, Kuczmarski MF, Miller ER 3rd, Zonderman AB, Evans MK, Powe NR. Dietary habits, poverty, and chronic kidney disease in an urban population. J Ren Nutr. 2015;25(2):103–10.

25. Lin J, Judd S, Le A, Ard J, Newsome BB, Howard G, et al. Associations of dietary fat with albuminuria and kidney dysfunction. Am J Clin Nutr. 2010;92(4):897–904.
26. Rebholz CM, Crews DC, Grams ME, Steffen LM, Levey AS, Miller ER 3rd, et al. DASH (dietary approaches to stop hypertension) diet and risk of subsequent kidney disease. Am J Kidney Dis. 2016;68(6):853–61.
27. Chang A, Van Horn L, Jacobs DR Jr, Liu K, Muntner P, Newsome B, et al. Lifestyle-related factors, obesity, and incident microalbuminuria: the CARDIA (Coronary Artery Risk Development in Young Adults) study. Am J Kidney Dis. 2013;62(2):267–75.
28. Lin J, Hu FB, Curhan GC. Associations of diet with albuminuria and kidney function decline. Clin J Am Soc Nephrol. 2010;5(5):836–43.
29. Liu Y, Kuczmarski MF, Miller ER 3rd, Nava MB, Zonderman AB, Evans MK, et al. Dietary habits and risk of kidney function decline in an urban population. J Ren Nutr. 2017;27(1):16–25.
30. Lin CK, Lin DJ, Yen CH, Chen SC, Chen CC, Wang TY, et al. Comparison of renal function and other health outcomes in vegetarians versus omnivores in Taiwan. J Health Popul Nutr. 2010;28(5):470–5.
31. Banerjee T, Liu Y, Crews D. Dietary patterns and CKD progression. Blood Purif. 2016;41(1–3):117–22.
32. Estruch R, Ros E, Salas-Salvadó J, et al. Primary prevention of cardiovascular disease with a Mediterranean diet supplemented with extra-virgin olive oil or nuts. N Engl J Med. 2018;378:e34.
33. Rees K, Hartley L, Flowers N, Clarke A, Hooper L, Thorogood M, et al. 'Mediterranean' dietary pattern for the primary prevention of cardiovascular disease. Cochrane Database Syst Rev. 2013;8:CD009825.
34. Sofi F, Cesari F, Abbate R, Gensini GF, Casini A. Adherence to Mediterranean diet and health status: meta-analysis. BMJ. 2008;337:a1344.
35. Trichopoulou A, Bamia C, Trichopoulos D. Anatomy of health effects of Mediterranean diet: Greek EPIC prospective cohort study. BMJ. 2009;338:b2337.
36. Khatri M, Moon YP, Scarmeas N, Gu Y, Gardener H, Cheung K, et al. The association between a Mediterranean-style diet and kidney function in the northern Manhattan study cohort. Clin J Am Soc Nephrol. 2014;9(11):1868–75.
37. Díaz-López A, Bulló M, Martínez-González MÁ, Guasch-Ferré M, Ros E, Basora J, et al. Effects of Mediterranean diets on kidney function: a report from the PREDIMED trial. Am J Kidney Dis. 2012;60(3):380–9.
38. Chauveau P, Combe C, Fouque D, Aparicio M. Vegetarianism: advantages and drawbacks in patients with chronic kidney diseases. J Ren Nutr. 2013;23(6):399–405.
39. Chauveau P, Koppe L, Combe C, Lasseur C, Trolonge S, Aparicio M. Vegetarian diets and chronic kidney disease. Nephrol Dial Transplant. 2019;34(2):199–207.
40. Haring B, Selvin E, Liang M, et al. Dietary protein sources and risk for incident chronic kidney disease: results from the Atherosclerosis Risk in Communities (ARIC) study. J Ren Nutr. 2017;27(4):233–42.
41. Foster MC, Hwang S-J, Massaro J, et al. Lifestyle factors and indices of kidney function in the Framingham heart study. Am J Nephrol. 2015;41(4–5):267–74.
42. Ma J, Jacques PF, Hwang SJ, Troy LM, McKeown NM, Chu AY, et al. Dietary guideline adherence index and kidney measures in the Framingham heart study. Am J Kidney Dis. 2016;68(5):703–15.
43. Reidlinger DP, Darzi J, Hall WL, Seed PT, Chowienczyk PJ, Sanders TA, et al. How effective are current dietary guidelines for cardiovascular disease prevention in healthy middle-aged and older men and women? A randomized controlled trial. Am J Clin Nutr. 2015;101(5):922–30.
44. Chan M, Kelly J, Tapsell L. Dietary modeling of foods for advanced CKD based on general healthy eating guidelines: what should be on the plate? Am J Kidney Dis. 2017;69(3):436–50.
45. K/DOQI working group. K/DOQI clinical practice guidelines on hypertension and antihypertensive agents in chronic kidney disease. Am J Kidney Dis. 2004;43(5 Suppl 1):S1–290.
46. National Kidney Foundation. KDOQI clinical practice guidelines and clinical practice recommendations for diabetes and chronic kidney disease. Am J Kidney Dis. 2007;49(2 Suppl 2):S1–S180.
47. Tyson CC, Lin P-H, Corsino L, Batch BC, Allen J, Sapp S, et al. Short-term effects of the DASH diet in adults with moderate chronic kidney disease: a pilot feeding study. Clin Kidney J. 2016;9(4):952–8.
48. Hannah J, Wells LM, Jones CH. The feasibility of using the Dietary Approaches to Stop Hypertension (DASH) diet in people with chronic kidney disease and hypertension. J Clin Nephrol Kidney Dis. 2018;3(1):1015.
49. De Lorenzo A, Noce A, Bigioni M, Calabrese V, Della Rocca DG, Di Daniele N, et al. The effects of Italian Mediterranean organic diet (IMOD) on health status. Curr Pharm Des. 2010;16(7):814–24.
50. Moe SM, Zidehsarai MP, Chambers MA, Jackman LA, Radcliffe JS, Trevino LL, et al. Vegetarian compared with meat dietary protein source and phosphorus homeostasis in chronic kidney disease. Clin J Am Soc Nephrol. 2011;6(2):257–64.
51. Schnorr SL, Candela M, Rampelli S, Centanni M, Consolandi C, Basaglia G, et al. Gut microbiome of the Hadza hunter-gatherers. Nat Commun. 2014;5:3654.
52. Evenepoel P, Meijers BK, Bammens BR, Verbeke K. Uremic toxins originating from colonic microbial metabolism. Kidney Int Suppl. 2009;114:S12–9.

53. den Besten G, van Eunen K, Groen AK, Venema K, Reijngoud DJ, Bakker BM. The role of short-chain fatty acids in the interplay between diet, gut microbiota, and host energy metabolism. J Lipid Res. 2013;54(9):2325–40.

54. Goraya N, Simoni J, Jo CH, Wesson DE. A comparison of treating metabolic acidosis in CKD stage 4 hypertensive kidney disease with fruits and vegetables or sodium bicarbonate. Clin J Am Soc Nephrol. 2013;8(3):371–81.

55. Calvo MS, Uribarri J. Contributions to total phosphorus intake: all sources considered. Semin Dial. 2013;26(1):54–61.

56. Saglimbene VM, Wong G, Ruospo M, et al. Fruit and vegetable intake and mortality in adults undergoing maintenance hemodialysis. Clin J Am Soc Nephrol. 2019;14(2):250–60.

57. Wai SN, Kelly JT, Johnson DJ, Campbell KL. Dietary patterns and clinical outcomes in chronic kidney disease: the CKD.QLD nutrition study. J Ren Nutr. 2016;27(3):175–82.

58. Krishnamurthy VM, Wei G, Baird BC, Murtaugh M, Chonchol MB, Raphael KL, et al. High dietary fiber intake is associated with decreased inflammation and all-cause mortality in patients with chronic kidney disease. Kidney Int. 2012;81(3):300–6.

59. Reynolds A, Mann J, Cummings J, Winter N, Mete E, Te Morenga L. Carbohydrate quality and human health: a series of systematic reviews and meta-analyses. Lancet. 2019;393(10170):434–45.

60. Chiavaroli L, Mirrahimi A, Sievenpiper JL, Jenkins DJ, Darling PB. Dietary fiber effects in chronic kidney disease: a systematic review and meta-analysis of controlled feeding trials. Eur J Clin Nutr. 2015;69(7):761–8.

61. Xu H, Sjogren P, Arnlov J, Banerjee T, Cederholm T, Risérus U, et al. A proinflammatory diet is associated with systemic inflammation and reduced kidney function in elderly adults. J Nutr. 2015;145(4):729–35.

62. Gopinath B, Harris DC, Flood VM, Burlutsky G, Brand-Miller J, Mitchell P. Carbohydrate nutrition is associated with the 5-year incidence of chronic kidney disease. J Nutr. 2011;141(3):433–9.

63. Xu H, Huang X, Risérus U, Krishnamurthy VM, Cederholm T, Arnlöv J, et al. Dietary fiber, kidney function, inflammation, and mortality risk. Clin J Am Soc Nephrol. 2014;9(12):2104–10.

64. Woodrow G. Con: the role of diet for people with advanced stage 5 CKD. Nephrol Dial Transplant. 2018;33(3):380–4.

65. Lew Q-LJ, Jafar TH, Koh HWL, Jin A, Chow KY, Yuan JM, et al. Red meat intake and risk of ESRD. J Am Soc Nephrol. 2016;28(1):304–12.

66. Tsuruya K, Fukuma S, Wakita T, Ninomiya T, Nagata M, Yoshida H, et al. Dietary patterns and clinical outcomes in hemodialysis patients in Japan: a cohort study. PLoS One. 2015;10(1):e0116677.

67. Knight EL, Stampfer MJ, Hankinson SE, Spiegelman D, Curhan GC. The impact of protein intake on renal function decline in women with normal renal function or mild renal insufficiency. Ann Intern Med. 2003;138(6):460–7.

68. Kelly JT, Carrero JJ. Dietary sources of protein and chronic kidney disease progression: the proof may be in the pattern. J Ren Nutr. 2017;27(4):221–4.

69. Luis D, Zlatkis K, Comenge B, García Z, Navarro JF, Lorenzo V, et al. Dietary quality and adherence to dietary recommendations in patients undergoing hemodialysis. J Ren Nutr. 2016;26(3):190–5.

70. Therrien M, Byham-Gray L, Denmark R, Beto J. Comparison of dietary intake among women on maintenance dialysis to a Women's Health Initiative cohort: results from the NKF-CRN second National Research Question Collaborative Study. J Ren Nutr. 2014;24(2):72–80.

71. Khoueiry G, Waked A, Goldman M, El-Charabaty E, Dunne E, Smith M, et al. Dietary intake in hemodialysis patients does not reflect a heart healthy diet. J Ren Nutr. 2011;21(6):438–47.

72. Luttrell KJ, Beto JA, Tangney CC, et al. Selected nutrition practices of women on hemodialysis and peritoneal dialysis: observations from the NKF-CRN second National Research Question Collaborative Study. J Ren Nutr. 2014;24(2):81–91.

73. Huang X, Lindholm B, Stenvinkel P, Carrero JJ. Dietary fat modification in patients with chronic kidney disease: n-3 fatty acids and beyond. J Nephrol. 2013;26(6):960–74.

74. Shapiro H, Theilla M, Attal-Singer J, Singer P. Effects of polyunsaturated fatty acid consumption in diabetic nephropathy. Nat Rev Nephrol. 2011;7(2):110–21.

75. Gopinath B, Harris DC, Flood VM, Burlutsky G, Mitchell P. Consumption of long-chain n-3 PUFA, α-linolenic acid and fish is associated with the prevalence of chronic kidney disease. Br J Nutr. 2011;105(9):1361–8.

76. Lee CC, Sharp SJ, Wexler DJ, Adler AI. Dietary intake of eicosapentaenoic and docosahexaenoic acid and diabetic nephropathy: cohort analysis of the diabetes control and complications trial. Diabetes Care. 2010;33(7):1454–6.

77. Hu J, Liu Z, Zhang H. Omega-3 fatty acid supplementation as an adjunctive therapy in the treatment of chronic kidney disease: a meta-analysis. Clinics (Sao Paulo). 2017;72(1):58–64.

78. Odermatt A. The Western-style diet: a major risk factor for impaired kidney function and chronic kidney disease. Am J Physiol Renal Physiol. 2011;301(5):F919–31.

79. Smyth A, O'Donnell MJ, Yusuf S, Clase CM, Teo KK, Canavan M, et al. Sodium intake and renal outcomes: a systematic review. Am J Hypertens. 2014;27(10):1277–84.

80. Joseph SV, Edirisinghe I, Burton-Freeman BM. Fruit polyphenols: a review of anti-inflammatory effects in humans. Crit Rev Food Sci Nutr. 2016;56(3):419–44.

81. Grassi D, Desideri G, Ferri C. Flavonoids: antioxidants against atherosclerosis. Nutrients. 2010;2(8):889–902.

82. Wang X, Ouyang Y, Liu J, Zhu M, Zhao G, Bao W, et al. Fruit and vegetable consumption and mortality from all causes, cardiovascular disease, and cancer: systematic review and dose-response meta-analysis of prospective cohort studies. BMJ. 2014;349:g4490.

83. Pakfetrat M, Akmali M, Malekmakan L, Dabaghimanesh M, Khorsand M. Role of turmeric in oxidative modulation in end-stage renal disease patients. Hemodial Int. 2015;19(1):124–31.

84. Janiques AGPR, Leal VO, Stockler-Pinto MB, Moreira NX, Mafra D. Effects of grape powder supplementation on inflammatory and antioxidant markers in hemodialysis patients: a randomized double-blind study. J Bras Nefrol. 2014;36(4):496–501.

85. Shema-Didi L, Kristal B, Ore L, Shapiro G, Geron R, Sela S. Pomegranate juice intake attenuates the increase in oxidative stress induced by intravenous iron during hemodialysis. Nutr Res. 2013;33(6):442–6.

86. Fallahzadeh MK, Dormanesh B, Sagheb MM, Roozbeh J, Vessal G, Pakfetrat M, et al. Effect of addition of silymarin to renin-angiotensin system inhibitors on proteinuria in type 2 diabetic patients with overt nephropathy: a randomized, double-blind, placebo-controlled trial. Am J Kidney Dis. 2012;60(6):896–903.

87. Turki K, Charradi K, Boukhalfa H, Belhaj M, Limam F, Aouani E. Grape seed powder improves renal failure of chronic kidney disease patients. EXCLI J. 2016;15:424–33. eCollection 2016

88. St-Jules DE, Goldfarb DS, Sevick MA. Nutrient non-equivalence: does restricting high-potassium plant foods help to prevent hyperkalemia in hemodialysis patients? J Ren Nutr. 2016;26(5):282–7.

89. Hayes C Jr, McLeod M, Robinson R. An extravenal mechanism for the maintenance of potassium balance in severe chronic renal failure. Trans Assoc Am Physicians. 1967;80:207–16.

90. Kidney Disease Outcomes Quality Initiative (K/DOQI). K/DOQI clinical practice guidelines on hypertension and antihypertensive agents in chronic kidney disease. Am J Kidney Dis. 2004;43(5 Suppl 1):S1–290.

91. Serra-Majem L, Bes-Rastrollo M, Román-Viñas B, Pfrimer K, Sánchez-Villegas A, Martínez-González MA. Dietary patterns and nutritional adequacy in a Mediterranean country. Br J Nutr. 2009;101(Suppl 2):S21–8.

92. American Heart Association Nutrition Committee, Lichtenstein AH, Appel LJ, Brands M, Carnethon M, Daniels S, et al. Diet and lifestyle recommendations revision 2006: a scientific statement from the American Heart Association Nutrition Committee. Circulation. 2006;114:82–96.

Chapter 32
Herbal and Other Natural Dietary Supplements

Diane Rigassio Radler

Keywords Kidney disease · Complementary medicine · Dietary supplements · Herbs · Botanicals

> **Key Points**
> - Some dietary supplements may offer protective benefits to kidneys.
> - Some dietary supplements may be associated with kidney dysfunction or drug interactions.
> - Dietary supplements may be sold without evidence of safety and efficacy.
> - Health professionals should engage in an open dialogue to encourage patients to disclose their interest in and their use of dietary supplements.

Introduction

Complementary or alternative approaches to healthcare are diverse medical and healthcare practices or strategies that are not considered to be part of conventional medicine [1]. "Complementary" approaches refer to practices that are adjunctive to conventional practice; conversely "alternative" refers to practices that are used instead of conventional practices; as evidence is established for safety and efficacy, the use of these strategies may evolve over time and be adopted into conventional healthcare referred to as integrative health [1]. The use of natural products is one type of complementary health approach for disease prevention, management, and treatment. Dietary supplements are considered part of the natural product category. People with kidney disease may wish to explore natural products; the focus of this chapter is with regard to non-vitamin, non-mineral dietary supplements and kidney disease.

Dietary Supplements

Plant-based medicines have been used for centuries and were instrumental in the evolution of many of the pharmaceutical therapies that exist today [2]. The availability and usage of dietary supplements have increased notably in the past two decades, with sales reported to be $46 billion in 2018 [3, 4].

D. R. Radler (✉)

Department of Clinical and Preventive Nutrition Sciences, Rutgers University, School of Health Professions, Newark, NJ, USA

e-mail: rigassdl@shp.rutgers.edu

© Springer Nature Switzerland AG 2020

J. D. Burrowes et al. (eds.), *Nutrition in Kidney Disease*, Nutrition and Health, https://doi.org/10.1007/978-3-030-44858-5_32

The American Botanical Council noted that sales of herbal products specifically continue to increase annually, and retail sales in 2017 exceeded $8 billion [5].

The surge in the availability and use of dietary supplements in the United States may be attributed to the Dietary Supplement Health and Education Act (DSHEA) of 1994 [6]. At that time, the Congress acknowledged that there may be a positive relationship between dietary practices, such as dietary supplements, and health promotion and disease prevention, which may translate into reduced healthcare burden. DSHEA amended the Food, Drug, and Cosmetic Act of 1958 to exclude dietary supplements from the premarket safety evaluations that food and drugs undergo. DSHEA mandated a definition of dietary supplements (Box 32.1) and guidelines for product claims and labels, including a disclaimer that the Food and Drug Administration (FDA) has not evaluated the product for safety or efficacy. DSHEA authorized FDA to establish good manufacturing practices (GMP) for the supplement industry and created the Office of Dietary Supplements to promote research and education regarding dietary supplements [6].

Box 32.1 Definition of Dietary Supplements [6]

"A product intended to supplement the diet to enhance health that contains one or more of the following:

- Vitamin, mineral, amino acid, herb or botanical
- Dietary substance to supplement the diet by increasing total dietary intake
- Concentrate, metabolite, constituent, extract or combination of any ingredient above
- Intended for ingestion as capsule, powder, gelcap and is not represented as a conventional food or as a sole item of a meal or the diet"

Efficacy and Safety of Dietary Supplements

Among the key issues concerning healthcare professionals regarding dietary supplements is the uncertainty over their efficacy and safety (Box 32.2). A natural source of a dietary supplement may differ according to species, soil, water, and growing conditions. Additionally, the rise in demand and availability, ease of obtaining products, and limited proof of efficacy and safety are cause for concern. With the ease of Internet searches for information, patients and clinicians must be wary of unsubstantiated claims and misinformation [7]. Moreover, in certain populations, such as persons diagnosed with kidney disease, dietary supplements may be contraindicated due to impaired renal function or possible drug interactions.

The FDA guidelines on GMP [8] provide consumers and clinicians some confidence in the quality of dietary supplements from reputable manufacturers that must uphold standards for quality and purity. There are also several independent monitoring agencies (Box 32.3) and independent certification programs that a manufacturer can seek to endorse the product. On a voluntary basis from the manufacturer, these independent organizations will evaluate the product for purity, accuracy of ingredient labeling, and manufacturing practices. One organization is the United States Pharmacopeia (USP) that evaluates products upon specified criteria and allows the manufacturers to use the designation, DSVP (Dietary Supplement Verification Program), if the product passes the rigorous testing. Another similar program is set up by the NSF International to obtain the right to use the NSF mark.

Box 32.2 Deciding for or Against the Use of Dietary Supplements
For
- Natural products are "natural."
- Many therapies have been used for centuries.
- May reduce the need for drugs and associated side effects when used properly.
- Other countries have been prescribing herbs safely for years.

Against
- Limited scientific testing.
- Sold without knowledge of action; active ingredient concentrations vary.
- May displace/enhance/interfere with current therapy.
- Herb-drug interactions.
- No federal regulation prior to sale.
- May be subject to misidentification and contamination.

Box 32.3 Websites for Independent Monitoring Agencies or Organization of Dietary Supplements
- MedWatch (http://www.fda.gov/medwatch).
- ConsumerLab: Independent evaluation with periodic reports; part of the report is available free, some by subscription (http://www.consumerlab.com).
- Dietary Supplement Verification Program (http://www.usp.org/usp-verification-services/usp-verified-dietary-supplements).
- NSF mark (http://www.nsf.org/consumer/dietary_supplements/dietary_certification.asp?program=DietarySup).

Dietary Supplements and Kidney Disease

The increasing use of complementary medicine and dietary supplements among patients with kidney disease worldwide has been documented [9–13]; hence, it warrants attention as a significant consideration in current healthcare practice. Although there is limited published literature on the actual patterns of use of dietary supplements by people with kidney disease, people may choose to use dietary supplements in an attempt to prevent further renal deterioration or may use them as an adjunct to mitigate side effects of the disease or treatments [14]. Supplement use may be classified as those with potential protective effects and those that should be avoided in kidney disease. Additional considerations include dietary supplements that may be toxic or contaminated and lead to kidney dysfunction and those that may have interactions with prescribed drugs.

Dietary Supplements with Potential Protective Effects

Preventing renal deterioration by using herbs and supplements would be a fortunate asset. Some countries may not have dialysis abundantly available, and traditional medicine using herbs may be one of the first choices in treatment [15]. Single herbs or formulations of several together may offer promising treatments. However, most of the published research is with animal studies; human applicability, safety, efficacy, and potential interaction with other medications must be explored. Astragalus (*Astragalus membranaceus*), an adaptogenic herb and antioxidant, may reduce proteinuria in glomerulonephritis [14, 16]. Traditional Chinese medicine uses astragalus often in combination with other herbs for its immune-enhancing potential; hence, individuals on immunosuppressants or those with autoimmune diseases should avoid its use [17]. The antioxidant properties of ginger (*Zingiber officinale*) may be linked to reduced inflammation in rats [18]. Other herbs such as milk thistle (*Silybum marianum*) and cordyceps (*Cordyceps sinensis*) may offer protection against nephrotoxic drugs [17].

Given that people with kidney disease often also have hypertension, diabetes, or hyperlipidemia, herbs and supplements with anti-inflammatory activity may be of interest in an attempt to mitigate cardiovascular risk factors [14]. Omega-3 fatty acids found in foods, mainly fish, are also available in the form of dietary supplements as anti-inflammatory agents. A systematic review article of 26 publications suggests that omega-3 fatty acids may be beneficial in reducing inflammation in kidney disease and other chronic diseases [19]. Evening primrose (*Oenothera biennis*) and borage (*Borago officinalis*) oil are sources of gamma-linolenic acid (GLA), an omega-6 fatty acid [17]. GLA may be converted to compounds that have anti-inflammatory properties. The judicious use of anti-inflammatory agents by people with kidney disease may be beneficial. Certainly side effects and drug interactions should be monitored and noted; fish oils can decrease platelet aggregation so large doses predispose a bleeding risk and may have additive effects with anticoagulant or antiplatelet medications [17].

The role of the human gut microbiome in kidney disease is of interest for disease severity and health consequences [20, 21]. Pre- and probiotics may modulate the microbiome in favor of reducing uremic toxins and mitigating their systemic effect. The main source of pre- and probiotics is from foods that may be challenging to consume on a typical renal diet, and dietary supplements delivering pre- and probiotics may have a role in chronic kidney disease management [22].

Dietary Supplements to Avoid in Kidney Disease

While there is still much research to be done with dietary supplements and specifically in populations with kidney disease, most supplements should be approached with caution. Published literature on case reports [23], with either positive or negative outcomes, may not be generalized to a larger population but should remind clinicians to engage in a discussion with patients about dietary supplements. Theoretical mechanisms of action need testing in vivo before the affirmation of use; both demonstrated and putative drug-herb interactions must be heeded.

Dandelion root (*Taraxacum officinale*) and Scotch broom (*Cytisus scoparius*) may have diuretic effects [17]. Parsley (*Carum petroselinum*), juniper (*Juniperus communis*), lovage (*Levisticum officinale*), and goldenrod (*Solidago virgaurea*) have constituents that irritate the kidney and increase renal blood flow and glomerular filtration, thus acting as aquaretics that increase water loss but not electrolyte excretion [17]. These herbs should be considered contraindicated in kidney disease.

Kidney disease may alter the pharmacokinetics of drugs. Given that dietary supplements are natural forms of active biochemical agents, and that often the active ingredient or the mechanism of action may not be fully understood in healthy individuals, people with kidney disease must use caution when considering the metabolism, distribution, and excretion of dietary supplements. For example, it is known that St. John's wort (*Hypericum perforatum*), which is used for mild depression, interferes with a metabolic pathway shared by many drugs [17]. When prescribed drugs and St. John's wort are used concomitantly, the blood concentration of the drug may be lower than expected and not therapeutic.

Table 32.1 Herbs with adverse renal effects [17, 25]

Herbs (scientific name)	Effect	Remark
Aristolochia (*Aristolochia auricularia*)	Renal fibrosis, carcinoma	Contains aristolochic acid which is nephrotoxic and carcinogenic
		FDA prohibits products containing aristolochic acid
		Other herbs such as asarabacca and costus root may be adulterated with aristolochic acid
Neem (*Azadirachta indica*)	Nephrotoxic	Leaf or seed oil may be nephrotoxic; flower, fruit, and twigs may be safe
Licorice (*Glycyrrhiza glabra*)	Hypernatremia, hypokalemia, edema	Numerous drug interactions
Senna (*Senna alexandrina*), cascara (*Rhamnus purshiana*)	Hypokalemia	Used as laxatives. Senna leaf is not for long-term use
Noni fruit (*Morinda citrifolia*)	Hyperkalemia	Fruit contains high concentration of potassium
Juniper berry (*Juniperus communis*), dandelion (*Taraxacum officinale*), asparagus tea (*Asparagus officinalis*), rupturewort (*Herniaria glabra*), Scotch broom (*Cytisus scoparius*), stinging nettle (*Urtica dioica*), uva ursi (*Arctostaphylos uva-ursi*)	Diuresis, electrolyte imbalance	May increase water loss without sodium excretion

Dietary Supplements and Kidney Dysfunction

Perhaps the most infamous case of herbs causing kidney dysfunction is the case of "Chinese herb nephropathy" or "aristolochic acid nephropathy." In an attempt at weight loss, a Belgian population took an herbal supplement with a misidentified herb containing aristolochic acid, a nephrotoxic and carcinogenic herb. It was later reported that numerous people who took the supplement needed dialysis or renal transplant and several developed cancer [24]. Other less common herbs implicated in kidney dysfunction have been reported and summarized [23]; refer to Table 32.1 for a list of herbs with adverse effects on the kidney. It would be prudent for practitioners with patient populations affiliated with healthcare practices of other cultures to familiarize themselves with particular regimens inherent in certain populations.

Considerations for Healthcare Providers

Conscientious healthcare providers understand the current science in health promotion and disease management and strive for the best possible outcomes in patient care [26]. Recognizing that patients may seek to include dietary supplements as a part of their healthcare regimen is vital for open communication and treatment. Healthcare providers must be willing to ask questions relative to dietary supplement use and be prepared to answer questions or dialogue the pros and cons of a given regimen. Often, however, the area of dietary supplements may be intimidating when faced with numerous supplements with uncommon names or formulations with several ingredients. Suggested approaches would be to identify those dietary supplements common to one's practice area, for example, in kidney disease, then research the evidence for safety and efficacy through either scientific publications or databases that synthesize the information into a quick, sound reference. Some resources are listed later in this chapter, including a free downloadable app with information on several popular herbs. Once the provider has background knowledge on the supplement, they are usually more comfortable dialoguing with the patient regarding dietary supplements. Likewise, a patient who perceives that their healthcare provider is willing to discuss the subject is more likely to disclose the truth about the contemplative or actual use. Pertinent information to discuss is what the patient wants to use and why. The "what" is relatively straightforward, but the "why" aspect may be more nebulous. Find out the source of the patient's information and identify the patient's expectations. Is the patient taking the dietary supplement to treat a side effect of the disease hoping that the supplement may cure the disease? Understanding the patient's issues and the safety and efficacy of the supplements leads to an open discussion to support or discourage their use.

The issues of safety and efficacy can be measured or assessed independently by first evaluating for evidence of efficacy, then evaluating for evidence of harm [26]. Where do the results of the assessment point to on an evidence-versus-harm scale? If there is some evidence of efficacy and no or minimal risk of harm, then the dietary supplement may be worthwhile, such as in the case of fish oil. On the contrary, if the evidence for harm outweighs any benefit, then the patient should be counseled on other therapies. If the patient understands the issues around dietary supplements and still intends to take one or some, healthcare providers may allow a trial period if the supplement is not harmful and the patient can afford the out-of-pocket expense. In that case, providers may advise the patient to start with one supplement at a time, monitor and report any side effects, allow 4–6 weeks to notice the desired effect, and report back to the provider all positive, negative, or neutral experiences. As expected with all patient contact, providers must document the dialogue and communicate the patient's actions with the healthcare team.

Conclusion

With the increase in use of dietary supplements, and the relative ease with which they may be marketed by manufacturers and purchased by consumers, healthcare providers need to be aware of common supplements and become cognizant of the safety concerns or interactions they may have with disease status and medication regimens. Healthcare providers can identify the notable dietary supplements that may be encountered in practice, and they can research the safety and efficacy issues with regard to their use or misuse. Honest, open communication with patients who may wish to explore the use of dietary supplements is essential for patient-clinician relations and optimal health outcomes.

Resources

Websites worth noting:

- American Botanical Council, http://www.herbalgram.org
- ConsumerLab (some free content; in-depth analysis by subscription), https://www.consumerlab.com/
- HerbList App, https://nccih.nih.gov/Health/HerbListApp?nav=govd
- National Center for Complementary and Integrative Health, http://nccih.nih.gov
- Natural Medicines, https://naturalmedicines.therapeuticresearch.com/
- NIH MedlinePlus, https://medlineplus.gov/druginfo/herb_All.html
- Office of Dietary Supplements, http://ods.od.nih.gov/

References

1. National Center for Complementary and Integrative Health. Complementary, Alternative, or Integrative Health: What's In a Name? Available from https://nccih.nih.gov/health/integrative-health#hed3.
2. Farnsworth NR, Akerele O, Bingel AS, Soejarto DD, Guo Z. Medicinal plants in therapy. Bull World Health Organ. 1985;63(6):965–81.
3. Nutrition Business Journal. 2019NBJ supplement business report2019. Available from https://www.nutritionbusinessjournal.com/reports/2019-nbj-supplement-business-report/.
4. Council for Responsible Nutrition. 2018.CRN Consumer Survey on Dietary Supplements2018. Available from: https://www.crnusa.org/CRNConsumerSurvey.
5. Smith TKK, Eckl V, Morton C, Stredney R. Herbal supplement sales in US increased 8.5% in 2017, topping $8 billion. HerbalGram. 2018;2018(119):62–71.
6. Office of Dietary Supplements. Dietary supplement health and education act of 1994. Available from https://ods.od.nih.gov/About/DSHEA_Wording.aspx.
7. Vamenta-Morris H, Dreisbach A, Shoemaker-Moyle M, Abdel-Rahman EM. Internet claims on dietary and herbal supplements in advanced nephropathy: truth or myth. Am J Nephrol. 2014;40(5):393–8.
8. Food and Drug Administration. Backgrounder on the final rule for current good manufacturing practices (CGMPs) for dietary supplements 2017. Available from https://www.fda.gov/food/current-good-manufacturing-practices-cgmps/backgrounder-final-rule-current-good-manufacturing-practices-cgmps-dietary-supplements.
9. Burrowes JD, Van Houten G. Use of alternative medicine by patients with stage 5 chronic kidney disease. Adv Chronic Kidney Dis. 2005;12(3):312–25.
10. Bahall M. Use of complementary and alternative medicine by patients with end-stage renal disease on haemodialysis in Trinidad: a descriptive study. BMC Complement Altern Med. 2017;17(1):250.
11. Osman NA, Hassanein SM, Leil MM, NasrAllah MM. Complementary and alternative medicine use among patients with chronic kidney disease and kidney transplant recipients. J Ren Nutr. 2015;25(6):466–71.
12. Jakimowicz-Tylicka M, Chmielewski M, Kuzmiuk-Glembin I, Skonieczny P, Dijakiewicz G, Zdrojewska G, et al. Dietary supplement use among patients with chronic kidney disease. Acta Biochim Pol. 2018;65(2):319–24.
13. Zyoud SH, Al-Jabi SW, Sweileh WM, Tabeeb GH, Ayaseh NA, Sawafta MN, et al. Use of complementary and alternative medicines in haemodialysis patients: a cross-sectional study from Palestine. BMC Complement Altern Med. 2016;16:204.
14. Markell MS. Potential benefits of complementary medicine modalities in patients with chronic kidney disease. Adv Chronic Kidney Dis. 2005;12(3):292–9.
15. Sabiu S, O'Neill FH, Ashafa AOT. The purview of phytotherapy in the management of kidney disorders: asystematic review on Nigeria and South Africa. Afr J Tradit Complement Altern Med. 2016;13(5):38–47.
16. Li X, Wang H. Chinese herbal medicine in the treatment of chronic kidney disease. Adv Chronic Kidney Dis. 2005;12(3):276–81.
17. Therapeutic Research Center. Natural medicines 2019. Available from www.naturalmedicines.com.
18. Ojewole JA. Analgesic, antiinflammatory and hypoglycaemic effects of ethanol extract of Zingiber officinale (Roscoe) rhizomes (Zingiberaceae) in mice and rats. Phytother Res. 2006;20(9):764–72.
19. Rangel-Huerta OD, Aguilera CM, Mesa MD, Gil A. Omega-3 long-chain polyunsaturated fatty acids supplementation on inflammatory biomakers: a systematic review of randomised clinical trials. Br J Nutr. 2012;107(Suppl 2):S159–70.
20. Kanbay M, Onal EM, Afsar B, Dagel T, Yerlikaya A, Covic A, et al. The crosstalk of gut microbiota and chronic kidney disease: role of inflammation, proteinuria, hypertension, and diabetes mellitus. Int Urol Nephrol. 2018;50(8):1453–66.
21. Simoes-Silva L, Araujo R, Pestana M, Soares-Silva I, Sampaio-Maia B. The microbiome in chronic kidney disease patients undergoing hemodialysis and peritoneal dialysis. Pharmacol Res. 2018;130:143–51.
22. Thongprayoon C, Kaewput W, Hatch ST, Bathini T, Sharma K, Wijarnpreecha K, et al. Effects of probiotics on inflammation and uremic toxins among patients on dialysis: asystematic review and meta-analysis. Dig Dis Sci. 2019;64(2):469–79.
23. Nauffal M, Gabardi S. Nephrotoxicity of natural products. Blood Purif. 2016;41(1–3):123–9.
24. Vanherweghem JL. Misuse of herbal remedies: the case of an outbreak of terminal renal failure in Belgium (Chinese herbs nephropathy). J Altern Complement Med. 1998;4(1):9–13.
25. Combest W, Newton M, Combest A, Kosier JH. Effects of herbal supplements on the kidney. Urol Nurs. 2005;25(5):381–6. 403
26. Rakel D. Using the evidence-versus-harm grading icons. In: Rakel D, editor. Integrative medicine. 4th ed. Philadelphia: Elsevier; 2018. p. xxv–xxvii.

Chapter 33
Vitamin and Trace Element Needs in Chronic Kidney Disease

Alison L. Steiber, Charles Chazot, and Joel D. Kopple

Keywords Vitamins · Minerals · Malnutrition · Dietary reference intake

> **Key Points**
> - Vitamin and trace element status may be altered in patients with chronic kidney disease.
> - Altered vitamin or trace element status may impact morbidity and mortality if untreated; thus, careful assessment and appropriate interventions must be conducted in this population.

Introduction

Malnutrition and the broader term of "protein–energy wasting" have the potential to impact not only macronutrient metabolism but also vitamin and trace element status in patients with chronic kidney disease (CKD). Nutrition professionals (often the registered dietitian nutritionist) use the Nutrition Care Process to assess, diagnose, intervene, and monitor their patients and clients. A thorough assessment is designed to understand three key items related to nutrition needs: (1) Has a nutrient deficiency been identified and is repletion necessary? (2) Is the diet inadequate to support the intake of key nutrients? (3) Are clinical conditions present that have or may cause an increased need in single or multiple nutrients? If any of these three factors are identified, the nutrition provider works with the healthcare team to determine how to prevent or treat a nutrient deficiency. Ideally, nutrition professionals use evidence-based nutrition practice guidelines as the foundation for their practice. However, guidelines are only as strong as the evidence used to create them. Therefore, it is imperative that research moves forward in nutrition to determine optimal nutrition care.

A. L. Steiber (✉)
Academy of Nutrition and Dietetics, Chicago, IL, USA
e-mail: asteiber@eatright.org

C. Chazot
NephroCare Tassin-Charcot, Sainte-Foy-lès-Lyon, France

J. D. Kopple
Professor Emeritus of Medicine and Public Health, University of California, Los Angeles, CA, USA

The Lundquist Institute for Biomedical Innovation at Harbor-UCLA Medical Center, Torrance, CA, USA

© Springer Nature Switzerland AG 2020
J. D. Burrowes et al. (eds.), *Nutrition in Kidney Disease*, Nutrition and Health,
https://doi.org/10.1007/978-3-030-44858-5_33

There is a paucity of evidence indicating that patients with CKD, on average, are inadequate in multiple nutrients and their clinical condition warrants increased nutrient intake. However, due to the high heterogeneity in the evidence, systematic reviews show little consensus in deficiency status and methods of treatment. While the systematic reviews show low evidence in vitamins and most minerals, there are examples of deficiency; vitamin K is just such an example of nutrient deficiency in CKD patients [1].

Data from the National Health and Nutrition Examination Survey (NHANES) [2] and the Modification of Diet in Renal Disease (MDRD) Study [3] showed that the daily ingestion of nutrients begins to decline as early as stage 3 CKD [2, 4, 5]. This reduction in intake may affect energy-producing nutrients (carbohydrates, protein, and fat), macrominerals, vitamins, and trace elements. However, more than intake alone affects vitamins and trace elements. Metabolic alterations in CKD patients may affect absorption, utilization, and excretion of micronutrients. Uremic toxicity, comorbidities, and finally the treatment of end-stage renal disease (ESRD) may all contribute to a heightened inflammatory status which affects the status of many micronutrients, especially those with antioxidant properties, such as vitamins C and E, retinol, and minerals such as selenium [2].

Whereas vitamin D nutrition has received substantial attention, less is written or known concerning the optimal intake of vitamins and trace elements in CKD. This lack of information may have important clinical consequences and lead to poor nutrition care. Clinicians may not recognize the risk of either inadequate intake or excessive body burden of nutrients and thus provide insufficient nutritional therapy or excessive supplementation of one or more vitamins or trace elements. Unfortunately, few vitamins, mineral, and trace elements have been extensively studied in the CKD population. Thus, the lower and upper ranges of body burden of these nutrients for their optimal metabolic functions are not known.

Three examples of nutrient alterations in advanced CKD patients are a high prevalence of deficiency with vitamin K, an increased need for vitamin B6 (pyridoxine hydrochloride) [6], and a reduced tolerance for vitamin A, due to excessive serum vitamin A levels and dietary intolerance to rather small increases in the intake of this vitamin [7]. In a study by Schlieper et al., the researchers determined which parameters predicted vitamin K status [1]. Patients with worsening vitamin K status had significantly lower body mass index (BMI), more years on dialysis, higher C-reactive protein (CRP) concentrations, and poorer survival [1]. Thus, those patients with lower body stores and higher inflammation had lower vitamin K serum concentrations and ultimately significantly increased risk of death [1]. This is an excellent example of why vitamin and mineral status should be assessed, problems identified and treated, and clinical symptoms monitored in the CKD population.

Determining the optimal nutritional status and recommended intake to maintain or replenish nutrient concentrations can be difficult and can require careful monitoring by knowledgeable nutrition providers. The purpose of this chapter is to assist nutrition providers to make more rational and informed clinical decisions, evidence-based where possible, regarding the vitamin and trace element status and nutritional needs of their CKD patients (Table 33.1).

Vitamin B1: Thiamin

Thiamin is a hydrophilic B vitamin involved with many metabolic functions such as serving as a cofactor for oxidative decarboxylation reactions. The dietary reference intake (DRI) for thiamin (age 50–70 years) is 1.2 and 1.1 mg/day for normal men and women, respectively [8]. Dietary sources of thiamin include pork, oat bran, whole grains, and enriched grains [9].

Thiamin and CKD: Dietary intake and nutritional status for thiamin in patients with CKD ($n = 14$) were assessed by Frank et al. [10]. Stages 4 and 5 CKD patients consumed an average of 1.26 mg of thiamin/day from the foods in their diet. The mean plasma thiamin concentration was 64.2 nmol/L,

Table 33.1 Recommendations/suggestions for daily vitamin supplement in patients with chronic kidney disease

Origin	Dietary reference intake [8, 33, 40]	Authors' suggestions	CARI [82]	Academy/KDOQI guidelines [12]	EBPG [83]	Academy/KDOQI guidelines [12]	Authors' suggestions	Authors' suggestions
	RDA in healthy subjects	Nephrotic syndrome	Nondialysis CKD patients	Nondialyzed CKD patients	MHD patients	MHD patients	MHD patients	CPD patients
Vitamin A	700–900 RE[a]	Up to RDA[b]		None	None	None	None[c]	None
Vitamin E	22.5 IU	Up to RDA[b]		None	400–800 IU	None	Up to the RDA[b]	400–800 IU
Vitamin K	80–120 µg	None		None	None	None	None[d]	None[d]
Vitamin B1	1.1–1.2 mg	Unknown[e]	>1 mg	Not specified	1.1–1.2 mg	Not specified	1.1–1.2 mg	1.1–1.2 mg
Riboflavin	1.1–1.3 mg	Unknown[e]	1–2 mg	Not specified	1.1–1.3 mg	Not specified	1.1–1.3 mg	1.1–1.3 mg
Vitamin B6	1.3–1.7 mg	5 mg	1.5–2 mg	Not specified	10 mg	Not specified	10 mg	10 mg[a]
Vitamin C	75–90 mg	75–90 mg		75–90 mg	75–90 mg	75–90 mg	75–90 mg	75–90 mg
Folic acid	400 µg	Unknown[e]		If clinical signs and symptoms	1 mg	If clinical signs and symptoms	1 mg	1 mg
Vitamin B12	2.4 µg	RDA			2.4 µg		2.4 µg	2.4 µg
Niacin	14–16 mg	Unknown[e]		Not specified	14–16 mg	Not specified	14–16 mg	14–16 mg
Biotin	30 µg	Unknown[e]		Not specified	30 µg	Not specified	30 µg	30 µg
Pantothenic acid	5 mg	Unknown[e]		Not specified	5 mg	Not specified	5 mg	5 mg

Adapted from Chazot et al. [84]

[a] Retinol equivalent

[b] For patients ingesting less than the DRI

[c] Recent data on vitamin A and survival question this usual recommendation

[d] 10 mg/d if prolonged antibiotic therapy or low food intake

[e] Insufficient data

and ETK-AC (erythrocyte transketolase activity coefficient, an indicator of thiamin adequacy) was 1.18 ± 0.19 (SD) (an ETK-AC indicating no deficiency is <1.20). ETK-AC has been regarded as a good functional indicator of thiamin status [11]. Thus, according to the data generated by Frank et al. [10], a substantial proportion of both CKD 4 and 5 patients had ETK-AC values greater than 1.20, indicating a thiamin-deficient status. While evidence does not indicate that all CKD patients are deficient in thiamin, it does suggest an increased risk and prevalence of insufficient or deficient concentrations in this population. Whether the DRI for normal adults is sufficient for patients with CKD is unknown. The recent systematic review by the Evidence Analysis Library of the Academy of Nutrition and Dietetics resulted in grade III evidence for thiamin supplementation, indicating that there is limited and unclear evidence for routine supplementation [12].

Vitamin B2: Riboflavin

Riboflavin is a water-soluble B vitamin with phosphorescent properties and promotes oxidation–reduction reactions. The DRI for riboflavin is 1.1 mg/day for women and 1.3 mg/day for men [8]. Some rich dietary sources of riboflavin are liver, duck, milk, eggs, mushrooms, spinach, chicken, and enriched grains [9].

Riboflavin and CKD: Porrini et al. [13] studied patients with advanced CKD who were not undergoing dialysis using the α-erythrocyte glutathione reductase stimulation index (α-EGR) to assess riboflavin status. In this study, 8% of patients were found to have elevated α-EGR, thus indicating riboflavin deficiency. When the prescribed protein intake of these patients was intentionally reduced to 1.0 or 0.6 g protein/kg/day, from the patients' usual intake, according to the research protocol, the prevalence of elevated α-EGR increased from 8% to 25% and 41%, respectively. The increased prevalence of elevated α-EGR was attributed to the fact that riboflavin is particularly abundant in foods containing animal proteins. Indeed, several works have recommended riboflavin supplements for CKD patients, especially when they ingest very low-protein diets (i.e., <0.6 g protein/kg/day) [5, 14, 15].

Niacin: Vitamin B3

Niacin is another water-soluble B vitamin that is ingested as either nicotinamide from animal sources or nicotinic acid from plant sources. These molecules are necessary cofactors for many oxidation–reduction reactions. Niacin also prevents and is the therapeutic agent for pellagra, which is a condition caused by niacin deficiency and often referred to by "the Ds": dermatitis, diarrhea, dementia, and death. Pellagra is associated with the chronic intake of low-riboflavin diets, alcoholism, and food faddism, and when untreated, maize is a primary staple of the diet [16]. The DRI for normal individuals is 14 mg/day for females and 16 mg/day for males [8]. Niacin is unusual in that it has an amino acid precursor, tryptophan; some of the tryptophan in the body is routinely converted to niacin. Thus, when niacin stores are low, the conversion of tryptophan can become a source of niacin. Primary food sources that are rich in niacin are meat, fish, legumes, coffee, and tea [9], all of which tend to be reduced in low-protein, low-phosphorus diets.

Niacin and CKD: It is possible that CKD patients who are prescribed low-protein diets (such as 0.6 g protein/kg/day) with phosphorus restriction (such as 800 mg/day) may be at increased risk for niacin deficiency due to the low niacin content of plant-based foods; thus, their dietary niacin intake may be quite low. However, the authors are unaware of any clinical trials that have examined the niacin intake of CKD patients and whether that amount is sufficient to maintain adequate niacin status.

Additionally, the niacin metabolite, nicotinamide, has been successfully used to reduce serum phosphorus concentrations in maintenance hemodialysis (MHD) patients using megadoses of niacin, 500–1500 mg/day given twice daily [17, 18].

The mechanisms of action involve the inhibition of the sodium/phosphorus type IIb cotransporter (NaPi-2b) and the type IIa cotransporter (NaPi-2a), which are the major transporters of inorganic phosphorus in the intestinal brush border, and in the proximal renal tubular epithelial cells of the kidneys, respectively [19, 20]. Therefore, it is likely that in nondialyzed CKD 3–5 patients, the action of nicotinamide on the NaPi-2b and NaPi-2a cotransporters not only will inhibit phosphorus absorption in the intestinal brush border but will also inhibit renal tubular phosphorus reabsorption and thereby increase phosphorus excretion in both feces and urine.

Nicotinamide use is associated with many side effects: most relevant are flushing; thrombocytopenia; hepatotoxicity (especially with sustained release doses); gastrointestinal symptoms such as diarrhea, vomiting, and constipation; and increased serum uric acid concentrations [20]. The increased serum uric acid may be of concern, because hyperuricemia has been associated with both hypertension and more rapid progression of renal failure [21]. In summary, while there is not sufficient evidence of niacin deficiency in CKD patients, those with chronically suboptimal dietary intake may benefit from a supplement at the DRI level to prevent deficiency.

Vitamin B6: Pyridoxine

Vitamin B6 exists in vivo as six compounds (i.e., pyridoxal, pyridoxine, pyridoxamine, and the 5′-phosphate derivatives of these three compounds). Pyridoxal-5′-phosphate (PLP) is a cofactor for many enzymes, particularly the ones involving amino acid metabolism. Possibly relevant to the anemia of CKD, PLP is a cofactor for (δ)-aminolevulinate synthase to initiate heme synthesis. The DRI for pyridoxine in men is 1.7 mg/day and for women is 1.5 mg/day [8]. Substantial dietary sources of vitamin B6 are liver, fish, meat, poultry, plums, bananas, plantains, barley, sweet potatoes, potatoes, and enriched grains [9].

B6 and CKD: Kopple et al. [6] conducted both dietary and biochemical assessments of pyridoxine status on patients with different stages of CKD. In a cross-sectional analysis, the amount of vitamin B6 consumed in foods declined as glomerular filtration rate (GFR) decreased, from 2.2 ± 0.8 (SD) mg/day in six patients with stages 3 and 4 CKD (serum creatinine from 2.1 to 3.5 mg/dL) to 1.2 ± 0.5 mg/day in seven nondialyzed patients with stages 4 and 5 CKD [6]. The mean intake of vitamin B6 for patients with severe CKD was significantly lower than the DRI for their age cohort. These declining intakes were reflected in the stimulation index of erythrocyte glutamic pyruvic transaminase (EGPT) activity. EGPT activity and the EGPT index are measurements of adequacy of body pyridoxine levels. An EGPT index greater than 1.25 is an indicator of vitamin B6 deficiency. The mean EGPT stimulation index rose (indicating vitamin B6 deficiency) inversely with the stage of CKD, where patients with higher GFR levels (CKD stages 3 and 4) had a mean EGPT index of 1.23 ± 0.09 (SD); CKD patients with lower GFR levels (stages 4 and 5) had a mean index of 1.30 ± 0.11. These were all significantly higher than the normal control values of 1.16 ± 0.06.

Podda et al. [22] found significantly lower serum PLP concentrations, 37.3 ± 51.7 versus 79.3 ± 65.6 pmol/mL, in patients with nephrotic syndrome as compared with healthy controls. The serum B6 values inversely correlated with the magnitude of proteinuria ($r = -0.41, p < 0.001$). These studies provide evidence that there are suboptimal levels of serum vitamin B6 in many patients with CKD.

Many medicines and other compounds can interfere with the actions or metabolism of vitamin B6 and may increase the likelihood that patients will develop B6 deficiency. This is especially likely to occur in CKD patients because their vitamin B6 intake is often low, they may have increased dietary needs for B6 [14], and it is likely that they may be prescribed some of these medicines. These interfering compounds include isoniazid, thyroxine, iproniazid, theophylline, hydralazine, caffeine, penicillamine, ethanol, and oral contraceptives. The data presented here suggests that patients at stage 3 CKD or higher are at increased risk for deficient concentrations of vitamin B6 and, therefore, should be supplemented adequately. It has been recommended by both the European Society of Parenteral and Enteral Nutrition (ESPEN) and Caring for Australians with Renal Impairment (CARI) guidelines that vitamin B6 be supplemented daily at a dose of 5 mg [23–25].

Folate

Folic acid is a pteroylmonoglutamic acid which provides methyl groups for pyrimidine and purine synthesis and is necessary for histidine catabolism and the conversion between glycine to serine and homocysteine to methionine, in addition to other processes. Deficiency of folic acid results in megaloblastic anemia. The DRI for both healthy males and females is 400 µg/day [8]. Dietary sources of folic acid are legumes, orange juice, spinach and other leafy greens, broccoli, beets, artichokes, papaya, and enriched grains [9].

Folic Acid and CKD: Low folate intake can be an important contributor to folate deficiency in CKD patients. The primary source of dietary folic acid is fresh green vegetables which, due to their high potassium content, are frequently restricted in the CKD diet. Medicines that interfere with folic acid and may lead to deficiency, particularly in people with low folate intakes, include barbiturates, primidone, cycloserine, pyrimethamine, diphenylhydantoin, triamterene, methotrexate, trimethoprim, Mysoline, pentamidine, salicylazosulfapyridine, and ethanol.

In advanced CKD (such as stages 4 and 5 prior to dialysis), the metabolism of folic acid or handling of its metabolites appears to be altered, although the cause and timing at which the alterations begin to occur are not well defined. Hannisdal et al. [26] compared the serum concentrations of folate and folic acid metabolites between healthy volunteers and nondialyzed patients with stages 3–5 CKD. Folate metabolites were analyzed by liquid chromatography–tandem mass spectrometry. The samples from patients with CKD had 22 to 30 times higher concentrations of folate metabolites than in sera from healthy volunteers [26]. These elevated serum metabolite levels may reflect impaired excretion rather than altered metabolism of folic acid.

The optimal or safe daily intake for folate for CKD patients prior to dialysis is unknown. Considering that there is currently no evidence for impaired folate activity or metabolism for nondialyzed people with stages 3–5 CKD, the daily intake for these individuals may be similar to that of people who do not have CKD. The recent evidence analysis library (EAL) systematic review which resulted in grade II evidence for folate indicated that while supplementation with folate does not decrease mortality in dialysis patients, it has been shown to decrease odds of CKD progression combined with all-cause mortality in patients with CKD stage 3 [12].

Cyanocobalamin: B12

Vitamin B12 is critical for two major reactions: (1) as a coenzyme in the reaction that converts homocysteine to methionine and (2) for the reaction that converts 1-methylmalonyl-CoA to succinyl-CoA [11]. B12 is unique because it requires an intrinsic factor for absorption by the brush border of the ileum [14]; therefore, patients with a history of stomach or bowel resection may, over time, become vitamin B12 deficient. The DRI for B12 is 2.4 µg/day for both men and women [8], and the primary dietary sources are liver, beef, chicken, eggs, trout, and salmon. Additionally, fortified foods, such as breakfast cereals, are also good sources of B12 [9].

B12 and CKD: In healthy adults, there is a 3- to 6-year body supply of B12 [11]. Therefore, if a healthy person consumed insufficient quantities of B12 for a short period of time (less than 3 years), they should not develop vitamin B12 deficiency. However, there are no data concerning the amount of B12 stored in the body in patients with CKD. A paucity of data has suggested that maintenance hemodialysis (MHD) patients respond favorably and quickly when they are supplemented with B12, even when the plasma values indicate normal ranges [27]. This may be related to the fact that plasma B12 concentrations are not a sensitive indicator of B12 status. Plasma methylmalonic acid and homocysteine are more sensitive indicators of B12 status.

Vitamin B12 is more abundant in high-protein foods. Thus, patients who consume low-protein or very low-protein diets for extended periods of time, for example, greater than 3 years, with no B12 supplementation, may become vitamin B12 deficient. Information on plasma and body levels of vitamin B12 is limited, and what data are available does not indicate that most or even many CKD patients are deficient. However, it may still be prudent to prescribe supplemental vitamin B12 equivalent to the DRI, i.e., about 3 µg/day, to CKD patients with prescribed diets low (0.6 g protein/day) or very low (0.3 g protein/day supplemented with keto acids and essential amino acids) in protein. However, the EAL systematic review on B12 resulted in grade III evidence with the conclusion being "Vitamin B12 supplementation increased vitamin B12 biomarkers, and there was evidence of a dose-response effect according to supplementation dosage. Most participants were vitamin B12 replete, but vitamin B12 status was not reported in all studies. Lack of comparison of results to a reference standard limits interpretation of findings" [12].

Homocysteine

Serum total homocysteine concentrations appear to be increased to roughly 1.5–2 times the upper limit of normal in the majority of stage 5 CKD patients [28]. While elevated homocysteine concentrations in the general, non-CKD population are associated with an increased incidence of adverse cardiovascular events and mortality [29], the relationship between this magnitude of elevated concentrations and adverse outcomes is less clear in CKD patients.

Hyperhomocysteinemia of this level has been associated with both increased and reduced mortality in the CKD population [30, 31], probably because of the interaction of serum homocysteine levels with protein–energy wasting.

Several clinical trials have tested treatment of stages 4 and 5 CKD patients with large doses of folic acid, pyridoxine HCl, and often vitamin B6 to reduce elevated plasma homocysteine levels. Perhaps the largest randomized prospective clinical trial with the longest follow-up concerning vitamins to lower homocysteine concentrations and improve clinical outcomes was the homocysteinemia in kidney and end-stage renal disease study (HOST) [28]. This was a randomized, double-blind, placebo-controlled trial conducted in 2056 Veterans Administration patients with stages 4 and 5 CKD who were not dialyzed ($n = 1305$) or who were undergoing MHD ($n = 751$) [28]. All patients were hyperhomocysteinemic (Hcy > 15 µmol/L) and they were randomized to receive daily treatment with 40 mg folic acid, 100 mg pyridoxine HCl, and 2 mg vitamin B12 or with placebo. Patients were treated for a mean of 4.5 years. Serum homocysteine levels decreased by 25.8% in the vitamin group ($p < 0.001$) as compared to the placebo group; however, there were no significant differences between the treatment group and the control group with regard to mortality, myocardial infarction, or amputations [28].

In a recently published study, 238 patients with diabetic nephropathy and nephrotic syndrome, stage 3 or earlier, were randomized to treatment with either placebo or a combination of folic acid 2.5 mg/day, pyridoxine HCl 25 mg/day, and vitamin B12 1 mg/day, for a mean of 31.9 months [32].

Patients randomized to vitamin treatment had a significantly faster decline in GFR (-16.5 ± 1.7 mL/min, mean change at 36 months) compared to patients receiving placebo (-10.7 ± 1.7 mL/min, $p = 0.045$). The patients taking the vitamins were significantly more likely to have a myocardial infarction, stroke, revascularization, or all-cause mortality [32].

Thus, there currently does not appear to be any clinical advantage to the routine use of megavitamin therapy to lower the modestly elevated serum homocysteine levels found in typical patients with advanced CKD.

Pantothenic Acid

Pantothenic acid is derived from pantothenate and is used in the synthesis of coenzyme A which is critical for many metabolic processes such as fatty acid oxidation, transport of proteins, and the formation of acetyl-CoA, a key molecule in energy metabolism [11]. There is inadequate information to determine a DRI for pantothenic acid for normal adults; however, the adequate intake (AI) level is set at 5 mg/day for men and women over 51 years of age [8]. Pantothenic acid appears to be ubiquitous in the food supply; the following foods are rich sources: beef, poultry, whole grains, potatoes, tomatoes, and broccoli [9].

Pantothenic Acid and CKD: There are currently no published reports demonstrating pantothenic acid deficiency in patients with CKD. Given the ubiquitous nature of pantothenic acid in the general food supply and the lack of evidence for insufficiency or deficiency in CKD patients, an intake beyond the AI level does not appear warranted.

Vitamin C

Vitamin C, or ascorbic acid, is a hydrophilic, six-carbon lactone that is capable of inhibiting the oxidation of other compounds by donating up to two electrons and, in the process, undergoing oxidation. Vitamin C scavenges reactive oxygen species in the body, thereby reducing the threat of cellular damage. The DRI for vitamin C is 75 mg/day for women and 90 mg/day for men [33]. Examples of dietary sources high in vitamin C are citrus fruits, berries, papaya, peppers, mangos, pineapple, broccoli, cauliflower, melons, greens, tomatoes, and tubers [9].

Vitamin C and CKD: Vitamin C intake is likely to be low in CKD patients because of dietary potassium restriction and because healthcare providers are often cautious in recommending vitamin C supplementation above the DRI due to the risk of increased oxalate production. Oxalate is a metabolite of both ascorbic acid and urine oxalate and is found in renal failure patients; serum oxalate may increase when individuals ingest supplemental ascorbic acid [14]. A direct correlation between serum ascorbic acid and serum oxalate concentrations has been reported in MHD patients. However, in a recent study of people without CKD who were at increased risk for oxalate formation, 500 mg/day of vitamin C did not increase 24-h urinary oxalate excretion [34]. To better assess the risk of supplemental ascorbic acid intakes, Chan et al. [35] conducted a study on the safety and efficacy of oral versus intravenous vitamin C administration in MHD patients and, not surprisingly, found no increase in the incidence of nephrolithiasis with 250 or 500 mg/day doses. Serum oxalate levels were not measured, and the possibility could not be ruled out that there might have been oxalate deposition in soft or other tissues.

Given the potential increase in oxidative stress due to uremic toxins and dialysis treatment, maintaining optimal concentrations of antioxidant status in CKD patients may improve clinical outcomes. In a study with peritoneal dialysis patients, ascorbic acid insufficiency and deficiency were demonstrated, respectively, in 74% and 44% of those individuals who were not receiving ascorbate supplements and in 22% and 17% of patients who were taking supplemental ascorbic acid, respectively [36]. A larger study by Zhang et al. [37] similarly demonstrated a high prevalence of vitamin C deficiency for both MHD and chronic peritoneal dialysis (CPD) patients who were not receiving ascorbic acid supplements, with 33% of patients deficient and 31% insufficient using plasma vitamin C values as the indicator. This study also showed an increased prevalence of clinical measures that are associated with suboptimal vitamin C status, such as elevated serum CRP and decreased serum prealbumin (transthyretin). Furthermore, in a recent meta-analysis where vitamin C was given at a dose of 500 mg to hemodialysis patients, this supplement was associated with an increase in hemoglobin levels and decreased doses of erythropoietin-stimulating agent [38]. The recent EAL systematic reviews on vitamin C showed limited evidence in the reduction of mortality, hospitalizations, and lipid parameters and limited evidence for increased quality of life [12].

Fat-Soluble Vitamins

Vitamin A

Vitamin A is a set of fat-soluble compounds classified as retinoids. Humans ingest preformed vitamin A (retinyl esters) or the vitamin A precursors, carotenoids. Retinal and retinoic acid (the acid form) are required for various reactions in the eye that support vision. Retinoic acid also promotes embryonic development, and retinoids are necessary for normal immune function. Carotenoids are composed of β-carotene, α-carotene, and β-cryptoxanthin [39] with β-carotene being the most common form of the carotenoids. β-Carotene can be converted to retinol; however, it has only approximately 50% of the activity of retinyl esters. The current recommended dietary allowance (RDA) for healthy men and women is 900 and 700 μg retinol activity equivalents (RAE)/day, respectively, and the upper safe limit is 3000 μg RAE/day [40]. Abundant dietary sources of vitamin A include liver, fish-liver oils, dairy products, butter, and eggs. β-Carotene is found in red- and yellow-colored fruits and vegetables such as cantaloupe, carrots, sweet potatoes, and winter squash and in dark-green leafy vegetables, such as spinach [9].

Vitamin A and CKD: A 2010 study in MHD patients and healthy controls compared lipid profiles, total antioxidant capacity, and vitamin A levels [41]. This study showed that both before and after a hemodialysis treatment, MHD patients had elevated serum values of vitamin A in comparison to the healthy controls (MHD patients, 133.2 ± 47.8 SD μg/dL before and 89.3 ± 39 μg/dL after hemodialysis; controls, 58.3 ± 11 μg/dL, $p < 0.05$). Potential mechanisms for the increased vitamin A levels include decreased catabolism of retinol-binding proteins. Frey et al. [42] showed that isoforms of retinol-binding protein 4 (the main transporter or retinol in blood) are increased in CKD, and this may partly explain elevated plasma concentrations in CKD patients. The NHANES III data demonstrated an association between elevated serum creatinine and elevated serum vitamin A concentrations [43]; this correlation was consistent across ethnicities and persisted after adjustment for confounding factors. This finding reinforces earlier studies that described elevated vitamin A levels in nondialyzed patients with CKD, ESRD patients, and kidney transplant recipients [44–46].

However, the story on vitamin A may be a bit more complicated. A recent cross-sectional analysis in peritoneal dialysis patients showed not only that these patients consume less vitamin A but that their vitamin A intake was associated with their serum levels of CRP, an inflammatory marker. Patients with high serum CRP had a significantly lower intake of vitamin A (207 vs. 522 μg/day) than those with a serum CRP within the normal range [47]. Furthermore, Espe et al. [7] demonstrated that patients with lower retinol status had significantly higher mortality. A similar relationship of serum vitamin A levels to mortality, both all cause and cardiovascular, was also found by Kalousova et al. [48].

Since serum vitamin A concentrations begin to increase when the serum creatinine starts to rise [42], there would seem to be no need to provide supplemental vitamin A for CKD patients, unless dietary intake is low or there is the unusual circumstance that serum retinol concentrations are below normal. This is consistent with the current recommendations against the need for supplemental vitamin A in CKD unless the patient is commonly ingesting less than the RDA for vitamin A [24]. In this latter circumstance, a supplement to increase vitamin A intake to the RDA can be given [14].

Vitamin E

Vitamin E is a fat-soluble vitamin that typically resides in cell membranes. It acts as an antioxidant, and it remains highly stable even after it scavenges free radicals. Vitamin E exists in four forms, α-tocopherol, β-tocopherol, γ-tocopherol, and δ-tocopherol; however, only α-tocopherol has an established RDA. The DRI for vitamin E (α-tocopherol) is 15 mg/day for both normal men and women [33]. Dietary sources of vitamin E are vegetable oils, unprocessed grains, nuts, fruits, vegetables, and meat [9].

Vitamin E and CKD: It has become increasingly evident that oxidative stress may act as a pathological agent in a number of disease states, and vitamin E has been considered as a potential treatment for this condition. Plasma vitamin E levels in CKD patients do not appear to be different from healthy controls [49, 50], even when dietary intake of vitamin E is reduced [50]. The results of clinical trials evaluating the effectiveness of vitamin E for the prevention of cardiovascular disease in people with CKD have been mixed.

Mann et al. [51] examined the outcomes in patients with mild–moderate kidney failure (serum creatinine, 1.4–2.3 mg/dL; approximately stage 3 CKD) and increased risk for cardiovascular events who were given 400 IU/day of vitamin E as part of the Heart Outcomes Prevention Evaluation (HOPE) trial. Patients with and without CKD in the HOPE trial were selected to be at higher risk for adverse cardiovascular events. Consistent with the findings in the HOPE trial, in patients who did not have CKD, there was no cardiovascular benefit to taking this dose of vitamin E. Moreover, the long-term use of this dose (400 IU/day or 363 mg/day) of supplemental vitamin E in individuals with or without CKD in the HOPE trial resulted in an increased incidence of heart failure, heart failure-related hospitalizations, and all-cause mortality (RR 1.13; 95% CI 1.01–1.26, $p = 0.03$ [39, 40]. This increased risk was associated with vitamin E intakes as low as 150 IU/day (136 mg/day) [52, 53].

Two studies examined vitamin E use as an antioxidant in MHD patients [54]. In the Boaz et al. [54] study, MHD patients ($n = 196$) were randomized to receive either an oral dose of vitamin E, 800 IU/day, or a placebo and followed for a median of 519 days. Treatment with vitamin E resulted in a reduction of the primary end point, a cardiovascular composite score (16% vs. 33%, $p = 0.014$). A more recent, but much smaller, study ($n = 80$) examined treatment with both silymarin and vitamin E for 21 days on plasma malondialdehyde (MDA), red blood cell glutathione peroxidase, and hemoglobin levels. Supplementation led to a significant decrease in MDA and an increase in red blood cell glutathione peroxidase and hemoglobin levels [55].

In the recent EAL systematic reviews, vitamin E was not shown to decrease mortality or cardiovascular outcomes in CKD patients in stages 1–5 [12].

Vitamin K

Vitamin K participates in post-translational carboxylation enabling the protein to bind to calcium and interact with other compounds. This is a necessary step for processes involving calcium interactions such as blood clotting and bone mineralization. The dietary form of vitamin K is phylloquinone.

Phylloquinone is absorbed in the jejunum and ileum and is primarily stored in the liver. Bacteria in the gut also produce vitamin K in the form of menaquinones which are absorbed from the distal bowel and stored in the liver. If vitamin K deficiency occurs, body proteins may be undercarboxylated. Carboxylation status of proteins, such as osteocalcin, can be measured and used to diagnose vitamin K deficiency. The normal AI for vitamin K is 90 µg/day for females and 120 µg/day for males. Formally, enough vitamin K was thought to be produced in the intestinal tract to prevent frank vitamin K deficiency even in the absence of dietary vitamin K intake. Newer evidence (see below) has led to a revision in this thinking. Dietary sources of vitamin K are green vegetables, cabbage, and plant oils [9].

Vitamin K and CKD: A decrease in dietary intake of vitamin K (phylloquinones) and/or a reduction in vitamin K production by gut bacteria can lower vitamin K levels. Antibiotics that suppress gut flora, and hence bacterial production of vitamin K, may increase the risk of vitamin K deficiency and impair blood clotting. This is especially likely to happen if the patient is also not eating or taking vitamin supplements and, therefore, has a low vitamin K intake. Two new studies have provided clinicians with evidence suggesting that a large proportion of patients with CKD may be deficient in vitamin K.

The first study by Holden et al. [56] in 172 patients with CKD stages 3–5 found that, depending on the vitamin K indicator used, 6% to 97% of patients were vitamin K deficient. When serum phylloquinone was used as a measure of adequate vitamin K status, a 6% deficiency was found in this population. However, when the measurement was the more *sensitive* marker, the percentage of the osteocalcin protein that is undercarboxylated (%ucOC), 60% of the patients were found to be deficient in vitamin K. Finally, when protein induced by vitamin K absence (PIVKA)-II, a less used but a potentially very accurate marker of vitamin K status, was measured, 97% of the patients were found to be deficient [56].

In the second study by Schlieper et al. [1], 64% of MHD patients ($n = 188$) were identified as deficient in vitamin K using PIVKA-II as an indicator. As mentioned at the beginning of this chapter, when MHD patients were categorized according to their serum desphospho-carboxylated matrix Gla-protein (MGP), those patients with serum values below 6139 pmol/L had significantly worse survival. Furthermore, when 17 patients were supplemented with oral doses of 135 µg/day of menaquinone-7 for 2 weeks, serum PIVKA-II decreased significantly, from 5.6 ± 3.2 to 3.4 ± 2.2 ng/mL, $p < 0.001$ [1].

These studies suggest that a large number of nondialyzed CKD patients as well as maintenance dialysis patients are deficient in vitamin K and may benefit from vitamin K supplements. Further studies need to be conducted to confirm the optimal doses and duration for such vitamin K supplements. In the recent EAL systematic reviews, vitamin K indicators are shown to improve in a dose-dependent manner with supplementation [12].

Minerals and Trace Elements

Many minerals, including iron, calcium, manganese, magnesium, chromium, copper, selenium, phosphorus, and zinc, are essential nutrients and necessary components to metabolism in healthy individuals and in CKD patients. However, some trace minerals when ingested can be nephrotoxic; these include arsenic [57], cadmium [58], chromium [59], germanium [60], lead [61], mercury [62], and silicon [62]. Supplements with these minerals should not be taken by CKD patients. Serum levels of some trace minerals appear to decline as kidney failure progresses; examples of these include calcium, copper, selenium, and zinc [63, 64]. It is noteworthy that copper, selenium, and zinc are all associated with lipid peroxidation, and patients with kidney failure can have augmented lipid peroxidation [65–67]. In a recent study by Guo et al. [68], chronic dialysis patients had significantly higher levels of MDA and superoxide dismutase (SOD) when compared with healthy controls, suggesting increased lipid peroxidation. The increased peroxidation may be attributed to uremic toxins, inflammatory and oxidant processes, nutrient imbalances, iron supplementation, or possibly other unrecognized factors [69].

Copper

Copper is a necessary cofactor for many enzymes including ferroxidases which facilitate iron binding to transferrin by changing its oxidation state. The DRI for copper is 900 µg/day for healthy individuals, and the upper safe limit for dietary intake is 10,000 µg/day. Abundant dietary sources of copper are organ meats, seafoods, nuts, seeds, whole grains, and cocoa.

Copper and CKD: Copper deficiency has been associated with cardiovascular dysfunction [70], and conversely, copper toxicity has been associated with lipid peroxidation and accelerated atherogenesis [71]. Very high serum copper levels may cause hemolysis. Yilmaz et al. [63] measured erythrocyte copper concentrations in patients at stages 1 through 5 CKD and found concentrations to be decreased as kidney failure progressed. In stage 1 CKD patients, the mean erythrocyte copper concentration was 0.9 ± 0.2 (SD) µg/mL. In stage 5 (not dialyzed) CKD, the mean concentration was 0.24 ± 0.7. These values were significantly lower than in the control group which had a mean erythrocyte copper concentration of 1.06 ± 0.14 µg/mL. In these same patients, serum MDA levels rose with increasing stages of CKD. At stage 1 CKD, MDA was 2.48 ± 0.49 nmol/mL as compared to stage 5 CKD, where the concentration was 8.06 ± 0.52 nmol/mL. Guo et al. [68] reported that continuous ambulatory peritoneal dialysis patients, had higher serum copper concentrations than did healthy controls (0.90 ± 0.25 vs. 0.53 ± 0.14 µg/mL, $p < 0.05$) and higher copper to zinc ratios (1.97 ± 1.31 vs. 0.67 ± 0.21, $p < 0.05$). As expected the peritoneal dialysis patients also had higher MDA concentrations (4.90 ± 2.12 vs. 2.24 ± 0.76 nmol/L, $p < 0.05$). We are unaware of any clinical trials that measure the effect of copper supplementation on MDA in CKD patients.

Molybdenum

Molybdenum is involved in the metabolism of purines, pyrimidines, pteridines, aldehydes, and oxidation [72]. Excessive intakes of molybdenum may be associated with hypercalcemia and hyperparathyroidism [73]. Interestingly, Smythe et al. [74] found significantly elevated molybdenum concentrations in the liver of uremic patients versus healthy control subjects (4.75 ± 2.05 µg/g vs. 3.52 ± 1.72, $p < 0.05$). However, at present there is insufficient evidence to indicate molybdenum supplementation or restriction is warranted in CKD patients. The DRI for molybdenum is 45 µg/day for men and women over the age of 30 years.

Magnesium

Magnesium is also a cofactor for many enzymes. The DRI for magnesium is 420 mg/day for men and 320 mg/day for women. Abundant dietary sources of magnesium are wheat bran, almonds, spinach, cashews, and soybeans.

Magnesium and CKD: There are some case study reports of patients with hypercalciuria and nephrocalcinosis who may have hypomagnesemia. These patients are characterized by low serum magnesium, normal to high urinary magnesium, high urinary calcium, and normal circulating calcium, potassium, and acid–base balance [75]. There is insufficient evidence to suggest a need for magnesium supplements for CKD patients except for rare cases of magnesium-losing disorders associated with kidney disease [75]. Endogenous magnesium is largely excreted by the kidneys, and in renal insufficiency, magnesium supplements could engender hypermagnesemia.

Manganese

Manganese is also a cofactor for enzymes and it is important in brain function, collagen synthesis, bone growth, urea synthesis, and glucose and lipid metabolism. The DRI for manganese is 2.3 mg/day for men and 1.8 mg/day for women with an upper safe limit of 11 mg/day. Major dietary sources of manganese are whole grains, nuts, leafy vegetables, and teas.

Manganese and CKD: One small study examined the relationship between serum manganese and neurological basal ganglia changes in MHD patients and observed that all five patients with these neurological disorders had elevated serum manganese as compared to controls [76]. The patients with elevated serum manganese were more likely to have pathological changes in the basal ganglia and, for example, Parkinson's symptoms. There are no published studies indicating abnormally low serum manganese concentrations in CKD patients.

Selenium

Selenium is a cofactor for such enzymes as glutathione peroxidase, 5′-deiodinase, and thioredoxin reductase and, as such, helps to protect cells against destruction by hydrogen peroxide and free radicals [77]. The DRI is 55 μg/day for both women and men. Major dietary sources are grains, meat, Brazil nuts, poultry, fish, and dairy products.

Selenium and CKD: Deficiency has been associated with many adverse side effects such as anemia, cancer, cardiovascular disease, immune dysfunction, and skeletal myopathy [14]. Smythe et al. [74] found differences between healthy normal subjects in Australia and the United States, with Australians having significantly lower selenium concentrations in all tissues measured. Additionally, in patients with advanced renal failure, these investigators found some organs with significantly lower concentrations of selenium (e.g., in the heart and lungs) but with significantly higher concentrations in the brain. Both whole blood and plasma selenium concentrations were significantly reduced in CKD patients as compared to healthy controls at the baseline of a clinical trial conducted by Zachara et al. [78]. In this study, the supplementation of CKD patients with 200 μg of selenium per day for 3 months resulted in marked increases in red cell and whole blood concentrations. Furthermore, baseline plasma glutathione peroxidase activity was 37% lower ($p < 0.0001$) than healthy controls at baseline, and, following supplementation, the activity of this enzyme increased by 15% ($p < 0.05$). Similar results were found by Yilmaz et al. [63]; they found selenium concentrations and glutathione peroxidase activity to significantly decline as the CKD stage rose. In a 2010 study, serum selenium concentrations were found to be below the normal range (60–120 μg/L) in 98.7% of MHD patients studied ($n = 81$, mean serum selenium $= 18.8 \pm 17.4$ μg/L) [79]. After supplementation with one Brazil nut per day (with an average selenium content of 290.5 μg per nut) for 3 months, the mean serum selenium concentration increased to $104 + 65$ μg/L, a change that was highly statistically significant ($p < 0.0001$) and which brought serum values to within the normal range. These studies indicate that selenium deficiency may not be uncommon in both nondialyzed CKD patients and MHD dialysis patients, and that supplementation can replete stores to normal values and increase glutathione peroxidase activity. While these results are of interest, the recent EAL systematic reviews on selenium supplementation in CKD patients did seem to improve interleukin-6 (IL-6), but had no other benefit in inflammatory markers and did not show any other benefit to comorbidities; however, the evidence was limited [12].

Zinc

Zinc is a cofactor for dozens of enzymes that facilitate the synthesis of large numbers of proteins as well as other compounds. Zinc is a necessary building block for hundreds of proteins; its function includes catalysis, regulation, and structural activities. The DRI for zinc is 8 mg/day for women and 11 mg/day for men. Zinc is found in foods with higher protein contents such as beef, liver, and poultry, and also whole grains.

Zinc and CKD: Piper [80] suggested that zinc supplementation may be necessary for patients fed very low-protein diets. However, Smythe et al. [74] found no significant difference in tissue concentrations of zinc between healthy controls and CKD patients. In contrast, McGregor [81] found decreased plasma zinc concentrations in CKD patients. Yilmaz [63] found a stepwise reduction in erythrocyte zinc levels with advancing stages of CKD. The recent EAL systematic reviews on zinc in CKD patients showed limited and unclear impact on most parameters, but did seem to increase high-density lipoprotein (HDL) cholesterol and serum albumin concentration [12].

Conclusion

Knowledge of vitamin and mineral requirements for patients with CKD remains incomplete. Given the data reviewed in this chapter, it would seem reasonable to state that many patients with CKD may be at risk for altered vitamin and mineral status. This may be particularly true for stages 4 and 5 CKD patients and MHD and CPD patients. Observational trials describing micronutrient status, dose–response pharmacological trials, and finally double-blind, randomized prospective clinical trials testing the effect of supplements with vitamins and trace elements need to be conducted before nutrient-specific recommendations for CKD patients can be generated with confidence. As suggested above, much work needs to be done to ascertain the sufficiently accurate and sensitive methods for determining nutritional adequacy for these nutrients. Until such time, micronutrient status, especially in those patients receiving low- or very low-protein diets, should be given careful consideration. Dietary, physical, and biochemical assessments should be routinely conducted in CKD patients as they approach stages 3 and below to ensure optimal nutritional care.

References

1. Schlieper G, Westenfeld R, Kruger T, Cranenburg EC, Magdeleyns EJ, Brandenburg VM, et al. Circulating non-phosphorylated carboxylated matrix gla protein predicts survival in ESRD. J Am Soc Nephrol. 2011;22(2):387–95.
2. Weiner DE, Tighiouart H, Elsayed EF, Griffith JL, Salem DN, Levey AS, et al. The relationship between nontraditional risk factors and outcomes in individuals with stage 3 to 4 CKD. Am J Kidney Dis. 2008;51(2):212–23.
3. Kopple JD, Greene T, Chumlea WC, Hollinger D, Maroni BJ, Merrill D, et al. Relationship between nutritional status and the glomerular filtration rate: results from the MDRD study. Kidney Int. 2000;57(4):1688–703.
4. Eustace JA, Astor B, Muntner PM, Ikizler TA, Coresh J. Prevalence of acidosis and inflammation and their association with low serum albumin in chronic kidney disease. Kidney Int. 2004;65(3):1031–40.
5. Kovesdy CP, Anderson JE, Kalantar-Zadeh K. Association of serum bicarbonate levels with mortality in patients with non-dialysis-dependent CKD. Nephrol Dial Transplant. 2009;24(4):1232–7.
6. Kopple JD, Mercurio K, Blumenkrantz MJ, Jones MR, Tallos J, Roberts C, et al. Daily requirement for pyridoxine supplements in chronic renal failure. Kidney Int. 1981;19(5):694–704.
7. Espe KM, Raila J, Henze A, Krane V, Schweigert FJ, Hocher B, et al. Impact of vitamin A on clinical outcomes in haemodialysis patients. Nephrol Dial Transplant. 2011;26(12):4054–61.
8. Institute of Medicine (U.S.). Standing Committee on the Scientific Evaluation of Dietary Reference Intakes, Institute of Medicine (U.S.). Panel on Folate Other B Vitamins and Choline, Institute of Medicine (U.S.). Subcommittee on

Upper Reference Levels of Nutrients. Dietary reference intakes for thiamin, riboflavin, niacin, vitamin B6, folate, vitamin B12, pantothenic acid, biotin, and choline. Washington, DC: National Academy Press; 1998.

9. Combs G. The vitamins, fundamental aspects in nutrition and health. New York: Academic; 1998.

10. Frank T, Czeche K, Bitsch R, Stein G. Assessment of thiamin status in chronic renal failure patients, transplant recipients and hemodialysis patients receiving a multivitamin supplementation. Int J Vitam Nutr Res. 2000;70(4):159–66.

11. Institute of Medicine. For thiamin, riboflavin, niacin, vitamin B6, folate, B12, pantothenic acid, biotin/choline. Washington, DC: National Academies Press; 2000.

12. Ikizler TA, Burrowes J, Byham-Gray L, Campbell K, Carrero JJ, Chan W, et al. KDOQI Nutrition in CKD Guideline Work Group. KDOQI clinical practice guideline for nutrition in CKD: 2020 update. Am J Kidney Dis. 2020; in press.

13. Porrini M, Simonetti P, Ciappellano S, Testolin G, Gentile MG, Manna G, et al. Thiamin, riboflavin and pyridoxine status in chronic renal insufficiency. Int J Vitam Nutr Res. 1989;59(3):304–8.

14. Joel D, Kopple SGM. Kopple and Massry's nutritional management of renal disease. 2nd ed. Philadelphia: Lippincott Williams & Wilkins; 2004.

15. Andreucci VE, Fissell RB, Bragg-Gresham JL, Ethier J, Greenwood R, Pauly M, et al. Dialysis Outcomes and Practice Patterns Study (DOPPS) data on medications in hemodialysis patients. Am J Kidney Dis. 2004;44(5 Suppl 2):61–7.

16. Seal AJ, Creeke PI, Dibari F, Cheung E, Kyroussis E, Semedo P, et al. Low and deficient niacin status and pellagra are endemic in postwar Angola. Am J Clin Nutr. 2007;85(1):218–24.

17. Takahashi Y, Tanaka A, Nakamura T, Fukuwatari T, Shibata K, Shimada N, et al. Nicotinamide suppresses hyperphosphatemia in hemodialysis patients. Kidney Int. 2004;65(3):1099–104.

18. Cheng SC, Young DO, Huang Y, Delmez JA, Coyne DW. A randomized, double-blind, placebo-controlled trial of niacinamide for reduction of phosphorus in hemodialysis patients. Clin J Am Soc Nephrol. 2008;3(4):1131–8.

19. Laroche M, Boyer JF. Phosphate diabetes, tubular phosphate reabsorption and phosphatonins. Joint Bone Spine. 2005;72(5):376–81.

20. Berns JS. Niacin and related compounds for treating hyperphosphatemia in dialysis patients. Semin Dial. 2008;21(3):203–5.

21. Feig DI. Uric acid and hypertension in adolescents. Semin Nephrol. 2005;25(1):32–8.

22. Podda GM, Lussana F, Moroni G, Faioni EM, Lombardi R, Fontana G, et al. Abnormalities of homocysteine and B vitamins in the nephrotic syndrome. Thromb Res. 2007;120(5):647–52.

23. Pollock C, McMahon L. The CARI guidelines. Biochemical and haematological targets guidelines. Haemoglobin. Nephrology. 2005;10(Suppl 4):S108–15.

24. Cano N, Fiaccadori E, Tesinsky P, Toigo G, Druml W, Kuhlmann M, et al. ESPEN guidelines on enteral nutrition: adult renal failure. Clin Nutr. 2006;25(2):295–310.

25. Pollock C, Voss D, Hodson E, Crompton C. The CARI guidelines. Nutrition and growth in kidney disease. Nephrology. 2005;10(Suppl 5):S177–230.

26. Hannisdal R, Ueland PM, Svardal A. Liquid chromatography-tandem mass spectrometry analysis of folate and folate catabolites in human serum. Clin Chem. 2009;55(6):1147–54.

27. Bastow MD, Woods HF, Walls J. Persistent anemia associated with reduced serum vitamin B12 levels in patients undergoing regular hemodialysis therapy. Clin Nephrol. 1979;11(3):133–5.

28. Jamison RL, Hartigan P, Kaufman JS, Goldfarb DS, Warren SR, Guarino PD, et al. Effect of homocysteine lowering on mortality and vascular disease in advanced chronic kidney disease and end-stage renal disease: a randomized controlled trial. JAMA. 2007;298(10):1163–70.

29. Menon V, Wang X, Greene T, Beck GJ, Kusek JW, Selhub J, et al. Homocysteine in chronic kidney disease: effect of low protein diet and repletion with B vitamins. Kidney Int. 2005;67(4):1539–46.

30. Suliman M, Stenvinkel P, Qureshi AR, Kalantar-Zadeh K, Barany P, Heimburger O, et al. The reverse epidemiology of plasma total homocysteine as a mortality risk factor is related to the impact of wasting and inflammation. Nephrol Dial Transplant. 2007;22(1):209–17.

31. Mallamaci F, Zoccali C, Tripepi G, Fermo I, Benedetto FA, Cataliotti A, et al. Hyperhomocysteinemia predicts cardiovascular outcomes in hemodialysis patients. Kidney Int. 2002;61(2):609–14.

32. House AA, Eliasziw M, Cattran DC, Churchill DN, Oliver MJ, Fine A, et al. Effect of B-vitamin therapy on progression of diabetic nephropathy: a randomized controlled trial. JAMA. 2010;303(16):1603–9.

33. Institute of Medicine (U.S.). Panel on Dietary Antioxidants and Related Compounds. Dietary reference intakes for vitamin C, vitamin E, selenium, and carotenoids: a report of the Panel on Dietary Antioxidants and Related Compounds, Subcommittees on Upper Reference Levels of Nutrients and of Interpretation and Use of Dietary Reference Intakes, and the Standing Committee on the Scientific Evaluation of Dietary Reference Intakes, Food and Nutrition Board, Institute of Medicine. Washington, DC: National Academy Press; 2000.

34. Moyad MA, Combs MA, Crowley DC, Baisley JE, Sharma P, Vrablic AS, et al. Vitamin C with metabolites reduce oxalate levels compared to ascorbic acid: a preliminary and novel clinical urologic finding. Urol Nurs. 2009;29(2):95–102.

35. Chan D, Irish A, Dogra G. Efficacy and safety of oral versus intravenous ascorbic acid for anaemia in haemodialysis patients. Nephrology (Carlton). 2005;10(4):336–40.

36. Singer R, Rhodes HC, Chin G, Kulkarni H, Ferrari P. High prevalence of ascorbate deficiency in an Australian peritoneal dialysis population. Nephrology (Carlton). 2008;13(1):17–22.

37. Zhang K, Liu L, Cheng X, Dong J, Geng Q, Zuo L. Low levels of vitamin C in dialysis patients is associated with decreased prealbumin and increased C-reactive protein. BMC Nephrol. 2011;12:18.

38. Deved V, Poyah P, James MT, Tonelli M, Manns BJ, Walsh M, et al. Ascorbic acid for anemia management in hemodialysis patients: a systematic review and meta-analysis. Am J Kidney Dis. 2009;54(6):1089–97.

39. Intakes CDR. Dietary reference intakes for vitamin C, vitamin E, selenium, and carotenoids. Washington, DC: National Academy Press; 2000.

40. Institute of Medicine (U.S.). Panel on Micronutrients. DRI: dietary reference intakes for vitamin A, vitamin K, arsenic, boron, chromium, copper, iodine, iron, manganese, molybdenum, nickel, silicon, vanadium, and zinc : a report of the Panel on Micronutrients … and the Standing Committee on the Scientific Evaluation of Dietary Reference Intakes, Food and Nutrition Board, Institute of Medicine. Washington, DC: National Academy Press; 2001.

41. Montazerifar F, Hashemi M, Karajibani M, Dikshit M. Hemodialysis alters lipid profiles, total antioxidant capacity, and vitamins A, E, and C concentrations in humans. J Med Food. 2010;13(6):1490–3.

42. Frey SK, Nagl B, Henze A, Raila J, Schlosser B, Berg T, et al. Isoforms of retinol binding protein 4 (RBP4) are increased in chronic diseases of the kidney but not of the liver. Lipids Health Dis. 2008;7:29.

43. Chen J, He J, Ogden LG, Batuman V, Whelton PK. Relationship of serum antioxidant vitamins to serum creatinine in the US population. Am J Kidney Dis. 2002;39(3):460–8.

44. Smith FR, Goodman DS. The effects of diseases of the liver, thyroid, and kidneys on the transport of vitamin a in human plasma. J Clin Invest. 1971;50(11):2426–36.

45. Yatzidis H, Digenis P, Fountas P. Hypervitaminosis A accompanying advanced chronic renal failure. Br Med J. 1975;3(5979):352–3.

46. Kelleher J, Humphrey CS, Homer D, Davison AM, Giles GR, Losowsky MS. Vitamin A and its transport proteins in patients with chronic renal failure receiving maintenance haemodialysis and after renal transplantation. Clin Sci (Lond). 1983;65(6):619–26.

47. Martin-Del-Campo F, Batis-Ruvalcaba C, Gonzalez-Espinoza L, Rojas-Campos E, Angel JR, Ruiz N, et al. Dietary micronutrient intake in peritoneal dialysis patients: relationship with nutrition and inflammation status. Perit Dial Int. 2012;32(2):183–91.

48. Kalousova M, Kubena AA, Kostirova M, Vinglerova M, Ing OM, Dusilova-Sulkova S, et al. Lower retinol levels as an independent predictor of mortality in long-term hemodialysis patients: a prospective observational cohort study. Am J Kidney Dis. 2010;56(3):513–21.

49. Karamouzis I, Sarafidis PA, Karamouzis M, Iliadis S, Haidich AB, Sioulis A, et al. Increase in oxidative stress but not in antioxidant capacity with advancing stages of chronic kidney disease. Am J Nephrol. 2008;28(3):397–404.

50. Galli F, Buoncristiani U, Conte C, Aisa C, Floridi A. Vitamin E in uremia and dialysis patients. Ann N Y Acad Sci. 2004;1031:348–51.

51. Mann JF, Lonn EM, Yi Q, Gerstein HC, Hoogwerf BJ, Pogue J, et al. Effects of vitamin E on cardiovascular outcomes in people with mild-to-moderate renal insufficiency: results of the HOPE study. Kidney Int. 2004;65(4):1375–80.

52. Lonn E, Bosch J, Yusuf S, Sheridan P, Pogue J, Arnold JM, et al. Effects of long-term vitamin E supplementation on cardiovascular events and cancer: a randomized controlled trial. JAMA. 2005;293(11):1338–47.

53. Miller ER III, Pastor-Barriuso R, Dalal D, Riemersma RA, Appel LJ, Guallar E. Meta-analysis: high-dosage vitamin E supplementation may increase all-cause mortality. Ann Intern Med. 2005;142(1):37–46.

54. Boaz M, Smetana S, Weinstein T, Matas Z, Gafter U, Iaina A, et al. Secondary prevention with antioxidants of cardiovascular disease in endstage renal disease (SPACE): randomised placebo-controlled trial. Lancet. 2000;356(9237):1213–8.

55. Roozbeh J, Shahriyari B, Akmali M, Vessal G, Pakfetrat M, Raees Jalali GA, et al. Comparative effects of silymarin and vitamin E supplementation on oxidative stress markers, and hemoglobin levels among patients on hemodialysis. Ren Fail. 2011;33(2):118–23.

56. Holden RM, Morton AR, Garland JS, Pavlov A, Day AG, Booth SL. Vitamins K and D status in stages 3–5 chronic kidney disease. Clin J Am Soc Nephrol. 2010;5(4):590–7.

57. Prasad GV, Rossi NF. Arsenic intoxication associated with tubulointerstitial nephritis. Am J Kidney Dis. 1995;26(2):373–6.

58. Griffin JL, Walker LA, Troke J, Osborn D, Shore RF, Nicholson JK. The initial pathogenesis of cadmium induced renal toxicity. FEBS Lett. 2000;478(1–2):147–50.

59. Dartsch PC, Hildenbrand S, Kimmel R, Schmahl FW. Investigations on the nephrotoxicity and hepatotoxicity of trivalent and hexavalent chromium compounds. Int Arch Occup Environ Health. 1998;71(Suppl):S40–5.

60. Takeuchi A, Yoshizawa N, Oshima S, Kubota T, Oshikawa Y, Akashi Y, et al. Nephrotoxicity of germanium compounds: report of a case and review of the literature. Nephron. 1992;60(4):436–42.

61. Staessen JA, Nawrot T, Hond ED, Thijs L, Fagard R, Hoppenbrouwers K, et al. Renal function, cytogenetic measurements, and sexual development in adolescents in relation to environmental pollutants: a feasibility study of biomarkers. Lancet. 2001;357(9269):1660–9.
62. Nuyts GD, Van Vlem E, Thys J, De Leersnijder D, D'Haese PC, Elseviers MM, et al. New occupational risk factors for chronic renal failure. Lancet. 1995;346(8966):7–11.
63. Yilmaz MI, Saglam M, Caglar K, Cakir E, Sonmez A, Ozgurtas T, et al. The determinants of endothelial dysfunction in CKD: oxidative stress and asymmetric dimethylarginine. Am J Kidney Dis. 2006;47(1):42–50.
64. Cuppari L, Carvalho AB, Draibe SA. Vitamin D status of chronic kidney disease patients living in a sunny country. J Ren Nutr. 2008;18(5):408–14.
65. Durak I, Akyol O, Basesme E, Canbolat O, Kavutcu M. Reduced erythrocyte defense mechanisms against free radical toxicity in patients with chronic renal failure. Nephron. 1994;66(1):76–80.
66. Mimic-Oka J, Simic T, Djukanovic L, Reljic Z, Davicevic Z. Alteration in plasma antioxidant capacity in various degrees of chronic renal failure. Clin Nephrol. 1999;51(4):233–41.
67. Richard MJ, Arnaud J, Jurkovitz C, Hachache T, Meftahi H, Laporte F, et al. Trace elements and lipid peroxidation abnormalities in patients with chronic renal failure. Nephron. 1991;57(1):10–5.
68. Guo CH, Chen PC, Yeh MS, Hsiung DY, Wang CL. Cu/Zn ratios are associated with nutritional status, oxidative stress, inflammation, and immune abnormalities in patients on peritoneal dialysis. Clin Biochem. 2011;44(4):275–80.
69. Mimic-Oka J, Savic-Radojevic A, Pljesa-Ercegovac M, Opacic M, Simic T, Dimkovic N, et al. Evaluation of oxidative stress after repeated intravenous iron supplementation. Ren Fail. 2005;27(3):345–51.
70. Klevay LM. Ischemic heart disease: nutrition or pharmacotherapy? J Trace Elem Electrolytes Health Dis. 1993;7(2):63–9.
71. Salonen JT, Salonen R. Ultrasound B-mode imaging in observational studies of atherosclerotic progression. Circulation. 1993;87(3 Suppl):II56–65.
72. Food and Nutrition Board Institute of Medicine. Molybdenum. In: Dietary reference intakes for vitamin A, vitamin K, boron, chromium, copper, iodine, iron, manganese, molybdenum, nickel, silicon, vanadium, and zinc. Washington, DC: National Academy Press; 2001. p. 420–41.
73. Hosokawa S, Yoshida O. Role of molybdenum in chronic hemodialysis patients. Int J Artif Organs. 1994;17(11):567–9.
74. Smythe WR, Alfrey AC, Craswell PW, Crouch CA, Ibels LS, Kubo H, et al. Trace element abnormalities in chronic uremia. Ann Intern Med. 1982;96(3):302–10.
75. Benigno V, Canonica CS, Bettinelli A, von Vigier RO, Truttmann AC, Bianchetti MG. Hypomagnesaemia-hypercalciuria-nephrocalcinosis: a report of nine cases and a review. Nephrol Dial Transplant. 2000;15(5):605–10.
76. da Silva CJ, da Rocha AJ, Jeronymo S, Mendes MF, Milani FT, Maia AC Jr, et al. A preliminary study revealing a new association in patients undergoing maintenance hemodialysis: manganism symptoms and T1 hyperintense changes in the basal ganglia. AJNR Am J Neuroradiol. 2007;28(8):1474–9.
77. Gropper S, Smith J, Groff J. Advanced nutrition and human metabolism. Belmont: Wadsworth Cengage Learning; 2009.
78. Zachara BA, Koterska D, Manitius J, Sadowski L, Dziedziczko A, Salak A, et al. Selenium supplementation on plasma glutathione peroxidase activity in patients with end-stage chronic renal failure. Biol Trace Elem Res. 2004;97(1):15–30.
79. Stockler-Pinto MB, Mafra D, Farage NE, Boaventura GT, Cozzolino SM. Effect of Brazil nut supplementation on the blood levels of selenium and glutathione peroxidase in hemodialysis patients. Nutrition. 2010;26(11–12):1065–9.
80. Piper CM. Very-low-protein diets in chronic renal failure: nutrient content and guidelines for supplementation. J Am Diet Assoc. 1985;85(10):1344–6.
81. McGregor DO, Dellow WJ, Lever M, George PM, Robson RA, Chambers ST. Dimethylglycine accumulates in uremia and predicts elevated plasma homocysteine concentrations. Kidney Int. 2001;59(6):2267–72.
82. Johnson DW, Atai E, Chan M, Phoon RKS, Scott C, Toussant ND, et al. KHA-CARI guideline: early chronic kidney disease: detection, prevention and management. Nephrology. 2013;18:340–50.
83. Fouque D, Vennegoor M, Wee PT, Wanner C, Basci A, Canaud B, et al. EBPG guideline on nutrition. Nephrol Dial Transplant. 2007;22(2):ii45–87.
84. Chazot C, et al. Vitamin metabolism and requirements in renal disease and renal failure. In: Kopple JD, Massry SG, Kalantar-Zadeh K, Fouque D, editors. Nutritional management of renal disease. 4th ed. Philadelphia: Elsevier; (in press).

Chapter 34
Factors Affecting Dietary Adherence and Strategies for Improving Adherence in Chronic Kidney Disease

Jerrilynn D. Burrowes

Keywords Dietary adherence · Dietary compliance · Chronic kidney disease · Nutrition counseling Nutrition education

Key Points
- Dietary adherence is a key component for successful treatment of chronic kidney disease.
- A patient's lifestyle, attitudes toward disease, socioeconomic status, culture, and social support may impact dietary adherence.
- Strategies for improving dietary adherence fit into one of three categories: educational, behavioral, and organizational.

Introduction

Medical nutrition therapy (MNT) is an integral component for successful treatment outcomes in patients with chronic kidney disease (CKD). Treatment requires adherence to a complex dietary prescription that changes throughout the stages of the disease. This chapter will review the factors (positive and negative) that may influence a patient's ability to follow the recommended diet prescription. Factors that may improve adherence include social support from family and/or caregivers and the health practitioner's knowledge of the patient's culture, food habits, beliefs, and practices. On the other hand, inhibitors of dietary adherence include the patient's lifestyle, attitude toward the disease, socioeconomic status, and cultural barriers. The health professional needs to understand these factors and implement strategies for achieving dietary adherence in CKD patients. This chapter will also provide evidence-based recommendations from the American Heart Association that the renal practitioner can apply to the CKD patient which may enhance adherence to the renal diet. Moreover, a brief comment about the use of technology to aid in achieving dietary adherence is included.

J. D. Burrowes (✉)
Department of Biomedical, Health and Nutritional Sciences, School of Health Professions and Nursing, Long Island University-Post, Brookville, NY, USA

© Springer Nature Switzerland AG 2020
J. D. Burrowes et al. (eds.), *Nutrition in Kidney Disease*, Nutrition and Health,
https://doi.org/10.1007/978-3-030-44858-5_34

Definitions

The terms adherence and compliance are often used interchangeably. The World Health Organization defines adherence as the extent to which a person's behavior (e.g., taking medications, following a diet, and/or executing lifestyle changes) corresponds with agreed or prescribed recommendations from a health-care provider [1]. Compliance suggests that the patient is passively following the practitioner's instructions and that the treatment plan is not based on a contract established between the patient and the practitioner [2]. Adherence is perceived as more neutral, emphasizing the self-regulatory actions of an individual. To the contrary, compliance devalues the patient's role in his/her health care; it is perceived as paternalistic, emphasizing obedience to a directive (e.g., "take this medication three times a day") [3]. The primary difference between the two terms is that adherence requires the patient's agreement with the recommendations, since the patient is an active collaborator with the practitioner in the treatment process. Throughout this chapter, the term adherence will be used since patients should be active participants in their health care.

Adherence is the single most important modifiable factor that compromises treatment outcome. It is also a primary determinant of the effectiveness of treatment because poor adherence attenuates optimum clinical benefit [4, 5]. The best treatment can be rendered ineffective by poor adherence [3]. Adherence also recognizes the patient's right to choose whether or not to follow advice [6]. On the other hand, nonadherence may be intentional (i.e., premeditated action against medical advice) or inadvertent (i.e., oversight by the patient) [7].

Dietary Adherence

Adherence to the diet prescription is critical for successful management of CKD. Poor dietary adherence places patients at risk for complications such as fluid overload, hyperkalemia, hyperphosphatemia, and malnutrition, to name a few. It may also complicate the patient-practitioner relationship and prevent an accurate assessment of the quality of care provided. In addition, patients with CKD usually have multiple comorbidities such as diabetes and cardiovascular disease, which may make their treatment regimen more complex and increase the likelihood of poor treatment outcomes [3]. For example, a dietary regimen such as the renal diabetes diet is more likely to be poorly adhered to because of the complexity of the diet.

Poor adherence wastes health-care resources, increases health-care expenditures, jeopardizes patient care, and increases morbidity and mortality risk [8]. Poor adherence to a dietary regimen usually goes undetected by health-care providers unless it is self-reported by the patient or until laboratory tests are obtained and reviewed. However, the latter monitor usually only reflects recent behavior in most instances [9]. Nonadherence can confuse the clinical picture and diagnostic process and may contribute to unnecessary testing and procedures, resulting in inappropriate regimen changes such as an increase in phosphate binders or changes in the dialysis prescription.

Factors Affecting Dietary Adherence

Dietary adherence is a multidimensional phenomenon determined by the interaction of several factors as shown in Table 34.1. Health professionals must understand how these factors influence adherence in order to develop strategies for achieving dietary adherence. Moreover, health professionals may help their patients overcome barriers to adherence by evaluating how they approach issues/challenges, how they provide advice, and, more importantly, how they involve patients in treatment decision-making [10].

Table 34.1 Barriers affecting dietary adherence to medical nutrition therapy for control of chronic kidney disease and strategies to improve adherence

Barriers affecting dietary adherence	What needs to be done
Social and economic factors	Assess social needs including shopping and meal preparation
	Assess family preparedness
Psychological factors	Assess the incidence of depression and the factors that contribute to depression
Health-care team and system-related factors	Engage in multidisciplinary care
	Improve patient/caregiver-practitioner relationship
	Provide training for health professionals on adherence
	Identify treatment goals and develop strategies to obtain them
	Provide continuing education for health professionals about the disease
	Provide continuous monitoring and reassessment of treatment
	Foster a nonjudgmental attitude and assistance
	Provide training in communication skills for health-care providers
	Reinforce desirable behavior
	Emphasize the value of the diet and the effects of adherence
Condition-related factors	Provide education on proper use of medications (e.g., phosphate binders)
	Keep the patient informed about the disease process and effective treatment options
	Provide in-depth nutrition education
Therapy-related factors	Simplify the treatment regimen
	Provide education on proper use of medications (e.g., phosphate binders)
	Improve patient/caregiver-health-care provider relationship
	Provide continuous feedback and support open communication
	Improve accessibility of the health professional to the patient and family
Patient-related factors	Provide behavior modification techniques
	Improve patient/caregiver-health-care provider relationship, considering the patient's beliefs and social and cultural norms
	Encourage self-management of disease and treatment
	Assess psychological needs
	Motivate patients to comply
	Increase patient's knowledge and understanding about the disease and the treatment regimen
	Reduce the complexity of the diet regimen
	Provide easy-to-read, simple education materials tailored for the patient
	Provide patient-centered education

Social and Economic Factors

Poverty, illiteracy, low level of education, unemployment, lack of effective social support networks, unstable living conditions, traveling a long distance to and from the treatment center, the high cost of transportation to the dialysis unit, the high cost of dialysis treatment and medication(s), cultural and lay beliefs about illness and treatment, and family dysfunction are some of the social and economic factors that affect adherence. Studies have shown that the cost of dialysis, particularly in developing nations, has been implicated in nonadherence to prescribed treatment regimens [11, 12]. Patient and family characteristics constitute additional sets of social factors that influence adherence. In fact, the attitude and support of the family are possibly the most important motivators for positive adherence [3]. Therefore, family members and/or significant others should be encouraged to attend nutrition counseling sessions with the patient to learn more about the condition and its treatment.

Psychological Factors

Depression is one of the most common psychological problems in CKD patients, which may result from stressors such as biochemical imbalance, physiological changes, neurological disturbances, and cognitive impairment [13]. The patients' response to these stressors may impact negatively on adjustment and response to treatment for CKD. DiMatteo et al. found that depressed patients were three times more likely to be nonadherent with treatment recommendations than non-depressed patients [14]. Irrational thoughts such as ignoring medical conditions, altered risk perceptions of behaviors, distorted views about controlling conditions, and using denial as a form of coping have also been reported to contribute to nonadherence [15].

Health-Care Team and System-Related Factors

Little research has been conducted on the effects of the health-care team and system-related factors on adherence. A good patient-practitioner relationship may improve adherence; however, there are many factors in this category that may have a negative effect on adherence. These include a lack of knowledge and training for health professionals on managing chronic kidney disease, overworked practitioners, lack of feedback on performance, short consultations with patients, and lack of knowledge about adherence and effective interventions for improving adherence [3]. Failure on the part of the health professionals to follow up with the patient about nonadherence, when it is detected, may enhance the negative behavior [16].

Condition-Related Factors

Illness-related demands faced by the patient such as the severity of symptoms, level of disability (e.g., physical, psychological, social, and vocational), rate of progression and severity of the disease, and the availability of effective treatments are examples of condition-related factors. The impact of these factors on adherence depends on how they influence the patients' risk perception, the importance of following the treatment, and the priority placed on adherence [3].

Therapy-Related Factors

The complexity of the medical regimen, the duration of treatment, previous treatment failures, frequent changes in the treatment prescription, immediate beneficial effects, negative side effects, and the availability of the health professionals to manage the side effects are examples of therapy-related factors that affect adherence [3]. A patient's ability to carry out the regimen as prescribed depends on the complexity of the regimen and the support systems available to assist the patient [9]. Dietary adherence is best achieved when the initial regimen is simple, with complexities introduced gradually. For example, nutrition education about the renal diet can begin with limiting high-potassium foods, whereas a more complex regimen may be to educate the patient about the renal diet exchange system. Furthermore, practical social difficulties such as not being able to coordinate the timing of phosphate binders with meals may also jeopardize adherence. Continuous reassurance by the practitioner may promote increased adherence when (and if) challenges arise.

Patient-Related Factors

The patient's knowledge, attitudes, beliefs, perceptions, and expectations represent patient-related factors that affect adherence. Knowledge and beliefs about the illness, motivation to manage it, confidence (self-efficacy) in the ability to engage in illness management behaviors, expectations regarding the outcome of treatment, and the consequences of poor adherence influence behavior [3]. A patient's motivation to adhere to a prescribed treatment regimen is influenced by the value placed on following the regimen (cost-benefit ratio) and the degree of confidence in being able to follow it [17]. Long-term regimens such as commitment to the renal diet require continuous adherence.

Oquendo and colleagues conducted an integrative review to identify the factors that contribute to diet adherence in patients receiving maintenance hemodialysis [18]. Among the 36 studies included in the review, they identified several intrinsic and extrinsic barriers and facilitators to diet adherence and also provided interventions to encourage adherence (Fig. 34.1). The lack of a gold standard to measure dietary adherence objectively makes obtaining an accurate assessment of adherence challenging. Some studies used laboratory and biometric markers (e.g., serum potassium or phosphorus levels or interdialytic fluid weight gains) or self-report questionnaires; not surprisingly, greater nonadherence was found among the studies using the latter tool [18].

Strategies for Achieving Dietary Adherence

Strategies to improve dietary adherence fit into one of three categories: educational, behavioral, and organizational [19–21]. Effective nutrition education is the first step in achieving dietary change. Education regarding the nutrition management of CKD should raise the patient's level of adherence to where it is

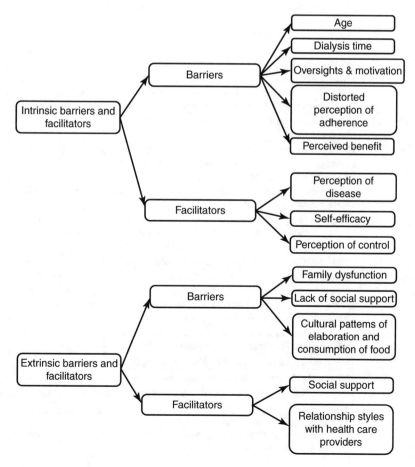

Fig. 34.1 Barriers to and facilitators of adherence to diet. (Reprinted from Oquendo et al. [18])

acceptable, but it is not sufficient to raise dietary adherence to the desired level [22], since education alone may not change attitude. However, nutrition education is better than no intervention at all.

Educational strategies rely on the transmission and dissemination of information and instructions with or without motivational appeal, with the intermediate objective of affecting a patient's knowledge and attitude [23]. Innovative educational activities such as interactive games and videos should be used. Nutrition information should be sensitive to the personal characteristics of the patient, including attitudes, cultural norms, beliefs, and reading/language skills [24]. Similarly, education alone is usually not sufficient to achieve long-term dietary adherence and sustain behavioral change. Webb and Byrd-Bredbenner suggest that nutrition education messages should be realistic, positive, easy to understand, and actionable [25]. A list of practical and effective strategies for increasing dietary adherence to nutritional advice is shown in Table 34.2. The American Heart Association has also developed evidence-based strategies to enhance adherence to dietary changes that can be applied to the renal patient [26] (Table 34.3).

Table 34.2 Practical and effective strategies to achieve dietary adherence

Improve communication	Adapt counseling style to each patient's needs
	Determine the best way to communicate with each patient and consider using communication aids (e.g., education materials with pictures) or use technology if the patient (and practitioner) are technologically savvy
	Determine the level of involvement the patient wants
	Ask open-ended questions and encourage patients to ask questions
	Listen more than talking
Increase patient involvement	Clearly explain the condition and the pros and cons of dietary adherence
	Clarify what the patient hopes the renal diet will achieve
	Listen to the patient (note any non-verbal cues) rather than making assumptions about the patients' understanding
	Help patients make decisions based on likely benefits of dietary adherence rather than misconceptions
	Accept that patients have the right to decide not to adhere to the diet if they have the capacity to, and have the information to make an informed decision. Dietary changes should allow for individual latitude in implementation
Understand the patient's perspective; simplify the message	Find out what patients know, believe, and understand about their condition and the need for a specialized diet
	Prioritize the message to be delivered. This decision will be based on the impact the changes will have on health outcomes. Radical dietary changes may lead to discouragement and nonadherence. For example, encouraging patients to eat a low-sodium diet immediately when they are accustomed to eating a lot of salt. This change needs to be made gradually (e.g., no added salt diet)
	Focus on one goal at a time to make nutrition education easier and success attainable. For example, emphasis on dietary protein intake will raise awareness and promote changes in other components of the diet (e.g., phosphorus intake)
	Work with objective data (e.g., monthly labs) to identify an achievable goal
Provide information and suggestions	Before recommending changes to the diet, offer patients clear, relevant information about their condition and the reason for changes to the diet. People need evidence that the changes they make will be effective. The monthly lab report and calculated interdialytic fluid weight gain can be used as evidence for change
	Patients need encouragement and reassurance that what they are doing is correct. Frequent follow-up, patient contact, and feedback are helpful
	Discuss information rather than just presenting it
	Offer individualized information that is easy to understand and free of jargon
	Provide recipes for fast, easy, and inexpensive prepared snacks that can be made readily available
	Encourage the patients to bring in family recipes for analysis to determine whether they "fit" within the renal diet. For recipes that are not "renal friendly," the dietitian may be able to suggest substitute ingredients

Table 34.3 Evidence-based strategies to enhance dietary changes based on the American Heart Association recommendations

Self-monitoring	Systematically observe and record one's behavior (e.g., food and beverages consumed). Consistency in self-monitoring is positively related to successful outcomes (e.g., better interdialytic weight gains and laboratory values)
Goal-setting	Teach patients the importance of setting goals for behavior change and have them be specific and attainable. Goals can target a change in intake (e.g., increase protein), specific foods (e.g., consume less high-sodium foods), or a behavior change (e.g., measure fluids for daily consumption). Give feedback on progress toward goal, use positive reinforcement for any effort, reevaluate goals and strategies, and problem-solve when progress to goal is absent
Relapse prevention	Teach patients to recognize situations that place them at risk for lapses from their dietary plan. They should learn how to use behavioral and cognitive strategies for handling these situations (e.g., remove the temptation(s) or convince them that the tempting food or beverage is not worth the outcome [e.g., high-phosphorus foods resulting in pruritus]). The dietitian should engage patients in strategies to sustain the diet while eating out
Reinforcement	Provide feedback on progress made toward the goal by acknowledging accomplishments and reinforcing confidence in the patient's capability of attaining a goal. Find any positive element that can be reinforced (e.g., interdialytic weight gains within recommended levels for the past 2 months)
Stimulus control	Patients should be aware of cues in the immediate and distant environment that can trigger behaviors, both healthy and unhealthy. The dietitian should counsel the patient to remove those stimuli and to restructure the home environment to minimize temptations (e.g., the patient should be advised to purchase no-sodium or low-sodium snacks and to make them visible and ready to eat around the house. Another example is to remove the salt shaker from the table.)
Social support	Patients should enlist the support of others in their environment and share their goals for behavior change. For example, patients should ask family members to keep high-sodium snacks out of the house and to remove the salt shaker from the table
Tailoring the regimen	The dietitian should be sensitive to the cultural practices and beliefs of diverse individuals when recommending dietary changes and also to be sensitive to literacy and financial constraints. For example, the dietitian should not ask patients of Hispanic descent to avoid consuming beans and rice, which is part of their culture. Patients should be taught how to fit beans and rice into the renal diet. This will help to promote adherence to the diet

Modified from VanHorn et al. [26]

Behavioral strategies are procedures that attempt to influence specific non-adherent behaviors directly through the use of techniques such as reminders, tailoring, contracting, self-monitoring, reinforcement, and family/peer support, but with information and instruction playing a secondary role [19]. However, behavioral strategies fail to maintain consistent change in the long-term [20]. Therefore, educational strategies should be continuous.

Lastly, organizational strategies focus primarily on the convenience of the dialysis unit and on the utilization of personnel for fostering dietary adherence [21]. Organizational changes can prevent or reduce adherence problems, often without the need for altering the practitioner's workloads or increasing budgets. Examples include making special appointments at odd hours or telephoning patients at home with abnormal lab results. This latter example may be more appropriate in a peritoneal dialysis clinic where the patients are seen less frequently than in the hemodialysis unit.

Use of Technology in Monitoring Dietary Adherence

In this age of advancing technology, the use of smartphones and mobile apps may be beneficial for self-monitoring dietary adherence. A personal digital assistant (PDA) device was used in three pilot studies with results showing limited applicability in self-monitoring diet and fluid intake in dialysis patients [27–29]. Studies of longer duration, with large sample sizes and strong study designs, are needed to determine whether electronic monitoring of dietary intake using the PDAs or other technology will promote dietary adherence.

Conclusion

Dietary adherence is a critical component for successful management of CKD. Several factors may inhibit or improve dietary adherence. Educational, behavioral, and organizational strategies may also improve adherence. Dietitians who educate patients with CKD and/or their family members need to be aware of these factors and the strategies that may improve or inhibit dietary adherence.

References

1. World Health Organization. Section I. World Health Organization. 2003. Available from https://www.who.int/chp/knowledge/publications/adherence_Section1.pdf.
2. Osterberg L, Blaschke T. Adherence to medication. N Engl J Med. 2005;353(5):487–97.
3. World Health Organization. Adherence to long term therapies: evidence for action. World Health Organization. 2003. Available from http://www.who.int/chp/knowledge/publications/adherence_report/en/.
4. World Health Organization. The World Health Report. Reducing risks, promoting healthy life. Geneva: World Health Organization; 2002. p. 2002.
5. Dunbar-Jacob J, Erlen JA, Schlenk EA, Ryan CM, Sereika SM, Doswell WM. Adherence in chronic disease. Annu Rev Nurs Res. 2000;18:48–90.
6. Cohen SM. Concept analysis of adherence in the context of cardiovascular risk reduction. Nurs Forum. 2009;44:25–36.
7. Clark S, Farrington K, Chilcot J. Nonadherence in dialysis patients: prevalence, measurement, outcome, and psychological determinants. Semin Dialysis. 2014;27(1):42–9.
8. DiMatteo MR. Variations in patients' adherence to medical recommendations. Med Care. 2004;42(3):200–9.
9. DiMatteo MR, Reiter RC, Gambone JC. Enhancing medication adherence through communication and informed collaborative choice. Health Commun. 1994;6(4):253–65.
10. Desroches S, Lapointe A, Ratté S, Gravel K, Légare F, Turcotte S. Interventions to enhance adherence to dietary advice for preventing and managing chronic diseases in adults. Cochrane Database Syst Rev. 2013;2:CD008722.
11. Chironda G, Manwere A, Nyamakura R, Chipfuwa T, Bhengu B. Perceived health status and adherence to haemodialysis by End Stage Renal Disease (ESRD) patients: a case of a central hospital in Zimbabwe. IOSR J Nurs Health Sci. 2014;22:31.
12. Alebiosu CO, Aodele OE. The global burden of chronic kidney disease and the way forward. Ethnic Dis. 2005;15:418.
13. Chironda G, Bhengu G. Contributing factors to non-adherence among chronic kidney disease (CKD) patients: a systematic review of literature. Med Clin Rev. 2016;2(4).
14. DiMatteo MR, Lepper HS, Croghan TW. Depression is a risk factor for noncompliance with medical treatment: meta-analysis of the effects of anxiety and depression on patient adherence. Arch Int Med. 2000;160:2101–7.
15. Williams ME. Management of diabetes in dialysis patients. Curr Diabetes Rep. 2009;9:466–72.
16. LaRosa JC. Poor compliance: the hidden risk factor. Curr Atheroscler Rep. 2000;2:1–4.
17. Miller W, Rollnick S. Motivational interviewing. New York: Guilford Press; 1999.
18. Oquendo LG, Asencio JMM, de las Nieves CB. Contributing factors for therapeutic diet adherence in patients receiving hemodialysis treatment: an integrative review. J Clin Nurs. 2017;26:3893–905.
19. Dunbar JM, Marshall GD, Hovell MF. Behavioral strategies for improving compliance. In: Haynes RB, Taylor DW, Sacket DL, editors. Compliance in health care. Baltimore: Johns Hopkins University Press; 1979. p. 174–90.
20. Leventhal H, Cameron L. Behavioral theories and the problem of compliance. Patient Educ Couns. 1987;10:117–38.
21. Gibson ES. Compliance and the organization of health services. In: Haynes RB, Taylor DW, Sacket DL, editors. Compliance in health care. Baltimore: Johns Hopkins University Press; 1979. p. 278–85.
22. Elliott WJ. Compliance strategies. Curr Opin Nephrol Hypertens. 1994;3:271–8.

23. Green LW. Educational strategies to improve compliance with therapeutic and preventive regimens: the recent evidence. In: Haynes RB, Taylor DW, Sacket DL, editors. Compliance in health care. Baltimore: Johns Hopkins University Press; 1979. p. 157–73.
24. Sherman AM, Bowen DJ, Vitolins M, Perri MG, Rosal MC, Sevick MA, et al. Dietary adherence: characteristics and interventions. Control Clin Trials. 2000;21:206S–11.
25. Webb D, Byrd-Bredbenner C. Overcoming consumer inertia to dietary guidance. Adv Nutr. 2015;65(4):391–6.
26. VanHorn L, Carson JS, Appel LJ, Burke LE, Economos C, Karmally W, et al. Recommended dietary pattern to achieve adherence to the American Heart Association/American College of Cardiology (AHA/ACC) guidelines. Circulation. 2016;134:e505–3329.
27. Welch J, Dowell S, Johnson CS. Feasibility of using a personal digital assistant to self-monitor diet and fluid intake: a pilot study. Nephrol Nurs J. 2007;34(1):43–8.
28. Stark S, Snetselaar L, Piraino B, Stone RA, Kim S, Hall B, et al. Personal digital assistant-based self-monitoring adherence rates in two dialysis dietary intervention pilot studies: balance-wise HD and balance-wise PD. J Ren Nutr. 2011;21(6):492–8.
29. Welch JL, Astroth KS, Perkins SM, Johnson CS, Connelly K, Siek K, et al. Using a mobile application to self-monitor diet and fluid intake among adults receiving hemodialysis. Res Nurs Health. 2013;36(3):284–98.

Chapter 35
Effective Communication and Counseling Approaches

Kathy K. Isoldi

Keywords Communication strategies · Cognitive behavioral therapy · Motivational interviewing Counseling strategies

Key Points
- Patients with chronic kidney disease experience several psychosocial detriments that may interfere with their readiness to make dietary and lifestyle changes.
- To achieve the best outcome, patients with chronic kidney disease should receive nutritional counseling in a supportive and engaging environment that focuses on empowerment and in increasing self-efficacy in managing food and lifestyle choices.
- It is essential that dietitians who counsel patients consider the stage of change each patient is exhibiting to provide stage-appropriate nutrition counseling.
- Combining the unique concepts and strategies of cognitive behavioral therapy and motivational interviewing have shown promise in promoting dietary adherence in patients who are prescribed dietary restrictions in the treatment of chronic kidney disease.
- Mining for "change talk" in ambivalent and resistant patients can promote forward progress.
- The emergence of new forms of patient communication offered by technological advances shows promise in supporting patient self-management.

Introduction

The prevalence of chronic kidney disease (CKD) has been rising over the past several decades and currently afflicts approximately 37 million American adults [1]. It was estimated in 2016 that 661,000 adults in the United States had kidney failure, with 468,000 receiving dialysis and 193,000 living with a functioning kidney transplant [2]. In addition to physical detriment, those with CKD also experience psychosocial detriments that influence how they view the dietary restrictions of the renal diet and their personal motivation aimed at self-care efforts [3–5]. Complicating life further for people with CKD are the psychological and social burdens that ripple toward the patient's expanded circle of family and friends, thereby creating a negative impact on an even greater number of individuals. These burdens undoubtedly influence the high prevalence of depression seen in patients with CKD, which is reported to be between 20% and 30% of patients [6, 7].

K. K. Isoldi (✉)
Nutrition Department, Long Island University, Brookville, NY, USA
e-mail: Kathy.isoldi@liu.edu

© Springer Nature Switzerland AG 2020
J. D. Burrowes et al. (eds.), *Nutrition in Kidney Disease*, Nutrition and Health,
https://doi.org/10.1007/978-3-030-44858-5_35

Research supports that the transition from CKD to end-stage renal disease (ESRD) may be slowed through dietary and lifestyle choices. In addition, individuals with ESRD may improve their longevity and quality of life by following an appropriate dietary protocol [8–11]. However, adherence to dietary restrictions in this population is low [12]. Researchers performed qualitative interviews with 16 patients receiving maintenance hemodialysis that led to the development and distribution of a survey to 156 similar patients. The results of this qualitative and quantitative study revealed that very few patients perceived any immediate positive effects from following their dietary restrictions. The researchers believe this may be one major reason for poor dietary adherence [4]. Clearly, there is a need for dietitians to guide patients with CKD to a better understanding about the influence of appropriate diet and lifestyle choices, as well as a need to confer a sense of empowerment to the patient with CKD.

It is essential that dietitians use effective strategies during nutrition counseling sessions to improve outcomes. Nutrition counseling approaches in the past have often involved education-based, directive style expert-centered guidance. More recently, patient-centered counseling approaches that focus on empowerment and shared decision-making have emerged and have shown improved patient outcomes [4, 13, 14]. The recommendation to use collaborative management in counseling patients with chronic illnesses has been suggested for over a decade [15]. However, implementing the theories of patient-centered, jointly owned planning in nutrition counseling has taken time to develop. Currently, dietitians have a communication and counseling toolbox filled with strategies to draw upon that serve to promote behavior change, ultimately improving patient health outcomes.

The use of the transtheoretical model (TTM) in guiding dietitians in identifying the stage of change each patient is experiencing has become a practical tool to use during the counseling process. Cognitive behavioral therapy (CBT) and motivational interviewing (MI) have also emerged as efficacious models to employ in promoting change in patient's food and lifestyle behaviors [4, 16–18]. This chapter will review techniques and strategies inherent in several models that can be used by dietitians while counseling patients with CKD to achieve increased dietary adherence, ultimately resulting in improved health outcomes, quality of life, and longevity.

The Transtheoretical Model

The onset of kidney disease does not wait for a patient to be ready to accept the diagnosis. Patients are often in need of guidance about changes in health and food behaviors that need to be taken even though they are not ready physically, psychologically, or emotionally to take action. Dietary nonadherence has been associated with incorrect matching of the proper counseling techniques with the stage of change the patient is exhibiting based on the principles of the transtheoretical model (TTM). If a patient arrives for guidance and is not ready to take action, and the counseling session amounts to a laundry list of what to do and what to eat, the likelihood of progress will be poor [19]. Patients often seeking help arrive at the dietitian's office or at the hemodialysis unit at different stages of readiness to change.

The TTM was first created by Prochaska and colleagues and, although it has received some criticism, the theory has revolutionized the way dietitians approach patient counseling. The essential elements of the TTM are basic to any discussion about behavior change. Briefly, the TTM is comprised of six stages: pre-contemplation, contemplation, preparation, action, maintenance, and relapse. The aim of the TTM is to guide the clinician in identifying a patient's stage of readiness to change and to offer guidance and counseling accordingly, with the ultimate goal of forward progress.

Patients in pre-contemplation do not see a link between their behaviors and health outcomes or negative consequences, and they are often reported as being in denial of the link between actions and health consequences. Patients in the contemplation stage report a known association between their behaviors and a negative consequence, but they cannot see how they can make the necessary changes to reap the benefits of change. In the stages of pre-contemplation and contemplation, patients are not ready to take action and make necessary changes. In the preparation stage, patients are cognizant of the need to make changes and they are ready to plan to make changes in food and health-related behaviors, usually within the next month. Patients in the action phase of the TTM are ready to take action immediately, or they are currently taking action to incorporate the changes needed to make lifestyle and/or dietary changes. During maintenance, patients focus on cementing the changes incorporated, and they maintain focus on all the behaviors implemented during the action phase. Finally, relapse occurs when a patient reverts back to his or her old, detrimental habits instead of moving forward or stabilizing in the maintenance phase. Research reports that the majority of patients who need to make dietary changes arrive for professional guidance while in either the pre-contemplation or contemplation stage [19, 20].

People who misunderstand the TTM assume that progress can only be made during the action phase. However, at each stage in the TTM, substantial progress can be made. Changes in thoughts and readiness to act are dynamic processes that include progress and regression. The role of the dietitian is to identify the stage the client is in, to work with strategies that are stage appropriate, and to guide the patient forward toward the next stage. In addition, the dietitian needs to work with the patient toward avoiding regression (or relapse). However, if relapse occurs, the dietitian should plan counseling techniques geared toward recovery, forgiveness, and movement forward toward the next stage of readiness [19, 20]. The following sections review several strategies useful in guiding patients in a forward motion and in cementing new behaviors. In addition, there are several questions that can be posed to patients that allow for the dietitian to evoke from patients their inner thoughts and concerns. See Table 35.1 for details on the TTM and how to proceed with counseling based upon stage of readiness.

Table 35.1 The transtheoretical model (stages of change) and counseling patients with CKD

Stage	Key elements	Patient comment	Appropriate action
Pre-contemplation	In denial Unable to accept need for change	"I don't see why I have to monitor my fruit intake. Fruit is healthy for you, right?"	Do not lecture the patient or make him/her see the truth Ask open-ended questions to move the conversation in a forward, positive direction, such as "What is your understanding about how eating high-potassium fruits affects your body?" Offer written material for the patient to read so you can discuss next time Suggest self-monitoring of food intake for future discussion
Contemplation	Knowing the need to change but feeling stuck Feeling ambivalent about why to change Pros and cons of change are equal	"I know that I have to watch my fluid intake in-between dialysis treatments, but I just can't do it. I try to plan ahead and avoid salty food, but then life gets in the way."	Help the patient explore the barriers and promote change talk Ask open-ended questions, such as "Can you tell me how you feel physically right before you begin dialysis?" Use the importance scale and have the client tell *you* why it is important to change Work on stress management Suggest self-monitoring fluid intake for the next week

(continued)

Table 35.1 (continued)

Stage	Key elements	Patient comment	Appropriate action
Preparation	Planning for change within the next month Commitment needs to be verbalized and/or reinforced	"I know I can change my diet and lower my phosphorus intake. I am committed to start next week as I am shopping for low-phosphorus foods for my home in a few days."	Help client with setting realistic goals Use confidence scale to gauge and increase confidence, as well as to identify barriers Suggest self-monitoring of food intake
Action	Actively and consistently incorporate the change	"I have been eating potatoes that have been soaked in water overnight for the past few weeks. It's easy now that I know what to do."	Use affirmations Modify goals—now that the potatoes are being managed, perhaps the patient is ready to take on another goal Work on social support and stimulus control
Maintenance	Patient has been successfully incorporating the change for ≥6 months	"I have been doing great for the last 8 months in making sure that I pre-measure my daily fluid allotment. My fluid gain in-between treatments has been consistently acceptable."	Be sure to use affirmations to support positive behaviors Work on relapse prevention Work on identifying high-risk situations to troubleshoot Support continued self-monitoring
Relapse	An expected, yet unplanned event whereby the patient had difficulty continuing to execute the healthy plan	"I really messed up. I forgot to eat my low-phosphorus, low-potassium, low-salt meal at home. I attended a party and was so hungry I lost control and ate many of the wrong foods. I felt awful and still feel awful."	Emphasize that lapses happen and are expected Use reflections to express understanding Help client see the benefits of forgiveness Support self-monitoring and stimulus control

Inquiries and Responding to Patients

During counseling sessions, dietitians can formulate several types of questions and responses to patients' comments that can influence the outcome of the session. Constructing questions and responses that allows for in-depth discussions can help to guide patients to a better understanding of potential obstacles that may interfere with meeting food-related behavior goals. In a rushed environment, dietitians may resort to formulating their questions based solely on obtaining facts about the patient in order to complete the nutrition assessment, and he or she may avoid questions that focus on exploring the patient's thoughts and concerns [20]. See Table 35.2 for examples of the different types of questions often used in nutrition counseling.

Closed-Ended Questions

Closed-ended questions are often formed to elicit a one-word response from the patient, and there may be times when it is appropriate to use closed-ended questions when speaking with a patient. For example, when time is limited and a patient needs information quickly, it may be appropriate to ask, "Do you need a list of potassium-rich foods to avoid before you leave the unit today?" However, closed-ended questions that are general in nature should be avoided during counseling such as "Are you following your renal diet?" or "Are you taking all of your medications?"

Table 35.2 Types of questions typically used during counseling

Type	Question	Comment
Closed-ended	"Do you avoid phosphorus-rich foods?"	Response from patient will offer very little insight into his/her actions and thoughts
	"Do you have a problem following your prescribed diet?"	The patient may feel disinterested or demoralized and not want to explore this topic. The question offers the patient the opportunity to just respond "No." Will not offer any insight
Leading	"Which phosphorus-rich foods do you avoid?"	Assumes patient is avoiding phosphorus-rich foods. Likely to result in an answer the patient thinks the dietitian wants to hear. Will not offer insights into patient's cognitions
	"What do you like about your new diet?"	Question makes the assumption that the patient has things about the diet that he or she likes. It does not allow the patient to express any dislike for the diet as the question *leads* the patient to address what is liked
Open-ended	"Can you tell me about the types of foods and beverages you usually eat on most days?"	No assumptions are embedded in the question. Creates the foundation for an honest conversation about current dietary intake
	"Can you share with me any difficulties you might be experiencing while following your renal diet?"	Offers a platform for an open dialogue for the patient. Offers the patient an opportunity to share his/her inner thoughts and concerns regarding the diet

There are several problems inherent in using too many closed-ended questions during a counseling session. For example, patients will not have the opportunity to express concerns and ambivalence or explore misunderstandings when closed-ended questions are posed. In addition, these types of questions may lead the patient to believe that the dietitian is disinterested in exploring issues that might be of concern to the patient [20].

Leading Questions

Leading questions implicitly express the dietitian's bias, and using this form of questioning will interfere with understanding what the patient is thinking and wants to share with the dietitian. When a patient is posed a leading question that infers professional bias, the patient may feel too embarrassed to respond honestly. Instead, the patient may answer the question to please the dietitian rather than express true feelings and opinions. Consider the following two versions of a question inquiring about daily food intake: (1) "Can you tell me what you ate for breakfast today?" or (2) "Can you tell me about the foods and beverages you ate after waking up today?" The first version of the question assumes that the patient eats breakfast, and this may not be true. The patient may be ashamed to admit that he or she skips breakfast and does not eat until lunchtime. In the second version of the question, the patient is asked to report on the first foods eaten upon waking. Asking the question in this way is more likely to result in an accurate response. Knowing that the patient skips breakfast is an important piece of dietary information and allows the dietitian to address this food behavior once it is revealed. Leading questions can interfere with an honest dialogue between the patient and the dietitian and should be avoided during nutrition counseling [20].

Open-Ended Questions

Open-ended questions have the greatest potential to promote collaboration and dynamic interviewing. These types of questions will open the door for the patient to express his or her thoughts, cognitions, fears, and concerns. It is under these circumstances that the dietitian can explore concerns with the patient and make substantial progress toward behavior change. Of course, the dietitian needs to be ready for a variety of responses—expected and unexpected. Therefore, using open-ended questioning when time does not permit and a proper discussion cannot occur can serve to be detrimental during the counseling process. The dietitian should ask primarily open-ended questions, and a sufficient amount of time should be given to the patient to express his or her concerns, as well as to promote an open dialogue.

Using open-ended questions also serves to promote in-depth discussions about diet and behavior change with those patients who are less likely, for a variety of reasons, to share their concerns [20]. Asking a patient "Can you please tell me how you are managing or coping with your new dietary restrictions?" will open the door for an important discussion regarding all the factors surrounding eating a limited diet. One way to gauge if a dietitian is using enough open-ended questions is to estimate the percentage of time during the counseling session that the patient is talking and compare this to how much time the dietitian is talking. Sessions that provide in-depth discussions with favorable outcomes result from the patient doing most of the talking.

Respond Using Reflective Listening

Reflective listening is a powerful communication technique that allows for clarification of messages sent and communicates to the patient that the dietitian is fully engaged and listening. The goal of this type of response is to reflect back to the patient what the dietitian believes he or she has heard the patient say. This serves to confirm messages received from the patient and to clarify their meaning, either stated or implied. Reflective listening can be simple reflections that constitute restating what has been said with little interpretation, or it can include interpretation of the feeling the dietitian believes is embedded in the patient's statement. More in-depth forms of reflective listening include amplified reflections that include the emotional feeling sensed by the dietitian, double-sided reflections that reveal the perceived ambivalence sensed, and reframing reflections that involves reframing the patient's statement to help him or her think differently about the situation. Reflective listening signals to patients that the dietitian understands and accepts their thoughts and concerns. In addition, it helps to generate discussions that will develop self-awareness about any ambivalence the patient may feel regarding the food and lifestyle changes recommended [21]. See Table 35.3 for examples of different types of reflective listening.

Table 35.3 Responding to the patient's concerns using reflective listening

The patient will say, "I know how important it is to lower the amount of potassium in my blood, but I can't seem to do it. I try, but it just isn't working. I can't do it!"	
Type of reflective listening	The nutrition professional may respond
Simple reflection Restating what is said, but changing the wording	"What I hear you saying is that you do not believe that you can lower your potassium."
Amplified reflection Reflecting emotional overtones	"What I think I hear you saying is that you would like to be able to reduce your potassium, but are feeling concerned and frustrated that you have not been able to achieve that as yet."
Two-sided reflection Revealing both sides of the patient's ambivalence	"So, on the one hand you are struggling to find a way to manage your potassium intake, but on the other hand you know how important it is to accomplish this task."
Reframing reflection Reframing to help the patient think differently about the situation	"I can hear your sense of frustration in trying to follow a diet to lower your serum potassium, and I wonder if you've considered looking into getting some support to help you with this task."

Social Learning Theory and Self-Efficacy

The social learning theory proposed by Albert Bandura [22] informs us that patients can learn within a social context by observing and modeling others [23]. Bandura has outlined four components that will increase the likelihood that one will learn the modeled behavior; these include attention, retention (remembering), reproduction (ability to imitate the behavior), and motivation (having a good reason to want to adopt the behavior) [23]. Application of the social learning theory during nutrition counseling might include the use of successful patient testimonials or demonstrations to help promote behavior change through modeling [16].

Bandura stresses the need to increase self-efficacy to promote behavior change [20, 22]. Self-efficacy is described as one's belief or confidence in being able to carry out a task [20]. Support for the use of social learning strategies to promote nutrition behavior change has not yet been strongly supported in research [16]. However, self-efficacy has been positively and strongly associated with several health indicators including improved blood glucose control, fewer depressive symptoms, and better quality of life in patients with chronic illness [24, 25]. Strategies aimed at improving self-efficacy in CKD patients are recommended. Self-efficacy can be influenced through a patient's physiological state, verbal persuasion received, vicarious experiences, and personal performance accomplishments [22]. Physiological states include discomfort, anxiety, and fear, which can detrimentally impact a patient's sense of self-efficacy. Positive verbal persuasion received from the dietitian will serve to promote a patient's self-efficacy. Similarly, patient group support meetings that include patients who adhere to the renal diet and who are doing well will serve as role models to others. However, the most effective way to improve self-efficacy is through performance accomplishments because it is based on personal mastery experiences [20, 22]. Therefore, helping patients with CKD set small, achievable goals will go a long way in improving self-efficacy through promoting a sense of personal performance accomplishment.

Behavior Modification and Cognitive Behavioral Therapy (CBT)

The basic tenets of behavior modification include the belief that behavior is influenced by the environment and, within that environment, behavior is driven by a series of positive and negative consequences. Food-related habits are formed by associated habits that are cemented over time. For example, the worker who comes home every night and eats dinner in front of the television is very likely to get hungry whenever he or she sits down to watch television. In this scenario, watching television becomes the unconditioned stimulus that will prompt eating, even in the absence of hunger. Behavior modification theory states that healthy behaviors can also be learned or conditioned/reinforced [20].

Behavioral theory and CBT interventions have the longest history in nutrition counseling and have been tested with the greatest frequency. The behavioral interventions are also referred to as behavior or lifestyle modification [16]. However, it is noteworthy that CBT focuses on promoting behavior change through modifying the patient's external factors (the environment) and internal factors (thoughts or cognitions). There is strong evidence supporting the use of behavior modification techniques to improve patient outcomes in changing food and lifestyle behaviors [16, 26]. Several strategies have been used to help guide patients toward positive change during behavior modification sessions. These include self-monitoring, social support, stress management, stimulus control, problem-solving, and reward strategies [16, 20]. See Table 35.4 for strategies to use to promote behavior change during nutrition counseling using the principles of CBT.

Table 35.4 Behavioral strategies useful in counseling

Strategy	Purpose	Example
Self-monitoring	To track food, behaviors, thoughts, or physical activity for patient self-revelation	Maintain a food log and/or a log of adherence to medication schedule Maintain a log of daily fluid intake Maintain a log of feelings associated with eating
Social support	To offer emotional support to the patient	Have a family member or friend join the patient during a counseling session to enhance understanding Offer/direct patient to group support meetings
Stress management	To target and reduce environmental stress	Use of relaxation techniques such as deep breathing or yoga to help reduce stress Encourage hobbies that the patient finds enjoyable
Stimulus control	To reduce social or environmental cues that trigger undesirable behavior	Have the patient limit sodium intake to help reduce the desire to drink fluids Remove high-potassium fruits and vegetables from the home Make acceptable food choices more visible in the home (e.g., acceptable fruits in the fruit bowl)
Problem-solving	To forecast trouble or handle current obstacles	Have patient make a list of obstacles that he or she is experiencing Conduct brainstorming sessions to plan ahead for challenging events, such as holiday and family parties Weigh the pros and cons of options available to address potential problems
Rewards	To support and encourage helpful and newly created health behaviors	Patient rewards self with a new book when the goal of not eating high-potassium fruits is maintained for 1 month Patient rewards self with an additional hour of reading time after going for a 30-minute walk

Cognitions

Cognitions are created through the processes of knowing through memory, remembering, and processing information [26]. They can be positive or negative in nature. Cognitions prompt self-talk that can move a patient forward or hold him or her back from trying something new. An example of positive self-talk emerges from a positive cognition and is displayed by saying to oneself, "I am strong enough to do this." On the contrary, saying "I knew I couldn't follow this new diet plan because I have no willpower" is an example of negative self-talk generated from negative cognitions. Cognitions are influenced by one's childhood and prior experiences [20]. In fact, cognitions about circumstances and life choices are very powerful in driving behavior. Encouraging positive cognitions and positive self-talk are fundamental to CBT [20, 26].

Cognitive Distortions

Cognitive distortions are negative and detrimental to personal growth and progress toward behavior change. They promote negative self-talk and hold patients back from making progress. A patient who is struggling to manage his or her renal diet may eat the wrong foods one day and feel discouraged and report, "I'm an idiot; I know what to eat and yet I made all the wrong choices." Self-talk that involves *negative labeling* can create a lack of confidence and reduce self-efficacy resulting in a lack of progress and possible regression [20].

Another common cognitive distortion is *all or nothing thinking* and occurs when patients believe that one error in their plan means that their whole plan has been ruined and that they should not bother attempting to do anything right. When this happens a patient may report, "I forgot to take my phosphate binders today so why bother trying to follow my diet. I might as well give up and eat what I want." If a patient voices a cognitive distortion, the dietitian needs to help the patient understand how this type of thinking interferes with progress, is unproductive, and is an irrational way to handle mistakes. An effective way to address cognitive distortions is through cognitive restructuring [16, 20].

Cognitive Restructuring

Cognitive restructuring is a process whereby the dietitian enhances the patient's awareness of his or her perceptions and reveals irrational (negative) cognitions held by the patient and helps to redirect (restructure) the thinking toward a rational (positive) cognition. In the process, patients are taught to turn negative self-talk into positive self-talk [16, 20]. For example, a patient who typically adheres to his or her diet states, "I am so angry at myself. I ate pizza for lunch and got so thirsty that I drank way too much soda. I drank so much that I had swelling in my legs all day yesterday. I just feel so discouraged right now." This represents an irrational thought. Just because the patient ate pizza and drank too much fluid one day should not make the patient angry with himself or herself. This situation presents an opportunity for the dietitian to discuss with the patient that occasional missteps with dietary restrictions occur and they can be overcome and must be forgiven. Using amplified reflective listening can help. The dietitian can respond, "I think I hear what you're saying, and you are really angry and frustrated with yourself for the choices you made for lunch yesterday. And even though you usually make the right choices this one event is enough to worry you and make you feel discouraged. Did I get that right?" Hopefully framing reflective listening in this way will prompt the discussion in a positive direction geared toward having the patient understand that one poor choice will not undo all the hard work and effort put forth during the majority of the week. The discussion can continue with a focus on what the patient can do to use the information learned to avoid eating pizza in the future. The negative self-talk can change to positive self-talk by helping the patient verbalize how well he or she has done in the past with diet adherence and how he or she can forgive the digression and be resilient following this event. After a few minutes of reflective listening and use of open-ended questions, the patient may even end the session by saying, "I guess I'm just human and not perfect. I know I can get back on track because I am strong and determined." Hence, the irrational thought has been reconstructed into a rational thought and negative self-talk has been transformed into positive self-talk. This ideal scenario does not always occur immediately, but may take time to evolve. The better the rapport between the dietitian and the patient, the quicker and more likely the transfer from negative to positive forward motion will occur.

Goal Setting

Goal setting is an essential component of behavior modification. Patients should be involved in setting their goals with the dietitian. This can be accomplished through setting SMART goals. SMART goals are *S*pecific, *M*easurable, *A*chievable, *R*ealistic/*R*elevant, and *T*imely. They need to be clearly understood and manageable for the patient. Patients who can achieve their goals are more likely to increase their self-efficacy, so it is wise to help patients choose goals that are manageable [20]. For example, after a consultation with the patient, both parties agree that the patient will keep a food log for three days during the following week (one weekend and two weekdays) and will record all foods and beverages consumed starting with the following Monday. This goal is specific, measurable, achievable, realistic/relevant, and timely, and both parties agree. Conversely, having the patient record all foods and beverages consumed every day of the week starting when the patient feels up to it is a goal that is both unrealistic (every day is too often for most patients) and does not give the patient a specific start date to begin logging food intake.

Motivational Interviewing

The presence of an illness such as CKD is not enough to motivate all patients to incorporate behavior changes. Research supports that patients with CKD who adhere to dietary restrictions experience less medical complications and improved quality of life, and it can increase their life expectancy by two decades or more [27]. However, studies report nonadherence with diet and/or fluid restrictions in 30–75% of patients [27, 28]. Durose and colleagues [27] found no association between dietary knowledge and improved adherence. It is clear that providing nutrition information and guidance is not enough to motivate patients with CKD to adhere to their prescribed diet. Patients need to be motivated to make the lasting changes needed.

Motivation is a complex concept that is influenced by conscious and unconscious processes [29]. The philosophy and strategies inherent in the theory of motivational interviewing (MI) have become appealing to dietitians who are working to guide patients toward behavior change [16, 30]. The concepts of MI were developed by Miller and Rollnick, working off the foundation of patient-centered counseling concepts that were first introduced by Rogers in 1951 [21]. MI techniques were first applied to treat individuals with drug and alcohol addictions. More recently, MI has been used in many counseling settings where behavior change is the desired outcome. It is aimed at helping patients explore and resolve their personal struggles with ambivalence about behavior change [18, 31].

Rollnick and colleagues describe MI as a gentle approach to counseling. In stark contrast to lecturing, the patient becomes an active participant in the process. Over time the goal is to create "change talk." During change talk the patient experiences a change in focus and reveals to himself or herself the reasons for making changes and will begin a self-dialogue that leads to motivation to take action. Change talk can be embedded within a monologue of "sustain talk," or reasons why one cannot take the steps toward change. Change talk displays the patients' reasons for change, which includes perceived desire, ability, reasons, and need for change. Four guiding principles are used while counseling patients to promote change talk; these principles are outlined using the acronym RULE [20, 31 32]:

1. *Resist the righting reflex*

   Dietitians are trained to help patients make the changes needed to stay healthy and improve their lives. However, while using MI, it is important to resist the urge to lead and to tell patients what the dietitian thinks is best for them to do. The dietitian should avoid arguing the case or trying to convince the patient how important it is to make the necessary changes. When a patient is ambivalent about change, pushing harder can result in greater resistance toward efforts aimed at persuasion. This creates a tug of war between the dietitian and the patient, rather than a respectful, collaborative effort. The patient's rebuttal to the dietitian's pleas for adherence further cements the patient's conviction that he or she cannot adhere to the dietary guidelines. The goal is for the patient to experience change in beliefs and to convince himself or herself how important it is to make the necessary changes.

2. *Understand and explore the patient's own motivations*

   The patient will respond strongly to his or her own thoughts and feelings. Helping a patient explore his or her reasons for wanting (or not wanting) to make dietary and lifestyle changes will result in progress. Amplified reflective listening and the use of open-ended questions during counseling will promote the exploration of the patient's source of motivation.

3. *Listen with empathy*

Patients will respond to thoughtful understanding. In addition to helping to establish rapport, shared understanding of the patient's struggles and obstacles can be a prelude to change talk. Patients with CKD have many fears and struggles to manage on a daily basis. Using reflective listening can amplify the message that the dietitian understands these burdens and is there to help the patient make changes, acknowledging the multitude of difficulties the patient is facing.

4. *Empower the patient, encouraging hope and optimism*

Exploring how patients can make a difference in their own lives and thereby offering empowerment can be very effective in making lasting changes. Outcomes are better when patients are actively involved in their own case. Patients ultimately become a consultant for the dietitian on how goals can best be met. The dietitian serves as a facilitator and encourages the patient to bring his or her expertise to the consultation.

To successfully execute the basic four tenets of the RULE philosophy of MI, it is suggested that dietitians use Open questions, Affirmations, Reflections, and Summaries (referred to as OARS). In addition to the use of open-ended questions and reflective listening during counseling, it is suggested that the dietitian highlight an individual's strength through the use of affirmations to promote self-efficacy in the patient with CKD. Telling a patient "You've done a wonderful job in lowering your serum phosphorus since last month" or "I can see how hard you are working on making the changes in your diet, and all your efforts are working" will help the patient with CKD feel confident and empowered. The dietitian can use affirmations while counseling all patients, even those who are struggling. For example, in the case where a patient is struggling to make progress in adhering to their potassium restriction, but has been unsuccessful, the dietitian can affirm effort with the following statement: "I know you have had difficulty lately in reducing your potassium intake, and your continued effort to move forward in improving your food choices reveals a strong determination."

Summaries provide opportunities for the dietitian to collect multiple change talk statements and to link them together to create a fuller picture for the patient or to link discrepant statements that capture ambivalence. Summary points can be used at any point during the counseling session. In the beginning it can be used to focus the patient on what has occurred since the last meeting, it can be used at the end of the session to summarize what has been accomplished during the session, or it can be used in the middle of the session to provide a path for progress [17]. For example, the dietitian may say, "Mrs. Conner, during today's session you have outlined all the right information about how you can lower your phosphorus intake and you have reported progress, but you still struggle with consistency. Where would you like to go from here? Would it be helpful if we continue with a discussion about some of the obstacles you are facing with being consistent with your low-phosphorus diet?"

Additional MI tools that promote progress during counseling sessions are the importance scale and confidence scale. These are simple tools but when used can offer a great amount of information. Using the importance scale with follow-up questions can get the patient talking about why certain dietary goals are important to them [18, 20, 32].

The following displays how the importance scale and follow-up questions can promote change talk during counseling:

Dietitian:	"On a scale of 1–10, with 1 being of little importance and 10 representing great importance, how important is it for you to maintain an acceptable potassium level?"
Patient:	"I would say about a 7."
Dietitian:	"So it sounds as if it is fairly important to you. I am sure that you have some obstacles, but can you tell me why you chose a 7 instead of a 4 or 5?"
Patient:	"I know that it's important to keep my potassium at a good level. I heard that if I don't it can affect my heart, and I want to stay healthy. I mean it's my heart and I only have one, right."

Dietitian: "Yes, I agree and am glad you see the value in maintaining a good potassium level. Would you like to discuss some strategies that can help with your potassium level?"

Patient: "That would make a lot of sense. I'd love to hear some suggestions."

Addressing any challenges or obstacles faced can be accomplished by using a different follow-up question as displayed below:

Dietitian: "On a scale of 1–10, with 1 being of little importance and 10 representing great importance, how important is it for you to maintain an acceptable potassium level?"

Patient: "I would say about a 7."

Dietitian: "So it sounds as if it is fairly important to you. I am sure that you have some obstacles, but can you tell me why you chose a 7 instead of an 8 or 9?"

Patient: "I know that it's important to keep my potassium at a good level, but I really have a hard time remembering this when I am eating. I eat first and think later. Also, I am not sure about the potassium content of all foods. I only know the biggest offenders to avoid, like bananas and mangos."

Dietitian: "I am so glad to hear about your challenges and obstacles. It's always helpful when you can identify what gets in your way. What do you think would help you overcome your obstacles?"

Patient: "I need to find a way to remember to think about a food's potassium content before I take my first bite. Do you have any suggestions to help me?"

In both scenarios the use of the importance scale and follow-up questions provides insight into the patient's thoughts and motivations for changing food-related behaviors. The verbalization of these thoughts by the patient is instrumental in promoting change talk and in cementing a plan of action that is borne through a shared effort [18, 20, 32]. This scale can also be used to gauge confidence and to promote improved confidence as well.

The following displays how the use of the confidence scale and follow-up questions can promote change talk during counseling:

Dietitian: "Now that we have discussed that you can keep index cards in your purse with the foods that you should avoid due to the high potassium content, on a scale of 1–10 how confident are you that you will be able to use this strategy?"

Patient: "I would choose a 7 in rating my confidence."

Dietitian: "That's good to hear. Can you tell me why you chose a 7 instead of a 5 or 6?"

Patient: "I chose a 7 because I think the plan is very reasonable and I should be able to follow through. I can go out about my day and have my plan with me in my purse. It's a simple solution that makes sense to me, but I have to remind myself to refer to the index cards when the time comes. That is one thing that I will have to work on."

Dietitian: "I am so happy to hear how confident you are and that you are ready to take the next step in addressing your potassium intake. I have some thoughts on how you might manage a prompt to help you remember to double-check your list before eating. Would you like to discuss some options?"

Patient: "Yes, I would really appreciate your suggestions as this remains an obstacle for me."

In reviewing the dialogue between the dietitian and the patient in the scenarios above, it is apparent that using the importance scale and confidence scale results in promoting forward motion in behavior change.

MI has been found to be effective in promoting positive change in a variety of health-related behaviors. In a systematic review of 72 studies, MI was found to outperform traditional advice giving in 80% of the studies reviewed [33]. Furthermore, Spahn and colleagues [16] report that MI was found to be a highly effective counseling strategy for diet and lifestyle modifications. A more recent systematic review focused on MI in weight loss interventions found that in more than one-half of the 24 randomized control studies included in the review, researchers reported successful outcome of at least 5% weight loss associated with participants who received a MI intervention [34]. Most studies investigating the benefits of MI were conducted on patients who were obese and had diabetes or cardiovascular disease. However, two studies published in 2011 and 2017 investigated the efficacy of using MI techniques in patients with CKD; both studies were conducted with small numbers of hemodialysis patients (29 and 18, respectively). The results revealed that MI delivered by MI-trained hemodialysis staff resulted in improvements in dialysis attendance and serum phosphorus and albumin levels. However, there was no effect on reducing interdialytic weight gain [32, 35]. These studies included few participants and were conducted for relatively short periods of time; however, researchers were optimistic that these studies show promise and that future research efforts conducted with a larger group of participants for longer periods of time may support the concept that MI is efficacious in counseling patients with CKD [32, 35].

Special Considerations for Patients Receiving Hemodialysis

Patients receiving hemodialysis typically dialyze thrice weekly, providing ample opportunity for the dietitian to meet with and build a rapport with patients, as well as to find an appropriate and/or convenient time for patients' sessions. However, most dialysis units do not offer privacy at the chair side and it can become quite noisy during counseling sessions. There may not be much that the dietitian can do to modify the setting, but closing a curtain and sitting in a chair or on a stool can help to make the session more private and personal. Moreover, sitting at the same eye level as the patient is desirable. It is useful to remember that the patient is immobilized by being connected to a dialysis machine for several hours. Under these circumstances, it is very important to consider the lack of power the patient has as he or she cannot get up and leave. The dietitian may stop by the patient's treatment area to discuss dietary and medication adherence issues when it appears to be most convenient for the clinician's schedule. However, this may not be the best time for the patient to discuss these issues. Checking in with the patient at treatment initiation and asking for permission to schedule an appointment later that day or during a subsequent session will express respect for the patient, and it will give the patient decision-making power about when a counseling session can take place. Finally, if absolute privacy is needed, a time can be arranged to meet with the patient in a private area before or after treatment.

Hemodialysis patients often have several components to their dietary restrictions. Addressing all components of the restriction at once can be overwhelming. Providing a focus on one component at a time and asking the patient to choose the component that he or she wants to discuss during that session (e.g., how to increase dietary intake of high-quality protein) may improve patient involvement and offer the patient the power of choice during the session [17]. These simple measures can go a long way in promoting positive, effective counseling sessions.

Future Directions

An investigation of patient needs revealed that patients with CKD report need for greater support from healthcare providers in executing a daily set of complex tasks [36]. There are more options today than ever before in reaching patients outside the clinic or doctor's office. Research has supported the use of computer-aided telehealth and mobile-enabled interventions in communicating health messages to promote and support self-management in those managing chronic diseases [37]. Research exploring the effect of mobile health on the adoption of healthy behaviors in patients with CKD is very limited; however, a new trial is underway comparing the effect of three technology-supported interventions in comparison to usual care in patients who are overweight and have type 2 diabetes mellitus and CKD (stages 1–4). The Healthy Hearts and Kidneys (HHK) study will investigate the interventional effects on dietary sodium intake, added dietary phosphorus, time spent exercising, and body weight outcomes in approximately 300 patients. Although the findings are not yet published, prior trials have shown promise in the use of technology-based outreach in supporting patients with chronic disease [38]. A recent survey study investigating the availability and acceptability of technology use in a sample of over 700 patients with CKD found that 89% had computer access and 84% owned a mobile phone. As expected, those younger than 60 years of age and who had achieved a higher level of education were most comfortable in using their mobile phone for complex communication. However, the researchers suggest that simple, less time-consuming technology that is more user-friendly will be the most likely to be adopted by the greatest majority of patients with chronic disease [39]. Clearly, there is great potential to connect, inform, and guide patients with CKD through various technology sources. However, technology-based healthcare is an evolving area of study and requires continued research to be able to best guide healthcare practitioners in the most effective measures to take to support patient self-management.

Conclusion

The prevalence of CKD is rising worldwide and dietitians are best poised to offer important, undoubtedly life-saving guidance to patients. However, nonadherence with dietary recommendations is common. Patient-centered counseling techniques fundamental to CBT and MI have been found to enhance patient outcomes for several chronic diseases, including CKD. Patients with CKD experience many physical and psychosocial detriments, and how the dietitian can best counsel to effectively lessen these burdens should be further explored to improve understanding, enhance change talk, and promote dietary adherence. Dietitians should explore the use of current technology options, once more evidence is available, to extend additional guidance and support outside the medical center or clinic.

Case Study

Mrs. Connor has been receiving hemodialysis for the past 6 months. She is a 48-year-old married woman and mother of a 12-year-old boy and a 14-year-old girl who have very active after-school schedules. In addition, she works full-time as a fifth-grade school teacher. She comes in for dialysis during the evening shifts to accommodate her home and work schedule. Mrs. Connor has been struggling with elevated serum potassium levels and also comes in with large interdialytic fluid weight gains. Her serum phosphorus is within normal limits, and she reports that she takes her phosphate-binding medications consistently. Additionally, she is very consistent in arriving for all scheduled dialysis treatments. She has met with the dietitian several times but always seems overwhelmed and distracted during the counseling time. She tells the dietitian, "I'm doing my best. I feel overwhelmed with all the responsibilities I have along with my restrictions on food and fluid. I want to bring down my potassium and better control my fluid intake, but I just don't know where to start. I do everything at home and I am responsible for 25 children at school who depend on me too. I come last on the list of priorities. If you just give me the instruction sheets I'll read over them."

Case Questions and Answers

1. What stage in the transtheoretical model stages of change is Mrs. Connor exhibiting in this case?
   Answer: Mrs. Connor is in the contemplation stage of the transtheoretical model. She knows that she needs to change her habits and restrict the potassium in her diet as well as lower her fluid intake. She is overwhelmed and the pros of making the changes are countered by the cons of not being able to make the time to care of her needs. This creates ambivalence and lack of progress.

2. Which type of reflective listening would you use to reflect back Mrs. Connor's comment about her challenges?
   Answer: All forms of reflective listening will help Mrs. Connor realize that the dietitian hears her and understands her issues and obstacles. However, her statements offer an opportunity for the dietitian to use a *two-sided reflection* to highlight her ambivalence. Reflecting, "I hear that on the one hand you are struggling with many daily responsibilities and cannot find the time to care for your needs, but on the other hand you see the value in addressing your dietary and fluid needs."

3. Would you suggest the use of cognitive restructuring in this case? If so, why or why not?
   Answer; Yes. Cognitive restructuring is an appropriate CBT strategy to use in this case. Mrs. Connor's comment "I come last on the list of priorities" is an irrational statement. She is managing so much for so many others, and if she does not take care of herself, then she cannot take care of others. She needs to make her needs a priority, especially while receiving hemodialysis. Using open-ended questions can help to get her talking about this irrational thought. Perhaps begin by asking "Who would take care of things if you were unable to do so?" or "Do you ever wonder how long you can continue working in this way without considering your needs?" might guide the conversation toward the understanding that she needs to take care of her needs first to be best equipped to help all who depend on her. Mrs. Connor would benefit from the dietitian highlighting that making herself a priority is not a selfish action, but a necessity.

4. Would you use the importance scale or confidence scale in this case? State the reasons for your choice.
   Answer: An *importance scale* is appropriate to use at this point. Mrs. Connor is not ready to take action and make plans for change as yet, so a confidence scale will not be useful. The dietitian may ask her, "On a scale of 1–10, with one being not important at all and 10 being very important, how important is it for you to lower your potassium intake?" This question can begin a discussion that addresses why she wants to make the change. If Mrs. Connor tells the dietitian why it's important to address the potassium in her diet, she will most likely listen to her own voice on the issue, and it avoids her feeling as if she is being lectured on the topic.

5. Assuming that Mrs. Connor says that she reports a "5" on the scale that you chose to use, how would you state your follow-up question, and why?
   Answer: Asking her *why she chose a 5 and not a 3 or 4* would prompt her to discuss why she thinks that lowering her potassium intake is so important. This discussion should help move her forward, perhaps towards the preparation stage where she is willing to consider planning to take action within the month.

6. What CBT strategies would be useful to use in this case?
   Answer: There are several CBT strategies that would be very useful in this case. Discussing *social support* will help Mrs. Connor get the help she might need from her family and friends. Perhaps her husband can assist with preparing low-potassium meals, and her children can help with chores at home. Mrs. Connor can ask her colleagues for support at work as well. She need not do everything herself. People are often happy to help others if they are asked and know what is needed to assist. *Problem-solving* will address how she can plan for her busy days with her dietary restrictions considered. Planning ahead to troubleshoot problems can change chaos into smoothly running procedures. *Stress management* will be essential to assist Mrs. Connor in helping her keep a level head and not feeling overwhelmed. Find the things that help her relax (e.g., meditation, going for a walk, reading a novel) and assist her in scheduling these relaxing activities into her daily schedule.

References

1. Centers for Disease Control and Prevention. Chronic Kidney Disease in the United States, 2019. Atlanta, GA: US Department of Health and Human Services, Centers for Disease Control and Prevention; 2019. https://www.cdc.gov/kidneydisease/publications-resources/2019-national-facts.html. Accessed 5 May 2020
2. National Institutes of Diabetes and Digestive and Kidney Diseases. Kidney disease statistics for the United States. 2016. Retrieved from https://www.niddk.nih.gov/health-information/health-statistics/kidney-disease. Accessed on 12 Feb 2019.
3. Tsay SL, Kee YC, Lee YC. Effects of an adaptation training programme for patients with end-stage renal disease. J Adv Nurs. 2005;50(1):39–46.
4. Krespi R, Bone M, Ahmad R, Worthington B, Salmon P. Haemodialysis patients' beliefs about renal failure and its treatment. Patient Educ Couns. 2004;53:189–96.
5. King N, Carroll C, Newton P, Dornan T. "You can't cure it so you have to endure it": the experience of adaptation to diabetic renal disease. Qual Health Res. 2002;12(3):329–46.
6. Fallon M. Depression in end-stage renal disease. J Psychosoc Nurs Ment Health Serv. 2011;49(8):30–4.
7. Mei-Chen L, Wu SFV, Nan-Chen H, Juin-Ming T. Self-management programs on eGFR, depression, and quality of life among patients with chronic kidney disease: a meta-analysis. Asian Nurs Res. 2016;10:255–62.
8. Cliffe M, Bloodworth LO, Jihani MM. Can malnutrition in predialysis patients be prevented by dietetic intervention? J Ren Nutr. 2001;11(3):161–5.
9. Mitch WE, Remuzzi G. Diets for patients with chronic kidney disease, still worth prescribing. J Am Soc Nephrol. 2004;15:234–7.
10. Akpele L, Bailey JL. Nutrition counseling improves serum albumin levels. J Ren Nutr. 2004;14(3):143–8.
11. Garneata L, Mircescu G. Nutritional intervention in uremia—myth or reality? J Ren Nutr. 2010;20:S31–4.
12. Khalil AA, Frazier SK, Lennie TA, Sawaya BP. Depressive symptoms and dietary adherence in patients with end-stage renal disease. J Ren Care. 2011;37(1):30.
13. Kaptein AA, van Dijk S, Broadbend E, Falzon L, Thong M, Dekker FW. Behavioural research in patients with end-stage renal disease: a review and research agenda. Patient Educ Couns. 2010;81:23–9.
14. Nygardh A, Malm D, Wikby K, Ahistrom G. The experience of empowerment in the patient-staff encounter: the patient's perspective. J Clin Nurs. 2012;21:897–904.
15. Van Korff VM, Gruman J, Schaefer J, Curry SJ, Wagner EH. Collaborative management of chronic illness. Ann Intern Med. 1997;127(12):1097–102.
16. Spahn JM, Reeves RS, Keim KS, Laquatra I, Kellogg M, Jortberg B, et al. State of the evidence regarding behavior change theories and strategies in nutrition counseling to facilitate health and food behavior change. J Am Diet Assoc. 2010;110:879–91.
17. Martino S. Motivational interviewing to engage patients in chronic kidney disease management. Blood Purif. 2011;31:77–81.
18. Naar S, Safren SA. Motivational interviewing and CBT: combining strategies for maximum effectiveness. New York/London: The Guilford Press; 2017.
19. Prochaska JO, Norcorss JC, DeClemente CC. Changing for good. New York: HarperCollins; 1994.
20. Holli BB, Beto JA. Nutrition counseling and education skills: a guide for professionals. 6th ed. New York: Lippincott, Williams & Wilkins; 2017.
21. Miller NH. Motivational interviewing as a prelude to coaching in healthcare settings. J Cardiovasc Nurs. 2010;25(3):247–51.
22. Bandura A. Self-efficacy: towards a unifying theory of behavior change. Psychol Rev. 1977;84(2):191–215.
23. Blackman MC, Kvaska CA. Nutrition psychology: improving dietary adherence. Boston: Jones and Bartlett Publishers; 2011.
24. Weng LC, Dai YT, Huang HL, Chiang YJ. Self-efficacy, self-care behaviors and quality of life of kidney transplant patients. J Adv Nurs. 2010;66(4):828–38.
25. Wells JR, Anderson ST. Self-efficacy and social support in African Americans diagnosed with end-stage renal disease. ABNF J. 2011;22(1):9–12.
26. Beck AT, Dozois DJA. Cognitive therapy: current status and future directions. Annu Rev Med. 2011;62:397–409.
27. Kugler C, Vlaminck H, Haverich A, Maes B. Nonadherence with diet and fluid restrictions among adults having hemodialysis. J Nurs Scholarsh. 2005;37(1):25–9.
28. Durose CL, Holdsworth M, Watson V, Przygrodzka F. Knowledge of dietary restrictions and the medical consequences of noncompliance by patients on hemodialysis are not predictive of dietary compliance. J Am Diet Assoc. 2004;104:35–41.
29. Tierney P, Hughes C, Hamilton S. Promoting health behaviour change in the cardiac patient. Br J Cardiac Nurs. 2011;6(3):126–30.
30. Karalis M, Wiesen K. Motivational interviewing. Nephrol Nurs J. 2007;34(3):336–8.

31. Rollnick S, Miller WR, Butler CC. Motivational interviewing in health care: helping patients change behavior. New York: Gilford Press; 2008.
32. Crown S, Vogel JA, Hurlock-Chorostecki C. Enhancing self-care management of interdialytic weight gain in patients on hemodialysis: a pilot using motivational interviewing. Nephrol Nurs J. 2017;41:49–55.
33. Rubak S, Sandboek A, Lauritzen T, Christensen B. Motivational interviewing: a systematic review and meta-analysis. Br J Gen Pract. 2005;55:305–12.
34. Barnes D, Ivezaj V. A systematic review of motivational interviewing for weight loss among adults in primary care. Obes Rev. 2015;16:304–18.
35. Cl R, Cronk NJ, Herron M. Motivational interviewing in dialysis adherence study. Nephrol Nurs J. 2011;38(3):229–36.
36. Haves K, Douglas C, Bonner A. Person-centered care in chronic disease: a cross-sectional study of patients' desires for self-management support. BMC Nephrol. 2017;18:17. https://doi.org/10.1186/s12882-016-0416-2.
37. Lynch CP, Williams JS, Ruggiero KJ, Knapp RG, Egede LE. Tablet-aided behavioral intervention effect on self-management skills (TABLETS) for diabetes. Trials. 2016;17:157. https://doi.org/10.1186/s13063-016-1243-2.
38. Sevick MA, Woolf K, Mattoo A, Katz SD, Li H, St. Jules DE, et al. The healthy hearts and kidneys (HHK) study: design of a 2x2 RCT of technology-supported self-monitoring and social cognitive theory-based counseling to engage overweight people with diabetes and chronic kidney disease in multiple lifestyle changes. Contemp Clin Trials. 2018;64:265–73.
39. Bonner A, Gillespie K, Campbell KL, Corones-Watkins K, Hayes G, Harvie B, et al. Evaluating the prevalence and opportunity for technology in chronic kidney disease patients: a cross-sectional study. BMC Nephrol. 2018;19:28. https://doi.org/10.1186/s12882-018-0830-8.

Chapter 36
Comparative Effectiveness Research and Renal Nutrition

Laura D. Byham-Gray

Keywords Outcomes research (OR) · Comparative effectiveness research (CER) · Patient-centered outcomes research (PCOR) · Kidney disease · Nutrition · Morbidity · Mortality · Evidence-based practice · Medical nutrition therapy · Dialysis Outcomes and Practice Patterns Study (DOPPS) Agency for Healthcare Research and Quality (AHRQ) · Patient-Centered Outcomes Research Initiative (PCORI)

> **Key Points**
> - To define the principles and processes of comparative effectiveness research
> - To discuss potential comparative effectiveness research projects in nutrition and kidney disease
> - To identify the role of nutrition in patient outcomes among individuals diagnosed with kidney disease

Introduction

Despite advances in medicine and technology, clinical outcomes among patients diagnosed with chronic kidney disease (CKD) have remained suboptimal. Historically, much of the focus in kidney disease had been on the burgeoning end-stage kidney disease (ESKD) population and the respective renal replacement therapies (RRTs) necessary for life maintenance, i.e., hemodialysis (HD), peritoneal dialysis (PD), and kidney transplantation. For the first time in decades, the incidence of individuals advancing to ESKD has slowed and may be related to the greater emphasis on early screening for CKD in primary care settings, leading to more timely and appropriate intervention(s) [1]. Capturing the patient once at stage 5 CKD may be too late to make meaningful changes in the factors associated with poorer outcomes.

This chapter will give a brief overview of the importance for studying the role that nutritional status has on key clinical outcomes in CKD, a clear description of comparative effectiveness research and its related methodology, as well as a discussion of clinical guidelines and their role in reducing practice variation.

L. D. Byham-Gray (✉)
Clinical and Preventive Nutrition Sciences, School of Health Professions, Rutgers University, Newark, NJ, USA
e-mail: laura.byham.gray@rutgers.edu

© Springer Nature Switzerland AG 2020
J. D. Burrowes et al. (eds.), *Nutrition in Kidney Disease*, Nutrition and Health,
https://doi.org/10.1007/978-3-030-44858-5_36

Challenges for Nutrition

The importance of nutrition in the treatment and management of CKD is unquestionable. The relationship between nutritional status and morbidity and mortality has been researched extensively. There are a multitude of outcomes across the spectrum of kidney disease that could and should be measured. For example, bone disease, diabetes, dyslipidemias, hypertension, dialysis adequacy, and anemia are all either directly or indirectly related to nutrition intervention. Understanding how nutritional status impacts morbidity and mortality is seemingly more difficult than studying either dialysis adequacy or anemia management. Protein-energy malnutrition or wasting is an independent contributor for mortality risk [2–6]. However, it remains unclear whether the malnutrition or wasting occurs over a period of time or as the result of a suboptimal status at the time of dialysis initiation, i.e., the association between malnutrition and death secondary to changes in nutritional status experienced over time or rather the presence of abnormalities at baseline [7, 8].

Multiple factors may explain the complexity of defining, treating, and reversing the malnutrition or wasting experienced and comprise both nutritional and non-nutritional components [9]. Nutritional status can be assessed and "diagnosed" by using anthropometric measures, biochemical indices, clinical symptoms, or dietary intake records separately or together; therein lies the difficulty, the lack of one single measure that provides a good estimate of nutritional status [10]. Compounding these challenges is the impact of metabolic aberrations and hemodynamic imbalances secondary to CKD that may falsely affect nutrition parameters; e.g., non-nutritional factors such as inflammation or hydration status may interfere with the reliability of measuring nutritional status through conventional means. Acknowledging the complexity of protein-energy malnutrition, the International Society of Renal Nutrition and Metabolism (ISRNM) convened an expert panel who proposed new nomenclature for protein-energy malnutrition with the intent of "systematically defin[ing] the diagnostic criteria" so that it will "clarify communication, enhance the effectiveness of patient care, and promote more incisive research in the field" [9]. The panel members recommended the term protein-energy wasting (PEW) instead of protein-energy malnutrition, since it incorporates a multifaceted explanation for the suboptimal nutritional status often experienced in CKD patients, and have offered guidance on how to best prevent or treat this syndrome [2, 11].

Nutrition intervention or medical nutrition therapy (MNT) does make a positive impact on patient health outcomes. Studies have reported the effectiveness of nutrition intervention for a number of clinical outcomes related to disease states/conditions such as diabetes, hyperlipidemia, cancer, unintentional weight loss, as well as outcomes related to cost and health-care utilization [12–20]. Researchers have also explored the impact of nutrition intervention (e.g., counseling or educational programs) on CKD patients [21–24]. Such literature is essential in determining how nutrition therapy or dietetic practice patterns can positively impact or influence patient health and outcomes.

Outcomes Research Defined

"The American health care delivery system is in need of fundamental change" is the opening statement to the Institute of Medicine's (IOM) report entitled *Crossing the Quality Chasm: A New Health Care System for the 21st Century, 2001* [25]. It is a provocative beginning for "what works and what doesn't work in health care" [26]. Thus, the goals for outcomes research, or rather comparative effectiveness research, are really to determine [27]: Which treatments are the most effective? Which providers give the best care? Which health plans are the most efficient? Which delivery systems provide the most patient-centered care? Who produces the best outcomes? Obviously, patients, providers, payers, and policymakers are all interested in the answers to the above questions. Thus, the Agency for Healthcare Research and Quality (AHRQ) was formulated with the specific charge to support outcomes research (OR) and thereby improve the quality of health care in the United States [28].

Outcomes research is often referred to as the "third revolution in health care" and is defined as "the process of obtaining data to measure the effect of a particular intervention on patient care" [26]. It has also been termed as "medical effectiveness research (MER)" or "outcomes effectiveness research (OER)." Most recently, the AHRQ has described outcomes research as "comparative effectiveness research" (CER) which is defined as "the generation and synthesis of evidence that compares the benefits and harms of alternative methods to prevent, diagnose, treat, and monitor a clinical condition or to improve the delivery of care. The purpose of CER is to assist consumers, clinicians, purchasers, and policymakers to make informed decisions that will improve health care at both the individual and population levels" [28]. In fact, the American Recovery and Reinvestment Act of 2009 (i.e., the economic stimulus package) provided significant funding for CER through the AHRQ's Effective Health Care Program which focused on key research priorities aimed at improving patient care and outcome. In 2010, with the passing of the Patient Protection and Affordable Care Act, the Patient-Centered Outcomes Research Institute (PCORI), comprising a 21-member board that included the directors from AHRQ and the National Institutes of Health (NIH), was formally devised to fund and promote CER that will "advanc[e] the quality and relevance of evidence concerning the manner in which diseases, disorders, and other health conditions can effectively and appropriately be prevented, diagnosed, treated, monitored, and managed through research and evidence synthesis" [29]. The PCORI includes an independent, federally appointed Methodology Committee who is charged with the mission of formulating the standards for patient-centered outcomes research (PCOR). The four general areas identified by the committee in which standards will be developed are [30]: (1) prioritizing research questions, (2) using appropriate study designs and analyses, (3) incorporating patient perspectives throughout the research continuum, and (4) fostering efficient dissemination and implementation of results. Integrating the patient's voice into the research process affords investigators with the unique opportunity to focus on research questions that matter the most to patients and their families. One example of how to engage stakeholders into the research process using deliberative panels has been recently published as a methodology paper in order to help guide other researchers [31]. Nonetheless, the continued existence of PCORI and the advent of PCOR are largely dependent on the future of the Affordable Care Act. Regardless of the acronym, outcomes research collects and analyzes data with the intent of aiding patients, health professionals, insurers, and administrators in the selection of suitable medical treatment options and setting health-care policy.

The benefits for conducting outcomes research are multiple [32]: it identifies best practices and improves the knowledge base of medical and health sciences, quantifies cost-effectiveness of therapeutic interventions, supplies the basis for practice guidelines, formulates methods for continuous quality improvement (CQI), and sets benchmarking thresholds, aids in market decisions, and provides accountability.

There is a distinction to be made between outcomes management and outcomes research; both are equally important for patient care. Outcomes management is the outcomes data routinely collected by practitioners, and it lays the groundwork for outcomes research [33]. Outcomes management allows the practitioner to participate in research at a more basic level, and it fosters further professional development in research skills. Outcomes research employs controlled research procedures. To assist practicing dietitians in the collection of data for the purpose of measuring effectiveness of care, the Academy of Nutrition and Dietetics Health Informatics Infrastructure (known as ANDHII®) has been designed and participation is strongly encouraged in key areas of research interest [34].

Seemingly, CQI or process improvement (PI) interfaces with outcomes management and outcomes research and can often represent an entrée into the conduction of CER [33]. CQI includes the analysis of the process(es), identification of key quality characteristics of the process, as well as the outcomes of interest. The measurements will often include data collection on key process variables rather than direct clinical care that are hypothesized to influence patient outcomes, such as frequency of contact, length of time between encounters, or when appointment scheduling occurs. Outcomes research, on the other hand, focuses closely on the impact of the treatment on patient outcome. Generally, outcomes projects lead to changes in practice standards. Quality of care is then measured according to such standards; this aspect represents CQI.

Types of Outcomes

Although categories in the literature may slightly vary, there are generally three "types of outcomes": clinical, patient-oriented, and economic (32). Clinical outcomes focus on health status outcomes and can include mortality, risk factors, changes in development or progression of symptoms, disease and its sequelae, and complications from treatment [26, 32]. Some examples of types of outcomes related to nutrition and CKD are provided in Table 36.1 [35]. Patient-oriented outcomes give attention to the consequences of interventions that are of concern to patients/families, such as survival, symptom relief, adverse effects of the condition or its treatment, functional status, quality of life (QoL), and satisfaction. Economic outcomes are related to indicators that reduce length of stay, minimize care costs, or maximize revenue generation. For example, if the practitioner wanted to study the effects of nutritional status on QoL (patient-oriented outcome), she/he would need to consult a number of validated tools to determine which one measured the constructs of interest.

Attributes of good outcome variables are "objective, precise, quantitative and translatable" [26]. Dhingra and Laski add that they should be "valid, reproducible, actionable, and comparable over geographic, demographic and temporal boundaries," allowing for benchmarking to occur [36]. Thus, one way to initiate more outcomes research in clinical practice, specifically in kidney disease, is to use the outcome measures published in evidence-based practice guidelines.

Table 36.1 Main types of outcome measures with nutrition-related examples cited

Clinical outcomes	Economic outcomes
Mortality rate	MNT reimbursement
Weight status	Length of stay
Body mass index	Hospitalizations
Subjective global assessment	Delays in CKD progression
Albumin or pre-albumin levels	Cost of enteral versus parenteral nutritional supplementation
Lean body mass	Cost-benefits of MNT versus other adjunctive therapies
C-reactive protein	
Normalized protein catabolic rate	
Interdialytic weight gains	
Patient-oriented outcomes	
Ability to live independently	
Perception of patient care received	
Health-related quality of life	
Symptom relief from early satiety	
Functional status	

Adapted from [35]

Evidence-Based Practice Guidelines

Variances in patient outcome and survival among industrialized countries (e.g., the United States, Europe, Canada, Australia, and Japan) were first recognized in 1989 at the Dallas symposium on morbidity and mortality of dialysis patients [37]. The United States reported the largest number of new patients with ESKD maintained on dialysis but also registered the highest crude mortality rate, ranging from 22% to 24%. Such results motivated several organizations and regulatory agencies (e.g., National Institutes of Health, Health Care Financing Administration, Kidney Physicians Association) to focus on efforts for improving the quality of care delivered to dialysis patients in the United States. This emphasis on "medical effectiveness" led to the creation of the Dialysis Outcomes Quality Initiative (DOQI) Project of the National Kidney Foundation (NKF) in 1995. To reflect a broader mission of improving the health status of patients across the spectrum of kidney disease, DOQI was later renamed in 1999 as the Kidney Disease Outcomes Quality Initiative (KDOQI). The first DOQI guidelines were released in 1997 with subsequent updates and topics expanded from dialysis adequacy, vascular access, and anemia to peritoneal dialysis, nutrition, CKD, dyslipidemia, bone disease, hypertension, and diabetes [38].

Concomitantly, other countries initiated their own system for creating and developing practice guidelines [39, 40]. For example, in addition to the United States [10, 41], there are three other international guidelines published on nutrition and CKD [42–44]. Although similar recommendations were established internationally, the target ranges or values for specific outcome measures and how the evidence was rated may be highly variable. A more uniform approach for evidence analysis was needed; therefore, the concept of KDIGO (which stands for Kidney Disease: Improving Global Outcomes) was conceived. Its mission is "to improve care and outcomes of kidney disease patients worldwide through promoting coordination, collaboration, and integration of initiatives to develop and implement clinical practice guidelines" [40]. Presently, there are several international clinical practice guidelines published on critical topics such as kidney transplantation, bone and mineral disorders, hepatitis C, and acute kidney injury, with these and others under constant review and development. While not part of the KDIGO initiative, there is a current international update to the original KDOQI Clinical Practice Guidelines for Nutrition being completed in collaboration with the Academy of Nutrition and Dietetics that is anticipated for publication in late 2020.

Implementation Science: Practice Guidelines and Patient Care

There is limited research whether practice guidelines actually affect clinical practice. Nonetheless, successful implementation of evidence-based guidelines can improve outcomes [45, 46]. Nonetheless, there are challenges to implementing guidelines into practice, often out of the practitioner's purview, and targeting a key guideline at first assists in early adoption [46]. For example, Burrowes et al. [47] surveyed renal dietitians about whether they implemented the 2000 KDOQI Nutrition Guidelines. The vast majority (92%) had integrated at least one guideline into practice, whereas only 5% had implemented all of them. Dietitians reported that they were unable to change their clinical practice according to the best evidence in all areas, as a number of barriers existed such as unavailable equipment or tools (e.g., computers, food models, and calipers), high patient-to-dietitian staffing ratios, or the lack of administrative support for change. In a study published 5 years later by Vergili and Wolf, it was evident that there was still substantial practice variation among renal dietitians in relation to the KDOQI Nutrition Guidelines [48]. Reasons given by the survey respondents included challenges within the practice setting as well as relevance of the guidelines published in 2000 to current practice. Thus, it is increasingly difficult to determine the impact of practice guidelines on patient outcomes if resources are lacking for their successful implementation. In order to overcome such barriers, the Academy of Nutrition and Dietetics has published a number of toolkits related to their clinical practice guidelines in nutrition including one on CKD, which provides several reliable indicators for measuring nutritional status and monitoring outcomes [49]. A useful initial outcomes research project may be to examine whether integrating such guidelines does impact care. It represents a relatively simple study design, and no investigations of this nature currently exist in nutrition and CKD.

Conclusion

The incidence of CKD patients is expanding in the United States, but sadly, poor outcomes prevail. The complexity of protein-energy malnutrition or wasting impedes its understanding, treatment, and subsequent elimination as a contributor toward the morbidity and mortality experienced in this specific patient population. The generation of evidence-based practice guidelines assists in positively affecting change in practice to optimize outcomes and serves as sources for measurable indicators in outcomes research. More research should concentrate on these areas of nutrition intervention in order to improve outcomes, provide direction for future study, and potentially create changes in clinical practice.

References

1. National Institutes of Health. U.S. Renal Data System 2018 Annual Data Report. Bethesda.
2. Etiology of the protein-energy wasting syndrome in chronic kidney disease: a consensus statement from the International Society of Renal Nutrition and Metabolism (ISRNM). J Ren Nutr. 2013;23(2):77–90. doi:https://doi.org/10.1053/j.jrn.2013.01.001.
3. Beddhu S, Chen X, Wei G, Raj D, Raphael KL, Boucher R, et al. Associations of protein-energy wasting syndrome criteria with body composition and mortality in the general and moderate chronic kidney disease populations in the United States. Kidney Int Rep. 2017;2(3):390–9. https://doi.org/10.1016/j.ekir.2017.01.002. Epub 2017/08/26. PubMed PMID: 28840197; PMCID: PMC5563827.
4. Kang SS, Chang JW, Park Y. Nutritional status predicts 10-year mortality in patients with end-stage renal disease on hemodialysis. Nutrients. 2017;9(4). doi: https://doi.org/10.3390/nu9040399. Epub 2017/04/20. PubMed PMID: 28420212; PMCID: PMC5409738.
5. Kovesdy CP, Kalantar-Zadeh K. Why is protein-energy wasting associated with mortality in chronic kidney disease? Semin Nephrol. 2009;29(1):3–14. Epub 2009/01/06. https://doi.org/10.1016/j.semnephrol.2008.10.002.
6. Segall L, Moscalu M, Hogas S, Mititiuc I, Nistor I, Veisa G, et al. Protein-energy wasting, as well as overweight and obesity, is a long-term risk factor for mortality in chronic hemodialysis patients. Int Urol Nephrol. 2014;46(3):615–21. Epub 2014/01/30. https://doi.org/10.1007/s11255-014-0650-0.
7. Stenvinkel P, Heimburger O, Paultre F, Diczfalusy U, Wang T, Berglund L. Strong association between malnutrition, inflammation, and atherosclerosis in chronic renal failure. Kidney Int. 1999;55(5):1899–911.
8. de Mutsert R, Grootendorst DC, Adelsson J, Boescholen EW, Kiedert RT, Deller FW. Excess mortality due to interaction between protein-energy wasting, inflammation, and cardiovascular disease in chronic dialysis patients. Nephrol Dial Transplant. 2008;23(9):2957–64.
9. Fouque D, Kalantar-Zadeh K, Kopple J, Cano N, Chauveau P, Cuppari L, et al. A proposed nomenclature and diagnostic criteria for protein-energy wasting in acute and chronic kidney disease. Kidney Int. 2008;73(4):391–8. Epub 2007/12/21. https://doi.org/10.1038/sj.ki.5002585.
10. National Kidney Foundation. Kidney Disease Dialysis Outcome Quality Initiative (K/DOQI) clinical practice guidelines for nutrition in chronic renal failure. Am J Kidney Dis. 2000;35(Suppl 2):S1–S140.
11. Ikizler T, Cano NJ, Franch H, Fouque D, Himmelfarb J, Kalantar-Zadeh K, et al. Prevention and treatment of protein energy wasting in chronic kidney disease patients: a consensus statement by the International Society of Renal Nutrition and Metabolism. Kidney Int. 2013;84(6):1096–107. https://doi.org/10.1038/ki.2013.147.
12. Delahanty L, Sonnenberg LA, Hayden D, Nathan DM. Clinical and cost outcomes of medical nutrition therapy in hypercholesterolemia: a controlled trial. J Am Diet Assoc. 2001;101:1012–23.

13. Franz M, Splett PL, Monk A. Cost-effectiveness of medical nutrition therapy provided by persons with non-insulin-dependent diabetes mellitus. J Am Diet Assoc. 1995;95:1018–24.

14. McGehee M, Johnson EQ, Rasmussen HM, Sahyoun N, Lynch MM, Carey M. Benefits and costs of medical nutrition therapy by registered dietitians for patients with hypercholesterolemia. J Am Diet Assoc. 1995;95:1041–3.

15. Splett P, Roth-Yousey LL, Vogelzang JL. Medical nutrition therapy for the prevention and treatment of unintentional weight loss in residential healthcare facilities. J Am Diet Assoc. 2003;103:352–62.

16. Parker AR, Byham-Gray L, Denmark R, Winkle PJ. The effect of medical nutrition therapy by a registered dietitian nutritionist in patients with prediabetes participating in a randomized controlled clinical research trial. J Acad Nutr Diet. 2014;114(11):1739–48. Epub 2014/09/15. https://doi.org/10.1016/j.jand.2014.07.020.

17. Lemon C, Lacey K, Lohse B, Hubacher DO, Klawitter B, Palta M. Outcomes monitoring of health, behavior, and quality of life after nutrition intervention in adults with type 2 diabetes. J Am Diet Assoc. 2004;104:1805–15.

18. Pavlovich W, Waters H, Weller W, Bass EB. Systematic review of literature on cost-effectiveness of nutrition services. J Am Diet Assoc. 2004;104:226–32.

19. Franz MJ, MacLeod J, Evert A, Brown C, Gradwell E, Handu D, Reppert A, Robinson M. Academy of nutrition and dietetics nutrition practice guideline for type 1 and type 2 diabetes in adults: systematic review of evidence for medical nutrition therapy effectiveness and recommendations for integration into the nutrition care process. J Acad Nutr Diet. 2017;117(10):1659–79. Epub 2017/05/24. https://doi.org/10.1016/j.jand.2017.03.022.

20. Suhl E, Anderson-Haynes SE, Mulla C, Patti ME. Medical nutrition therapy for post-bariatric hypoglycemia: practical insights. Surg Obes Relat Dis. 2017;13(5):888–96. https://doi.org/10.1016/j.soard.2017.01.025. Epub 2017/04/11. PubMed PMID: 28392017; PMCID: PMC5469688.

21. Medical nutrition therapy improves primary nutrition outcomes in adults with CKD: a systematic review. J Ren Nutr. 2019;29(3):263. doi:https://doi.org/10.1053/j.jrn.2019.03.072.

22. Beto JA, Ramirez WE, Bansal VK. Medical nutrition therapy in adults with chronic kidney disease: integrating evidence and consensus into practice for the generalist registered dietitian nutritionist. J Acad Nutr Diet. 2014;114(7):1077–87. Epub 2014/03/04. https://doi.org/10.1016/j.jand.2013.12.009.

23. Yu PY. Nutritional status of peritoneal dialysis (PD) patients after medical nutrition therapy at Singapore General Hospital PD Centre. J Ren Nutr. 2010;20(2):139. https://doi.org/10.1053/j.jrn.2010.01.038.

24. de Waal D, Heaslip E, Callas P. Medical nutrition therapy for chronic kidney disease improves biomarkers and slows time to dialysis. J Ren Nutr. 2016;26(1):1–9. https://doi.org/10.1053/j.jrn.2015.08.002.

25. Institute of Medicine. Crossing the quality chasm: a new health system for the 21st century. Washington, DC: National Academies Press; 2001.

26. Murphy W, Hand R. Outcomes research and economic analysis. In: Van Horn L, Beto J, editors. Research: successful approaches. 3rd ed. Chicago: Academy of Nutrition and Dietetics; 2019.

27. Iezzoni L. Risk adjustment for measuring health care outcomes. Chicago: Health Administration Press; 2003.

28. Agency for Healthcare Research and Quality. Comparative effectiveness research. Available from https://www.ahrq.gov/. Accessed 9 Aug 2019.

29. The Patient Protection and Affordable Care Act (PPACA), Pub. L. No. 111-148, 124 Stat. 119, March 23, 2010.

30. Selby J, Beal AC, Frank L. The Patient-Centered Outcomes Research Institute (PCORI) national priorities for Research and Initial Research Agenda. JAMA. 2012;307(15):1583–4.

31. Byham-Gray L, Peters, E., Rothpletz-Puglia, P. Stakeholder Engagement. J Ren Nutr. 2019; [in press].

32. Kane R, Radosevich DM. Conducting health outcomes research. Boston: Jones & Bartlett Publishers; 2011.

33. Academy of Nutrition and Dietetics. Nutrition care process. Available from https://www.ncpro.org/nutrition-care-process. Accessed 29 July 2019.

34. Academy of Nutrition and Dietetics. Academy of Nutrition and Dietetics Health Informatics Infrastructure (ANDII). Available from https://www.eatrightpro.org/research/projects-tools-and-initiatives/andhii. Accessed 29 July 2019.

35. Schiller M, Moore C. Practical approaches to outcomes evaluation. Top Clin Nutr. 1999;14(2):1–12.

36. Dhingra H, Laski ME. Outcomes research in dialysis. Semin Nephrol. 2003;23:295–305.

37. Hull A, Parker T. Proceedings from the morbidity, mortality, and prescription of dialysis symposium. Dallas, Texas. September 15-17, 1989. Am J Kidney Dis. 1990;15:365–83.

38. National Kidney Foundation. Kidney disease outcomes quality initiative. Available from https://www.kidney.org/professionals/guidelines. Accessed 1 Aug 2019.

39. Port F, Eknoyan G. The Dialysis Outcomes and Practice Patterns Study (DOPPS) and the Kidney Disease Outcomes Quality Initiative (K/DOQI): a cooperative initiative to improve outcomes for hemodialysis patients worldwide. Am J Kidney Dis. 2004;44(5, Suppl 2):S1–6.

40. Kidney Disease-Improving Global Outcomes (KDIGO). Practice guidelines. Available from https://kdigo.org/guidelines/. Accessed 1 Aug 2019.

41. Academy of Nutrition and Dietetics. Chronic kidney disease evidence-based nutrition practice guideline. 2010. Available from http://andevidencelibrary.com/topic.cfm?cat=3927. Accessed 9 Oct 2019.

42. Cano NJ, Aparicio M, Brunori G, Carrero JJ, Cianciaruso B, Fiaccadori E, et al. ESPEN. ESPEN Guidelines on Parenteral Nutrition: adult renal failure. Clin Nutr. 2009;28(4):401–14. https://doi.org/10.1016/j.clnu.2009.05.016. Epub 2009 Jun 17

43. Pollock C, Voss D, Hodson E, Crompton C. Caring for Australasians with Renal Impairment (CARI) Guidelines. Nutrition and growth in kidney disease. Nephrology (Carlton). 2005;10(Suppl 5):S177–230.

44. Fouque D, Vennegoor M, Ter Wee P, Wanner C, Basci A, Canaud B, et al. EBPG on nutrition. Nephrol Dial Transplant. 2007;22(suppl_2):ii45–87. https://doi.org/10.1093/ndt/gfm020.

45. Kirk MA, Kelley C, Yankey N, Birken SA, Abadie B, Damschroder L. A systematic review of the use of the consolidated framework for implementation research. Implement Sci. 2016;11(1):72.

46. Damschroder LJ, Aron DC, Keith RE, Kirsh SR, Alexander JA, Lowery JC. Fostering implementation of health services research findings into practice: a consolidated framework for advancing implementation science. Implement Sci. 2009;4(50). https://doi.org/10.1186/1748-5908-4-50.

47. Burrowes J, Russell GB, Rocco MV. Multiple factors affect renal dietitians' use of the NKF K/DOQI adult nutrition guidelines. J Ren Nutr. 2005;15:407–26.

48. Vergili JM, Wolf RL. Nutrition practices of renal dietitians in hemodialysis centers throughout the United States: a descriptive study. J Ren Nutr. 2010;20(1):8.e1–8.e16. https://doi.org/10.1053/j.jrn.2009.06.019.

49. Academy of Nutrition and Dietetics. Toolkits. Available from https://www.eatrightstore.org/product-type/toolkits?pageSize=20&pageIndex=2&sortBy=namedesc. Accessed 1 Aug 2019.

Chapter 37
Suggested Resources for the Practitioner

Melissa Prest

Keywords Nutrition practice guidelines · Nutritional assessment tools · Nutrition education resources Potassium sources · Phosphorus sources · Phosphorus additives · Oxalate

Key Points
- To find information on topics related to kidney disease and related fields
- To access information in a systematic and well-defined manner
- To share information and to distribute it to those persons who are in need and will benefit from this knowledge
- To identify the vast number of resources available

Introduction

This chapter provides a compilation of professional resources that may be of benefit for the practitioner. Its primary goal is to be an accessible reference for the practitioner who treats patients with chronic kidney disease (CKD). The chapter is organized in four basic sections: (1) evidence-based practice guidelines in chronic kidney disease, (2) diet-related resources and food lists, (3) critical tools for conducting nutrition assessments and delivering quality care, and (4) Internet websites and applications. The majority of the information in this chapter augments topics already presented and discussed in earlier chapters.

Evidence-Based Practice Guidelines

Practitioners in CKD have several evidence-based practice guidelines at their disposal that will assist them in evaluating the patient's nutritional status and making appropriate clinical decisions for delivery of care. These include guidelines published by the Academy of Nutrition and Dietetics (Academy), the National Kidney Foundation (NKF), and the Kidney Disease: Improving Global Outcomes (KDIGO). The following highlights the key nutrition-related guidelines for the CKD population.

The editors acknowledge June Leung Fung's contribution to this chapter in *Nutrition in Kidney Disease, Second Edition*, Nutrition and Health, DOI 10.1007/978-1-62703-685-6_1, © Springer Science+Business Media New York 2014.

M. Prest (✉)
National Kidney Foundation of Illinois, Chicago, IL, USA

Academy of Nutrition and Dietetics Evidence Analysis Library (EAL)

The EAL is a resource of systematic reviews related to pertinent nutrition topics that is free to individuals who are members of the Academy of Nutrition and Dietetics. Non-members are also able to access the guidelines for an annual subscription fee. The guidelines are available online at https://www.andeal.org/ and in the NutriGuides Mobile App, which is accessible at https://www.andeal.org/nutriguides. Currently, there are dozens of evidenced-based guidelines, many of which may be of benefit to the renal practitioner. The most pertinent topics include chronic kidney disease (CKD), adult weight management (AWM), diabetes types 1 and 2, diabetes (type 2) prevention, dietary fatty acids, disorders of lipid metabolism (DLM), fiber, hypertension (HTN), nutrition counseling, sodium, telenutrition, and vegetarian nutrition (VEG).

The 2010 CKD guidelines by the Academy are intended for use by Registered Dietitian Nutritionists (RDN) who provide medical nutrition therapy (MNT) to adults with CKD who are not receiving renal replacement therapy. The Work Group's recommendations were derived from systematic reviews and were intended to not overlap with the existing evidenced-based guidelines for persons receiving maintenance hemodialysis from the NKF-Kidney Disease Outcomes Quality Initiative (KDOQI) [1].

KDOQI Clinical Practice Guidelines

The NKF and their appointed Work Groups, as part of KDOQI, have published a number of practice guidelines related to topics of dialysis adequacy, cardiovascular disease, anemia, bone disease, and, of course, nutrition, as well as many others. The reader may access the guidelines at the NKF website (www.kidney.org) for routine updates and full explanation and details of each practice guideline. Due to space limitations, only the links to various clinical practice guidelines that may be of interest to the reader are presented below:

- Diabetes and CKD (2012 update): https://www.ajkd.org/article/S0272-6386(12)00957-2/pdf [2]
- Nutrition in Children with CKD (2008 update): http://kidneyfoundation.cachefly.net/professionals/KDOQI/guidelines_ped_ckd/index.htm [3]

KDOQI Clinical Practice Guideline for Nutrition in CKD: 2020 Update

The Work Group for this collaborative project was a diverse group of renal nutrition experts (physicians, RDNs (or international equivalents), researchers, and methodologists) from around the globe (i.e., Australia, Brazil, France, Hong Kong, Switzerland, Sweden, the United Kingdom, and the United States) [4].

KDIGO Clinical Practice Guidelines

- Anemia in CKD (2012): https://kdigo.org/guidelines/anemia-in-ckd/ [5]
- Blood Pressure in CKD (2012): https://kdigo.org/guidelines/blood-pressure-in-ckd/ [6]
- CKD Mineral and Bone Disorder (MBD) (2017): https://kdigo.org/guidelines/ckd-mbd/ [7]

- Diabetes and CKD: https://kdigo.org/guidelines/diabetes-ckd/ [8]
- Lipids in CKD (2013): https://kdigo.org/guidelines/lipids-in-ckd/ [9]

Diet-Related Resources and Food Lists

Dietitians assist in translating research in nutrition and CKD to patients and their caregivers. A number of resources are available to help with this process in clinical practice, and a few are provided within this section. The *Journal of Renal Nutrition*, the official journal of the Council on Renal Nutrition of the National Kidney Foundation, includes patient education and product update sections within most of the issues. Additionally, the National Institute of Diabetes and Digestive and Kidney Diseases (NIDDK) National Kidney Disease Education Program (NKDEP) provides patient education resources in English and Spanish (https://www.niddk.nih.gov/health-information/communication-programs/nkdep) [10].

The following sections comprise several tables that cover the nutrition composition of foods for various stages of CKD; food sources of potassium, phosphorus, and oxalate; examples of high biological value protein sources; and renal micronutrient supplements. Many of the tables in this edition remain as originally compiled by June Leung Fung, PhD, RD.

Nutrient Composition of Foods

Tables 37.1 and 37.2 present the calories, protein, sodium, potassium, and phosphorus composition of foods for people with CKD stages 3–5 [11].

Table 37.1 Nutrition composition of foods (per serving) for people with stage 3 or 4 chronic kidney disease

Foods	Protein (g)	Calories (kcal)	Sodium (mg)	Potassium (mg)	Phosphorus (mg)	Example
Protein						
High	6–8	50–100	20–150	50–150	50–100	1 oz beef, chicken, fish
High phosphorus	6–8	50–100	20–150	50–350	100–300	1 oz organ meats
High sodium	6–8	50–100	200–450	50–150	50–100	¼ c cottage cheese
Vegetable						
Low K+	2–3	10–100	0–50	20–150	10–70	1 c cabbage
Medium K+	2–3	10–100	0–50	150–250	10–70	½ c beets
High K+	2–3	10–100	0–50	250–550	10–70	¼ whole avocado
Fruit						
Low K+	0–1	20–100	0–10	20–150	1–20	One medium apple
Medium K+	0–1	20–100	0–10	150–250	1–20	½ c medium peach
High K+	0–1	20–100	0–10	250–550	1–20	Two apricot halves
Dairy/high phosphorus	2–3	50–200	150–400	10–100	100–200	1 c sherbet
Breads/cereals	2–3	50–200	0–150	10–100	10–70	½ small sweet roll, no nuts
Free calories	0–1	100–150	0–100	0–100	0–100	1 (3 oz) popsicle

Adapted from Renal Practice Group of the American Dietetic Association [11]. With permission © Academy of Nutrition and Dietetics (formerly the American Dietetic Association)
c cup, *K* + potassium, *oz* ounce

Table 37.2 Nutrition composition of foods (per serving) for people with stage 5 chronic kidney disease

Foods	Protein (g)	Calories (kcal)	Sodium (mg)	Potassium (mg)	Phosphorus (mg)	Example
Protein						
Animal	6–8	50–100	20–150	50–150	50–100	1 oz beef, chicken, fish
Animal (with higher Na^{2+} or PO$_4$– contents)	6–8	50–100	200–500	50–150	100–300	1 oz sardines
Fruit/vegetable						
Low K$^+$	0–3	10–100	1–50	20–150	0–70	1 c lettuce or ½ c grape juice
Medium K$^+$	0–3	10–100	1–50	150–250	0–70	½ c cooked broccoli or two tbsp raisins
High K$^+$	0–3	10–100	1–50	250–550	0–70	One medium tomato or one small nectarine
Dairy/high PO$_4$ –	2–8	100–400	30–300	50–400	100–120	½ c milk
Breads/cereals	2–3	50–200	0–150	10–100	10–70	½ small bagel
Free calories	0–1	100–150	0–100	0–100	0–100	Four pieces hard candy

Adapted from Renal Practice Group of the American Dietetic Association [11]. With permission © Academy of Nutrition and Dietetics (formerly the American Dietetic Association)

c cup, *K$^+$* potassium, *Na^{2+}* sodium, *PO$_4$–*, phosphorus, *oz* ounce, *tbsp* tablespoon

Food Sources of Potassium

The NKF's Potassium and Your CKD Diet patient education material comprises lists of foods that are both high and low in potassium. This material can be found at http://www.kidney.org/atoz/content/potassium#

Food Sources of Phosphorus

A listing of foods high in phosphorus and better alternative food choices are provided on the NKF's Phosphorus and Your CKD Diet information health guide at https://www.kidney.org/atoz/content/phosphorus. Table 37.3 lists the phosphorus and protein content of common foods [12]. Additional literature and listing of dietary phosphorus, protein, and potassium content of food items ranked by phosphorus to protein ratio categories have been published and can be accessed at http://cjasn.asn-journals.org/content/5/3/519.full.pdf+html [13].

Phosphate-based food additives can affect the diets of those with CKD and care is taken to limit the intake of foods containing these additives. Table 37.4 displays the most common phosphate additives, their use, and food products in which they are found [14].

Protein Quality in Foods

Education and monitoring of protein restriction in patients with CKD not receiving maintenance dialysis and adequate protein intake in patients with CKD stages 3–5 are important in the care of this population. Table 37.5 presents the biologic values of animal- and plant-based foods.

Table 37.3 Phosphorus and protein content of common foods

Food	Amount	Phosphorus (mg)	Protein (g)	Phos (mg)/protein (g)
Beans, legumes, tofu				
Kidney beans, black beans	1 cup	245	15	16.3
Refried beans, lima beans	1 cup	215	15	14.3
Navy beans	1 cup	290	16	18.1
Soybeans, boiled	1 cup	420	29	14.4
Soybeans, roasted	1 cup	625	60	10.4
Tofu, firm	100 g	75	6	12.5
Tofu, soft	100 g	55	4	13.8
Cheese				
Cheddar cheese	1 oz	145	7	20.7
Mozzarella cheese	1 oz	140	7	20.0
Swiss cheese	1 oz	170	8	21.3
Cottage cheese, 1% fat	1 cup	150	14	10.7
Cottage cheese, 2% fat	1 cup	340	31	11.0
Cream cheese	2 tbsp	30	2	15.0
Cream, milk, yogurt				
Half and half cream	1 cup	230	7	33.0
Heavy cream	1 cup	150	5	29.8
Sour cream	2 tbsp	30	1	30.0
Buttermilk	1 cup	220	8	27.5
Nonfat milk	1 cup	250	8	31.3
1% milk	1 cup	235	8	29.4
2% milk	1 cup	230	8	29.0
Whole milk	1 cup	230	8	28.7
Low fat yogurt	1 cup	340	12	28.3
Regular yogurt	1 cup	215	8	26.9
Fish and seafood				
Blue crab	3 oz	175	17	10.3
Dungeness crab	3 oz	150	19	8.0
King crab	3 oz	240	16	15
Halibut	3 oz	215	23	9.3
Oysters	3 oz	195	13	15
Salmon	3 oz	270	21	12.8
Shrimp	3 oz	115	18	6.4
Meat, poultry, eggs				
Beef liver	3 oz	390	23	17.0
Top sirloin	3 oz	200	25	8.0
Chicken breast	3 oz	195	27	7.2
Chicken thigh	3 oz	150	22	6.8
Egg	1 large	85	7	12.1
Ham	3 oz	240	19	12.6
Lamb chop	3 oz	190	22	8.6
Pork loin	3 oz	145	22	6.6
Turkey	3 oz	190	27	7.0
Veal loin	3 oz	190	22	8.6
Nuts and nut butters				
Almonds	1 oz	140	6	23.3

(continued)

Table 37.3 (continued)

Food	Amount	Phosphorus (mg)	Protein (g)	Phos (mg)/protein (g)
Macadamia	1 oz	55	2	27.5
Peanuts, roasted	1 oz	150	8	18.8
Peanut butter	2 tbsp	110	8	13.8
Walnuts	1 oz	100	4	25.0
Fast foods				
Bean/cheese burrito	2 small	180	15	12.0
Breakfast biscuit (egg, cheese, bacon)	1 serving	460	16	28.8
Cheeseburger	1 serving	310	28	11.0
Chicken sandwich	1 serving	405	29	14.0
Pepperoni pizza	1 slice	225	16	14.0
Other foods				
Beer	12 oz	40	1	40
Milk chocolate	1 oz	60	2	30
Semisweet chocolate	1 oz	35	1	35
Coffee	1 cup	2	0	
Colas	12 oz	45	0	
Lemon lime soda	12 oz	0	0	
Lemonade	1 cup	5	0.5	10
Root beer	12 oz	0	0	
Tea	1 cup	2	0	

Adapted from National Kidney Foundation [12]. With permission from Elsevier Limited

Table 37.4 Common phosphate additives in foods

Phosphate additive common name	Uses	Products
Dicalcium phosphate anhydrous	Dough conditioner; mineral source	Bakery mixes; yeast-raised bakery products; cereals; dry powder beverages; flour; food bars; infant food; milk-based beverages; multivitamin tablets; yogurts. Used in powder form as an abrasive in toothpaste
Dicalcium phosphate dihydrous	Leavening agent; mineral source	Bakery mixes; cereals; dry powder beverages; flour; food bars; infant food; milk-based beverages; multivitamin tablets; yogurt
Dipotassium phosphate	Buffer; nutrient in yeast culturing; sequestrant	Casein-based creamers; processed cheese; meat products; mineral supplements; nondairy creamers; starter cultures; yeast-containing products
Disodium phosphate anhydrous	Absorbent; alkalinity source; buffering agent; emulsifier; fortification; pH control agent; protein modifier; sequestrant; stabilizer; thickener Is used to adjust pH of cereal and pasta products to maintain quality color in final product. Accelerates the cook time of pasta and quick cooking cereals	Cereal, cooked and dry breakfast; cheese, imitation and processed; cream; gelatin; half and half; ice cream; infant food; instant cheesecake; instant pudding; isotonic drinks; milk, condensed, evaporated, flavored, and nonfat dry milk powders; pasta; starch; vitamin capsules; whipped topping
Disodium phosphate dihydrous	Same as disodium phosphate anhydrous	Same as disodium phosphate anhydrous
Magnesium phosphate	Dietary supplement; flow aid; nutritional source of magnesium and phosphorous; pH control agent	Magnesium source in infant formulas and diet beverages

Table 37.4 (continued)

Phosphate additive common name	Uses	Products
Monocalcium phosphate monohydrate	Acidulant for foods and beverages; dietary supplement; firming agent in canning; leavening acid; nutrient; thickener; yeast food dough conditioner Calcium source for fortification or enrichment	Baking powder; biscuits; cakes; cake mixes; donuts; canned fruit; muffins; pudding; canned and frozen vegetables
Monopotassium phosphate	Acidulant; buffering agent; coloring; leavening agent; nutrient source; pH control agent; stabilizer; whipping properties	Beverages: dry powder and isotonic; bread; dough; egg products; mineral supplements; starter cultures; yeast cultures
Monopotassium phosphate anhydrous	Buffering agent; color enhancer; dry acidulant; emulsifier; flavor enhancer (tartness); gelling agent; leavening agent; protein modifier; sequestrant	Beverages, cola, dry powder, and isotonic; egg, yolks and liquid egg mixtures; gelatin; instant cheesecake; instant pudding
Monosodium phosphate	Color stabilizer; whipping properties	Egg products
Pentasodium triphosphate	Buffering agent; coagulant; curing agent; dispersing agent; emulsifier; flavor enhancer; humectants; moisture retention; pH control; reduces oxidation; sequestrant; stabilizer; texturizer; thickener	Meat; poultry; seafood
Phosphoric acid	Acidulant; buffering agent; flavor enhancer; pH control agent; sequestrant; stabilizer; synergist; thickener	Carbonated and noncarbonated beverages; cottage cheese
Sodium acid pyrophosphate	Acidulant; buffering agent; coagulant; dispersing agent; emulsifier; formulation aid; humectant; leavening agent; pH control agent; protein modifier; processing aid; sequestrant; stabilizer; synergist; texturizer; thickener	Baking powder; cake donuts; cake mixes; canned crab; cheese: imitation and processed; refrigerated dough; icing and frostings; processed meat including bologna, chicken and chicken products, and hot dogs; nondairy creamers; processed potatoes; seafood; canned tuna
Sodium hexametaphosphate	Buffering agent; color stabilizer; curing agent; deflocculant; dough strengthener; emulsifier; firming agent; flavor enhancer; flavoring agent; humectant; neutral salt; nutrient supplement; processing aid; sequestrant; stabilizer; surface-active agent; synergist; texturizer; thickener	Processed cheese; egg products; meat; poultry; cheese; seafood; sour cream; table syrups; canned and frozen vegetables; vegetable proteins; whey; whipped toppings
Sodium tripolyphosphate	Emulsifier; flavor enhancer; mechanical peeling of shrimp; moisture binding; stabilizer; texture modification	Fish; meats: chicken, corned beef, ham, roast beef, bologna, hot dogs, and sausage; scallops; shrimp; canned or frozen vegetables
Tetrapotassium pyrophosphate	Alkalinity source; antioxidant; buffering agent; coagulant; dispersing agent; nutrient source; pH control agent; protein modifier; sequestrant; texturizer	Processed cheese; milk powders
Tetrasodium pyrophosphate	Buffer; color agent; emulsifying agent; protein modifier; provides "meltability: in processed cheese; quickens cooking time of cooked breakfast cereals; stabilizer; thickener"	Cheese: processed and imitation cheese; isotonic beverages; cooked breakfast cereals; pudding
Tricalcium phosphate	Fortification; prevents caking; reduction in cooking time	Cooked cereal; dry drink mixes; fruit juices; soy beverages
Tripotassium phosphate	Alkalinity source; buffering agent; emulsifier; nutrient; protein modifier; stabilizer	Cereals; processed cheese; bread and dough conditioners; dairy products; isotonic beverages; starter cultures

Source: Summary of Phosphate Citations [14]

Table 37.5 Biologic values of selected animal and vegetable foods

Foods	Biologic value range (%)[a]
Red beans, lentils	45
Wheat flour, wheat gluten, bean (avg), baker's yeast	50–59
Sesame seed, white rice, black beans, peas, kale, cooked oatmeal, butter beans, wheat (avg), lima beans, brewer's yeast, chick peas, coconut	60–69
Sunflower seeds, cheddar cheese, sardines, brown rice, soybeans, potatoes, wheat germ, beef, veal, chicken, pork, shrimp, fish (avg), rye, buckwheat	70–79
Mushrooms, casein, barley, cod, haddock, milk, lobster	80–89
Egg	>90

Developed by Joni Pagenkemper. *Source*: Food and Agriculture Organization of the United Nations [15]
[a]Adequate protein quality >60 adults, >70 children

Additional biologic values of certain foods can be found in the FAO Amino Acid Content of Foods and Biological Data on Proteins [15].

Oxalates in Food

For populations in which dietary oxalates are of concern, Table 37.6 lists high and moderate oxalate contents of common foods [16].

Vitamin Recommendations and Supplementation in CKD

Patients with CKD have altered vitamin metabolism, and they are thought to have increased requirements for some vitamins. Table 37.7 presents the Dietary Reference Intakes for vitamins and their suggested recommendations for various stages of CKD [17–22]. Table 37.8 lists the micronutrient content of currently available specially formulated renal vitamins.

Assessment Tools

As discussed in Chaps. 4–7 on nutrition assessment, there are typically four components to conducting a comprehensive nutrition assessment: (1) anthropometrics, (2) biochemical indices, (3) clinical symptomatology, and (4) dietary intake data. The reader is encouraged to consult the KDOQI clinical practice guidelines for additional information on nutrition assessment in CKD [4].

As stated in the KDOQI Guideline, the seven-point subjective global assessment (SGA) is a valid and reliable tool for assessing nutritional status in adults receiving maintenance dialysis [4]. In 1994, SGA was presented at the annual meeting of the American Society of Nephrology. Since that time, it has been used in growing numbers of dialysis clinics as another tool to assess the nutritional status of patients receiving maintenance dialysis. SGA is simple, subjective, and hands on [23, 24].

SGA is a score-based assessment based on medical history and a physical assessment. Its ratings have been found to be highly predictive of outcome as well as correlate strongly with other subjective and objective measures of nutrition [23–25]. While it was originally used to categorize surgical

Table 37.6 Food sources of oxalate

High oxalate content (≥10 mg)	Moderate oxalate content (5–9 mg)
Avocado	Fresh figs
Dates	Canned cherries
Grapefruit	Artichokes
Kiwi	Asparagus
Orange	Carrots, cooked
Raspberries	Hot chili peppers
Tangerine	Chili powder
Canned and dried pineapple	Brewer's yeast
Dried prunes	Mixed vegetables, frozen
Bamboo shoots	Oriental vegetables, frozen
Beets	Soybeans
Fava beans	String beans
Navy beans	Tomato, fresh
Okra	Chocolate milk
Olives	Blueberry muffins
Parsnip	Biscuits (plain or buttermilk)
Red kidney beans	Bran muffins
Refried beans	Bran muffin low fat
Rhubarb	Cracked wheat bread
Rutabaga	English muffin
Spinach, cooked	English muffin multi-grain
Spinach, raw	English muffin wheat
Tomato sauce	Low-fat muffins
Turnip	Rye bread
Yams	Popcorn
Dried figs	Pretzels, hard
Carrots, raw	Tortillas, corn
Celery, cooked	Tortillas, flour
Collards	White bread
French fries (homemade or fast food)	Wheat bran bread
Baked potato with skin	Whole oat bread
Mashed potatoes	Whole wheat bread
Potato chips	Prune juice
Potato salad	Pies
Sweet potatoes	
French toast	
English muffin whole wheat	
Pancakes (homemade)	
Pancakes (mix)	
All-purpose flour	
Brown rice, cooked	
Brown rice flour	
Buckwheat groats	
Bulgur, cooked	
Cocoa powder	
Corn grits	
Cornmeal	
Couscous	
Lasagna	
Millet, cooked	
Miso	
Rice bran	

(continued)

Table 37.6 (continued)

High oxalate content (≥10 mg)	Moderate oxalate content (5–9 mg)
Soy flour	
Wheat berries	
Wheat flour, whole grain	
Spaghetti	
White rice flour	
Tofu	
Soy burgers	
Chocolate	
Carrot juice	
Hot chocolate (homemade)	
Lemonade (frozen from concentrate)	
Tea, brewed	
Tomato juice	
Almonds	
Candies with nuts	
Cashews	
Peanuts and peanut butter	
Pistachios	
Mixed nuts (with peanuts)	
Pumpkin seeds	
Trail mix	
Tahini	
Walnuts	
Pecans	
Sunflower seeds	
Brownies	
Cake	

Source: United States Department of Agriculture, Human Nutrition Information Service. Agriculture Handbook Number 8–11, Composition of Foods: Vegetables and Vegetable Products. Revised August 1984
Oxalate Content of Foods [16]

Table 37.7 Daily vitamin recommendations for CKD

Vitamin	Dietary Reference Intakes[a]	Predialysis CKD	Maintenance HD/PD
Vitamin C	75–90 mg/day	60–100 mg/day	60–100 mg/day
Thiamin (B1)	1.1–1.2 mg/day	1.5 mg/day	1.5 mg/day
Riboflavin (B2)	1.1–1.3 mg/day	1.8 mg/day	1.1–1.3 mg/day
Niacin	14–16 mg/day	14–20 mg/day	14–20 mg/day
Vitamin B6	1.3–1.7 mg/day	5 mg/day	10 mg/day
Vitamin B12	2.4 μg/day	2–3 μg/day	2–3 μg/day
Folic acid	0.4 mg/day	1 mg/day	1 mg/day
Pantothenic acid	5 mg/day	5 mg/day	5 mg/day
Biotin	30 μg/day	30–100 μg/day	30–100 μg/day
Vitamin A	700–900 μg/day	700–900 μg/day	700–900 μg/day
Vitamin E	15 mg/day	15 mg/day	15 mg/day
Vitamin K	90–120 μg/day	90–120 μg/day	90–120 μg/day

[a]Dietary Reference Intakes for adults >18 years. Sources: see Refs. [17–22]
CKD chronic kidney disease; *HD* hemodialysis; *PD* peritoneal dialysis

Table 37.8 Renal micronutrient supplement comparison chart

Product	Vitamin C (mg)	Thiamin (mg)	Riboflavin (mg)	Niacin (mg)	B6 (mg)	B12 (µg)	Folic acid (mg)	Pantothenic acid (mg)	Biotin (µg)	Vitamin D[a] (IU)	Vitamin E (IU)	Zn (mg)	Fe[b] (mg)	Se (µg)
Dialyvite® 800	60	1.5	1.7	20	10	6	0.8	10	300	–	–	–	–	–
Dialyvite® 60 Chewable		1.5	1.7	20	10	6	0.8	10	300	–	–	–	–	–
Dialyvite® 800 with zinc	60	1.5	1.7	20	10	6	0.8	10	300	–	–	50	–	–
Dialyvite® 800 with zinc 15	60	1.5	1.7	20	10	6	0.8	10	300	–	–	15	–	–
Dialyvite® 800 with iron	60	1.5	1.7	20	10	6	0.8	10	300	–	–	–	29	–
Dialyvite® 800 Ultra D	60	1.5	1.7	20	10	6	0.8	10	300	2000	30	15	–	70
Dialyvite® 800 Plus D Chewable	60	1.5	1.7	20	10	6	0.8	10	300	2000	–	–	–	–
Dialyvite® Rx	100	1.5	1.7	20	10	6	1	10	300	–	–	–	–	–
Dialyvite® Rx with zinc	100	1.5	1.7	20	10	6	1	10	300	–	–	50	–	–
Dialyvite® 3000 Rx	100	1.5	1.7	20	25	1	3	10	300	–	30	15	–	70
Dialyvite® 5000 Rx	100	1.5	1.7	20	50	2	5	10	300	–	30	25	–	70
Dialyvite® Supreme D Rx	100	1.5	1.7	20	25	1	3	10	300	2000	30	15	–	70
Diatx® ZN	60	1.5	1.7	20	50	2	5	10	300	–	–	25	–	–
Folbee Plus®	60	1.5	1.5	20	50	1	5	10	300	–	–	–	–	–
Folbee Plus® CZ	60	1.5	1.5	20	50	2	5	10	300	–	–	25	–	–
Healthy Factor	60	1.5	1.7	20	10	6	0.8	10	300	–	–	–	–	–
Nephrocaps®	100	1.5	1.7	20	10	6	1	5	150	–	–	–	–	–
Nephron FA®	40	1.5	1.7	20	10	6	1	10	300	–	–	–	66	–
Nephronex® (liquid)	60	1.5	1.7	20	10	10	0.9	10	30	–	–	–	–	–
Nephrovite®	60	1.5	1.7	20	10	6	0.8	10	300	–	–	–	–	–
Nephrovite® Rx	60	1.5	1.7	20	10	6	1	10	300	–	–	–	–	–
NephPlex® Rx	60	1.5	1.7	20	10	6	1	10	300	–	–	12.5	–	–
ProRenal® Vital	60	1.5	2	20	10	2.4	0.8	5	30	1000	–	8	8	55

(continued)

Table 37.8 (continued)

Product	Vitamin C (mg)	Thiamin (mg)	Riboflavin (mg)	Niacin (mg)	B6 (mg)	B12 (µg)	Folic acid (mg)	Pantothenic acid (mg)	Biotin (µg)	Vitamin D[a] (IU)	Vitamin E (IU)	Zn (mg)	Fe[b] (mg)	Se (µg)
ProRenal®+D with Omega-3	60	1.5	2	20	10	2.4	0.8	5	30	1000	10	8	8	55
PS Nephro Aid®	60	1.5	1.7	20	20	1	2	5	300	–	–	–	–	–
Renal Caps®	100	1.5	1.7	20	10	6	1	5	150	–	–	–	–	–
RenaPlex®	60	1.5	1.7	20	10	6	0.8	10	300	–	–	15	–	–
RenaPlex® D	60	1.5	1.7	20	10	6	0.8	10	300	2000	35	15	–	70
Rena-Vite®	60	1.5	1.7	20	10	6	0.8	10	300	–	–	–	–	–
Rena-Vite Rx®	60	1.5	1.7	20	10	6	1	10	300	–	–	15	–	–
Renal Tab I	125	12.5	7.5	50	20	12.5	1	30	300	–	15	15	–	–
Renal Tab II	60	1.5	1.7	20	10	6	1	10	300					
Renal Tab Zn	60	1.5	1.7	20	10	6	1	10	300			15		
Renal Tab Zn + D	60	1.5	1.7	20	10	6	1	10	300	1000		15		
Reno Caps	100	1.5	1.7	20	10	6	1	5	150	–	–	–	–	–

All Dialyvite® supplements are registered trademarks of Hillestad Pharmaceuticals USA, Inc., Woodruff, WI

Diatx® Zn is a registered trademark of Centrix Pharmaceutical, Inc., Birmingham, AL

Folbee Plus® and Folbee Plus® CZ are registered trademarks of Breckenridge Pharmaceuticals, Inc. Boca Raton, FL

Healthy Factor is a product of Healthy Factor, Arbor Vitae, WI

Nephrocaps® is a registered trademark of Valeant Pharmaceuticals International, Inc., Quebec, Canada

Nephron FA®, NephPlex® Rx, RenaPlex®, and RenaPlex® D are registered trademarks of Nephro-Tech Inc., Shawnee, KS

Nephronex® is a registered trademark of Llorens Pharmaceutical, Miami, FL

Nephrovite® and Nephrovite® Rx are registered trademarks of Watson Pharmaceuticals, Inc., Parsippany, NJ

ProRenal® Vital and ProRenal®+D with Omega-3 are registered trademarks of Nephroceuticals, LLC, Beavercreek, OH

PS Nephro Aid® is a registered trademark of Physician Select Vitamins, Pearland, TX

Renal Caps® is a registered trademark of Cypress Pharmaceuticals, Inc., Madison, WI

Rena-Vite® and Rena-Vite® Rx are registered trademarks of Cypress Pharmaceutical, Inc., Madison, MS

Renal Tab I, II, Zn, Zn + D are products of Renalab, Templeton, CA

Reno Caps is a product of Nnodum Pharmaceuticals, Cincinnati, OH

[a]Vitamin D in the form of cholecalciferol

[b]Elemental iron

patients, it is now recognized as a valid and reliable nutritional assessment tool for dialysis patients [26–32]. Studies in patients with CKD have also shown the predictive capability of survival outcomes and correlations of SGA with anthropometric and other outcome measures [27–32]. The medical history includes progression of weight change, dietary intake, gastrointestinal symptoms, physiological functioning, and a simple analysis of metabolic stress. The physiological assessment includes loss of subcutaneous fat and muscle mass and edema. Originally, patients were evaluated as (A) well-nourished, (B) mild to moderately malnourished, or (C) severely malnourished [23, 24]. This ABC rating has been changed to a seven-point scale [29] which are as follows:

1. 6 or 7 = mildly nutritional risk to well-nourished
2. 3, 4, or 5 = mild to moderately malnourished
3. 1 or 2 = severely malnourished

Healthcare professionals should be trained on SGA methods prior to using it in practice.

As an alternative to SGA, the Malnutrition inflammation Score (MIS) is a fully quantified assessment developed for use in patients with CKD [33]. The KDOQI Work Group recommends that the MIS may be used to assess nutritional status in adults with CKD on maintenance hemodialysis and post-transplant [4]. The following link takes the reader to the Abbott Nutrition Health Institute and a presentation about the MIS by the nephrologist, Dr. Kamyar Kalantar-Zadeh (https://anhi.org/conferences/biomarkers-of-malnutrition/ckd-and-inflammation-score).

Internet Sites

There are a plethora of websites that provide resources and online tools that may be useful for the renal practitioner. Table 37.9 includes a select few.

Table 37.9 Online resources and tools

Academy of Nutrition and Dietetics	www.eatright.org
American Association of Kidney Patients (AAKP)	www.aakp.org
American Diabetes Association (ADA)	www.diabetes.org
American Kidney Fund (AKF)	www.akfinc.org
Centers for Medicare & Medicaid Services (CMS)	www.cms.gov
Council of Renal Nutrition (CRN)	www.kidney.org/professionals/CRN/
Council of Nephrology Social Workers (CNSW)	www.kidney.org/professionals/CNSW/
Council of Nephrology Nurses & Technicians (CNNT)	www.kidney.org/professionals/CNNT/
DaVita Kidney Care	www.davita.com
Fresenius Kidney Care (FKC)	https://www.freseniuskidneycare.com/
Hypertension, Dialysis and Clinical Nephrology	www.hdcn.com
Kidney School	www.kidneyschool.org
Life Options Rehabilitation Program	www.lifeoptions.org
National Institute of Diabetes and Digestive and Kidney Diseases (NIDDK)	www.niddk.nih.gov
National Kidney Disease Education Program (NKDEP)	www.nkdep.nih.gov
National Kidney Foundation (NKF)	www.kidney.org
The Nephron Information Center	http://nephron.com/
Renal Dietitians Dietetic Practice Group (RPG) of the Academy of Nutrition and Dietetics	www.renalnutrition.org
RenalWEB-Vortex Website of the Dialysis World	www.renalweb.com
USDA Dietary Reference Intakes (DRI) Calculator for Healthcare Professionals	https://www.nal.usda.gov/fnic/dri-calculator/
United States Renal Data System (USRDS)	www.usrds.org

Mobile Apps

With the increasing use of smartphones and tablets, a growing number of mobile apps are available that practitioners and clients can use to manage care and treatment. However, choosing an app can be challenging because the scientific evidence is limited for commercially available apps. As with all print and Internet resources available, mobile apps should be reviewed and used with appropriate professional and clinical judgment. The NKF has an APP center that includes links to various apps that can be used on Androids, iPads, and/or iPhones. The link can be found at https://www.kidney.org/apps. Below are some links to apps the reader may find useful:

- CRN Pocket Guide to Nutrition Assessment in the patient with CKD. This app supports the 5th edition of the Pocket Guide: https://www.kidney.org/apps/professionals/crn-pocket-guide-nutrition-assessment-patient-ckd-mobile-app
- *Journal of Renal Nutrition (JRN)*. Keep up to date with advances in the science and practice of renal nutrition: https://www.kidney.org/apps/professionals/journal-renal-nutrition-jrn-app
- *American Journal of Kidney Disease (AJKD)*. Keep up to date with the advances in the science and practice of nephrology: https://www.kidney.org/apps/professionals/ajkd-american-journal-kidney-diseases
- *Advances in Chronic Kidney Disease (ACKD)*. Stay current on the latest professional research for chronic kidney disease: https://www.kidney.org/apps/professionals/advances-chronic-kidney-disease-ackd
- *CKD Care: An Interactive Guide for Clinicians*. This app allows medical professionals to estimate kidney function using an estimated glomerular filtration rate (eGFR) calculator and provides care guidelines based on multiple parameters entered by the user. This clinical tool offers succinct, patient-specific strategies that define diagnosis and guide management: https://www.kidney.org/apps/professionals/ckd-care-interactive-guide-clinicians
- H2Overload: Fluid Control for Heart-Kidney Health. This app is designed for people who need to limit their fluid intake, especially people with hyponatremia, kidney failure, or heart disease: https://www.kidney.org/apps/patients/h2overload-fluid-control-heart-kidney-health
- *Gout Central*: Empowers patients with the most essential tools and information for controlling gout and protecting their kidneys. Guidance is provided on the optimal use of nutrition, lifestyle, and medication for the prevention and treatment of gout flares: https://www.kidney.org/apps/patients/gout-central
- *My Food Coach by NKF*: Designed to help the consumer understand and manage personalized nutrition requirements: https://appadvice.com/game/app/my-food-coach/785222447.
- *Relative Risk, Monitoring and Referral in Patients with CKD*: Summarizes new science that explains how estimated glomerular filtration rate (eGFR) and urinary albumin-to-creatinine ratio (ACR) are independent risk factors for adverse outcomes: https://www.kidney.org/apps/professionals/relative-risk-monitoring-and-referral-patients-ckd
- *Screening for Albuminuria in Patients with Diabetes*. A quick pocket tool to help medical professionals assess and treat albuminuria in persons with diabetes: https://www.kidney.org/apps/professionals/screening-albuminuria-patients-diabetes
- *Care After Kidney Transplant*: A consumer app created to help patients stay healthy post kidney transplant: https://www.kidney.org/apps/patients/care-after-kidney-transplant-app
- *eGFR Calculator*: Helps medical professionals estimate kidney function using five separate eGFR calculators: https://www.kidney.org/apps/professionals/egfr-calculator
- MySugr – My Diabetes Tracker. Allows the user to keep diabetes data under control (e.g., blood sugar tracker, carb logger, and estimated HbA1c) – all at a glance: https://apps.apple.com/us/app/mysugr-diabetes-tracker-log/id516509211

- American Diabetes Association Standards of Medical Care. Includes the full standards of care narrative and interactive tools accessing the most referenced algorithms: https://professional.diabetes.org/content-page/standards-care-app-1

Conclusion

This chapter represents a collection of resources that are required for clinical practice in nutrition and kidney disease. It does not contain an exhaustive list of tools, but should serve to assist the practitioner in locating critical pieces of information necessary for appropriate delivery of care for patients with kidney disease.

References

1. Chronic Kidney Disease. Academy of nutrition and dietetics evidence analysis library website. https://www.andeal.org/. Updated on May 10, 2019. Accessed 17 Dec 2019.
2. KDOQI clinical practice guideline for diabetes and CKD: 2012 update. Am J Kidney Dis. 2012;60(5):850–86.
3. KDOQI Work Group. KDOQI clinical practice guideline for nutrition in children with chronic kidney disease: 2008 update. Am J Kidney Dis. 2009;53 Suppl 2:S11–104.
4. Ikizler TA, Burrowes J, Byham-Gray L, Campbell K, Carrero JJ, Chan W, et al. KDOQI Nutrition in CKD Guideline Work Group. KDOQI clinical practice guideline for nutrition in CKD: 2020 update. Am J Kidney Dis. 2020; in press.
5. Anemia in CKD. Kidney disease improving global outcomes website. Published August 2012. https://kdigo.org/guidelines/anemia-in-ckd/. Accessed 19 Dec 2019.
6. Blood Pressure in CKD. Kidney disease improving global outcomes website. Published December 2012. https://kdigo.org/guidelines/blood-pressure-in-ckd/. Accessed 19 Dec 2019.
7. CKD Mineral and Bone Disorder (MBD). Kidney disease improving global outcomes website. Published July 2017. https://kdigo.org/guidelines/ckd-mbd/. Accessed 19 Dec 2019.
8. Diabetes and CKD. Kidney Disease improving global outcomes website. https://kdigo.org/guidelines/diabetes-ckd/. Accessed 19 Dec 2019.
9. Lipids in CKD. Kidney disease improving global outcomes website. Published November 2013. https://kdigo.org/guidelines/lipids-in-ckd/. Accessed 19 Dec 2019.
10. National Kidney Disease Education Program. National Institute of Diabetes and Digestive and Kidney Diseases website. https://www.niddk.nih.gov/health-information/communication-programs/nkdep. Accessed 23 Dec 2019.
11. Renal Practice Group of the American Dietetic Association. National renal diet professional guide. 2nd ed. Chicago: American Dietetic Association; 2002.
12. National Kidney Foundation. K/DOQI clinical practice guidelines for bone metabolism and disease in chronic kidney disease. Am J Kidney Dis. 2003;42 Suppl 3:S1–201.
13. Kalantar-Zadeh K, Gutekunst L, Mehrotra R, Kovesdy CP, Bross R, Shinaberger CS, Noori N, Hirschberg R, Benner D, Nissenson AR, Kopple JD. Understanding sources of dietary phosphorus in the treatment of patients with chronic kidney disease. Clin J Am Soc Nephrol. 2010;5:519–30.
14. Summary of Phosphate Citations. International food additives council. https://www.foodingredientfacts.org/summary-phosphate-citations/. Accessed 19 Dec 2019.
15. Amino acid content of foods and biological data on proteins. Food and agriculture organization of the United Nations website. Update published 1981. http://www.fao.org/3/AC854T/AC854T00.htm#TOC. Accessed 19 Dec 2019.
16. Oxalate Content of Foods. Harvard T.H. Chan School of Public Health Nutrition Department's File Download Site website. Published March 13, 2017. https://regepi.bwh.harvard.edu/health/Oxalate/files. Accessed on 19 Dec 2019.
17. Institute of Medicine, Food and Nutrition Board. Dietary reference intakes for thiamin, riboflavin, niacin, vitamin B6, folate, vitamin B12, pantothenic acid, biotin, and choline. Washington, DC: National Academies Press; 1998.
18. Institute of Medicine, Food and Nutrition Board. Dietary reference intakes for vitamin C, vitamin E, selenium, and carotenoids. Washington, DC: The National Academies Press; 2000.

19. Institute of Medicine, Food and Nutrition Board, Dietary reference intakes for vitamin A, vitamin K, arsenic, boron, chromium, copper, iodine, iron, manganese, molybdenum, nickel, silicon, vanadium, and zinc. Washington, DC: The National Academies Press; 2001.

20. Kopple JD, Massry SG, editors. Nutritional management of renal disease. Philadelphia: Lippincott Williams & Wilkins; 2004.

21. Mitch WE, Klahr S, editors. Handbook of nutrition and the kidney. 5th ed. Philadelphia: Lippincott Williams & Wilkins; 2005.

22. Steiber AL, Kopple JD. Vitamin status and needs for people with stages 3–5 chronic kidney disease. J Ren Nutr. 2011;21:355–68.

23. Detsky AS, McLaughlin JR, Baker JP, Johnston N, Whittaker S, Mendelson RA, Jeejeebhoy KN. What is subjective global assessment? JPEN J Parenter Enteral Nutr. 1987;11:8–13.

24. Jeejeebhoy KN, Detsky AS, Baker JP. Assessment of nutritional status. JPEN J Parenter Enteral Nutr. 1990;14:193S–6.

25. Baker JP, Detsky AS, Wesson DE, Wolman SL, Stewart S, Whitewa J, Langer B, Jeejeebhoy KN. Nutritional assessment: a comparison of clinical judgment and objective measurements. N Engl J Med. 1982;306:969–72.

26. Young GA, Kopple JD, Lindholm B, Vonesh EF, De Vecchi A, Scalamogna A, Castelnova C, Oreopoulos DG, Anderson GH, Bergstrom J, DiChiro J, Gentile D, Nissenson A, Sakhrani L, Brownjohn AM, Nolph KD, Prowant BF, Algrim CE, Martis L, Serkes KD. Nutritional assessment of continuous ambulatory peritoneal dialysis patients: an international study. Am J Kidney Dis. 1991;17:462–71.

27. Enia G, Sicuso C, Alati G, Zoccali C. Subjective global assessment of nutrition in dialysis patients. Nephrol Dial Transplant. 1993;8:1094–8.

28. Fenton SSA, Johnston N, Delmore T, Detsky AS, Whitewall J, O'Sullhan R, Cattran C, Richardson RMA, Jeejeebhoy KN. Nutrition assessment of continuous ambulatory peritoneal dialysis patients. Trans Am Soc Artif Intern Organs. 1987;33:650–3.

29. Canada-USA (CANUSA) Peritoneal Dialysis Study Group. Adequacy of dialysis and nutrition in continuous peritoneal dialysis: association with clinical outcomes. J Am Soc Nephrol. 1996;7:198–207.

30. Visser R, Dekker FW, Boeschoten EW, Stevens P, Krediet RT. Reliability of the 7-point subjective global assessment scale in assessing nutritional status of dialysis patients. Adv Perit Dial. 1999;15:222–5.

31. Steiber A, Leon JB, Secker D, McCarthy M, McCann L, Serra M, Sehgal AR, Kalantar-Zadeh K. Multicenter study of the validity and reliability of subjective global assessment in the hemodialysis population. J Ren Nutr. 2007;17:336–42.

32. Steiber AL, Kalantar-Zadeh K, Secker D, McCarthy M, Sehgal A, McCann L. Subjective global assessment in chronic kidney disease: a review. J Ren Nutr. 2004;14:191–200.

33. Kalantar-Zadeh K, Kopple JD, Block G, Humphreys MH. A malnutrition-inflammation score is correlated with morbidity and mortality in maintenance hemodialysis patients. Am J Kidney Dis. 2001;38:1251–63.

Index

© Springer Nature Switzerland AG 2020
J. D. Burrowes et al. (eds.), *Nutrition in Kidney Disease*, Nutrition and Health,
https://doi.org/10.1007/978-3-030-44858-5

Printed in the United States
by Baker & Taylor Publisher Services